BOTTOM LINE'S
ULTIMATE HEALING

EXPANDED EDITION

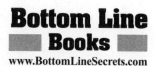
Bottom Line Books
www.BottomLineSecrets.com

Contents

5 • CURES THAT COST PENNIES

6 • HEALTH ALERTS

7 • EASY PAIN RELIEF

12 • HEART AND STROKE HELP

13 • DIABETES AND OTHER DISEASES

19 • SURPRISING FOOD CURES

Expanded Edition Preface

We are proud to bring you *Bottom Line's Ultimate Healing*. We trust that you'll find the latest discoveries, best treatments and money-saving solutions to your health concerns.

Whether it's cancer prevention, new heart therapies, breakthrough arthritis treatments or cutting-edge nutritional advice, our editors talk to the people—from medical doctors to consumer health advocates—who are creating the true innovations in health care.

How do we find all these top-notch medical professionals? Over the past two decades, we have built a network of literally thousands of leading physicians in both alternative and conventional medicine. They are affiliated with the premier medical institutions and the best universities throughout the world. We read the important medical journals and follow the latest research that is reported at medical conferences. And we regularly talk to our advisors in major teaching hospitals, private practices and government health agencies.

Bottom Line's Ultimate Healing is a result of our ongoing research and contact with these experts, and is a distillation of their latest findings and advice. We trust that you will enjoy the presentation and glean new, helpful and affordable information about the health topics that concern you and your family.

As a reader of a Bottom Line Book, please be assured that you are receiving reliable and well-researched information from a trusted source.

But, please use prudence in health matters. Always speak to your physician before taking vitamins, supplements or over-the-counter medication…changing your diet…or beginning an exercise program. If you experience side effects from any regimen, contact your doctor immediately.

The Editors, Bottom Line Books, Stamford, CT.

1

Smart Consumer

Get Your Drugs at Half Off—Or Even Free

 nyone who takes prescription medication on a regular basis knows how pricey drugs can be. Over a seven-year period (1999–2006), medication costs rose by nearly 54%, on average, in the United States.

Fortunately, there are places where you can buy your drugs for less—or sometimes even get them for free. The key is knowing where to look.

Important: Although most low-cost drug programs have income eligibility requirements, do not assume that you won't be accepted into a program just because your income is officially too high. Many programs will consider applications case-by-case.

Best resources for finding low-cost or free medications…

DRUG DISCOUNT NETWORKS

Some groups connect patients to public and private assistance programs that provide discounted or free drugs to eligible patients. *These include…*

•**Partnership for Prescription Assistance** (888-477-2669, *www.pparx.org*). This collaborative network of professional medical organizations, including the American Academy of Family Physicians and the National Medical Association, and private groups, such as the National Alliance for Hispanic Health, links patients to more than 475 public and private patient assistance programs that offer more than 2,500 drugs at reduced cost or no charge. Income qualifications vary by state. (Some programs look at patients' assets rather than income.)

•**Together Rx program** (800-444-4106, *www.togetherrxaccess.com*). Backed by a consortium of pharmaceutical companies, including

Edward Jardini, MD, a family physician at Twin Cities Community Hospital in Templeton, California, where he has served as chair of the pharmacy and therapeutics committee. He is the author of *How to Save on Prescription Drugs: 20 Cost-Saving Methods.* Celestial Arts. *www. howtosaveondrugs.com.*

Abbott, Novartis and Pfizer, this program provides a 25% to 40% discount on more than 300 brand-name and generic prescription drugs. The program targets people who don't have prescription drug coverage with annual incomes of $30,000 or less for individuals…$40,000 for a family of two…and up to $70,000 for a family of five.

PHARMACEUTICAL PATIENT-ASSISTANCE PROGRAMS

Major pharmaceutical companies have their own patient-assistance programs that offer many —though not all—drugs at a discount, or even for free, to people who cannot afford them.

Eligibility requirements vary—even families earning up to $70,000 a year can qualify. Not all companies ask for proof of income, and some will consider applications on a case-by-case basis.

To obtain a free copy of *Directory of Prescription Drug Patient Assistance Programs,* call the Partnership for Prescription Assistance at 800-762-4636. *Among the pharmaceutical companies with programs…*

•**Abbott Patient Assistance Program,** (800-222-6885, *www.abbott.com*).

•**AstraZeneca's AZ & Me Prescription Savings Program** (800-292-6363, *www.astrazeneca-us.com*).

•**Lilly Cares Patient Assistance Program** (Eli Lilly) (800-545-6962, *www.lillycares.com*).

•**Merck Patient Assistance Program** (800-727-5400, *www.merck.com/merckhelps/patientassistance/home.html*).

•**Novartis Patient Assistance Foundation** (800-277-2254, *www.pharma.us.novartis.com*).

•**Pfizer Helpful Answers** (866-776-3700, *www.pfizerhelpfulanswers.com*).

•**Roche Labs Patient Assistant Foundation** (877-757-6243, *www.rocheusa.com/programs/patientassist.asp*).

•**Schering-Plough Cares** (800-656-9485, *www.schering-plough.com/schering_plough/pc/sp_cares.jsp*).

•**Wyeth Pharmaceutical Patient Assistance Program** (800-568-9938, *www.wyeth.com*).

Some pharmaceutical companies also offer coupons that can be printed from their Web sites, as well as discount card programs offering savings on some of their most popular products. Check the drug manufacturer's Web site for details.

There are a number of ways to dramatically reduce your medication costs. Unfortunately, most drug-discount programs don't advertise their services, so few people are aware of all the available options. Some programs even waive income eligibility requirements.

Among the best resources…

PHARMACY BENEFIT MANAGERS

Because of their size, large companies that act as third-party managers of prescription drug programs can provide discounted medications. *Ones to consider…*

•**Caremark: RxSavings Plus** (877-673-3688, *www.rxsavingsplus.com*). This program offers a card that is accepted at 57,000 US pharmacies and provides an average savings of 20%. You can use the card as long as you're not receiving insurance reimbursement, including Medicare. For up to a 50% discount, order a 90-day supply by mail.

•**Express Scripts: Rx Outreach** (800-769-3880, *www.rxoutreach.com*). Designed for low-income patients, this program sets annual income limits of less than $31,200 for most individuals or less than $42,000 a year for couples. A 90-day supply of medications costs from $15 to $135, depending on the drug. Supplies of 180 days also available.

GOVERNMENT PROGRAMS

Federal, state and local governments also offer eligible patients access to low-cost drugs…

•**US Department of Veterans Affairs** (877-222-8387, *www.va.gov*). For people who were honorably discharged from active duty in a branch of the military, the VA will provide prescription drugs at a cost of $8 a month. The prescription must be written by a doctor in a VA clinic. To qualify, you must fill out application form *10-10EZ* (available at local VA offices and medical centers or on-line at *www.va.gov/health eligibility/application*) and provide a copy of your discharge document.

The VA also offers a separate health-care program, called CHAMPVA, for family members of a veteran who has a permanent disability or who died in the line of duty or due to a service-connected disability—as long as they're not eligible for TRICARE (see below).

•**TRICARE** (800-538-9552, *www.tricare.mil*). TRICARE is a healthcare benefit for active-duty service members, reserve members, retired uniformed armed services members, their families and survivors. Widows and widowers of active-duty members also may qualify unless they remarry. The plan includes prescription coverage.

If the medication is obtained at a military treatment facility, it is free.

•**National Conference of State Legislatures** (*www.ncsl.org/programs/health/drugaid. htm#discount*). As of late 2008, at least 42 states had established some type of program to provide prescription drug coverage or subsidies to low-income older adults or disabled persons who do not qualify for Medicaid. The programs vary widely—and the information is available through state departments of health or social services.

PATIENT ADVOCACY GROUPS

Some groups charge a set fee to help patients find free or low-cost medications. This works well for people who don't want to deal with the application process required for most drug-assistance programs.

•**Free Medicine Foundation** (573-996-3333, *www.freemedicine.com*). This group will search for programs that can provide your drugs for little or no charge. The onetime fee of $10 is reimbursed if the group fails to find your medication for free. The service is available to people with incomes up to $80,000 for a family of four…$52,800 for couples…and $39,200 for individuals.

•**IPS** (727-521-2646, *www.ipsc.cc*). A onetime registration fee of $25 is required for this program, and each prescription (usually three months' worth of medication) costs $20.

MASS-MARKET RETAILERS

Some large retail stores, such as Walmart, Target, Costco and Kmart, offer low-price prescriptions on generic and some brand-name medications. Walmart, for instance, offers a program that covers mostly generic drugs at a cost of $4 for a 30-day supply and $10 for a 90-day supply. For information, go to store Web sites or ask at your local store's pharmacy.

■ **More from Edward Jardini, MD…**

Smart Ways to Slash the Cost of Prescription Drugs

The high cost of prescription medication creates a heavy financial burden for many Americans. According to a study in *American Journal of Medicine,* an estimated one in five Americans over the age of 50 with a chronic health problem has been forced to cut back on essentials—including food—to pay for prescription drugs. Nearly one in five has had to skip doses of prescribed medications to save money.

High deductibles and copayments mean that these problems can affect even people who have prescription drug coverage through health insurance.

But there are ways to reduce out-of-pocket prescription drug costs…

•**Decline free samples.** Receiving things for free sounds like a wonderful money-saver—but accepting free samples to start a new long-term treatment could cost you a bundle. Pharmaceutical companies typically supply doctors with free samples of expensive new drugs with which they are trying to win market share from lower-cost, better proven alternatives. These free sample drugs often require long-term use, so receiving the first dose for free will mean much less to your bottom line than the hefty price you will pay for subsequent doses.

Unless your doctor has reason to believe that this drug is better for you than the alternatives, say, "No, thank you, Doctor. Keep the samples. Just give me a prescription for a trusted medication that's within my budget."

Exception: Free samples will save you money if your doctor is willing to give you enough samples for a complete course of treatment. Though uncommon, this might be possible with, say, an antihistamine for a case of hives or an antibiotic for an infection.

•**Split tablets.** You may know that splitting tablets can save you money. But most people, including doctors, don't realize just how much you can save. Most prescription drugs are sold in a range of dosages. There might be a 20-milligram (mg) pill, a 40-mg pill and an 80-mg pill.

The higher-dose pills usually are a relative bargain, per milligram of medication, compared with lower-dose pills. In other words, an 80-mg pill will almost always cost substantially less than twice the price of a 40-mg pill and less than four times the price of a 20-mg pill. In some cases, pills of different dosages are priced exactly the same.

Example: The 20-mg, 40-mg and 80-mg versions of the cholesterol medication Lipitor cost the same per pill.

Whenever you are prescribed an expensive medication, ask your doctor if it would be possible for him/her to prescribe half-tablet doses of pills twice as strong as you need—half an 80-mg tablet rather than one 40-mg tablet, for example. Most doctors aren't very familiar with medication prices, so you might have to explain that this could save you a lot of money. Pill-splitting devices, sold at pharmacies, can help you divide pills accurately.

Caution: Certain types of pills, including capsules, gelcaps and extended-release tablets, cannot be split safely. Discuss any plans you have to split pills with your doctor and pharmacist.

•**Apply to pharmaceutical company patient-assistance programs.** Most major pharmaceutical companies will supply their drugs for free to patients who are unable to afford them. These underpublicized, underutilized assistance programs are not necessarily restricted to people who are very poor. Families making as much as $70,000 per year can qualify for the most liberal programs. Other pharmaceutical company programs cap income at $40,000 or less, but exceptions may be made or applicants may be allowed to deduct the cost of medical expenses when determining their annual income. Income, not assets, is used to determine need, so retirees often qualify even if they have considerable savings.

There is no downside to applying. Look for details and an application on the pharmaceutical company's Web site or call its 800 number.

Attention veterans: Anyone who has been honorably discharged from the military following active service can obtain many prescription drugs for $8 per month per prescription through the US Department of Veterans Affairs' health care system. Contact the VA for more information on health-care eligibility (877-222-8387, *www.va.gov*).

•**Ask your doctor to prescribe a cheaper alternative** to a name-brand drug. Most people know that generic versions of expensive prescription pharmaceuticals are just as effective at a fraction of the cost.

Examples: The generic equivalents of the popular drugs Ambien, Prozac, Soma, Xanax and Zantac can cost as little as 10% as much as the name brands.

However, you may not realize that there are less expensive medications within the same class of drugs that might be equally effective for you.

Example: Beta-blockers are a class of drug used to treat high blood pressure. Though all beta-blockers are very similar, a three-month supply of Zebeta costs about $242...a three-month supply of Inderal is closer to $80. Even generic versions of these drugs differ substantially in price—$90 for a three-month supply of the generic version of Zebeta...only $11 for generic Inderal.

Sometimes it is possible to switch to a different, cheaper class of drugs without any health consequences. New classes of drugs are heavily marketed, but that does not mean they are any better than older, cheaper drugs that treat the same problems. Ask your doctor whether there is evidence that the expensive new class of drug he/she wants to prescribe will be any more effective for you than a drug from an older, less expensive class.

•**Don't ask your doctor for advertised drugs.** Pharmaceutical companies now market prescription medications directly to consumers. Asking your doctor about an advertised drug could be bad for both your financial and physical health. Not only are heavily advertised prescription drugs usually very expensive, research suggests that mentioning advertised drugs to your doctor could lead to prescriptions that you do not need.

•Don't use insurance for very low-cost drugs. Patients who have prescription drug coverage typically use this insurance every time they purchase medication. When these prescriptions are for low-cost generic drugs, however, their copayments can exceed the cost of purchasing the drugs out-of-pocket. Ask your pharmacist the cash cost of a generic drug before producing your insurance card.

Example: I prescribed one-half tablet per day of *hydrochlorothiazide,* a high blood pressure medication, to a patient. This patient used his prescription drug plan to buy the medication, paying a $10 copayment each month, for a total cost of $120 per year. These pills would have cost him only around a nickel apiece had he paid cash—approximately $10 per year.

Also, check Walmart and Target for their $4 prescription drug plans.

Easy Ways to Cut Your Drug Costs

Marvin D. Shepherd, PhD, director of the Center for Pharmacoeconomic Studies and professor and division head of the Pharmacy Administration Division at the College of Pharmacy, University of Texas, Austin.

S everal years ago, the average American (some with drug coverage, some without) spent approximately $487 on prescription drugs. Adults age 75 and older spent about $1,028.

Although the increasing costs of drug development continue to drive drug costs up, most people can save *at least* 50%.

Secret: Smart shopping, plus inside information on how to get the most medication for your money.

Whether you pay for drugs out-of-pocket or have drug coverage, here's the top money-saving advice…

PRICE SHOP

Prescription drug prices can vary by 25% or more from one pharmacy to the next. Don't assume that big chains have the best prices. Some smaller pharmacies scout out the cheapest drug wholesalers and pass the savings to consumers.

Smart idea: Price shop by phone. Call in the evening or weekday afternoons when pharmacists are typically less busy.

BUY ON-LINE

You can save anywhere from 20% to 50% buying drugs from on-line pharmacies, which have low overhead costs. It's a smart strategy for patients with chronic conditions, such as arthritis or high cholesterol, who use large quantities of the same drugs over time.

For computer users, the most reliable on-line pharmacies include Medco, *www.medcohealth. com*…and *www.drugstore.com*.

Important: Buy only from on-line pharmacies that display the Verified Internet Pharmacy Practice Sites (VIPPS) seal. This means that the company has been inspected and accredited by the National Association of Boards of Pharmacy. Also, avoid on-line pharmacies that don't require a prescription. This is a sign that the company may be foreign or sells drugs illegally.

REQUEST OLDER DRUGS

Doctors don't admit it, but they're just as likely as patients to be influenced by slick drug marketing campaigns. Studies have shown that doctors are more likely to prescribe new drugs than older ones—even when there's clear evidence that the older drugs are just as effective and much less expensive.

Example: Millions of Americans with osteoarthritis switched to COX-2 inhibitors, such as *celecoxib* (Celebrex) when this class of drugs was introduced. For most patients, COX 2 inhibitors are no more effective than aspirin, acetaminophen or ibuprofen. Now studies show that these drugs may even increase risk for heart attack or stroke. What's more, a single dose of a COX-2 inhibitor might cost more than $2, compared with pennies for aspirin.

Smart idea: Ask your doctor to write prescriptions for older, less-expensive drugs unless there's a compelling medical reason to take a newer medication.

GENERIC DRUGS

The average price of a brand-name prescription in 2007 was $119.51, compared with $34.34

for a generic, according to the National Association of Chain Drug Stores. That's a difference of 248%.

If your doctor prescribes a brand-name drug, your pharmacist is permitted under state law to substitute a less-expensive generic.

To find out if a generic is available: Go to the FDA's Web site, *www.fda.gov/cder/ob/default.htm,* for a list of all FDA-approved drugs and generic equivalents. Or use a drug reference book, such as *Physicians' Desk Reference* (Thomson) or *The Pill Book* (Bantam), available in bookstores and libraries.

DRUG DISCOUNT CARDS

The Medicare Prescription Drug, Improvement, and Modernization Act of 2003 gave people on Medicare the right to acquire drug discount cards as of January, 2006.

In addition, some pharmaceutical companies have their own plans for low-income or uninsured people that offer discounts of 10% to 40%.

To find out about medication discounts offered by pharmaceutical companies, go to the Pharmaceutical Research and Manufacturers of America's Web site, *www.phrma.org.*

To order the group's *Directory of PhRMA Member Company Patient Assistance Programs,* call 800-762-4636 or download if free from *www.pparx.org.*

Other major discount cards…

•**Together Rx Access,** 800-444-4106, *www.togetherrxaccess.com.*

Income ceiling: $30,000 for singles, $10,000 for each additional family member, $40,000 for couples.

•**US Pharmaceutical Group's Nations Health Discount Prescription Plan,** 800-977-0351, *www.nationshealth.com.*

Income ceiling: None.

BUY IN BULK

Check with your insurance plan to see if you can get a 90-day supply of your medications. You may be able to save co-pay charges and dispensing fee charges.

Caution: Buy drugs in bulk only if you've already been taking them and know they work for you.

SPLIT PILLS

You can double the quantity of the doses in a single prescription by getting a higher-strength tablet and using a pill splitter to cut the pills into halves. A 100-mg tablet often costs about the same as a 50-mg tablet of the same drug.

Important: Capsules cannot be split. Pills with enteric coatings or other time-release mechanisms also should not be split. Ask your doctor or pharmacist if your pills can be split.

Do not use a kitchen knife to split your pills. Use a pill splitter, sold in pharmacies and on-line for about $5.

Examples: EZY Dose Tablet Cutter and Deluxe Tablet Cutter.

The High Cost of Drug Samples?

Rebecca Shannonhouse, editor of the *Bottom Line/Health* newsletters, Boardroom Inc., 281 Tresser Blvd., Stamford, Connecticut 06901.

The free drug samples that many people get from their doctors can save them money and trips to the pharmacy. But there's a catch—your drug bill might wind up being higher in the long run.

Study finding: Patients who never received free drug samples had estimated out-of-pocket prescription costs of $178 over six months, while those who had received free samples for six months paid $212 for the six-month period following receipt of the freebies.

The study was not designed to identify the cause of the disparity, says Anirban Basu, PhD, a University of Chicago assistant professor and coauthor of the study. However, a likely explanation is that once patients receive free samples of a new, expensive medication, they're apt to keep taking it. Free drug samples can be a boon if you don't have health insurance. *Samples also can work well for…*

•**Short-term prescriptions,** such as those for some antibiotics or pain relievers.

•**Drugs that require a "test drive."** For some conditions—depression, for example—patients may need to try a number of drugs before finding the right one. Similarly, a patient may need to find out if a therapeutic approach—say, the particular class of blood pressure drug—is effective.

•**Short-term prescriptions, such as those for some antibiotics or pain relievers.**

•**Drugs that require a "test drive."** For some conditions—depression, for example—patients may need to try a number of drugs before finding the right one. Similarly, a patient may need to find out if a therapeutic approach —say, the use of a particular class of blood pressure drug—is effective.

Smart idea: If you need to continue a drug after trying a free sample, ask your doctor if you can switch to a similar, but older and less-expensive, medication.

Another option: Ask for a 60- to 90-day prescription (rather than 30 days) to save out-of-pocket costs.

■ ■ ■ ■

Get Medicare to Cover More

U*sing Your Medicare Drug Plan: What to Do If Your Medicine Isn't Covered,* a booklet available from the Federal Citizen Information Center and YourPharmacyBenefit.org, will inform you about all your options, including how to appeal a denial of coverage. The booklet guides you through the process and provides tips on how to handle your situation. To obtain your free copy, go on-line to *www.pueblo. gsa.gov* and look up publication #520R or enter "drug plan" in the search box…or call 888-878-3256.

Note: There is a $2 service fee for orders placed by phone.

What You Need to Know About Overseas Medical Care

Charles B. Inlander is a consumer advocate and health-care consultant based in Fogelsville, Pennsylvania. He was the founding president of the nonprofit People's Medical Society, a consumer advocacy organization active in the 1980s and 1990s, and is the author of more than 20 books, including *Take This Book to the Hospital with You: A Consumer Guide to Surviving Your Hospital Stay.* St. Martin's.

I n years past, medical tourism referred mainly to the practice of bringing people from foreign countries to the US for high-quality medical care. In recent years, the term has assumed a new definition, as US citizens leave the country for more affordable surgery and other treatments. Hundreds of thousands of Americans are seeking foreign medical care each year, and this trend is expected to grow as US insurance companies consider covering off-shore medicine. *But before you jump on a plane, here are some important points to consider…*

•**Is it safe?** Americans have long assumed that foreign medical care is more dangerous than that offered here at home. But high-quality medical care can be found in many places throughout the world. The Joint Commission, the private group that accredits hospitals in the US, has an international branch (*www.jointcom missioninternational.org*) that accredits foreign hospitals. If you are thinking about going abroad for medical care, make sure that the facility you are considering has been accredited by the joint commission. Also, check on the training of the doctors who would be caring for you. Look for physicians who were educated at US medical schools and completed a residency in their area of specialty at a US hospital. This is not a guarantee that you will receive high-quality care, but it does give you some reassurance because it is easier to check the reputation of medical schools and residency programs in the US.

•**Will I really save money?** MedSolution (*www.medsolution.com*), a Canadian medical-tourism firm, released these cost comparisons: Hip replacement—$40,000 in North America, $15,000 in France and $5,800 in India…coronary angioplasty—$35,000 in North America, $18,400 in France and $3,700 in India. Many people going abroad for face-lifts and other cosmetic procedures are paying about 30% to 50% of US prices.

•**Do I have all the facts?** Its usually best to use a medical-tourism firm. To find one, search the term medical tourism on the Internet. The firm you select will ask for your medical records to review, and you will then be matched with a doctor and hospital. These firms handle all the details, including travel and hotel arrangements. But make sure you get references for the firm (check for complaints with the Better Business Bureau or the attorney generals office in the firms home state) as well as the hospital and doctors they recommend to you (ask the firm for contact information for patients treated at these medical facilities).

Buyer beware: If something goes wrong with your overseas medical care, emergency treatment will be provided (your insurance probably won't cover the cost, though). Also, you have no legal recourse in the US against the overseas provider. Each country has its own malpractice laws. Most are not as protective as those in the US. Very few foreign hospitals or doctors will be of much help to you once you return to the US. Make sure that you have a doctor here who is ready to provide follow-up care.

■ ■ ■ ■

Lowering Drug Costs

Now you can get a personalized report on programs you qualify for that can help you reduce your prescription drug costs. The National Council on Aging has created a Web site that will provide the report directly to you.

How it works: You enter your personal information and more than 1,550 programs in all 50 states are searched through to find benefits that you qualify for. Prescription drugs are included. Visit *www.benefitscheckup.org*.

How to Save Up to 50% on Prescriptions

Randall S. Stafford, MD, PhD, associate professor of medicine, Stanford Prevention Research Center, Stanford School of Medicine, Stanford, California. His study was published in *The American Journal of Managed Care*, 666 Plainsboro Rd., Plainsboro, New Jersey 08536. *www.ajmc.com*.

Reduce your medication costs by asking your doctor to prescribe *twice* your usual drug dosage. Cut the pills in half using a pill splitter, sold in most drugstores. Take one-half of a pill as your normal dosage. Because a double dosage of a prescription drug usually costs only slightly more than the prescribed amount, this practice can reduce the price of some medications by up to 50%.

Important: Not all drugs can be safely halved. Ask your pharmacist for advice. *Here are 11 commonly used medications that can be split...*

Drug	Brand Name	Condition	Estimated Savings
Atorvastatin	Lipitor	High cholesterol	49%
Pravastatin	Pravachol	High cholesterol	23%
Doxazosin	Cardura	Hypertension, prostate enlargement	46%
Lisinopril	Zestril	Congestive heart failure, hypertension	38%
Sildenafil	Viagra	Impotence	50%
Citalopram	Celexa	Depression	46%
Paroxetine	Paxil	Depression, anxiety	46%
Nefazodone	Serzone	Depression	49%
Sertraline	Zoloft	Depression	46%
Olanzapine	Zyprexa	Schizophrenia, bipolar disorder	31%
Clonazepam	Klonopin	Panic disorder, epilepsy	41%

The Right Way to Save on Medicine from Canada

Gary Passmore, spokesperson for Congress of California Seniors, a nonprofit senior advocacy group based in Sacramento.

The sky-high cost of prescription drugs in the United States has prompted about one million Americans to buy from Canadian pharmacies. Prescription drugs cost less in Canada than in the US because Canada—like most industrialized countries—has price controls to keep down drug prices. America does not have such price controls.

For Americans who have chronic conditions requiring long-term prescriptions that are not covered by insurance, ordering drugs from north of the border can cut the cost of medications by half—and sometimes even more.

But is it safe? For answers, Gary Passmore, who has toured Canadian pharmacies for the Congress of California Seniors, a senior advocacy group, was interviewed.

KEEPING IMPORTED PRESCRIPTIONS LEGAL

Why isn't it legal for Americans to order prescription medications from Canada?

According to federal law, the US Food and Drug Administration (FDA) must approve the safety of all pharmaceuticals brought into the country and certify the safety of the companies that handle and sell them. For the past decade, through both the Clinton and Bush administrations, the US government has declined to provide the necessary certification for Canadian pharmacies.

Do Americans risk prosecution when they import prescription drugs?

No, not if they do so within reason. While the FDA refuses to take steps to make importing prescription drugs legal, the US Customs Department will not take action against individual Americans who import prescription drugs for their own personal use—if they have valid prescriptions and bring in no more than a 90-day supply. This is according to a statement made before the Senate by former FDA Associate Commissioner William K. Hubbard. This applies to drugs sent through the mail or driven across the border. (To avoid problems, bring your prescription with you if you intend to drive.)

The US government says that importing Canadian pharmaceuticals poses safety risks. Are Canadian drugs truly less safe than American drugs?

Health Canada (the Canadian department of health) is as rigorous in its inspections of pharmaceutical makers and distributors as the FDA. The only reason the US government is claiming that there are safety issues is that the pharmaceutical industry has considerable power in Congress and wants Americans to buy drugs at higher prices.

CHOOSE THE RIGHT PHARMACY

How should Americans select a Canadian pharmacy?

I advise sticking with pharmacies that belong to the Canadian International Pharmacy Association (CIPA). They are listed on CIPA's Web site, *www.ciparx.ca*.

I have met with CIPA's leadership, and I'm convinced that it is committed to maintaining high professional standards.

How much can an American save by ordering drugs from Canada? Is it important to shop around?

The savings vary by drug and with fluctuations in the exchange rate between the US dollar and the Canadian dollar. Generally, you can save between 40% and 80%, even after you account for shipping charges.

Certainly, you should shop around and check the prices at a few different pharmacies—but don't expect prices to vary much because the Canadian government regulates how much pharmaceutical companies can charge.

FUTURE POLICY

Is there any chance that the US government will start cracking down on citizens who import their prescription drugs from Canada?

It is unlikely that the US will start arresting people at the border. No politician wants to be seen locking up grandmothers who can't afford to buy their medications at home.

The greater risk to this savings opportunity is that the Canadian pharmaceutical system could be stretched beyond its limit.

Ordering from Canada is not a long-term solution to our nation's high drug-price problem. The American government is going to have to come up with a better way to make affordable pharmaceuticals available.

Advantages of Buying Drugs Abroad

Cynthia M. Ronan, MD, OB/GYN at Griffin Hospital, 300 Seymour Ave., Suite 108, Derby, Connecticut 06418.

Many drugs that require a prescription in the US are sold over-the-counter in other countries.

Even when a medication requires a prescription, most foreign doctors will give you one if you say you have a prescription in the US.

Rules about prescriptions are much looser abroad. In Latin America, for instance, doctors commonly write large-quantity (100 tablets plus), *refillable* prescriptions for drugs that, in the US, require a new prescription to be written each time the drug is dispensed.

Outside the US, you can buy some medications that aren't available here, even with a prescription.

Also more readily available abroad: Drugs that are experimental.

There are many people in the US who suffer from fatal and very serious diseases. They are often turned down for experimental treatment.

Reasons: There are manufacturers' restrictions on which patients are eligible for experimentation and there is potential for enormous losses from lawsuits.

Treatment using interferon for malignant forms of leukemia and melanoma are also available abroad.

Risks: Side effects and proper dosages of experimental medications aren't fully known. That's one of the reasons the Food and Drug Administration hasn't approved them for general use.

■■■■

Beware of Internet Drugs

Fake drugs have slipped into drug markets in the US. The risk of buying mislabeled, adulterated or inactive drugs is higher if you buy on the Internet or in foreign countries. High-priced drugs, which usually are prescribed for serious conditions—such as *epoetin* (Procrit) for anemia—are likely candidates to be counterfeited.

To protect yourself: Ask your pharmacist if he purchases drugs from distributors who are licensed by the Food and Drug Administration (FDA) and if he inspects drug packaging. If you buy from the Internet, make sure the pharmacy displays the Verified Internet Pharmacy Practice Sites (VIPPS) seal of the National Association of Boards of Pharmacy.

Mitchel C. Rothholz, RPh, chief of staff, American Pharmacists Association, Washington, DC. *www.aphanet.org.*

Are Bargain Medicines Really Safe?

Jack Rosenberg, PharmD, PhD, professor of pharmacy practice and pharmacology, International Drug Information Center, Long Island University, New York.

It is a painful reality in America—health care and prescription medications cost a bundle. Many Americans—especially seniors who take multiple medications—are tempted to buy cheap prescription medications in Canada or over the Internet. But are these drugs safe?

The answer depends upon whom you ask.

THE OFFICIAL POINT OF VIEW

Under a law passed in 1987, it generally is illegal for anyone other than the manufacturer to import drugs into the US. The US Food and Drug Administration (FDA) warns that imported medication may be outdated, contaminated, counterfeit or contain too much or too little of the active ingredient.

Not surprisingly, pharmaceutical companies agree with this official point of view. Ironically, however, the fact is that we already import a huge quantity of drugs from other countries. While drug manufacturers publicly worry about the safety of medications from abroad, they have quietly relocated many of their own factories to foreign shores to take advantage of cheaper labor costs. The difference is that these plants are considered safe because they are inspected by the FDA.

PLAYING WITH FIRE

While everyone agrees that we want safe drugs, problems arise because of the pharmaceutical industry's unbalanced pricing structure. American consumers currently pay the world's highest prices for drugs, while price controls and shrewd bargaining compel manufacturers to sell the same drugs for far less money in foreign markets. This makes imported drugs a great bargain.

Unfortunately, when you buy imported drugs that have not been inspected by the FDA, you're playing with fire. Ten percent of drugs worldwide may be counterfeit, according to the World Health Organization (WHO). Without FDA inspection, there is usually no way to tell whether a drug is real or fake.

There also is no way to know how imported drugs have been stored. It was reported that in one sting operation, the FDA discovered that a Canadian supplier mistakenly shipped insulin, which requires refrigeration, at room temperature.

CONSUMERS SEEK A MORE ECONOMICAL ALTERNATIVE

Safe or not, legal or not, seniors in border states from Maine to Washington organize regular bus trips to Canada to purchase prescription medications. In just one trip, they collectively save thousands of dollars. Moreover, American consumers tend to trust the safety of Canadian drugs, which are regulated much like the drugs in our own country. (This is clearly not the case with all imported medications.) If you are set on visiting a Canadian pharmacy, you can first check to see if it is accredited at *www.napra. org*, Canada's National Association of Pharmacy Regulatory Authorities.

In a new trend that extends beyond individuals, several cities and states around the country also have expressed interest in buying drugs from abroad. In open defiance of the FDA, the city of Springfield, Massachusetts, imported drugs from Canada for its workers and retirees, and at least two states—Illinois and California—considered the possibility of doing so as well.

EXERCISE CARE ON THE INTERNET

Another tempting alternative is shopping on the Internet. Both domestic and imported drugs are available on-line. If you spend much time on the Web, chances are you are already bombarded with e-mail opportunities to buy prescription drugs.

On the Internet, it's "buyer beware." Although it's very tempting when you see an ad for a drug you're taking at a significant discount, you must be careful.

Which sites are safe? *The FDA offers the following suggestions…*

•**Check with the Verified Internet Pharmacy Practice Sites (VIPPS)** (*http://vipps.nabp. net/verify.asp*) to determine whether the Web site is a licensed pharmacy in good standing.

•**Don't use sites that offer to prescribe a prescription drug for the first time without verification** that you have had a physical exam or that will sell a prescription drug without a prescription.

•**Avoid sites that do not provide a US address** and phone number to contact if there is a problem.

•**Steer clear of foreign sites,** sites that advertise "new cures" or "amazing results" and sites that claim the government or researchers have conspired to suppress a product.

SAFER ALTERNATIVES

Many states offer discounted-drug plans to seniors with limited incomes. Call your local office for the aging to inquire about your particular state's policies. There are also options that guarantee health insurance to all children of low-income parents. Contact your local or state authorities for details. Finally, if you are having difficulty with prescription bills, talk to your doctor. Most pharmaceutical companies offer discounts to those who can't otherwise afford their medications.

Are You Shopping at the Right Pharmacy?

Charles B. Inlander is a consumer advocate and health-care consultant based in Fogelsville, Pennsylvania. He was the founding president of the nonprofit People's Medical Society, a consumer advocacy organization active in the 1980s and 1990s, and is the author of more than 20 books, including *Take This Book to the Hospital with You: A Consumer Guide to Surviving Your Hospital Stay.* St. Martin's.

Twenty years ago, your community most likely had an independent neighborhood pharmacy and, possibly, a chain drugstore. Today, supermarkets, discount stores and mail-order and Internet companies also sell prescription drugs. *What you need to know about each...*

•**Independent neighborhood pharmacy.** Because these pharmacies rely heavily on return business, they usually provide excellent service. However, the cost of prescriptions at independent neighborhood pharmacies is usually 15% to 20% higher than in other settings. That's because they cannot buy drugs in the same volume as chain drugstores or other larger outlets.

Special case: If your medication needs to be compounded (customized for an individual patient), the independent neighborhood pharmacy probably is the place to go. Few chain drugstores, discount stores or mail-order companies provide this service.

My recommendation: If personalized service is more important than cost, the independent neighborhood pharmacy may be right for you.

•**Chain drugstores.** CVS, Rite Aid, Longs and Walgreens are the dominant players in the pharmacy business. Chains provide many services that consumers like. Many stores are open 24 hours a day and have drive-up windows for convenience. Their computer systems help track potential drug interactions and let you fill prescriptions at almost any of their stores without additional paperwork. Chains also accept most insurance plans, something a neighborhood pharmacy cannot always afford to do. Because they buy in volume, their prices tend to be low.

My recommendation: Chains are best if you want to be able to fill your prescriptions at multiple locations.

•**Supermarkets and discount stores.** This is perhaps the fastest-growing segment of the retail prescription drug sector. Kroger and Walmart are the big names here. They sell convenience. You simply drop off your prescription when you come in to shop and pick it up on your way out. Because prescription drugs are more profitable than food and most other items, they often are deeply discounted to get you into the store.

My recommendation: For the lowest-priced retail outlets, go to supermarkets and discount stores.

•**Mail-order and on-line drugstores.** These most often are your cheapest source of prescription drugs, thanks to low overhead. Service, of course, is not personal. There are many mail-order companies, including Walgreens Health Initiatives (877-422-7718, *www.mywhi. com*), and on-line retailers, such as Drugstore. com (800-378-4786, *www.drugstore.com*).

My recommendation: If you buy medications for a chronic health condition, mail-order and on-line drugstores are typically the best choice, since they offer 90-day supplies of drugs at a lower price.

■ **More from Charles B. Inlander...**

How to Pay *Much* Less For Health Care

Most people never think about negotiating fees with a doctor or other health-care provider. Negotiating is something we do with a car dealer or at a flea market. But the truth is, doctors and hospitals negotiate fees with insurance companies and the government all the time. So why not with you? If you have health insurance, you can save by negotiating such health-care fees as copayments. If you are uninsured or need a medical treatment that is not covered by your insurance, you can save even more. *How to negotiate fees for health care and medical products...*

•**Don't be afraid to ask.** Most doctors are willing to lower their fees for people with limited budgets who may not have health insurance (or only very basic coverage). But you must initiate the negotiation.

My advice: If the quoted fee is more than you can pay, ask if some other payment arrangement, such as paying in monthly installments, can be made or if the fee can be lowered.

What you might say: "What is the fee for this treatment/service? Unfortunately, I can't afford that. Can we negotiate?" If you have been treated by the health-care provider for many years, mention your loyal patronage.

•**Talk to the right person.** In a report published in *U.S. News & World Report*, a hospital's chief financial officer (CFO) noted that it is common for hospitals to reduce charges by 30% for needy or uninsured patients who contact the CFO directly. He noted that most hospitals give large health insurers discounts of 60% or more, so deals with individual patients are still profitable to the facility.

My advice: Always negotiate with a decision-maker. For fee reductions at a hospital, before you receive surgery or any other treatment, call the hospital and ask the operator to connect you to the office of the CFO or the assistant CFO—one of them must sign off on all of the hospital's financial negotiations. At a doctor's office, talk directly to the doctor about lower fees—not the nurse, office manager or receptionist.

What you might say to a doctor or hospital CFO: "What does Medicare pay you for the service or treatment I am going to get? Will you accept the same payment from me?"

•**Request a discount on medical products.** Several years ago, I took a friend to a hearing-aid shop, and we negotiated 40% off the *lowest* quoted price. Since most stores that sell hearing aids, wheelchairs and other types of durable medical equipment are privately owned, and typically mark up products by 50% to 100%, you usually can strike a good bargain with the owner.

My advice: Shop around before negotiating and don't forget to check prices on the Internet. Then start by offering 20% less than the best price you found elsewhere. Offer to pay in cash rather than by credit card or check—this saves the merchant a processing fee.

The worst that can happen if you try to negotiate a medical fee is that your request will be turned down. But chances are you'll save a tidy sum with little effort on your part.

How to Get Health Care Regardless of Your Ability to Pay

http://findahealthcenter.hrsa.gov.

Here are some places to look for free or reduced-cost health care, if you are beyond your insurance limits or have very low income.

•**Community health centers provide health care regardless of your ability to pay and even if you have no health insurance.** To find the closest community health center, go to *http://findahealthcenter.hrsa.gov.*

If you don't have internet access, call your city or county government to find a community health center. Phone the center for information or for an appointment.

•**Hill-Burton Facilities.** About 200 health care facilities nationwide are obligated to provide free or reduced-cost care to people with very low incomes who are unable to pay. They are known as Hill-Burton obligated facilities after the law that created them. Each facility chooses which services it will provide at no or lowered cost and who will receive them. Eligibility is based on family size and income. You may apply at a Hill-Burton obligated facility for free or reduced-cost care either before or after you receive care. Be sure to follow the application's guidelines carefully. To find one, call the Hill-Burton Hotline (800) 638-0742; (800) 492-0359 in Maryland.

•**State medical assistance program**s help people with incomes under certain limits pay for prescription medications, visits to the doctor, hospitalizations, and insurance premiums. Each program is different and not all states have medical assistance programs. Contact your local department of social services or a local hospital's social worker to see if your s tate has a program and if you might be eligible to apply.

•**The National Breast and Cervical Cancer Early Detection Program** for low-income women helps them afford mammograms and Pap tests. Find a free or low-cost mammogram and Pap test in your State.

Contact: Centers for Disease Control and Prevention, Division of Cancer Prevention and Control, 4770 Buford Hwy, NE, MS K-64, Atlanta, GA 30341-3717. Call (800) CDC-INFO; TTY (888) 232-6348; fax (770) 488-4760; E-mail *cdcinfo@cdc.gov*.

• **Veterans Medical Benefits provide care to enrolled veterans.** If you served in the military and were discharged in other than dishonorable conditions, you are probably eligible. For more information, see the US Department of Veteran Affairs web site *http://www.va.gov.*

VA Benefits: (800) 827-1000.

Health care benefits: (877) 222-8387.

How to Cut Costs of Chronic Conditions

David Nganele, founder of Harmony Health Communications, where he developed award-winning disease-management programs in cooperation with doctors, drug companies and community groups. He is author of several books, including *The Best Healthcare for Less.* Wiley.

A chronic disease can be financially devastating even for someone who has health insurance. Benefit limits often are reached before the condition is under control.

People without insurance may be forced to borrow money or sell assets when faced with such conditions as recurring cancers, heart disease, depression and diabetes.

Making lifestyle changes—quitting smoking, improving your diet and exercising—can reduce the need for medication for many conditions. In addition, sufferers can eliminate some costs entirely by understanding how hospitals, drug companies and doctors do business. *Most effective cost-saving strategies...*

AT-HOME CARE

•**Become an expert.** Learning all you can about your illness may help you discover lower-cost treatments and aspects of the condition that even your doctor may not know about. You'll also benefit psychologically from putting yourself in charge instead of relying solely on your doctor.

•**Contact associations specializing in your condition.** They can help you to locate low-cost treatment centers and suggest ways to prevent your condition from worsening.

Example: Adding supplemental chromium, magnesium and vanadium to your diet may help with diabetes.

Associations for several common illnesses...

•American Cancer Society, 800-227-2345, *www.cancer.org.*

•American Diabetes Association, 800-342-2383, *www.diabetes.org.*

•American Heart Association, 800-242-8721, *www.americanheart.org.*

•American Kidney Fund, 800-638-8299, *www.kidneyfund.org.*

•Depression and Bipolar Support Alliance, 800-826-3632, *www.dbsalliance.org.*

If you're unsure of the appropriate organization, contact the American Medical Association for a referral (800-621-8335, *www.ama-assn.org*).

•**Investigate alternative treatments,** such as acupuncture and biofeedback. Many now are covered by insurance. Even if they're not, they may cost less and be more effective than conventional treatments. For information, contact the federal government's National Center for Complementary and Alternative Medicine at 888-644-6226, *www.nccam.nih.gov.*

•**Buy drugs in large quantities to save on copayments.** Most insurers charge a copayment for each prescription, regardless of the drug's cost. Copayments today can be as high as $50.

Ask your doctor to write 90-day prescriptions, instead of 30-day. You will reduce your copayment by two-thirds.

Example: If you take eight prescription medicines—not unusual for someone with a chronic condition—and have a $30 copayment, your cost will fall by $1,920, or two-thirds—from $2,880 (8 x $30 x 12) to $960 (8 x $30 x 4).

If your insurance company won't allow more than a 30-day supply of a drug from a local pharmacy, ask your health insurer if it uses a mail-order drug service. They typically supply 90-day quantities. Most insurers prefer that you order by mail because it holds down their costs.

•**Ask your doctors for free samples.** Pharmaceutical companies give away billions of dollars worth of samples for doctors to pass on to patients. Don't be embarrassed to ask. If your doctor doesn't have samples, ask him to prescribe generic drugs. For all but a very small percentage of patients, generics are just as effective as brand-name drugs. If you do have insurance, you may have a smaller copayment with generic drugs.

Example: A patient who suffers from depression and doesn't have drug coverage typically pays about $943 for 90 capsules of Prozac in 40-milligram (mg) strength. The generic equivalent represents a saving of 70% or more.

•**Take part in a clinical trial.** Each year, thousands of people with chronic ailments receive free treatment by taking part in trials designed to assess new drugs and procedures. The drug industry or National Institutes of Health (800-411-1222, *www.nih.gov*) coordinates most of these trials.

Important: Participants are given a consent form explaining the trial. Read it, and ask questions before signing.

Some trials are *open*—all the participants are given the medicine being tested and are informed about the results of the trial at each stage.

Other trials are *double-blind*—some participants are given the treatment while others receive a placebo. This prevents test results from being skewed by psychological factors. Patients—and often the doctors who administer the drug—aren't told who has received the drug and who has received the placebo.

Despite the risk that you won't receive any treatment, don't rule out a double-blind trial. If you take part in one, you have about a 50-50 chance of receiving cutting-edge medication.

Even if you get the placebo, doctors typically take you out of the trial if your condition worsens, so you can resume treatment on your own.

HOSPITAL-BASED CARE

•**When you are hospitalized, put your primary-care physician in charge.** Doctors who are unfamiliar with your health history might recommend costly, unnecessary procedures.

Primary physicians, as a rule, recommend fewer procedures than other doctors at a hospital. Your primary doctor already is familiar with your condition and may have tried a variety of treatments for you in the past.

You might even ask your primary physician to help check your hospital bill for inaccuracies. As a patient with a chronic illness, you need to be vigilant about not reaching insurance policy limits sooner than necessary.

•**Consider treatment at a teaching or government-run hospital or clinic.** These institutions usually charge patients according to their ability to pay. They can make sense for people with limited incomes, especially those who lack insurance or have passed their insurance limit.

Information: Health Resources and Services Administration, 800-400-2742, *www.hrsa.gov*.

•**Negotiate with the hospital and other providers.** Pay what you can now, and work out a payment plan for the rest. Or ask for a fee reduction. A hospital or doctor nearly always will compromise because reducing the bill may be cheaper than paying a collection agency or not collecting at all.

•**Get the opinion of more than one doctor before any procedure.** Second opinions increase your chance of finding less expensive—and perhaps more effective—treatment.

Example: Cancer treatments vary greatly in cost and outcome. Since few doctors are experts in all procedures, it's best to weigh the options with different specialists.

Many chronic disease sufferers don't get more than one opinion because they think that their insurance will not pay for a second opinion. In fact, most policies will pay for two or three consultations as long as the doctors are in the insurer's network of approved physicians.

■ ■ ■ ■

On-Line Help

Information on low-cost health services is available on-line. The *American Cancer Society* Web site (*www.cancer.org*) has links to information about free cancer screenings. *Lions Clubs International* (*www.lionsclubs.org*) offers free vision screenings and recycled glasses to those in need. The *Health Resources and Services Administratioin* (*ask.hrsa.gov/pc*) gives information on low-cost medical clinics. *The National Kidney Foundation* (*www.kidney.org/news/keep/index. cfm*) lists free kidney screenings nationwide.

AARP Bulletin, 601 E St. NW, Washington, DC 20049

Free Medical Tests

Jim Miller, an advocate for senior citizens, writes "Savvy Senior," a weekly information column syndicated in 400 newspapers nationwide. Based in Norman, Oklahoma, he offers a free senior newswire service. To sign up, go to *www.savvysenior.org.*

In addition to a nutritious diet, regular exercise and not smoking, health screenings are the best way to stay healthy as you age. But for the 45.7 million Americans living without health insurance and millions more who are underinsured, health screenings may be a luxury they can't afford.

Fortunately, free or low-cost health screenings for a wide range of medical conditions are provided through various national, state and local organizations, government agencies and even businesses.

The best way to find these screenings in your area is by calling the health department of your city, county or state. Also check with hospitals, pharmacies, senior centers and your "area agency on aging."

National and local health associations that focus on particular diseases also may help you. For example, to search for free or low-cost cancer screenings, call the American Cancer Society (800-227-2345) or the National Cancer Institute (800-422-6237).

Other national and regional screening programs and services...

CARDIOVASCULAR DISEASE

•**Legs for Life.** This program offers free screenings for *peripheral arterial disease* (PAD), a "hardening of the arteries" condition that affects an estimated 8 million to 10 million Americans. Individuals with PAD have much greater risk for heart attack, stroke and even leg amputation. Some screening sites also can test for related diseases, such as abdominal aortic aneurysm and carotid artery disease. Most screenings take place in September and require an appointment. 800-488-7284, *www.legsforlife.org.*

•**Society for Vascular Surgery** offers a list of 21 clinics and health-care facilities around the country that provide a variety of free or low-cost vascular screenings. *www.vascularweb.org* (click on "Patients and Families," then "Vascular Screenings").

•**WISEWOMAN Program.** For low-income, uninsured and underinsured women between the ages of 40 and 64, the Centers for Disease Control and Prevention (CDC) offers free blood pressure and cholesterol tests in 20 states. Some sites also offer testing for diabetes and osteoporosis. 800-232-4636, *www.cdc.gov/wisewoman.*

•**Sister to Sister Foundation** sponsors National Women's Healthy Heart Fairs in 18 major cities around the country. The fairs offer women free screenings for blood pressure, body mass index (BMI), cholesterol, glucose (blood sugar), triglycerides (blood fats) and waist circumference. 888-718-8033, *www.sistertosister.org.*

SKIN CANCER

•**American Academy of Dermatology** offers free skin cancer screenings by volunteer dermatologists across the US. 888-462-3376, *www.aad.org/public/exams/screenings.*

•**Skin Cancer Foundation** is nowoperating a nationwide "Road to Healthy Skin Tour" that started in May and runs through October. 800-754-6490, *www.skincancer.org.*

BREAST AND CERVICAL CANCER

•**National Breast and Cervical Cancer Early Detection Program.** This CDC program is for low-income, uninsured and underinsured women. It offers free or low-cost mammograms and Pap tests year-round in all 50 states, the District of Columbia and five US territories. 800-232-4636, *www.cdc.gov/cancer/nbccedp*.

•**National Mammography Day.** On the third Friday of October every year (October 16 in 2009), hundreds of hospitals and clinics across the country offer free or low-cost mammograms to women in need. To locate a screening site, visit the National Breast Cancer Awareness Month Web site at *www.nbcam.org* (click on "Find a Mammography Center Near You"). Then call the site to find out if it is offering free screenings.

PROSTATE CANCER

•**Prostate Cancer Awareness Week.** Each year, during the third full week of September (September 20 through 26 in 2009), the Prostate Cancer Educational Council coordinates with hundreds of sites across America to offer free or low-cost screenings to all men over age 45 and to high-risk men (African-Americans and men who have a family history of the disease) over age 40. The screening consists of a prostate-specific antigen (PSA) blood test and digital rectal exam. 866-477-6788, *www.pcaw.org*.

•**ZERO–The Project to End Prostate Cancer** and The Drive Against Prostate Cancer offer free screenings from mobile screening units that tour the country. 888-245-9455, *www.fightprostatecancer.org*.

COLORECTAL CANCER

•**CDC** currently offers five programs that provide free or low-cost colon and rectal cancer screenings to people ages 50 and older who have no insurance and low incomes. The programs are in Baltimore (866-632-6566)…St. Louis (314-879-6392)…King, Clallam and Jefferson counties in Washington (800-756-5437)…Nebraska (800-532-2227)…and Suffolk County, New York (631-444-7644). *www.cdc.gov/cancer/colorectal*.

•**Colorectal Cancer Coalition** offers free information about colorectal cancer research, free or low-cost screenings, diagnosis and treatment options. 877-427-2111.

KIDNEY DISEASE

•**Kidney Early Evaluation Program** (KEEP). Sponsored by the National Kidney Foundation, this program offers free screenings for those at elevated risk, including adults with high blood pressure, diabetes or a family history of kidney disease. It also offers free screenings in at least 20 cities on World Kidney Day, the second Thursday in March (March 11 in 2010). 800-622-9010, *www.keeponline.org*.

•**American Kidney Fund** offers free kidney screenings to anyone age 18 and older in the Atlanta, Chicago, New York City and Washington, DC, metropolitan areas. 866-300-2900, *www.kidneyfund.org*.

ASTHMA

•**American College of Allergy, Asthma & Immunology** sponsors free asthma screenings, mostly done in May, in more than 250 locations across the US as part of National Asthma and Allergy Awareness Month. *www.acaai.org* (click on "Patient Education").

MEMORY

•**National Memory Screening Day.** On the third Tuesday in November (November 16 in 2009), the Alzheimer's Foundation of America offers free, confidential memory screenings. 866-232-8484, *www.nationalmemoryscreening.org*.

VISION

•**Prevent Blindness America** offers free vision screenings in 21 states and the District of Columbia. 800-331-2020, *www.preventblindness.org*.

MENTAL HEALTH

•**National Depression Screening Day.** On October 8, 2009, Screening for Mental Health Inc. offers free confidential screenings nationwide for depression, suicide risk, bipolar disorder, chronic anxiety and posttraumatic stress disorder. *http://mentalhealthscreening.org*.

SEXUALLY TRANSMITTED DISEASES

Most health departments and many hospitals and other health-care facilities provide free or low-cost screenings for HIV, AIDS and other sexually transmitted diseases. 800-458-5231, *www.hivtest.org*.

The national retail pharmacy chain Walgreens is sponsoring a free health-screening program across the US called Take Care Health Tour. This 300-city, 12-month tour offers six free screenings —cholesterol…blood pressure…bone density… glucose levels…body mass index…and waist circumference. 866-484-8687, *www.walgreens.com/about/community/wellness/tour.jsp.*

■ **More from Jim Miller…**

Low-Cost Doctor Care

There are a variety of programs and services that provide free or low-cost medical care…

•**Health centers.** Federally funded by the Health Resources and Services Administration (HRSA), these health centers provide low-cost health and dental care. You pay what you can afford based on your income. 888-275-4772, *http://findahealthcenter.hrsa.gov.*

•**Hill-Burton Facilities.** There are more than 200 Hill-Burton health-care facili-ties around the country that offer free or reduced-cost health care. Eligibility standards vary by facility, but most require your income to be at or below two times the US poverty guideline (see *http://aspe.hhs.gov/poverty/08poverty.shtml*). 800-638-0742 (800-492-0359 for Maryland residents), *www.hrsa.gov/billburton.*

•**Free clinics.** Nationwide, there are privately funded, non-profit, community-based clinics that typically provide care to those in need at little or no cost. To locate one in your area, call your local hospital or visit *www.freemedicalcamps.com.*

•**Indian Health Service (IHS).** An agency within the Department of Health and Human Service, IHS provides free medical care to approximately 3.3 million American Indians and Alaska Natives. *www.ihs.gov.*

•**Remote Area Medical.** A nonprofit, all-volunteer, charitable organization that provides free health, dental and eye care to uninsured or underinsured people in rural remote areas of the country. *www.ramusa.org.*

•**EyeCare America.** This program, coordinated by the American Academy of Ophthalmology, provides a medical eye exam and up to one year of treatment at no out-of-pocket expense for seniors and diabetics. 800-222-3937, *www.eyecareamerica.org.*

•**Mission Cataract USA** provides free cataract surgery to people of all ages who don't have Medicare, Medicaid or private insurance and have no other means to pay. 800-343-7265, *www.missioncataractusa.org.*

•**Vision USA.** Coordinated by the American Optometric Association (AOA), Vision USA provides free eye-care services to uninsured and low-income workers and their families who have no other means of obtaining care. 800-766-4466, *www.aoa.org.*

•**New Eyes for the Needy.** A not-for-profit eyeglass program that accepts donations of used prescription eyeglasses and distributes them to people in need. 973-376-4903, *www.neweyesfortheneedy.org.*

•**Lions Club.** Your local Lions Club can help you find free or discounted eye-care and eyeglasses programs, including the Give the Gift of Sight program (*www.givethegiftofsight.org*), along with other local services. Call 800-747-4448 to get the number of your state Lions Club office, which can refer you to your community representative, or visit *www.lionsclubs.org.*

■ **And finally from Jim Miller…**

Low-Cost or Even Free Vision Care

Free or discounted vision care is available for people with limited incomes. *Check out these helpful resources…*

•**EyeCare America's Seniors EyeCare Program.** Coordinated by the American Academy of Ophthalmology, this program provides free medical eye care to all US citizens age 65 and older who have not seen an ophthalmologist in three or more years and who don't have coverage through an HMO or the Veterans Administration. Programs include a diabetes and glaucoma eye-care program.* 800-222-3937, *www. eyecareamerica.org.*

• **Knights Templar Eye Foundation.** This charitable foundation provides financial assistance for eye care to any citizen who needs surgery if they are unable to pay and don't qualify for other programs. 847-490-3838, *www.knights templar.org/ktef.* Knights Templar also cosponsors the EyeCare America program above.

• **Mission Cataract USA.** Coordinated by the Volunteer Eye Surgeons' Association, this program provides free cataract surgery to people of all ages who don't have Medicare, Medicaid or private insurance and have no other means to pay. 800-343-7265, *www.missioncataractusa.org.*

• **Vision USA.** Coordinated by the American Optometric Association (AOA), Vision USA provides free eye-care services to uninsured and lower-income workers and their families who have no means of obtaining care. 800-766-4466, *www.aoa.org.*

• **New Eyes for the Needy.** This international program distributes new prescription eyeglasses to people with limited incomes. 973-376-4903, *www.neweyesfortheneedy.org.*

• **Local Lions Clubs.** This is a top referral resource for eye-care and eyeglasses programs that are available in your area. Programs and eligibility requirements vary by community. Phone your local Lions Club chapter or contact Lions Clubs International, 800-747-4448, *www.lionsclubs.org.*

• **"Give the Gift of Sight" program.** Sponsored by the Luxottica Group and in partnership with Lions Clubs International, this program provides free screening and glasses to people who can't afford them. 513-765-6000, *www. givethegiftofsight.com,* or contact LensCrafters. To find a nearby store, call 800-541-5367 or visit *www.lenscrafters.com.*

*Offers subject to change.

■ ■ ■ ■

Free or Low-Cost Flu Shots Available

Free or low-cost flu shots are available at an increasing number of locations, including county health departments and pharmacies. At most of these locations, however, the shots are offered for only a very limited time. The American Lung Association's on-line Flu Clinic Locator (*www.flucliniclocator.org*) can search for upcoming flu shot clinics in your area so you don't miss your chance.

Virtually everyone should get a flu shot each year, particularly those over age 50…between ages 2 and 18…suffering from a chronic lung or heart problem…or in regular contact with someone who falls into any of these increased-risk categories. The shot usually becomes available in late September. Flu and flu complications kill about 36,000 Americans each year.

Norman Edelman, MD, chief medical officer, American Lung Association, and professor of medicine, State University of New York at Stony Brook.

Low-Cost Health Care Options for Children

Concerns about the economy are making escalating medical care costs a greater challenge than ever…especially when it comes to health care for the whole family. This isn't just about children of the unemployed. Businesses are increasingly passing on the burden of skyrocketing insurance premiums to employees in the form of higher deductibles and co-pays, and many middle-class Americans now worry that their health care benefits will be cut or lost.

The good news is that health care resources are available at low cost, and in some cases even for free, to support families and help ensure that no child falls between the health care cracks. While there are those who may never have thought about seeking out these programs, economic pressure may require revisiting that decision, and many people may be surprised that they do in fact qualify for assistance. *Here's how to look for and access options from low-cost health care to free vaccinations…*

FEDERALLY FUNDED HEALTH CENTERS
When money is tight, these centers care for both children and adults—whether or not you have health insurance. Fees are based on income. Services may include free or reduced-cost

check-ups, immunizations, medical and mental health treatment, dental care and prescription drugs. To locate a federally funded center near you, go to *http://findahealthcenter.hrsa.gov* and type in your address, or call 1-888-Ask-HRSA. Centers are available in most metropolitan and many rural areas. For example, there are seven health centers listed for Oklahoma City, Oklahoma, and Montpelier, Vermont…22 for Houston, Texas…and 188 for Chicago. Requirements for being able to use these centers vary.

MEDICAID AND WIC

Medicaid and WIC (the Special Supplemental Nutrition Program for Women, Infants and Children) are government-administered programs for low-income families. Each state sets its own guidelines regarding eligibility and services. At *http://www.aap.org/advocacy/staccess.htm,* the American Academy of Pediatrics offers fact sheets to explain Medicaid benefits for children on a state-by-state basis. Learn more about WIC—which provides nutritional assistance and health care referrals to low-income pregnant, postpartum and nursing women, infants and children up to age five—at *http://www.fns. usda.gov/wic/aboutwic.*

INSURE KIDS NOW

Every state has a health insurance program for infants, children and teens. Families who earn too much to qualify for Medicaid but too little to afford private insurance may be eligible for their State's Children's Health Insurance Program (SCHIP). While eligibility varies, in most states uninsured children 18 and younger whose families earn on average up to $34,000 a year (for a family of four) are eligible. For little or no cost, insurance covers doctor visits, immunizations, emergency room visits, hospitalizations and more. To learn how to enroll, visit the Web site of the US Department of Health & Human Services at *http://www.insurekidsnow. gov* and click on "Your State's Program," or call 1-877-KIDS-NOW.

THE VACCINES FOR CHILDREN (VFC) PROGRAM

This federal entitlement program, enacted in 1994, helps families of children who do not otherwise have access to immunizations. To prevent disease outbreaks, vaccines are made available at no charge or a small fee for eligible children. For instance, after Hurricane Katrina, all children displaced by the storm were made eligible, whether they were staying at shelters, hotels or with family and friends, and regardless of their prior health insurance coverage status. More information about the VFC program is available at *http://www.cdc.gov/vaccines/programs/vfc.*

COMMUNITY-BASED HEALTH CARE OPTIONS

Currently this type of coverage varies widely, town by town, state by state, but most communities subsidize some level of services, such as immunizations and hearing and vision screening for low-income children. Your local health department is the best source of information about free or low-cost community-based health care in your area. You can also look into low-cost community health care providers at the state health agencies at the US Food and Drug Administration's Web site, *http://www.fda.gov/ oca/sthealth.htm.*

SIMPLE AS ABC: GO BACK TO SCHOOL

Often your best bet is to investigate available services through your child's school. Since public schools typically require certain immunizations and annual check-ups, it is in their best interest—as well as that of your child—to put mechanisms into place to ensure that all children have access to them. Find out if your school district offers some form of gratis or discounted health care for students, such as immunizations and medical and dental check-ups. Some schools even have their own clinics. For details, call the school office, school nurse, PTA rep or parent coordinator, or contact your local board of education. Find out if local colleges also underwrite health clinics and free immunization programs, providing an array of health services to the student body at no or low cost.

In some cases, school districts take matters a step further, and also sponsor additional health care coverage for sports team members. Find out if they supply only very basic coverage, or go the whole nine yards. For example, a state-funded program called PlaySafe Sports Medicine Program provides on-the-field doctors and athletic trainers from the University of California, San Francisco at all public high school football games in San Francisco. Some universities may also offer supplemental medical coverage for athletes for any injuries sustained while playing.

In short, when it comes to keeping your child healthy, you're not alone. Help is out there on federal, state and community levels to enable you to meet this goal. (The uninsured.org is also a good place for information on a state-by-state basis.) *Take advantage of it...*

•*http://www.amsa.org/cph/CHIPfact.cfm*

•*http://findahealthcenter.hrsa.gov/*

•*http://www.cms.hhs.gov/LowCost HealthInsFamChild/*

•*http://www.insurekidsnow.gov*

•*http://www.aap.org/advocacy/washing/ elections/med_factsheet_pub.htm*

•*http://www.fns.usda.gov/wic/aboutwic*

•*http://www.fda.gov/oca/sthealth.htm*

How to Get Dental Care For Less Money

Jordan Braverman, MPH, former director of legislative and health policy analysis at Georgetown University's Health Policy Institute, Washington, DC. He is author of several books on health-care policy and financing, including *Your Money & Your Health*. Prometheus.

Dental care is rarely covered by Medicare ...few retirees have dental insurance... and those who have dental insurance often find that their coverage is very limited.

Dental bills average around $677 per year for the typical senior, and a major procedure, such as a root canal or a dental implant, can push that tab into four or even five figures.

Exception: Medicare usually will pay dental bills if they are related to a medical incident that requires a hospital stay, such as jaw reconstruction following a car accident.

Some resources that could help you dramatically reduce your dental bills or even provide dental care for free...

HEALTH INSURANCE

Insurance can help pay dental bills. *Options to consider...*

•**Dental insurance.** If you have access to subsidized group dental insurance through an employer or former employer, it likely is worth having. If not, the case for dental insurance is less compelling.

Dental insurance typically features copayments as high as 50%...annual benefit caps in the low four figures...often long waiting periods before expensive procedures are covered...and usually only 80% coverage if your dentist is out of network.

Dental insurance premiums for seniors are about $430 per year for individual plans. That's a steep price for such limited coverage, but not necessarily an awful deal if you have reason to believe that you will require significant dental work within a few years, perhaps because your dentist has warned you that a major procedure cannot be put off too much longer.

If you do decide to sign up for dental insurance, consider the policies offered through AARP. Rates on AARP dental policies often are a bit lower than what comparable individual dental coverage would cost elsewhere.

More information: Visit *www3.deltadental ins.com/aarp*.

If you do have dental insurance, confirm that your dentist will accept it before agreeing to any procedure. Work with him/her to get the most out of the insurance if he does.

Example: If the dental work you require is not an emergency and significantly exceeds your coverage's annual benefits cap, ask your dentist if the work—and the bill—could be spread out over two or more plan years.

•**Private health insurance.** If you do not have dental insurance but have private health insurance in addition to Medicare, this health insurance could include some basic dental benefits. Read the plan literature or call the insurance company's customer service department to find out.

•**Medical flexible spending accounts (FSAs).** FSAs can substantially trim the effective cost of dental care by allowing patients to pay for health-care bills—including dental bills—with pretax dollars. Unfortunately for retirees, FSAs are available only to employees whose employers offer FSAs as part of their benefits packages.

HAGGLING

Dentists' bills often are negotiable—but only if you discuss costs before having the dental work done. Ask if you can get a senior discount or a cash discount if you pay in cash. Either of these appeals could net you savings of 5% to 10%.

Call other dentists' offices to ask their prices for the procedure. If you find a better rate, tell your dentist that you are on a tight budget and ask if he can match the lower price.

Get a second opinion before agreeing to any major procedure. There's a chance that your dentist could be recommending an expensive procedure that is not necessary. Have your dental files, including the most recent test results and X-rays, forwarded to the dentist who will provide this second opinion so that you do not have to pay to have these repeated. You will have to pay for the second opinion, but the cost of a simple office visit is so much lower than the cost of an elaborate dental procedure that it can be a smart investment if there is any chance that the original dentist was wrong.

IF YOU HAVE A LIMITED INCOME

You probably can get dental care even if your financial resources are very limited...

•**Medicaid.** Medicaid is available only to those with low incomes and limited assets. Eligibility rules and program benefits vary by state. In most states, Medicaid provides at least basic dental care for those living near or below the poverty line.

To find out if you qualify, contact your state's Medicaid Office. (Visit *www.benefits.gov*, select Medicaid/Medicare from the Benefits Quick Search menu, then choose your home state. Or call 800-333-4636 for a contact phone number for your state's Medicaid office.)

Helpful: Nursing homes are legally required to arrange for dental care for residents who use Medicaid to pay for their stays. That typically means that they must either bring a dentist to the nursing home or transport the resident to a dentist's office to receive care.

•**Local and state dental associations.** Many have programs that provide dental services for free or reduced rates to those in financial need. Services are provided by dentists who volunteer their time. Eligibility requirements vary.

State and local dental associations can be found on the Web site of the American Dental Association (ADA)—at *www.ada.org*, select "Dental Organizations" off the menu, then check both the "Constituent (State) Directory" and the "Component (Local) Directory" to find relevant associations. Or call the ADA at 312-440-2500 and ask for your state dental association's phone number.

Example: The Connecticut Dental Association sponsors an annual "Mission of Mercy" program that provides free cleanings, extractions and fillings on a first-come, first-served basis. Unlike most programs of this sort, Connecticut's Mission of Mercy does not require proof of limited income. The next event is scheduled for April 17 and 18, 2009, in New Haven. See the Connecticut Dental Association's Web site for more information (*www.csda.com/ctmom/ctmom4.html*).

•**Public or nonprofit dental clinics.** Available in many regions, these typically charge very low rates, perhaps linked to the patients' ability to pay. In some cases, treatment is free.

Your area Agency on Aging should be able to direct you to any dental clinics in your region and might know of other local low-cost dental options for seniors. (Call the US Administration on Aging's Eldercare Locator, 800-677-1116, or use the Locator on the Web at *www.eldercare.gov* to find your local Agency on Aging if you cannot locate it in your phone book.) Your local or state dental association also might know of area clinics.

MONEY-SAVING OPTIONS

If you are too well off to qualify for low-income dental programs, consider these options...

•**Local dental colleges.** Performed for perhaps half the usual cost, the work is done by dental students under the supervision of qualified instructors. The quality of the dental care tends to be good...however, a dental school might not provide a full range of dental services.

The American Dental Education Association Web site can help you find dental schools in your region. (At *www.adea.org*, click "About ADEA" then "Who We Are," and "Predoctoral Dental Education Programs.") Typing "dental schools" and the name of your state into Google.com also can help you find any schools in your region.

•**Retail dental centers.** Usually located in shopping malls, they typically charge 10% to 20% less than traditional dentists' offices.

Free Health Care! Call These Health and Crisis Hotlines

Gretchen Phillips, MD, a hospitalist (specialist in inpatient medicine) and family physician at Fairview Lakes Medical Center in Wyoming, Minnesota, with long-standing interest in urgent care and women's health. She is the host of the regional radio programs *Fairview On Call with Dr. Gretchen Phillips. www.doctorgretchen.com.*

When a woman is diagnosed with a serious disease or faces a personal or mental-health crisis, help can be as close as the nearest telephone. *Health helplines* provide information from national organizations on specific medical conditions…give referrals to treatment facilities…and suggest coping strategies. *Crisis hotlines* operate around the clock, providing emotional support and step-by-step guidelines on how to handle a crisis.

More hotlines: Check the government Web site *http://healthhotlines.nlm.nih.gov.*

CRISIS SITUATION

•**Domestic Violence** National Domestic Violence Hotline, 800-799-SAFE (800-799-7233), *www.ndvh.org.*

•**Sexual Assault** National Sexual Assault Hotline, 800-656-HOPE (800-656-4673), *www.rainn.org.*

•**Suicidal Intentions** National Suicide Prevention Lifeline, 800-273-TALK (800-273-8255), *www.suicidepreventionlifeline.org.*

GENERAL HEALTH

•**Arthritis** Arthritis Foundation, 800-283-7800, *www.arthritis.org*

•**Breast Cancer** Susan G. Komen for the Cure, 877-GO-KOMEN (877-465-6636), *www.komen.org.*

•**Cancer** American Cancer Society, 800-ACS-2345 (800-227-2345), *www.cancer.org.*

•**Diabetes** American Diabetes Association, 800-342-2383, *www.diabetes.org.*

•**Headache/Migraine** American Headache Society, 800-255-ACHE (800-255-2243), *www.americanheadachesociety.org.*

•**Heart Disease** American Heart Association, 800-AHA-USA-1 (800-242-8721), *www.americanheart.org.*

•**Ovarian Cancer** Gilda Radner Familial Ovarian Cancer Registry, 800-OVARIAN (800-682-7426), *www.ovariancancer.com.*

•**Pain** American Chronic Pain Association, 800-533-3231, *www.theacpa.org.*

MENTAL HEALTH

•**Alcoholism/Drug Addiction** National Council on Alcoholism and Drug Dependence, 800-NCA-CALL (800-622-2255), *www.ncadd.org*

•**Alzheimer's Disease** Alzheimer's Foundation of America, 866-AFA-8484 (866-232-8484), *www.alzfdn.org.*

•**Depression/Bipolar Disorder** Depression and Bipolar Support Alliance, 800-826-3632, *www.dbsalliance.org.*

•**Grief/End of Life** Caring Connections, 800-658-8898, *www.caringinfo.org.*

CAREGIVING

•**Family Care Providers** National Family Caregivers Association, 800-896-3650, *www.thefamilycaregiver.org.*

•**Hospice** Hospice Education Institute, 800-331-1620, *www.hospiceworld.org.*

•**Senior Care** Department of Health and Human Services Eldercare Locator, 800-677-1116, *www.eldercare.gov.*

Reliable Answers to Your Health Questions

Trisha Torrey, a patient advocate, health columnist and radio talk show host based in Baldwinsville, New York. She became a patient advocate after being falsely diagnosed with cancer in 2004. Trisha is the founder of the Web sites *www.EveryPatientsAdvocate.com* and *www.diagknowsis.org,* and an expert in patient empowerment for About.com (*http://patients.About.com*).

Until the Internet became so widely used, finding a medical specialist or getting a health question answered usually required time-consuming research at the library or an appointment with your doctor.

Now: With a few computer keystrokes, people who have access to the Internet can find literally thousands of health-related Web sites. But much of this information is misleading or simply incorrect—and answers to some health questions require the training of a skilled physician. *Reliable health information that's free of charge on-line...*

1. Secrets to living with medical conditions. Let's say you're wondering how to get through a long movie when you have arthritis, what to say to a friend with cancer or how to tell your boss about your diabetes. These kinds of questions are ideal to ask at on-line health forums, where you can get input on problems that you might want to discuss with a friend—if only you had one who had been in a similar situation.

How on-line health forums work: People with access to the Internet can share their experiences and advice on a "message board" where others who log on to the same Web site are able to read the messages and respond to them, if they so desire. Keep in mind that the people who post comments on these message boards are not medical professionals. They are patients and caregivers who are speaking from their own experience.

Good sites: HealthBoards (*www.healthboards. com*) offers more than 150 message boards on a variety of health topics and medical conditions ...Daily Strength (*www.dailystrength.org*) provides access to more than 500 on-line support groups dedicated to physical health issues, such as cancer or diabetes, mental health issues, including depression and anxiety, and personal challenges, such as bereavement or dieting. Some Web sites sponsored by organizations that focus on specific diseases, such as the American Cancer Society (*www.cancer.org*) or the Leukemia & Lymphoma Society (*www.leukemia-lymphoma.org*), also offer on-line message boards.

Important: Communications posted on an on-line health forum's message board are anonymous, so any information or advice that involves specific treatment recommendations or medical products should always be verified with a medical professional. When participating in these forums, do not provide identifying details, such as your last name, phone number or address. It's okay to provide your first name and city or state.

2. What a medical symptom may mean. Most medical symptoms are best evaluated by a doctor, but there may be times—for example, when you're waiting for a scheduled doctor appointment to arrive—that it's useful to consult Web sites that give a list of possible causes for specific symptoms.

This type of on-line tool—often known as a "Symptom Checker"—allows you to select a body part, such as the legs, then choose from a list of symptoms. When you click on a specific symptom, such as ankle pain, the Web site takes you through a list of questions to identify the most likely causes of your symptom—for example, ankle pain may be due to an acute problem such as an ankle fracture or strain or a chronic condition such as rheumatoid arthritis. Familiarizing yourself with the range of possible causes for your symptom can allow you to ask more informed questions when you do see your doctor.

Good sites: Symptom-checking tools are available at WebMD.com (*www.symptoms.webmd.com*), Mayoclinic.com (go to *www.mayoclinic.com* and search for "symptom checker") and About.com (*www.symptomchecker.about.com*), which provides health information from the Harvard Medical School.

Important: The results generated by on-line symptom-checking tools are by no means conclusive. Such information may help you narrow the possible causes of your symptom, but you should rely only on a trained physician for an actual diagnosis.

3. The credentials of specific doctors. Your neighbor may have had a good experience with his orthopedist, but is this doctor the best one to perform your hip surgery? It's important to check the credentials of a doctor you may have heard about or read about.

At a minimum, a doctor should be licensed, the basic credential issued by each state. The Federation of State Medical Boards Web site (*www.fsmb.org/directory_smb.html*) provides a directory of state boards that allows you to confirm that a particular doctor is licensed to practice.

Also, check whether a doctor is board-certified in his/her medical specialty, which ensures that the physician has met minimum competency and continuing education requirements. To confirm this information for medical doctors (MDs), go to the American Board of Medical Specialties (ABMS) Web site (*www.abms.org*). After you register an e-mail address and create a password, you can search for the information according to the doctor's name. If you're inquiring about a doctor of osteopathy (a licensed physician whose training focuses on preventive health care and the musculoskeletal system's role in causing illness or injury), consult the American Osteopathic Association (800-621-1773, *www.osteopathic.org*).

Important: Be wary of Web sites that invite patients to comment on a doctor's performance. Anyone—including friends of the physician or irate former patients—can submit reviews that are either overly flattering or unfairly critical.

4. Information on medications and supplements. Your doctor and pharmacist are good resources, but there also are several helpful Web sites devoted to the proper use of medications and supplements.

Best sites: The Physicians' Desk Reference (PDR) Web site (*www.pdrhealth.com*) provides important details on prescription and over-the-counter (OTC) drugs as well as herbal remedies and dietary supplements. The site explains the condition for which a drug or supplement may be prescribed, how best to take it and whether it may interact with foods or other medications.

This Web site also has photographs of pills so you can confirm what a pill should look like at a specific dosage—for example, a pill containing a 10-mg dosage of the osteoporosis drug *alendronate* (Fosamax) is white and oval, while the same medication in a 40-mg dosage is white and triangular.

If you can't find a particular medication listed at the PDR Web site or if you're taking an expensive brand-name drug and want to see whether it's available in a less expensive generic equivalent, check the Food and Drug Administration's Electronic Orange book at *www.fda.gov/cder/ob*.

For a list of additional Web sites that provide information on medications and supplements, consult the resource library on my Web site (*www.diagknowsis.org*), which gives information on how to research medical diagnoses and treatments, along with links to credible health Web sites.

HOW TO PROTECT YOURSELF

Even though the Internet can be a tremendous source of information, you need to be cautious—especially when you have questions about your health. *My advice...*

•**Do *not* rely on the Internet for a medical diagnosis.** Trying to diagnose yourself with information gathered from Web sites is dangerous. What's more, credible Web sites are careful to avoid giving diagnoses because of liability issues.

•***Do* not pay money to get medical advice on-line.** A Web site could claim that a medical professional with outstanding credentials is offering the advice, but you cannot be sure—due to the remote nature of the Internet—who is answering your question.

•**Do make sure that you're consulting credible Web sites.** Look for Web sites that are backed by major medical institutions, such as the Mayo Clinic (*www.mayoclinic.com*) or the Cleveland Clinic (*http://my.clevelandclinic.org*)...organizations that focus on specific diseases, such as the American Diabetes Association (*www.diabetes.org*) or the American Stroke Association (*www.strokeassociation.org*)...or government agencies, such as the National Institutes of Health (*www.nlm.nih.gov*).

Helpful: Look for the "HONcode" accreditation from the Health on the Net Foundation in Switzerland, which guides lay users and medical professionals to reliable sources of health-care information on-line. This accreditation ensures that the Web site has been deemed a reliable source of health information and meets standards including those related to the qualification of the authorities cited on the site, privacy of personal data submitted by a visitor to the site and financial disclosures of funding sources.

Surprising Perks in Health Insurance Plans

Sam Gibbs, senior vice president of sales of eHealth-Insurance Services, Inc., where consumers can compare health insurance plans and apply for and purchase health insurance on-line. eHealthInsurance is not aligned with any particular health insurance provider. *www.ehealth insurance.com.*

Your health insurance might offer unexpected savings. Some group and individual health insurers have negotiated special discounts on behalf of their members on products and services, such as gym memberships and even elective plastic surgery. These discounts are not always well publicized, and many plan members do not even realize they exist. Read your health insurance company's mailings or visit its Web site to see if there are any special discounts through your plan.

These discounts typically are categorized as "perks" rather than plan benefits, which means insurance companies can alter or discontinue them without first notifying plan members. Contact your insurance provider or the company featured in the offer to confirm that a discount is still in effect before trying to take advantage of it. Also ask if any special rules or limitations apply.

COMMON DISCOUNTS

Among the benefits found in many health insurance plans...

•**Fitness club memberships.** Many health plans offer a discount of 10% to 20% or more off the cost of gym membership. This discount usually is available only at select national fitness chains. Some plans also include discounts at yoga studios...or discounts on the purchase of fitness equipment from participating retailers.

•**Naturopathic treatments.** Some insurance companies cover these treatments. Those that don't may offer discounts of 20% or more on acupuncture, chiropractic services, massage therapy and hypnotherapy.

Example: Most Anthem Blue Cross of California members can get these discounts simply by showing their membership cards at participating providers.

•**Weight-loss programs.** Savings of 20% or more off membership in national weight-loss chains, such as Jenny Craig, are common. Even the special low-calorie meals required by some weight-loss programs might be discounted.

•**Quit-smoking programs.** Insurance plans often cover quit-smoking programs in part or in whole. Discounts might be available on nicotine patches, gum and related products.

OTHER PERKS

These perks turn up only occasionally in health insurance plans, but they are worth watching for...

•**Cosmetic surgery and dentistry.** Cosmetic procedures typically are not covered by health insurance, but some plans do offer special negotiated rates on elective surgery at participating providers. Covered procedures could include Botox injections, face-lifts and tooth whitening. The savings often are 20% or more off standard rates.

•**Vision correction.** Some insurance companies offer discounts on eyeglasses, contact lenses, even laser surgery.

Example: Golden Rule (owned by United-Healthcare) offers 10% to 40% savings on eye exams, eyeglasses, contact lenses and LASIK laser eye surgery to their members through an affiliation with the Federation of American Consumers and Travelers.

•**Prescription and nonprescription drug coverage without a drug plan.** Even if your health plan does not include drug coverage, there might be a discount of 10% or more if you purchase your drugs at a "featured" or "partner" drugstore.

•**Vitamins and supplements.** Discounts of as much as 40% to 50% sometimes are available.

You will need to buy your vitamins through a designated provider to receive these savings.

•**Book discounts.** Some insurance plans have partnered with on-line book sellers to offer discounts of 5 % or 10% on "featured" books. These books typically focus on health or wellness topics.

•**Travel discounts.** Some major health insurers have negotiated discount rates for their members at hotel chains, car rental chains and amusement parks. Savings of 10% to 20% are typical. Read the discount terms carefully—in some cases, members must provide special discount codes or reserve their discount rates in advance...while, in other cases, members simply show their insurance plan membership cards upon arrival.

Example: Members of Golden Rule can get 20% discounts at participating Choice Hotels International, such as Comfort Suites and Econo Lodge...100% off Magellan's Travel Supplies... and car-rental discounts.

■ ■ ■ ■

Free Eldercare

A free eldercare-services hotline can refer you to local agencies that may help meet your needs. Help is available for problems involving medical care, taxes, the law, investments, housing, transportation and much more. The Eldercare Locator service (*www.eldercare.gov*) is funded by the US Administration on Aging. Call 800-677-1116.

Veterans' Benefits You May Not Know About

Christopher Michel, a former naval flight officer and founder of Military.com, America's largest military membership organization, located in San Francisco. He is author of *The Military Advantage: A Comprehensive Guide to Your Military & Veterans Benefits*. Simon & Schuster.

No country in the world offers more benefits to those who have served in its armed forces than the United States.

Some of the benefits are available only to active service members or military retirees (those who have retired after at least 20 years of service), but many are offered to all of America's 24 million veterans and their families.

There are programs that offer benefits to veterans for home loans, education, careers, travel and discount programs. Look on the Web at *military.com* for further details.

MEDICAL BENEFITS

The Department of Veteran's Affairs is required by law to provide eligible veterans with "needed" hospital care and outpatient care. VA defines "needed" as care or service that will promote, preserve and restore health. This includes treatment, supplies and services, such as physical exams and immunizations. The decision of "need" will be based on the judgment of the vet's health-care provider at the VA and in accordance with generally accepted standards of clinical practice. There are also VA clinical health programs that vets may be eligible for, including treatment for blindness rehabilitation, Agent Orange exposure and HIV/AIDS.

Veterans' dependents are also eligible for these VA health-care programs in many cases. Final eligibility depends on several factors for each program. These factors include the nature of a veteran's discharge from military service (e.g., honorable, other than honorable, dishonorable), length of service, service-connected disabilities, income level and available VA resources, among others. Generally, the vet must be enrolled in the VA health-care system—there are more than 1,400 VA facilities throughout the country—to receive benefits.

More information: Visit the United States Department of Veterans Affairs site (*www.va.gov/healtheligibility/eligibility/PriorityGroupsAll.asp*).

BURIAL BENEFITS, TOO

Veterans are eligible for free burial in any of 131 VA national cemeteries, space permitting. Veterans' spouses are also eligible. The cemetery plot, headstone, transportation of the remains, burial with military honors, if requested, and grave upkeep are provided by the government at no charge. The casket and other funeral home expenses remain the responsibility of the family.

More information: Call the VA at 800-827-1000 for more information. You will need a copy of the vet's discharge papers. Burial at Arlington National Cemetery is subject to greater restrictions. For more information call 703-607-8585. If a vet prefers to be buried in a private cemetery, the VA still can provide a free headstone. Call the VA for more details, or visit Military.com and submit VA Form 40-1330.

■ ■ ■ ■

Medicare Caution

Medicare does not cover medicines prescribed for off-label use, even if a doctor determines that the drugs are medically necessary. A medicine is prescribed off-label when a doctor believes it will help a patient, even though the patient's condition is not one for which the drug has been approved by the Food and Drug Administration.

Self-defense: If your doctor says a drug is medically necessary and Medicare refuses to cover it, appeal the decision by calling the Medicare Rights Center hotline (800-333-4114).

Deane Beebe, public affairs director, Medicare Rights Center, 520 Eighth Ave., New York City 10018.

When a Medicare Claim Is Denied…How to Fight Back and Win

Judith Stein, JD, founder and executive director of the Center for Medicare Advocacy, Inc., a nonprofit advocacy organization that provides assistance with the Medicare system. It is based in Willimantic, Connecticut, with an office in Washington, DC. *www.medicareadvocacy.org.*

Many seniors assume that they have no choice but to pay when their Medicare claims are declined in whole or in part. In fact, denied or underpaid claims can be appealed—and more than half of these appeals are successful.

When your Medicare claim is denied or approved for less than the full amount, you have 120 days to request a "redetermination" of the decision. The *Medicare Redetermination Request Form* (Form CMS-20027) is available on the Medicare and Medicaid Web site (*www.cms.hhs.gov/cmsforms/downloads/cms20027.pdf*) or by calling 800-633-4227.

The written claim denial that you originally received includes instructions for where and how to submit this form. The claim denial includes an explanation as to why your claim was denied or why payment for your treatment wasn't covered in full. You will need to contest this explanation to win your appeal. Ask your doctor to write a letter responding to the points raised in the denial and explaining why the health care is necessary. Include a copy of this letter with your appeals form, and keep a copy for your records.

Common reasons for denial of treatment and how to fight them…

Reason for Denial: The treatment, prescription or medical service is unlikely to cause your health condition to improve. (The denial likely falls into this category if the notice you received includes words or phrases such as "stable," "chronic," "not improving" or "no restorative potential.")

How to fight: The Medicare program is required to look at your total condition and health-care needs, not just a specific diagnosis or your chance for full or partial recovery. Ask your doctor to write a letter explaining why the medical care is needed.

Example: Medicare denied home health care to a patient with Lou Gehrig's disease, an incurable degenerative condition, because the care would not help her improve. The patient successfully appealed, arguing—with her doctor's help—that while having a nurse visit her home would not improve her condition, it could slow the disease's progression and is needed to otherwise care for her various health issues.

Reason for Denial: You are likely to require care for a very long time…or have already received treatment for a very long time without a resolution of the problem.

How to fight: Point out that Medicare coverage is not limited to treatments that work quickly. As long as your doctor continues to order this treatment for you, Medicare should continue to cover it. Include a letter from your doctor explaining that the treatment is having some positive effect or expressing an expectation that it will. (Medicare rules do limit how many days' coverage is available in a nursing home or a hospital but not for home care.)

Reason for Denial: You do not qualify for Medicare-covered home care because you are not homebound.

How to fight: According to Medicare rules, "homebound" does not mean that you are completely unable to leave your home, nor does it mean that you are confined to a bed. You can be considered homebound even if you leave your home to obtain medical care or attend occasional family gatherings. You must require assistance and considerable effort to get out of the house.

Ask your care provider (which could be a family member, a home health professional or a doctor) to write a letter describing in detail how difficult it is for you to leave your home, and include this with the appeals form.

Reason for Denial: The dosage level of a prescription is greater than the dosage normally prescribed...or the drug prescribed is not normally prescribed for your health problem.

How to fight: Have your doctor write a letter explaining why the unusual dosage or drug is medically necessary for you. If possible, have the doctor cite published reports of similar usage.

Example: Your doctor might explain that you are allergic to the drug normally prescribed for your health problem.

Reason for Denial: Technical errors were made in the original Medicare claim. The rejection might cite a "coding error" or "incorrect Medicare recipient number."

How to fight: Ask the health-care provider that submitted the claim to correct the problem and resubmit.

DON'T GIVE UP

If your Medicare appeal is denied, you have the right to file as many as four more appeals. Your odds of success improve the further you pursue the fight. While the initial "redetermination" appeal is made to the same group that initially denied your claim, later appeals are made to increasingly independent arbiters.

Appeal #2: You have 180 days from the date your redetermination request is denied to request that a Qualified Independent Contractor (QIC) make a "reconsideration determination." You will have to complete the Medicare Reconsideration Request Form (Form CMS-20033, available at *www.cms.hhs.gov/cmsforms/down loads/CMS20033.pdf*).

If the redetermination denial includes any reasons for denial not mentioned earlier, ask your doctor to write a new letter. Otherwise, attach a copy of your doctor's earlier letter.

Appeal #3: If your second appeal is denied as well and the amount in dispute is at least $120, then you have 60 days to file a third appeal, this time with an Administrative Law Judge (ALJ) of the US Department of Health and Human Services. Filing instructions are included with the denial.

ALJ appeals are presented to the judge via telephone (or videoconference if you have the necessary technology). At the beginning of the hearing, confirm that the judge has a copy of any letters of support written by your doctors. Then explain your situation and why you require the care in dispute.

Helpful: Judges are supposed to rule based on the evidence and the law, but they are human. It never hurts to remind the judge that you are living on a fixed income and that you would face major financial problems or even health problems if Medicare fails to pay this bill and/or approve the treatment.

Appeal #4: If the judge turns down your third appeal, you have 60 days to request that the Medicare Appeals Council (MAC) review the decision. The ALJ denial will include instructions on how to do this.

Appeal #5: If the MAC turns down your appeal, you have 60 days to determine if you wish to hire an attorney and file a judicial review in Federal District Court. The amount in dispute must be greater than $1,180 to qualify. (This amount may change each year.) For more information, contact the US Department of Health and Human Services at 877-696-6775 or *www.hhs.gov/omha*.

How to Get Your Health Insurer to Pay Up

William M. Shernoff, JD, senior and managing partner of the law firm Shernoff Bidart Darras & Echeverria LLP, Claremont, California. The firm represents policyholders who have been treated unfairly by insurers or HMOs. Shernoff established the consumer law program at the University of Wisconsin, Madison, and is author of several books, including *Fight Back and Win: How to Get HMOs and Health Insurance to Pay Up*. Capital. *www.sbd-law.com*.

You pay your health insurance policy premiums without fail—but that doesn't mean your insurance company will be as reliable when you make a claim. It is very possible that your claim will be improperly denied.

Very few people bother to fight these denials. That's unfortunate, because policyholders who intelligently contest health insurance claims denials often get them reversed.

If a seemingly valid health insurance claim you make is denied in whole or in part, ask the insurance company to send you a full explanation of why it was denied (or accepted for only a lesser amount). *Then follow these steps to get your claim covered...*

STEP 1: Enlist support. If you have a group health policy, ask the group benefits administrator to help you contest the denial. If you purchased an individual policy through an independent insurance agent, ask this agent to help. Not only do benefits administrators and insurance agents have experience with these matters, they have clout with the insurers. An insurance company might relent to an administrator's or agent's request to pay a claim simply to avoid losing future business.

STEP 2: Write a letter to the insurer requesting a formal review of the denial and explaining why you believe it is incorrect. Get the name of the person to write to from your benefits administrator or agent. Send this letter via certified mail, return receipt requested.

Cite the insurance company's own literature if it seems to contradict the argument made in the denial. If the policy literature is vague or confusing—it often is—do not accept the insurance company's position that it means what it says it means. In most states, the courts interpret insurance policy provisions as a layperson would understand them, not as a corporate lawyer would interpret them.

Example: Your insurance company refuses to pay for your home care following a serious accident, arguing that the care you received was "custodial" care, which is not covered, rather than "skilled" care, which is. If you received what the average person would consider skilled care and your policy does not specifically define these terms in a way that defends the insurer's position, the law is likely on your side.

Some common reasons for claims denials and possible responses...

•**The procedure was not medically necessary.** Ask your doctor to write a letter to the insurer explaining why the procedure was necessary in your case.

•**The procedure was experimental.** Ask your doctor to write a letter to the insurer noting that Medicare or other insurers cover the procedure or citing statistics showing that it is widely used.

•**There was a filing error, such as a missed deadline.** In most states, the insurer cannot legally deny your claim because of a technical filing mistake unless it can show that it was harmed by this mistake.

•**The bill exceeds "reasonable and customary" charges.** Ask your doctor if there were special circumstances in your case that would justify higher costs. If there were, have him/her write a letter to the insurer describing them. Another option is to call other medical facilities in the region and ask what they charge for the procedure. Insurers often rely on old data or data from other parts of the country when they set these "reasonable and customary" estimates. If you can establish that your doctor did not charge more than others in your region do, the insurer might back down.

***STEP 3:* If your letter doesn't work, repeat your argument in a letter to the manager** or supervisor of the insurance company's claims department. Get the name of the individual from your claims representative. Work your way up the corporate ladder. You may need to convince only one person to agree with you for your denial to be reversed.

Remain calm and polite. Contesting an insurance claim denial is frustrating, but insurance company employees are more likely to take your side if they like you. Write down the name of any person you speak to, as well as the date and time and what you were told.

***STEP 4:* Contact your state's department of insurance,** and ask what it can do to help you. The quality and power of state insurance departments vary significantly. Some help policyholders stand up to unfair insurance company practices or conduct independent reviews of denied claims.

Example: California's Department of Managed Health Care offer "independent medical reviews" of denied health insurance claims. Approximately 40% of those reviewed are decided in the patient's favor.

Simply involving your state's department of insurance may be enough to convince an insurer that it is easier to pay your claim than fight it.

***STEP 5:* Call the media.** Local TV news programs and newspapers love stories about people being treated unfairly by big health insurance companies. Insurers despise this bad press and sometimes relent when reporters call. Determine which local reporters cover human-interest stories of this sort, contact them and ask if they would be interested in your story.

***STEP 6:* Go to court.** If your claim is in the low four figures or less, it might qualify for small-claims court. If it is larger, you will need to hire an attorney. If your case appears strong, there will be plenty of attorneys willing to take it on a contingency basis (they get paid only if they win or settle).

Hiring an attorney makes the most sense when the insurance company's unfair claim denial has interfered with your medical treatment and endangered your health. Juries often award substantial damages when this occurs.

■ **More from William M. Shernoff, JD...**

If Your Insurance Company Tries to Drop You

If you have an individual health insurance policy, *not a group health plan*, having a claim unjustly denied is not the only risk. If you develop an expensive health problem, your insurance company might attempt to retroactively terminate your coverage, a process known as "rescission."

When you file a major claim, your insurer could have an investigator examine your original policy application. If the investigator finds even the smallest error, the insurer may use this as an excuse to rescind your policy even if the application error has nothing to do with the current claim.

Example: Blue Cross of California canceled the policy of a woman who needed surgery to remove her gallbladder and refused to pay her $60,000 medical bills. The insurer argued that the woman's husband had failed to note on the couple's original policy application that he once had an elevated cholesterol reading.

States are beginning to enact rules to protect policyholders from this tactic, but for now, the danger remains. *To minimize your risk...*

•**Take your time with health insurance applications.** If possible, obtain a copy of your health records from your doctor and use these to fill out the form, rather than rely on your memory.

•**Contact the insurance company for clarification** if a question on the application is confusing. Don't provide an answer until you truly understand the question.

•**Include your medical providers' contact information on the application form.** If the insurer later attempts to rescind your policy, you can argue in court that you didn't intentionally hide anything and that the insurer should have contacted your doctors.

The Secret to Winning a Personal Injury Claim

Evan K. Aidman, principal of the law offices of Evan K. Aidman in Ardmore, Pennsylvania. He has 25 years of experience in personal injury law and is author of *Winning Your Personal Injury Claim*. Sourcebooks. *www. legalaidman.com.*

If you are injured due to someone else's negligence, it might be possible to receive compensation for your medical bills, lost wages and perhaps even for your pain and suffering, through either an insurance settlement or the courts.

Types of accidents that could be someone else's fault include car accidents...slip-and-fall accidents...dog bites...medical malpractice... and accidents caused by defective products.

LIKELIHOOD OF WINNING

There are only a few situations in which it can be relatively easy to receive compensation for injuries...

•**If you are injured on the property of someone who has homeowner's insurance.** This insurance likely contains a "no-fault" medical component that will pay your medical bills up to the policy limits even if the accident was your fault. Ask the home owner to contact his/her insurer.

Similarly, your own auto insurance may have "no fault" protection that covers medical bills and lost wages regardless of fault in an auto accident.

•**If your insurance claim is less than $5,000.** Insurance companies often do not aggressively fight injury claims less than this amount.

Otherwise, do not expect it to be easy to recover your losses. Insurance companies have become extremely aggressive in fighting injury claims in recent years, and personal injury cases are more difficult to win in court. You will have to prove that your injuries and your financial losses are as significant as you claim and that the person, business or government entity you blame for your injuries truly is legally responsible.

Also, there might be no point in pursuing a case if the individual responsible for your accident has no insurance and few assets. Still, a lawyer might be able to track down hidden assets or find other defendants with deeper pockets who share legal responsibility.

Example: The home owner whose uneven sidewalk you tripped over has no insurance. Perhaps the local municipality is legally responsible for ensuring that local residents maintain their sidewalks. If your lawyer can show it failed to do so, the municipality could be liable.

IMPORTANT STEPS

If you are ever injured in an accident, do the following...

•**Watch your words at the scene of an accident.** Do not say anything that implies that you were wholly or even partially responsible or that you could have done something to avoid the accident.

If you believe you are injured, say this and request medical help. If you do not feel hurt, do not say that you feel fine. Say only that you're not certain yet whether you are hurt. It is very common to not notice injuries or register pain until many hours after an accident, when the initial shock has worn off. Certain injuries are not apparent until days later. An insurance company or jury is more likely to meet your claims of injury with skepticism if you initially say you were unhurt.

Helpful: If the manager of a business in which you are injured asks you to fill out a form about your accident, politely decline and say that you will take the form home and fill it out later. This will help ensure that you say nothing that could hurt the claim.

•**Ask any witnesses what they saw.** If their version of events confirms that someone other than you was at fault, take the witnesses' names and phone numbers. If you are too injured to take down names, ask someone else on the scene to do so for you.

•**Write down any statements, such as apologies or admissions of mistakes, made by the person at fault for your accident.**

Example: You fall on a loose tile in a store and break your hip. The store owner says, "I'm so sorry. I've been meaning to fix that." If others hear these statements, ask them to sign and date a note detailing what they heard.

•**Take photos of the accident scene from many angles and distances.** Take these pictures as soon as possible—if you have a cell phone with a built-in digital camera, you can do so almost immediately. The longer you wait, the greater the odds the conditions will change.

Examples: The ice you slipped on could melt or be cleared…the uneven sidewalk you tripped on could be fixed in hours if the property owner responsible for it races to conceal all evidence of the problem.

•**Take photos of your injuries soon after the accident**—and again several days later if bruises have become more visible. The worse your injuries look in photos, the more difficult it will be for an insurance company or defense attorney to claim that you are exaggerating.

•**Schedule an appointment with your doctor** if your injuries were not severe enough to require an immediate visit to the emergency room. This creates an official medical record of the injuries.

•**Send a brief letter laying out the basic facts of the accident to the responsible party's insurance company.** Send copies of your medical bills and reports, as well as the police report and witness statements. State what you would like to be compensated for (medical bills, lost wages, etc.).

•**Go to court.** If the responsible party's insurance company does not offer a settlement that you consider acceptable, you will have to go to small claims court (if the amount is within the limits your state specifies) or hire an attorney who specializes in personal injury law. Try to find a lawyer with at least a decade of experience who is respected by insurance companies and other local attorneys, not one known simply for his television ads. A local attorney with a different specialty might be able to provide a referral.

■ **More from Evan K. Aidman…**

Common Personal Injury Cases

Different personal injury situations often require different approaches. *What you need to know to handle these situations…*

•**Auto accidents.** Auto accidents are one of the most common ways to get hurt because of someone else's mistake. There is a specific procedure for handling auto accidents. Typically, the police are summoned to the scene to produce an accident report…then the driver's auto insurance company is contacted to work out a settlement. An injured party might contact an attorney if he or she is not satisfied with the insurance company settlement offer.

Do not agree with the at-fault driver if he wants to keep the police and insurance companies out of the matter. Do not sign anything sent to you by your insurance company or the other driver's insurance company until you are certain of the extent of your injuries—you might sign away your right to have any future medical bills covered.

•**Slip-and-fall cases.** You will need to prove that your fall was caused by negligence on the part of the home owner, business or government entity responsible for maintaining the property (with the exception of no-fault medical homeowner's insurance claims). There might be no negligence if the dangerous condition that led to your fall did not exist until shortly before your accident.

Examples: If you slipped on the ice in the parking lot outside a store, you must show that the ice was there long enough that the retailer should have known about it and removed it…If you tripped on an uneven sidewalk, you must prove that the sidewalk had been in disrepair for an extended time. Testimony from neighbors and other witnesses can be very helpful.

The credibility of the person who is injured is the single most important factor in a slip-and-fall case. An insurance settlement or victory in court is much more likely if the victim does not exaggerate his injuries and has no history of filing frivolous lawsuits.

•**Dog bites.** A dog-bite lawsuit or insurance claim is most likely to be successful if you can show that the dog has a history of biting…that the breed is known for aggressiveness…or that the owner failed to keep the dog under reasonable control.

Example: A pit bull is allowed to roam free through a neighborhood and bites a woman while she is in her own backyard.

• **Medical malpractice.** These cases tend to be expensive and difficult to win. The fact that a medical procedure failed to deliver the desired result is not on its own enough to establish malpractice. You must show that the quality of the care provided was below the standard of care in the community.

Example: Laser eye surgery may result in poor night vision. This is not necessarily malpractice unless a medical expert hired by the victim's attorney can show that the doctor mismeasured the eye or made some other mistake in treatment, such as operating on a person for whom the surgery is not appropriate.

• **Product liability.** If your efforts to reach a settlement with the company or business fail and you decide to go to court, you will need an expert to testify that your injury was due to a defect in the design, manufacture or maintenance of the product, not your own misuse of it. Expert witnesses don't come cheap, so these cases should not to be attempted lightly.

• **Food poisoning.** Food poisoning cases are often not worth pursuing. Even if you suspect that a particular restaurant meal was to blame, it's very difficult to prove and food poisoning typically passes in a day or so. The exception is life-threatening infections, such as salmonella or *E. coli.*

Do You Really Need That Medical Test?

Charles B. Inlander is a consumer advocate and health-care consultant based in Fogelsville, Pennsylvania. He was the founding president of the nonprofit People's Medical Society, a consumer advocacy organization active in the 1980s and 1990s, and is the author of more than 20 books, including *Take This Book to the Hospital with You: A Consumer Guide to Surviving Your Hospital Stay.* St. Martin's.

A recent study found that an adult American's chances of having an unnecessary medical test at his/her next checkup is

at least 43%. And a report in *The New England Journal of Medicine* suggested that up to 2% of all cancer cases come from overexposure to radiation from too many diagnostic computed tomography (CT) scans. These reports—and many more like them—have raised a red flag about the overuse of unnecessary and/or risky testing. Of course you should not use any of these reports as an excuse for not having a test that might save your life, but it is important to understand why a test is being recommended. *Questions to ask your doctor…*

• **Do I really need the test?** This seems like an obvious question, but many people fail to ask it. Federal guidelines advise against such common medical tests as urinalysis, electrocardiograms (ECGs) and even routine chest X-rays unless you have symptoms that may be related to the urinary tract, heart or lungs, respectively. Yet one or more of those tests is often ordered for patients during annual checkups even though they have no associated symptoms. After asking your doctor to explain why he wants you to have a particular test, find out if he suspects a specific problem—and, if so, whether other follow-up tests may be necessary.

• **What are the risks associated with the test?** Many medical tests have some level of risk. For example, a CT scan of the stomach exposes a person to 50 times more radiation than a conventional stomach X-ray. The more radiation you have over a lifetime, the higher your risk for some types of cancer, including malignancies of the lungs and liver. If you're having a biopsy of the prostate gland, you should know that the procedure can cause infection or bleeding into the urethra or bladder. When asking your doctor about the risks associated with each test, find out whether there are less risky alternatives to the test that is being proposed. For example, one possible alternative to a prostate biopsy is a new special color-prostate sonogram (ultrasound). Let your doctor know if you have had negative effects from any previous tests, such as bleeding or infections.

Helpful: Tell your doctor if you have had exposure to other CT scans or X-rays in the past. *Questions to ask yourself…*

•**Are my fears preventing me from getting a necessary test?** While medical tests are not always comfortable, it's important to weigh the potential discomfort and/or risks against the benefits. For example, a recent report has shown that fewer women are getting mammograms than in years past. It cited the pain and discomfort associated with the test as the probable reason. Yet mammograms have been shown to be the primary reason that breast cancer deaths have declined in the US. Do not let your fear of the possible discomfort and/or risks associated with a medical test cloud your assessment of its benefits.

•**Do I have all the facts?** If you ask the right questions, do a little research and weigh the test's risks against its benefits, you can trust that the decision you and your doctor make will be the right one.

Medical Scams, Cons And Rip-Offs

Chuck Whitlock, a journalist whose work exposing scams has been featured on many television programs, including *Inside Edition* and *Extra*. He is author of several books about scams, including *MediScams: Dangerous Medical Practices and Health Care Frauds*. St. Martin's Griffin. *www.chuckwhitlock.com.*

Bogus "miracle cures" and quack physicians probably have been around as long as the health-care profession. Con artists prey upon the unhealthy because sick people may be so desperate to find a cure that they will try any possible treatment, however expensive and farfetched.

These snake oil salesmen have been on the rise in recent years, as our aging population has more medical problems...millions of underinsured and uninsured Americans search for health-care options that they can afford...and the surging popularity of "alternative medicine" makes unscientific treatments seem more mainstream.

Sometimes it's obvious when a claim is fraudulent—but certain scams and unethical practices are difficult to spot...

SCAMS

•**Cheap health insurance.** Many of the more than 45.7 million Americans who are without health insurance are desperate to find affordable coverage. Disreputable insurance companies offer these people exactly what they want—health insurance at a low price, sometimes as little as $50 per month.

Most buyers are so thrilled to find insurance they can afford that they don't pay attention to the fine print. Many of these policies have huge deductibles, scant benefits and other restrictions that make them virtually worthless.

Most policyholders do not discover the problems until they have a serious health condition and receive the bill.

What to do: Look for a policy that covers doctor visits and protects against a major medical expense. A way to spot-check the quality of a policy is to look at the benefits for hospital stays. A good policy should pay $500 or more per day for the hospital room, with additional coverage for other hospital costs. An inadequate policy might provide only $100 a day.

Wise: Contact your state's insurance commissioner to find out if complaints have been filed against the company. Blue Cross/Blue Shield offers many reputable plans, and Kaiser Permanente has a good reputation for a health maintenance organization (HMO).

•**Natural appetite suppressants.** Unscrupulous marketers claim that there are natural supplements that help you lose weight—but these supplements don't work or have dangerous side effects. The most heavily promoted "appetite suppressants" include ephedra, garcinia cambogia and hoodia.

Ephedra is an herbal stimulant, and like other stimulants, it does suppress appetite but at the price of increased heart rate, nervousness and agitation. In large doses, ephedra has killed people, and the FDA has pulled it off the market, though it's still available on the Web.

Garcinia cambogia (a fruit from Asia) and hoodia (from a succulent African plant) are not stimulants and seem to be safe—but they don't work. No studies have shown them to be effective.

What to do: The only reliable cures for excess weight are consuming fewer calories and getting more exercise.

•**Organ transplants in developing countries.** America's organ donation program can't keep pace with the demand for transplants. For patients languishing on waiting lists, flying to a developing country where organs can be purchased on the black market might seem viable. Before you board a plane to India, the Philippines, Hungary or Russia and agree to pay $1,000 to $100,000 for an organ, consider that you're putting yourself in the hands of people who are more interested in taking your money than saving your life.

These people might find an organ for you—but you might not receive it until you've been milked for many times the agreed-upon price. Some patients are told at the last minute that someone else will pay more for the organ, which might or might not be true. To get the organ, you have to top this other offer. Even when patients do get their organs, their transplants often are performed according to medical standards that are not as strict as they are in the US.

What to do: Talk to your doctor about the best options.

UNETHICAL PRACTICES

•**Bonuses from HMOs and PPOs to doctors who skip useful tests.** HMOs and preferred provider organizations (PPOs) often give cash bonuses to doctors who don't perform pricey tests—even when those tests are in the patient's best interest. They are essentially bribing doctors to scam their patients.

Example: Your HMO or PPO doctor tells you that he/she is going to spare you the invasive thallium stress test (where radioactive dye is injected into your bloodstream) and perform a routine treadmill test without thallium, though the thallium test is warranted.

What to do: When your HMO or PPO doctor tells you that you have a particular health condition, research that condition on a reliable Internet Web site, such as WebMD.com or MayoClinic.com. If the site mentions a test that your doctor has not performed, ask him why it was skipped. If the doctor's response seems evasive, consider getting a second opinion.

•**Unqualified plastic surgeon.** Many doctors have switched to plastic surgery in recent years, drawn by the lucrative nature of the specialty and its lower reliance on insurance payments. (Most plastic surgery procedures are elective and not covered by insurance.) No law or regulation prevents doctors from changing their specialty to plastic surgery—even if they have no background or training in this field. Patients likely have no idea that they are trusting their lives and appearances to what are essentially unqualified, untrained novices.

What to do: If you're considering plastic surgery, ask the surgeon…

Are you board-certified in plastic surgery? He/she should be.

At what hospital do you have physician's privileges? A general hospital is fine, but a university hospital is even better—university hospitals tend to have very high standards.

Who will be handling my anesthesia? Don't trust a plastic surgeon who says he'll handle it himself. He may be trying to cut corners and putting your health at risk in the process.

Beware: Medical Identity Theft Is on the Rise

Joy Pritts, JD, founding director of the Center on Medical Record Rights and Privacy at Georgetown University's Health Policy Institute, Washington, DC. She has testified before Congress on privacy and the use of medical information, and is the prime author of *Your Medical Record Rights,* a series of publications available free on-line that explain patients' rights to their medical records in each of the 50 states and DC. *http://ihcrp.georgetown.edu/privacy/records.html.*

A growing form of identity theft known as medical ID theft can devastate victims' finances. It also can compromise their medical records—and even put their health at risk.

With medical ID theft, criminals access victims' medical records rather than their bank or credit records. Medical records contain victims' Social Security numbers and credit card numbers (assuming that the victims have used credit cards to pay medical charges), so the criminal can make fraudulent charges and open accounts in victims' names, just as with standard ID theft.

The difference is that medical identity thieves also gain access to victims' health insurance policy information and medical histories. They can use this information to forge insurance ID cards that can be sold to uninsured people in need of expensive medical treatments.

The ID thief's "customers" receive medical treatment under the victim's name, Social Security number and health insurance policy, then disappear. Bills for co-payments or uncovered procedures are sent to the victim, who must sort out the mess.

GROWING PROBLEM

Medical identity theft currently is less common than standard financial identity theft—but it is becoming more common, in part because many health-care facilities do a poor job of protecting patient records. At least 13% of health-care providers have experienced a data breach, according to a 2008 survey. The ongoing digitalization of medical records will only make it easier for tech-savvy thieves to steal medical identities.

For victims, dealing with medical identity theft can be even more daunting than dealing with conventional identity theft. Victims not only must convince service providers and collection agencies that bills are fraudulent and repair their damaged credit histories, they also must correct the inaccurate medical information that is now part of their health records.

If someone else's medical problems are mixed in with your records, you could have difficulty obtaining life insurance or individual health insurance. The inaccurate medical history could cause a health-care provider to supply treatments or medications that are inappropriate for you, potentially endangering your health, even your life.

Medical ID theft even could lead to blackmail if medical records contain details about sensitive health conditions that patients don't want others to know about.

PREVENTING MEDICAL ID THEFT

It's important to guard your health insurance identification number just as closely as you do your Social Security and credit card numbers. Never leave your insurance card where it can be seen or lend it out, even to a seemingly helpful neighbor who offers to pick up your prescription.

Also, do not post your insurance identification number next to your phone or read the number out loud to a pharmacist if other customers are within earshot. Shred insurance documents before throwing them away.

Unfortunately, there is nothing you can do to prevent your medical records from being stolen from a hospital or doctor's office. *However, you can limit the potential damage if a theft does occur by taking these six steps...*

1. Open and read all medical bills and "Explanation of Benefits" (EOB) statements from your health insurer as soon as they reach you. If these describe treatments that you did not receive or name doctors or medical facilities that you don't remember visiting, immediately contact your insurance company or the health-care facility and request additional details.

2. If you're convinced that a bill or insurance statement refers to treatment you did not receive, ask to speak to the employee in charge of investigating fraud or medical ID theft at your insurance company and at the medical facility involved. Inform these individuals that there is a treatment in your records that was not provided to you and that you are the victim of either medical identity theft or a billing error.

Follow up your phone calls with letters sent directly to these employees via registered mail with return receipts requested. In your letters, describe the situation once again, then ask for any bills to be voided and your medical records to be amended to state that you did not have this health problem and did not receive this treatment.

Important: Americans have the right under federal Health Insurance Portability and Accountability Act (HIPAA) rules to have any inaccuracies in their health records amended, but not to have inaccurate information completely removed, even in cases of medical identity theft. Medical service providers argue that if inaccurate information were completely removed from patients' files, health-care providers could be sued for improper treatments that they had prescribed in good faith based on the now-deleted information.

3. Report the ID theft to the police in the town in which the medical services were rendered and to that state's attorney general's office. Most police departments do not pursue identity thieves with much vigor, but reporting the crime could at least provide you with a copy of a police report, which you can send to bill collectors who contact you.

4. Contact every health-care provider you use, explain what has occurred and ask if the erroneous information has found its way into that provider's records. If it has, request that the records be corrected. If possible, provide some evidence of the crime, such as a copy of the police report or a letter from your health-care provider or insurance company. There is no centralized medical record bureau to correct errors.

5. Call the major credit bureaus to report the fraud and set up fraud alerts, just as you would with any case of identity theft. The three credit bureaus to contact are Equifax (888-766-0008,

www.equifax.com)...Experian (888-397-3742, *www.experian.com*)...and TransUnion (800-680-7289, *www.transunion.com*).

Request free copies of your credit reports, and make sure no fraudulent new accounts have been opened in your name.

If you have ever used a credit or debit card to pay a medical bill, the thief could have your account information. Contact your card issuers, ask to review recent activity for suspicious charges, then cancel the cards and request replacements.

6. Scan your medical records for errors every few years, assuming that it is not too expensive to do so. Inaccuracies are distressingly common, even without identity theft.

Patients have a legal right to receive a copy of their medical records from any doctor's office or hospital where they received treatment, but first ask how much this will cost. Some states allow medical facilities to charge fees, which could be $1 per page or more for potentially hundreds of pages of records.

2

Best Health Care

Get Better Care from Your Doctor

Even people who are ordinarily savvy consumers lose their normal assertiveness at the examining room door—just when it's needed most.

The average internist sees 22 to 28 patients a day. In hectic medical environments, doctors barely have time to discuss their patients' major symptoms and complaints, much less minor health problems.

Traps to avoid...

***Trap 1:* Wasting time during the exam.** Most patients can provide a doctor with all the pertinent information in about 90 seconds—if they're mentally organized and make sure the doctor actually hears what they're saying.

Research shows that doctors interrupt patients, on average, after 23 seconds—and only 2% of patients get a chance to finish their opening statements.

Many people know to write down their symptoms and/or complaints ahead of time. But they make long, complicated lists that aren't much help during a short exam.

Helpful: Limit your written list to three main points—and keep the sentences short.

Example: "I've been having pain in my lower back," "I haven't been sleeping well" and "I'm having trouble with urination."

Hand a copy of the list to your doctor when he/she comes into the examining room. Reading a list while you're talking makes it easier for the doctor to process the information...and it ensures that you don't forget key points.

***Trap 2:* Not getting a second opinion.** Even though most people agree that second opinions are a good idea, only 20% of patients

Mehmet C. Oz, MD, director of the Cardiovascular Institute and Complimentary Medicine Program at New York-Presbyterian Medical Center and professor and vice chairman and professor of surgery at Columbia University, both in New York City, is coauthor of *You: The Smart Patient: An Insider's Handbook for Getting the Best Treatment.* Free Press.

actually seek them out—often because they are afraid of offending their doctors.

Getting a second opinion doesn't mean that you don't trust your doctor, or that his recommendations aren't valid. It just means that you're wisely exploring other treatment choices. One study found that 33% of second opinions resulted in a significant change in treatment. Health insurers usually pay for second opinions, especially for important procedures. It's a good idea to submit your request in writing to your insurer.

When to seek a second opinion…

•**If your doctor recommends any kind of surgery.**

•**If you have a condition that's uncommon or that's outside your doctor's main area of expertise.**

•**If a treatment doesn't seem to be working.** A patient with high blood pressure, for example, should show improvement within a few weeks. If that doesn't occur, a drug combination suggested by a different doctor might work better.

Useful: Use the Internet to look for scientific papers that have been written about your health problem. When you find a relevant study, write down the first author and last author listed at the end. The first author will be the doctor who did most of the research. The last author is usually the supervising physician. Both are good choices for a second opinion. Doctors who write papers for medical journals are usually among the country's top experts. Even if these doctors are not based in your area, they can probably provide a second opinion by phone if your doctor sends reports, test results, X-rays, etc.

Trap 3: **Not educating yourself on your condition.** Patients who do their research have basic knowledge that allows them to use their appointment time much more productively. Rather than wasting time discussing, say, the anatomy of the heart, you can inquire about the specifics of various treatments—for example, whether one class of drugs is better than another, different types of surgery, etc.

Important: When conducting research, Internet sites with URLs that end with ".edu" (educational institutions) or ".gov" (US government agencies) are among the most reliable.

My favorite is *www.pubmed.gov*, sponsored by the US National Library of Medicine and the National Institutes of Health.

Other research strategies…

•**Check when the information was updated.** Medical information that's more than two years old is ancient. Anything newer than that generally is timely.

•**Rely on Web sites that don't include advertising.** They are usually more reliable than those that do.

•**Don't trust information that suggests only one treatment plan.** That's often a tip-off that the information is biased and unreliable.

If you don't have time to do your own research, consider using a fee-based medical research service, such as The Health Resource, Inc. (800-949-0090, *www.thehealthresource.com*).

Trap 4: **Not understanding how to take your medication.** Only about half of all prescriptions are filled or taken correctly. In addition, medication errors—especially not identifying dangerous drug interactions—are among the most common preventable mistakes.

Smart idea: Go to the same pharmacy every time—and get to know the pharmacists. Someone who knows your health history is more likely to catch potential problems. The pharmacist might look at a new prescription and say something like, "You've never taken anything like this before. Let me call the doctor and check."

Other advice…

•**Choose a pharmacy that uses cross-checking software and medication-monitoring technology,** which checks for any potential drug interactions. (Just ask the staff if they use this technology.)

•**Ask your doctor to write detailed notes for you on the drug(s) you're taking.** Make sure you know the dose, when you're supposed to take it and how to take it (on an empty stomach, for example) and whether there are possible interactions with other drugs.

•**Inquire about age-related side effects.** A large study at Duke University found that more than 20% of older patients were given prescriptions for drugs that could cause serious side effects in people age 65 or older.

What Nurses Know—And Doctors Don't Tell You

Patricia Carroll, RN, quality-management coordinator, Franciscan Home Care and Hospice Care in Meriden, Connecticut, is the author of *What Nurses Know and Doctors Don't Have Time to Tell You: Practical Wisdom for Everyday Home Health Care*. Perigee.

M edical doctors are trained to treat illness, injury and disease with medication, surgery and/or hospitalization—but they rarely have time to give detailed self-care advice.

Nurses are usually the best people to offer this type of advice and help patients avoid dangerous medical mistakes.

Common mistakes...

•**Relying on an ear thermometer.** Ear thermometers use an infrared beam to gauge the temperature of the eardrum. They are accurate when trained nurses use them on unconscious patients, who aren't moving. Getting an accurate reading on a conscious patient, who is almost certain to move slightly, is less likely. When a patient moves, the infrared beam may shift off the eardrum, making the reading unreliable.

Rectal thermometers are still the gold standard for getting an accurate temperature reading. Digital oral thermometers also are reliable. But, according to a study conducted at the University of Virginia Health System, you should not eat or drink anything for 15 to 25 minutes before taking the reading.

Forehead thermometers gauge the temperature in the temporal artery, which supplies blood to the temple and scalp, and are considered less reliable because proper placement and use can be tricky. Follow label instructions carefully.

•**Using silverware to measure liquid medicines.** Daily doses of certain medications —for example, anticonvulsant drugs, such as *phenytoin* (Dilantin)—must be measured precisely because there is a narrow range between optimal and toxic doses. Liquid drug doses are prescribed in milliliters but often are translated into teaspoons and tablespoons for convenience. However, the size of silverware teaspoons and tablespoons varies widely.

Ask your health-care provider to skip this translation. Measure out your prescribed dose in milliliters in a needleless syringe or a dosing spoon (a plastic device with a spoon on one end and measurements along the handle).

Check with your health-care provider for a needleless syringe. Or buy a dosing spoon, available at a drugstore for about $2. If you're not sure how to use these devices, ask a pharmacist or nurse for a demonstration.

•**Storing medicine in the bathroom medicine cabinet.** The humidity that commonly develops in a bathroom with a shower or bathtub increases the chances that your prescription or over-the-counter (OTC) drugs will break down quickly, losing their efficacy and possibly causing unwanted side effects, such as stomach upset or skin rash.

A box, placed in a linen closet near the bathroom, is the best place for your drugs because it keeps the medication cool and dry. (If you have children in your home, place the box on the top shelf, where it is out of reach.)

•**Taking pain relievers that contain caffeine instead of getting it from coffee.** The OTC pain reliever Excedrin contains *acetaminophen*, aspirin and caffeine. Anacin, another OTC pain reliever, contains aspirin and caffeine. These drugs cost up to three times more than plain aspirin or acetaminophen.

Caffeine is added because aspirin and acetaminophen are absorbed up to 40% faster when taken with caffeine. However, a cup of caffeinated coffee contains about 135 mg of caffeine—compared with 64 mg to 130 mg per dose of pain reliever—and works just as well. Black tea, which contains 40 mg to 70 mg of caffeine per cup, also can be used.

If you use aspirin or acetaminophen, take it with a cup of coffee or tea in the morning to boost the drug's absorption. To avoid unwanted side effects, such as restlessness, do *not* drink coffee or tea at night.

Many people with arthritis suffer the most severe pain when they wake in the morning. Taking a pain reliever without caffeine allows you to take it at bedtime so it lasts until morning, without keeping you up at night.

What Your Doctor Should Ask You—But Won't

Leo Galland, MD, director, Foundation for Integrated Medicine, New York City. His latest book is *The Fat Resistance Diet*. Broadway. *www.fatresistancediet.com*. Dr. Galland is a recipient of the Linus Pauling Award.

In the US, the typical doctor's office visit lasts seven to 10 minutes. During that time, the doctor reviews your medical history, asks questions about your symptoms, performs an exam and orders tests, if necessary.

This approach can be effective for emergencies or acute illnesses, such as earaches, bronchitis or chest pain. It doesn't work as well for chronic diseases, such as diabetes, arthritis, asthma or fatigue.

Reason: Doctors don't ask questions that reveal the key facts about a person's life that can significantly affect the development and progression of disease.

Example: One of my patients had severe rheumatoid arthritis. She failed to improve even with the latest, most powerful drugs. None of her doctors thought to ask about her diet, which was triggering the release of inflammatory chemicals that exacerbated her symptoms.

I ask my patients to complete a 20-page questionnaire before their initial visit with me. In many cases, their answers give important clues to an accurate diagnosis. Even if your doctor doesn't ask the questions listed below, you should bring up these issues with him/her during your appointment.

Questions your doctor should ask—but many do not…

1. Have you ever felt better after avoiding particular foods? Up to 40% of *healthy* Americans report having an intolerance to one or more foods.

Why it matters: Millions of Americans react to wheat, dairy or other specific foods or food groups. Food intolerance is a frequent cause of diarrhea and other digestive problems. It also can cause fatigue and headache. Patients often suffer for years without being accurately diagnosed. The quality of a person's diet can have a significant impact on the risk for chronic or recurrent disease…energy levels, mood and body weight…recovery from infection…and the control of chronic disorders such as diabetes and high blood pressure.

What you can do: If you have unexplained symptoms, such as headache or diarrhea, keep a food diary to record everything you eat and drink over a three-day period, including spices and condiments such as pepper and mustard. The most common culprits are milk products, wheat, corn, yeast, sugar, artificial colors and flavors and spices. Eliminate a suspected problem food from your diet for five to seven days. Do your symptoms improve when you avoid the food? Do they get worse when you reintroduce it? If you find a problem food, ask your doctor whether you may have a food intolerance.

2. What are the major sources of stress in your life? Our bodies' nerves, hormones and immune cells work together to help us cope with emotional stress. In people who suffer chronic stress, this network becomes overwhelmed and stops working efficiently.

Why it matters: The body is designed to respond to stress and often benefits by becoming stronger. However, when people experience high levels of stress on a daily basis, the cost of responding to stress exceeds the benefit. This results in an increased risk for cardiovascular disease, infection, depression and other illnesses.

What you can do: It's impossible to eliminate stress altogether, but we all can learn to manage it more efficiently. For example, daily exercise—30 minutes of walking at a moderate to brisk pace—diminishes the effects of stress-related hormones.

3. Do you feel close to your family and/or friends? Doctors are often reluctant (or too busy) to ask about patients' personal lives. However, personal relationships are among the most important factors in preventing and treating disease.

Why it matters: Patients who are diagnosed with serious illnesses, including cancer and heart disease, live longer when they have a strong social network. Research also shows that people who are active in their communities or close to family and friends are less likely to get sick in the first place. A social support network also eases depression and protects you from the effects of daily stress.

What you can do: Take stock of your relationships with other people and nourish them by spending time with people you care about. If you are isolated, get involved in activities that help others.

4. How much personal control do you believe you have over your health? There are two primary ways that you can approach your health—you can rely on your doctor to tell you what to do…or you can actively participate in your health care.

Why it matters: Research shows that people are healthier and have better medical outcomes when they take responsibility for their own care…make important lifestyle changes… and generally put themselves in charge of their own health.

What you can do: The first step is to motivate yourself and make a commitment to yourself and those you love that you will be proactive in advocating for your own health. The second step is to learn what you can about the health conditions that affect you.

5. Do you have physical problems or certain personality traits that remind you of someone in your family? Your family medical history can help identify diseases that you may be predisposed to develop. Family history is an especially important risk factor for depression, heart disease, diabetes, high blood pressure and allergic and autoimmune disorders. Most cancers are not due to genetic risk factors, but to environmental exposures or diet.

Why it matters: A family history of a disease doesn't mean that you will develop that illness—but knowing your history, or just noticing similarities, makes it easier to predict and prevent future problems. For example, if you suffer from unexplained fatigue, weight gain or mood disturbances, and there is a history of thyroid problems in a close family member, such as a parent or sibling, your symptoms may be thyroid-related.

What you can do: Maintain a family tree that includes the health status and cause of death of grandparents, parents, aunts, uncles and siblings —and show it to your doctor.

ER Doctor Answers 12 Curious Health Questions

Billy Goldberg, MD, assistant professor and assistant director department of emergency medicine, New York University Medical Center, both in New York City, is co-author of *Why Do Men Fall Asleep After Sex? More Questions You'd Only Ask a Doctor After Your Third Whiskey Sour.* Three Rivers.

We all have little things that we would like to ask our doctors—but we don't want to waste their time or we're too embarrassed to ask. *Here, an emergency room physician answers those questions…*

•Do carrots improve vision?

There is only a grain of truth to this—carrots are a good source of vitamin A, a lack of which can lead to blindness. However, most people get enough vitamin A in their diets with or without carrots.

The story that carrots really improve vision was started by Britain's Royal Air Force during World War II. The Brits didn't want Germany to figure out that they had developed improved radar systems, so they spread the word that the unprecedented nighttime accuracy of British fighter pilots was the result of eyesight sharpened by carrot consumption. Though the war has been over for 60 years, the carrot cover story remains widely believed.

Consuming excessive amounts of vitamin A in supplement form won't give you superior vision, but it could cause toxicity, with symptoms such as hair loss, fatigue and headaches.

•Why do men have nipples?

During the early weeks of embryonic development, both men and women are designed on the female template. Not until about six weeks after conception do male embryos begin to show male characteristics. By that point, males have nipples.

Men also have a small amount of breast tissue, which means it is possible for them to develop breast cancer. Men account for approximately one in every 100 cases of breast cancer. The first sign of male breast cancer usually is a breast lump, the same as it is for a woman.

•Why does urine smell funny after we eat asparagus?

Asparagus contains *mercaptan*, a sulfur compound that also is found in onions, garlic, rotten eggs and the secretions of skunks. In the case of asparagus, the odor isn't produced until the compound has been broken down by digestive enzymes. Interestingly, not everyone has the gene for the enzyme that breaks down mercaptan, so some people can consume asparagus without having their urine smell afterward. A study in *British Journal of Clinical Pharmacology* found that less than half of British people tested produced the odor, while all French people tested did.

•Does cracking knuckles lead to arthritis?

There's no connection. Knuckle cracking is relatively harmless—the loud noise is just bubbles popping in the synovial fluid surrounding the joint. Long-term knuckle cracking might stretch the ligaments surrounding the joint, causing a slight decrease in grip strength, but this isn't likely to become a significant problem.

•Why do we cry when we slice onions?

Cutting into an onion causes enzymes and amino acids in the onion to react together in a way that forms sulfenic acids. These sulfenic acids release a chemical called *syn-propanethial-S-oxide* into the air, which comes in contact with the nerve fibers of our corneas and stimulates our tear glands.

Attempts have been made to develop tear-free onions, but it turns out that when you remove the enzymes that lead to crying, you also remove the onion's flavor. Research continues, however, and a flavorful, tear-free onion might be available someday.

For the moment, the best ways to reduce onion tears are to chop under a steady stream of water or wear goggles.

•Why do we tend to feel hungry again only an hour or so after eating Chinese food?

Chinese food emphasizes white rice and noodles. These low-protein, high-carbohydrate foods cause blood sugar to peak, then fall quickly, leaving us hungry again. To avoid this, select Chinese dishes that contain lots of protein, such as chicken, beef, tofu and fish.

•What causes canker sores?

Canker sores, known to doctors as *recurrent apthous ulcers*, are among the most common oral disease—yet we still don't know exactly what causes them.

Canker sores, which occur inside the mouth, are different from cold sores, which appear on the lips. Cold sores are caused by the herpes virus and are contagious. Canker sores are not contagious. Unfortunately, there is no treatment for canker sores.

•Do microwave ovens cause cancer?

There is no evidence that modern microwave ovens are capable of causing cancer. This relatively common fear springs from the fact that microwaves use radiation to cook. But while ionizing radiation, such as X-rays, can cause molecular damage, microwaves use nonionizing radiation, which does not, according to all evidence.

If nonionizing radiation did indeed cause cancer, we would have much bigger problems than our microwave ovens—all visible light is nonionizing radiation.

•Why does hair turn gray as we get older?

We lose hair color because the pigment cells in our hair follicles die off as we get older. The age at which this occurs is determined largely by heredity, though smoking or vitamin deficiency can speed up the process.

•Why do cucumber slices often soothe puffy eyes?

Cucumbers are 90% water, and that water is likely to be nicely chilled when the vegetable has been stored in the refrigerator. The cold water constricts the blood vessels around the eyes and the puffiness decreases.

If cucumbers don't do the job, try black tea bags soaked in cold water. Not only will the cold water work, the tannic acid in the tea can help reduce swelling as well.

•Why do some people have "innie" belly buttons while others have "outies"?

There's a widespread misconception that the type of belly button you have is determined by the type of knot the doctor tied after you were delivered. I believed this myself—until I delivered my first baby and realized that no knot was involved. Clips are used to clamp off the umbilical cord, then it's cut. The type of belly button you're left with is just a matter of chance, determined by how you heal when the remainder of the umbilical cord dries up and falls off.

Some belly buttons do turn from innies to outies later in life, but that's usually due to hernias in the belly button region.

•Is it true that eating poppy seeds can make you fail a drug test?

Some drug tests do indeed label poppy seed fans as heroin addicts. The same plant that produces poppy seeds also is the source of opium, from which heroin is produced. As little as one teaspoon of poppy seeds might be enough to cause a positive test.

If you know that you're going to have to take a drug test, avoid poppy seeds for about five days. If you have failed a drug test and think that poppy seeds are responsible, there are more precise drug tests that can differentiate between heroin and poppy seeds, so it might be possible to retest your urine sample and prove your innocence.

■ ■ ■ ■

Screening Tests

Many medical tests become unnecessary as we get older. A test should be ordered only if the potential benefit outweighs the potential harm. For many older people who are in only fair or poor health, certain tests are likely to cause more harm, discomfort and anxiety than the diseases they might detect.

Example: Prostate-specific antigen (PSA) screening, which may detect prostate cancer, is not recommended for men with a life expectancy of less than 10 years. Older men in poor health will probably experience only the adverse effects of the screening, such as psychological distress, additional procedures due to false-positive results and/or the complications of treating clinically insignificant prostate cancer.

Self-defense: Ask your doctor about the benefits before getting tested for any condition.

Louise C. Walter, MD, associate professor of geriatrics, University of California, San Francisco, and staff physician at San Francisco VA Medical Center.

Serious Conditions Doctors Misdiagnose

Vicki Rackner, MD, a surgeon and clinical instructor at the University of Washington School of Medicine in Seattle, is the author of *The Biggest Skeleton in Your Doctor's Closet.* Medical Bridges. *www.drvicki.org.*

Each year, up to 40% of Americans who are seen in an emergency room or intensive care unit are misdiagnosed. In some cases, a patient's condition is correctly diagnosed, and appropriate treatment is administered later. In other cases, the time that is lost through a misdiagnosis can be life-threatening.

Example: A patient who has painful abdominal cramping may be diagnosed with "gastroenteritis" (inflammation of the gastrointestinal tract) when the real culprit is a potentially fatal bowel obstruction.

Important: Listen to your intuition, but don't try to self-diagnose your problem. Get a complete evaluation from your doctor and a second opinion, if desired.

Often-misdiagnosed conditions…

Wrong diagnosis: **Gastroenteritis.** Gastroenteritis can be caused by ingesting food or water contaminated with a virus (Norwalk virus, adenovirus)…a bacterium (Salmonella, Escherichia coli)…a parasite (Giardia)…rare microorganisms (amoebas or parasitic worms)… or a food allergy. Gastroenteritis can result in cramping, vomiting and/or diarrhea.

But these symptoms also can characterize bowel obstruction (commonly caused by scar tissue from previous abdominal or pelvic surgery) …appendicitis…gallbladder disease…or antibiotic-associated colitis.

Self-defense: Do not accept a diagnosis of "gastroenteritis" if your symptoms include…

•**Crampy abdominal pain that comes and goes.** This could indicate a bowel obstruction.

•**Pain that begins around the navel and migrates to the lower right abdomen.** This could be appendicitis.

•**Sudden pain in the upper-right abdomen after eating a high-fat meal.** This symptom could be due to a gallbladder attack.

•**Severe diarrhea, abdominal pain and/or fever.** These symptoms could be caused by pseudomembranous colitis, an inflammatory condition of the colon that occurs in some people who have used antibiotics. It's usually caused by overgrowth of the bacterium *Clostridium difficile.*

To diagnose your condition correctly, your doctor should take a thorough medical history and perform a physical exam. Tests may include blood work, X-rays and an ultrasound or computed tomography (CT) scan.

***Wrong diagnosis:* Migraine.** More than 45 million people seek medical care each year for headaches. Many have a true migraine, a severe headache often accompanied by nausea, vomiting and/or extreme sensitivity to light and sound. Others have a tension or cluster headache.

In rare cases, a headache can signal a potentially serious condition, such as a stroke…a ruptured brain aneurysm (a weakened blood vessel that has burst)…a contusion (bruising of the brain)…a concussion (a head injury that can cause headache, confusion and amnesia)…a subdural hematoma (bleeding from veins between the outer and middle layers of tissue covering the brain, usually following a head injury)…a brain tumor…meningitis (a bacterial or viral infection of the membrane that surrounds the spinal cord and brain)…or a sinus infection.

Self-defense: Do not accept a diagnosis of "migraine" if your symptoms include…

•**Headache with confusion, weakness on one side of the body, double vision and/or trouble speaking.** This could indicate a stroke.

•**"The worst headache of my life" or a headache that "hits like a lightning bolt."** These are signs of a possible stroke or ruptured brain aneurysm.

•**Headache that gets worse after coughing, exertion, straining or sudden movement.** This can indicate a ruptured brain aneurysm.

•**Headache after a head injury, especially if the headache gets worse over the next day or two.** It could be a brain injury, such as a contusion, concussion or subdural hematoma.

•**New headache pain or changes in headache pattern** (location, intensity or frequency), especially in people age 55 or older. This could signal a brain tumor.

•**Headache with a fever, stiff neck and/or rash.** These are red flags for meningitis.

•**Headache after a recent sore throat, cold or flu.** This could indicate a sinus infection.

Ask your doctor whether you should be seen by a neurologist. Tests may include blood work, a CT or magnetic resonance imaging (MRI) scan, sinus X-rays or a spinal tap, in which a sample of the fluid that surrounds the brain and spinal cord is withdrawn with a needle and sent to a lab for analysis.

***Wrong diagnosis:* Muscle strain.** Muscle strain often is diagnosed when a person overexerts himself/herself and then experiences pain and/or swelling.

Among the more serious conditions characterized by these symptoms are an infection…or an aortic dissection (a potentially fatal condition in which the inner layer of the wall of the aorta, the main artery of the body, tears).

Self-defense: Do not accept a diagnosis of "muscle strain" if your symptoms include…

•**Fever and/or a joint that is red and hot.** These are red flags for infectious arthritis (infection of the tissues of a joint).

•**A "ripping" or "tearing" sensation in the upper back.** This commonly occurs in patients who have suffered an aortic dissection.

An evaluation may include X-rays, a CT or MRI scan, blood tests and/or arthrocentesis (removal of joint fluid that is analyzed for bacteria, other microorganisms or gouty crystals).

***Wrong diagnosis:* Pleurisy.** Pleurisy is an inflammation of the pleura, the lining of the lung and inner chest wall. This condition is often diagnosed when a sharp chest pain occurs during inhalation.

But chest pain also accompanies heart attack and pulmonary embolism (a blood clot that travels from a leg to the lungs). In addition, pleurisy usually has an underlying cause—such as influenza, pneumonia or fractured ribs—which doctors sometimes fail to identify.

Self-defense: Do not accept a diagnosis of "pleurisy" if your symptoms also include…

•**Shortness of breath, numbness in your arm and/or sweating.** These are all symptoms of a heart attack. In women, heart attack symptoms may include jaw pain, indigestion, back pain and/or fatigue.

•**Rapid heart rate, shortness of breath and/or sharp chest pain that worsens with deep breathing.** These could be red flags for a potentially fatal pulmonary embolism.

Your doctor may order a chest X-ray, electrocardiogram (EKG) or lung scan to look for blood clots.

Wrong diagnosis: Rash. Rashes are often harmless immune responses to a substance that a person touches or eats. They usually go away on their own or when treated with over-the-counter cortisone cream.

But rashes also can be due to a bacterial or viral infection.

Self-defense: Do not accept a diagnosis of "rash" if your symptoms also include…

•**Fever, chills, severe headache, aches and pains.** This can indicate an infection, such as Rocky Mountain spotted fever or scarlet fever.

•**Fatigue, muscle and joint stiffness and a bull's-eye–shaped rash.** These are some signs of Lyme disease.

•**Chills, fever, nausea and/or fluid-filled blisters in a band on one side of the body.** These are signs of shingles.

Your doctor will perform a physical exam and order a blood test and/or other tests, if necessary.

Read This Before You Have "Minor" Surgery

Hector Vila, Jr., MD, assistant professor of oncology and anesthesiology, H. Lee Moffitt Cancer Center & Research Institute, Tampa, Florida.
Archives of Surgery.

Having plastic surgery, endoscopies and other minor surgeries in a doctor's office is risky, a study says.

"Our research compared adverse outcomes and deaths in physicians' offices with those in ambulatory surgical centers," explains study author Dr. Hector Vila, Jr., assistant professor of oncology and anesthesiology at the H. Lee Moffitt Cancer Center & Research Institute in Tampa, Florida. "We found a much higher death rate and a much higher injury rate when surgery was done in the physician's office," he adds.

THE STUDY

Vila and his colleagues studied all the deaths and injuries during surgery in doctors' offices reported to the Florida Board of Medicine from 2000 through 2002. They looked at similar data from ambulatory surgical centers during 2000, reported to the Florida Agency for Health Care Administration.

The study included all types of outpatient surgeries. Vila says most surgeries were plastic surgeries and endoscopies, a procedure using a fiber optic scope to look at the intestinal tract.

Vila's team found that the injury rate in doctors' offices was 66 per 100,000 operations, compared with five per 100,000 surgeries in ambulatory surgical centers. For death, the corresponding numbers were nine per 100,000 in doctors' offices and less than one per 100,000 in ambulatory surgical centers.

The researchers note that if all procedures had been done in surgical centers, approximately 43 injuries and six deaths would have been prevented each year. Vila believes that this problem is not confined to Florida.

CHECK THEIR CREDENTIALS

There are many reasons for the dramatic difference in death and injury rates, Vila says, including a lack of equipment and personnel, a lack of set procedures and the inability to deal with emergencies. "Sometimes it's the [lack of] credentials of the people performing the procedure or administering the anesthesia," Vila adds.

"To work in a hospital, a physician has to apply for privileges, but a private physician can do whatever he or she wants in their office," Vila says.

In addition, office surgeries are much cheaper than those done in ambulatory surgery centers.

Patients concerned with safety need to ask several questions before deciding to have surgery in their doctor's office, Vila advises.

"You should ask your doctor if he has the same standards as those used in the hospital or ambulatory surgical center. Are the physicians board-certified in the specialty that normally performs this procedure? Do they have the same equipment? Do they have emergency resuscitative equipment? Who is going to be giving the anesthesia? And, where will you be taken if there is an emergency?

"If you are unsure, then you should consider having your surgery in an ambulatory surgical center," Vila says.

The American College of Surgeons offers more information about surgical procedures and risk at *www.facs.org*. Click on "Public and Press."

4 Common Surgeries You May Not Need

Charles B. Inlander is a consumer advocate and health-care consultant based in Fogelsville, Pennsylvania. He was the founding president of the nonprofit People's Medical Society, a consumer advocacy organization active in the 1980s and 1990s, and is the author of more than 20 books, including *Take This Book to the Hospital with You: A Consumer Guide to Surviving Your Hospital Stay.* St. Martin's.

Few things are worse than having an unnecessary surgical procedure. Yet every year, millions of Americans have operations they do not need. In fact, the Congressional Committee on Energy and Commerce reports that 20% of all surgeries performed in the US are unnecessary. *Surgeries you may not need...*

•**Prostate removal.** The most common treatment for prostate cancer is removal of the prostate gland, but clinical studies show that the operation is of little benefit to men who have a life expectancy of 10 years or less because the cancer grows very slowly. This means that most men over age 75 have nothing to gain and may suffer from side effects of the surgery, such as incontinence and infection. Regardless of a man's age, he should seek several medical opinions (including that of a urologist who does not perform surgery).

•**Cataract removal.** More than a decade ago, the Agency for Healthcare Policy and Research warned that many of the operations performed to remove a cataract were not necessary. The National Institutes for Health suggests that cataract removal is best performed if your vision has been reduced to at least 20/150—even with glasses. Yet each year, hundreds of thousands of Americans have the surgery even though their eyesight is far better than that. In many cases, surgery will not improve sight and can cause infection. For a more impartial view, get a second opinion from an optometrist (a health-care provider licensed to provide a broad range of eye-care services), rather than a surgical ophthalmologist (a medical doctor who specializes in eye disease).

•**Gallbladder removal.** Since the late 1980s, the number of gallbladder surgeries has increased by 40%. The reason is the advent of minimally invasive laparoscopic surgery. This procedure can be done in an outpatient setting and is quicker (conventional surgery typically requires three days in the hospital), more convenient and more profitable for doctors. But it is often not necessary. Before agreeing to gallbladder removal consult an experienced internist about nonsurgical options, such as a special diet or the gallstone-dissolving medication *ursodiol* (Actigall).

•**Wisdom tooth extraction.** This is the granddaddy of all unnecessary surgeries, as about half of all wisdom tooth extractions are unnecessary. For decades, major dental organizations and journals have criticized the removal of wisdom teeth that are symptom free. To protect yourself, any time a dentist recommends having your wisdom teeth removed, get a second opinion from another dentist. If wisdom teeth are impacted, infected or are causing other teeth to shift, surgery may be necessary. But many times they will not cause any problems, and you can save yourself a lot of time, money and pain.

"Full-Body" CT Scans

Mark A. Stengler, ND, naturopathic physician in private practice, La Jolla, California...adjunct associate clinical professor at the National College of Natural Medicine, Portland, Oregon...author of many books, including *The Natural Physician's Healing Therapies* and coauthor of *Prescription for Natural Cures* (both from Bottom Line Books)...and author of the *Bottom Line/Natural Healing* newsletter.

It wasn't so long ago that a Cat scan—a computerized X-ray technique, also called a CT (for "computed tomography") scan—seemed very exotic. In fact, if you're age 35 or older, there were no CT scanners in clinical use when you were born. Today, of course, CT scans are commonplace.

Now there's an even more advanced, and highly touted, version—electron beam computed tomography (EBCT), often (erroneously) referred to as a full-body scan. EBCT scans examine the abdominal cavity and chest (including coronary arteries and lungs). These scans are available in cities nationwide and are being promoted as a way to detect coronary artery disease and other abnormalities, including tumors and aneurysms in the chest, abdomen and pelvic area. In many states, a prescription is not required to get a scan. Even if you're healthy, you can just contact an imaging center and ask—and pay—for the test. The idea is to find trouble before any symptoms appear.

EBCT scans use very rapidly processed X-rays that capture images in a fraction of a second. This allows for clear, freeze-frame pictures of the heart and arteries while the heart is beating. Images are captured from many angles, allowing a three-dimensional view of the heart as well as other organs and systems.

The test is painless. While the patient lies on a table, an overhead scan machine takes images in an open environment—not in an enclosed space as with some other CT and magnetic resonance imaging (MRI) scans. Testing usually takes 10 to 15 minutes. Typically, a center's radiologist or cardiologist determines if there are any visible abnormalities and reviews the results with the patient within minutes. Upon your request, a copy of the report and images can be sent to your primary care doctor.

One purpose of an EBCT scan is to determine the amount of calcium buildup in the lining of the arteries, including the coronary arteries. Several studies, including one conducted at the respected Cooper Institute in Dallas and published in the *American Journal of Epidemiology*, have shown a correlation between the degree of calcification and the severity of hardening of the arteries, known as atherosclerosis. A low level of calcium buildup in the arteries means that your risk for coronary artery disease is low. A high level means that you are at higher risk for cardiovascular problems in the future.

There are a few downsides to EBCT scans. One is the radiation exposure from the X-rays—which can be two to 10 times more than that of a standard X-ray. Radiation is a known risk factor

for cancer (although the risk appears small with occasional scans). The EBCT scan also may result in "false positives"—meaning that doctors may spot a suspected lesion that requires follow-up tests, possibly even an invasive biopsy, and it may turn out to be nothing serious. Lastly, many insurance companies don't cover EBCT preventive screening. Scan costs start at $500 and can go as high as $1,700 or more.

Despite the financial cost, I do recommend that people age 40 and older get a preventive EBCT screening. If the results are normal, then follow up with another in five to 10 years. The test is even more important for those with a strong family history of heart disease or cancer. While EBCT scanning is not foolproof, it can help detect life-threatening diseases that are best treated with early intervention.

■ ■ ■ ■

Future Hospitals

New hospitals under construction will likely have only private rooms.

Reason: Patients in private rooms have up to 45% lower risk for hospital-acquired ("nosocomial") infections than patients who share hospital rooms.

Richard A. Van Enk, PhD, director, infection control and epidemiology, Bronson Methodist Hospital, Kalamazoo, Michigan, and leader of a study of infection rates in private rooms, published in *The Architecture of Hospitals*. NAI.

Hospitals' Hidden Killers: Blood Clots

Steven Deitelzweig, MD, chairman, department of hospital medicine and vice president of medical affairs, Ochsner Health System, New Orleans.

Samuel Goldhaber, MD, staff cardiologist, director of Anticoagulation Service, director, Venous Thromboembolism Research Group, Brigham and Women's Hospital and professor of medicine, Harvard Medical School, both in Boston.

Doctors at the Ochsner Clinic Foundation in New Orleans have started a campaign against hidden conditions that are responsible for 10% of all hospital deaths each year.

One of these conditions is *deep vein thrombosis* (DVT), which occurs when a blood clot forms in the leg and blocks the flow of blood. This can lead to potentially life-threatening pulmonary embolisms, which are caused when a clot breaks free, travels upward through the body and lodges in a lung. If the clot is large enough, it can cause sudden death.

Approximately 600,000 Americans develop pulmonary embolisms every year, and about 60,000 people die from them. The American College of Chest Physicians says it may be the most preventable cause of hospital death.

WHO'S AT RISK?

People hospitalized for long periods of time are particularly at risk because blood can collect in their legs and increase the probability of a clot forming.

Air travelers can also be prone to the condition because of the long hours spent cramped in a seat, experts say.

Those with cancer, chronic heart or respiratory failure, and an inherited or acquired predisposition to clotting and varicose veins also have an increased risk. So do people who are obese, as well as women who are pregnant or are using birth control pills or hormone-replacement therapy.

Symptoms of DVT can include leg pain, swelling, tenderness, discoloration or redness. Often, though, there are no symptoms.

Dr. Samuel Goldhaber, director of the Venous Thromboembolism Research Group, says the conditions are difficult to diagnose.

WHAT CAN BE DONE

Dr. Steven Deitelzweig, Ochsner's chairman of the department of hospital medicine, and his colleagues have developed a clinical assessment tool to help identify people who are at risk for developing DVT. The various risk factors—obesity, heart failure, infections, lung problems, prolonged immobility—are put on a grid. Everyone admitted to the hospital is assessed and put in a category of low, medium or high risk.

People who have two risk factors get treated with nonpharmacological devices, such as compression stockings.

If a person has at least three risk factors, or two risk factors and a history of stroke or cancer, they get at least one blood-thinning drug.

Choose the Best Hospital for Your Health

Charles B. Inlander is a consumer advocate and health-care consultant based in Fogelsville, Pennsylvania. He was the founding president of the nonprofit People's Medical Society, a consumer advocacy organization active in the 1980s and 1990s, and is the author of more than 20 books, including *Take This Book to the Hospital with You: A Consumer Guide to Surviving Your Hospital Stay*. St. Martin's.

If you assume that hospitals are roughly equivalent in the quality of care they offer, you could be making a deadly mistake. Most people are not aware of the differences among the various types of hospitals. *What you should know...*

There are two major categories of hospitals—specialty hospitals and general hospitals.

•**Specialty hospitals** focus on either one type of medical condition, such as cancer or eye problems, or deal exclusively with a specific category of patients, such as women or children.

Advantage: Greater access to applicable new technology and treatment techniques.

Disadvantage: Since not all communities have specialty hospitals, you may have to travel a great distance to use one.

Best used for: Complicated problems, such as major heart surgery, or rare conditions, such as certain cancers.

•**General hospitals** deal with a wide variety of medical conditions.

Advantage: General hospitals are better equipped to handle unexpected medical situations that may occur in the course of treatment.

Disadvantage: They may not be expert in rare or unique problems.

A general hospital can be a community hospital or a medical center...

•**Community hospitals** typically have fewer than 250 beds but are fully equipped to handle most medical conditions.

Advantage: Because they have fewer patients and shorter lengths of stay, on average, community hospitals have lower infection rates than larger hospitals.

Disadvantage: They may not have as many highly trained specialists.

Best used for: Routine treatment and surgery, such as appendectomy.

•**Medical centers** are large institutions that are typically, though not always, affiliated with universities.

Advantage: Medical centers offer state-of-the-art intensive care and coronary care.

Disadvantage: Because medical centers typically have sicker patients who get less personalized attention, higher infection rates are often reported at these facilities.

Best used for: Complicated conditions requiring medical experts in a number of specialties —for example, cardiology and endocrinology —and/or rare conditions that require comprehensive diagnostic services.

Community hospitals and medical centers can be classified as teaching or nonteaching facilities...

•**Teaching hospitals** provide teaching programs for medical students, interns (students still in training) and residents (doctors learning specialties).

Advantage: Access to cutting-edge technology and renowned expertise (that's why students come there).

Disadvantage: Students are learning on you! Therefore, you are often treated as a condition, not a person. There are no studies indicating that teaching hospitals are better than nonteaching hospitals, so choose the type of facility that best meets your needs.

•**Nonteaching hospitals** are strictly care facilities.

Advantage: Less intrusive care.

Disadvantage: Usually fewer specialties are offered.

Best used for: People who are being treated for non-life-threatening conditions.

How to Complain About Your Doctor Or Hospital

Charles B. Inlander is a consumer advocate and health-care consultant based in Fogelsville, Pennsylvania. He was the founding president of the nonprofit People's Medical Society, a consumer advocacy organization active in the 1980s and 1990s, and is the author of more than 20 books, including *Take This Book to the Hospital with You: A Consumer Guide to Surviving Your Hospital Stay.* St. Martin's.

In my 40 years of helping consumers with health-care problems, the number-one reason that people have contacted me is to find out where to file a complaint about a doctor, hospital, nurse or pharmacist. In most cases, the individual is not interested in filing a medical malpractice lawsuit. Rather, he/she simply wants to report shoddy business practices, including billing problems, or poor health care.

Filing a complaint is relatively easy. But knowing where to file can be tricky. All complaints are investigated. Results vary from state to state, and from board to board, but you will be notified of the outcome, which could include suspension or revocation of the health-care provider's license. *Here's how and where to file a complaint when you have a gripe against a health-care practitioner or a facility...*

•**State licensing board.** If you have a complaint against a doctor, contact the state medical licensing board in the state where the problem occurred. All doctors must be licensed by the state in which they practice. You can find the address, phone number and Web site of the medical licensing board in your state at *www.aimmembers.org/boarddirectory.*

Filing a complaint against a nurse or a pharmacist also is done at the state level. The National Council of State Boards of Nursing lists all the boards and their contact information at *www.ncsbn.org.* Click "Boards of Nursing" on their home page. The National Association of Boards of Pharmacy also lists each state board at *www.nabp.net*. Click "Boards of Pharmacy" on the home page. Hospitals and nursing homes are usually licensed by a division of a state's health department. If you do not have access to a computer, call your state's governor's office for the phone number of the board you are trying to reach.

•**Attorney general's office.** If you have a complaint about a doctor's bill or you suspect fraudulent billing, you also should file a complaint with your state's attorney general's office. You can find contact information from the National Association of Attorneys General at *http://www.naag.org/attorneys_general.php*. The attorney general investigates and litigates all business and criminal charges that might need to be brought against a licensed doctor or facility. The attorney general's office may refer some criminal complaints to your local district attorney's office.

•**Medicare.** If you are a Medicare or Medicaid beneficiary and have a complaint against a doctor or hospital for matters relating to your insurance, call Medicare at 800-633-4227 to file your complaint. They will pass it along to the appropriate government agency.

All complaints should be made in writing. To ensure a proper investigation, include the full name of the offending party...tell where, when and what time the incident occurred...and include statements of witnesses, if available. Also include copies of bills and other pertinent paperwork, if requested.

■ ■ ■ ■

Longer ER Waits

Emergency room waiting times are getting longer. Because of rising patient volume, the average amount of time a patient waited to see a physician in the ER increased from 38 minutes in 1997 to 56 minutes in 2006 (the most recent statistics available). According to the National Center for Health Statistics, more than 119.2 million visits were made to emergency departments, doctors' offices and hospital outpatient centers in 2006.

National Center for Health Statistics, Hyattsville, Maryland.

How to Stay Safe In the Hospital

David J. Sherer, MD, a board-certified anesthesiologist in clinical practice in Falls Church, Virginia, is author of *Dr. David Sherer's Hospital Survival Guide: 100+ Ways to Make Your Hospital Stay Safe and Comfortable.* Claren.

As many as 195,000 patients die each year in US hospitals because of medical errors, according to a study by HealthGrades, a leading health-care rating company. Here's how to stay safe next time you're in the hospital. If you're too incapacitated by your illness or injury to do these things for yourself, a family member can do many of them for you.

1. Keep a list of prescribed medications with dosages. You can get this list from the attending physician (the doctor in charge of your case), an intern, resident or nurse. Receiving the wrong medication is one of the most common—and dangerous—hospital errors. When a hospital staff member hands you a pill or starts to hook an intravenous (IV) bag to your arm, ask what you're being given. *If the drug isn't on the list of medications you have been prescribed...*

•Ask "What does this treat?" If the answer isn't a condition that you think you have, double-check that the drug provider knows your name and birthday, to confirm you're the patient he/she thinks you are.

•Make sure it's not a drug with a similar name. If you've been prescribed Zantac and someone's trying to give you Xanax or you take Celebrex but the nurse shows up with Cerebyx, someone may have misheard the instructions and provided the wrong medication.

Also, if it is a drug you've been prescribed but you previously received a different dosage, make sure the change was intentional.

2. Label yourself. If you're in the hospital for an operation on a limb, a lung or anything else that you have more than one of on or in your body, use a marker or ballpoint pen to write "this arm," "this leg" or just "yes" on the side that should go under the knife, so there is no confusion in the operating room. (At some hospitals, your surgeon will sign his initials to the body part in advance of your operation.) Don't use an

"X" to mark the spot, because an "X" is ambiguous—it could be misinterpreted as "not here."

•If you're allergic to any medications, make a sign to this effect and post it over your hospital bed. *Example:* "Allergic to Penicillin."

3. Schedule your hospital stay wisely. New interns, residents and medical school students begin assignments at teaching hospitals in early July. If possible, postpone elective procedures until a different time, when young medical professionals have more experience.

If you can't avoid a July stay in a teaching hospital, be wary about what you let interns and medical students do. If one wants to draw blood, insert a catheter or perform another common hospital task, ask how many times he/she has done it before. If the answer doesn't fill you with confidence, insist that a nurse or resident take over.

Important: Also, at any time of the year, try to schedule your surgery for early in the day. By the end of a long day, even the most skilled surgeons aren't at the top of their game. Also, because patients aren't allowed to eat or drink before surgery, a late operation means extra hours of hunger, thirst and worry.

4. Get to know the staff. A wide range of doctors, nurses, physician's assistants, interns, residents, orderlies and others might be involved in your care. Whenever a new face arrives, politely ask his name and what his role is, unless his name tag makes this obvious, then engage in some friendly conversation.

Helpful: If you make a personal connection with everyone involved in your care, it reduces the odds that you'll be mistaken for a different patient with potentially dangerous results. It also increases the odds that you'll get prompt care. Because most hospital patients are preoccupied with their health problems, the few who remain composed, personable and interested in the hospital staff often are treated more favorably.

5. Know who should do what. Find out when you can expect your attending physician to visit your bedside, and save any questions you have until then. Answers you receive from anyone else might not be definitive.

Don't let a UAP (also known as unlicensed assistive personnel or nurse assistant) insert an IV or catheter, change a sterile dressing, give you a shot or feed you through a tube. Such tasks should be handled by trained medical staff, such as a registered nurse. Check the person's name tag. If there's no designation, such as RN, ask what his training is.

6. Select the right surgeon. Unless it is an emergency, you shouldn't necessarily settle for the first surgeon you're sent to. *When you meet with a surgeon for a consultation, ask...*

•Are you board-certified in this specialty? Or check this on the Web site of the American Board of Medical Specialties (*www.abms.org*). You will have to register, but it is free.

•How many times have you performed this exact procedure? You want someone who has done it hundreds or even thousands of times. If the procedure is rare, you at least want a surgeon who performs it dozens of times per year.

7. Find the right hospital. If your surgeon has privileges at more than one hospital in your area, the annual "America's Best Hospitals" of *U.S. News & World Report* (*www.usnews.com* and click on "Health" and then "Best Hospitals" at left) can help you decide which facility is best for a given procedure. Be aware that your health insurance might limit you to a particular hospital or restrict your choice of surgeons.

8. Plan for the unexpected *before* you wind up in a hospital. Ask your doctor now which emergency room in your region he considers the best, assuming that there's more than one. (Of course, in situations where every second counts, the closest ER is almost always the best choice.)

9. Speak up. Make no effort to conceal your pain in a crowded emergency room—the ER staff might equate a quiet patient with a low-priority medical problem and treat others ahead of you. If you must wait, let the staff know if the pain gets worse...you have trouble breathing ...feel increasingly lightheaded...or lose feeling in, or control over, part of your body.

10. Encourage bedside visitors. Visitors don't just keep you company in the hospital. They can keep an eye on the quality of your care when you're unable to do so yourself. And because hospital employees know that family members keep an eye on what's going on, more visitors tend to mean more attention from the staff.

11. Warn your anesthesiologist of any loose teeth. A loose tooth could be knocked out during intubation (when a breathing tube is placed in your windpipe), causing a potentially serious infection if the tooth reaches your lungs. Also, ask your doctor about removing any dentures or artificial teeth before you're taken to the operating room.

■ ■ ■ ■

Insurance for High Risk

Thirty-four states guarantee health insurance to residents through high-risk pools. Rules vary.

Caution: Three states popular with retirees —Arizona, Florida and Nevada—don't have open high-risk pools. If you want to move to one of these states or a state without a high-risk pool, be sure you have private insurance or wait until you qualify for Medicare.

Details at *www.selfemployedcountry.org.*

Bruce Abbe, former vice president of public affairs, Communicating for America, Fergus Falls, Minnesota.

Survive a Trip to the Emergency Room

Joel Cohen, MD, medical director of MD RoomService and DoctorCare, a house call practice in Phoenix and Scottsdale, Arizona. He has practiced emergency care and internal medicine for more than 15 years and is author of *ER: Enter at Your Own Risk—How to Avoid Dangers Inside Emergency Rooms.* New Horizon.

To experience true chaos, just visit an emergency room. Through those metal doors is a busy, often disorganized place that can be hazardous to your health.

ERs are overcrowded and understaffed. You may be treated by an overworked medical student, an exhausted intern or a doctor trained in a field unrelated to your problem.

Obtaining high-quality emergency care fast can be vital after an accident or when a chronic illness, such as heart disease or asthma, suddenly becomes life threatening. But in a surprising number of situations, you'll have enough leeway to *choose* your ER.

Key: Know how to go to the right place at the right time for the right reasons—and be treated by the right caregiver. *Here's how...*

PREPARATION IS IMPORTANT

Get ready for the ER visit that you hope you'll never need. *Do your homework...*

• **Visit all ERs within 30 minutes of your home.** If your condition demands exceptional treatment, arriving in a half hour may be better than being transferred from another hospital later.

Look around. Would you feel well cared for?

Snowbird alert: If you have multiple homes or travel to the same places frequently, also do this exercise in these locations.

• **Identify facilities geared to your health problems.**

Example: If you have a heart condition, locate the ER with the best cardiac service. Your ultimate plan will be to ask an ambulance driver to take you there if your condition, such as symptoms of a mild heart attack, permits.

It surprises many people to learn that you often can get an ambulance crew to take you to the hospital of your choice. If the ambulance must go elsewhere or your condition demands faster treatment, the paramedic will say so.

Find the best ERs: Ask your primary care doctor, pulmonologist, cardiologist or other specialist where to find local high-level trauma or teaching hospitals. Ask the public relations departments at nearby hospitals for brochures promoting the hospitals' areas of expertise. Read hospital Web sites. Consult Castle Connolly Medical Ltd., a guide to top doctors and hospitals (212-367-8400, *www.castleconnolly.com*).

Cost: $24.95 for a one-year membership.

• **Wear a tag, necklace or bracelet identifying your medical status.**

Examples: Diabetes, medication allergies, need for dialysis. Wearing this information on a medical alert tag will help ensure that you receive appropriate care. Also, medical personnel will be able to retrieve your health information by calling the tag sponsor.

Information: MedicAlert (888-633-4298, *www.medicalert.org*)...Bodyguard Medical I.D. Tags (800-383-7790, *www.medicalidtags.com*).

KEEP THESE ER AIDS IN YOUR WALLET

Regularly update information that could be life-saving in the ER. *Don't leave home without a…*

•**List of your drug allergies** (or the statement "no known drug allergies").

•**List of all current medications,** prescription and nonprescription (herbs, vitamins, antacids), including dose and reason.

•**Health insurance and/or Medicare card.**

•**Miniature copy of your baseline electrocardiogram** (ECG), laminated. Take your ECG readout to a copy place, reduce it to wallet size and cover it with self-stick clear plastic sheets, sold at stationery and office supply stores.

Why: Comparing a new ECG with an old one can increase accuracy in diagnosing heart problems.

•**Research your health insurance plan's emergency coverage.** Must you report an ER visit within 24 hours? What if you're out of town or taken to an out-of-plan hospital? Having this information on hand will save precious time when admitted to an ER.

•**Maintain a relationship with a trusted physician.** In an emergency, your doctor may help you decide whether an ER visit is warranted …meet you there or consult by phone…recommend a specialist if you need one…find you a local doctor if you're out of town.

KNOW WHEN TO GO

For flu, a twisted ankle, longtime bad back or repeat kidney stone pain, call your doctor for an appointment. Consider going to a good walk-in urgent-care center (their quality varies tremendously) if your doctor isn't available and your insurance covers it. If you can, avoid ERs on Mondays and on Friday and Saturday nights, the busiest times.

Do head for the ER if you're experiencing unbearable or worst-ever pain…profuse bleeding…unfamiliar or severe chest pain, shortness of breath or abdominal pain…sudden arm or leg numbness or weakness…any other signs of a stroke or heart attack (see below).

STEALTH SYMPTOMS

If you are having a stroke or heart attack, the sooner you reach an ER that has the appropriate technology and expertise, the better. When given within about three hours for stroke, six hours for a heart attack, clot-busting drugs may save your life or reduce disability. Optimal stroke treatment can make the difference between paralysis and a little weakness.

Little-known symptom: In older women, shortness of breath is a more common primary heart attack symptom than chest pain.

Other subtle heart symptoms: Weakness …fatigue…unfamiliar indigestion…jaw or upper back pain.

Information: American Heart Association (800-242-8721, *www.americanheart.org*)…National Heart, Lung, and Blood Institute (301-592-8573, *www.nhlbi.nih.gov/actintime*).

Subtle stroke symptoms: Severe headache… facial tingling…drooping mouth…unexplained dizziness.

Information: American Stroke Association (888-478-7653, *www.strokeassociation.org*).

THE BEST CARE ONCE THERE

At the ER, contribute to the quality of your care. *Be sure to…*

•**Enter riding.** Patients arriving by ambulance get much faster attention than walk-ins. Don't let a friend drive you unless waiting for an ambulance would take too long.

•**Focus on one or two chief complaints.** The more vague you are, the less seriously your problem will be taken.

Example: Mention the new sharp pain in your side, not your arthritic hip.

•**Help the staff to help you.** Don't accept every test or treatment suggested without a discussion. Ask the doctor treating you in the ER to help you decide whether the potential gains of any proposed intervention justify possible risks.

•**Identify yourself and your circumstances often.** Ask what you're being given and why. To a nurse adding medication to your IV line, say, "Do you know about my drug allergies?" Don't assume that everyone has read your chart.

•**Be wary.** Reject medications and prescriptions proposed without logical, compelling reasons. Refuse any risky or unnecessary test or treatment.

Reasons: Older people are especially vulnerable to complications from invasive procedures… standard adult drug dosages can be too strong for older people.

If you are sensitive to drugs or you have kidney or liver problems, tell every ER staff member who treats you.

•**Don't leave too soon.** An ER staff eager to "clear the board" may want to send you home although you feel the same as or worse than when you arrived. Explain that you still feel bad. Ask the person discharging you, "Are you an attending physician here? Will you discuss my case with my family doctor?" You can also ask to speak to the attending physician yourself, but he/she may not be available.

TAKE AN ADVOCATE

It's hard to advocate for yourself in the midst of a health emergency. A relative, friend or neighbor can make sure your needs are met...scrutinize your care...discuss options...make phone calls...take detailed notes. Staff are more vigilant when someone is watching.

Your advocate can request the business card of every doctor who sees you...the name of every nurse who treats you...the name of every test that you're given. You may need these details later in the day or for your records.

Self-defense: With an "ER buddy," visit ERs together and compare notes. Show each other where your relevant medical papers are kept, such as health-care proxies naming the person who can make health decisions for you. Agree to accompany each other to the ER if needed.

Avoid Deadly Errors in the Hospital

Michael F. Roizen, MD, chief wellness officer at the Cleveland Clinic, Ohio, is coauthor of *YOU: The Smart Patient* (Free Press). Dr. Roizen has cowritten *YOU: The Owner's Manual* (Collins), and served on the boards of five nonprofit foundations. He is former chair of a Food and Drug Administration advisory committee and has published over 160 peer-reviewed papers.

The hospital is one of the most dangerous places you'll ever go. Patients are exposed to bacteria and viruses...subjected to tests and procedures with high risks...and given drugs that should be closely monitored—but sometimes aren't.

Over 100,000 Americans die annually from hospital errors. Although patients can't control everything that happens in the hospital, they can lower their risks more than they realize.

Example: Use only a hospital that's accredited by The Joint Commission. Accreditation means the hospital is evaluated every three years to ensure that it meets the best standards in cleanliness, infection control, drug administration guidelines, etc. To check, go to *www.qualitycheck.org*, or call 630-792-5800. *Other ways to stay safe...*

PICK THE BEST HOSPITAL

Teaching hospitals affiliated with major medical universities tend to have the latest technology and best-trained staff. If you require major surgery (such as a transplant operation) or have a life-threatening condition (such as an aortic aneurysm or pancreatic cancer), a teaching hospital is your best option. Smaller hospitals are fine for patients with "routine" health problems, such as pneumonia or a broken leg.

Warning: In the summer months, teaching hospitals are largely staffed by new residents and interns. Their lack of experience can adversely affect patient care. If you can, avoid teaching hospitals during the first two weeks of July, when the new school year begins. *Other points to consider...*

•**Is it a "magnet" hospital?** Medical centers with outstanding nursing programs earn this designation from the American Nurses Credentialing Center (800-284-2378, *www.nursecredentialing.org*). Patients in these hospitals benefit from improved care...less staff turnover...and high-quality physicians, who are more likely to work at a hospital with magnet status.

•**Are there full-time *intensivists* and *hospitalists*?** Intensivists are doctors who specialize in treating critically ill patients. Hospitalists are doctors who treat only hospital patients. Both types of specialists provide superior hospital care and don't maintain private practices "on the side."

•**How often does the hospital perform the procedure you're undergoing?** The best outcomes usually occur at hospitals where a given procedure is performed most often, on average.

Examples: A top-flight hospital will perform at least 500 open-heart procedures annually…100 carotid-artery grafts or surgeries …and 25 mastectomies.

CHOOSE THE BEST SURGEON

Only use a surgeon who is board certified in the specialty related to your operation—neurosurgery, cardiac surgery, etc. Look for the letters "FACS" (Fellow, American College of Surgeons) after his/ her name. This means that the surgeon has been evaluated for competence and ethical standards.

Helpful: Call the hospital anesthesiology department, and ask one of the anesthesiologists which surgeon he would pick. (Anesthesiologists often are free between 3 pm and 5 pm.) They know all the surgeons and have no reason not to give a straight answer.

Once you have some recommendations, choose a surgeon who does only a few types of procedures. Research has shown that surgeons who specialize—in nerve-sparing prostate surgery, for example—have better results and fewer complications than the national average.

Caution: Don't shave your surgical site before surgery. You'll wind up with thousands of invisible nicks that increase the risk for infection. Let the operating room staff do it. They use special creams that prevent nicks.

Important: Ask the anesthesiologist to provide a blanket (if it won't get in the way) to keep you warm during surgery. Patients who maintain normothermia (normal body temperature) have a lower risk for infection and other complications.

PREVENT HOSPITAL INFECTIONS

Each year, an estimated 2 million hospital patients develop an infection. With the emergence of antibiotic-resistant bacteria, even a minor initial infection can be fatal.

We all know the importance of hand washing, so insist that visitors (including nurses and doctors) wash their hands before touching you. A quick rinse doesn't help. Studies show that you must wash vigorously with soap and warm water for at least 15 to 20 seconds to remove all bacteria. As an alternative, hand-sanitizing gel, which is now located outside many hospital rooms, may be used by visitors.

Other self-defense strategies…

•**Keep a bottle of hand-sanitizing gel at your bedside.** Use this hand cleanser yourself before eating.

•**Beware of the TV remote control.** One study found that remote controls in hospitals have three times more bacteria than doorknobs or nurse call buttons. To protect yourself, cover the TV remote with a new hospital glove. You'll still be able to change the channels.

•**Ask about the stethoscope.** Doctors and nurses are supposed to clean their stethoscopes with alcohol between patients—but some get too busy and forget. Uncleaned stethoscopes have been linked to hospital infections.

DRUG PROTECTION

Drug mistakes—giving the wrong drug, a dangerous drug combination or the wrong dose—often occur in hospitals. Ask your primary care doctor to supervise all of your health care, including drug prescriptions. If that isn't possible, ask one of the hospitalists to do it. Patients with one supervising doctor face fewer risks.

Each time you're given medication: Show your ID bracelet. To ensure that you're getting the right drug (medical test or procedure), ask the nurse to check your ID wrist bracelet.

Also, ask the nurse to tell you what each drug is and why you're taking it. Don't take a drug unless you're sure it's the one that you're supposed to be taking. If you're receiving a medical test or procedure, confirm that it's the correct one.

Finally, ask a family member or friend to help monitor your daily care. This is especially important if the patient is not able to do so.

Are You Being Overcharged for Medical Care?

Sid Kirchheimer, an investigative reporter and author of the "Scam Alert" column in AARP Bulletin, is author of *Scam Proof Your Life: 377 Smart Ways to Protect You & Your Family from Ripoffs, Bogus Deals & Other Consumer Headaches.* Sterling.

Three-quarters of hospital bills have overcharges, and the average overcharge is about $1,000. Doctors, too, are handing inflated bills to patients.

Good news: It's simple to fight back.

If your health insurance completely covers hospital and doctor visits, these steps might not be necessary, though making the extra effort to eliminate overcharges can help bring down medical costs for everyone. Also, be aware that your insurance coverage might not be as comprehensive as you think—call your insurance carrier or review the exclusions section of your policy.

DOCTORS' BILLS

To avoid paying more than you should...

• **Negotiate.** If you have no health insurance, ask your doctor for a discount. Only 13% of patients ever make this request, but when they do, the majority secure a lower price, according to a survey of 2,118 adults conducted by Harris Interactive.

Ask the doctor in person. Requests made by phone or to an office assistant rarely work.

Keep in mind that insurance companies typically pay doctors one-half to two-thirds of the billed amount. If you will be paying out-of-pocket, you can offer to pay somewhere in that range when negotiating a price.

• **Get blood tests done at a lab.** When your doctor does a blood test, he/she charges you for the office visit...plus an added fee for drawing your blood...plus the amount a lab charges to run the test.

Ask the doctor to waive his fees, or go directly to a lab to have the test done and pay only for the test (ask the doctor to supply any necessary paperwork).

Look in your local yellow pages under "Laboratories—Clinical, Medical, Diagnostic" or "Laboratories—Testing" for labs in your area.

• **Don't pay for the follow-up visit.** When you see a doctor about a health problem, you often have to see him again a few weeks later to confirm that the treatment was successful. Chances are, your doctor will look you over for a few seconds during this follow-up, pronounce you well—then bill you another $50 to $100 for the second appointment.

During your initial appointment, tell the doctor that you're paying out-of-pocket and ask if he'll waive or reduce the charge for the follow-up visit, assuming that it takes only a moment.

Many doctors will agree to this, particularly for regular patients.

• **Confirm that tests are necessary.** Doctors often order unnecessary medical tests out of fear that not conducting these tests might open the door for negligence lawsuits later. Unless your health insurance is picking up the entire bill, question whether recommended tests—including MRIs, CAT scans and X-rays—really are necessary. Ask what these tests will determine.

HOSPITAL OVERCHARGES

Here's how to spot overbilling on hospital statements...

• **Ask for a daily itemized bill.** When you check into the hospital, tell the staff member who takes down your insurance information that you want an itemized bill brought to your bed every day. Hospitals are required to provide this upon request.

When you receive these daily bills, review each listing (or ask a family member to do so for you). Were you billed for two doctor visits yesterday even though you saw a doctor only once? Were you billed for tests that you don't recall getting? Are there vague entries, such as "miscellaneous costs" or "lab fees?" Are there listings you can't understand? Tell the nurse you would like to speak with the hospital's patient advocate, then ask the advocate to explain any charge that isn't clear. You might be appalled by what you're told.

Examples: Some hospitals have been known to call a box of tissues a $12 "mucus recovery system" and a bag of ice cubes a $30 "thermal therapy kit."

Save the daily bills so you can reconcile them later with the final bill.

If the patient advocate won't help remove the mistakes and reduce egregious overcharges from your bill, hire an independent medical billing advocate. He/she will examine your bill and fight to remove any overcharges, usually in exchange for a percentage—typically 35%—of the amount he saves you.

To find a medical billing advocate: Contact Medical Billing Advocates of America (540-387-5870, *www.billadvocates.com*)...American Medical Bill Review (530-221-4759, *www.ambr. com*)...or Edward R. Waxman & Associates (877-679-7224, *www.hospitalbillauditing.com*).

•**Bypass the hospital pharmacy.** Hospitals dramatically overcharge for drugs. A patient might be billed $5 to $10 for a pill that retails for 10 cents elsewhere.

If you are taking medications on an ongoing basis and are not fully covered by insurance, bring your drugs with you to the hospital.

When you consult with your doctor prior to entering the hospital, find out which drugs you're likely to be given during your stay. Ask the doctor to write you prescriptions so that you can buy these drugs at your local pharmacy in advance and avoid the hospital markup. Even if your doctor won't do this, you can bring any nonprescription pills you're told you'll need, such as vitamins.

If you must get drugs through the hospital pharmacy and your insurance isn't footing the bill, ask your doctor to specify generics whenever possible. When you get your itemized daily bill, double-check that you weren't charged for brand-name drugs instead.

•**Watch for double billing.** Hospitals often bill patients twice for certain things. If your bill lists sheets and pillows, ask the hospital's patient advocate if these items are included in your daily room rate. If you're billed for the scrubs, masks and gloves worn by surgical staff, find out if these were included in your bill for operating room time.

Also double-check the times on your operating room bill. Hospitals charge from $20 to $90 for every minute you're in the operating room, so if the time you spent in surgery is padded even a little, it will add a lot to your bill. Your anesthesia records will say how long your operation really lasted.

•**Don't pay for your last day.** Hospital patients are charged the full day's room rate for the day they check in—even if they arrive at 11:59 pm. In exchange, patients are not supposed to be charged for their last day, but hospitals often try to bill for the final day anyway. Sometimes these last-day room bills are simply removed when you complain, but there are hospitals that insist the last-day charge is legitimate for patients who aren't discharged by a certain hour, often noon.

During your hospitalization, ask the hospital's patient advocate whether you'll be billed for your room on the final day of your stay. If the answer is, "Yes, if you're not out by a certain hour," ask your doctor on the next-to-last day of your stay to give you your final checkup and discharge the following morning, rather than waiting until the afternoon. If the doctor says this doesn't fit his schedule, tell the patient advocate that you shouldn't have to pay because the delay is the doctor's fault.

Quality Medical Care at Great Savings

Rudy Rupak is a cofounder of PlanetHospital, a foreign medical-treatment company based in Calabasas, California, that arranges affordable surgeries overseas and offers free evaluations to those seeking surgery abroad.

More and more Americans are traveling to Europe, the Far East and Mexico for medical treatment.

Key reason: Low prices on top-quality care.

In the past, this kind of medical tourism has been associated with elective plastic surgery and experimental treatments not available in the US. But last year, more than 55,000 Americans went abroad for necessary but nonemergency operations, such as angioplasty, knee replacement and cataract surgery.* Less expensive labor and administrative costs make foreign treatment 50% to 75% cheaper. That can be a bargain even with the additional costs of airfare and accommodations. *Costs of medical procedures vary widely, within the US and internationally, but here are a few examples...*

•**Cataract surgery** in the US costs about $3,000 an eye...in Eastern Europe, it costs $1,200 an eye.

•**Repairing a herniated disk** in the US can range from $30,000 to $90,000...in Bangkok, Thailand, it starts at $3,500.

•**A total knee replacement** in the US is about $48,000...in India, $5,500.

•**Angioplasty** in the US, around $80,000...in Singapore, $15,000.

•**Root canal** in the US can range from $500 to $900...in Mexico, less than $300.

*US insurance companies currently do not pay for overseas surgery if it is not an emergency.

FINDING THE BEST

Flying thousands of miles from home for an operation is not for everyone, but it's worth exploring if you don't have adequate health insurance. Of course, you would want to use only top-quality foreign hospitals and physicians. *Here's how to find them...*

•**Start by word of mouth.** Ask friends and associates who have had medical procedures overseas for recommendations. Also ask doctors who specialize in the type of surgery you need.

•**Check with Partners Harvard Medical International** (PHMI). This is a self-supporting, not-for-profit subsidiary of Harvard Medical School. Its role is to extend internationally the school's tradition of improving the quality of health care. PHMI is affiliated with more than 50 programs in more than 30 countries. (617-535-6400, *www.hmi.hms.harvard.edu*)

•**Contact the Joint Commission International** (JCI), the global arm of the institution that accredits US hospitals. JCI hospitals have to meet rigorous standards of patient care, medication safety and infection control. (630-268-2900, *www.jointcommissioninternational.org*)

•**Choose a hospital with an international patient coordinator** on staff. He/she will help you coordinate doctor's appointments, diagnostics and treatment at the hospital, as well as arrange postoperative recuperation. He also can help with practical matters, such as airport pickup, currency exchange, hospital meal choices and interpreters if necessary.

•**Ask the foreign doctor/hospital for references** from Americans who have had the same type of treatment.

TOP FOREIGN HOSPITALS

These are foreign hospitals I would trust for myself and my family...

•**India.**

•*Apollo Hospitals.* Has hospitals in Delhi, Chennai and Hyderabad that cater to foreigners and specialize in heart-related procedures.

•*Wockhardt Hospitals Group.* Has hospitals in Mumbai (formerly Bombay) and Bangalore that specialize in heart, eye, bone, brain and spinal surgery. Associated with Harvard Medical International. *www.wockhardthospitals.net.*

•*The Max Hospital.* Has a specialty branch in New Delhi, which offers state-of-the-art surgery for brain and pituitary tumors, aneurysms and vascular malformations. *www.maxhealthcare.in.*

•**Thailand.**

•*Bumrungrad International.* Bangkok's leading health-care institution. Specialties include endocrinology, nephrology and neurology. *www.bumrungrad.com.*

•*Samitivej Hospitals.* Has branches in Bangkok and Chonburi. Specialties include cardiac and cancer surgery. *www.samitivej.co.th/index_en.aspx.*

•**Singapore.**

•*Parkway Health Hospital.* Three hospitals specializing in cardiac surgery and neurosurgery—East Shore, Gleneagles and Mount Elizabeth. *www.ipac.sg/en.*

•**Belgium.**

•*ANCA Clinic.* Ghent specializes in hip-related surgery. *www.hip-clinic.com.*

•**Mexico.**

•*Hospitales Angeles.* Has 17 hospitals in cities such as Tijuana and Juarez. Specializes in neurosurgery and dental surgery. *www.mediks.com* (site is in Spanish only).

GETTING QUALITY CARE

•**Ask for a full diagnosis** from your own doctor first. Develop a treatment plan you both feel comfortable with. Your doctor should be willing to forward all diagnostic information and communicate with the foreign surgeon to discuss your condition. Once you arrive, the foreign doctor also will evaluate you prior to surgery.

•**Bring a family member or friend.** You need someone for emotional support and to serve as your advocate. That person should bring with him/her your health-care power of attorney, which will be honored by international hospitals. This document allows him to make health decisions for you if you are unable to communicate your own wishes.

While a second person doubles the cost of the airfare, most foreign hospitals will allow a companion to stay as a guest in your room for no extra charge.

•**Know the costs.** Most international hospitals and/or health-care providers expect 50% of their fee to book the surgery and the rest of the cost of treatment at the time of admission. If complications prevent you from returning home immediately, hospitals will accommodate you longer, but ask for the rates so that you can plan accordingly. Also, you should be able to change any airfare you book multiple times with minimal penalty.

Important: Check with your insurance company to make sure it will pay for the treatment of any complications once you arrive home.

•**Confirm that the hospital gives you the same rights** that you have in the US. Reputable hospitals and surgeons will guarantee these rights in writing before you travel overseas. *You should have the right to…*

•Receive complete and current information concerning your diagnosis, treatment and prognosis in terms that you can understand, including serious side effects or risks, problems related to recovery and the likelihood of success.

•Have access to all information contained in your medical records.

•Accept or refuse any treatment and be informed of the consequences of any such refusal.

•Request consultation with the hospital ethics/oversight committee regarding complaints and ethical issues involved in your care.

•Be transferred to another facility at your request or when it is medically appropriate.

•Examine your bill and receive an explanation of the charges.

•**Understand that your legal rights are limited** if medical malpractice is committed overseas. You cannot sue in American courts, and most foreign countries strictly limit malpractice damage awards.

Helpful: If your overseas doctor has a medical board certification in the US, you can complain to the board and seek sanctions.

■ ■ ■ ■

Interim Health Coverage

Between jobs and need health coverage? Your cheapest option might be a short-term policy, says insurance expert Bob Hurley. It is almost always less expensive than federally regulated COBRA, which extends your former employer's coverage.

To compare prices: Shop at sites such as *Insurance.com* and *eHealthInsurance.com*.

Important: If you have a preexisting condition, get COBRA and then see if you can get a short-term policy. After you get one, cancel COBRA.

Bob Hurley is senior vice president of carrier relations at eHealthInsurance, a leading site for finding, comparing and buying health insurance, Mountain View, California. *www.ehealthinsurance.com.*

How to Speed Your Recovery in the Hospital

Marjory Abrams, publisher, *Bottom Line* newsletters, Boardroom Inc., 281 Tresser Blvd., Stamford, Connecticut 06901.

A friend who just finished a two-week hospital stay after orthopedic surgery learned firsthand how much a patient can do to help—or occasionally hinder—recovery.

Take the simple act of breathing, for example. Pam Hagan, RN, notes that when patients are sedentary, lung secretions may build up, resulting in pneumonia. Pam, a nurse for more than 25 years and the chief programs officer for the American Nurses Association (*www.nursingworld.org*), encourages patients to cough frequently and vigorously—even if they don't feel the need.

Some hospital patients are given an inspirometer to help with breathing. Request it if you're not given one. The deeper you breathe, the higher the ball in the inspirometer rises. Use it often—your lungs will thank you for it.

Pam also urges patients confined to bed to flex their feet, do ankle rotations and perform other simple exercises. Ask a nurse or a physical therapist for suggestions.

Other things you can do…

•**Ring for assistance getting out of bed.** More than a million falls occur each year in US hospitals, at least 30% resulting in moderate to severe injuries. The biggest risks are falling when attempting to get to the bathroom or in the bathroom. Ask for help before the need is urgent. Painkillers, diuretics, laxatives, sedatives and other drugs can increase the risk of falling.

Also helpful: Keep the bed in a low position. Drink to stay hydrated—to help prevent blood clots and increase the flow of secretions.

•**Eat nutritiously.** Poor nutrition can suppress the immune system, increasing the likelihood of medical complications. Pam encourages patients to request foods they like, as long as they comply with doctor-ordered limitations on salt and other restrictions. Ask to speak with the hospital dietitian if you have concerns. *Among the situations you may encounter...*

•**If you don't like what you get**—the meal, the flavor of your protein shake—request something else.

•**If you are hungry between meals** or want more of something, ask. My friend ate voluminous amounts of plain yogurt—which wasn't even on the menu.

Pam notes that sleep is a great healer, but hospital patients often don't get enough. *To get better shut-eye...*

•**Wear earplugs and/or an eye mask.**

•**Ask your night nurse to help you** into a comfortable sleeping position and turn off lights.

•**Make the nursing staff aware of your normal sleep schedule.** They may be able to adjust the timing of your medications or other nighttime interruptions.

•**If you feel you need a sleeping pill, ask your physician for one.** Talk with the nursing staff about pain medication, too. Day or night, preventing pain is easier than relieving it.

Have you noticed how frequently the word "ask" appears on this page? Optimal recovery requires a partnership between hospital professionals and patients. Communication is key.

■■■■

Hospital Care at Home

Treatments that were previously done only in a hospital, such as intravenous therapy or certain antibiotic therapies, now can be done at home by nurses, we hear from health-care advocate Charles Inlander. This may be useful for some patients who require careful short-term monitoring—for example, elderly people with chronic conditions, such as congestive heart failure and chronic obstructive pulmonary disease.

Advantages of home care: Greater comfort and less chance of infection. This type of care costs less than in-hospital care, but Medicare will pay for only a limited time, based on a doctor's orders.

Charles B. Inlander is a consumer advocate and health-care consultant based in Fogelsville, Pennsylvania. He was the founding president of the nonprofit People's Medical Society, a consumer advocacy organization active in the 1980s and 1990s, and is the author of more than 20 books, including Take This Book to the Hospital with You: A Consumer Guide to Surviving Your Hospital Stay. *St. Martin's.*

How to Find a Top "Alternative" Doc

Andrew L. Rubman, ND, and Susan Gordon, PhD. Dr. Rubman is director of the Southbury Clinic for Traditional Medicines in Southbury, Connecticut. Dr. Gordon is the clinic's research director.

A federal survey of more than 31,000 Americans found that 36% use some form of alternative or complementary medicine. But finding a capable practitioner is tricky.

Chiropractors, naturopathic doctors (NDs), acupuncturists and massage therapists are required to complete formal training and may be subject to state oversight. But many specialties in alternative or complementary medicine, such as herbal medicine and aromatherapy, have minimal—and in some cases, no—training requirements. *How to find a qualified practitioner...*

•**Start with an ND.** Naturopathy is a medical system that utilizes herbs, homeopathy, physical manipulation and many other modalities. Practitioners believe that the body has an innate ability to heal...that prevention should be emphasized...and that natural treatments usually are preferable to drugs and/or invasive procedures.

NDs attend a four-year, graduate-level program. There are four schools in the US that offer this type of program.* The programs include

*National College of Natural Medicine, Portland, Oregon...Bastyr University, Kenmore, Washington...Southwest College of Naturopathic Medicine, Tempe, Arizona...University of Bridgeport, Bridgeport, Connecticut.

many of the same courses taught in conventional medical schools, with an added emphasis on nutrition, preventive care and natural treatments.

In most states, you can use an ND as your primary care physician. He/she can order blood and imaging tests, take a medical history and perform clinical exams. Some states allow naturopathic physicians to prescribe drugs and perform minor surgery. Many insurance plans cover a naturopathic doctor's services—check with your provider.

Important: A naturopath is not the same as a naturopathic doctor. In many states, NDs have to complete standardized board exams to earn a license to practice. Naturopaths (sometimes called "traditional naturopaths") aren't licensed. Their education may consist of correspondence courses or an apprenticeship—or they may be self-taught.

•**Stick with older approaches.** Therapies that have been practiced for a long time are more likely to be effective than newer, trendy therapies. Traditional Chinese Medicine, for example, has been utilized for thousands of years.

Also, chiropractic, founded in 1895, has been thoroughly researched and is used by many medical specialists, including physical therapists and orthopedic physicians.

Some older approaches fall into a gray zone. For example, I can't say for sure that homeopathy works, but I'm not sure that it doesn't work.

•**Seek out evidence.** An alternative practitioner should be able to defend his specialty. Does the specialty have a peer-reviewed journal? Has the technique been tested in placebo-controlled, double-blind trials (where neither the study subjects nor the researchers know which participants are receiving placebos)?

A lack of scientific studies does not necessarily mean that a particular therapy doesn't work. Research is enormously expensive. The cost of developing a new drug, for example, can easily exceed $1 billion. Large organizations, including academic centers and pharmaceutical companies, can afford the investment. Alternative practitioners often cannot. But a practitioner should be able to recommend a place you can look for more information—an on-line journal, papers by other practitioners in the field, etc.

•**Ask about training.** Ask practitioners where (and how long) they trained, how many years they have been in practice and whether they can provide the names of other patients and/or medical professionals who can recommend them.

Try to find a practitioner who specializes in your health issue(s). A naturopathic physician might specialize in endocrinology or gastrointestinal disorders. An herbalist might have extensive experience with women's health issues.

•**Look for a practitioner who gives referrals.** A competent practitioner is willing to refer patients to other practitioners, including mainstream MDs and specialists. I routinely refer patients to chiropractors, neurologists, gastroenterologists, etc. Avoid any holistic/alternative practitioner who refuses to communicate with—or refer patients to—conventional doctors.

Also, look for a practitioner who recognizes the value of laboratory and imaging tests. Every practitioner should know when to refer patients for testing and understand how to interpret and utilize test results.

To find a practitioner: The following organizations can help you locate an alternative practitioner in your area…

•The American Association of Naturopathic Physicians, 866-538-2267, *www.naturopathic.org.*

•American College for Advancement in Medicine, 888-439-6891, *www.acamnet.org.*

•American Holistic Medical Association, 216-292-6644, *www.holisticmedicine.org.*

6 Steps to Stay Out of The Hospital

Mary D. Naylor, PhD, RN, the Marian S. Ware Professor in Gerontology and director of the New Courtland Center for Transitions and Health at the University of Pennsylvania School of Nursing in Philadelphia. She is cofounder of Living Independently for Elders (*www.lifeupenn.org*), which provides health, day-care and other services designed to help older adults remain in their homes and communities.

More than half of general hospital admissions involve adults age 65 and older—many of whom are hospitalized repeatedly for complications from chronic conditions, such as heart disease, high blood pressure and diabetes.

Problem: Even a short hospitalization of two or three days often precipitates a serious health decline—primarily due to the high rate of hospital-acquired infections and medication errors.

Solution: As many as one-third of repeat hospitalizations among older adults are preventable. Mary D. Naylor, PhD, RN, is a leading researcher at the University of Pennsylvania who has studied the problem of frequent hospitalizations among older adults for nearly two decades. *Naylor's advice...*

STEP 1:
BE AWARE OF YOUR WARNING SIGNS

Patients who know what symptoms to watch for are far more likely to seek prompt medical attention at a doctor's office. This often can remedy a potential problem without emergency room or hospital care.

Example: Fluid retention (in the feet, legs or abdomen) is one of the first signs of heart failure (inadequate pumping action of the heart) that is poorly controlled. This usually can be reversed by changing a drug or adjusting a prescribed dosage.

Self-defense: Ask your health-care provider to list early symptoms of any chronic conditions you may have and the best ways to watch for these changes. Write down the symptoms and keep them in a conspicuous location, such as on your refrigerator.

STEP 2:
DON'T SETTLE FOR A STANDARD DISCHARGE

When a patient is discharged from a hospital, he/she is given basic instructions for ongoing care. But this process is rarely adequate.

Self-defense: Don't leave the hospital until you and/or a family member completely understand your next steps. Before discharge, find out which medications you received that day, when the next dose is due and any changes that require filling a new prescription or increasing or decreasing the dosage taken before you were admitted.

You also need to know how soon you should see your doctor after discharge. Insist on getting the name and phone number of someone you can contact—including after-hours—if you have questions. Ideally, this will be one of the doctors or nurses who is most familiar with your medical history.

STEP 3:
DO MEDICATION CHECKS

Medication errors (such as being given the wrong medication or no dosage instructions) are a main cause of repeat hospital admissions. Potentially dangerous drugs, such as *warfarin* (Coumadin) or other types of blood-thinning medication, are among the drugs most commonly involved in repeat hospitalizations.

When researchers at the University of Pennsylvania tracked patients after their discharge from the hospital, they found a 70% error rate in medication use. For example, some patients were given inaccurate information about medication types or doses...or drugs that were discontinued when patients entered the hospital weren't always restarted once they left.

Self-defense: Keep an up-to-date list of your medications (including over-the-counter drugs) and supplements where family members can find it if you go to the hospital unexpectedly. In the hospital, post a list of your medications beside your bed in the hospital. Every time you see a new doctor, ask him to review the list.

Helpful: Don't throw away your older lists. Compare older medication lists with the newest one. If there's been a change in a drug or dose, ask your doctor about it to ensure that it's not a mistake.

STEP 4:
PREVENT FALLS

Falls account for about 1.8 million emergency room visits and 16,000 deaths annually in the US. People who fall, especially older adults, often experience a cascade of complications—for example, a bone fracture can lead to extended periods of immobility that increases risk for pneumonia, which often requires hospitalization.

Self-defense: If you're age 70 or older, get a comprehensive assessment from a geriatrician once a year.* He will look at fall risk factors, such as muscle strength, balance and vision changes.

*To find a geriatrician in your area, contact the American Geriatrics Society's Foundation for Health in Aging, 800-563-4916, *www.healthinaging.org.*

Helpful: Improve your muscle strength with regular exercise such as walking or swimming. Specific exercises that improve balance include one-legged stands, in which you stand on each leg (near a counter so you can catch yourself if you lose your balance) for 30 seconds several times a day.

STEP 5:
ASK FOR A MENTAL ASSESSMENT

Most doctors don't routinely check for mental changes.

Recent study: When University of Pennsylvania research assistants went to a number of hospitals to conduct rigorous cognitive assessments, they found that more than one-third of older patients admitted for complications from chronic diseases had some degree of cognitive impairment (primarily memory loss). Of those patients, 65% had never been identified as having memory problems, which increases a person's risk for making the kinds of mistakes (such as forgetting to take medication) that can lead to hospitalization.

Self-defense: Ask your primary care provider whether you should see a geriatrician or neurologist to have your cognitive functioning evaluated. Testing, which takes about 10 to 20 minutes, typically involves measuring your ability to complete simple memory and/or motor tasks.

STEP 6:
EAT WELL

Malnutrition and dehydration are common in older adults and can result in gradual declines in mental and physical functioning.

Self-defense: Get a nutritional assessment from your health-care team. Also, keep a diary in which you write down everything you eat and drink, as well as your eating patterns (for example, time of day) and settings, for one to two weeks.

People who do nothing more than eat nutritiously and drink enough fluids are far less likely to require hospitalization—or to suffer complications from underlying chronic diseases.

▪ ▪ ▪ ▪

Don't Let ERs Get Your Cash

Advance payment cannot be demanded at emergency rooms prior to treatment. Some hospitals have been asking for credit cards before emergency treatment starts to ensure payment later. If this happens to you, ask for the payment demand in writing on hospital letterhead and signed by the person requesting the payment, specifying how much money the hospital wants before treatment. This should get the hospital to stop asking—federal law forbids demands for advance emergency room payment.

Nora Johnson, medical advocate, Med-X, a company that specializes in medical billing errors, Caldwell, West Virginia.

What You Must Know Now About Long-Term Care

Joseph L. Matthews, JD, a San Francisco–based attorney specializing in issues relating to seniors. He is author of numerous books, including Long-Term Care: How to Plan & Pay for It. *Nolo.*

The average cost of a private room in a nursing home today is nearly $77,380 per year, according to the 2008 MetLife Market Survey of Nursing Home & Assisted Living Costs. Top facilities can cost well into six figures a year. Recently revised government rules make it more difficult than ever to obtain Medicaid assistance to pay these bills.

Most people never require an extended nursing home stay, but for those who do, the result can be financial devastation. By understanding the ways you can finance long-term care, you can reduce the chances that it will have such a devastating impact on your finances.

How to decide which options are the best for you...

LONG-TERM-CARE INSURANCE

Insurance that pays long-term-care bills sounds like a "no brainer" idea—until you take a close look at the details. These policies cost thousands of dollars a year. You may pay premiums for decades before coverage is needed, if it is ever never needed at all...and the premiums can increase significantly over the years, even with a so-called "fixed-rate" policy. For these reasons, long-term-care insurance generally is not an effective investment. Also, collecting on the policies is often difficult. Between 2003 and 2006, complaints to state regulators over denied claims soared 74%.

So why even consider this form of insurance? If you would sleep better at night knowing that a long stay in a long-term-care facility would not deplete your assets, consider purchasing a policy.

However, as a rule of thumb, if coverage costs in excess of 5% of the combined total of your pension, Social Security, retirement plan distributions and any other income, it is too expensive, because you would be sacrificing too much elsewhere in your retirement budget. Speak with a financial planner to determine your projected monthly budget in retirement.

Despite the drawbacks, the popularity of these long-term-care policies has grown. Total premiums collected have jumped 21%, from $8.2 billion in 2004 to a total of $10 billion in 2007.

The best time to consider long-term-care insurance is when you are between the ages of 50 and 65 and still healthy—any sooner and you would have to pay premiums for too many years...any later and the annual premiums would become so expensive that you probably would be better off paying for long-term care out of pocket. (Most insurance companies charge sharply higher premiums for people over age 60 or 65.)

For information on how to choose a policy, see the following article.

MEDICAID

Half of all nursing home residents depend on Medicaid, the government health insurance program for the poor, to pay for their stays. (Some states have different names for Medicaid, such as Medi-Cal in California, and Medicaid laws vary from state to state.) Unfortunately, Medicaid will not pick up your nursing home bills until you have depleted virtually all of your assets. In the past, many people who thought that they were likely to need a nursing home stay in coming years gave their assets to their children, making themselves poor enough to qualify for Medicaid.

New, stricter rules make this much more difficult. Any assets given away or sold for less than their true value within five years of applying for Medicaid are included in calculations of your

wealth, and that could delay the date on which you qualify for Medicaid.

Medicaid recipients are allowed to own a car, a burial plot, a limited amount of life insurance, a wedding ring and a few other possessions. A recipient can keep his/her home if his spouse is living in it.

Many nursing homes will not be available to you if you use Medicaid to pay for long-term care. Those with the strongest reputations and highest demand for beds often don't accept Medicaid as payment...or have space for only a few Medicaid patients.

On the bright side, once you are in a nursing home, you cannot legally be forced to leave just because you have run out of money. Even facilities that do not accept Medicaid patients still must let you pay with Medicaid once you have been accepted, should you outlive your assets or a long-term-care insurance policy. (You might, however, be demoted to smaller or less appealing accommodations after Medicaid starts paying your bill.)

VA FACILITIES

The Veterans Administration (VA) operates a large number of surprisingly well-funded and well-run long-term-care facilities. They are free for former military personnel—but because millions of former service people are in need of nursing home care, demand far exceeds supply.

The VA has a complex formula for determining which applicants are accepted into its facilities. Top priority is given to veterans suffering service-related disabilities...those in extreme financial need...and retired career service people. Veterans should contact the VA (877-222-8387, *www.va.gov/directory*) as soon as it becomes apparent that a stay in a long-term-care facility is likely in the future.

OTHER TYPES OF CARE

Twenty years ago, nursing homes were virtually the only option. Today, there is a range of long-term-care facilities. *Most of them are less expensive than nursing homes, and they may be covered by long-term-care insurance...*

•**Independent-living residences** are small apartments that provide limited assistance as needed and cost less than assisted-living facilities. Twenty-four-hour security and emergency response systems are usually provided.

•**Assisted-living facilities** cost perhaps one-third to one-half less than nursing homes. They do not provide 24-hour care, but their services, including assistance with transportation and shopping, bathing and eating, are sufficient for many seniors.

•**Continuing-care retirement communities.** Some senior-care facilities have different types of accommodations ranging from senior residences to nursing home care on one site. Residents move from one level of care to the next as their needs dictate.

PAYING OUT OF POCKET

If you choose not to buy long-term-care insurance…have too much money to qualify for Medicaid…and are not eligible for VA care, you likely will have to pay for long-term care out of your own pocket. To stretch your money, depend on in-home care from family members for as long as possible before resorting to professional care. Some seniors postpone their nursing home stays by months or years with the assistance of spouses or adult children. Discuss this with your family before your health deteriorates.

If you must move to a long-term-care facility, do not pay for more assistance than you actually need. Consider independent living and assisted living first.

If you have only enough assets to pay for three to six months of long-term care, consider moving into a nursing home even if an assisted-living facility or independent-living residence would be sufficient for your needs, particularly if you have a degenerative condition. Once you are in a nursing home, you cannot legally be kicked out for lack of funds. For a free on-line guide to long-term care insurance, go to Caring.com and put "long-term care" in the search window.

■ **More from Joseph L. Matthews…**

Selecting a Long-Term-Care Policy

If you do decide to purchase long-term-care insurance, be sure to buy from an established insurance company. Certainly a very familiar company name is a good sign, but also check the company's financial strength. The best insurance companies earn grades of AAA or AA from Standard & Poor's. *Long-term-care coverage should include…*

•**Long exclusion period.** To reduce the cost of coverage, select a policy with a 90-day to six-month "exclusion period." This means that if you ever need care, you would have to pay out of pocket for this period before the benefits begin. Your premiums would be as much as one-third lower than with a 30-day exclusion period, the most common exclusion option.

•**Inflation protection.** This protection is best when it is linked to increases in the actual cost of living, not to an arbitrary preset inflation rate.

•**Premium protection.** Select a policy that does not allow your insurance company to raise your premium unless it also raises the premium for everyone holding the same policy. Insurance companies must apply to state regulators for this type of premium raise, making excessive increases less likely (though still possible).

•**Payout flexibility.** Your policy should pay for home care, assisted-living care and nursing home care.

•**Minimal impairment to trigger coverage.** A good policy will offer benefits when you cannot perform two or three daily living tasks, while a poor one might require four or five.

•**At least three years of coverage.** An extended stay in a facility is unlikely, but the purpose of insurance is to protect against unlikely but financially crippling scenarios.

You Don't Have to Suffer "Medical Loneliness"

Charles B. Inlander is a consumer advocate and health-care consultant based in Fogelsville, Pennsylvania. He was the founding president of the nonprofit People's Medical Society, a consumer advocacy organization active in the 1980s and 1990s, and is the author of more than 20 books, including *Take This Book to the Hospital with You: A Consumer Guide to Surviving Your Hospital Stay.* St. Martin's.

About 10 years ago, at the age of 50, a former college fraternity brother of mine suffered a severe stroke that left him partially paralyzed. All of his friends were very concerned. But as time passed, most of us lost touch with him. We didn't realize how his world had fallen apart. He could not work and had to go on disability. He and his wife divorced. Health bills and other expenses accumulated. He was alone and overwhelmed.

About four months ago, in desperation, he called another fraternity brother to ask for help. In a period of two weeks, more than 90 of our fellow fraternity brothers paid all his bills, set up a financial plan to cover his expenses and created a schedule for us to see him regularly.

Any serious medical condition—whether it's cancer, diabetes, Parkinson's disease or some other major health issue—is life-altering. Too often, however, the enormity of dealing with a medical problem leads a person to withdraw, as my fraternity brother did, from society, one's friends and favorite activities. That's a mistake because studies show that staying as active as possible and interacting with friends and family can help a person feel better and stay healthier longer.

Here's my advice for dealing with what I call "medical loneliness"…

•**Don't let your medical condition define you.** Hospital staff often refer to patients based on their medical conditions—for example, the "gallbladder in room 204." As consumers, we often do it to ourselves by letting our disease or condition dominate our lives. But no matter how serious the health problem, you are a lot more than your medical circumstance. Having diabetes, for example, doesn't mean you cannot go out to eat. It just means that you must watch what you eat. Being treated for cancer might sap your energy, but you can still enjoy going out occasionally to a movie. Do the best you can to control the disease or condition, but do not let it control you.

•**Learn the secret to staying connected.** People with serious medical conditions often become isolated because their health issues are their main topic of conversation. If you like baseball, talk about baseball. Brag about your grandchildren or talk politics. If you limit conversations to your medical issues, both you and your friends or family members will end up feeling bad.

•**Find the right self-help group.** There are more than 700,000 self-help groups in the US. These groups, which are usually founded and run by people who have been diagnosed with a particular medical condition, help others who have a similar problem connect with one another (online or in person) to discuss everything from the daily challenges they share to treatments that work and those that don't work. These groups not only provide help, but also keep you in touch with the outside world, even if you are confined to home. To find a group near you, contact the American Self-Help Group Clearinghouse at *www.mentalhelp.net/selfhelp.*

3

Simple Healers

Coffee…Chocolate and More Surprising Ways to Live Longer

Many of the proven strategies for living longer—such as restricting calories and exercising on a regular basis—can feel like punishment for some people.

Fortunately, there are many enjoyable ways to stay healthy—but doctors don't recommend these strategies as often as they should. Research has shown that activities nearly everyone enjoys can literally add years to a person's life.

Fun-filled ways to live longer…

1. Get the right kind of sleep. Studies have found that people who get deep, restorative sleep typically live three years longer than those who don't. During deep sleep, the body normally produces higher levels of *melatonin*, a hormone that improves immunity and reduces the risk for infections as well as cancer. Deep sleep also increases levels of growth hormone, which improves energy and helps promote a healthy weight.

Good news: You don't have to sleep uninterrupted through the night to get the benefits of deep sleep, as long as you complete a series of at least 90-minute sleep cycles—each one beginning with light sleep (stages 1 and 2)…progressing through deeper sleep (stages 3 and 4) …and then into the deepest stage, known as rapid eye movement (REM) sleep. As long as you complete this 90-minute cycle several times a night, it doesn't matter if you wake up a time or two.

2. Enjoy your coffee. Many people assume that coffee—unlike green tea, for example—isn't a healthful beverage. But that's not true. Studies have found that caffeinated and decaffeinated coffee are a main source of antioxidants in the average American's diet.

Michael F. Roizen, MD, chief wellness officer at the Cleveland Clinic, Ohio. Dr. Roizen has cowritten *YOU: The Owner's Manual* (Collins), and served on the boards of five nonprofit foundations. He is former chair of a Food and Drug Administration advisory committee.

Research has shown that caffeinated coffee decreases the risk for Parkinson's and Alzheimer's diseases by 30% to 40%—health benefits that are largely attributed to the beverage's caffeine. (Decaffeinated coffee does not offer these same benefits.) The caffeine in coffee also is good for cognitive health.

Important: Caffeinated coffee may cause several side effects, such as blood pressure spikes, abnormal heartbeat, anxiety and gastric upset.

My recommendation: If you do not experience any of these side effects, and you enjoy drinking coffee, have as many cups of caffeinated coffee as you like. If you do experience side effects, you may prefer to drink decaffeinated coffee. Even though it does not have the health benefits previously described, studies show that decaffeinated coffee may help fight type 2 diabetes.

3. Go dancing. Men and women who get optimal amounts of physical activity—about 30 minutes a day, seven days a week—can make their "RealAges" (the "biological ages" of their bodies, based on lifestyle and behaviors) 6.4 years younger.

Many types of dancing give a superb physical workout. Ballroom and square dancing are particularly good for cognitive health. They involve both physical and mental stimulation (in order to execute the appropriate dance steps) and may help reduce the risk for dementia. Aim to dance at least 30 minutes a day.

4. Do some singing. Whether you lend your voice to a choir or merely sing for pleasure in the shower, singing improves immunity and elevates levels of hormones known as *endorphins* and *dopamine*—both of which reduce stress and activate the brain's pleasure centers. Studies have shown that singing helps people with asthma…reduces stress hormones…and may temporarily help improve memory in patients with Alzheimer's disease.

5. Continue learning. People who take pleasure in expanding their minds—for example, by learning to paint, attending lectures or doing puzzles—can make their RealAges about 2.5 years younger.

Studies have shown that people with higher levels of education, and those who continue learning throughout life, form more connections between brain cells, making them less likely to experience later-life memory loss.

6. Eat some chocolate. The powerful antioxidants known as *flavonoids* in dark chocolate increase levels of the body's *nitric oxide* (NO), a gas that dilates arteries and can help reduce blood pressure in people with hypertension.

This is particularly helpful for people over age 50, because age-related buildup of fatty deposits in the arteries (atherosclerosis) reduces natural levels of NO.

My recommendation: Eat one-half ounce of dark chocolate (at least 70% cocoa) twice daily. Don't overindulge in chocolate—it is high in calories.

Other good flavonoid sources include brewed black or green tea…red wine…dark grape juice…strawberries, cranberries and apples… and brussels sprouts and onions.

7. Find opportunities to laugh. People who laugh—and who make others laugh—tend to have better immunity than people who are humor-impaired. Telling a joke is also a good way to improve your memory. It requires the teller—as well as the listener—to pay attention, and we laugh when we expect one outcome but are surprised by a different one. Psychologists call this "conceptual blending."

Benefit: Jokes and riddles challenge the brain, improve memory and can help delay the onset of cognitive decline. In addition, laughter is a well-known stress reducer. People who are calmer and more relaxed have lower levels of heart disease and cancer.

8. Have more sex. Men and women who have sex (that results in orgasm) an average of twice a week have arteries with greater elasticity (which helps prevent hardening of the arteries). Overall, those who have sex twice a week have lower rates of mortality and a RealAge that's about two years younger than their calendar age. Men and women who have sex daily, on average, are biologically eight years younger than those who have it once a week.

9. Rest more often. Everyone enjoys taking a break from life's stresses. Research shows that people who give themselves time to relax (thus minimizing the effects of stress) can live up to eight years longer.

Stress reducers—such as meditating, taking long walks, watching the sunset—can add years to your life. Yoga is particularly good. It lowers blood pressure, heart rate and stress hormones, and increases levels of dopamine and the "feel good" hormone *serotonin*. Aim for about 10 minutes daily of a stress-reduction activity.

10. Get a pet. People who own pets can make themselves an average of one year younger. Studies show that taking care of and bonding with a pet reduces depression and blood pressure.

After a heart attack, people with pets have a one-year survival rate of 94%, compared with 72% for people who don't have pets. Studies show that dog owners, who live about three years longer, tend to be a little healthier than those with other pets—in part because they get regular exercise when they walk their dogs.

How to Undo Bad Health Habits

Davis Liu, MD, a board-certified family physician with the Permanente Medical Group in northern California. He has a degree from the Wharton School, University of Pennsylvania, Philadelphia, and is an expert in evaluating health-care policy. He is author of *Stay Healthy, Live Longer, Spend Wisely.* Stetho.

We all know that we should eat right, exercise and not smoke. But lesser-known—and sometimes seemingly minor—choices also can affect our health and longevity. *Some of the most important—and overlooked—health issues include...*

NOT HAVING A PRIMARY DOCTOR

Millions of Americans don't have a primary-care physician, the gatekeeper to their overall care. Get one. A primary-care physician reviews your records at every visit...recommends screening tests...and coordinates care when you're seeing more than one doctor.

Studies have consistently shown that adults with a primary-care physician have lower health-care costs and are less likely to die than those who use a specialist. A primary-care doctor can help you navigate the confusing health-care system. One health plan found that 41% of all referrals to specialists were made by the patients themselves, and 60% of those self-referrals were to the wrong specialists.

POOR CHECKUP PREPARATION

The average office visit is about 17 minutes, and one study found that doctors usually interrupt patients within the first 23 seconds.

Much of what doctors learn about a patient's health comes from listening to the patient, so you must take responsibility. Before walking into a doctor's office, decide what you want to talk about. Limit your topics to no more than four items—that's about all that can be adequately covered in the time period—and start with the most important one. *For each item, tell the doctor about the Four Ws...*

•**When the problem began,** when it occurs and when it last occurred.

•**What activities, treatments or behaviors** seem to make the problem better or worse... what the problem feels like (sharp pain, comes and goes, etc.)...and what other problems/ symptoms seem to be associated with it.

•**Where in the body** the problem began and whether it moves to different locations in the body.

•**Why you're seeing the doctor.** You probably want to know if the problem is serious or if you need to change your behavior or medications. Maybe the problem is interfering with your lifestyle or family members are worried about you. This is important information.

INATTENTION

A study at the Mayo Clinic found that patients remember less than half of what physicians tell them.

Solution: Take notes during office visits, or ask a friend or family member to come along and take notes for you. To remember the most important details, use the acronym DATE. Make sure you fully understand the *Diagnosis*...whether you need *Additional tests*/procedures...what the *Treatment* plan is...and when you need to return for further *Evaluation*.

UNNECESSARY DRUGS

Doctors are just as influenced by drug-company marketing as anyone. They're likely to prescribe a newer—and higher-priced—drug when an older medication would work just as well. They also tend to prescribe drugs when no medication is required.

Example: In 2000, Merck, the pharmaceutical company, spent millions promoting Vioxx, a new anti-inflammatory drug that was less likely to cause stomach bleeding and ulcers than older drugs. It was good for a select group of patients, but millions of Americans without gastrointestinal risk factors also were given Vioxx—which was found to increase the risk for heart attack, and was eventually withdrawn from the market.

Before accepting any prescription, ask your doctor if the medication is really necessary...if the medication has been proved effective for your condition...and if there are less expensive alternatives that work just as well.

NOT GETTING VACCINATIONS

Few adults get all of the recommended immunizations. For example, 72% of Americans 65 years and older are vaccinated for the flu, even though 36,000 people (90% of whom are 65 and older) in the US die annually from flu-related complications. *In addition to an annual flu shot, ask your doctor about the following vaccines...*

•**Tetanus** protects against a bacterium found in soil and animal feces that is fatal in more than 10% of cases. A booster dose is given once every 10 years (assuming adequate childhood immunization).

•**Meningococcal,** given once by injection, prevents meningitis, a serious brain inflammation. The vaccine is recommended for those living in group settings, such as dormitories and nursing homes, and for international travelers.

•**Pneumococcal,** a one-time vaccine usually given at age 65, protects against a bacterium

that causes pneumonia, blood infections and many other diseases.

For more information about vaccines, go to *www.cdc.gov/vaccines* or call 800-232-4636.

Avoid Global Warming Health Hazards

Georges Benjamin, MD, an internist who serves as executive director of the American Public Health Association, *www.apha.org*, and professorial lecturer at George Washington University School of Public Health and Health Services, both in Washington, DC. He is former secretary of the Maryland Department of Health and Mental Hygiene with an expertise in emergency preparedness.

The World Health Organization estimates that 150,000 deaths annually, mostly in Africa and Asia, are caused by climate change—primarily related to increases in the planet's surface temperature (commonly known as global warming). The death toll is expected to double in the next 20 to 30 years.

Latest development: Health implications are also starting to be felt in the US.

LUNG DISEASES

Higher temperatures cause an increase in ground-level ozone, a gas that irritates the airways and increases the risk for asthma and other lung diseases—and exacerbates symptoms in those who already have any pulmonary disorder.

What to do: If you or a family member has a pulmonary condition or you're healthy but planning to spend a good deal of time outdoors, check the daily air quality forecast. It's available online at Enviro Flash (*www.enviroflash.info*), a program sponsored by the Environmental Protection Agency.

HAY FEVER AND MOLD

The increase in the atmospheric gas carbon dioxide (CO_2) can stimulate pollen-producing plants to release more pollen, which exacerbates symptoms in people with hay fever as well as asthma. Rising temperatures and CO_2 levels also increase the growth of molds, which attach to pollutants in the atmosphere and more readily enter the lungs.

What to do: If you or a family member has allergies or asthma, check daily pollen reports. The National Allergy Bureau (*www.aaaai.org/nab*) provides daily pollen and mold counts from about 69 counting stations throughout the US. Limit your time outdoors on "high pollen" days.

HEATSTROKE

We're seeing more heat waves nationally. In areas that once had just a few hot days a year, now there might be stretches of four, five or six days of temperatures that are 10 degrees or more above average high temperatures for a region. Heat can be deadly, particularly for the elderly.

Older adults don't sweat as much, so they're less able to dissipate heat.

Result: Their body temperature can rise to dangerous levels—and stay there.

People with impaired mobility or those taking diuretics (which promote the excretion of fluids) have a very high risk for heat-related conditions, such as heatstroke (a potentially deadly condition that causes raised body temperature and loss of consciousness). People who are overheated often feel weak, making them less able to get up for a drink of water. The combination of low fluid intake and decreased sweating is extremely dangerous.

What to do: Anyone at risk for overheating (as previously described) should have access to an air conditioner or, at a minimum, a fan. If mobility is an issue, fill a pitcher of cool water and keep it nearby. If you have difficulty getting around, consider buying an alert bracelet so you can summon help in an emergency. Even if you're in good health, drink two to four glasses of cool water per hour in extreme heat or while physically active.

MOSQUITO-BORNE DISEASES

Worldwide, 350 million to 500 million people get malaria (an infectious disease that causes high fever and chills) every year, and more than 1 million die from it.

Malaria and other mosquito-borne diseases haven't been a significant threat in the US since the early 1950s, following a successful eradication program using drainage, removal of mosquito breeding sites and pesticides. But that could change with global warming. Warmer temperatures allow mosquito populations to proliferate. According to the most recent CDC data, 1,278 cases of malaria, including seven deaths, were reported in the US in 2003.

Right now, there's an epidemic of dengue fever (a mosquito-borne infectious disease that causes severe joint pain, headache, fever and rash) in South America. If temperatures continue to rise in the US, an increase in dengue fever (cases have been reported in Hawaii) will almost certainly occur here. A similar increase in West Nile virus (a mosquito-borne illness that causes flu-like symptoms) also could occur in the US.

What to do: To reduce mosquito populations, remove breeding sites. After it rains, look for places where water accumulates—for example, in flowerpots—and dump it out as soon as possible. Cover barbecue grills and other outdoor water "traps." Maintain rain gutters so that there is no standing water. Mosquitoes are attracted to as little as one teaspoon of standing water, and their eggs typically hatch within 48 hours.

Also helpful: Keep fish in backyard ponds. Many species, including mosquitofish and bitterlings, eat mosquito larvae. If you live in a warm, damp area where mosquitoes proliferate, wear long sleeves and pants whenever possible, and/or use a repellent, such as one containing DEET or picaridin. Or stay indoors during the early morning and at dusk, when mosquitoes are most active.

WATERBORNE INFECTIONS

With global warming, extreme storms and floods are likely to occur more often. These pose obvious risks for those in coastal areas—but inland regions aren't necessarily safe.

Drowning and/or water damage are obvious concerns. A bigger issue is water quality. Many metropolitan areas have sewage systems that can't handle severe downpours—water from the sewers can overflow into clean water supplies, causing outbreaks of potentially fatal bacterial infections.

What to do: Following severe downpours or floods, tune in to news channels for up-to-date reports on water quality. If there are concerns about water quality, keep a stockpile of bottled water…boil (for at least one full minute) water used for cooking, cleaning and bathing…and wash your hands often with soap and disinfected water.

How Your Mind Can Heal Your Body

Bernie Siegel, MD, is a pioneer in mind-body medicine and the founder of Exceptional Cancer Patients (*www.ecap-online.org*), a nonprofit organization that provides resources and programs based on mind-body-spirit medicine. He is also the author of many books and audio programs, including *Love, Medicine and Miracles* (Harper), *Help Me to Heal* (Hay House) and the CD *Healing Meditations: Enhance Your Immune System and Find the Key to Good Health* (Hay House).

Words are powerful tools—especially for people who are dealing with any kind of illness. Doctors often tell cancer patients, for example, that their treatment is designed to "kill," "destroy" or "attack" cancer cells. All of this is good and well if these words make a patient feel more powerful. But all too often, this approach has the opposite effect and makes those who are ill feel that they are at war with their own bodies—and their health suffers as a result. Why does this happen?

THE PROCESS

Even if you are "assaulting" an illness—be it cancer, heart disease, diabetes or any other serious ailment—your body is designed to shift into a self-protection mode in the midst of this assault. When threatened, our bodies release stress hormones to fuel a quick escape from whatever is endangering us, and our immune function (one of the keys to overcoming virtually all types of illness) becomes suppressed. Some people feel energized by a good fight, and they approach their health challenge with the precision of a sergeant leading his/her troops. Others, on the other hand, feel completely at odds with such an approach.

This was the case for Dave, a Quaker friend of mine who developed cancer. His oncologist told him, "I am going to kill your cancer." Dave

quietly responded, "I am a Quaker. I don't kill anything," and he walked out the door.

Dave ended up consulting a different doctor for his cancer treatment and worked with me on alternative therapies that included imagery and therapeutic drawing. Because the aggressive words used by his initial doctor felt so wrong to Dave, he began a regular practice of visualization that included images of his white cells "carrying away"—rather than destroying—his cancer cells.

I also introduced Dave to drawing, which gave him an opportunity to conceptualize and reproduce images of the healing he sought for his body. You don't need any artistic skill to benefit from therapeutic drawing. It's designed to help patients grapple with questions and fears about their illnesses and their treatment options. Dave lived 12 years after his doctor had given him one to two years to live.

THE PROOF

If you think all of this sounds unscientific, I don't blame you. When I first became involved in mind-body medicine more than 30 years ago, I was skeptical, too. I was a surgeon, and I believed that the scalpel was all-powerful. Then I began examining the evidence and could no longer deny how our minds—and mental well-being—can affect our response to illness. It's been shown that women who have lung cancer or melanoma tend to live longer than men who have the same type of malignancy. We know that this is not a result of female hormones—studies also show that married men who have prostate or bladder cancer generally live longer than single men who have the same cancers. According to my observations, it's all about having positive connections with others. In fact, I am firmly convinced that women are more likely than men to have strong emotional connections that can literally extend their lives.

THE POWER OF WILL

This point is illustrated by a woman I once knew who was a devoted mother at the time of her cancer diagnosis. "I have nine kids, and I can't die until they are all married and out of the house," she told me. Twenty-three years later, when her last child left the house, her cancer returned and soon proved to be fatal. I have seen similar stories in the hundreds of cancer patients I have known and worked with over the years. What saddened me about the woman with nine children is that she no longer felt that her life had meaning once all of them had left the house.

DO IT YOURSELF

So before you embark on a new medical treatment, ask yourself two important questions…

1. *Does my mind feel at ease with the type of therapy I am considering—or am I simply complying with my doctor's wishes?* If the treatment doesn't feel right, is there a way that I can mentally frame it differently? Even a treatment that has potentially unpleasant side effects, such as chemotherapy, can feel "right" if it is undertaken in the spirit of extending a life that has meaning. The treatment becomes a "labor pain of self-birth"—seen in this way, the side effects are diminished when you're undergoing the therapy to give yourself a new life.

2. *Is there anything I can do to live my life more fully in the midst of my health challenge?* Staying mentally healthy is an invaluable tool. When you heal your life and find peace of mind, your body is much more likely to get the message, too.

■ ■ ■ ■

Don't Get Mad—Get Healthy

Inability to control anger can slow down the natural healing process.

Recent finding: Patients with experimentally induced blisters on their forearms who ranked low on anger control scales measured by psychological tests healed less quickly than patients who had more control over the expression of their anger. Patients who frequently had outbursts of anger or who could not stop themselves from losing their temper were four times more likely to heal slowly.

Possible reason: People who fail to hold in anger secrete more of the stress hormone cortisol, which may slow wound healing.

Janice Kiecolt-Glaser, PhD, and Jean-Philippe Gouin, MPS, psychologists, University of Ohio, Columbus, and leaders of a study of 98 people, published in *Brain, Behaviour, and Immunity.*

Write Your Way to Good Health

Kathleen Adams, director of The Center for Journal Therapy, a consulting and training organization based in Wheat Ridge, Colorado. She is author of six books on journaling, including *Journal to the Self.* Grand Central. She has been keeping a journal since she was 10 years old and still writes in her journal for a half-hour at least four times a week. *www.journaltherapy.com.*

Writing in a journal is not just a way to keep track of daily life—it actually can make you happier, more successful, even healthier.

Example: A study published in *The Journal of the American Medical Association* found that writing about stressful experiences in a journal relieves stress and thus increases the body's immune response, reducing the impact of chronic conditions, such as rheumatoid arthritis and asthma.

You can write in a journal longhand or type it on a computer, whichever feels more comfortable to you. What you write in your journal depends in part on what you hope to achieve.

Trap: People who write only about difficult life circumstances in their journals sometimes find that the process makes them feel worse, not better. If this happens to you, each time you write about a painful problem, make sure you also write about something that gives you pleasure or something for which you are grateful.

Seven effective journaling strategies…

UNSENT LETTERS

Useful if you…are angry or unhappy with someone in your life. Or if you are feeling grief or loneliness following a divorce or the death of someone close to you.

What to do: Write brutally honest letters expressing exactly how you feel—but do not send these letters. Leave them in your journal or tear them up. Venting your emotions on paper helps you feel better and allows you to explore issues calmly and productively.

Example: Margaret was furious with her husband because he was working late and they had to cancel out on a dinner with friends—again. She wrote him a letter telling him how she felt. Upon completion, she read it over once and ripped it into small pieces. Venting her rage on paper allowed her to sit calmly in the living room reading a book until he came home. Then Margaret handed him the pieces of her letter and asked for a problem-solving talk.

THE FIVE-MINUTE SPRINT

Useful if you…feel stressed or overwhelmed.

What to do: Set a timer, and sit down to write in your journal for five minutes—even the busiest people can spare this much time each day. Write about what is at the forefront of your mind now…what tasks you most need to get done…and how you can prioritize your responsibilities. Writing these things makes most people feel more in control and less overwhelmed by most situations.

Example: After a client meeting that didn't go well, an executive grabbed a legal pad and wrote fast about what to do next. At the end of five minutes, he had brainstormed three creative options to get the project back on track.

LISTING

Useful if you…suffer from depression or low self-esteem or are feeling overwhelmed.

What to do: If you are feeling depressed, take a few minutes each day to list three to five things for which you are grateful—or three to five pleasant experiences or encounters that you had since your last journal entry.

If you feel overwhelmed, list the most pleasant sights or moments you experience each day. This will help calm you as you take more notice of the wonderful aspects of the world around you.

If you suffer from low self-esteem, list a few things—even small things—that you accomplished or felt proud of today.

Example: After several weeks of listing on-the-job achievements and successes each day, a financial analyst felt confident enough to ask for a larger bonus.

EMOTIONAL RELEASE

Useful if you…feel that you have not recovered from an emotionally difficult or stressful event in your past and/or if you suffer from a chronic health problem aggravated by stress, such as rheumatoid arthritis or asthma.

What to do: Use a four-day strategy, writing for 15 to 20 minutes a day (if you just can't find that much time, 10 minutes is acceptable). This process was designed by James W. Pennebaker, PhD, of the University of Texas at Austin, to help people leave behind the heavy burdens of past stresses that they might otherwise lug around for the rest of their lives. Pennebaker's process not only reduces stress, it also frees the immune system from the rigors of dealing with this stress, leaving your body better able to cope with health problems.

Day One: Write about the most emotionally difficult or stressful event of your life. Write what happened and how it made you feel when it occurred.

Day Two: Write more about this story—what else happened that you did not include in the first journal entry? What other details can you remember? What other emotions did you experience along the way?

Day Three: Write about how this difficult event shaped you and made you the person you are today. Consider what it means to live with the feelings that you have about this episode.

Day Four: Write about where you can go from here. What is next for you? Does this painful event lead you anywhere? Do you want to go down this path…or would you prefer to simply let the incident go?

Example: A fired executive wrote about losing his job. In the process, he realized how much he had pulled away from his wife. He then suggested to her that they go on weekly "date nights" to set the marriage back on track.

DIALOGUE

Useful if you…are interested in improving your relationships…are painfully shy…and/or suffer from chronic pain, such as back pain.

What to do: Journal therapy pioneer Ira Progoff, PhD, now deceased, advised patients to write down both sides of imagined dialogues in their journals. Write "Me," then what you would like to say to someone. Then write the other party's name, followed by what you believe would be his/her response. Make an honest effort to consider the situation from this other party's perspective, and write what he actually might say. Continue this written dialogue until you have "discussed" the matter fully. The result will look like a movie script.

This process will feel contrived at first, but stay with it. It can help build your confidence for actual conversations, and it can help you better understand other people's viewpoints, which can increase your empathy and negotiation skills. This technique can be particularly effective when used after the unsent letter technique, previously discussed.

To help with chronic pain, including back pain, use this technique to tap into your innate understanding of your own body.

Example: If you suffer from chronic pain, write a dialogue between you and your back.

"Me: My back hurts again. Is there anything I can do to feel better?"

"Back: You don't get enough exercise. Maybe building up your strength would help."

WEIGHT CONTROL

Useful if you are trying to lose weight.

What to do: Formal diet plans often recommend recording every calorie consumed to increase awareness of what one is eating. Perhaps even more valuable, a diet journal can improve your awareness of how your emotions influence your eating habits. Write about what you are feeling when you overeat. Are you actually hungry...or are you snacking to ease boredom, anxieties or depression? List other strategies in your journal that could make you feel better.

Examples: Pet my dog...take a walk...call a friend...read a novel...go to the gym...take a bath.

Next time you feel bad and want a food treat, refer to this journal list and choose an alternative from your feel-good list instead. Afterward, write in the journal about how great this alternative made you feel.

Example: "I felt bad about work, so I treated myself to an evening reading a mystery novel. I enjoyed it so much, I'm going to pick up another mystery tomorrow."

CAPTURED MOMENTS

Useful for stress, anxiety or depression.

What to do: Pick a single moment of beauty or pleasure each day, freeze it in your mind, then write a few paragraphs about it later.

Example: Write about the beauty of a tree you saw or the joyousness of a child's laugh.

•**Write from your senses.** What did the tree look like? How did it smell and feel? What sound did the leaves make in the breeze? Use big, flowery, expressive words that you would not use in real life. This technique forces us to take heed of moments of beauty and pleasure that we might otherwise ignore and allows us to luxuriate in these moments later.

■ ■ ■ ■

Helping Makes You Healthy

Volunteering improves your health. Volunteering creates a sense of belonging and can relieve depression and chronic pain and reduce risk for heart attack and stroke.

To find an opportunity: Check at your house of worship, or with *VolunteerMatch.org* (415-241-6868, *www.volunteermatch.org*), United Way of America (703-836-7112, *www.liveunited. org/volunteer*) and the American Red Cross (800-733-2767, *www.redcross.org/services*).

Other ways to volunteer: Shop or run errands for an elderly neighbor...offer a ride... cook a meal for a friend in need.

Sarah M. Speck, MD, medical director, Center for Cardiovascular Wellness, Swedish Medical Center, Seattle.

■ ■ ■ ■

Fitness Beats Thinness

An important study compared the effects of fitness and obesity on longevity by tracking 2,600 people over age 60 for 12 years.

Findings: Overweight or obese people judged physically fit by performance on a treadmill had a lower death rate than those who had normal body weight but were not fit.

Importance: It's best to be fit and not overweight, but if you are obese, moderate exercise can improve your health. Increasing fitness from the level of the "bottom fifth" to the next-lowest fifth reduced mortality risk by 50%.

Steven Blair, PED, professor, department of exercise science, University of South Carolina, Columbia.

Massage Away Pain And Boost Your Immunity

Ben E. Benjamin, PhD, who maintains a private massage practice in Cambridge, Massachusetts. His books include *The Ethics of Touch* (Lippincott Williams & Wilkins) and *Exercise Without Injury*. MTI.

A good massage can be much more than just a relaxing treat. Research shows that a number of massage therapies can be used to alleviate various types of pain (such as headache, backache and knee pain), relieve chronic tension and boost immunity.

What you should know about the four most popular types of massage…

SWEDISH

Swedish massage uses a variety of movements, such as long, sweeping strokes as well as kneading strokes over muscles, to help move blood through the body. This increases circulation and gently reduces muscle tension.

Best used for: Mild insomnia, headache, anxiety, stress and muscle tension.

SHIATSU

Shiatsu—Japanese for "finger pressure"—uses acupressure points along pathways in the body (meridians) to move a form of energy known as "qi" (pronounced "chee"). Shiatsu aims to prevent disease with consistent and fluid movements that open channels of energy. Some massage therapists use their elbows, knees and feet in addition to thumb pressure, which may be very light or strong and deep.

Best used for: Headache, insomnia, low back pain, postoperative pain and low energy.

ORTHOPEDIC

Musculoskeletal pain occurs when a joint, muscle, tendon (tough bundle of fibers that attaches muscle to bone) or ligament (connective tissue that joins two bones at a joint) becomes swollen, inflamed and/or torn.

Even seemingly harmless activities, such as sleeping in an awkward position, bending in an unusual way or sitting at a computer for long periods, can cause the damage.

With orthopedic massage, a therapist uses his/her hands or fingers to end this pain-causing cycle by focusing on adhesive scar tissue that forms in response to the initial damage. Orthopedic massage can be mildly uncomfortable but should not be painful.

Best used for: Low back pain, knee pain, and strained muscles, tendons and ligaments.

MYOFASCIAL RELEASE

The *fascia* is a connective tissue that surrounds muscles, joints, nerves, blood vessels and internal organs. Ordinarily relaxed and pliable, fasciae develop adhesive scar tissue after an injury and become a source of tension throughout the body.

Myofascial release (also known as deep-tissue work) involves a combination of deep and gentle pressure designed to affect not only the deeper structures of the musculoskeletal system, such as the spine and joints, but also the skin and muscles. To apply proper pressure, the therapist may use his fingertips, knuckles or elbows.

Best used for: Fatigue, stiffness, recovery from accidents and/or chronic poor posture.

■ **More from Ben E. Benjamin, PhD…**

Massage Essentials

Body massage is available at many health clubs and spas as well as medical centers and hospitals. Most massages last 30 to 60 minutes with prices ranging from about $50 to $150 per hour. Health insurance may cover all or part of the cost of massage therapy with a doctor's referral.

•**Massage is generally considered safe for most people.** However, massage should be avoided by people who have deep vein thrombosis, bleeding disorders, fever, varicose veins, osteoporosis, a recent fracture, open wounds or who have had recent surgery (unless approved by a physician).

Until recently, many medical experts warned cancer patients to avoid massage for fear of stimulating growth or spread of a malignancy. Now, this belief has been debunked and massage is generally considered safe for cancer patients, who often experience energy-boosting and/or stress-relieving benefits. If you have cancer, however, you should still check with your doctor before you receive massage. In some cases, it can damage tissue that is fragile due to radiation treatments and/or chemotherapy.

•**When selecting a massage therapist,** choose someone who is licensed by his/her municipality or state and certified by a national certifying agency. These qualifications will ensure that the practitioner has at least 500 hours of training. You can also seek a referral from the American Massage Therapy Association, 877-905-2700, *www.amtamassage.org*...or the Associated Bodywork & Massage Professionals, 800-458-2267, *www.abmp.com.*

The Healing Powers Of Touch

Tiffany M. Field, PhD, director of the Touch Research Institute (*www.miami.edu/touch-research*) at the University of Miami School of Medicine. She has participated in more than 100 studies on the effects of massage therapy on many medical and psychological conditions. She is the author of *Touch.* MIT Press.

Nearly 60% of doctors in the US recommend massage for some patients—almost twice as many as recommended it five years ago.

Why the dramatic increase?

For years, therapeutic massage was recommended primarily for musculoskeletal conditions, such as arthritis, low back pain and muscle tension. Now, credible research shows that massage has benefits that most doctors never expected. *What we now know...*

WHY MASSAGE HELPS

Scientists now have evidence that massage affects virtually every major body function—from immunity to lung and brain function—and

confers health benefits through a variety of mechanisms.

Even though massage therapists are usually trained in one or more massage techniques, such as Swedish, Shiatsu and deep tissue massage, there is no evidence that one technique is better than another for most conditions.

Studies indicate that the application of moderate pressure—firm enough to make an indentation in the skin—is the key to massage's health benefits. By stimulating *pressure receptors* under the skin, massage activates different branches of the *vagus nerve,* which regulates blood pressure, heart rate and many other physiological functions.

Massage also...

•**Reduces levels of stress hormones, such as cortisol.** This is important for pain relief, easing depression and increasing energy levels. Reductions in cortisol also enhance immune function, including the ability of natural killer cells to target viruses and cancer cells.

•**Enhances deeper sleep stages** (known as *delta sleep),* which helps reduce levels of a brain chemical, known as *substance P*, that is related to the sensation of pain.

Massage is now used to treat...

HIGH BLOOD PRESSURE

Patients with elevated blood pressure often have high levels of stress hormones. Massage not only lowers levels of these hormones but also stimulates the branch of the vagus nerve that leads to the heart. Stimulating the nerve decreases heart rate and lowers blood pressure.

In one study, adults with hypertension were given 10 half-hour massages over five weeks. They showed a statistically significant decrease in diastolic (bottom number) blood pressure and reported less depression and anxiety—common problems in patients being treated for hypertension.

CARPAL TUNNEL SYNDROME

The *median nerve* in the wrist passes through a narrow opening (the carpal tunnel) on the palm side of the wrist. Swelling or inflammation of the nerve, usually caused by repetitive movements such as typing or using a screwdriver, can result in chronic tingling, numbness and/or pain in the thumb as well as the index and middle fingers. Researchers at Baylor University Medical Center have reported that even gripping the steering wheel of a car for long hours may lead to carpal tunnel syndrome.

A daily self-massage can reduce pain and promote an increase in *nerve-conduction velocity*, a measure of nerve health.

15-minute self-massage: Using moderate pressure, stroke from the wrist to the elbow and back down on both sides of the forearm. Next, apply a wringing motion to the same area. Using the thumb and index finger, stroke the entire forearm and the hand in a circular or back-and-forth motion. Finish by rolling the skin with the thumb and index finger, moving across the hand and up both sides of the forearm.

BURNS

Serious burns are among the most painful wounds. The standard treatments—including brushing away debris and cleaning the area—can be excruciatingly painful. Massage done before the skin is brushed appears to elevate the pain threshold of burn patients—perhaps by increasing levels of the brain chemical *serotonin*.

Example: If one hand is burned, another person can vigorously rub the patient's *other* hand. This activation of skin receptors, in effect, blocks the feeling of pain related to the burn.

PAIN

Studies show that massage curbs back pain, migraine and cancer pain. It may do this by reducing the pain-promoting chemical substance P as well as the stress hormone cortisol.

Key findings: In three separate studies, patients with back pain were treated either with massage or a sham treatment (a massage with insufficient pressure to provide any benefit). Patients in both groups were treated twice weekly for 20 minutes. Those in the massage group consistently had less pain and better range of motion than patients in the sham group.

Massage also seems to help post-surgical pain. In a pilot study, researchers at Cedars-Sinai Medical Center in Los Angeles found that patients who received massages after heart-bypass surgery had less pain and fewer muscle spasms than those who didn't get massages.

To find a massage therapist, consult the American Massage Therapy Association, 877-905-2700, *www.amtamassage.org.*

■ **More from Tiffany M. Field, PhD...**

At-Home Massage

If you are unable to receive a professional massage, you can get some of the same benefits at home. It's easy for your spouse, another family member or a friend to give you a massage by following some basic guidelines...*

•**The part of the body that gets massaged isn't that important.** For most conditions, rubbing *any* part of the body—such as the back, arms or shoulders—is effective. When moderate pressure to the skin is applied, the body undergoes physiological changes that help curb pain and other common ailments.

•**Don't worry about massage strokes.** The health benefits of massage typically occur regardless of the type of hand movements used, such as up and down or in circles. Using a variety of strokes can make a massage more interesting but doesn't necessarily affect the results.

•**Use massage oil** (available at health-food stores and pharmacies). Most people find this more comfortable than a "dry" massage.

*If you have a chronic medical condition, check with your doctor first.

Feel-Good Exercises You Can Do in Bed

Genie Tartell, DC, RN, a New York City–based chiropractor and registered nurse who focuses on physical rehabilitation. She is coauthor of *Get Fit in Bed*. New Harbinger.

Think about the last time you really stretched your body. Didn't you feel great afterward?

Unfortunately, most people—including many who are physically active—don't do enough to improve their muscle tone, flexibility and strength. To help people incorporate a simple workout regimen into their daily routines, I have devised a program that can be performed in a comfortable setting you are bound to visit each day—your bed.

These bed exercises not only increase your strength, flexibility and endurance, but also stimulate production of the mood-enhancing brain chemical *serotonin*, leaving you feeling calm and relaxed. As a result, most people find that they sleep better when they do these exercises at night, and feel invigorated if they do the routine in the morning.

The following exercises are designed for anyone but are particularly helpful for people who are confined to bed (while recovering from an illness or injury) and for those unable to find time during the day to exercise. They can be completed in just 10 minutes a day.

Important: When performing each movement, breathe in slowly for a count of four... hold for a count of one...then exhale through pursed lips for a count of four.

ALTERNATE LEG LENGTHENER

Purpose: Tones and stretches the spine and pelvis, which bears much of the upper body's weight.

What to do: While lying on your back with your body centered on the bed and your hips and legs flat on the bed, stretch your right leg forward by pushing with the heel of your right foot. Return your leg to the starting position. Do the same stretch with your left leg. Repeat five times with each leg.

HIP SIDE TO SIDE

Purpose: Tones and stretches the hips and low back.

What to do: While lying on your back with your hips flat on the bed, rock your hips gently —as far as comfortable—to the right and then to the left. Keep your upper body stable. Repeat five times in each direction.

ARMS-SHOULDER SEESAW

Purpose: Tones and stretches the shoulders and upper back.

What to do: While lying on your back, place your arms at your sides. Slide your right arm and shoulder toward your right foot. Next, raise your right shoulder toward your head, while at the same time sliding your left arm and shoulder toward your left foot. Then raise your left shoulder toward your head, while lowering your right arm and shoulder toward your right foot. Repeat five times on each side, moving your shoulders up and down like a seesaw.

ARMS TOWARD THE HEADBOARD

Purpose: Stretches the shoulders and rib cage, allowing for deeper, more relaxed breathing.

What to do: While lying on your back, extend your arms behind your head. Stretch your right arm toward the headboard of your bed or the wall behind you. Return your right arm to your side and then extend your left arm behind you. Repeat five times on each side.

ELBOW-KNEE PISTON

Purpose: Strengthens your abdominal muscles while increasing your heart rate (improves heart muscle strength and endurance).

What to do: While lying on your back, raise your knees and, using your stomach muscles, lift your upper body toward them. Bend your arms so that your elbows are pointing at your knees. Bring your left elbow toward your right knee, then return to the starting position. Then bring your right elbow toward your left knee, maintaining a continuous pumping motion. Repeat six times.

COBRA

Purpose: Builds upper body strength (important for daily activities such as bathing and cooking).

What to do: Lie on your stomach with your elbows bent and palms flat on the bed next to your shoulders. Fully straighten your arms to lift your upper body so that it curves into a cobra-like position. Hold for a few seconds, then return to the starting position. Repeat three times.

MODIFIED BOW

Purpose: Tones and strengthens the back and improves muscular coordination.

What to do: Lie on your stomach with your arms at your sides. Raise your legs and upper body simultaneously (only to a level that is comfortable), then reach back with your arms as if you are trying to touch your raised feet. Hold for a few seconds, then return to the starting position. Repeat three times.

SWIMMING IN BED

Purpose: Strengthens the arms and legs, while increasing heart rate and stimulating blood flow throughout the body.

What to do: While lying on your stomach, move one arm forward, then move it back while moving the other arm forward, simultaneously kicking your legs. Repeat 20 times, counting each arm movement as one repetition.

BRIDGE

Purpose: Cools down the body and directs blood flow away from the legs to the heart, reducing risk for blood clots in the legs.

What to do: Lie on your back with your knees bent, feet flat on the bed and your arms at your sides. Tighten your buttock muscles as you lift your pelvis toward the ceiling—until your pelvis is in line with your thighs. Then gently lower your body back to the bed. Repeat five times.

Important: If you think any of these exercises may be too strenuous for you, check with your doctor before trying them.

Illustrations by Shawn Banner.

■ ■ ■ ■

Don't Laugh—It Works!

Laughter yoga combines traditional yoga stretches and poses with exercise designed to make people laugh. In terms of cardiovascular benefits, one minute of laughter (about 100 giggles) is the equivalent of six to 10 minutes on a rowing machine. Laughter has aerobic benefits and can help lower blood pressure, lift mood and boost immunity. To find a class near you, call 212-956-5920 or go to *www.laughteryoga.org.*

Alex Eingorn, DC, laughter-yoga instructor and director, Better Laugh Laughter Club, New York, *www.better laugh.us.*

Harness Your Body's Healing Power

Roger Jahnke, OMD, a board-certified doctor of oriental medicine and author of *The Healer Within* (Harper SanFrancisco). He is director and chief instructor of the Institute of Integral Qigong and Tai Chi in Santa Barbara, California. *www.instituteofintegralqigongandtaichi.org.*

The Chinese wellness system qigong (chee-GONG) combines four ancient practices, all meant to harness the body's self-healing powers. The basics are easy to learn and easy on the body, and they can be done at home. Here are samples of qigong movements and methods. Practice each daily to generate vitality and promote healing.

BODY MOVEMENT

Slow, gentle exercises build awareness of posture…increase strength, endurance and flexibility…and unlike vigorous exercises, do not cause injury or consume internal resources (such as energy) to fuel muscles.

•**Gentle bending of the spine.** Stand with feet shoulder-width apart, knees slightly bent. Inhaling, raise arms above head, elbows slightly bent and palms facing skyward…tip head back and tilt the pelvis, arching back slightly. On the exhalation, bend elbows and bring arms down in front of you, hands fisted and pressed together…tuck chin to chest, tilt the pelvis under and round your back. Repeat five to 10 times.

BREATH PRACTICE

Deep breathing sends more oxygen-rich blood toward tissues…and "pumps" lymph fluid through the lymphatic system, a major part of the immune system.

•**Gathering breath.** Sit with hands in your lap. Inhaling through the nose, move hands outward and upward, scooping up healing energy, until hands are just above face level, palms toward you and elbows slightly bent. Exhaling slowly, bring hands toward you, then downward past the chest and navel. Repeat five to 10 times.

MASSAGE

Reflexes refer to areas of the body that are separated physically, yet linked via acupuncture and energy channels. Self-massage of points on the hands, ears and feet has a healing effect on the organs, joints or tissues to which these reflexes connect.

•**Healing hand massage.** Grasp your left hand with your right hand, thumb against the palm and fingers on the back of the hand. Starting gently and gradually increasing the pressure, knead your left hand, including fingers and wrist. Spend extra time on any sore points—these areas are linked to body functions and organs that are not operating optimally. Continue for three to five minutes, then switch hands.

MEDITATION

Stress overstimulates the nervous system and exhausts the adrenal glands (which secrete stress hormones). Meditation counteracts stress, enhancing healing brain chemicals and hormones.

•**Qigong meditation.** Stand, sit or lie comfortably. Inhale fully, imagining you are drawing in *qi* (vitality) from the universe through hundreds of energy gates (acupuncture points) all over your body's surface. Exhale slowly, visualizing healing resources circulating inside you. Continue for five to 15 minutes, mentally directing the healing flow to wherever your body needs it most.

Illustrations by Shawn Banner.

The Perfect Exercise

Gabe Mirkin, MD, a Kensington, Maryland–based physician who specializes in sports medicine. He is the author of eight books, including *The Healthy Heart Miracle*. HarperCollins. Dr. Mirkin and his wife, Diana, ride their tandem bike more than 200 miles weekly.

Physical activity has unequivocally been shown to be one of the best ways to ensure a long, healthy life. But which type of activity is best?

Walking is ideal, according to many medical experts. But for many people, cycling may be even better. Like vigorous walking, cycling reduces risk for heart attack and stroke. However, cycling is generally much easier on a person's joints—so it's an excellent choice if you are overweight or have back problems or arthritis.

If you're age 50 or older: Get an exercise stress test (to measure the heart's electrical impulses during physical activity) before beginning any new exercise program.

HOW TO START

I tell my patients to start with a stationary "spinning-based" bike (now available at many health clubs), in which the resistance comes from a weighted flywheel. This type of bike lets you control the pedaling resistance manually (by changing tension on the flywheel), which is more precise and gradual than the control you have when using a computerized bike. This is important because it allows you to better control the degree to which your leg muscles are taxed.

If you want to buy a spinning-based bike for home use, dozens of good models are available, starting at about $700. The best ones have at least a 40-pound flywheel. Stationary flywheel bikes are available in recumbent (with back support) as well as upright models.

Stationary bike workouts...

•**Beginner.** Start by pedaling for 10 minutes at a very low resistance (one that requires you to exert little pressure on the pedals). Next, increase your workouts by five minutes per week until you can ride comfortably for 30 minutes uninterrupted.

•**Intermediate.** Once you can ride for 30 minutes at more than 60 revolutions per minute, consider adding fitness-building workouts to your program. Start with five to 10 minutes of easy cycling, then gradually increase the resistance until you feel a burning sensation in your leg muscles (due to fatigue).

When you feel the "burn," immediately turn the resistance down so that you're pedaling very easily. Continue pedaling at a low resistance until your muscles are recovered, then repeat the process. Continue for 10 to 20 minutes, then finish by pedaling at a low resistance for a five-minute cooldown. Each fitness-building workout should be followed by as many easy "recovery" workouts (entire sessions that consist of low-resistance cycling) as needed on subsequent days.

How this process works: By bringing your leg muscles to the brink of fatigue (with the "burn"), you're actually damaging your muscle fibers slightly. Your muscle fibers then repair themselves and become stronger during recovery days. Many people perform one hard workout per week followed by six easy recovery workouts.

•**Advanced.** As you become more fit, you can gradually increase the length of your workouts to 60 minutes or more. Be sure that your muscles are fully recovered before each fitness-building workout.

A CYCLING PROGRAM

After you reach an intermediate level of stationary cycling, you'll be ready to also bike outdoors. Outdoor cycling should follow the steps used for stationary cycling—whenever your pedaling rate becomes slower than one full revolution per second, switch immediately to a lower gear.

Helpful: For people who don't want to share the road with cars, many communities now have cycling trails. Never ride a bike without wearing a bike helmet.

Ideally, your bike should have at least 14 gears.

Reason: As with stationary cycling, you want to be able to adjust your resistance level. More gears allow you to do this more precisely.

Hundreds of good bike models are available, starting at prices as low as $200. To avoid injuring your knees, make sure that your seat is adjusted so that the knee is slightly bent when the corresponding pedal is at its lowest point. Men should install a "noseless" seat that won't press against the pelvic nerves (this can lead to discomfort or, in some cases, impotence). Noseless seats are available at bike shops and online.

Smart idea: If you plan to ride primarily with your spouse or another partner, consider purchasing a tandem bike that both riders pedal at the same rate. My wife, who is age 66, and I, at 73, have been riding a tandem for years and love it. You can get a good tandem bike for less than $2,000.

To find a bicycling class near you, consult the League of American Bicyclists (202-822-1333, *www.bikeleague.org*).

The Easiest Step to Better Health

Rebecca Shannonhouse, editor of the *Bottom Line/Health* newsletters, Boardroom Inc., 281 Tresser Blvd., Stamford, Connecticut 06901.

If you are looking for one simple action you can take to improve your health in the coming year, consider getting (and using) a pedometer throughout your day.

Most people have heard of these small devices, which measure the number of steps and/or the distance the wearer walks each day.

But a new study published in the *Journal of the American Medical Association* shows that a pedometer can have a greater impact on one's activity level and overall health than researchers had ever imagined.

After reviewing 26 studies, including a total of 2,767 men and women, researchers found that participants who used pedometers walked approximately 2,200 *additional steps*—a little over a mile—per day. This equates to an impressive 27% increase in activity level.

In addition, the study shows that the systolic (top number) blood pressure of pedometer users dropped by 3.8 mm Hg. (Each 2 mm Hg reduction translates into a 10% reduction in death from stroke.)

Having a specific daily step goal and recording results in a diary each day also increased activity levels. Most health experts recommend that healthy adults walk 10,000 steps (about five miles) per day.

Pedometers are widely available at sporting-goods and discount stores for as little as $13 to $20. You also can purchase pedometers at Step Into Health, 800-929-9775, *www.stepintohealth. com*...or Sports Unlimited Inc., 800-693-6368, *www.sportsunlimitedinc.com*.

I've owned a pedometer for several years—and have given many away as gifts. Clipping on one of these little devices may well give a big boost to your health.

Five Simple Ways to Fight Weight Gain

JoAnn E. Manson, MD, DrPH, is a professor of medicine and women's health at Harvard Medical School and chief of the division of preventive medicine at Brigham and Women's Hospital, both in Boston. A lead investigator for two important studies on women's health, Dr. Manson is coauthor of *Hot Flashes, Hormones & Your Health*. McGraw-Hill.

The statistics are scary—62% of American women are now overweight, and more than half of these women are obese. Everyone knows that too much food and too little exercise lead to weight gain—but to reach and maintain a healthy weight, it's important to recognize lesser-known culprits...

•**Stress.** When we're stressed, our adrenal glands release the hormone *cortisol,* which boosts activity of the enzyme *lipoprotein lipase*, causing the body to store extra fat.

Smart: Make exercise a priority—it triggers the release of soothing brain chemicals called *endorphins*. Talk to your doctor if you suffer from depression or an anxiety disorder, as these also are linked to elevated levels of cortisol.

•**Sleep deprivation.** The average American sleeps fewer than seven hours per weeknight—and many of us log six hours or less. In surveys, overweight people generally report sleeping less than slim people do.

Theories: Sleep deprivation may slow carbohydrate metabolism...increase cortisol levels ...reduce the hunger-suppressing hormone *leptin*...and increase the appetite-stimulating hormone *ghrelin*.

Solutions: Avoid late-evening meals and caffeine...turn off telephones (including cell phones) at night...get the computer and TV out of the bedroom...and maintain a consistent bedtime that allows for eight hours of rest.

•**Stillness.** Obese people tend to sit still (literally), spending, on average, 2.5 fewer hours per day pacing and fidgeting than lean people do.

Surprising: These seemingly insignificant movements burn about 350 calories per day—preventing a gain of about 36 pounds per year. A tendency towards stillness may be genetically determined, but long hours at a desk or in a car exacerbate the situation.

Good habit: Don't sit when you can stand or ride when you can walk.

•**Fat friends and family.** Our chances of becoming obese may rise by 57% if a close friend becomes obese...40% if a sibling becomes obese...and 37% if a spouse becomes obese.

One reason: When judgments are based on comparison with others, a loved one's obesity may shift our perception of an acceptable weight.

Best: Ask loved ones to start a weight-loss program with you, and avoid picking up their bad habits.

•**Diet composition.** High-glycemic foods rapidly increase blood sugar levels, triggering a surge of the hormone *insulin*. These foods may be more likely to cause weight gain, independent of their calorie content, because insulin increases fat storage and prevents fat breakdown in the body.

Slenderizing: Limit high-glycemic foods, such as white bread, pasta, sugary cereals, baked goods and soda. Eat more low-glycemic foods—fruits, vegetables, legumes and whole grains—which stabilize blood sugar.

Sinus Infections: Nothing to Sneeze At

Ralph B. Metson, MD, clinical professor of otology and laryngology (diseases of the ear and throat) at Harvard Medical School and director of the rhinology fellowship program (concerning the nose) at the Massachusetts Eye and Ear Infirmary, both in Boston. He is coauthor of *The Harvard Medical School Guide to Healing Your Sinuses*. McGraw-Hill.

It's bad enough when a cold or an allergic reaction to dust or pet dander leads to the pain and congestion of *acute sinusitis* (infection of the sinuses that lasts no more than four weeks). But for an estimated 30 to 40 million

Americans, sinusitis is a chronic problem that takes a surprisingly serious toll on energy levels and quality of life.

The sad thing is that much of this suffering is *not* necessary. With a proper understanding of what causes sinusitis and appropriate preventive steps, you can get the upper hand against this all-too-common medical problem.

WHAT IS SINUSITIS?

Sinusitis is an infection of the mucous membrane-lined air spaces (sinuses) in the bones of the forehead and on each side of the nose.

Common symptoms include nasal congestion, mucous discharge from the nose, facial pain and headache. Lesser-known symptoms include bad breath, aching in the upper jaw and teeth, sore throat, ear pain and fatigue.

THE INSIDE STORY

The nasal cavity and sinuses are lined with membranes containing cells that produce mucus (up to eight ounces daily). Airborne irritants, such as dust, pollen and pet dander, are trapped by the mucus in the sinuses and moved into the nasal cavity through tiny openings called *ostia,* so that the mucus (and irritants) can then be swallowed or expelled by blowing the nose.

Trouble starts when the area inside the nose where the ostia drain becomes blocked as a result of a cold, allergy or some other condition. Mucus then becomes trapped in the sinuses—creating a perfect environment for bacteria to flourish and infection to develop.

Pressure in the sinuses builds, making it hard to breathe, and infected mucus turns a thick, cloudy green or yellow. If a culture determines that the infection is bacterial, an antibiotic will probably be prescribed to quell the infection. Viral infections usually improve on their own. For people with chronic sinusitis, such episodes recur four or more times a year, often requiring prolonged, repeated antibiotic therapy—or even surgery to open the blocked sinus drainage passages.

OVERLOOKED TRIGGERS

Next to the common cold, allergies are the second most common cause of sinusitis, playing a role in about one-third of chronic sinusitis cases. With this type of sinusitis, the inflammatory response triggered by the allergen blocks the flow of mucus from the sinuses and sets the stage for infection. Skin testing by an allergist can often identify the allergens involved, and dust control, allergy shots and antihistamine drugs, such as *loratadine* (Claritin) and *fexofenadine* (Allegra), can help alleviate the sinus problem.

However, few doctors recognize that allergic-type reactions to *food* also can be involved. Most often, this is caused by certain alcoholic beverages, such as red wine, whiskey and certain beers. The alcohol itself is not to blame, but rather the constituents of alcoholic drinks called *congeners*—these substances provide taste and aroma to alcohol, but they can inflame sensitive mucous membranes when they are ingested during drinking.

My advice: If your sinus symptoms worsen the day after consuming certain alcoholic beverages, such as merlot or pinot noir, try switching to white wine, clear spirits (vodka or gin, for example) or lighter beers.

For some sinusitis sufferers, symptoms are aggravated by foods containing milk. To find out if you are milk sensitive, eliminate all dairy products from your diet for three weeks. If milk and other dairy products are a trigger, your symptoms will noticeably improve.

KEEP YOUR NOSE CLEAN

Simply keeping the nose clear of mucus that contains bacteria and allergen particles is one of the most effective ways to prevent and relieve sinusitis. Nasal irrigation—a safe, simple practice you can do at home—is more efficient than nose blowing for clearing mucus.

Caution: Vigorous nose blowing can force bacteria-filled mucus back into the sinuses.

Nasal irrigation requires only a rubber bulb syringe (the kind used to clean an infant's nose and widely available at mass market retailers for about $5).

What to do: Mix about a teaspoon of salt with eight ounces of warm water. Fill the syringe with the salt water, gently squeeze it into one nostril, and let it run out that nostril. Repeat the process, first in one nostril and then the other until all the water is gone, twice daily. If the mixture stings or burns, try more or less salt, to match the salinity of the mucus. Adding one-half teaspoon of baking soda can make the solution more soothing—it helps adjust the irrigant to the pH (level of acidity and alkalinity) of mucus.

Other options: A plastic squeeze bottle specially designed to fit the nose (available at drugstores for about $5 to $10) or a neti pot (a cup-sized container with a spout at one end, a style that has been used in India for centuries to clear nasal passages). Squeeze bottles come prefilled with saline (a salt and water solution) or with premeasured packets that you mix with tap water. Neti pots are available at some drugstores and most health-food stores for about $15. The neti pot is gentler than the bulb syringe or squeeze bottle, but may not be forceful enough if mucus is thick.

Important: If you've never done nasal irrigation before, it may seem unsettling the first few times—it will remind you of getting water up your nose when swimming. But most people get used to it quickly and find it worth the brief initial discomfort.

My advice: Irrigate twice daily around the same time you brush your teeth. Be sure to rinse the irrigation tool between uses.

Some people find saline nasal sprays, such as Simply Saline or Xlear nasal wash (available at drugstores for about $5 to $13), to be easier to use than nasal irrigation methods. Nasal sprays can relieve nasal dryness and may loosen mucus, but a recent study at the University of Michigan found them to be significantly less effective than irrigation in reducing sinusitis symptoms.

BREATHE EASIER

Some people with sinus problems also develop crusty deposits (composed of dried mucus) inside the nose, particularly in winter when nasal membranes are dried out by indoor heating. Crusts can further obstruct breathing already reduced by sinusitis congestion.

My advice: To fight multiplying bacteria that can grow on nasal crusts, apply an over-the-counter antibiotic ointment, such as Bacitracin or Neosporin, twice daily on the inside of the nose. Use of a humidifier, especially during the winter, also can help reduce indoor dryness.

For some sinusitis sufferers, obstruction is worsened by a narrowing of the *nasal valve*—

an area of soft tissue in the middle of the nose that tends to collapse when you inhale. Nasal tapes, such as Breathe Right nasal strips, which fit across the top of the nose and lift the sides, can keep the valve from closing, allowing you to breathe more freely. These products are available at most drugstores for about $16.

IMPROVED TREATMENTS

Sinus surgery becomes an option when infections are frequent despite medical treatment, including antibiotics and allergy medications. Surgery aims to correct anatomical obstructions in the nose and sinuses. For example, a narrow sinus opening may be enlarged or an obstruction, such as a polyp (a usually benign growth), may be removed.

Endoscopic surgery, using a thin tube to insert miniaturized instruments into the sinus passages via the nostrils, has improved the outcome of sinus operations.

The latest innovation, *image-guided surgery,* adds to the precision—it is similar to global positioning technology (the guidance systems drivers use) and helps locate the exact site that needs repair. This technology enables a surgeon to monitor the location of instruments during the procedure—and is helpful in difficult cases, such as those involving patients who have extensive disease or who have undergone previous sinus surgery.

■ ■ ■ ■

Faster Allergy Relief On the Horizon

A burst of carbon dioxide into the nose relieves congestion and other nasal symptoms within 10 minutes, and keeps working for 24 hours. The treatment—not yet FDA-approved—may be an effective alternative to steroid sprays.

Creighton University, Omaha, Nebraska, *www.creighton.edu.*

■ ■ ■ ■

Surprise Strengthener

Magnesium makes you stronger, according to Ligia J. Dominguez, MD.

New finding: In a study of 1,138 men and women, participants with the highest blood levels of magnesium were stronger (based on tests for handgrip strength and power in leg muscles) than those with the lowest levels.

Theory: Magnesium is essential to the body's cellular energy production, thereby promoting optimal muscle performance.

Self-defense: To get the recommended intake of magnesium (420 mg daily for men age 31 or older…320 mg daily for women age 31 or older), eat such foods as dark green, leafy vegetables, navy beans and pumpkin seeds.

Ligia J. Dominguez, MD, researcher, geriatric unit, University of Palermo, Italy.

The Music Cure—It Can Ease Pain, Lower Blood Pressure, Relieve Asthma, More

Barbara Reuer, PhD, founder and clinical training director of MusicWorx of California, a music-therapy consulting agency in San Diego. *www.musicworxofcali fornia.com*. She is past president of the American Music Therapy Association and has worked in medical and psychiatric settings for more than 30 years.

Music has been used for healing for thousands of years—and numerous recent studies confirm its healing powers. It can reduce pain and anxiety and improve blood pressure and breathing. It even can help infants in neonatal intensive care units gain weight faster. *Here's how you can use music to improve your mental and physical health…*

PAIN RELIEF

Music therapy can relieve pain and decrease the need for painkilling drugs. It seems to be most effective for short-term pain, such as during dental procedures, after surgery, etc. A study published in *European Journal of Anesthesiology* reported that postsurgical patients who listened to music required less morphine.

It also helps some types of chronic pain. A study published in *Journal of Advanced Nursing* found that listening to music for an hour a day reduced chronic pain by up to 21% and depression by up to 25%.

How it helps: People in pain can't focus on opposing sensations simultaneously. Listening to music helps block the perception of pain signals and reduces anxiety, which can heighten pain.

Recommended: When you're in pain, practice deep breathing while listening to a favorite piece of relaxing music. Ask your doctor to play calming background music during painful procedures. If a music therapist is available during the procedure, he/she might play music while guiding you through a visualization exercise (such as imagining a peaceful scene) or encouraging you to breathe more deeply.

HEART HELP

Music therapy is used in some coronary care units to lower blood pressure and heart rate. Music also lowers levels of stress hormones (such as cortisol) that may increase the risk for a heart attack.

Recommended: At least once a day, listen to music that you find relaxing. Pay attention to the melodies, rhythms and words…think about what the music means to you…and notice the physical signs of relaxation.

STROKE AND PARKINSON'S

A type of therapy called *neurologic music therapy* can help patients with neurological deficits that are caused by stroke, Parkinson's disease, etc.

Example: Parkinson's patients often walk with an uneven gait, which makes it difficult for them to get around and increases the risk for falls. With rhythmic auditory stimulation, therapists play music (or use a metronome) during walking exercises. This helps the brain stimulate skeletal muscles and coordinate movements, creating a more even stride.

The same technique is used with stroke patients, who often lose control of one side of the body. The unaffected brain hemisphere processes the music, "translating" the beat into physical movements. A music therapist, along with a physical therapist, can determine a patient's gait pattern and use music at certain tempos to help the patient improve his gait.

Singing also is helpful. Stroke patients who have lost the ability to speak sometimes can sing. A music therapist can use singing exercises to help patients recover speech skills.

DEMENTIA RELIEF

People with advanced Alzheimer's disease or other forms of dementia often are closed off in a private world. They may be confused and/or hostile. Playing music that was popular in their youth will sometimes make them more "present"…make it easier for them to remember the past…and will even evoke a positive emotional response.

How it helps: The moments of lucidity provoked by music can reduce anxiety and make patients feel better. The sessions can be conducted when family members are present. This gives them a chance to reconnect, at least briefly, with loved ones.

BETTER BREATHING

In addition to listening to music, active music-making can be an effective component of music therapy. People who sing or play a wind instrument gain additional strength/flexibility in muscles in the chest wall. Improved muscle flexibility, called *elastance*, allows them to take deeper breaths with less fatigue.

Example: It's common for patients with asthma or chronic obstructive pulmonary disease (COPD) to take unusually shallow breaths. Singing or playing a wind instrument trains them to breathe more deeply…helps clear mucus from the lungs…and helps establish normal breathing rhythms. One study found that children who completed singing exercises had increased peak respiratory flow rates, a measure of lung health.

Recommended: Learn to play the harmonica. It's often used to help pulmonary patients exercise the chest-wall muscles and develop good breath control. Playing the harmonica requires a slow breath in and out, so it enables patients to focus on their breathing in a way that improves respiratory function. Harmonicas and instruction books can be found at most music stores.

EMERGING CLINICAL PRACTICE

There are now approximately 70 four-year degree programs approved by the American Music Therapy Association (AMTA). There are about 5,000 board-certified music therapists who work in hospitals, pain clinics, hospice settings, etc.

How it works: A doctor, nurse or social worker may request music therapy for patients on a case-by-case basis. The therapist meets with the patient and assesses his/her needs. Is the patient depressed, in pain or anxious? Is he having trouble walking or breathing? The therapist then decides how the patient can benefit—physically and emotionally—from the treatments.

To find a music therapist, go to the AMTA site, *www.musictherapy.org.*

RESOURCES

Many music stores offer therapeutic music CDs and cassettes and may have a section labeled "health," "new age," "wellness," etc. Try to sample the music first to make sure you like it. Personal preference is important—if you find the music unpleasant, it won't be helpful to you. Good Web sites for therapeutic music include *www.rhythmic medicine.com* and *www.innerpeacemusic.com.*

Astounding Stories of Mind/Body Cures

Joan Borysenko, PhD, cofounder and former director of the mind-body clinical programs at two Harvard Medical School hospitals, now merged as Boston's Beth Israel Deaconess Medical Center. Based in Boulder, Colorado, she runs workshops and conducts lectures on mind-body healing. An updated 20th anniversary edition of her *Minding the Body, Mending the Mind* was released in 2007. Da Capo. *www.joanborysenko.com.*

On occasion, a health problem that was expected to be permanent or fatal instead disappears without medical intervention. The limited research that has been done suggests that the reason why one person recovers when most others do not might have as much to do with the mind as the body.

Joan Borysenko, PhD, a former Harvard medical scientist, is a renowned expert in the field of mind/body healing. *She relayed these true stories of spontaneous healing…*

MIND/BODY CURE

In 1985, Alice Epstein, a sociology doctoral student at the University of Massachusetts, was diagnosed with kidney cancer. One of her kidneys was removed, but it was no use—the cancer had spread to her lungs, and treatment was impossible. Epstein was told she had only a few more months to live.

With no way to treat the physical problem, Epstein and her psychology-professor husband decided to treat her mind. Epstein used meditation to reduce her stress, and psychotherapy to deal with the angry, unhappy component of her personality. Within six weeks, tests showed that her cancer was going into remission. Her progress slowed when she took time off from the intensive psychotherapy but resumed once the psychotherapy resumed. The cancer eventually disappeared. Epstein earned her PhD and is still alive today, more than 20 years later.

•**What may have happened.** Eliminating stress and anger will not cure every disease, but it can trigger a host of biochemical changes in the body—including providing a boost to the immune system. It is possible that Epstein's aggressive mental treatments played a role in her return to physical health.

A VISION IN LOURDES

Nearly 150 years ago, a teenage girl in Lourdes, France, reported seeing a vision of the Virgin Mary. Ever since, the waters in that area have been credited with healing powers. Most of these incidents involve cancer, multiple sclerosis and other diseases that occasionally go into remission, even without a visit to Lourdes.

The 1908 case of Marie Bire is more interesting. The 41-year-old French woman was blind as a result of optic atrophy—the degeneration of her optic nerve. According to medical science, it should not have been possible for optic nerves to recover from such a condition.

At Lourdes, the blind Bire attended Mass and received Holy Communion. Then, as the Blessed Sacrament in procession was passing the place where she sat, she suddenly regained her sight. Ten doctors examined Bire. They all found that her optic nerves were still withered but that she could see.

•**What may have happened.** We do not have to believe in divine miracles to believe that Bire's faith might have played a role in her recovery. Studies have found that depending upon the medical condition, between 30% and 50% of people respond to placebos. If you tell these people that you have given them pain-killers, their brain activity will show that they actually feel less pain.

CONFIDENCE DESPITE THE ODDS

In 1975, Ian Gawler, a 24-year-old Australian veterinarian and decathlete, learned that he had bone cancer in his right leg. The leg was amputated, but the cancer reappeared later that year and spread throughout his body. In 1976, Gawler was given two weeks to live. No one had ever been known to recover from such an advanced case of this form of cancer. As a doctor, Gawler knew that the reasonable response was to prepare for death. Instead, he remained certain that he would recover. He focused on meditation, positive thinking and a natural diet.

Gawler did recover. He founded and is now therapeutic director of The Gawler Foundation (*www.gawler.org*), which provides support for others suffering from serious illnesses. The foundation stresses healthy food, meditation and belief in recovery.

•**What may have happened.** We cannot simply imagine cancer away, but there is reason to think that believing in the desired health outcome might improve the odds that it will occur.

SURROUNDED BY LOVE

Fifty years ago, the outlook was bleak for those suffering psychotic hallucinations. Today's pharmaceuticals and cognitive behavior therapy were not yet available. Recovery was very rare.

That was bad news for one previously healthy 10-year-old girl growing up in the 1950s. Her nightmares had entered her waking life—she saw snakes, scorpions and headhunters. The girl believed that these tormentors were going to kill her family and that the only way she could stop them was to repeat obsessive-compulsive behaviors, such as scraping the inside of her mouth with her fingernails, reading books only upside down and backward, rereading each sentence three times and erasing everything she wrote three times before continuing. The girl eventually was pulled from school and lived each day in a landscape of terror.

For months, she prayed intensely for a cure. One day during these prayers, she suddenly felt surrounded by love and wisdom, as though she were being held in the arms of God. Her fear instantly disappeared, and she stopped her obsessive-compulsive behavior cold turkey. Within days, all of her symptoms were gone, never to return.

I was that little girl. The experience sparked my lifelong interest in psychology and spirituality.

•**What may have happened.** Most people with mental disorders cannot just pray their way to recovery. Still, it is worth noting that many people who experience spontaneous healing also experience a transformative spiritual episode similar to mine—a single moment when they feel aided by a loving, powerful outside force.

Medical Miracles Really Do Happen

Larry Dossey, MD, executive editor of *Explore: The Journal of Science and Healing* and the former executive editor of the journal *Alternative Therapies in Health and Medicine*. He is the author of 10 books, including *Healing Words* and *Prayer Is Good Medicine* (both HarperOne) and *The Extraordinary Healing Power of Ordinary Things* (Harmony).

Most of us have heard of people who recover from diseases that were considered incurable. The phenomenon, referred to in medical literature as spontaneous remission, occurs when serious, often deadly illnesses such as cancer quickly and inexplicably—some would even say miraculously—disappear.

No one knows exactly how often such cases occur. Approximately 3,500 medically documented cases of seeming miracles—based on reports from doctors in America and around the world dating to 1967—have appeared in 800 peer-reviewed medical journals and cover all major illnesses, including cancer, heart disease, diabetes and arthritis.*

To find out more about medically documented "miracles"—and what they might mean for improving everyday health and healing—*Bottom Line/Health* spoke to Larry Dossey, MD, former cochair of the National Institutes of Health's Mind/Body Panel and the author of *The Extraordinary Healing Power of Ordinary Things* (Harmony), which includes an essay on medical miracles…

•**What is a "medically documented miracle"?** The word *miracle* is from the Latin *mirari,* meaning to look at in awe. For me, a medical miracle is an awe-inspiring healing event—a disease that goes away suddenly, unexpectedly and completely.

Attempts have been made to define and medically document miracle-type cures. For example, in 1954, the Catholic Church established the International Medical Committee of Lourdes, a panel that includes dozens of experts from the European medical community. These doctors decide whether a cure reported by a person who has visited the healing shrine at Lourdes in southwestern France is an "authentic" miracle, using rigorous criteria, including a permanent remission of the disease. As of 2008, the committee had documented 67 cases.

•**Have any of your patients ever experienced this type of healing?** Early in my career, I had an elderly patient with cancer in both lungs that had spread throughout his body. We had no medical therapies for this type of cancer, but during visiting hours, people from his church stood near his bed, praying and singing gospel music. I expected him to die within days, and when he asked to go home, I respected his wishes and discharged him.

About a year later, this patient was back in the hospital—this time with a bad case of the flu. I went to the radiology department to look at his current chest X-ray, and it was completely normal. I thought that in the past year he must have had a dramatic response to additional therapy

*These cases are found in *Spontaneous Remission: An Annotated Bibliography* (The Institute of Noetic Sciences). An on-line version of the bibliography is available at *www.noetic.org.*

of some kind, but he hadn't undergone any therapy. To me, this was a true miracle cure.

•**Are religious and supernatural influences believed to play a role in most medical miracles?** Many medical miracles occur in a religious, spiritual or supernatural context—people pray to God, or to saints or rely on what they believe to be the healing energies of the universe. Perhaps some unknown mind-body process is triggered by belief. But even this is pure speculation—because atheists and agnostics also experience what seem to be miracle cures.

Not knowing why something works is not necessarily a problem. Throughout the history of medicine, we often have known that a treatment works before we understand how it works. Aspirin and penicillin are two examples. We can add miracle-type cures to that list. Perhaps science will someday explain these occurrences. For now, they remain inexplicable.

•**How do people who experience these cures explain their recoveries?** In interviews conducted for a book called *Remarkable Recovery* (Riverhead), individuals whose illnesses were reversed pointed to a variety of factors they thought played an important role in their healing.

Paradoxically, the two most commonly cited factors seem like opposites—75% attributed the recovery to a "belief in a positive outcome," while 71% said it was based on "acceptance of the disease." This shows that there is no one "personality type" that experiences miracle-type healings.

Sixty-eight percent believed that prayer was responsible, followed by meditation and faith. Self-help regimens, including exercise, music and singing, were also cited.

•**Some doctors believe that telling patients about miracle-type cures instills "false hope." What do you think?** Yes, some doctors may believe that speaking about medically documented miracles promotes "false hope" in seriously ill patients. But I would say that not informing and educating patients about this possibility promotes "false pessimism"—a negative viewpoint that is not justified by the facts. Documented miracle cures are a fact of medical history. For someone

who is ill, that knowledge can provide comfort and consolation.

An Effective Treatment For Healing Head to Toe

Timothy McCall, MD, an internist, medical editor of *Yoga Journal* and author of *Examining Your Doctor* (Citadel Press) and *Yoga as Medicine* (Bantam). *www.drmccall.com.*

Yoga is one of the most underutilized and underrated medical therapies in the US. Until recently, it was extremely rare for American medical doctors to prescribe yoga—most are not knowledgeable about its wide array of health benefits.

WHAT IS YOGA?

Yoga is a holistic system of exercise and controlled breathing aimed at optimizing physical and mental well-being. Yoga stretches all muscle groups while gently squeezing internal organs—a practice that lowers blood pressure and breathing rate and increases cardiac efficiency. It also builds strength, flexibility, balance and is perhaps the best overall system for stress reduction ever invented.

What you may not know: More than 100 scientific studies show that yoga can improve health problems ranging from heart disease to insomnia…diabetes to arthritis…and cancer to bronchitis.

As a medical doctor who has practiced yoga for 14 years, I firmly believe that it is the most powerful system of overall health and well-being that I have ever seen. By promoting overall health, yoga increases the benefits you may derive from conventional and/or other alternative/complementary therapies—and may even eliminate your need for medication.

HOW YOGA HELPS

While yoga isn't a cure-all, studies suggest that virtually all health problems respond positively to yoga.

Landmark research: When 2,700 people suffering from a variety of ailments practiced yoga (for at least two hours a week for one year or longer), it helped 96% of those with back disorders…94% of those with heart disease …90% of those with cancer…90% of those with arthritis…88% of those with bronchitis or asthma …and 86% of those with diabetes.

What's responsible for all these salutary effects? Yoga, which is practiced by children as well as adults well into their 80s and 90s, helps with such a wide range of medical conditions because of its many different mechanisms of action. *Yoga can…*

•**Increase flexibility,** strengthen muscles and improve posture and balance.

•**Boost immunity** by reducing levels of the stress hormone *cortisol* and increasing the circulation of *lymph* (a fluid rich in lymphocytes and other immune cells).

•**Enhance lung function** by using slower and deeper breathing that promotes oxygenation of tissues.

•**Strengthen bones** and nourish the cartilage in spinal discs and joints by improving range of motion, helping to deliver nutrients to the cartilage.

•**Condition the heart and circulatory system,** lower elevated blood sugars and artery-damaging high blood pressure and improve levels of cholesterol and triglycerides (blood fats).

•**Relieve pain** due to conditions such as arthritis, back problems, fibromyalgia and carpal tunnel syndrome, by reducing muscle spasms, improving the alignment of bones in joints and teaching people to separate pain from their emotional response to the pain.

•**Improve brain function** by changing the levels of neurotransmitters (brain chemicals) and activating an area of the brain (the left prefrontal cortex) that studies suggest is associated with happiness and resiliency to stress.

GETTING THE BENEFITS

There are a variety of ways to maximize the effectiveness and safety of yoga therapy. *My advice…*

•**Talk to your doctor.** Certain yoga practices are not recommended for people who suffer from specific medical conditions.

Example: People who have diabetic retinopathy (damage to the retina as a result of diabetes) should avoid upside-down poses such as a shoulder stand and headstand, because these poses can increase pressure on the blood vessels in the eyes.

Helpful: When you visit your doctor, bring a book with photos of yoga poses that reflect the yoga style that you are considering. Since your doctor may not be aware of all possible contraindications, be sure to also discuss your concerns with your yoga teacher.

•**Choose the right type of instruction.** Yoga therapy ideally is tailored to the individual based on the evaluation of an experienced yoga teacher. While large group yoga classes can be great preventive medicine for people who are relatively fit and flexible, those with chronic medical conditions are usually better off working with a teacher privately or in a small group (two to four students). The cost of private lessons ranges from about $40 to $100 or more an hour. Group classes range from about $10 to $20 a session.

Helpful: If you're not sure whether a class is right for you, call or e-mail the teacher before you attend and explain your situation. If the class doesn't fit your needs, ask for a recommendation for another class or teacher.

•**Find an experienced teacher.** Some styles of yoga require teachers to undergo 200 to 500 hours of training to be certified. However, there is no universal accrediting organization.*

Warning: Some yoga teachers may have completed only a weekend training course to become "certified." Before attending a yoga class, ask the instructor how long he/she trained. (At least 200 hours is standard.)

•**Pay attention to your body.** If you experience sharp pain when you do a yoga posture, stop. If you perform a breathing exercise and feel short of breath, stop. In either case, tell the teacher as soon as possible—during or after the class.

•**Practice regularly.** The key to success with yoga is steady practice—once a day is ideal—even if it's only for 10 or 15 minutes. Yoga works

*To find a yoga instructor near you, go to the Web site of the International Association of Yoga Therapists, *www.iayt.org.*

well as part of an overall fitness program that in-cludes aerobic exercise and strength training.

Helpful: Set a goal for daily practice and make an appointment with yourself, just as you would make plans to meet a friend for lunch.

•**Be patient.** Most drugs work fast, but the longer you take them, the less effective they tend to become. Yoga is not a quick fix. But the lon-ger you practice it, the more effective it tends to become. Yoga is slow—but strong—medicine.

That doesn't mean you won't see immediate results. It's well known among yoga teachers that people starting yoga make quicker progress with health problems than people who have been practicing for a long time. Just a little bit of added flexibility, strength and balance can make a huge difference in how you function day to day—by reducing back pain, for exam-ple, or helping you climb stairs more easily.

And some yoga techniques can help you *in-stantly* in stress-provoking situations, such as getting stuck in traffic.

Example: Counting silently, inhale for three seconds and exhale for six seconds, for a single breath. Take a few normal breaths, then repeat the first sequence, breathing smoothly. In a few breaths, you should start to feel calmer.

■ **More from Timothy McCall, MD…**

What Yoga Style Is Right for You?

Several styles of yoga are practiced in the US. *Among the most common…*

•**Iyengar yoga** strives for precise body align-ment and uses bolsters, blocks and other props to provide support to help prevent injury.

Good for: People with back pain, arthritis or any condition in which body alignment may play a role.

•**Viniyoga yoga** focuses heavily on breath and postures are gentle, so the risk for injury is very low.

Good for: People with chronic diseases, such as diabetes, high blood pressure, heart disease or cancer.

•**Integral yoga** is a gentle approach that in-corporates basic poses with breathing exercises

as well as meditation and discussions of ancient yoga texts.

Good for: Chronic diseases, such as heart disease or cancer.

•**Anusara yoga** is a fast-growing style com-bining the anatomical awareness of Iyengar yoga with an emphasis on positive reinforcement.

Good for: People with back pain.

The term *hatha* yoga is used to describe a variety of styles, including Iyengar and Integral. If a teacher uses this term, ask which styles of yoga he/she finds most influential.

Your Secret Weapon for Better Health

Gary B. Huffnagle, PhD, professor of internal medi-cine, microbiology and immunology, University of Michigan Medical School, Ann Arbor. His research on probiotics has appeared in leading scientific journals. He is also the author of *The Probiotics Revolution*. Bantam.

The small and large intestines (gut) do most of the work involved in digesting the 20 tons of food that the average person consumes in a lifetime. This process involves trillions of bacteria—some of them harmful and others beneficial.

What you may not know: While the gut is most commonly associated with digestion, it's estimated that at least 60% of a person's im-mune system is located there. "Good" bacteria protect against the growth of harmful bacteria to help prevent infections, such as vaginal yeast infections and urinary tract infections.

Probiotic bacteria (a subset of good bacte-ria) also secrete substances that act on intestinal muscles and help regulate motility (the intestinal contractions that move food and waste through the intestine at the proper rate).

Because these good bacteria play a key role in preventing infections as well as keeping the di-gestive system functioning properly, "probiotics" —dietary supplements or foods that contain ben-eficial bacteria or yeasts similar to those found in the human gut—have become increasingly popular, particularly among people who take antibiotics.

Reason: Antibiotics kill not only harmful microorganisms that cause disease, but also the body's beneficial bacteria, sometimes leading to gas, cramping and such conditions as diarrhea. People who take antibiotics regularly may have permanent reductions in probiotic organisms unless they replenish the body's natural supply. For most people, the occasional use of antibiotics—such as a 10-day course—is unlikely to cause lasting problems.

WHEN SUPPLEMENTS HELP

Probiotics are live microorganisms. Two of the most beneficial types of probiotics—*Lactobacilli* and *Bifida* organisms—thrive in the naturally acidic environments of the digestive tract's stomach and small intestine.

Probiotics are often recommended for digestion (to help reduce such problems as gas, bloating, constipation and diarrhea), but they appear to be equally important—if not more so—for the immune system.

Probiotics in the intestine stimulate production of white blood cells known as regulatory *T cells*, which help fight inflammation associated with such disorders as eczema, seasonal allergies and inflammatory bowel disease (IBD), a condition in which the bowel becomes inflamed, often resulting in abdominal cramps and diarrhea.

Probiotics also help prevent and treat diarrhea related to *Clostridium difficile* infection.

There are many dozens of species of probiotic organisms. The most reliable probiotic formulations now available in the US are in capsule form. Most probiotic capsules should be refrigerated.

Two highly effective products are used primarily for digestive problems. *Use the one that most closely matches your symptoms…**

•**Culturelle.** Studies over the past 30 years have shown that *Lactobacillus* GG (the active organism in this product) reduces the severity and duration of traveler's diarrhea, as well as diarrhea associated with antibiotic therapy.

*If you have an immune deficiency, talk to your doctor before taking probiotics.

Typical dose: One to two daily supplements (each containing 30 billion organisms), taken at the onset of diarrhea. Continue for one week after symptoms stop. To prevent antibiotic-related diarrhea, take the supplements during antibiotic therapy and for at least one week afterward.

Important: To ensure optimal effectiveness of the antibiotic, do not take it at the same time of day you are taking the probiotic.

•**Align** has *Bifidobacterium infantis* 35624, an organism shown in studies to decrease symptoms of irritable bowel syndrome (IBS), a condition that causes diarrhea and/or constipation and other digestive problems.

Typical dose: One capsule (containing one billion live organisms) daily—taken indefinitely if symptoms are ongoing. If bowel symptoms are associated with stomach flu, take the probiotic supplement during symptoms and continue for one week after they subside.

IMMUNE-BOOSTING BENEFITS

To ensure that your immune system is working at its best, it's a good idea to take probiotic supplements and/or to eat foods containing probiotics daily even if you don't have a particular condition that you're trying to treat.

To boost immunity, look for probiotic supplements and foods that contain the bacterium *Lactobacillus casei* or several probiotic bacteria strains.

My favorite multistrain supplements are Jarro-Dophilus EPS and Theralac. Follow the dosage instructions on the label.

Helpful: Probiotics are stimulated by soluble dietary fiber, so they're more likely to proliferate in the intestine when you also eat complex carbohydrates, such as legumes, vegetables and whole grains. These foods contain "prebiotics," which provide the nutrition that probiotics need to multiply.

PROBIOTIC FOODS

In the last few years, food manufacturers have begun to promote probiotic-enriched foods, such as the low-fat yogurt Activia and the probiotic dairy drink DanActive (both by Dannon). These products contain the well-researched probiotic bacteria *Bifidobacterium animalis* and L. casei, respectively.

95

When these foods are bought in a grocery store and analyzed in a laboratory, they consistently contain about the same number of active organisms as listed on the labels.

Other probiotic food products...

•**Yogurt.**

Best choices: Foods with the "Live & Active cultures" seal from the National Yogurt Association. These refrigerated products must contain at least 100 million live bacteria per gram at the time of their manufacture.

•**Aged cheeses,** such as cheddar or blue cheese, typically contain three billion to 10 billion organisms per serving. Generally, the longer a cheese is aged, the higher the probiotic load.

•**Kefir,** a type of fermented milk, usually has at least three billion organisms per serving.

Caution: Aged cheeses and kefir should be avoided by people who have food sensitivities to milk products.

Relief at Your Fingertips

Michael Reed Gach, PhD, founder of the Acupressure Institute in Berkeley, California. He is author of self-healing instructional DVDs and CDs and many books, including *Acupressure's Potent Points* (Bantam), *Acupressure for Lovers* (Bantam), *Arthritis Relief at Your Fingertips* (Warner) and coauthor of *Acupressure for Emotional Healing* (Bantam). *www.acupressure.com.*

You've probably heard of acupuncture, but there's something similar that you can do yourself—no needles involved—called *acupressure.* Acupressure can alleviate many physical, mental and emotional problems in only a few minutes—and it is free.

Acupressure involves stimulating acupoints on the body with fingertips or knuckles and is based on the principles of acupuncture, an ancient healing technique used by practitioners of Traditional Chinese Medicine (TCM). The acupoints often have ancient descriptive names, such as "Joining the Valley" and "Mind Clearing." Acupressure increases blood flow to the treated area and triggers the release of *endorphins,* pain-relieving brain chemicals.

Here are the acupressure techniques for various health problems. Unless otherwise noted, daily acupressure sessions, three times a day, are the best way to relieve a temporary or chronic problem.

ARTHRITIS PAIN

Joining the Valley is a truly amazing acupoint because it can relieve arthritis pain anywhere in the body.

Location: In the webbing between the thumb and index finger, at the highest spot of the muscle when the thumb and index finger are brought close together.

What to do: Rhythmically squeeze the acupoint. As you're squeezing, place the side of your hand that is closest to the little finger on your thigh or a tabletop. Apply pressure in the webbing as you press downward. This allows you to angle more deeply into the point, increasing the benefits.

Also good for: Headache, toothache, hangover, hay fever symptoms, constipation.

Caution: This point is forbidden for pregnant women because its stimulation can cause premature contraction in the uterus.

MEMORY PROBLEMS

The *Mind Clearing* acupoints are for improving recall instantly—for example, when you have forgotten a name or gone to the supermarket without your shopping list.

Location: One finger width (about one-half inch) directly above the center of each eyebrow.

What to do: Gently place your right thumb above your right eyebrow and your middle fingertip above the eyebrow on the left side. Hold very gently. You should feel a slight dip or indentation in the bone structure—the acupoints on both sides are in the dip. Press the indentation very lightly, hold and breathe deeply. After a minute or two, you'll experience more mental clarity and sharper memory.

LOWER BACK PAIN

To help prevent and relieve lower back pain, practice this exercise for one minute three times a day. You can do it standing or sitting.

Location: Place the backs of your hands against your lower back, about one inch outside the spine.

What to do: Briskly rub your hands up and down—about three inches up and six inches down—using the friction to create heat in your lower back.

If you're doing the technique correctly, you'll need to breathe deeply to sustain the vigorous rubbing, and you'll break out in a slight sweat.

Also good for: Food cravings, especially sugar cravings, chronic fatigue, sexual problems, chills, phobias and fibromyalgia symptoms.

EMOTIONAL UPSET

The *Inner Gate* acupoint can reduce emotional upset—such as anxiety, depression and irritability—in two to three minutes.

Location: On the inner side of the forearm, three finger widths up from the center of the wrist crease, in between two thick tendons.

What to do: Place your thumb on the point and your fingers directly behind the outside of the forearm between the two bones. Squeeze in slowly and firmly, hold for two to three minutes, breathing deeply. Repeat on the other arm for the same amount of time.

Also good for: Carpal tunnel syndrome, insomnia, indigestion and nausea.

COLDS AND FLU

If you think you're about to get a cold or flu, stimulating the *Heavenly Rejuvenation* acupoint may prevent infection.

Location: On the shoulders, midway between the base of the neck and the outside of the shoulders, one-half inch below the top of the shoulders.

What to do: There are two ways to stimulate this point…

•**Curving your fingers,** hook your right hand on your right shoulder and your left hand on your left shoulder. You also can use your fingers on your opposite shoulder, which may be easier. With your fingertips, firmly press the point and take three slow, deep breaths.

•**If you don't have the flexibility to perform the first technique…**lie down on your back, on a firm mattress or carpeted floor, with your knees bent and feet on the floor as close to your buttocks as possible. Bring your hands above your head, and rest the backs of your hands on the floor beside or above your head. Inhale and lift up your pelvis, pressing your feet against the floor to assist the lift. The higher your pelvis, the more weight will be transferred onto your shoulders, stimulating the acupoint. Hold this posture for one minute, taking long, slow, deep breaths, with your eyes closed. Lower your pelvis, and rest for three minutes.

Also good for: Nervous tension, stiff neck, high fever, chills, shoulder aches and irritability.

INSOMNIA

The acupoints *Calm Sleep* and *Joyful Sleep*—on the outer and inner ankles—can help relieve insomnia. Use these acupressure points whenever you want to deeply relax and sleep better.

Calm

Joyful

Location: Calm Sleep is in the first indentation below the outer anklebone. *Joyful Sleep* is directly below the inside of the anklebone, in a slight indentation.

What to do: Place your thumb on one side of your ankle and your fingers on the other, and press firmly. If you're on the right spot, it will be slightly sore. Hold for two minutes, breathing deeply. Repeat on the other ankle. Do this again if you still are having trouble sleeping or if you wake up.

HEADACHES

The acupoints *Gates of Consciousness* relieve a tension headache or migraine.

Location: Underneath the base of your skull to either side of your spine, about three to four inches apart, depending on the size of your head.

Illustrations courtesy of Michael Reed Gach, PhD.

What to do: Using your fingers, thumbs or knuckles, press the points under the base of your skull.

At the same time, slowly tilt your head back so that the angle of your head relaxes your neck muscles. Press forward (toward your throat), upward (underneath the base of your skull) and slightly inward, angling the pressure toward the center of your brain. Continue to apply pressure for two minutes, breathing.

Also good for: Neck pain, insomnia, high blood pressure.

■ **More from Michael Reed Gach, PhD...**

Acupressure Basics

Unless otherwise noted, use your middle finger, with your index and ring fingers for support. Firmly and gradually, apply stationary pressure directly on the acupoint for about three minutes.

•**Firmly** means using an amount of pressure that causes a sensation between pleasure and pain—pressure that "hurts good." If the pressure is applied too fast or too hard, the point will hurt. If the pressure is too soft, you won't get the full benefit.

•**Gradually** means moving your finger into and out of the point in super-slow motion. Applying and releasing finger pressure allow the tissue to respond and relax, promoting healing.

•**Stationary** means you are not rubbing or massaging the area.

•**Directly** means at a 90-degree angle from the surface of the skin. If you are pulling the skin, the angle of pressure is incorrect.

•**When you apply pressure,** lean your weight toward the point. If your hands are weak or it hurts your fingers when you apply pressure, try using your knuckles. You also can use a tool, such as a golf ball or pencil eraser.

•**Breathe** slowly and deeply while you apply pressure. This helps release pain and tension.

4

Everyday Ailments

Natural Ways to Guard Against Colds, Flu—And Worse

Even people who pay close attention to their health often could be doing more to boost their immunity. Your body's immune system consists of specialized cells and chemicals that kill and/or inactivate viruses and other invaders. When viruses invade your body, they not only can trigger colds and the flu, but also Epstein-Barr infections (which have been implicated in hepatitis and certain cancers) and severe acute respiratory syndrome (SARS).

Latest development: Immunity researchers are confirming the profound importance of eating a healthful diet—and finding other helpful ways for you to protect yourself from viruses.

BEST DEFENSE

Some people forget that good nutrition is as important for strong viral immunity as it is for the health of your heart and arteries. And despite all the talk about eating healthfully, most people fall short in at least one key food group.

Best immunity-boosting diet…

• **Complex carbohydrates** should account for about 50% to 60% of your daily calories.

Good choices: Whole grains, such as brown and basmati rice, and legumes.

• **Vegetables and fruits** (preferably organic) —have one or two servings at each meal.

Good choices: Papaya, pineapple or peaches with breakfast…garden salad, with fresh tomatoes with lunch…and steamed carrots and broccoli with dinner.

• **Fats** should account for 20% to 25% of your daily calories. Choose unsaturated oils that are rich in omega-3 fatty acids.

J.E. Williams, doctor of oriental medicine (OMD) and past academic dean of East West College of Natural Medicine in Sarasota, Florida, is the author of *Viral Immunity: A 10-Step Plan to Enhance Your Immunity Against Viral Disease Using Natural Medicines.* Hampton Roads. He is a member of the American Academy of Anti-Aging Medicine and a Fellow of the American Association of Integrative Medicine.

Good sources: Cold-water fish, such as salmon, mackerel and sardines...avocados...nuts (particularly walnuts and almonds) and seeds (particularly flax).

•**Protein** should make up about 20% of your daily diet.

Good choices: Protein from animal sources, such as fish, poultry, lean meat, low-fat milk and eggs. The vegetable protein found in grains and legumes (beans) also is nourishing. However, if you eat mostly plant-based proteins, take 12 g daily of whey protein (milk protein without fats or lactose) as a supplement.

If it's difficult to maintain this daily diet, I recommend taking supplements to compensate for any missing nutrients. In addition to a daily multivitamin, take 200 mg to 500 mg of vitamin C...200 international units (IU) of vitamin E...200 micrograms (mcg) of selenium...and 15 mg of zinc.

IMMUNITY-BOOSTING LIFESTYLE

Other ways to maximize your body's virus-fighting power...

•**Avoid fried foods.** Even an occasional serving of french fries or fried chicken can compromise your body's immunity. That's because fats are oxidized during the frying process, creating compounds that damage all cells, including those that fight viruses.

My advice: For optimal benefit from a generally healthful diet, avoid all fried foods. Grill (with low heat), boil, steam or bake your food instead.

•**Limit alcohol consumption.** Alcohol can depress immune function. Studies have linked excessive alcohol to susceptibility to lung infections, including bacterial pneumonia and tuberculosis.

My advice: Drink alcohol in moderation (up to one drink daily for women...two for men)—or not at all.

•**Drink pure water.** Most people don't consume enough water—or the right type. Water is one of the simplest ways to effectively flush toxins from the body and introduce the minerals as well as trace minerals that have been shown to support immune function.

Even though some experts don't believe that it's necessary to drink as many as eight eight-ounce glasses of water daily, I stand by this advice. If you exercise—even if you don't sweat—you need even more water because greater amounts of it are lost from the lungs due to exhalation. During winter, excessively heated rooms also deplete water from your body.

My advice: Don't include soda, juice or other sugary beverages in your daily water quota. Drink pure spring water, such as Evian or Volvic, or filtered tap water. It helps flush viruses from your body without the immune-depressing effects of sugar and other additives.

•**Get enough sleep.** A study published in *Nature Reviews Immunology* showed that insufficient sleep inhibits the production of chemicals, such as cytokines, which help boost the body's immunity. Not surprisingly, sleep deprivation is associated with increased rates of infection.

My advice: Most people need at least eight hours of sleep a night to restore normal body functions. If you feel rundown or are battling the early stages of a cold or other viral infection, try to get even more sleep.

Important: Just being in bed for eight hours does not count if you're having trouble falling asleep or are waking up during the night. If this occurs, ask your doctor for advice on improving the quality of your sleep.

•**Exercise—but not too much.** Regular exercise has been shown to neutralize inflammatory chemicals and improve the function of the body's natural killer cells—both key players in viral immunity.

But overly strenuous workouts, such as running a marathon, can have the opposite effect, triggering the production of cortisol, adrenaline and other stress hormones that suppress immune function and increase your odds of contracting an infection.

My advice: Up to one hour a day of moderate exercise (such as brisk walking, bicycling or swimming) is right for most people. Let your body be your guide—if you feel exhausted and generally worse after you exercise, cut back.

•**Take a sauna.** Dangerous chemicals from the environment, including the pesticides that we consume in nonorganic foods, cause an imbalance in the immune cells that fight viral infections. A sauna helps your body to release these chemicals via perspiration.

My advice: Take a dry sauna once or twice weekly. Don't exceed 20 minutes, and drink at least an extra quart of pure water to compensate for what you lose through perspiration.

Caution: Saunas may not be safe for people over age 65 or anyone who is weak or has a fever.

IMMUNITY-BOOSTING PLANTS

The leaves, stems and roots of some plants are concentrated sources of powerful antiviral compounds. Unless you have a chronic viral infection, such as chronic hepatitis, it's usually best not to take these on a regular basis.

However, if you're under considerable stress, feel rundown or are exposed to viral illnesses, consider taking one or more of the following supplements throughout cold and flu season…*

•**Astragalus.** Prized in Chinese medicine for its ability to restore the body's energy, this herb strengthens antiviral defenses by stimulating the production of interferon, a substance that inhibits viral growth.

Typical dose: As a tea, drink one cup twice daily. To prepare: Simmer 30 g of dried astragalus root in one cup of water for 20 minutes. Or take two to three 500-mg capsules twice daily.

•**Ginseng.** This herb is known as an energy tonic, but it also stimulates the immune system.

Typical dose: Take a 250-mg capsule twice daily (choose a standardized extract containing 30% of the active ingredient ginsenosides per 250 mg).

Caution: Don't take ginseng if you have high blood pressure, a fever or an active infection. This herb also should be avoided by people who take a monoamine oxidase inhibitor (MAOI) antidepressant, such as *phenelzine* (Nardil) or *tranylcypromine* (Parnate) or blood thinners such as *warfarin* (Coumadin).

•**Acemannan.** This aloe vera extract has been shown to increase the activity of virus-killing T-cells and stimulate the release of interleukin-1, an important immune system messenger chemical. Acemannan is available at most health-food stores in a product called Manapol, manufactured by Carrington Labs.

Typical dose: One 80-mg capsule one to three times daily.

*If you use prescription medication, are pregnant, nursing or have a chronic disease, such as diabetes or heart, liver or kidney disease, do not take any of these supplements without consulting your doctor.

Doctor's Warning on Steroidal Inhalers

Richard Firshein, DO, director of the Firshein Center for Comprehensive Medicine in New York City and author of *Reversing Asthma* (Grand Central) and *Your Asthma-Free Child* (Avery). Dr. Firshein has also written *The Nutraceutical Revolution* (Riverhead), was honored by the American Medical Association for work with asthmatic children, and is the founder and creator of *DrCity.com*.

Currently, steroidal inhalers are a standard treatment for asthma in children. Yet a study in *The New England Journal of Medicine* reported that these drugs have no long-term impact on the progression of asthma or on lung function in preschoolers. While symptoms were controlled during treatment, benefits disappeared when treatment was halted. Additionally, steroids have many dangerous side effects, with children in the study experiencing slowed growth when using steroidal inhalers. Bad for children. Bad for adults. What else to do?

Richard Firshein, DO, director of the Firshein Center for Comprehensive Medicine in New York City, explains his expert's take on steroids and safer, natural alternatives. He acknowledges that inhaled steroids are not a panacea, but they do play a helpful role when symptoms are particularly troublesome. For example, if a child is experiencing a high level of inflammation and/or wheezing and missing many school days, Dr. Firshein is apt to prescribe a corticosteroid inhaler for short-term use. However, he does not recommend these drugs on a long-term basis, and emphasized that his first line of defense is to prevent symptoms naturally. Patients with long-term asthma should consider Singulair or a bronchodilator on an "as needed" basis, he says.

BUILD A STRONG FOUNDATION

Asthma has many triggers. Among its possible triggers are airborne pollutants, secondhand smoke, allergens (dust mites, animal dander, mold, chemicals, foods, etc.) and cold air.

Also: Aspirin and NSAIDs can trigger an attack, as can a viral infection. To prevent asthma symptoms from occurring in the first place, rather than simply responding to them, Dr. Firshein stresses that you must make healthful changes—changes that reduce the exposure to the things that trigger asthma, and changes that strengthen the body's immune system to resist those triggers. That advice applies not only to children with asthma, but to asthma sufferers of all ages. Allergy shots have also been shown to reduce the sensitivity to allergy triggers such as dust, dust mites, pollen and pet dander.

To build a foundation, Dr. Firshein suggests...

•**Closely monitor your environment.** Go through your house carefully and remove possible triggers. For example, eliminate dust collectors such as wall-to-wall carpeting and heavy drapes...install an air filter to clean household air...frequently wash non-allergenic bedding and non-allergenic pillow and mattress covers ...use a dehumidifier in damp basements and bathrooms and bedrooms...and avoid using air fresheners. Additionally, do not neglect school or work environments, where we spend so many hours of our lives. It's equally important to eliminate triggers here. Parents should speak directly to principals and teachers about a child's allergy triggers and have emergency procedures in place, should an attack occur.

•**Keep an eye on diet.** Dr. Firshein is particularly concerned with asthmatic children eating junk food, which he compares to an adult with heart disease eating fat-laden cheeseburgers and fries. He points out that junk foods promote inflammation, which promotes asthma. Instead, follow an anti-inflammatory diet rich in nutrient-dense whole foods such as fresh fruits and veggies (berries are especially rich in inflammation-fighting antioxidants), fish, nuts and seeds. Whenever possible, go with organic products.

•**Take immune-boosting supplements.** In particular, Dr. Firshein recommends vitamin C (1,000 mg), magnesium (500 mg), fish oil and a good multivitamin. When using inhaled steroids, which may compromise the bones, he also recommends a calcium-magnesium supplement (1,200 mg of calcium) for added protection.

Note: Dosages should be reduced in children by 50% to 75% of an adult dosage. In general, he finds that children respond much more rapidly to multivitamins than adults, allowing them to catch fewer colds and miss fewer school/work days, and gain heartier immunity overall with relatively simple supplementation.

•**Learn to breathe easy.** The Firshein Technique for Asthma Breathing is a series of exercises that teach children to stabilize their asthma. He finds that children above age five do particularly well with breathing exercises. Asthma sufferers often feel nervous and out of control when they approach a situation that they know brings on symptoms, such as exercise or cold air. These breathing exercises give individuals a sense of control over a situation, and also strengthen muscles in the diaphragm, which is crucial to controlling asthma.

Dr. Firshein recommends these simple exercises when encountering potential triggers...

•Breathe in through the nose for a count of five, and breathe out through the mouth for a count of seven.

•Next, breathe in deeply, and then blow out the air in a burst like you're blowing out a candle. This strengthens the lungs and diaphragm, explains Dr. Firshein.

•Now use your stomach. Lie down, and as you breathe in through the nose, consciously make your stomach expand. As you exhale through the mouth, return to your normal position.

•Try a rocking motion while standing, breathing in and rocking to one side then breathing out while rocking to the other side. Then switch. Air gets trapped in the lungs of people with asthma, so they cannot take in enough new oxygen, observes Dr. Firshein. Rocking back and forth helps the body use the ribcage more to expel the stale air so there's more room in the lungs.

•Get plenty of exercise. Exercise is doubly important for the asthmatic child, says Dr. Firshein. Breathing exercises work by reducing stress, improving oxygen intake and by strengthening the muscles that are used in respiration. If exercise is a trigger of asthma symptoms, the physician should closely monitor the exercise program. In some cases, breathing exercises may ease and prevent attacks. Using a peak flow meter is the most effective way to monitor breathing at home.

HOW TO INHALE STEROIDS CORRECTLY

If you or your child must take steroids for a period of time, Dr. Firshein recommends a safer way to go about using them. Spacing devices provide an effective way of maximizing medication and minimizing deposits in the mouth. He cautions that steroids in dry powder form are difficult to inhale, with often as much as 90% of the powdered medication ending up in the mouth. When you swallow this, you are apt to experience greater side effects and less effectiveness. To reduce side effects, following inhalation, rinse your mouth thoroughly.

A BETTER WAY

With side effects from steroids being so severe and their effectiveness being so limited, they should only be used when they are truly necessary. Using simple strategies that build a strong foundation for your health can lower risk of asthma attacks and cut back on the medication required to control them.

Good News for Asthmatics! Lower Doses of Steroids Work Just as Well

Neil C. Thomson, MD, professor of respiratory medicine, University of Glasgow, Scotland.

John J. Costa, MD, assistant clinical professor of medicine, Brigham and Women's Hospital, Harvard Medical School, Boston.

BMJ (British Medical Journal).

If you're among the 15% of all asthmatics who take high dosages of inhaled steroids, you may not need as much medicine as you think to keep your disease in check.

A Scottish study shows that patients with chronic, severe asthma can sharply reduce their dosages of inhaled steroids (to cut the risk of side effects) and still keep their condition under control.

The study was the first carefully controlled trial to show that this "step-down" approach works in chronic, severe cases of asthma.

Inhaled steroids are the recommended treatment for chronic asthma, but they are accompanied by a number of side effects, including weakened bones and eye problems, such as cataracts and glaucoma. For these reasons, doctors prefer to keep the dosage at a minimum.

The study included 259 adult asthma patients with symptoms severe enough to require an average of 1,400 micrograms per day of *beclomethasone*, or equivalent amounts of other steroids.

For the study, 130 patients began taking half of their previous dosage, while 129 continued their old dosage. As is common in such controlled studies, none of the patients were told how much they were taking.

After one year, results were as good for the reduced-dosage patients as they were for the higher-dosage patients, according to Dr. Neil C. Thomson, professor of respiratory medicine at the University of Glasgow, and leader of the study.

DOCTORS SHOULD FOLLOW UP ON TREATMENT

"The study is a welcome reminder that doctors treating asthma patients should look toward reducing steroid dosage," says Dr. John J. Costa, assistant clinical professor of medicine at Brigham and Women's Hospital in Boston.

Often, asthma patients go to their doctors when the disease flares up, and higher doses are prescribed to bring things back to normal, he says.

"The importance of this is to remind practitioners that often they see asthmatics and decide that a certain amount of medicine is needed to address what is going on at that moment. It may not be the amount of medicine needed when the patient is not in the middle of a flare-up," Costa says. "The doctor should follow up to see if it is possible to reduce the dosage."

■ ■ ■ ■

Inhaler Ban

Some asthma inhalers have been banned by the US Food and Drug Administration as of the end of 2008. Inhalers that use atmosphere-damaging chlorofluorocarbons (CFCs) to dispense the medication *albuterol* will no longer be produced, marketed or sold in the US.

Karen Mahoney, medical officer, US Food and Drug Administration, Rockville, Maryland.

Drug-Free Asthma Busters

Richard Firshein, DO, director of the Firshein Center for Comprehensive Medicine in New York City and author of *Reversing Asthma* (Grand Central) and *Your Asthma-Free Child* (Avery). Dr. Firshein has also written *The Nutraceutical Revolution* (Riverhead), was honored by the American Medical Association for work with asthmatic children, and is the founder and creator of *DrCity.com*.

L iving with asthma does not have to be a life sentence with the drug companies. There are natural health-building ways to breathe free, drug free.

For the 20 to 40 million Americans who suffer from asthma, life can be very scary. In addition to dealing with debilitating and frightening attacks, many sufferers experience unpleasant side effects from the medications used to control the illness. "I've seen patients shaking, anxious, jittery, unable to concentrate and even complaining of chest pain—and they don't know it's their asthma medication," says New York City-based family physician Richard Firshein, DO, who specializes in complementary medicine. What's worse, some of the remedies fail to address the underlying causes, so sufferers continue to experience attacks.

The good news is that drug-free treatments abound, and they really work. "Alternative traditional therapies not only reduce or eliminate the need for medications, they also improve people's quality of life quite dramatically," says Dr. Firshein, author of *Reversing Asthma* (Grand Central).

Managing asthma, an allergic inflammation of the lungs, is increasingly important. The number of cases in this country is rising at an alarming rate—it has more than doubled just in the last 20 years.

Dr. Firshein calls on an arsenal of natural remedies and includes the manipulation of diet and environment and the addition of supplements, breathing exercises and acupuncture to help his patients live drug-free.

EXAMINE YOUR DIET

Asthma is a disease of inflammation, so it's especially important for sufferers to avoid foods that are triggers. Excessive sugar and salt are prime culprits, as are heavily processed foods that contain all kinds of chemicals.

In addition, individual asthmatics may find that they have other individual food allergies that trigger asthma attacks. To determine the problematic fare, Dr. Firshein recommends doing a "rotation diet" in which you avoid one of the major allergens—milk, corn, soy, wheat, eggs or nuts—for a four- to five-day period and see if symptoms abate. After you omit one item, reintroduce the food and see if you feel worse. When you have completed one food, try the next. "It's not foolproof," says Dr. Firshein, "but if you do it long enough, you might realize that you're only allergic to one or two things. Then you can feel so much better simply by avoiding those items," he says.

Dr. Firshein also recommends identifying your personal allergens with one of two tests—skin testing or a blood test called the radioallergosorbent test (RAST). In this test, substances known to trigger allergies are added to the blood sample and then the level of allergy antibodies is measured. The levels will be high if there is an allergic reaction. One of these tests, along with the rotation diet, should determine 80% of triggers, Dr. Firshein says.

NUTRITIONAL SHORTFALLS

Dr. Firshein, who also is author of *The Nutraceutical Revolution* (Riverhead), recommends talking to a doctor who specializes in nutrition about taking a well-balanced antioxidant, one that contains moderate amounts of vitamins A, C and E, the B vitamins, selenium and others. Several studies have drawn connections between low levels of antioxidants and higher levels of asthma. For example, many asthmatics have been shown to be deficient in magnesium, which acts as a natural bronchodilator. In other research, vitamin C has been found to reduce exercise-induced asthma.

TRY BREATHING

Most people don't know how to breathe properly. They breathe shallowly, allowing their chest to rise and fall with each breath. Abdominal breathing—using the diaphragm to draw air in and out—is, according to Dr. Firshein, "one of the most effective ways to strengthen weakened lungs and control attacks. Using your diaphragm helps you relax and gain control over your breathing, improving oxygenation," he says. "It can make a substantial difference."

With asthma, he explains, the problem is not that air can't get into the lungs—it is that it can't get out. The following breathing exercise helps constricted lungs pump air out more efficiently. "It's like a Heimlich maneuver for asthma sufferers, a natural bronchodilator," he says. *Do it for 10 minutes once or twice a day...*

1. Start by getting into a relaxed state of mind, by using meditation or imagining yourself lounging on a beach.

2. Breathe in deeply and visualize your stomach, not your chest, expanding. You even can place one hand on your stomach and one on your chest to ensure that your body is following along.

3. Start counting out your breaths—inhale on three counts, exhale on six counts. Blow air out through pursed lips.

This breathing technique is taught as "pranayama" by instructors in hatha yoga. It is the art of yogic breathing.

GO UNDER THE NEEDLE

The 1996 National Institutes of Health (NIH) Consensus Statement on Acupuncture found strong evidence that acupuncture can treat asthma effectively. Kim Jobst, MD, of Oxford University reports in an article for the *Journal of Alternative and Complementary Medicine* that, at the request of the NIH, he collected all the research on acupuncture and chronic lung diseases. Of the 16 studies he reviewed, he found that acupuncture was effective—reducing attacks and doses of drugs—in 62% of cases. Other research, including data from *The Journal of Traditional Chinese Medicine*, puts the success rate at closer to 85% or higher.

Dr. Firshein finds acupuncture to be an important part of any nonconventional treatment for asthma because it's helpful in maintaining proper lung function. It may work by stimulating certain responsive parts of the body's nervous system, which then transmit signals along the nerves and also produce biochemicals that influence other cells of the body. The nervous system also is linked to the hormonal system by way of the adrenal glands.

CONTROL YOUR ENVIRONMENT

Most asthmatics already know this, but it's good to mention that your home can have many triggers. Go through your house room by room to eliminate potential allergens, such as smoke, dust mites, mold, pet dander and water or chimney leaks. Also, install a carbon monoxide detector.

"It's very exciting to have all these different modalities for treating asthma," Dr. Firshein says. "It gives people a lot of options, a lot of choices, and they don't feel as threatened by the condition. They feel that they can do something to help themselves." Most important, these techniques look to cure the underlying ailments rather than simply suppress symptoms. Consider adding a physician formally schooled in these nonconventional modalities who can cooperate with your allergist or pulmonologist. It is a much more effective strategy for long-term health.

■■■■

Allergy Nation

Most Americans test positive for sensitivity to one or more allergens. The most common allergen is dust mites—27% of those tested responded positively.

Reacting to an allergen doesn't necessarily mean that you will develop allergies, but there is a strong correlation between the two.

Samuel Arbes, DDS, MPH, PhD, researcher, Rho, Inc. Chapel Hill, North Carolina, and leader of a survey of 10,500 individuals, reported in *Journal of Allergy and Clinical Immunology.*

Natural Therapies to Fight the Flu

Jamison Starbuck, ND, a naturopathic physician in family practice in Missoula, Montana. She is past president of the American Association of Naturopathic Physicians.

During the worst flu pandemic in history, the 1918 Spanish flu, naturopathic treatments—including hygiene, nutrition and homeopathy—saved more lives than conventional medicine. To create your own naturopathic flu defense, follow these steps...*

*To learn more natural flu-prevention strategies, read the book *Flu: Alternative Treatments and Prevention* by Randall Neustaedter, OMD. North Atlantic.

•**Be vigilant about hand-washing and hydration.** The flu virus enters your body via your respiratory tract, typically when you inhale infected droplets from a sick person's sneeze or cough. Try to keep your distance from people who are sneezing and coughing. The virus also can be transmitted if you touch an infected droplet or mucus from a sick person and then rub your eyes, nose or mouth. If the virus can attach itself to the walls of your nose, throat and/or lungs, it will stay there and multiply. Hand-washing before eating and after visiting any public place will lessen your exposure. Adequate hydration (½ ounce of water per pound of body weight daily) keeps your mucous membranes moist, which makes it more difficult for viruses to attach.

•**Boost your immunity.** Research shows that eating fruits, vegetables and grains boosts your immunity, while a diet rich in sugar, fats and salt increases your risk of getting sick.

During flu season, also take these: B-complex (find a supplement that contains at least 50 mg of vitamin B-6 and 800 micrograms of folic acid)…2,000 mg of vitamin C…and 2,000 mg of fish oil.

Caution: Do not take fish oil if you take *warfarin* (Coumadin) or another blood thinner.

•**Use a homeopathic remedy.** Several homeopathic flu-prevention remedies, such as Mucococcinum, Oscillococcinum and Influenzinum 200C, are available at health-food stores or through holistic practitioners. At the beginning of flu season, take one dose per the label instructions under the tongue once a week for three weeks. Then continue with one dose once every three weeks for the rest of the winter.

In my 20 years of practice, I have seen individually prescribed homeopathic remedies successfully treat the flu. If you get it, visit a practitioner trained in homeopathy in your area. You can find one on the National Center for Homeopathy Web site, *http://nationalcenterforhomeopathy.org*, or consult The American Association of Naturopathic Physicians, 866-538-2267, *www.naturopathic.org*.

•**Do not be afraid.** Fear causes stress, which lowers immunity. Speak to your doctor about your flu risk. Natural therapy is effective for most healthy people. A flu shot may be recommended for older adults and people with compromised immunity.

■ **More from Jamison Starbuck, ND…**

Cure for Stomach Flu

Doctor, this is my third bout this winter! What can I do to get over it for good?" Ken was in obvious distress, holding his belly and rocking back and forth. Ken had "stomach flu"—a catchall phrase for *gastroenteritis,* an acute inflammation of the lining of the stomach and intestines characterized by nausea, vomiting, abdominal discomfort and diarrhea. It is usually caused by a viral or bacterial infection. He was suffering yet another episode of these acute symptoms after following the advice of his medical doctor. Now he was ready to try a natural approach.

When medical doctors treat gastroenteritis, they recommend bed rest, bland food and lots of fluids. They typically prescribe antibiotics when patients have high fevers. After a few days of symptoms, most people recover—or so they think. If gastroenteritis is treated conventionally, you may fail to *fully* recover.

Here's why: The organisms that cause the infection also inflame intestinal membranes, and vomiting and diarrhea may have eliminated both the "bad" and "good" bacteria found in the intestines. This is a setup to make you more susceptible to repeat infections.

My naturopathic approach…

•**Limit your diet.** To rest the gastrointestinal tract and speed healing, drink chicken or vegetable broth and eat baked apples and/or pears (the pectin in these fruits soothes the stomach and helps stop the diarrhea) until your symptoms abate. Avoid dehydration by consuming at least 72 ounces of water per day while you have the flu. Also, drink chamomile, peppermint, ginger, black or green tea. These teas have antinausea and antivomiting properties. Make a strong tea using two tea bags per 12 ounces of water. Drink three to six cups daily, preferably on an empty stomach.

•**Use a mustard poultice.** This will relieve nausea and vomiting.

What to do: Combine one tablespoon of mustard powder with one cup of flour. Stir in enough water to make a smooth paste. Saturate a piece of cotton cloth about the size of a face-cloth with hot water from the faucet, wring it out and spread the paste over the cloth. Place it (paste-side up) over your abdomen. Cover with a dry cotton cloth, and then a hot water bottle or heating pad. Leave the poultice in place for 30 minutes. Apply twice a day.

•**Take an herbal tincture.** Clinical trials confirm that the herbs Oregon grape root and geranium have antimicrobial properties, while slippery elm and licorice reduce inflammation and promote tissue growth in the intestine. Make a mixture of equal parts of these tinctures, which are sold individually at most health-food stores. Take 60 drops of the combined tinctures in two ounces of water, on an empty stomach, four times per day for up to five days.

•**Try probiotics.** *Lactobacillus acidophilus* and *Bifidobacterium bifidum* replenish "friendly" bacteria in the bowels. Probiotics are available at health-food stores in powder, liquid or capsules. Take 10 billion colony-forming units (CFUs) each of L. acidophilus and B. bifidum in four divided doses daily for the duration of the illness and for three weeks after your symptoms have resolved.

■■■■

New Flu Test

A test diagnoses flu the same day, says Katherine A. Poehling, MD. That is especially important for older people and those with compromised immune systems or chronic diseases, and it could help prevent complications.

Cost for the test: About $20. Antiviral medicines generally shorten the course of the flu by one day if taken within 48 hours of initial symptoms. The best defense against flu is vaccination.

Katherine A. Poehling, MD, pediatrician in Winston Salem, North Carolina. She was leader of a study of influenza in more than 4,500 preschoolers, published in *The New England Journal of Medicine.*

■■■■

Statins vs. Flu

Statins may fight bird flu. Cholesterol-lowering drugs, including Zocor and Lipitor, may be effective for treating inflammation and fluid buildup associated with avian flu.

Also being investigated: The asthma drug albuterol, which may potentially remove fluid from the air sacs of the lungs.

Jeffrey R. Jacobson, MD, assistant professor of medicine, pulmonary and critical care medicine, University of Chicago.

■■■■

Legionnaires' Look-Out

Legionnaires' disease is on the rise, warns Janet E. Stout, PhD. This respiratory infection is caused by a bacteria most often found in the water-distribution and air-conditioning systems of large buildings and cruise ships. More than 20,000 cases occur nationwide each year. About one-quarter of those afflicted die. Symptoms—high fever, cough, headache and diarrhea—are similar to those of other illnesses, so the disease may go untreated until it is too late for antibiotics to work.

Self-defense: If you experience symptoms and recently have been in a hospital or hotel or on a cruise ship, ask to be tested for the disease.

Janet E. Stout, PhD, is microbiologist at Veterans Affairs Medical Center, Pittsburgh, the Special Pathogens Unit, and research assistant professor, Division of Infectious Diseases, University of Pittsburgh School of Medicine.

■■■■

Honey-Biotic?

Honey acts as a natural antibiotic, according to Peter Molan, PhD.

How it works: Honey's natural acidity creates an inhospitable environment for germs… and it contains a small amount of germ-killing hydrogen peroxide.

Important: Heat can destroy honey's beneficial properties, so buy the raw and unpasteurized kind. Honey can be used on most wounds. If you have a puncture wound, consult your doctor.

What to do: Work one tablespoon of warmed honey into a four-inch by four-inch gauze pad, then place it on the wound. Change the dressing at least twice daily until the wound heals.

Caution: Infants younger than age one should not eat honey.

Peter Molan, PhD, professor of biological sciences, University of Waikato, Hamilton, New Zealand.

■ ■ ■ ■

Antibiotics vs. Viruses

Bronchitis can't be cured with antibiotics, according to recent research.

Bronchitis sufferers who were otherwise healthy did not get better any faster by taking antibiotics.

Possible reason: Most bronchitis infections are caused by viruses, which antibiotics don't fight.

Best treatment: Drink lots of fluids, and take pain and fever relievers, such as *acetaminophen*.

Paul Little, MD, professor of primary care research, University of Southampton, Highfield, England, and author of a study of 640 bronchitis patients, published in *The Journal of the American Medical Association*.

■ ■ ■ ■

Tick Fever Help

Rocky Mountain spotted fever can be spread by the common brown dog tick. Until recently, it was thought that only two less common ticks could transmit the disease, which is found across the country and has a fatality rate as high as 20% when untreated. Rocky Mountain spotted fever is especially severe in children. Symptoms, including fever, nausea, vomiting, muscle pain, lack of appetite, severe headache and a rash, appear one to two weeks after infection.

Good news: Antibiotics are effective when given early.

Linda J. Demma, PhD, senior epidemiologist, Food-borne Disease Action Surveillance Network, Centers for Disease Control and Prevention, Atlanta, and leader of a study of tick transmission of Rocky Mountain spotted fever, published in *The New England Journal of Medicine*.

■ ■ ■ ■

Allergy Alert

Allergies can cause surprising symptoms. Any part of the body can become swollen or inflamed. A person can feel lethargic or cranky...have mood changes, joint pain, an irritable bowel or intestinal cramps. Look for triggers—a specific place or time when symptoms occur, such as at work, after consuming certain foods or beverages or after exposure to inhalants, such as pollen. If you can't figure out the triggers on your own, see an allergist.

Thomas Brunoski, MD, is a specialist in food and environmental allergies and nutritional medicine, Westport, Connecticut.

Winter Ailments: Folk Remedies for Colds, Coughs and Flu

Joan Wilen and Lydia Wilen are folk-remedy experts based in New York City. The sisters are coauthors of many books, including *Bottom Line's Healing Remedies: Over 1,000 Astounding Ways to Heal Arthritis, Asthma, High Blood Pressure, Varicose Veins, Warts and More!* Bottom Line Books. *www.BottomLineSecrets.com.*

Not every winter illness requires a trip to the doctor's office. The following time-tested folk remedies offer effective, inexpensive treatments for minor health complaints.

Important: Consult your doctor if your condition persists or grows worse.

COLDS

The average adult contracts between two and four colds each year, mostly between September and May. *Medical science has no cure for these highly contagious viral infections, but the following folk remedies can help ward off colds, ease symptoms and possibly shorten a cold's duration...*

•**Garlic.** Garlic contains *allicin*, which has been shown to reduce the severity of a cold. Eat four cloves of freshly crushed raw garlic three times a day until you have recovered.

•**Cinnamon, sage and bay.** Cinnamon contains compounds believed to reduce congestion. Sage can help sooth sore throats. Some Native American cultures have used bay leaves to clear breathing passages. Steep one-half teaspoon each of cinnamon and sage with a bay leaf in six ounces of hot water. Strain and add one tablespoon of lemon juice. Lemon helps reduce mucus buildup. If you like your tea sweet, add some honey.

•**Chicken soup.** The Mayo Clinic has said in its health newsletter that chicken soup can be an excellent treatment for head colds and other viral respiratory infections for which antibiotics are not helpful.

FLU

Influenza is a potentially serious viral infection. People often mistake colds for the flu. Colds take hold gradually and are not usually accompanied by severe aches or a fever. The onset of the flu is sudden, and symptoms include fever, severe muscle aches and fatigue.

•**Garlic and cognac.** A shot of cognac is a popular flu remedy in Germany, where it's thought to ease symptoms and help the body cleanse itself. Garlic helps clear mucus, among other potential benefits. Peel and dice a half-pound of garlic. Add one quart of 90-proof cognac, and seal the mixture in an airtight bottle. Store in a cool, dark place for two weeks. Strain out the garlic, and reseal the liquid in the bottle. Prepare a new batch each year.

To treat the flu: Add 20 drops to eight ounces of water. Drink threes glasses a day, one before each meal.

For prevention: Use 10 to 15 drops, instead of 20, per glass in flu season.

Important: This treatment is not advisable for people who have drinking problems or for children.

•**Sauerkraut.** Sauerkraut's concentration of lactic acid bacteria may weaken infections. Have two tablespoons of sauerkraut juice or about one-half cup of sauerkraut each day during flu season to reduce the chances of infection.

SORE THROATS

Experiment with these remedies until you find what works best for you…

•**Apple cider vinegar.** Vinegar is a powerful anti-inflammatory, and its acidity might help kill the bacteria that cause some sore throats. Add two teaspoons of apple cider vinegar to six ounces of warm water. Gargle with a mouthful, spit it out, then drink a mouthful. Continue this until the mixture is gone. Rinse your mouth with water to prevent the vinegar from eroding your teeth. Repeat the vinegar gargle every hour for as long as your sore throat persists.

•**Sage.** Sage is an anti-inflammatory. Add one teaspoon of dried sage to one six-ounce cup of boiling water. Steep for three to five minutes, strain, then gargle and swallow.

•**Lemon and honey.** Honey coats the throat, while lemon can temporarily reduce the mucus buildup that often accompanies a sore throat. Squeeze one lemon, add a teaspoon of honey and drink. Repeat every two hours.

•**Tongue stretching.** Stick out your tongue for 30 seconds, relax it for a few seconds, then repeat four times. This is believed to increase blood flow to the throat, speeding the healing process.

COUGHS

Try these folk remedies to figure out which works best for you…

•**Lemon, honey and olive oil.** Honey and olive oil coat and soothe, while lemon reduces mucus. Heat one cup of honey, a half cup of olive oil and the juice of one lemon over a medium flame for five minutes. Turn off the heat, and stir for two minutes to blend the ingredients. Consume one teaspoon of the mixture every two hours.

•**Vinegar and cayenne pepper.** Cayenne pepper contains *capsaicin*, a proven painkiller, while vinegar serves as an anti-inflammatory. Add a half cup of apple cider vinegar and one teaspoon of cayenne pepper to one-half cup of water. Add honey if desired. Take one tablespoon when your cough acts up and another tablespoon before bed.

•**Horseradish and honey.** Horseradish can help loosen mucus, while honey coats the throat. Grate one teaspoon of fresh, peeled horseradish into two teaspoons of honey. Consume one teaspoon every two to three hours.

•**Ginger.** Ginger is an anti-inflammatory that contains gingerols, which provide pain-reducing and sedative benefits. Chew a piece of fresh, peeled gingerroot when you feel the cough acting up, usually in the evening before bed. Chew until the ginger loses its kick.

•**Licorice root tea.** Licorice relieves the pain of irritated mucous membranes. Drink licorice root tea as long as your cough persists.

Note: Don't try licorice root if you have high blood pressure or kidney problems.

Say Good-Bye to Hay Fever: Natural Remedies That Work

Mark A. Stengler, ND, naturopathic physician in private practice, La Jolla, California…adjunct associate clinical professor at the National College of Natural Medicine, Portland, Oregon…author of many books, including *The Natural Physician's Healing Therapies* and coauthor of *Prescription for Natural Cures* (both from Bottom Line Books)…and author of the *Bottom Line/Natural Healing* newsletter.

Oh, the sneezing! About 50 million Americans suffer from upper respiratory tract symptoms due to airborne allergies. One of the most common is hay fever, which results from a reaction to pollen.

Pollen enters the nasal cavity and triggers a cascade of reactions that lead to the release of *histamine* and other inflammatory chemicals. This can cause sneezing, coughing and postnasal drip, a runny or congested nose and itchy, watery, red eyes with dark circles underneath. Hay fever can keep you awake at night, making you feel fatigued and generally terrible all day long.

The most widespread pollen allergen is ragweed. One plant can generate a million grains of pollen a day. Other offenders include sagebrush, redroot pigweed, lamb's quarter, Russian thistle (tumbleweed) and English plantain.

Even if none of the plants that cause hay fever are found in your area, you are still susceptible to exposure because the small, light, dry pollen grains are easily transported by wind. Scientists have found ragweed pollen two miles high in the air and up to 400 miles away from its original source.

PREVENTION STRATEGIES

Pollen season occurs during the spring, summer and fall, when pollen is released by trees, grasses and weeds. Pollen counts tend to be highest in the morning, especially on warm, dry, breezy days, and lowest during cool, rainy periods. The pollen concentration is available for most urban areas—check your newspaper. Another resource for pollen counts is the American Academy of Allergy, Asthma & Immunology's National Allergy Bureau at *www.aaaai.org/nab*. You can monitor pollen levels and plan accordingly. For example, allergy sufferers should try to stay indoors with the windows closed when pollen levels are high.

You can wear a dust and pollen mask designed to stop pollen from entering the nasal passageways (available at most pharmacies). You can use a high-efficiency particulate air (HEPA) purifier in your house, especially in your bedroom since pollen counts increase during the night.

DRUG THERAPIES

Several pharmaceutical medications can be used to treat hay fever, all of which can have side effects.

We all know about antihistamines, which are used to control excess mucus and reduce itching and sneezing. Examples include the prescription drugs *fexofenadine* (Allegra), *desloratadine* (Clarinex) and *cetirizine* (Zyrtec) and the over-the-counter (OTC) medications *loratadine* (Claritin) and *diphenhydramine* (Benadryl). *Cromolyn sodium* (Nasalcrom) is an OTC nasal spray antihistamine.

Potential side effects of oral medications include drowsiness and impaired coordination. The nasal spray can cause nasal irritation, nosebleeds, sinus pain, tightness in chest, wheezing and fever.

Decongestants are used for nasal congestion. A common OTC oral form is *pseudoephedrine* (Sudafed). *Phenylephrine* (NeoSynephrine, Sinex) is a widely used nasal spray. Decongestants may raise blood pressure, cause insomnia and anxiety. They should be avoided by people with high blood pressure and/or glaucoma (they can increase the eye's intraocular pressure). Decongestants should be taken for only a few days—long-term use causes increased blood vessel constriction, which worsens blood pressure.

Corticosteroid treatments contain small doses of steroids to reduce nasal inflammation and swelling. They prevent and treat most allergy symptoms. Common examples of prescription nasal corticosteroids include *fluticasone* (Flonase), *mometasone* (Nasonex) and *triamcinolone* (Nasacort). These nasal corticosteroid sprays can cause fungal infection of the sinuses and mouth.

Sometimes oral steroids are used for severe allergies. These are very powerful prescription medicines that should be used for only a short time (up to a few weeks). Short-term side effects may include weight gain, water retention, high blood pressure, mood swings and depression. Long-term side effects include increased risk for diabetes, cataracts, osteoporosis and muscle weakness.

I know firsthand the miseries of hay fever. *Fortunately, the natural approaches I describe below have worked extremely well for me and for my patients...*

NASAL RINSE

An effective technique for people prone to hay fever and/or sinusitis is nasal irrigation. This involves rinsing the nasal passages with a warm saline solution to reduce the concentration of pollen, dust and other allergens. It also helps to clear excess mucus from the nasal passageways. This is typically done with a neti pot, a small ceramic container with a narrow spout that allows you to pour water into your nostrils and sinus cavities. Neti pots are available at health-food stores for about $15.

To use a neti pot, mix one-quarter teaspoon of salt in a cup of warm water. Pour the solution into the neti pot. Tilt your head to the side, and insert the spout into the upper nostril. The solution will flow into the upper nostril and out the lower nostril. After a few seconds, remove the pot. With your head still tilted, blow through both nostrils. Do not cover one side of your nose—this will force the mucus and bacteria up into your sinuses. Repeat the rinse on the other side. It's messy, but it works. Use once

daily for low-grade allergies and twice daily for acute allergies.

An easier alternative is Sinus Rinse. You open a packet of premeasured saline and baking soda, pour it into the bottle that comes with the kit and add warm water. Push the tip of the bottle into one nostril, and squeeze the bottle so the solution comes out the other nostril. Repeat with the other nostril. Do this once or twice daily. A kit containing 50 premixed packets is available from Allergy Solutions for $12.95 (800-491-4300, *www.allergysolution.com*).

Important: To avoid introducing bacteria into your nasal passageways, clean the tip of the neti pot (or Sinus Rinse bottle) with alcohol between uses.

HOMEOPATHIC HELP

Homeopathy treats hay fever by desensitizing the immune system to the offending pollen(s)—or the symptoms they trigger. This is based on the principle that "like cures like"—that is, substances that cause allergy symptoms can be used in a highly diluted form to alleviate those same symptoms.

For example, ragweed, oak and grasses can be taken as individual remedies or as part of a combination remedy. If you know that you are allergic to ragweed pollen, you can take homeopathic ragweed to minimize your response. An allergist can do skin testing to determine which allergens affect you.

Homeopathic remedies are somewhat similar to conventional allergy shots, in which minute doses of the substances you're allergic to are injected under the skin. The advantage of the homeopathic approach is that it is convenient (it requires dissolving some pellets or a liquid solution under your tongue) and relatively inexpensive ($10 to $20 a month).

Researchers at the Southwest College of Naturopathic Medicine and Health Sciences in Tempe, Arizona, conducted a four-week, double-blind clinical trial comparing homeopathic preparations with a placebo during the regional allergy season from February to May. Participants included 40 men and women, ages 26 to 63, diagnosed with moderate to severe seasonal allergy symptoms. Those taking the homeopathic preparations had a 38% reduction in symptoms, such as watery eyes and sneezing, compared with a 26% decline for those using the placebo.

There are two homeopathic remedies that I recommend for the treatment of hay fever. Which one you take depends on your symptoms. They are available at most health-food stores. The dosage is two pellets of a 30C potency twice daily.

•**Allium cepa** (from onion) is for those with watery and burning eyes…runny nose… sneezing.

•**Euphrasia** (from the eyebright plant) is for hay fever that mainly affects only the eyes, causing burning, tearing and redness.

If you don't know which homeopathic remedy to use, try Sabadil Allergy by Boiron, available at health-food stores for about $10. This formula contains six remedies commonly used for hay fever. The typical dose is two tablets dissolved in the mouth every 15 minutes for one hour, then two pellets three times daily.

CHOOSING SUPPLEMENTS

The right supplements also help control hay fever. *My recommendations…*

•**Quercetin,** a type of plant pigment known as a flavonoid, is nature's antihistamine, with anti-inflammatory and antioxidant properties. It is found in onions, apples and green tea. It works best at a starting dosage of 1,000 mg three times daily for five days, followed by a maintenance dosage of 500 mg two or three times daily. Quercetin is very safe, and side effects are uncommon. Quercetin also works well when combined with vitamin C, which may help reduce allergy symptoms in some individuals. A typical dose for hay fever is 3,000 mg to 5,000 mg of vitamin C daily. Reduce the dosage if you develop loose stools. If you have a history of kidney stones, consult your doctor before taking vitamin C supplements.

•**Stinging nettle leaf** is a popular herbal treatment for the relief of hay fever. I have seen it help some patients when used at the first sign of hay fever symptoms. A randomized, double-blind study conducted at the National College of Naturopathic Medicine in Portland, Oregon, involved 69 people with hay fever who took 300 mg of a stinging nettle leaf supplement or a placebo daily. Researchers found that after one week, 58% of those who took stinging nettle leaf had a reduction in symptoms, such as sneezing and itchy eyes, compared with 37% of those who received a placebo.

Interestingly, nettle leaves are a natural source of vitamin C and quercetin. Stinging nettle leaf supplements should be avoided by those with kidney disease because they have a diuretic (water-excreting) effect. The type of stinging nettle leaf used in the study mentioned above is available from Eclectic Institute and can be found at health-food stores.

•**N-acetylcysteine** (NAC) is a great supplement to use if you are suffering from postnasal drip or coughing as the result of mucous formation. I find that 500 mg twice daily is helpful for patients. Side effects, such as nausea, constipation and diarrhea, are rare.

GETTING STARTED

When using homeopathic remedies and supplements, it's best to start two weeks before allergy season and then continue until the end of the season if the treatment is helping. Try quercetin first. If you do not get relief within one week, try stinging nettle leaf, NAC and/or a homeopathic treatment.

A book that I especially like is *Sinus Survival: A Self-Help Guide*, by Rob Ivker, DO (Tarcher).

Uncommon Knowledge About the Common Cold

William Schaffner, MD, chairman of the department of preventive medicine at Vanderbilt University School of Medicine, Nashville, is editor of the *Journal of Infectious Diseases*. He is president-elect of the National Foundation for Infectious Diseases Board of Directors.

The average American gets more than 100 colds in his/her lifetime, and scientists have amassed lots of information about the common cold. But misinformation still is widely circulated as fact.

Take the following quiz to see how much you really know about the common cold…

•*True or False?* **Colds are mainly spread by coughs and sneezes.**

False: The viruses that cause colds usually are spread by hand-to-hand, hand-to-nose or hand-to-object contact. The *rhinovirus*, the most common cold virus, flourishes in mucous membranes. Someone infected with the virus rubs his nose or eyes, picking up the virus on his fingers. He then touches you or deposits the virus on another surface (doorknob, telephone, etc.).

The virus can survive for 24 to 48 hours, so it can be readily picked up by the next person who comes along.

•*True or False?* **People with colds are highly contagious before they experience symptoms.**

True: You're most contagious in the 24 hours before symptoms start. You may feel healthy, but the virus is incubating—and spreading. Colds often are transmitted during this period because people who are infected aren't yet staying home—and other people aren't avoiding them the way they would someone who is coughing or sneezing.

•*True or False?* **Antimicrobial soap kills cold viruses.**

False: Antimicrobial soap kills bacteria, not the viruses that cause colds. The best protection against colds is to wash your hands often with warm, soapy water. It takes about a minute of washing to remove viruses from your hands.

Waterless alcohol-based hand sanitizers can be helpful when soap and water aren't available. Hand sanitizers such as Purell and Nexcare kill cold viruses, as do disposable alcohol towelettes.

•*True or False?* **Being cold increases the risk of getting a cold.**

False: Generations of moms have said, "Bundle up or you'll catch a cold"—but the best current evidence indicates that Mom was wrong.

In one well-regarded study, scientists divided volunteers into a "warm" group and a group that was damp and chilled. They exposed people in both groups to cold viruses. There was no difference in the incidence of subsequent colds between the two groups.

Opposing view: In a study reported in *Journal of Family Practice*, scientists did find an increase in colds in volunteers who soaked their feet in icy water for 20 minutes. This wasn't a controlled experiment, however. The scientists didn't know, for example, if the volunteers who got sick had more contact with people who already had colds than those who didn't get sick.

Cold weather brings an increase in colds, but being cold doesn't seem to be a factor.

•*True or False?* **Vitamin C has been proven to reduce the duration and/or severity of colds.**

False: Ever since the publication of Linus Pauling's book *Vitamin C and the Common Cold*, millions of Americans have attempted to prevent and/or treat colds by taking enormous amounts of vitamin C—as much as 1,000 milligrams (mg) every few hours. Since then, many studies have looked at the connection between colds and vitamin C. Most have been inconclusive—and many showed no benefit at all.

In large doses, vitamin C inhibits the effects of *histamine*, a body chemical that causes sniffles and other cold symptoms, but studies have not shown that it prevents colds.

Caution: Vitamin C is cleared through the kidneys. Taking large amounts can cause the vitamin to crystallize and result in kidney stones. Drink more water than usual if you decide to take extra vitamin C—and don't exceed 250 mg to 500 mg daily.

•*True or False?* **Yellow or green mucus indicates a serious infection.**

False: People who develop yellow or greenish mucus often rush to their doctors to ask for antibiotics because they believe that discolored mucus indicates a serious bacterial infection.

Colds can cause either clear, watery mucus or mucus that's thick and discolored. The coloration means that there's inflammation and more white blood cells. These immune cells are present in both viral and bacterial infections. Discolored mucus isn't a useful way to distinguish one from the other—and it doesn't mean that your cold is more serious or that it will last longer.

•*True or False?* **We get fewer colds as we get older.**

True: There are approximately 200 different viruses that cause colds. Each time your immune system is exposed to one of these viruses, it develops antibodies that make you immune to that particular strain. By the time you reach your 60s or 70s and have a lifetime of colds behind you, you have developed immunity to many—but not all—of the circulating cold viruses.

•*True or False?* **Stress increases the likelihood of getting a cold.**

False: There are theoretical reasons to think that emotional stress could increase the risk of getting a cold, but it has never been shown conclusively.

Studies have shown that chronic stress decreases the immune system's ability to suppress infections. But stress is ubiquitous—nearly everyone reports having stress in the days or weeks before a survey—so it's difficult to link it with illness.

•*True or False?* **Hot tea eases cold symptoms.**

True: Black and green tea both contain theophylline, a mild bronchodilator. Drinking tea when you have a cold may open the airways and make breathing easier. The heat and steam from the liquid also thin mucus and ease congestion.

Chicken soup also is a traditional remedy for colds—but don't expect too much. Though it provides extra fluids and the steam eases congestion, chicken soup cannot cure a cold, despite what many people think.

■ ■ ■ ■

Bacteria Threat

Common bacteria may cause blindness, says a noted ophthalmologist.

Recent study: The bacteria that causes respiratory infections, *Chlamydia pneumoniae*, was found in six of nine samples from patients who had age-related macular degeneration, the leading cause of blindness in people age 55 and older in the US. C. pneumoniae also has been linked to coronary artery disease, heart attack and cerebrovascular disease (related to the blood supply to the brain).

Theory: The bacteria cause inflammation, a factor in the development of macular degeneration.

Self-defense: Eat a heart-healthy diet, and avoid smoking.

Joan W. Miller, MD, is professor and chair, department of ophthalmology, Harvard Medical School, and chief of Ophthalmology at the Massachusetts Eye and Ear Infirmary, Boston. She is senior author of a study, published in *Graefe's Archive for Clinical and Experimental Ophthalmology.*

Exercise Can Improve Immunity

David Nieman, Dr.PH, director, Health, Leisure and Exercise Sciences, Appalachian State University, Boone, North Carolina. Dr. Nieman was president of the International Society of Exercise Immunology for two terms, and is the author of nine books, including *Nutritional Assessment*. McGraw-Hill. He has also contributed over 200 peer-reviewed articles in books and journals.

If you want to avoid a nasty cold this winter, go for a nice, brisk walk. Studies have shown that people who walk briskly for 45 minutes most days of the week have just half the number of sick days caused by colds or sore throats as non-exercisers. David Nieman, Dr.PH, director of the Appalachian State University Health, Leisure and Exercise Sciences in Boone, North Carolina, has researched the impact of exercise on human cells for more than 20 years.

EXERCISE AND IMMUNE BOOSTING

Dr. Nieman says that moderate aerobic exercise creates favorable immune changes, including improvements in the killer T-cell function and improved immune system surveillance, which is the body's ability to detect and defend against bugs. This improvement is triggered every time you exercise and lasts for one to three hours after the activity. The key, says Dr. Nieman, is frequency. Even though the change is just hours a day, over time it becomes protective. If you prefer, say, three 15-minute segments instead of 45 minutes, Dr. Nieman says it is probably equally effective as a cold fighter, but he can't confirm that until he completes research, now under way.

TOO MUCH OF A GOOD THING

Dr. Nieman does have one important caveat about exercise, however—beware of the more-must-be-better trap. Overexercising, which is 90-plus minutes per day or running 60 or more miles a week, increases vulnerability to illness. Marathon runners, for example, are six times more likely to get ill in the one to two weeks following a race because excessive exercise suppresses the immune system. Dr. Nieman says that it pops back up to normal quickly, but to get around the suppressed immunity period, superathletes need to be particularly careful to follow the rules of good health—avoid exposure to germs, eat healthfully and get enough sleep. In fact, studies have proven that lack of sleep as well as rapid weight loss and stress cause immune suppression.

Should you continue exercising if you are getting or have a cold or the flu? Not if you have fever, aches and pains that are symptomatic of flu or other systemic illnesses. Heavy exercising will make symptoms worse and last longer, says Dr. Nieman. In the case of a simple cold, though, exercise is neutral—it will neither hurt nor help you.

As to the old saw that cold weather can increase vulnerability to colds and flu, Dr. Nieman says it's unlikely, assuming that your body is not cold, so dress warmly.

His advice: Get out and move whatever the season—there is every reason to believe you are doing yourself a favor.

■■■■

Moderate Exercise May Fight Colds

Researchers studied 115 women who were sedentary and either overweight or obese. Half performed moderate exercise, such as brisk walking, for 30 to 45 minutes five days a week. The other half attended a once-weekly 45-minute stretching class.

Result: Over 12 months, 48% of the stretchers had at least one cold, compared with only 30% of the exercisers.

Theory: Moderate exercise temporarily increases white blood cell production, which may help guard against infection.

Cornelia Ulrich, PhD, associate member/associate professor, Fred Hutchinson Cancer Center, Seattle.

■■■■

Inoculations for Adults

Have a chickenpox vaccination if you have not had the disease, or aren't sure if you've had it. Get hepatitis B shots if you have been sexually active with more than one partner in the past six months. Have a flu shot annually after age 49 and a pneumoccocal shot once after age 64. Be vaccinated against measles, mumps and rubella if you were born in 1957 or later and have not had measles or mumps, or are not sure whether you had the diseases or a vaccination. Get a tetanus and diphtheria shot once every 10 years.

Raymond A. Strikas, MD, a preventive medicine specialist practicing in Atlanta and former associate director for adult immunization, National Immunization Program, Centers for Disease Control and Prevention, Atlanta.

■■■■

Unstuffy Nose

Relieve a stuffy nose by alternately thrusting your tongue against the roof of your mouth, then pressing one finger between your eyebrows. This causes the vomer and ethmoid bones to move up and down, which helps loosen congestion. After 20 seconds or so, your sinuses will start to drain.

Lisa DeStefano, DO, a neuromusculoskeletal medicine specialist, Michigan State University, DOP, a medical group practice in East Lansing.

■■■■

The Strep Attack

The most effective strep-throat treatment is a group of antibiotics called *cephalosporins*, sold as Cefpodoxime and Cefdinir. They work better in four to five days than *penicillin* or *amoxicillin* in 10 days.

Children given penicillin were back at the doctor within three weeks 25% of the time… those treated with amoxicillin went back 18% of the time. Only 7% of children treated with cephalosporins saw the doctor a second time.

Michael Pichichero, MD, professor of microbiology and immunology, University of Rochester Medical Center, Rochester, New York, and leader of a review of treatment of more than 11,000 children with strep throat, reported in Interscience Conference on Antimicrobial Agents and Chemotherapy proceedings.

Immunity Boosters: Proven Ways to Stay Healthy

Michael F. Roizen, MD, chief wellness officer at the Cleveland Clinic, Ohio, is coauthor of *YOU: The Smart Patient* (Free Press). Dr. Roizen has cowritten *YOU: The Owner's Manual* (Collins), and served on the boards of five nonprofit foundations. He is former chair of a Food and Drug Administration advisory committee and has published over 160 peer-reviewed papers.

It's amazing that we're not sick all the time. We are attacked more than 100 million times a day by viruses, bacteria and other disease-causing organisms. Our hands alone harbor up to two million germs. The only reason we're not continually sick is that the immune system is remarkably effective at recognizing and fighting threats.

Many harmful organisms are blocked by barriers, such as skin and mucous membranes, that prevent harmful organisms from getting into the body.

Those that get past the initial barriers are spotted by antibodies and attacked by a barrage of immune cells. The antibodies "remember" individual pathogens and attack and neutralize them during subsequent exposures.

FLAWS IN THE SYSTEM

The immune system isn't perfect, however. Immune cells aren't always effective—due to nutritional deficiencies, emotional stress and aging.

If the immune system has never been exposed to a particular virus or bacterium, it may not be able to mount an effective defense. Also, viruses and bacteria can develop their own defenses, which make them harder to detect and eliminate. In addition, the immune system can mistake healthy tissues for foreign invaders and launch an attack. This is what happens in autoimmune diseases, such as lupus.

Almost half of all deaths are due to infection or other immune-related problems. Even some cancers are caused by infectious organisms that break down the immune system.

Here's how to build up your immune system…

IMMUNITY BOOSTERS

Limiting exposure to harmful organisms is one of the best preventive measures. Wash your hands after you shake hands or touch surfaces that others have touched. Avoid people who are sneezing or coughing. These measures alone can significantly cut infection from colds or flu.

Also helpful…

•**Stay social.** People with active social lives and those who participate in religious or community groups are less likely to experience depression than those without social ties. Depression reduces immune response, mainly by inhibiting the activity of "attack" cells called T and B cells.

Get professional help if you're experiencing depression. The majority of depressed patients who receive medication or therapy improve within three months—and nearly all of them improve within six months.

•**Exercise daily—but don't overdo it.** People who get regular exercise and take care of themselves in other ways—eating nutritious meals, not smoking, etc.—can improve immune response. Symptoms of depression also can be reduced by exercise. Thirty minutes a day is optimal for most people.

Caution: Exercising more than two hours daily actually causes immunity to decline.

•**Manage stress.** Not only does stress weaken immunity, but poor responses to stress—such as smoking, not eating healthfully and not exercising—are linked to infection. Not getting enough sleep is both a cause and a result of stress and can impair the activity of infection-fighting T cells and B cells.

Stress reducers: Set aside 20 minutes to listen to music or meditate…breathe deeply for a few minutes…go for a walk or engage in other exercise.

•**Get enough omega-3s.** The omega-3 fatty acids in nuts and fish have been shown to reduce depression and improve immunity. Have one-quarter cup of walnuts daily…three servings of fish weekly…or take two grams of a fish oil supplement daily.

•**Boost vitamin C.** Studies indicate that vitamin C may prevent infection by boosting levels of T cells and B cells. The optimal dosage is 500 milligrams (mg) twice daily. You can get this much vitamin C with several daily servings of vitamin C–rich foods, such as tomatoes, bell peppers and citrus fruits—or you can take a supplement.

•**Favor flavonoids.** These vitamin-like substances in fruits, vegetables and whole grains minimize age-related declines in immune function. You need about 31 mg of flavonoids daily.

Best sources: Cranberry juice (13 mg per eight-ounce glass)…tomato juice (7.2 mg per eight-ounce glass)…apples (4.2 mg per medium apple)…strawberries (4.2 mg per cup)…broccoli (4.2 mg per cup)…onions (3 mg per small onion)…red wine (3 mg per five-ounce glass).

•**Avoid sugar.** Sugary foods, such as candy, cakes, cookies, etc., can drive blood glucose levels above 250 milli-moles per liter of blood (a normal level is between 65 and 140). Elevated blood sugar impairs the ability of immune cells to destroy bacteria.

How to Stop Staph

Jay R. Kostman, MD, chief, infectious diseases division, Penn Presbyterian Medical Center, Philadelphia.

Staph infections used to be a hospital-based problem, treatable with available antibiotics. Now they occur with increasing frequency outside of the hospital. The new, antibiotic-resistant strain of staph is known as MRSA, methicillin-resistant Staphylococcus Aureus. It is resistant to antibiotics such as *penicillin* and *amoxicillin* and it turns ordinary scrapes and cuts into potentially fatal problems.

According to Jay Kostman, MD, chief, infectious diseases division at the Penn Presbyterian Medical Center in Philadelphia, many common wound infections that would have responded to routine antibiotics are now MRSA infections, and they resist traditional treatment. Staph bacteria are everywhere, including on the body, but they're harmless unless there is a break in the skin. In places where people gather and literally rub shoulders, and sometimes towels (think gyms, Jacuzzis and locker rooms), a cut, scrape or even a rug burn can be an invitation for the bacteria to hop in and cause trouble.

Athletic teams, children at camp and toddlers in day-care centers in close quarters are all vulnerable to the possibility of MRSA infection. It can also result from everyday falls on a sidewalk—or anywhere that provides an opportunity for the bacteria to penetrate the outer layers of the skin to the underlying tissue, perhaps eventually entering the blood stream.

HOW TO PROTECT YOURSELF

The first and best precaution is to cleanse all wounds thoroughly, even small ones. Cover with a bandage to keep the area clean, until healed. Dr. Kostman advises to wash minor cuts with soap and water or an antibacterial soap. A topical antibiotic such as Neosporin may be applied after cleaning, but OTC ointments should be used sparingly, as bacteria are becoming resistant to these everyday antidotes. For deeper injuries, seek medical attention immediately.

As a rule, careful cleaning protects against infection. But watch the wound as it heals to be sure no infection sets in, says Dr. Kostman. *Watch for these changes, which might signal infection…*

•**Pain or tenderness** at the site of the wound.

•**Fever,** even a slight one.

•**Redness around the wound** (especially red streaks running up from the wound site).

•**Drainage of pus.**

If any symptoms develop, see your doctor right away to be tested for MRSA or other bacteria. Several types of antibiotics are effective for MRSA. These include *trimethoprim, sulfamethoxazole* (Bactrim), *clindamycin* (Cleocin), and *linezolid* (Zyvox) or *vancomycin* (Vancocin). These medications must be taken for up to two weeks.

MRSA infections can both develop and escalate, including into a bloodstream infection, startlingly fast, sometimes in hours. This kind of rapidly moving infection is a medical emergency—do not wait for the next morning to call the doctor...get to the ER right away. Danger signals include a fever that reaches 102 degrees and is accompanied by shaking, chills, severe muscle aches and pains and altered thinking. Other infections may remain localized, says Dr. Kostman, typically showing up as an abscess with extreme tenderness and redness, similar in appearance to a boil.

Even after minor cuts and scrapes, remain vigilant for some time, because MRSA infection can develop even a few weeks later. As a rule, says Dr. Kostman, the danger of infection decreases sharply once a wound has closed, but even then it takes some time to be completely clear of risk.

"Handy" Guide to Your Health— Look at Your Nails

Jamison Starbuck, ND, a naturopathic physician in family practice in Missoula, Montana. She is past president of the American Association of Naturopathic Physicians.

Since the time of Hippocrates, most doctors have examined patients' fingernails during routine physical exams. That's because the fingernail is an important window through which an astute physician can see signs of some diseases and even clues about a person's nutritional status, lifestyle and emotional health.

Fingernails should be strong, with a light pink color to the nail bed (the skin on which the nail rests). A few white spots and/or lines are usually due to injury to the nail bed and are harmless. However, if you have any of the conditions described below, see your physician for an evaluation and treatment, such as the use of medication and/or supplements. *What to look for...*

•**Brittle, dry, splitting nails,** with deep longitudinal (from the cuticle to the fingernail tip) ridges, can indicate thyroid disease, usually hypothyroidism (an underactive thyroid). It also can be a sign of a mineral deficiency, particularly calcium or zinc.

•**Nails loosening or separating from the nail bed** can indicate hyperthyroidism (an overactive thyroid). This condition also can be a sign of psoriasis (a chronic skin disease) or a reaction to synthetic nails or a nail injury.

•**Nail pitting** (deep depressions) can indicate psoriasis, psoriatic arthritis (a condition with symptoms of both arthritis and psoriasis) or chronic dermatitis (skin rash). Nail pitting also can be seen in people with *alopecia areata*, an autoimmune disease that causes sudden patchy hair loss, usually in the scalp or beard.

•**Nails curved around enlarged fingertips** (known as clubbing) can be a harmless condition that runs in families, or it can be a sign of low oxygen in the blood, a common marker for chronic lung disease.

•**Hollowed or dipped nails** (known as spoon nails) are often associated with an iron deficiency. A three-year-old boy I recently saw had 10 tiny scooped-out fingernails that could have each contained a drop of water.

•**Opaque (white) nails** with a dark band at the fingertip (known as Terry's nails) can be a harmless sign of aging, or it can indicate cardiac disease, particularly congestive heart failure.

•**Yellow nails** can be due to nicotine stains, bacterial infection, fungus in the nail and nail bed, chronic bronchitis or lymphedema (swelling and congestion of the lymph system).

•**Bitten nails** can indicate anxiety, severe stress or compulsive behavior.

The best way to keep your nails healthy is to keep them clean, trim and warm. Don't pick at hangnails. Clip them. Limit nail polish remover use to twice a month (it dries nails and makes them more brittle). Protect your nails from harsh chemicals by wearing gloves and avoiding the use of synthetic nails. With normal growth, an injured nail will be replaced in four to six months.

When Hiccups Are Serious—And 10 Ways To Stop Them

Anil Minocha, MD, is professor of medicine, Louisiana State University and VA Medical Center. He is author of the *Handbook of Digestive Diseases*. Slack Incorporated. *http://minochahealth.typepad.com.*

Charles Osborne, an Iowa farmer, holds the world record for the longest bout of hiccups. He started hiccupping in 1922 (at rates up to 40 times a minute) and didn't stop until shortly before his death about 68 years later.

Fortunately, hiccups such as this are rare—though almost everyone gets the hiccups sometimes. They usually disappear on their own within a few minutes, causing nothing more than mild discomfort—or a little embarrassment if the "hic" pops out at an inappropriate time. But they can be the sign of a serious problem.

ANATOMY OF A HICCUP

Hiccups are caused by an involuntary spasm of the diaphragm, the dome-shaped muscle that separates the chest from the abdomen and is largely responsible for breathing. The spasms are thought to be triggered by activation (or irritation) of the phrenic or vagus nerves, which carry signals to the brain from the diaphragm and other respiratory muscles.

Most hiccup cycles are brief. Something stimulates the nerve pathways...the diaphragm contracts...and vocal cords briefly close and open, causing the "hic" sound. Though bouts of hiccups can be uncomfortable, they become a health concern only when they're persistent (lasting longer than 48 hours) or intractable (lasting two months or more).

WHEN TO WORRY

Persistent hiccups aren't necessarily a serious symptom, but they do tend to occur in people with an underlying medical problem. *Examples...*

•**Metabolic or kidney disorders.** These can cause abnormal levels of *electrolytes* (minerals that conduct electrical signals), an increase in waste products or abnormal levels of carbon dioxide in the blood, each of which can cause persistent hiccups in some people.

•**An irritation of nerves in the inner ear,** sometimes caused by a foreign body (often a hair) that presses against the eardrum.

•**Gastroesophageal reflux disease** (GERD). Frequent heartburn can irritate nerves in the esophagus and respiratory system, causing frequent hiccups.

•**An infection or tumor** in the brain or spinal cord.

Anyone who has severe or frequent hiccups that don't go away within 48 hours should see a doctor. In addition to taking a medical history and performing a physical exam (including an ear exam), the doctor will probably order blood tests to check for infection or metabolic disorders. He/she also may order a chest CT scan to look for a tumor or abnormalities affecting the diaphragm or the vagus or phrenic nerves.

PREVENTION

Hiccups often can be prevented. *Best steps...*

•**Don't overeat.** Excessively large meals cause the stomach to distend. It then pushes against the diaphragm and may irritate the phrenic nerves.

•**Take care of heartburn.** People who treat heartburn with medications, such as *omeprazole* (Prilosec), often have a reduction in hiccups.

•**Drink water or juice** instead of carbonated beverages. The carbon dioxide in colas, beer and other carbonated beverages can cause the stomach to expand and exert pressure on the diaphragm.

•**Manage stress.** People who experience a lot of emotional stress tend to "gulp" air, some of which passes through the esophagus into the stomach, causing stomach distension. Stress reducers include deep-breathing exercises... relaxation techniques, such as meditation and yoga...and regular exercise.

Also helpful: Patients with chronic stress sometimes improve when they take a low-dose antidepressant at bedtime. Drugs such as *imipramine* (Tofranil) or *amitriptyline* (Elavil) can improve sleep and reduce stress, even in those without depression. Talk to your doctor if you feel chronically stressed out.

•**Drink body-temperature liquids.** Any sudden change in temperature—from drinking hot or cold beverages, walking from a warm room into the cold or switching from hot to cold water in the shower—can trigger hiccups.

•**Avoid alcohol, spicy foods and tobacco.** Alcohol relaxes the diaphragm and makes it more sensitive to hiccup triggers. Smoking and some foods—especially spicy foods—can irritate the nerves that control normal contractions of your diaphragm.

•**Ask about medications.** A variety of prescription drugs have been used to prevent hiccups. These include *nifedipine* (Adalat, Procardia), used to treat high blood pressure...*baclofen* (Kemstro, Lioresal), a muscle relaxant...and *diazepam* (Valium), a sedative. Because these drugs can have significant side effects, doctors recommend them only for patients with severe hiccups who aren't helped by other measures.

HOME REMEDIES

Folklore is filled with hiccup remedies. None have been adequately studied in clinical trials, but some do appear to help, such as eating a spoonful of sugar or having someone startle you. *Other remedies...*

•**Drink water through a straw while** holding your ears closed with your fingers. This appears to interrupt the "arc" of nervous signals that travel from the diaphragm to the brain. Gargling, which activates the throat muscles, may have a similar effect.

•**Take a deep breath, hold it for as long** as you comfortably can, then breathe out. The respiratory muscles aren't working when you hold your breath. This can reduce the transmission of the nerve signals that trigger hiccups.

•**Breathe into a paper bag for about a minute.** It increases blood levels of carbon dioxide, which seems to reduce hiccups in some people. It's also good during periods of stress. It focuses your attention on something other than the stressful situation and can help reduce the swallowing and gulping of air.

•**Try acupressure.** Rest the heels of the palms on both cheekbones while placing the hands over the eyes. Massage the temples by pulling the thumbs in toward the palm. After massaging, remove the hands from the eyes and lightly press the tip of the nose with a fingertip.

Best Way to Beat Wintertime Bugs

Mark A. Stengler, ND, naturopathic physician in private practice, La Jolla, California...adjunct associate clinical professor at the National College of Natural Medicine, Portland, Oregon...author of many books, including *The Natural Physician's Healing Therapies* and coauthor of *Prescription for Natural Cures* (both from Bottom Line Books)...and author of the *Bottom Line/Natural Healing* newsletter.

In winter, we spend more time indoors...and in close contact with one another. This gives cold and flu viruses an ideal opportunity to spread themselves around and make people miserable. However, you *can* get through the cold months without becoming sick.

Key: Supercharging your immune system so that it is strong enough to withstand the barrage of wintertime bugs.

THE BETA GLUCAN BOOST

One of the most thoroughly researched and effective substances for strengthening the immune system is *beta glucan*—a fiber-type *polysaccharide* (complex sugar) naturally found in most yeasts, some mushrooms, oats, barley and rye. Chinese and Japanese healers have used mushrooms for more than 2,000 years—but only in the last few decades have we realized that beta glucan is partially responsible for mushrooms' beneficial effects.

There are many types of beta glucan, and they vary in molecular structure, biological activity and health benefits.

Example: Oat-derived beta glucan lowers cholesterol by mixing with cholesterol-based bile acids in the digestive tract, which are then excreted, causing the body to pull cholesterol from the bloodstream to replace the bile acids. It also helps control blood glucose (sugar) levels in diabetes, perhaps by lowering the rate at which food breaks down and glucose is released into the bloodstream.

When it comes to strengthening immunity, though, a unique superstar is the beta glucan from baker's yeast. This is *beta-1,3/1,6 glucan* or *whole glucan particle 3-6,* often referred to by the brand name WGP 3-6. Of the more than 800 studies on beta glucan, many have focused on WGP 3-6 and its role in promoting good health.

Dozens of studies have established that beta glucan from baker's yeast boosts the immune system's effectiveness against…

●**Cancer.** One problem for cancer patients is that radiation as well as chemotherapy inhibit production of disease-fighting white blood cells. WGP 3-6 supplements raise white blood cell counts during and after treatment. When WGP 3-6 is used with *monoclonal antibody therapy*—in which antibodies attach to cancer cells to better target and destroy them during chemotherapy and/or radiation—tumors shrink more and patient survival times increase.

●**Postoperative and antibiotic-resistant infections.** A study in *Archives of Surgery* showed that surgical patients who took a type of beta glucan similar to WGP 3-6 were 39% less likely to get postoperative infections than patients who did not take it. A 1998 animal study on antibiotic-resistant strains of bacteria, including *staphylococci,* showed that beta glucan combined with antibiotics resulted in a synergistic reaction so powerful that eight to 20 times more bacteria than usual were required to cause infection.

●**Anthrax.** In a 2003 study, mice were given a daily oral dose of WGP 3-6 for one week before being infected with anthrax. All of the mice treated with WGP 3-6 survived, while half of the untreated mice died. In separate tests, among mice infected first and then given WGP 3-6 for 10 days, 80% to 90% survived, compared with just 30% of untreated mice.

CHOOSING AND USING BETA GLUCAN

Though beta glucan is found in some yeast foods, it is not possible to eat enough to get significant immune benefits. Also, the yeast cell includes the carbohydrate *mannan* and the protein *mannoprotein,* which can interfere with immune-stimulating effects, cause digestive problems and/or trigger allergic reactions, such as skin rashes. That's why it is best to get WGP 3-6 through supplements.

Choose a brand that is highly purified to remove mannan and mannoprotein. I like ImmunotiX 3-6, made by Xymogen (800-647-6100, *www.xymogen.com*). Its main ingredient, the WGP 3-6 product made by Biothera, appears to be very safe. ImmunotiX 3-6 is available from health-care practitioners and costs $83 for 60 500-mg capsules.

Buyer beware: Some health-food stores carry beta glucan supplements that are only minimally processed. These products contain mannan and mannoprotein, and so do not provide the same health benefits as purified WGP 3-6.

Also: In many brands, beta glucan comprises only 10% to 30% of the product—so you would need to take up to 10 pills to get the same benefits as from one capsule of ImmunotiX, which is nearly 100% WGP 3-6.

The appropriate dose of WGP 3-6 depends on your health status, so follow the guidelines below. Dosages listed are for teens and adults. For children ages two to 12, halve the dosages by giving WGP 3-6 half as often (do not cut the pills). I have seen no studies on WGP 3-6 use in children younger than age two.

●**For a general immune system boost**—500 mg of WGP 3-6 once a day during the winter.

●**People who frequently are exposed to infectious agents** (for instance, health-care providers and schoolteachers)—500 mg twice daily during winter.

●**Adults age 65 and older**—500 mg twice daily during winter.

●**Athletes training intensely and anyone under stress**—500 mg twice daily for as long as the situation continues.

●**Cancer patients** (except those on immuno-suppressant drugs)—500 mg twice daily during treatment and for five years after, under an oncologist's supervision.

●**For any active infection, including a cold or flu**—500 mg four times daily, starting as soon as symptoms begin and continuing until symptoms are gone.

Caution: If you have an autoimmune disease, such as lupus or rheumatoid arthritis, take WGP 3-6 only under a doctor's guidance because, in

■ ■ ■ ■

theory, it might overstimulate your immune system and worsen your condition. Do not take WGP 3-6 if you have an active or a chronic yeast infection (because the product is made from yeast and might exacerbate symptoms)...if you are a transplant patient taking immunosuppressive medication...or if you are pregnant or breast-feeding (as a general precaution).

VACCINATION CONCERNS

While too few people seem to know about the health benefits of beta glucan, nearly everyone has heard of—and has questions about—the flu shot. The decision on whether or not to get vaccinated against the flu must be made on an individual basis.

Flu shots contain several inactive (killed) flu viruses that stimulate the immune system to produce antibodies against the flu. If you are at heightened risk for suffering severe effects of flu, speak with your doctor about the pros and cons of vaccination.

Limitation: The FDA and vaccine manufacturers must predict which flu virus strains are most likely to appear the next winter. If their estimates are wrong, the vaccine offers little protection. In contrast, natural therapies strengthen the immune system overall and so fight all strains.

If you don't fall into a high-risk category and are relatively healthy, I suggest skipping the flu shot and instead using natural immune boosters. These include WGP 3-6...the herbs echinacea and astragalus...high-potency multivitamin supplements plus additional vitamin C and vitamin D...and the homeopathic medicine *influenzinum,* which is made from various flu viruses and helps prevent flu by strengthening the immune system's protective response.

My main concern about the flu shot is *thimerosal,* a preservative that has been eliminated from most vaccines for childhood diseases yet still is used in most flu shots.

Problem: Thimerosal contains mercury, and mercury can damage the central nervous system and kidneys. A typical flu shot contains 25 micrograms (mcg) of mercury. In addition, the flu shot poses a risk for allergic reactions—especially for people who are allergic to eggs, because it contains egg protein. There also is a very slight risk of contracting Guillain-Barré syndrome, a rare nervous system disorder. More common side effects include pain at the injection site, muscle aches, fever and fatigue.

Safer: The vaccine *FluZone* (go to *www.fluzone.com* for more information), approved for adults and for children age six months and older. Just be sure to get the single-dose, prefilled syringe, which requires no preservatives and contains no thimerosal.

Caution: The formula used in a multidose vial of FluZone does contain thimerosal and has 25 mcg of mercury per dose. FluZone should not be used if you are allergic to eggs...have a bleeding disorder, such as hemophilia...or take blood-thinning medication, such as aspirin or *warfarin* (Coumadin).

Another option is the flu vaccine *Fluarix* (*www.fluarix.com*), which also comes as a single-use, prefilled syringe and contains only a minute trace of thimerosal—less than 1 mcg. Not all conventional doctors provide it, so you may need to get it from a holistic health-care practitioner. Cost is equivalent to that of the standard shot, and health insurance may or may not cover it. Fluarix is approved for adults age 18 years and older. It should not be used by anyone who is allergic to eggs or who has had a prior severe reaction to a flu vaccine.

The nasal spray flu vaccine *FluMist* (*www.flumist.com*) is thimerosal-free. However, because FluMist has attenuated (weakened) live viruses rather than inactive viruses, it has a slight risk of causing the flu and is appropriate only for healthy people ages two to 49. Side effects include nasal congestion, sore throat and/or fever. FluMist should not be used by pregnant women...children or teens on long-term aspirin therapy...anyone with asthma...Guillain-Barré patients...people who have severely compromised immunity, such as organ transplant recipients and AIDS patients...or anyone allergic to eggs. FluMist is sold over the counter, though not all pharmacies carry it. It is somewhat more expensive than the standard flu shot. Insurance sometimes covers it.

Whether or not you opt for the flu shot, do tell your friends about beta glucan. The more people who are protected against winter illnesses, the fewer people there will be to spread flu viruses.

Dental Plaque Can Cause Pneumonia

Dental plaque, which is composed mostly of germs, and gum disease have been found to be connected to heart disease and other maladies as a result of germs entering the bloodstream from the mouth. Studies now indicate they may contribute to pneumonia as well, due to germs moving from mouth to lungs.

At greatest risk are patients on ventilators—as a ventilator pushes air into the lungs, it can push germs from the mouth with it. Between 10% and 25% of patients on ventilators come down with pneumonia.

Self-defense: Brush and floss regularly to prevent plaque buildup and gum disease, and see your dentist if they do develop.

Harvard Health Letter, 10 Shattuck St., Boston 02115.

■ ■ ■ ■

Easy Tick Removal

The *Tick Key* is a small metal device that you can attach to a key chain or dog collar. Place the tear-shaped opening over a tick, then pull to dislodge the tick.

Great for anyone who spends time outdoors.

Cost: $5. 203-228-7923, *http://thetickkey.com*.

5

Cures That Cost Pennies

Research Proves Music Lowers Blood Pressure And More!

Everyone has benefited from the soothing effect of listening to a favorite piece of music. But until recently, there was little scientific evidence to support its effectiveness in helping to combat specific health problems.

Now: A growing body of research is finding that music can affect key areas of the brain that help regulate specific physiological functions necessary for good health. The best choice of music and the time spent listening depends on an individual's needs and preferences. *Medical conditions that can be improved by listening to appropriate music...*

HIGH BLOOD PRESSURE

The *hypothalamus* helps control the autonomic nervous system, which regulates our breathing, heartbeat and other automatic responses in the body. It also is linked to emotional activity.

How music helps: When a person listens to music that stimulates positive memories and/or images, the activity of the hypothalamus helps slow a person's heart and respiration rates as well as blood pressure.

Scientific evidence: In a study published in the *British Journal of Health Psychology*, 75 adults performed a stressful three-minute math problem. Afterward, they were randomly assigned to sit in silence or listen to classical, jazz or popular music. Those who heard classical selections had significantly lower systolic (top number) blood pressure levels. Blood pressure did not significantly improve in people who listened to the other selections.

Suzanne B. Hanser, EdD, chair of the music therapy department at Berklee College of Music in Boston and past president of the American Music Therapy Association and the World Federation of Music Therapy, is a research associate at the Dana-Farber Cancer Institute, an affiliate of Harvard Medical School, where she investigates medical applications of music therapy.

What to do: Observe how you respond to different types of music. Match your state of mind to the tempo and dynamics.

Example: If you are agitated, listen to something with a strong, fast beat, then gradually switch to slower and softer music. This can reduce stress and lower blood pressure.

INSOMNIA

Although healthy adults typically fall asleep within 30 minutes, adults age 50 and older often have more trouble falling—and staying—asleep.

How music helps: Soft, restful music can act as a sedative by reducing the amount of the stress-related neurotransmitter noradrenaline that circulates in the bloodstream.

Scientific evidence: Sixty people ages 60 to 83 who reported sleep difficulties took part in a study at Tzu-Chi General Hospital in Taiwan. After three weeks, researchers found a 35% improvement in sleep quality, length of sleep, daytime dysfunction and sleep disturbances in subjects who listened to slow, soft music at night. The most effective types of music used in the study were piano versions of popular "oldies," New Age, harp, classical and slow jazz.

What to do: Make sure your bedroom temperature is comfortably cool, then lie in bed at your usual bedtime, with the lights out (light interferes with the production of the sleep hormone *melatonin*) and your eyes closed while listening to music. Experiment with different types of music until you discover what's relaxing for you. (Earphones are optional.) If you wake during the night, try listening to music again.

PAIN

Listening to music does not eliminate pain, but it can help distract your brain by creating a secondary stimulus that diverts your attention from the feeling of discomfort.

Scientific evidence: In a 14-day study published in the *Journal of Advanced Nursing,* 66 older adults with osteoarthritis pain sat quietly for 20 minutes daily, while another group listened to music. Those who listened to music reported a significant decrease in pain.

What to do: For pain reduction, it's important to identify music that engages you—that is, it should elicit memories and/or make you want to tap your foot, sway or even dance. Singing, which requires deep breathing, or using a simple percussion instrument (such as chimes or a drum), which does not require playing specific notes, also helps.

Best Natural Ways to Calm a Cough

Jamison Starbuck, ND, a naturopathic physician in family practice in Missoula, Montana. She is past president of the American Association of Naturopathic Physicians.

Many Americans are quick to try over-the-counter cough syrups, but most coughs will get better without *any* treatment. In most cases, coughing is simply the body's attempt to clear irritants (dust, pollen or pet dander) or infectious agents (viruses and bacteria) from the airways. It is a very effective process that usually stops on its own when the job is done.

If you have a cough with a cold or sore throat, your doctor may tell you to stay home (to avoid infecting others) and let the cough run its course.

Caution: If you have a fever over 101°F, chest pain, shortness of breath, sputum that is pink or contains flecks of blood…or if your cough persists for more than a week without these symptoms, see a doctor immediately. You could have pneumonia, chronic bronchitis or another serious illness. *Otherwise, consider trying these natural medicines…*

•**Honey-orange-lemon syrup.** This soothes the throat and reduces the cough reflex.

What to do: After washing them, cut three oranges and two lemons into quarters. Put the fruit with rinds into a pan and add one cup of honey and enough water to just cover the fruit. Simmer, covered, until the fruit has become very soft (usually about two hours). Remove the fruit pieces, store the liquid in a glass jar and refrigerate. Take one tablespoon every three hours.

Alternative: An herbal cough syrup that contains honey and wild cherry bark…zinc lozenges…or slippery elm lozenges.

•**Onion poultice.** The beneficial compounds in this remedy help ease inflammation associated with a cough.

What to do: Chop up one large yellow onion and gently sauté it in vegetable oil until transparent. Then add two tablespoons of apple cider vinegar and one-half cup of cornmeal. Cover and let it sit for five minutes. Place a 12" x 12" piece of clean flannel or soft cotton under hot tap water and wring it out. Have a dry second piece of cloth, a hot water bottle or heating pad, and a helper nearby. Lie down (facedown and barebacked) with pillows under your face and chest. Your helper should put the moist, warm flannel over your back, from the shoulders to the mid-back (over your lungs). He/she should then spread the onion/vinegar/cornmeal mix over the wet cloth and cover it with the dry cloth. A hot water bottle or heating pad (set at moderate heat) should be placed on top of the dry cloth. If you are suffering from a cough, applying this remedy for 20 minutes at night will help you get a good night's sleep.

Alternative: Vicks VapoRub ointment or cream, applied to the back or chest.

•**Hydration.** Soothing herbal tea can both hydrate you and curb coughing.

What to do: Mix together herbs that help thin mucus and make it easier to cough up from the respiratory tract—elecampane, marsh mallow root, mullein, wild cherry bark and anise—in equal amounts. Add one tablespoon of the herbal mix to 12 ounces of water. Gently simmer, covered, for six minutes. Strain, sweeten with honey and sip up to four cups daily.

Alternative: A premixed blend containing some or all of these herbs.

■ ■ ■ ■

Are Saunas Good for Your Health?

Saunas promote relaxation and alleviate nasal congestion. They may ease soreness and fatigue after exertion by increasing blood flow to muscles…and may help the body sweat out toxins.

Caution: Saunas dilate blood vessels, affecting blood flow—so if you have high blood pressure or take drugs that affect the heart (such as beta-blockers), use a sauna only under a doctor's guidance.

Leo Galland, MD, director, Foundation for Integrated Medicine, New York City. His latest book is *The Fat Resistance Diet*. Broadway. *www.fatresistancediet.com*. Dr. Galland is a recipient of the Linus Pauling Award.

_____

Think Thin, Get Thin

Judith S. Beck, PhD, director of the Beck Institute for Cognitive Therapy and Research in Bala Cynwyd, Pennsylvania (*www.beckinstitute.org*). She is a clinical associate professor of psychology in psychiatry at the University of Pennsylvania, Philadelphia, and past president of the Academy of Cognitive Therapy, Bala Cynwyd. Her books include *The Beck Diet Solution: Train Your Brain to Think Like a Thin Person* (Oxmoor House) and *Cognitive Therapy: Basics and Beyond* (Guilford).

_____

You try and try again, but dieting just doesn't work for you? Don't berate yourself for failing to slim down. Ingrained patterns of negative thinking can sabotage your best intentions and make it tough to stick to a weight-loss plan.

Fact: When you decided to learn to play tennis or use a computer, you needed to master new skills. Dieting works the same way, though the mastery you need is primarily psychological. An approach called *cognitive therapy* (CT) can teach you the skills necessary to follow any nutritious weight-loss regimen you may choose —and to shed weight permanently.

The key: Learning to think like a thin person.

HOW IT WORKS

A form of talk therapy, CT was pioneered in the 1960s by my father, psychiatrist Aaron Beck, MD. Through CT, a person learns specific techniques for changing distorted, self-defeating thinking patterns that lead to negative emotions and harmful behavior. More than 400 research studies have shown CT to be effective for relieving depression, anxiety, insomnia, substance abuse and eating disorders.

For weight loss, CT works by taking the emotion out of eating and changing the negative thoughts that can lead to failure.

Evidence of success: In a Swedish study of 105 people, obese participants who attended CT group sessions lost an average of 19 pounds in 10 weeks—and in the 18 months that followed, they lost an average of four more pounds. Members of a control group who did not use CT gained an average of five pounds.

For about 20 years, I have been using CT with my psychiatric patients who want to lose weight, and the results have been excellent. My experience is personal, too. In 1995, I used CT techniques myself to lose 15 pounds, which I have kept off ever since.

PLANNING AHEAD

Very simply, to lose weight permanently, you need to allocate time to planning meals, buying and preparing foods, eating mindfully and exercising regularly. If you think you cannot do that, ask yourself what's more important—planning ahead and losing weight…or eating whenever the urge strikes and gaining weight. The choice is yours.

CT can be used with any healthful, well-balanced weight-loss plan. Your doctor can suggest several appropriate options. Select one that fits your lifestyle and is flexible enough to suit a variety of situations, and that includes foods you enjoy and can prepare easily.

Feel free to modify a plan in advance to incorporate favorite foods, so you won't feel deprived.

Example: I eat whatever type of treat I want—but only after dinner and only in an amount that does not exceed 300 calories. Knowing that I can have my best-loved snacks in the early evening makes it easy to resist temptations during the day.

SELF-SABOTAGING THOUGHTS

To successfully use CT for weight loss, recognize one important fact—eating is not automatic. Before we bite into anything, we first have a thought about eating it—and that thought leads to the act of eating or not eating. By identifying such triggering thoughts, we can learn to avoid missteps.

You may wonder, *Why should I have to be conscious of thoughts that pop into my head, when so many people stay thin with no apparent effort?* The answer is that most thin people do think about restricting their eating, but they do this so habitually and matter-of-factly that they may scarcely be aware of the process. You can learn to think like that—but for it to become a habit, you first must consciously practice.

Consider the common sabotaging thoughts below. Challenge each diet-defeating thought with the corresponding truth, and eventually the appropriate responses will spring to your mind automatically.

Sabotaging thought: I can't resist eating this food.

Appropriate response: If I really want this food, I can eat it tomorrow as part of a planned meal or snack.

Sabotage: I feel stressed out, and I need to eat something.

Response: Eating makes me feel better momentarily, but afterward I feel bad about blowing my diet. I can combat stress better by taking a walk or phoning a friend.

Sabotage: I know I shouldn't eat this, but I don't care.

Response: I do care because I want to lose weight. Besides, I'm having lunch in an hour.

Sabotage: It's okay to eat that food just this once.

Response: If I give in now, I may give in next time, too—and end up overeating. It's better to stick to my diet so I can slim down.

Sabotage: I'm hungry, so I should eat.

Response: I'm not hungry, I'm just bored. I'll read until dinnertime. By then, I really will be hungry, so my meal will taste even better.

Sabotage: I ate something that I shouldn't. My diet is ruined for today, so I might as well splurge now and start over tomorrow.

Response: In a week, this one small mistake won't matter. But if I stop trying to stick to my diet, I will gain weight.

Give yourself due credit whenever you dispel a sabotaging thought. A mental pat on the back —*I'm proud of myself for not eating that doughnut*—reinforces your new positive thought patterns.

Best Natural Remedies For Allergies

Jamison Starbuck, ND, a naturopathic physician in family practice in Missoula, Montana. She is past president of the American Association of Naturopathic Physicians.

I treat a lot of people who are miserable because of seasonal allergies—they suffer from itchy eyes and throat, sneezing and a runny nose. Seasonal allergies typically result from exposure to allergens, such as pollen from grass, trees and ragweed. But there's another type of allergy that can affect people year-round. Dust, feathers and animal dander are the most common causes of these so-called "perennial" allergies.

Regardless of the trigger, an allergy is an immune disorder. When an airborne irritant, such as pollen or dust, is inhaled, the body recognizes it as a harmful substance. This activates the body's defensive response, which leads not only to sneezing and a runny nose but also to watery eyes, sinus congestion and/or ear pain. When the body is under assault from allergens, the immune system works hard. That's why for some people, the only sign of seasonal allergies is lethargy (extreme physical and mental sluggishness).

When allergies are treated with medication (such as antihistamines and corticosteroids), symptoms are *temporarily* relieved. Allergy shots can reduce allergic reactions in some people but, like medication, they do not cure the problem. *To address the root cause of allergies, try my natural allergy-fighting regimen (products are available at most health-food stores)...*

•**Get more flavonoids.** These powerful antioxidants strengthen the cells in your upper respiratory tract (particularly the membranes of your nose), which helps protect your body from the ill effects of inhaled irritants. Take 300 mg each of supplements containing the flavonoids *quercetin* and *hesperidin* four times daily during allergy season. Fruits—particularly citrus and berries—are rich in flavonoids. Eat them daily. Organic fresh fruits are best.

*Check with your doctor before taking any of these supplements.

•**Reduce stress.** Researchers at the University of Texas Medical School in Houston have linked worsening allergy symptoms to anxiety, depression and psychological stress. That's because chronic stress triggers immune dysfunction, weakening the body's ability to defend against irritants. If you have allergies, review what causes stress in your life and take steps to remedy these situations, especially during allergy season.

•**Take herbs.** *Adaptogen* herbs help the body "adapt" to stress, generally by supporting adrenal gland health. I recommend astragalus and borage for allergy season. Mix one-eighth teaspoon each of a tincture of astragalus and a tincture of borage in two ounces of water and take 15 minutes before or after meals, twice daily throughout allergy season.

•**Drink tea.** To safely relieve allergy symptoms, try flavonoid-rich elderflower tea, which reduces nasal and sinus congestion, fights sneezing and relieves watery eyes. Pour one cup of boiling water over two teaspoons of dried elderflower blossoms (or an elderflower teabag) and steep for 10 minutes. Strain and drink hot (add lemon and/or honey, if you like) three times daily until symptoms improve.

■ ■ ■ ■

Free Help for Allergies

Allergy alerts and pollen counts are available anytime at the American Academy of Allergy, Asthma & Immunology's free Web site, *www.aaaai.org* (click on "Pollen Counts"). Click on your region for a list of all national allergy bureau locations, where measurements of pollen and mold are taken.

Helpful: Sign up for a free account at the site to view each pollen count in detail.

Example: If you are allergic to pollen from oak trees but not maple trees, you can find out which specific type of tree has a high count each day.

Martha V. White, MD, director of research, Institute for Asthma and Allergy, Wheaton, Maryland.

■ ■ ■ ■

Kick Out Foot Fungus

Avoid foot fungus. Never go barefoot in shared bathrooms—wear flip-flops, even when showering. Scrub your feet during a shower, then dry them thoroughly, especially between the toes. Wear socks made of cotton or other natural fibers. Change socks often if your feet sweat a lot. Avoid tight shoes—they cause excess perspiration, which can increase fungus growth. Check feet and toenails for flaky skin, itchiness between toes and/or on the bottom of feet, thickening of nails and discoloration. Have a doctor treat any of these problems.

Oliver Zong, DPM, podiatrist and foot surgeon, NYC Foot Care, New York City.

Natural Ways to Improve Digestive Health

Jamison Starbuck, ND, a naturopathic physician in family practice in Missoula, Montana. She is past president of the American Association of Naturopathic Physicians.

Though sometimes overlooked by doctors, gastrointestinal (GI) health is fundamental to overall wellness. The GI tract, also known as the "gut," allows us to draw nourishment from our food and eliminate toxins. A variety of medications claim to promote intestinal health, but I prefer my own eight-step natural approach, which is both inexpensive and easy to follow. Add one new step each day. If you're like most people, your GI tract will be healthier within two weeks. *My advice…*

1. Avoid foods that cause indigestion. Indigestion is your body's way of telling you that a certain food is not readily digestible. Instead of trying to *make* a food digestible by taking drugs, choose foods that you can easily digest, such as fish, brown rice and steamed vegetables.

2. Shortly after awakening in the morning, drink an eight-ounce glass of room-temperature water. This "wakes up" the GI tract, preparing you for both digestion and elimination. Repeat this step five to 10 minutes *before* each meal. Avoid iced beverages, including water, with meals and 15 minutes before and afterward. Some research suggests that cold beverages decrease the secretion of digestive enzymes.

3. Squeeze fresh lemon or sprinkle vinegar on your food. For most people, one-half teaspoon of lemon or vinegar per meal fights indigestion by increasing stomach acidity and improving the digestion of fats.

4. Take a 15-minute walk after meals. Doing so will improve your digestion and elimination. If you can't do this after every meal, do so following the largest meal of the day.

5. Practice simple home hydrotherapy. This practice increases blood flow to your intestines, which helps them function properly.

What to do: Finish your daily shower or bath with a 30-second spray of cool or cold water to your entire abdomen. Towel dry with brisk strokes immediately after the cool water spray.

Caution: If you have a history of stroke, check with your doctor before trying hydrotherapy.

6. Drink chamomile or peppermint tea after dinner. These herbs soothe the lining of the stomach and intestines. Add one tea bag or two teaspoons of loose herb to eight ounces of water.

7. Use foot reflexology to relieve intestinal pain. Massaging reflexology points on the feet is thought to help increase blood flow to and improve the function of corresponding organs or body parts.

What to do: Whenever you have GI discomfort, firmly massage (for five to seven minutes) with your thumb and forefinger the outside portion of the middle one-third of the soles of the feet. According to reflexologists, this area corresponds to the colon. Your strokes should move toward the heel.

8. Never eat when you are stressed. Our bodies are not designed to simultaneously manage both stress and digestion. Studies show that just a few moments of relaxation, such as deep breathing or prayer, before a meal will improve the digestive process.

Home Remedies That Work Better Than Drugs

Lydia Wilen and Joan Wilen are folk-remedy experts based in New York City. The sisters are coauthors of many books, including *Bottom Line's Healing Remedies: Over 1,000 Astounding Ways to Heal Arthritis, Asthma, High Blood Pressure, Varicose Veins, Warts* and More! (Bottom Line Books, 800-678-5835, *www.BottomLine Secrets.com/store*).

The Wilen sisters have been using home remedies all their lives, and for the last quarter of a century, they've been researching and writing about them as well.

They may not always be able to explain why the remedies work—but they work. All use ingredients readily available in most kitchens, supermarkets or health-food stores. Of course, always check with your doctor before taking any dietary supplement or herb.

SORE THROAT

At the first sign of a sore or scratchy throat, mix two teaspoons of *apple cider vinegar* in six-to-eight ounces of warm water. Take a mouthful, gargle with it and spit it out—then swallow a mouthful. Repeat the gargle/swallow pattern until there's nothing left in the glass. Do this every hour until your throat is better. We usually feel better within two or three hours.

COLDS

We eat *chicken soup* when we feel a cold coming on. Aside from it being a comfort food, it helps prevent a cold from becoming full-blown and/or it shortens the duration of one. We either prepare the soup from scratch, adding lots of veggies (carrots, onions, parsnip, celery, string beans) or we do the next best thing—buy packaged soup found in the supermarket's frozen food section, then add vegetables. In either case, we add the most potent and health-restoring ingredient—garlic. To derive the full healing powers of garlic, add one or two finely minced raw cloves after the warmed soup is in the bowl.

STOP BLEEDING

A simple first-aid procedure to stop a minor cut or gash from bleeding is to cover the cut with *cayenne pepper* from your spice cabinet. Gently pour on the pepper. Yes, it will sting. And yes, the bleeding will stop quickly.

DIARRHEA

If you must be away from a restroom, prepare *slippery elm tea* (we use the inner bark powder available at health-food stores). Pour eight ounces of just-boiled water over a heaping teaspoon of the powder. Let it steep for about eight minutes, then strain the liquid into a mug and drink it. It works quickly. For severe cases, do not strain it—just drink this soothing, gloppy tea.

HEARTBURN

We use our mother's remedy. As soon as the burning starts, eat a palmful of *almonds*—that's about one ounce—and the heartburn stops immediately. Our mom used dry-roasted almonds. We buy raw almond slivers.

STY

A sty is an inflamed swelling on the eyelid. This classic folk remedy sounds ridiculous but has worked for us many times. The minute you feel as though you're getting a sty, take a *14-carat gold ring* (wash it first) and rub it several times across your eyelid every 15 minutes or so, until that "styish" feeling disappears…along with the sty. In our experience, it works right away.

BURNED FINGERTIPS

Ever reach for a pot handle that's surprisingly hot? How about grabbing the wrong side of a plugged-in iron? We have a unique way of treating these minor first-degree burns, where the skin is painful and red but unbroken. It's a form of *acupressure*. Place your thumb on the back side of your earlobe, and the burned fingertips on the front side of the same earlobe. Press firmly. After a minute, the pain is gone.

INSOMNIA

Our new best friends are nuts—in this case, *walnuts*. They're rich in *serotonin*, the brain chemical that calms anxiety and allows us to turn off the pressures of the day to get a good night's sleep. Eat a palmful (one ounce) of raw walnuts before going to bed. It's important to chew each mouthful thoroughly, until the nut pieces are ground down.

The Power of Probiotics To Fight Disease

Gary B. Huffnagle, PhD, professor of internal medicine, microbiology and immunology at University of Michigan Medical School in Ann Arbor. His research on probiotics has appeared in leading scientific journals. He is coauthor, with Sarah Wernick, of *The Probiotics Revolution*. Bantam.

Probiotics are emerging as a key to overall wellness. These beneficial bacteria, which reside in the digestive tract, are naturally present in certain foods, such as yogurt and aged cheese. *While it's not clear exactly how probiotics do it, clinical studies show that they can help prevent or treat many health problems, including...*

•**Digestive distress.** Numerous studies show that probiotics promote the overall health of the intestinal lining and can reduce the duration and severity of viral and bacterial diarrhea. A diet rich in probiotics also can be effective for cases of inflammatory bowel disease (IBD)—an autoimmune condition that includes ulcerative colitis and Crohn's disease—because these microbes encourage a healthier immune system. According to one study, the probiotic *Lactobacillus* GG increased the time between ulcerative colitis attacks. Probiotics also keep the level of the bacterium *Helicobacter pylori* (normally present in the stomach) under control, thereby reducing the chance of developing ulcers.

•**Chronic immune/inflammatory problems.** An overactive immune system can cause autoimmune disorders, such as rheumatoid arthritis and multiple sclerosis, as well as eczema, asthma, allergies and other conditions. In simplest terms, the body identifies a harmless molecule as a dangerous one and sends the immune system on the attack. Probiotics can counter this offensive by encouraging the development of regulatory *T cells* (which can call off the battle) and stimulating *B cells* (found in the intestinal tract) to make *secretory IgA*—antibodies that identify molecules as harmless.

•**Cancer.** Preliminary studies indicate that probiotics break down carcinogens in food and make them harmless. Also, their support of the body's immune system gives it the strength necessary to identify and destroy abnormal cells without harming the normal ones.

•**Tooth decay and gum disease.** It's theorized that the probiotics in plain yogurt keep the level of *Streptococcus mutans* (linked to tooth decay) and *Porphyromonas gingivalis* (linked to gum disease) under control.

•**Adverse effects of medications.** Probiotics can repopulate the good bacteria in the intestines that are destroyed by antibiotics. Other medications that can upset the probiotic balance include oral antifungal medications...antacids...nonsteroidal anti-inflammatory drugs (NSAIDs), such as aspirin and ibuprofen...and any medication that lists constipation as a side effect.

TYPES OF PROBIOTICS

There are a several types of probiotics offering different health benefits...

•**Bifidobacterium**—may reduce allergic response to food...strengthens the immune system...can reduce incidence of gastroenteritis (irritation and inflammation of the stomach and intestines) and infantile colic.

•**Streptococcus thermophilus**—strengthens the immune system...can reduce incidence of colic.

•**Lactobacillus**—may reduce allergic responses to food...strengthens the immune system...reduces risk for ulcers...may prevent IBD. *Specific species...*

•L. acidophilus—reduces risk for ulcers...prevents antibiotic-induced diarrhea...may help prevent kidney stones.

•L. casei—strengthens the immune system...reduces risk for ulcers...reduces allergic response to food.

•L. reuteri—reduces fever and diarrhea in infants...may prevent IBD.

BEST FOOD SOURCES

Probiotics need a steady source of healthy foods to thrive, ideally from *prebiotics*. Prebiotics are nondigestible dietary fibers, such as those found in fruits, vegetables and whole grains, that stimulate the growth of good bacteria.

A diet that emphasizes high amounts of fat or sugar gives harmful microbes the edge, making it more difficult for probiotics to thrive. In addition to eating healthfully overall, you can increase your probiotic population by eating certain foods. *Aim for two servings a day of probiotic-rich foods...*

•**Yogurt** is probably the most familiar probiotic food source, but you need to choose a product with live bacteria. Look for the "Live & Active Cultures" seal from the National Yogurt Association (NYA), which means that the yogurt contains at least 100 million bacteria per gram at the time of manufacture. Or look for phrases such as "Contains active yogurt cultures" or "Contains living yogurt cultures." Beware of brands with the words "Made with active cultures" on the label—they may have been heat-treated after fermentation, which kills the bacteria.

All yogurts with live bacteria contain the probiotics *Lactobacillus bulgaricus* (for general digestive health) and *Streptococcus thermophilus*. Other probiotics also may be included, such as *L. acidophilus, L. casei* and *L. reuteri*. As for flavoring, avoid the high-sugar varieties. Instead, add your own fruits and sweeteners (preferably honey, which is believed to be a prebiotic), or mix sweetened forms with plain yogurt to reduce the sugar content. Adding low-sugar granola or other cereals to the yogurt increases taste and fiber.

•**Aged (fermented) cheeses** contain probiotics, with the amount ranging from three billion to 10 billion bacteria per 1.5-ounce serving. Generally speaking, the longer the cheese has aged, the more probiotics it contains—aged Parmesan and Romano are high in probiotics. One-and-a-half ounces of cheese daily provides your system with valuable probiotics and calcium without pushing your fat intake over a healthy level.

•**Kefir** is a fermented milk drink. Eight ounces provides an estimated three billion to 10 billion bacteria. For specific information, check the label or consult the individual producer's Web site.

•**Pickles and sauerkraut** that are produced by a traditional fermentation process rather than by chemical treatment can contain varying amounts of probiotics. Select pickles packed in brine and sauerkraut that is fermented in salt. Be aware that heating destroys live healthful bacteria.

SUPPLEMENTS

It can be hard to get enough probiotics from food, especially if you're trying to combat a health problem. Supplements are available at many pharmacies and health-food stores. Generally, it's best to look for a supplement that includes both the *Lactobacillus* and *Bifidobacterium* groups. As for dosage amounts, three billion to five billion colony-forming units (CFU) per day maintains good health, while six billion to 10 billion CFU per day help address a specific health concern, such as digestive problems, allergies, etc. Increase the amount to 20 billion to 30 billion CFU per day for mild-to-moderate health conditions (diarrhea or eczema, for example). For more serious medical conditions, take supplements under medical supervision.

Choose your supplier carefully. Is the stock replenished frequently? Are the probiotics refrigerated? When ordering by mail, avoid shipments sent during the hottest time of the year, because heat can degrade the quality. Opt for capsules or single-use packets. Take them with food or drink (preferably a calcium source, which fosters probiotics), and keep them cool and dry.

Some people may initially experience some digestive upset, such as gas or bloating, when they start taking probiotics, but that typically goes away within a week. You also can cut back on the amount of probiotics that you initially take and then slowly increase the dose.

Caution: There are certain circumstances when your physician needs to be consulted before you add probiotic supplements to your regular nutritional plan.

Examples: Do not take probiotics without medical supervision if you are immunocompromised...critically ill...undergoing chemotherapy or radiation...are under care for a serious digestive tract disorder...or ever have had an adverse reaction to a probiotic formulation.

Natural Cures for an Ailing Immune System

Jamison Starbuck, ND, a naturopathic physician in family practice in Missoula, Montana. She is past president of the American Association of Naturopathic Physicians.

The immune system is remarkable in its ability to help fight off infections and a wide variety of serious illnesses ranging from flu to staph infections. When our defenses go awry, however, our health can be threatened in a number of ways. For unknown reasons, the body's immune system can attack a part of itself, resulting in autoimmune disease.

Examples: Systemic lupus erythematosus (commonly known as lupus) can affect the kidneys, skin and blood vessels. With Crohn's disease, the immune system strikes the bowel. In patients who have rheumatoid arthritis, the joints are assaulted.

When a patient is diagnosed with an autoimmune disease, conventional doctors generally begin treatment with medication. For lupus and Crohn's disease, *prednisone* (a steroid drug) is commonly used. For rheumatoid arthritis, medications typically include nonsteroidal anti-inflammatory drugs (NSAIDs), corticosteroids and, most recently, drugs called *tumor necrosis factor inhibitors*, such as *etanercept* (Enbrel) and *infliximab* (Remicade). While these medications reduce symptoms, they can cause potentially serious side effects, such as liver damage and hypertension. That's why I prefer to treat symptoms naturally whenever possible, reserving strong medications for flare-ups. *My advice for people with autoimmune disease...*

• **Eat an anti-inflammatory diet.** Limit meat and poultry to two meals per day and no more than three to four ounces per meal. Also consume at least five one-half cup servings of vegetables daily...one cup of a whole grain, such as brown rice or millet, and/or legumes, such as lentils or split peas...a small handful of nuts... and two or more pieces of fruit.

• **Take an omega-3 supplement.** For most of my patients with an autoimmune disease, I recommend a daily dose of 2,800 mg of an inflammation-fighting omega-3 fish oil, 50% of which should be *eicosapentaenoic acid* (EPA), a fatty acid shown to have strong immune-supportive effects. Omega-3 oils should always be taken with food because they are more readily digested.

• **Limit your exposure to environmental pollutants and drugs.** Both appear to trigger autoimmune disease in sensitive individuals. Substances that are known to cause this reaction in some people include mercury, cadmium, pesticides, anticonvulsant medications, beta-blockers (taken for heart disease) and estrogens (taken for menopausal symptoms). Talk to your doctor about getting tested for heavy metal toxicity and about taking only those prescription medications that he/she feels are absolutely necessary.

• **Take a vitamin D supplement daily.** An increasing body of scientific evidence links vitamin D deficiency with autoimmune disease. Researchers theorize that vitamin D helps regulate immune cell activity in the body.

My recommendation: A supplement containing 800 international units (IU) to 1,200 IU of vitamin D daily.

Pharmacist Prescribes Natural Remedies Better Than Drugs

Suzy Cohen, RPh, a registered practicing pharmacist for 20 years and author of *The 24-Hour Pharmacist.* Collins. Her syndicated newspaper column, "Dear Pharmacist," reaches more than 24 million readers. Based in Florida, she is a member of the Association of Natural Medicine Pharmacists and the American Holistic Health Association. *www.dearpharmacist.com.*

As a pharmacist for almost two decades, Suzy Cohen knows the importance of medication—but she also has learned to "think outside the pill" and recommend natural options that often are just as good or better at promoting health without the risk of dangerous side effects.

133

Here are the remedies she recommends most often. All are free of significant side effects unless otherwise noted, but always talk with your doctor before using any supplements.

TEA TREE OIL FOR WOUNDS

This oil kills germs, reduces pain and helps wounds heal more quickly. You can use it in place of antibiotic ointment for minor cuts, scratches and burns...to treat toenail fungus... and, when diluted, as a gargle to kill the germs that cause sore throat.

How it works: It's a strong antiseptic that kills bacteria as well as fungi.

How to use: Moisten a cotton ball or swab with one or two drops of the oil, and apply it to the area two to three times daily until it heals.

For a gargle for sore throat: Mix a few drops in a cup of water, gargle and spit it out.

Caution: Do not swallow it.

GINGER FOR NAUSEA

Studies have shown that ginger can relieve nausea—due to pregnancy, seasickness, etc.—as well as or better than over-the-counter drugs.

In one study, published in *The Lancet,* volunteers were given either ginger or Dramamine (a nausea-preventing drug), then were seated in a chair designed to trigger motion sickness. Those given ginger were able to withstand the motion 57% longer than those given the drug.

How to use: Put one teaspoon of peeled, grated fresh gingerroot in a cup of boiling water. Let it steep for 10 minutes, then drink (you can filter out the ginger if you want). Or chew and swallow a piece of crystallized ginger, sold in health-food stores.

Caution: Ginger can increase the risk of bleeding when taken with blood-thinning drugs, such as *warfarin* (Coumadin).

RHODIOLA ROSEA FOR STRESS

This herb acts like a natural form of Valium by reducing physical and emotional stress. The supplement is made from the root of the Siberian plant.

How it works: Herbalists classify Rhodiola as an *adaptogen,* a class of herbs that "sense" chemicals in the body and either raise or lower them. It normalizes levels of brain chemicals that

affect mood, such as *monoamines* and *beta-endorphins,* which help counter the effects of stress. Rhodiola also may increase *serotonin,* which enhances feelings of well-being.

How to use: During times of stress, take 100 milligrams (mg) of rhodiola rosea in capsule form, two to three times daily. It's best taken on a cyclical basis—two months on, two weeks off.

CALCIUM PLUS MAGNESIUM FOR CRAMPS

People who experience frequent and/or painful menstrual or muscle cramps often have a deficiency of calcium and magnesium.

How it works: Calcium and magnesium regulate the contraction and relaxation of muscles.

How to use: Before going to bed, take 500 mg to 600 mg of calcium, along with 150 mg to 200 mg of magnesium (using the chelate or glycinate forms—check the label). Combination formulas are easy to find and fine to use.

For menstrual problems, start 10 days before you expect your period to begin each month and continue until your period is complete.

GABA FOR INSOMNIA

Gamma-aminobutyric acid (GABA) is a neurotransmitter (mood-related brain chemical) that is naturally present in the body. It's taken in supplement form to reduce insomnia, as well as anxiety and depression.

How it works: GABA is an inhibitory neurotransmitter that slows activity in the brain and makes it easier to fall asleep.

How to use: Take 500 mg to 1,000 mg one hour before bedtime if you have trouble getting to sleep. If your problem is that you wake in the middle of the night and can't get back to sleep, take it then. Don't exceed recommended doses on the package. Do this for two weeks. If it doesn't help, talk to your doctor.

Caution: Combining GABA with prescription or over-the-counter sleep aids can cause excessive sedation.

CAPSAICIN CREAM FOR PAIN

Capsaicin is the chemical compound that puts the "hot" in chili peppers. It is effective for easing muscle aches, back and joint pain and nerve pain caused by the herpes Zoster virus (shingles —known medically as post-herpetic neuralgia).

How it works: When applied as a cream, it causes nerve cells to empty their reservoirs of *substance P,* a pain-causing chemical. This results in less pain from the underlying disorder.

How to use: Start with a 0.025% concentration. Apply it two to three times daily—the initial burning sensation diminishes with continued use. If needed, you can always buy the stronger 0.075% concentration—but it's best to work your way up to this strength.

Caution: Wear latex gloves when applying capsaicin—and wash your hands thoroughly after using to prevent residual cream from getting into the eyes, nose, etc. Don't use if you are pregnant or planning to become pregnant.

PROBIOTICS FOR DIGESTIVE DISCOMFORT

A healthy digestive tract contains trillions of bacteria, many of which have beneficial effects. These so-called "good" (probiotic) organisms promote digestive health, improve immunity and aid in the synthesis of B vitamins, among many other functions.

How they work: Probiotic supplements replenish beneficial bacteria and crowd out harmful organisms that can cause gas, bloating, diarrhea and other digestive problems.

How to use: Take a daily supplement of at least 10 billion organisms that contains a variety of living organisms, such as *L. bulgaricus, L. bifida* and *B. longum.* Some yogurts contain these live active cultures, but avoid those that contain sugar or artificial sweeteners.

BIOTIN FOR CRACKED NAILS

The B vitamin biotin is the only nutrient that has been shown to improve nail health in generally healthy adults. People with a deficiency of biotin often have fragile nails that crack easily.

How it works: Biotin is absorbed by the nail matrix, the part under the fingernail where nail cells are generated.

How to use: Take 2,000 micrograms (mcg) to 4,000 mcg of biotin daily, as well as a B-complex supplement. Most people will notice an improvement in nail strength and thickness in one to two months.

Low-Cost Cures for Headache, Stomach Upset, Flu and More!

Edward Shalts, MD, DHt, has been practicing homeopathy for 25 years. Currently in private homeopathic and holistic practice in New York City. He also is vice president of the National Center for Homeopathy and author of two books—*The American Institute of Homeopathy Handbook for Parents* (Jossey-Bass) and *Easy Homeopathy* (McGraw-Hill). *www.homeopathynewyork.com.*

Homeopathy is a type of treatment that can be used for a wide range of ailments. It uses minute doses of natural substances to stimulate the body's self-healing response. There is controversy within the medical community about whether homeopathy works, but I have found that it can quickly resolve a health issue when the correct remedy is matched to a specific set of symptoms.

The right homeopathic remedy can shorten the duration of symptoms, with relief often beginning in as little as 15 minutes. It also can help prevent relatively benign conditions from evolving into more dangerous ones. It can reduce the dosage of conventional medication required to manage some chronic diseases or eliminate the need for medication altogether. Unlike conventional drugs, which have the potential to produce unpleasant side effects, homeopathic remedies are exceedingly safe.

Important dosage information: For the following remedies, a dose is three pills (pellets) of 30C concentration unless otherwise noted. Allow the pills to dissolve under your tongue. *Also, unless otherwise noted, follow these instructions...*

•**If you don't notice any change in symptoms** after 30 minutes, don't repeat the dose. Try another homeopathic remedy or conventional medicine.

•**If you feel somewhat better** after 30 minutes but not completely better, repeat the dose.

•**If your symptoms have improved dramatically,** don't take another dose unless the problem comes back.

The rule of thumb is to take no more than three doses at 30-minute intervals over two hours—if that doesn't work, talk to your doctor. Also, talk

135

to your doctor before taking any medication or supplement.

All remedies mentioned here are available at most health-food stores and many pharmacies.

COLD OR FLU

•**Oscillococcinum.** A remedy produced by Boiron. Use at the first sign of a cold or flu. Instructions are printed on the package.

DIARRHEA

If the remedy is working, episodes become progressively less frequent. Take after each episode of diarrhea.

•**Arsenicum album.** For any case of diarrhea, including from food poisoning.

•**Podophyllum.** For explosive diarrhea that leaves you weak after each stool.

HEADACHE

•**Iris versicolor.** Frequently indicated for classic migraine headaches that begin with visual aura and end with vomiting. It also is for blurry vision, and sometimes even blindness during headache. Take every 15 minutes, a maximum of three times. Stop if there is a significant improvement earlier.

HERPES ZOSTER (SHINGLES)

Take one of these remedies twice a day for three days. If there is no effect or you feel worse, discontinue.

•**Apis mellifica.** For shingles lesions on the face.

•**Arsenicum album.** For burning pain.

•**Ranunculus bulbosus.** The remedy of choice for shingles on the left side of the chest.

INDIGESTION

Take either of the following three times a day for one day. Stop if the condition improves earlier. Also, discontinue if there is no effect after three doses.

•**Nux vomica.** For indigestion from overeating in general, along with irritability and cramping pains.

•**Arsenicum album.** For indigestion from eating too much fruit.

INSECT BITES AND STINGS

Take either remedy below every 15 minutes for a total of three times.

•**Apis mellifica.** For stings and bites from bees and other small insects, such as spiders. The site of the bite is typically hot to the touch, red and swollen.

•**Ledum palustre.** For stings and bites by large insects (wasps, for example). The site of the bite is cold to the touch and has a bluish tinge.

MOTION SICKNESS

Take either remedy below a maximum of three times, at 15- to 20-minute intervals.

•**Cocculus indicus.** Works best if your symptoms are worse in open air.

•**Tabacum.** Useful if you turn pale (almost green) or if you feel better in fresh air.

POISON IVY/POISON OAK

•**Poison Ivy Pills.** This product is made by Washington Homeopathic Products. Follow label directions. Most patients find it effective if started at the first sign of trouble.

SPRAINS AND STRAINS

Take any of the remedies listed below three times a day for two to three days. Discontinue after three days.

•**Arnica montana.** For a sore, bruised feeling. Often indicated for people who have overexercised after a long break.

•**Bryonia alba.** For ankle sprains and strains.

•**Rhus toxicodendron.** The most frequently recommended remedy for these conditions. You also can apply Rhus tox ointment twice a day.

WRIST CONDITIONS

•**Ruta graveolens.** A specific remedy for wrist problems. Take three times a day for three days. For long-standing wrist strain, take three 12C pellets once a day every day for a month.

■ **More from Edward Shalts...**

Homeopathy for Mental Strain

If a person is under mental strain, the best treatment is to deal with the initial cause. *As a temporary measure, try the following...*

STRESS

●**Nux vomica.** For overworked, stressed-out, career-oriented people. Also for anger in people who work many hours in a row and are on edge and whose nerves feel raw. Take the dose. Repeat after 15 minutes, then again after another 15 minutes.

ANXIETY

●**Aconitum napellus.** For panic.

●**Argentum nitricum.** For restless anxiety.

●**Gelsemium sempervirens.** For the patient who feels paralyzed from anxiety, wants to be left alone.

GRIEF

●**Ignatia amara.** Take three 200C pellets immediately after the bad news. On the first day, it can be repeated two more times. Then one dose a day for three more days.

MENTAL FATIGUE/EXHAUSTION

●**Picricum acidum.** For exhaustion after long studies, such as cramming for exams or other intellectual strain. Take once a day for three days.

The Best Healing Herbs

David Hoffmann, a clinical medical herbalist based in Sonoma County, California, a fellow of Britain's National Institute of Medical Herbalists and one of the founding members of the American Herbalists Guild. He is the author of 17 books, including *Herbal Prescriptions After 50.* Healing Arts.

Anyone who has taken prescription drugs is well aware that these medications can not only be costly, but they also can cause a variety of uncomfortable or even dangerous side effects, such as excessive bleeding, headache, nausea and dizziness.

Recently reported problem: A study of 150,000 older adults (who are among the heaviest users of prescription medications) found that 29% were taking at least one inappropriate drug—including medications that were ineffective or even dangerous.

Often-overlooked alternative to drugs: Herbal medicine. Herbs should not be substituted for all prescription medications, but the careful use of medicinal plants can improve overall health and reduce or eliminate the need for some medications—as well as the risks for drug-related side effects.*

Common conditions—and the best herbal treatments…

CHRONIC BRONCHITIS

As many as 9.1 million Americans are diagnosed each year with chronic bronchitis (a mucus-producing cough that occurs on most days of the month at least three months of the year).

Best herbal treatment: **Horehound** (leaves and flowering tops). It relaxes the bronchi (airways that connect the windpipe to the lungs) and makes it easier to expel mucus.

How to use: Add 1 milliliter (ml) to 2 ml of horehound tincture (concentrated liquid) to one ounce of hot or cold water. Drink this amount three times daily during bronchitis flare-ups.

Important: Most herbs are available in various forms, such as dry leaf, capsules and powders, but tinctures are convenient, among the quickest to be absorbed and have a long shelf life.

HEARTBURN

When acid from the stomach backs up into the esophagus, the result is often heartburn (a burning pain behind the breastbone).

Best herbal treatment: **Marshmallow root.** It coats and soothes the esophageal lining.

How to use: Make an infusion by adding one heaping teaspoon of powdered marshmallow root to a cup of cold water and letting it sit at room temperature for 12 hours. Drink the entire mixture when heartburn occurs. If you get heartburn more than three times a week, drink one infusion in the morning and another at bedtime until the heartburn eases. If you make more than one cup in advance, you can refrigerate the unused portion for 24 hours.

Important: Do not use hot water. It will provide only about one-fourth of the soothing mucilage (lubricating substance) of a cold-water infusion.

*See your doctor before using medicinal herbs—especially if you take any medications, have a chronic medical condition or are pregnant or nursing.

HYPERTENSION

High blood pressure (hypertension) is among the main causes of heart attack and stroke. Prescription medications usually are required for this condition, but herbal therapy can sometimes allow patients to take lower doses of blood pressure–lowering drugs.

Important: Check with your doctor before trying herbs for hypertension. Because the potential complications of hypertension are serious, everyone with this condition should be under a doctor's care.

Best herbal treatment: **Hawthorn** (berries). This herbal therapy dilates arteries (which allows blood to circulate with less force)…and strengthens the cardiovascular system, in part by enhancing the activity of cells in the heart muscle. In Germany, hawthorn is widely recommended by doctors for cardiovascular disease.

How to use: Add 1 ml to 2 ml of hawthorn tincture to one ounce of hot or cold water. Drink this amount three times daily.

Alternative: Drink hot tea (two to three times daily) that combines hawthorn with linden flowers, an herb that has a mild antihypertensive effect. Such tea bags are available at most health-food stores.

INSOMNIA

Stress, poor sleep habits and health problems that cause pain are common causes of insomnia (an inability to fall asleep or remain asleep).

Best herbal treatment: **Passion flower** (leaves or whole plant). Its depressant effect on the central nervous system helps promote restful sleep.

How to use: Add 1 ml to 4 ml of passion-flower tincture to one ounce of cold water, or make an infusion by pouring one cup of boiling water over one teaspoon of dried passionflower and letting it sit for 15 minutes. Drink the entire tincture mixture or infusion at bedtime when you suffer from insomnia.

Caution: People who take drugs with sedative effects, such as certain antihistamines, anti-anxiety medications and insomnia supplements or drugs, should not use passionflower, which can increase these sedative effects.

IRRITABLE BOWEL SYNDROME

Alternating bouts of constipation and diarrhea are characteristic of irritable bowel syndrome (IBS).

Best herbal treatment: **Yarrow** (leaves and other parts that grow aboveground) for the diarrhea phase…**mugwort** (leaves) for constipation. These herbs also are effective for episodes of diarrhea and constipation that are not related to IBS.

Yarrow contains *tannins*, substances that reduce the amount of water released by the intestinal lining. Mugwort is a bitter herb that promotes the intestinal contractions needed for bowel movements.

How to use: Add 1 ml to 2 ml of yarrow or mugwort tincture to one ounce of hot or cold water. Drink this amount three times daily when you have diarrhea or constipation.

OSTEOARTHRITIS

Age-related changes in the joints are the primary cause of osteoarthritis. Most patients can get temporary relief with pain relievers, such as *ibuprofen* (Advil), but these drugs often cause side effects, such as gastrointestinal bleeding.

Best herbal treatment: **Black mustard** (for external use) and **meadowsweet** (for internal use). A poultice of black mustard causes mild, temporary inflammation that stimulates circulation—good for muscle and/or joint pain.

How to use: Make a black-mustard poultice by grinding the seeds in a coffee grinder and mixing one-half cup of the mustard powder with one cup of flour. Add enough hot water to make a paste. Spread the mixture on a piece of heavy brown paper, cotton or muslin that has been soaked in hot water, then cover it with a second piece of dry material. Lay the moist side of the poultice across the painful area, leaving it on for 15 to 30 minutes once daily.

Caution: Consult a doctor before using the poultice on a young child, or on anyone who is age 70 or older or seriously ill.

Meadowsweet is a pain reliever that contains aspirin-like chemicals called *salicylates*.

How to use: Add 1 ml to 2 ml of meadowsweet tincture to one ounce of hot or cold water. Drink this amount three times daily until symptoms subside.

PERIODONTAL DISEASE

Bacterial buildup in the spaces between the teeth and gums leads to periodontal (gum) disease—the most common cause of tooth loss in older adults. Gum infection has been linked to an increased risk for heart attack and stroke. Regular dental care and cleanings (at least annually) are essential.

Best herbal treatment: Goldenseal and/or myrrh. Goldenseal acts as a topical antibiotic. Myrrh strengthens mucous membranes. Start treatment when you first notice gum tenderness and/or bleeding—the first signs of periodontal disease.

How to use: Mix equal amounts of goldenseal and myrrh tinctures. Use a very fine paintbrush to apply the mixture to the gum line. Leave it on as long as you can—the taste is unpleasant—then rinse your mouth with water and spit it out. Repeat two or three times daily.

SKIN DRYNESS

Declines in the activity of oil-producing glands make skin dryness a common complaint after age 50.

Best herbal treatment: Gentian. It's a bitter herb that stimulates the oil-producing *exocrine* glands in the skin.

How to use: Add 1 ml to 2 ml of tincture to one ounce of hot or cold water. Drink this amount three times daily, until your skin's condition improves.

Natural Remedies to Treat And Prevent Heart Disease

Gary Null, PhD, consumer health advocate and educator for more than 30 years, is a nationally syndicated talk show host and author of more than 70 books, including *Complete Encyclopedia of Natural Healing*. Bottom Line. He is adjunct professor at Fairleigh Dickinson University, Teaneck, NJ, and research director of Institute of Applied Biology, New York City.

Heart disease is America's number-one killer. Yet heart disease, which is primarily caused by inflammation and an accumulation of plaque in the coronary arteries, is one of the most preventable of all illnesses.

The key is to make lifestyle changes and take natural supplements. In fact, there is scientific evidence that people who already are suffering from heart problems can reverse the effects of the disease.

Here are three all-natural programs—one for general heart health, another for high cholesterol, a third for high blood pressure. Choose one, two or all three programs.

If you are doing more than one at a time, don't double or triple up on supplements. Take no more than the highest amount called for in one program. All the supplements listed are available at most health-food stores.

Regular aerobic exercise is part of each of these programs, and I offer advice on getting the most out of exercise at the end of this article.

Important: Review these programs, including supplement dosages, with your doctor. Natural remedies are not a substitute for standard or conventional treatment but are meant to be done in conjunction with whatever your primary doctor or cardiologist recommends.

GENERAL HEART HEALTH

Your body needs certain nutrients to counteract the effects of internal inflammation on the coronary arteries…

•**Coenzyme Q10,** one of my favorites, is a superstar in protecting the heart. It increases oxygenation to the heart and helps prevent recurrences in people who have had a heart attack.

Recommendation: 100 mg to 300 mg daily.

•**Omega-3 fatty acids** decrease the growth rate of atherosclerotic plaque, which can lead to atherosclerosis, known as hardening of the arteries. Omega-3s also reduce the risk of arrhythmias, which can lead to sudden cardiac death.

Recommendation: 3,000 mg daily.

•**L-carnitine** helps transport long-chain fatty acids, which bring energy to the heart and aid in prevention of heart disease, high blood pressure and other cardiovascular diseases.

Recommendation: 500 mg to 1,000 mg daily.

•**Vitamin E,** which has *tocotrienols* and *gamma tocopherol*, is an antioxidant that helps protect cells against damage.

139

Recommendation: 200 international units (IU) to 400 IU daily. Consult your doctor.

•**Cayenne pepper** contains the active ingredient capsaicin, a natural blood thinner that helps prevent heart attacks and strokes.

Dosage: Sprinkle regularly on food.

Caution: Check with your doctor if you are on a blood-thinning medication, such as *warfarin* (Coumadin).

•**Hawthorn berry** relaxes blood vessels, enhances circulation and helps prevent arterial hardening.

Recommendation: 100 mg twice daily.

REDUCE CHOLESTEROL

Elevated levels of cholesterol are a major marker for heart attacks. Cholesterol provides the raw material for plaque, a fatty substance that builds up inside arteries and clogs them.

Optimal levels: A combined blood cholesterol count under 200 mg/dL, with LDL levels (often referred to as "bad" cholesterol) under 70 mg/dL and HDL levels ("good" cholesterol) over 45 mg/dL.

•**L-carnosine** is an amino acid found naturally in the body. This antioxidant helps rejuvenate cells and protect them from premature aging.

Recommendation: 500 mg to 1,000 mg daily.

•**Niacin/vitamin B3,** also known as nicotinic acid, lowers LDL cholesterol and raises HDL cholesterol.

Recommendation: 100 mg daily.

•**Shiitake mushrooms** speed up the processing of cholesterol in the liver and stimulate the immune system.

Recommendation: One-half to one cup of shiitake mushrooms daily. I like them lightly sautéed in olive oil.

•**Fruits and fruit juices** are rich in *phytonutrients*, which are powerful antioxidants.

Recommendation: Two to three servings daily. Look for juices that have no added sugar.

Best: Tart cherry, pomegranate, wild blueberry.

LOWER HIGH BLOOD PRESSURE

Prolonged high blood pressure (hypertension) damages the lining of the arteries that supply blood to the heart. This can lead to atherosclerosis.

Optimal blood pressure levels: A systolic rate (the top number) under 115 mm/Hg and a diastolic rate (the bottom number) under 75 mm/Hg.

•**Calcium citrate and magnesium.** This combination supplement promotes relaxation of the muscles, including the heart.

Recommendation: 1,500 mg daily.

•**Garlic** lowers blood pressure by thinning the blood, thus enhancing circulation.

Recommendation: Two to three cloves daily. It is easiest to digest when sautéed until translucent (not brown). Or take a 1,000-mg garlic supplement, but check with your doctor if you are on a blood-thinning drug.

•**Potassium** is needed for electrolyte balance, especially if you take certain blood pressure medications. Check with your doctor.

Recommendation: 500 mg daily.

•**Green vegetable juices,** especially those from spinach, broccoli and kale, help thin the blood, lowering blood pressure. You can buy them at health-food stores or make them yourself with a vegetable juicer (add a pear or an apple if you like a sweeter taste).

Recommendation: Two to three six-ounce servings daily. Check with your doctor if you are on blood-thinning medication.

EXERCISE

Regular aerobic exercise, such as fast walking, reduces cholesterol, increases circulation and keeps arteries healthy. *To get the most out of exercise...*

•**Work up to 45 minutes of aerobic exercise four times a week.** This can take several months. Get a clean bill of health from your doctor before starting.

•**Take your pulse.** Take it before you exercise, then immediately upon stopping, then every five minutes until your pulse has returned to its pre-exercise level. You know you are in shape if your pulse returns to its pre-exercise level in less than five minutes.

•**When you walk or jog, keep your feet as close to the ground as possible, almost as if you're shuffling.** The higher the knee comes off the ground, the greater the pressure and the risk of injury when your leg comes down.

Save Over $70 a Month on Heart-Healthy Fish Oil

Mark A. Stengler, ND, naturopathic physician in private practice, La Jolla, California...adjunct associate clinical professor at the National College of Natural Medicine, Portland, Oregon...author of many books, including *The Natural Physician's Healing Therapies* and coauthor of *Prescription for Natural Cures* (both from Bottom Line Books)...and author of the *Bottom Line/Natural Healing* newsletter.

Fish oil supplements have been sold over the counter (OTC) in health-food stores for years. But ever since the FDA approved a prescription brand called Lovaza (formerly Omacor) in 2004, patients have been asking if they should toss their OTC fish oil in favor of this new product. That would be a mistake.

Lovaza's manufacturer, Reliant Pharmaceuticals (now owned by GlaxoSmithKline), obtained FDA approval by conducting a clinical trial showing that the product reduces blood levels of triglycerides (fats) and thereby lowers a person's risk for cardiovascular disease. Laws prohibit OTC supplement manufacturers from making specific health claims unless the product is FDA-approved—which means Lovaza is the only fish oil that can advertise its triglyceride-lowering effects.

Fact: Any good-quality OTC fish oil product, used at the right dosage, can lower triglycerides and provide numerous other health benefits—at a fraction of Lovaza whopping cost of $180 for 120 capsules.

Do the math: Suppose you want to take about 1,600 mg per day of a combination of the two most beneficial components of fish oil —*docosahexaenoic acid* (DHA) and *eicosapentaenoic acid* (EPA). You would take two capsules daily of Lovaza, at a cost per month of $79. You could get an equal amount of DHA/EPA by taking three capsules daily of the reputable OTC brand Nordic Naturals Omega-3 (800-662-2544, *www.nordicnaturals.com*), at a cost per month of about $27 on-line to $43 retail...while the per-month cost of the brand Natural Factors RxOmega-3 Factors would be just $14 on-line (at various sites, including *www.webvitamins.com,* 800-919-9122) to $27 retail. Even if your health insurance covers Lovaza—which it may not—your out-of-pocket prescription co-pay could exceed the cost of a quality OTC brand.

WHAT'S ESSENTIAL ABOUT FISH OIL?

Fish oil is an unbeatable source of omega-3s, one type of the *essential fatty acids* (EFAs), which the body needs but cannot make on its own and therefore must get through diet. Of the six different forms of omega-3s, the most beneficial are DHA and EPA, which are abundant in fish oil. A second type of EFAs are the omega-6s.

Together, omega-3s and omega-6s serve the body in many ways. As vital structural components of cell membranes, EFAs affect the health of all of our cells, particularly those found in the eyes, skin, brain, nervous system and cardiovascular system. EFAs also help to regulate metabolism, hormone production, blood pressure and blood clotting...strengthen the immune system ...and combat tissue-damaging inflammation.

To function properly, omega-3s and omega-6s must be in balance with each other, ideally at a ratio of from one-to-three to one-to-four in favor of omega-6s.

Problem: Many people consume 10 times as many omega-6s as omega-3s. Vegetable oils and grains, including corn—all common in processed and packaged foods—are loaded with omega-6s. These ingredients also are used in feed given to livestock, so they get into our bodies when we eat meat and poultry. Omega-6s are not harmful in and of themselves—but when they overwhelm omega-3s, they increase the risk for chronic inflammation, cardiovascular disease, diabetes, autoimmune diseases (including lupus and psoriasis), mood disorders and perhaps even some cancers.

THE POWER OF OMEGA-3s

Hundreds of studies demonstrate how omega-3s fight various diseases. *Among them...*

- **Cardiovascular disease.**
- **Cognitive and mental disorders.**
- **Arthritis.**
- **Cancer.**
- **Retinal problems.**

SENSIBLE DIET & SUPPLEMENT GUIDE

Flaxseeds and walnuts, as well as canola, soybean and walnut oils, contain small amounts of the omega-3 *alpha-linolenic acid* (ALA), which the body converts to EPA and DHA. However, the richest food sources of EPA and DHA are cold-water fish—particularly salmon, herring, anchovies and sardines. Halibut, mackerel and tuna (including canned) also have omega-3s, but I recommend eating them no more than once a month due to concerns about mercury contamination.

I think wild fish are preferable to farm-raised fish. Instead of living far out to sea, farm-raised fish live near shore—and so are more likely to be contaminated with man-made pollutants. Some farmed fish may have more omega-3s, depending on their diet, but many are fed grains that disproportionately raise their omega-6 content. I advise limiting consumption of farmed fish to one serving monthly.

Consumer savvy: When fish is wild, the fish sellers usually highlight that fact.

Due to our contaminated food supply, the best way to get enough omega-3s generally is to supplement with fish oil. Reputable supplement brands usually undergo independent testing to verify purity and potency. Fish oil supplements are available in liquid or gel capsule form. The liquid usually provides a higher concentration per dose, costs less and is available flavored with lemon or orange to reduce the fishy taste. Even so, most people prefer gel capsules, which have no taste.

For some people, fish oil triggers unpleasant bouts of belching and/or nausea. To minimize this, take fish oil with meals and in divided doses. If the problem persists, try enteric-coated capsules—their harder casing keeps capsules from opening until they reach the small intestine, preventing stomach gassiness and upset. A good economical brand is Fisol Enteric-Coated Fish Oil by Nature's Way (800-962-8873, *www. naturesway.com*).

Note: Despite its high price, prescription Omacor is not enteric-coated.

Fish oil capsules often come in 1,000-mg doses, but this may refer to the weight of the oil rather than the amount of DHA and EPA they provide.

Smart: Check labels to see how many capsules you must take daily to get the standard dose of 500 mg to 1,000 mg of combined DHA and EPA (usually manufactured at a 1.5-to-1 ratio favoring EPA). Start with the lower dose, and if you are satisfied with the effects—such as the level of improvement in mild joint pain—stick with it. Otherwise, after six weeks, increase to the higher dose. Take 2,000 mg to 3,000 mg daily if you have any risk factors for cardiovascular disease, such as high cholesterol or triglycerides, hypertension, atherosclerosis or irregular heartbeat…are at high risk for cancer (for instance, due to family history)…or have arthritis or Alzheimer's.

Freshness is important. When fish oil turns rancid, it undergoes a chemical change called *oxidation*—so you end up swallowing health-damaging molecules called free radicals. *To prevent this…*

• **Choose a fish oil that includes an antioxidant,** such as vitamin E or rosemary extract, which prevents rancidity. The brands I have recommended contain antioxidants.

• **If your fish oil brand has no antioxidant,** prevent the oxidation reaction from occurring within your body's cells by also taking a daily multivitamin that contains vitamin E or by taking a separate daily supplement of vitamin E, usually sold in capsules of 200 international units (IU) to 400 IU. Ask your doctor.

• **Check the expiration date before you buy.**

• **Select a product that comes in an opaque container,** which filters out oil-degrading light.

• **Refrigerate after opening.**

• **To guard against rancidity,** take note if a liquid product develops an "off" taste. Check capsules monthly by cutting into one and taking a whiff or taste. If the oil has a strong odor or very unpleasant flavor, discard the rest and buy a fresh supply.

SUPPLEMENT SAFETY

Fish oil generally is safe for everyone—but these guidelines help to prevent potential problems.

• **Get your doctor's approval before taking fish oil if you…**

• Use blood-thinning medication, such as aspirin, *warfarin* (Coumadin) or *clopidogrel* (Plavix).

Fish oil thins the blood and reduces clotting, so you may need a lower dose of medication.

•Are pregnant or nursing. Fish oil is beneficial during pregnancy—yet as a general precaution, discuss all your nutritional supplements (and OTC drugs) with your obstetrician.

•**Switch to a different brand if you develop a skin rash.** This uncommon side effect may result from a sensitivity to the oil's preservatives or to the type of fish from which a particular brand is derived.

•**Take fish oil along with garlic if your LDL "bad" cholesterol level rises** after you start taking fish oil. This effect, which is rare and not well-understood, can be countered by taking 1,200 mg of aged garlic extract daily.

•**Stop taking fish oil 10 days prior to scheduled surgery** (including dental surgery but not regular cleanings) to prevent excessive bleeding. Start taking it again one week after surgery, with your doctor's approval.

Free Way to Help Your Heart, Boost Memory And More!

Sara Mednick, PhD, associate professor, department of psychiatry, University of California, San Diego. Dr. Mednick is author of *Take A Nap!* Workman.

What if there were a safe, nontoxic, simple, *free* way to increase your alertness…boost your creativity…improve your memory…*reduce your stress*…and *even reduce your risk for heart disease*, all in just 20 minutes a day? There is. It's called a nap.

NAPPING WITHOUT GUILT

In our work-driven, activity-driven society, the hardest part of taking a nap is getting past that little voice in your head telling you that napping is a sign of laziness.

Reality: People who nap tend to be more productive, not less.

When you allow yourself that brief period of rest and refreshment, you wake up alert and energized, ready to be active for the rest of the day. The time you spend sleeping is more than made up for by the improved work or activity time a nap can give you.

Instead of a nap, you could just have coffee or another form of caffeine to perk yourself up, but a nap is a better idea. Caffeine makes you more alert, but it doesn't give you any of the other benefits of napping.

Example: Napping enhances performance on a wide range of memory tests. Studies show that a 90-minute nap is as good as a full night's sleep for improving memory.

THE SLEEP CYCLE

To understand why napping can be so valuable, it helps to understand the basic concept of the sleep cycle and how it applies to both nighttime sleeping and daytime napping.

Through the night, your sleep moves through a consistent pattern of four distinct phases…

•**Stage 1.** This occurs when you're just falling asleep and generally lasts for only a few minutes. Your structured thinking gradually gives way to dreamlike imagery.

•**Stage 2.** After you've fallen asleep, stage 2 sleep takes over. During this time, many parts of your brain are less active, but stage 2 sleep is the sleep that restores alertness and helps consolidate motor learning—anything that involves muscle movements such as dancing or driving.

•**Stage 3.** When you move into stage 3 sleep, your brain waves slow down, so much so that this stage is also called slow-wave sleep (SWS). In SWS, your body repairs itself because growth hormone is secreted during this phase, which helps with muscle fiber growth and repair as well as bone growth—basically, the antidote to cortisol, a stress hormone—and consolidates memory, such as new information you've just learned (a phone number, for example) so that you'll remember it.

•**Stage 4.** During stage 4, you move into rapid eye movement (REM) sleep, or dreaming. REM sleep is when you consolidate more complex information and learning, such as a vocabulary list in a foreign language.

In the course of the night, you generally go through stage 1 sleep only once, just as you fall asleep. After that, you cycle through stage 2, stage 3 (SWS) and stage 4 (REM) sleep several times through the night. Each cycle takes about 90 minutes. Of that, about 60% is spent in stage 2 sleep. The amount of time spent in SWS and REM sleep varies through the cycles.

YOUR OPTIMUM NAP

Most people feel a natural lull in their energy levels sometime during the afternoon. That's the natural time for napping—and in many countries, the traditional siesta happens then. Ideally, because one sleep cycle takes about 90 minutes, you would nap for that long and awaken feeling refreshed and alert.

Not too many of us can manage a full 90 minutes in the middle of the day, however, and not everyone feels the need to nap that long. *To choose the best nap length for you, decide what you want to get from your nap...*

•**Stage 2 nap.** Reduces sleepiness, heightens alertness, increases concentration, enhances motor performance and elevates mood.

Sleep for: 15 to 20 minutes.

•**Stage 3 (SWS) nap.** Clears away useless information, improves conscious memory recall and restores and repairs tissues.

Sleep for: 60 minutes.

•**Stage 4 (REM sleep) nap.** Increases creativity, improves perceptual and sensory processing, and improves memory for complex information.

Sleep for: 90 minutes.

The best time for your nap depends on several factors, including when you woke up and what type of sleep you want to get from your nap.

NAPPING AND YOUR HEALTH

We know that lack of sleep is definitely bad for your health, but is napping good for it? That has actually been a hotly debated question. Over the years, some studies seemed to show that people who often napped had a greater risk for death, especially from heart disease.

A recent Harvard University study, however, strongly suggests the opposite. In the study, more than 23,000 people in Greece were followed for an average of 6.3 years. None of the individuals had a history of heart disease, stroke or cancer at the start of the study, and they ranged in age from 20 to 86. The results showed that the people who regularly napped for at least 30 minutes at least three times a week had a 37% lower risk for death from heart disease than the non-nappers.

Taking a nap in the afternoon doesn't usually affect a person's ability to get to sleep at his/her normal bedtime or to sleep for the normal number of hours at night. In fact, many people who start taking daytime naps report that they fall asleep more easily at bedtime and feel more refreshed in the morning.

Exception: Don't nap within two to three hours of your usual bedtime—it could keep you from getting to sleep on schedule.

SLEEP AND AGE

Older adults often find themselves waking up earlier than they used to and having trouble getting back to sleep. Shifting to an earlier wake-up time—and feeling the need for an earlier bedtime—is a natural part of the changes in body rhythm that come with aging. Rather than fighting your body's normal needs, accept them. A great way to make up for the lost sleep and help yourself stay up later? Take a nap!

■ ■ ■ ■

Nap for Heart Health

To reduce risk of death from coronary heart disease, take a midday nap.

Study: People who napped for about a half hour at least three times a week had a 37% lower risk of dying from heart attacks or other heart problems than those who did not nap. Individuals who took naps of any duration had a 34% lower risk of dying from heart disease.

Dimitrios Trichopoulos, MD, PhD, professor, department of epidemiology, Harvard School of Public Health, Boston.

Take Time To Nap

William A. Anthony, PhD, executive director of Boston University's Center for Psychiatric Rehabilitation, and the author of *The Art of Napping*. Larson.

According to the National Sleep Foundation, about 62% of Americans get sleepy in the afternoon at least three days a week—but our fast-paced culture discourages the habit of napping. That may be a mistake.

Our natural sleep pattern includes a significant drop in body temperature and alertness at night, as well as a similar (if less dramatic) drop at midday.

Recent research suggests that those who take 10- to 20-minute naps score better on cognitive tests. These people also have more energy, are involved in fewer accidents and, generally, are healthier—napping is believed to reduce stress, pulse rate and hypertension, improvements that promote cardiovascular health.

Naps are not a substitute for sleeping well at night. If you feel tired when you awaken in the morning, see your doctor for advice. And don't nap for too long—30 minutes or more makes people groggy when they wake up.

Best: A daily *power nap* lasting 15 or 20 minutes. That's just long enough to satisfy the body's need for rest, without interfering with nighttime sleep. Enjoy!

6

Health Alerts

Symptoms You Should Never Ignore

We all experience troublesome symptoms from time to time, such as fatigue or digestive upset. These usually indicate mild conditions, but they can be a sign of dangerous problems. Complicating matters is that some symptoms are more likely to be serious for men, others for women. Symptoms and what they can mean…

DANGEROUS SYMPTOMS FOR MEN

Symptom: Shoulder pain.

Could be: Coronary artery disease.

Many men are sedentary during the week, then overdo it on weekends—and blame sudden shoulder pain on muscle strain. But shoulder pain that comes on suddenly often is a sign of coronary artery disease. In some cases, this is the only symptom. More often, men also will report that they are experiencing occasional shortness of breath and possibly subtle chest pain.

Important: Call 911 or get to an emergency room immediately if shoulder pain comes on suddenly for no obvious reason—or if it's accompanied by other symptoms. You could be having a heart attack.

Also: Ask your doctor, before an emergency arises, if you should take aspirin if you are having symptoms of a heart attack. Aspirin (chewed and swallowed) can reduce the severity of a heart attack.

Symptom: Persistent foot and hip pain.

Could be: Prostate cancer.

Nearly everyone experiences joint pain on occasion. It's usually due to overuse injuries or relatively mild "wear and tear" arthritis—joint pain that gets more common with age.

J. Edward Hill, MD, past president of the American Medical Association, board member of the Mississippi Department of Health and an adviser for the American Medical Association, *Family Medical Guide* (Wiley), is a family physician and a faculty member at the Family Medicine Residency Center, North Mississippi Medical Center, Tupelo.

However, a man who experiences joint pain that doesn't improve after a few days with the usual treatments, such as rest and over-the-counter analgesics, should get a complete checkup. This is especially important if the pain starts in the foot or ankle, then extends to the hip. It could indicate that prostate cancer has started to spread. Any delay could be life-threatening.

Also important: Men should see a doctor immediately if they notice any change in their urine or urinary habits—difficulty urinating, blood in the urine, etc. Men often assume that this is due to normal, age-related changes in the prostate gland—but changes in urinary habits also can indicate early-stage prostate cancer.

DANGEROUS SYMPTOMS FOR WOMEN

Symptoms: Slight numbness in an arm or leg, transient loss of balance, intermittent blurred vision.

Could be: Multiple sclerosis (MS).

Numbness, balance difficulties and vision changes are classic signs of MS, a disease that affects women about twice as often as men. Women often ignore the symptoms because they tend to come and go quickly—and they may occur so rarely that they don't seem serious. Many patients with MS report having symptoms up to seven years before being diagnosed.

MS symptoms usually get worse over time. Women who get early treatment—with drugs such as beta interferons, for example—usually have a marked reduction in symptoms and retain their ability to live normal lives.

Symptom: Minor abdominal/pelvic pain that comes and goes.

Could be: Ovarian cancer.

Most women of child-bearing age experience occasional discomfort in the abdomen or pelvic region. It's usually due to digestive distress or menstruation, but it also can be an early sign of ovarian cancer. The discomfort usually lasts a few days, then goes away for weeks or months. Because the pain tends to be minor and intermittent, most women ignore it—even when it occurs over the course of months or years.

Other possible symptoms of ovarian cancer: Abdominal swelling or bloating...indigestion and/or nausea...and/or urinary urgency.

The discomfort of menstrual or digestive conditions tends to occur in a predictable fashion—for example, at a certain time of the month or after eating certain foods. With ovarian cancer, the discomfort gets more persistent and severe as the cancer grows.

Important: Women experiencing this kind of pain should see a doctor right away. Ovarian cancer can be successfully treated when it is detected in the early stages. Because it causes only minor symptoms—or no symptoms at all, in some cases—only about 29% of patients are diagnosed before the cancer has spread. At that point, treatments are much less likely to be effective.

Symptoms: Unusual fatigue, shortness of breath.

Could be: Heart disease.

A woman's symptoms of heart disease or a heart attack are typically different than a man's. Women are unlikely to experience crushing chest pain or pain radiating down one or both arms. Instead, they are more likely to experience fatigue, difficulty breathing, pressure or pain in the upper abdomen or symptoms resembling indigestion.

A woman with heart disease may get short of breath or feel exhausted all the time. If you suspect you are having a heart attack, call for emergency medical help immediately.

Also: Ask your doctor, before an emergency arises, if you should take aspirin if you are having symptoms of a heart attack. Aspirin (chewed and swallowed) can reduce the severity of a heart attack.

■ ■ ■ ■

The Lowdown on Bedbugs

Bedbugs—small nocturnal insects that feed on human and animal blood—are a growing problem in hotels in the US and abroad, as well as in apartment houses, dormitories, sleep-away camps and other places.

Unlike mosquitoes, bedbugs don't transmit disease—but their bites can cause irritation and discomfort. They do not attach themselves to people. They move from place to place via luggage, clothing and other items.

To protect yourself...

When staying away from home: Pull back the bed sheets, and check the mattress seams and tufts. Look for live bugs that are about one-quarter to one-half-inch long and vary in color from reddish brown to nearly transparent.

Also: Check for light brown, translucent molted skins…and pin-sized black spots (excrement). If possible, pull back the fabric headboard and inspect it, too. If signs are present, ask for another room.

Helpful: Keep your luggage in the bathroom until you have checked the bed.

When you return home: Leave luggage outside until you have inspected each item.

At home: If you find bedbugs on an article of clothing, comforters or other linens, wash them in 150° water. You may also want to call an exterminator.

Caution: Do not bring used furniture or mattresses into your home.

Dini M. Miller, PhD, associate professor of entomology, Virginia Tech, Blacksburg, Virginia. Virginia Tech raises bedbugs for research.

Organ Transplants Can Also Transfer Disease

Rona MacKie, MD, honorary senior research fellow, University of Glasgow, Scotland.

Daniel G. Coit, MD, co-leader of the melanoma disease management team, Memorial Sloan-Kettering Cancer Center, New York City.

Robert A. Fisher, MD, professor of surgery, and director, Liver Transplant Programs, Virginia Commonwealth University Medical Center, Richmond.

The New England Journal of Medicine.

Sixteen years after a Scottish woman was diagnosed with melanoma, the deadly cancer was transferred to two more people via the woman's donated kidneys. Although the transplant surgeons should have checked the Scottish woman's background, they could not reach her primary care physician.

That incident and similar ones have resulted in stricter controls in some hospitals for organ transplants.

EXPERT OPINIONS

"It's very worrisome," says Dr. Rona MacKie, professor of dermatology at the University of Glasgow in Scotland. "The amazing thing about this patient is the gap between having the melanoma diagnosed and giving her kidneys."

The time gap was twice as long as any other case, which testifies to the resilience of tumor cells, MacKie says.

Although other cancers have been transferred with a transplanted organ, melanoma seems to be particularly dangerous.

"There is a significant risk in patients with melanoma, even after 10 or 15 years. It's not the same with other cancers," says Dr. Robert Fisher, director of the liver transplant program at Virginia Commonwealth University Medical Center.

Caution: People who have had invasive melanoma should not donate organs. In fact, they are already prohibited from donating blood, according to the American Red Cross.

THE TRANSPLANTS

In May 1998, a woman in Glasgow finally received the kidney that would enable her to go off dialysis. She seemed well until a year and a half later, when a routine mammography turned up a spot on the woman's left breast.

A biopsy uncovered something unusual: Secondary melanoma but no primary site. Secondary cancers are those that have spread from another part of the body. MacKie said there was no evidence of a primary melanoma, which is usually attached to a tumor.

Four months later, a second transplant patient arrived at the same hospital with a lump in his kidney that turned out—again—to be secondary melanoma with no indication of a primary site. His transplant and the woman's transplant were done only 24 hours apart.

The donor in both cases turned out to be the same person, a 62-year-old woman who had been treated for melanoma in 1982. After treatment, her doctors considered her cured of the cancer. She died 16 years later, ostensibly of a hemorrhage.

Both kidney recipients had the organs removed and were treated for melanoma, but only one survived.

HOW DID IT HAPPEN?

Although how this happened will never be known because an autopsy was not performed on the donor, two scenarios emerge as possibilities, says Dr. Daniel G. Coit, co-leader of the melanoma disease management team at Memorial Sloan-Kettering Cancer Center in New York City.

One scenario is that the donor actually died of undetected metastatic melanoma. The second is that individual melanoma cells were lurking in her body, waiting for the opportunity to flourish.

MacKie prefers the second scenario, and believes the cancer cells were lying dormant in the kidneys. Because transplant patients take immunosuppressant drugs to minimize the chances that the donated organ will be rejected, the weakened immune system may have encouraged the cancer growth.

Nicotine Vaccine Helps Smokers Quit

Kim D. Janda, PhD, professor of chemistry, The Scripps Research Institute, La Jolla, California. Dr. Janda is the recipient of an NIH First Award.
Journal of the American Chemical Society.

A nicotine vaccine shows promise in ending nicotine addiction and helping smokers kick the habit, researchers say.

The vaccine allows the immune system to provide potent antibodies to remove nicotine from the body before it reaches the brain, says lead researcher Kim D. Janda, a professor of chemistry at The Scripps Research Institute in La Jolla, California.

The vaccine could act as a crutch for people trying to stop smoking by preventing nicotine from reaching the brain, Janda says.

FURTHER STUDY NEEDED

The next step in the development of this new vaccine is to do more studies; it has only been tested in mice and rats. Once the researchers have more evidence that the vaccine is safe, it will be ready for clinical human trials.

The vaccine is designed to help smokers during the critical first 90 days of smoking cessation, when many relapse.

Epilepsy Drug Helps Alcoholics

Bankole A. Johnson, MD, PhD, DSc, former professor of psychiatry and pharmacology, deputy chairman of research and director of the South Texas Addiction Research and Technology Center, University of Texas Health Science Center, San Antonio. Dr. Johnson is currently professor and chairman of psychiatry and neurobehavioral sciences at the University of Virginia, Charlottesville.
The Lancet.

I n what could be a breakthrough in the treatment of alcoholism, researchers say an antiseizure drug dramatically reduced drinking among alcoholics.

Alcoholics who took *topiramate* were six times as likely as those who took a placebo to abstain from drinking for at least four consecutive weeks during a 12-week study, say researchers at the University of Texas Health Science Center in San Antonio. Topiramate is a drug that the US Food and Drug Administration (FDA) approved for the treatment of epileptic and other seizures.

The study also found that those who took the placebo were four times as likely as those who took topiramate to drink heavily for 28 consecutive days.

PROMISING IMPLICATIONS

The dramatic results suggest that the drug may be more effective than any others currently being used to treat alcoholics, says lead researcher Dr. Bankole A. Johnson.

"The critical factor here is not only were all [of the subjects] heavily dependent on alcohol, but they were all still drinking heavily," says Johnson, director of the Health Science Center's South Texas Addiction Research and Technology Center.

Researchers defined drinking heavily as more than five drinks per day for men and more than four for women.

Johnson says existing drugs for alcoholism —*disulfiram* (Antabuse), which makes patients sick if they drink, and *naltrexone* (Depde), which blocks the pleasure sensations from alcohol—are designed mainly to prevent a relapse among alcoholics who stop drinking.

Topiramate helps alcoholics quit by blocking the "high" from alcohol while reducing withdrawal symptoms and cravings, Johnson says.

Your Dental Visit Can Save Your Life

Alan Winter, DDS, a periodontist in private practice and clinical assistant professor of periodontology and implant dentistry at the New York University College of Dentistry, both in New York City, has published more than a dozen medical journal articles on gum disease.

If you think that regular dental exams are just for your teeth and gums and aren't very important, you could be putting yourself in danger. Dentists are able to identify signs of a variety of serious diseases that affect other parts of the body.

Important finding: About 78% of periodontists (dentists who specialize in the diagnosis and treatment of gum disease) have referred patients age 60 or older to be evaluated for diabetes, and 21% have made referrals for osteoporosis, according to a poll conducted by the American Academy of Periodontology. All dentists are trained to identify these diseases and others.

How can an oral exam yield such crucial health information? While you're sitting in the dentist's chair to be treated for tooth or gum problems, your dentist is also checking for signs of cancer and other diseases. By monitoring changes in your gum tissue, your dentist can look for oral manifestations of diseases or other serious health problems.

Adults should get dental exams at least twice a year, or three to four times if they have gum (periodontal) disease. During a thorough exam, a dentist inspects all the soft tissues, including the gums, tongue, palate and throat, and feels (palpates) the patient's neck and under the chin. Signs of possible health problems include ulcerations, thickened tissue, pigmentation changes and abnormal color or consistency of gums and other soft tissues.

No one should consider a dental exam an adequate screening of overall physical health. However, your dentist can serve as a valuable adjunct to your other doctors in helping to spot signs of serious medical conditions.

CANCER

Dentists can spot possible malignancies that form in the gums, palate, cheek or other soft tissues. They also can identify tumors in the jawbone, which either originated there or metastasized (spread) from the breasts, bones, lungs or elsewhere in the body.

Warning signs: A newly formed lesion (open sore) or bump anywhere in the mouth that doesn't go away after seven to 10 days… swelling of the gums…teeth that suddenly become loose…and/or nonspecific oral pain that doesn't seem to be related to a tooth problem. Less commonly, a cancerous lesion in the jawbone may be seen on an X-ray, but many people who have cancer that has spread to the jaw are already being treated by an oncologist or surgeon. On rare occasions, a dentist may be the first to identify such a metastasis.

Self-defense: If you have a bump or lesion that doesn't heal in seven to 10 days without treatment, see your dentist. He/she will decide whether you should see a specialist, such as a periodontist, oral surgeon or ear, nose and throat specialist.

Important: Although some bumps and lesions are cancerous, most are benign and due to canker sores, routine gum problems, root canal problems—or they are the result of trauma, such as hitting your gum with the head of your toothbrush. To reach a proper diagnosis, your dentist will do a thorough examination, get a detailed medical history and may even take a biopsy.

DIABETES

Periodontal disease develops over a period of years. If a dentist sees gum breakdown that is more rapid than expected or there has been extreme bone loss that can't be explained, diabetes should be suspected.

Warning signs: Poor healing after oral surgery, inflammation in the gums and other periodontal problems. These may be signs of diabetes or diabetes that is not well controlled. Such problems can occur because diabetes suppresses the immune system, which impairs the infection-fighting function of white blood cells.

Self-defense: If your dentist suspects diabetes, you should see your primary care doctor or an endocrinologist for a glucose tolerance test.

OSTEOPOROSIS

Most people associate osteoporosis with bone loss in the spine or hips, but it also can occur in the jawbone.

Warning sign: On an X-ray, the jawbone will look less dense than it should.

Self-defense: Follow up with your primary care doctor. A bone-density test may be needed.

Caution: Bisphosphonate drugs, such as *alendronate* (Fosamax), have been linked to osteonecrosis of the jaw—death of areas of jawbone. Most reports of this side effect are associated with bisphosphonates taken intravenously by cancer patients whose malignancy has spread to their bones, but a handful of cases have involved people who took the oral form of the medication.

A LINK TO HEART DISEASE

Contrary to what many people believe, dentists cannot diagnose heart disease based on the appearance of a person's gums. Much has been written about a possible link between gum disease and heart disease. However, the research that showed a connection was retrospective—that is, it reviewed the characteristics of a particular group.

One such study was conducted by Robert Genco, PhD, professor at the State University of New York at Buffalo, and colleagues at the University of North Carolina at Chapel Hill. The researchers noted that cumulative evidence supports—but does not prove—an association between periodontal infection and cardiovascular disease. In a recent Finnish study, people with gum disease were found to be 1.6 times more likely to suffer a stroke.

Additional research is needed to determine whether gum disease is, in fact, a risk factor for cardiovascular disease. In the meantime, it makes sense to keep your gums healthy to help minimize the possible risk for heart disease. Studies have shown that people with heart disease are more likely to smoke, not exercise regularly and/or have poor diets.

Dentists often send people with diagnosed heart disease for a cardiovascular evaluation.

Reason: These patients need to get medical clearance for dental surgery. During these evaluations, the cardiologist checks the patient's blood pressure, use of blood thinners and overall risk for heart attack and stroke. A cardiovascular evaluation also helps determine which anesthetic to use—an additive used in some anesthesia can stimulate the heart.

No More Eyestrain

Mark A. Stengler, ND, naturopathic physician in private practice, La Jolla, California...adjunct associate clinical professor at the National College of Natural Medicine, Portland, Oregon...author of many books, including *The Natural Physician's Healing Therapies* and coauthor of *Prescription for Natural Cures* (both from Bottom Line Books)...and author of the *Bottom Line/Natural Healing* newsletter.

Anyone who spends extended time at a computer (an hour or more without a break) is vulnerable to blurred vision, red eyes, difficulty seeing long distances and headaches.

One of the first steps is to eliminate glare by tilting the screen away from light or getting an antiglare screen. These screens ($20 to over $100) are sold at office-supply and computer-accessory stores. Face your monitor away from windows and other bright light sources, and place it so the middle of the screen is slightly below eye level (about 20 degrees).

Take a five-minute break every 45 to 60 minutes to relax your eyes and body. Get up and walk around, and look away from bright light. Then sit in a relaxed position—for example, with your back straight and your hands on your knees, and take deep breaths. Perform a "cupping" technique to relax the eye muscles—place your cupped hands over your closed eyes, fingers resting on your forehead. Leave your hands there for one to two minutes while you relax.

The herbal extract bilberry (available at health-food stores and pharmacies) improves circulation to the eyes and reduces the redness and irritation that many people experience from computer use. Take 320 mg daily of a 25% *anthocyanoside* extract. For best results, take bilberry indefinitely.

Cell Phone Dangers

Rebecca Shannonhouse, editor of the *Bottom Line/Health* newsletters, Boardroom Inc., 281 Tresser Blvd., Stamford, Connecticut 06901.

There are more than 255 million cell-phone users in the US—and researchers are now beginning to identify some of the associated risks.

While studies have shown that there appears to be no increase in the risk for brain cancer among cell-phone users, these devices may not be safe in all circumstances.

Driving while talking on a cell phone is dangerous—even if you're using a "hands-free" model. A study indicates that motorists who talk on any type of cell phone show the same kind and degree of impairment—such as slowed reaction times—as drunken drivers.

People engaged in cell-phone conversations experience "inattention blindness"—even though they're looking at the road and traffic, their ability to process information drops by as much as 50%, explains Frank Drews, PhD, associate professor of psychology at the University of Utah in Salt Lake City and coauthor of the study.

Some people argue that other distractions, such as putting on makeup or talking to a passenger, are equally risky, but Drews doesn't buy it. "I've never seen a driver putting on makeup in the car—but at least every fourth or fifth driver is on a cell phone."

Meanwhile, in London, a 15-year-old girl suffered severe injuries after being struck by lightning while talking on her cell phone. People struck by lightning are often not critically injured, but holding a cell phone to the ear during a storm can provide a conduit that allows electricity—more than 100 million volts, in some cases—to flow into the body.

These recent developments show that it pays to think before you pick up a cell phone.

■ ■ ■ ■

Recycle Cell Phones

Cell phones contain toxic substances that can contaminate water and soil. Lead, mercury and other potentially dangerous elements are used in the manufacture of cell phones.

Best: Don't throw away an old cell phone. Instead, talk to your service provider or a third-party cell-phone recycler, such as Collective Good (*www.collectivegood.com*), about recycling it.

Samuel A. Simon, founder, Telecommunications Research and Action Center, Washington, DC.

Keep Your Shoulders Safe from Injury

Kevin D. Plancher, MD, a leading orthopedic surgeon and sports medicine specialist based in Greenwich, Connecticut, is associate clinical professor of orthopedics at Albert Einstein College of Medicine and attending physician at Beth Israel Hospital, both in New York City.

The shoulder is one of the most mobile joints in the body, capable of moving up to 180 degrees in a variety of planes, such as front to back and across the body. This versatility of movement aids performance in many activities and sports but leaves the shoulder uniquely vulnerable to painful and often debilitating injuries. In fact, shoulder problems account for 35% to 40% of all orthopedic injuries.

Shoulder troubles among athletes are common —but everyone is vulnerable. Even daily activities, such as household chores and yard work, can put tremendous strain on the shoulder joint.

Example: When carrying heavy boxes, people typically hold them well in front of the body, sometimes shoulder height or higher. These positions strain the shoulder and can result in soreness—or, in some cases, even permanent damage.

The most common shoulder injuries include *rotator cuff tears* (damage to the muscles/tendons that connect the upper arm bone, or humerus, to the shoulder blade)...*dislocations* (in which the humerus separates from the socket)...and *impingement syndrome* (the tendons of the rotator cuff get trapped between the roof of the shoulder, or acromion, and the head of the humerus).

Some injuries, such as a partial rotator cuff tear, near dislocation and impingement syndrome, improve when treated with ice for 20 minutes every three to four waking hours (do not put ice directly on the skin—use a towel) and/or over-the-counter anti-inflammatories, such as *ibuprofen* (Advil) or *naproxen* (Aleve). Follow label directions.

If these strategies don't relieve your acute shoulder pain within 72 hours, see an orthopedist or other sports medicine-trained physician. You may need a prescription painkiller, such as *hydrocodone* and *acetaminophen* (Vicodin) or *acetaminophen* and *codeine* (Tylenol with codeine)...physical therapy...and/or surgery to correct the problem.

Even though shoulder injuries can occur during virtually any activity that requires overhead or extensive shoulder movements, overexertion during exercise is still the most common trigger. The changes associated with aging, such as loss of muscle mass and diminished tendon flexibility, increase the risk for such joint damage.

Most common traps—and how to avoid them...

Trap 1: **Intermittent exercise.** Injuries often occur after people take a hiatus from a sport or start a new exercise or activity—for example, in the spring, when people who have been sedentary all winter spend long hours on the tennis court or working in the yard.

Muscles have "memory"—when skeletal muscle activity is repeated, the muscles remember that activity and can continue to perform at that level. That's why people who exercise regularly are not as prone to injury as "weekend warriors" (sedentary people who exceed their muscle memory on weekends).

Muscles and tendons require a longer warm-up time if you don't exercise daily. A good way to prepare includes five minutes of a gentle version of the exercise you're planning to perform.

Example: Walking before jogging...simulating a tennis serve...swinging a golf club without hitting a ball.

My recommendation: Before exercising, also be sure to stretch your shoulders. To do this, take a long towel and place it over your shoulder. Grip the top end with your right hand, and the bottom end with your left hand. Pull it up and down 10 to 15 times, bringing your right elbow up toward the ceiling. Switch sides and repeat. This rotational stretch works the main muscles in the shoulders and helps prevent many injuries, including rotator cuff tears.

Important: Stretching before and after exercise is particularly important for people age 40 and older, regardless of their overall activity level. Stretching and warming up before exercise gets muscles ready for the activity. Stretching after exercise increases blood flow to help muscles heal and recover.

Trap 2: **Lifting weights overhead.** This is among the most popular exercises for strengthening the shoulders. It's also one of the most dangerous. Lifting heavy weights straight overhead while standing—often called a military press—exerts tremendous stress on the shoulders. This exercise is a common cause of impingement.

My recommendation: Use the incline press (which allows you to lift weights overhead while lying on an incline). It works the same muscles, but without placing so much stress on the shoulders. Even patients with a history of impingement usually can do incline lifts without discomfort or risk.

Trap 3: **Hands out of sight.** Studies show that when the hands and/or fingers are out of your peripheral line of vision when doing strength training, the benefits of the exercise are minimized and the risk for injury to shoulder muscles is greatly increased.

Example: You'll often see people lowering the bar on a pull-down machine behind the

Illustration by Shawn Banner.

head. It's during that phase in motion (when the hands disappear from sight) that the risk for subluxation (movement of the shoulder out of the joint) increases.

My recommendation: When exercising, always keep your hands in your direct or peripheral line of vision when looking straight ahead. When doing pull-downs, lower the bar in front of your head.

Trap 4: **Too-wide grip.** Most upper-body exercise equipment includes some sort of bar with handles. The handles are typically positioned for a man of average height, shoulder-spread and reach length. For women and smaller men, the handle grips are usually too far apart. This puts excessive stress on the rotator cuff, which can cause damage and/or possible dislocation of the shoulder joint.

My recommendation: Grip the bars on exercise equipment no more than shoulder-width apart, regardless of where the handles are. The narrower grip reduces shoulder stress.

Trap 5: **Overtraining.** Performing exercises that work the same muscles every day leads to injuries, because muscle fibers don't have a chance to recover.

My recommendation: Give the shoulders time to recover by doing a different kind of workout—aerobics, weight-lifting, sports, etc.—every other day. On weekends, pick an activity you haven't done during the week. If you were sedentary, vary the workout (for example, work the upper body for a half hour and then the lower body for a half hour). Giving specific muscles a day of rest promotes muscle healing and faster recovery—and reduces risk for soreness or injuries.

RED FLAGS

If you experience any of the following signs of shoulder injury—or any kind of acute shoulder pain and/or restricted movement for more than a few days—see an orthopedic physician…

•**Pain** when you are putting on a coat or when you're reaching around to the backseat of a car could be signs of impingement or rotator cuff irritation.

•**Inability to lift your arm** from your side and raise an object above shoulder height without arching your back. This can indicate a serious rotator cuff tear.

•**Inability to sleep on one shoulder** due to pain. It is often a sign of early-stage rotator cuff damage.

•**Pain when reaching for objects overhead.** This can indicate impingement or other shoulder problems.

Caution: If you experience severe shoulder pain, go to the hospital right away. You could have a dislocated shoulder.

A Doctor Explains How To Stay Safe in Your Yard

Richard O'Brien, MD, spokesman for the American College of Emergency Physicians, is an emergency physician at Moses Taylor Hospital, Scranton, Pennsylvania.

The combination of warm weather and outdoor activities sends millions of Americans to emergency rooms each summer. Most of their injuries could have been prevented. *Here, an emergency room physician reveals the biggest dangers and how to avoid them…*

LAWN MOWERS

The lawn mower is probably the most dangerous tool around the house. A nine-year study published in *Annals of Emergency Medicine* reports an annual average of 74,000 emergency room visits due to lawn mower injuries. Most injuries are caused by debris flying into the bodies or eyes of lawn mower operators and bystanders. About one-third of lawn mower-related hospitalizations are due to injuries from the blades, including the loss of toes and/or fingers.

Self-defense: Remove twigs, sticks and rocks before mowing. Keep bystanders, especially children, away from the mower. Wear shoes—not sandals—long pants and safety goggles while mowing. Don't depend on glasses or sunglasses to protect eyes—they won't prevent debris from entering at the sides.

Also, wear hearing protection (ear plugs, ear mufflers, etc.). Don't use an iPod or similar portable music device—you really have to crank up the volume to hear the music, which can result in permanent hearing damage.

ELECTRIC HEDGE TRIMMERS

I see at least one patient a month who has been hurt by a hedge trimmer. It can cut off a finger instantly or cause a nasty injury—crushing tissue and bone—that is very difficult to repair.

Self-defense: Wear heavy leather or canvas gloves, sturdy shoes and long pants when using a trimmer. Don't overreach—you may lose your balance. Turn off the trimmer and unplug it before trying to clear it of stuck debris.

GARAGE DOORS

Some manual and electric garage doors have large, heavy springs on each side. A spring that suddenly loosens can hit your head with the force of a swinging baseball bat. A spring also can take off a finger.

Self-defense: Never attempt to repair or replace a garage door yourself. Hire an experienced professional to do it.

TICK BITES

Lyme disease gets most of the headlines, but ticks carry many other diseases, including ehrlichiosis and Rocky Mountain spotted fever, both bacterial infections that can cause fatigue, fever, severe muscle pain and headaches—and also can be life-threatening.

Self-defense: Removing a tick from your skin within 12 to 24 hours almost guarantees that you won't get sick. Grip the tick close to the skin with tweezers and pull it out. If part of the tick remains in the skin, try your best to remove it. If you're not able to remove it all, see a doctor. Wash the area well, and apply an antibiotic ointment to prevent infection.

If you're spending time in grassy or wooded areas, you can prevent most tick bites by using an insect repellent that contains DEET. Apply the repellent to exposed skin and clothing. A non-DEET repellent, Picaridin, is useful for people whose skin is sensitive to DEET. Also wear closed shoes rather than sandals…tuck long pants into socks…and wear a long-sleeved shirt, tucked in.

POISON IVY, OAK AND SUMAC

All of these plants contain *urushiol*, an oily substance that can cause an itchy rash in people who are sensitive to it. (To view the plants so you can identify them, go to *www.poisonivy.aesir.com.*) As little as one-billionth of a gram of urushiol can cause the rash—so even brushing against one of these plants is a problem. The oil also can get on tools, gloves and clothing and stays active indefinitely, so it must be washed off.

Self-defense: If your skin comes into contact with one of the "poisons," wash the area immediately with soap and water. If you're outside and don't have access to soap or water, splash the area with any liquid—soda, beer, etc. If a rash develops, apply hydrocortisone ointment, available at drugstores. If the rash worsens, see a doctor.

CYCLING

Each year, bicycle accidents result in more than half a million visits to emergency rooms. More than 800 bicyclists die annually, many from head injuries.

Self-defense: Always wear a helmet, even if you (or your children) are riding close to home. Studies indicate that helmets are up to 85% effective in preventing head injuries. Helmets with visors are helpful for preventing facial lacerations. Be sure the helmet fits properly and is buckled snugly.

Warning: Most cycling deaths occur between 6 pm and 9 pm, when visibility is diminished. Wear reflective clothing to make yourself more visible.

SWIMMING

Drowning is one of the leading causes of accidental death in the US.

Reasons: People overestimate their swimming ability…panic in deep water or fast currents …or consume large amounts of alcohol before entering the water.

Self-defense: Enter unfamiliar water feet first to prevent head and neck injuries. Don't depend on flotation devices—they can fail and sink. Never drink alcohol before or while swimming.

Danger for women: The bacteria that cause urinary tract infections thrive in moist environments. Women who sit around in wet swimsuits give these organisms an opportunity to proliferate and migrate into the urethra—and possibly up into the kidneys, resulting in a potentially life-threatening infection. Change into dry clothing after you're done swimming. Also, drink lots of water—it increases urination, which helps flush bacteria from the urethra.

Protect Your Home from Dangerous Toxins

Mitchell Gaynor, MD, assistant clinical professor of medicine at Weill Medical College of Cornell University, and founder and president of Gaynor Integrative Oncology, both in New York City, is the author of *Nurture Nature/Nurture Health: Your Health and the Environment.* Nurture Nature.

As long as you breathe, eat and drink, you can't entirely escape environmental toxins. Research on the risks associated with these toxins is ongoing, but many scientists believe that existing evidence suggests that toxic buildup in our bodies contributes to the development of Parkinson's disease and may increase risk for some types of cancer and other serious conditions. A Centers for Disease Control and Prevention study that tested 10,000 men and women for the presence of 116 chemicals, including phthalates and dioxin, found that most Americans carried some combination of these toxins in small amounts in their blood.

TOXICITY IN THE HOME

Household sources of toxins that are under investigation...

•**Home furnishings.** *Polybrominated diphenylethers* (PBDEs), common ingredients in flame retardants that are used to treat upholstered chairs and sofas, foam mattresses and cushions, may be carcinogenic. PBDEs also may disrupt thyroid function and brain development.

What to do: When buying foam mattresses, upholstered furniture, etc., ask whether PBDEs were used during manufacturing.

•**Pressed wood and fiberboard,** which often are used in furniture and shelving, are common sources of *formaldehyde*, a gaseous compound that is used as a disinfectant. Formaldehyde has been found to be a probable carcinogen.

What to do: Look for solid-wood products or those carrying the seal of the American National Standards Institute (ANSI), which certifies that the item is low in formaldehyde emissions.

To find furniture and other products that are low in potentially dangerous chemical emissions, consult the Greenguard Environmental Institute, a nonprofit, independent organization that certifies low-emitting products, 800-427-9681, *www.greenguard.org.*

•**Cleaning products.** Most people use a wide variety of cleaning products, many of which contain toxic chemicals. Chlorine bleach is potentially carcinogenic and can damage the respiratory system. Among its by-products are *chlorinated hydrocarbons, chloroform* and *trihalomethanes*, all of which act like weak estrogens and cause breast cells to divide more rapidly. These by-products have been shown to cause breast tumors in animals.

What to do: Use commercial cleansers that are free of chlorine and most chemicals. Seventh Generation and Sun & Earth are two brands that are widely available at health-food stores.

Or use natural cleaning alternatives—baking soda to scrub sinks, tubs and toilets...white distilled vinegar in a pump-spray bottle to clean mirrors and windows. If you must use chlorine-containing cleaners, make sure the room is well-ventilated.

•**Pesticides.** Research has shown that pesticides increase risk for Parkinson's disease—and may be a cause of some cancers.

What to do: Use baits and traps instead of sprays. Try organic alternatives to toxic bug killers, including oil sprays, such as Sharpshooter, an all-natural insect killer containing plant oils...Burnout II, a natural herbicide that contains vinegar, clove and lemon...and corn gluten meal, a natural weed killer. All of these products are available at most garden centers that carry organic products.

For more information on pesticides and other toxic household products, visit the Web site of EarthShare (a nationwide network of environmental organizations) at *www.earthshare.org.*

•**Cosmetics.** *Para-phenylenediamine*, a chemical found in some dark hair dyes, increases risk for bladder cancer in humans, according to a study in the journal *Carcinogenesis. Other toxic ingredients used in cosmetics...*

•*Phthalates*, typically used as a solvent and plastic softener, have been linked to cancer and to birth defects of the male reproductive system. They are found in many shampoos and other hair products, cosmetics, deodorants and nail polish. To learn more about phthalates and get a list of products that contain them, go to a reliable Web site of several consumer environmental groups at *www.safecosmetics.org.*

•*Talc*, in talcum powder, has been linked to a 60% increase in the risk for ovarian cancer in women who use it in the genital area.

•*Propylene glycol*, an ingredient found in some moisturizing products and skin creams, is absorbed through the skin, and high levels may damage the kidneys and liver.

What to do: Read labels carefully. By law, cosmetic ingredients must be listed on the label, starting with those in largest amounts. Choose all-natural alternatives, such as products made with olive oil, safflower oil or oatmeal, whenever possible. To find hair products, lotions, deodorants and other products from companies that have replaced or are replacing toxic ingredients, go to *www.safecosmetics.org* (look for safe companies).

SELF-DEFENSE

Antioxidants such as vitamins C and E are known to promote health by scavenging free radicals (harmful by-products of metabolism), which damage our cells and contribute to cancer and other diseases.

But antioxidants have another role that is possibly even more important in protecting against environmental toxins. Antioxidants stimulate an area of the DNA called the *antioxidant responsive element* (ARE), which activates a gene that produces detoxifying enzymes. This is the body's way of breaking down carcinogens and other toxins.

In addition to commonly known antioxidant sources, such as brightly colored produce (carrots, beets, kale and tomatoes), be sure your diet contains...

•**Cruciferous vegetables,** such as cauliflower and brussels sprouts, which contain *sulforaphane*, a potent enzyme inducer.

•**Green tea,** an antioxidant source that is 20 times more potent than vitamin E, according to the American Chemical Society. Drink two to five cups daily.

•**Rosemary,** a source of *carnosol*, which has antioxidant and anticarcinogenic properties. Use rosemary in cooking, or drink one cup of rosemary tea daily.

•**Curry,** which contains curcumin and turmeric, two potent cancer-fighting herbs. Cook with curry three times a week.

Avoid Germs in Public Bathrooms

Use the first stall—it tends to be the least popular. Flush the toilet with your foot, then leave the stall quickly to avoid airborne bacteria. To be sure you are washing your hands long enough, sing the song *Happy Birthday to You* to yourself twice. Wash with comfortably lukewarm water—hotter water does not kill more germs. Use a paper towel to turn off the faucet and pull the door handle so that you don't pick up more germs after cleaning your hands.

Philip M. Tierno, Jr., PhD, director and adjunct associate professor of microbiology, New York University Medical Center, New York City, and author of The Secret Life of Germs. *Atria.*

Hospital Bed Warning

Hospital beds can trap patients between the rails and the mattress. Since 1985, more than 400 frail patients have become wedged in beds and died.

Self-defense: Check with the manufacturer to make sure that the bed meets current standards and that the parts fit together snugly. Read the Food and Drug Administration's safety recommendations at *www.fda.gov/cdrh/beds*, or order the brochure "A Guide to Bed Safety" at 888-463-6332.

Larry G. Kessler, ScD, director, USFDA Office of Science and Engineering Laboratories, Rockville, Maryland.

Calming Scents

Certain scents reduce road rage. Drivers exposed to the smell of cinnamon and peppermint reported feeling less frustrated. Add two drops of peppermint and cinnamon oil to two cotton balls...wrap the cotton balls in a piece of cheesecloth...and put it under the car seat. The scent will last about a week.

Bryan Raudenbush, PhD, LPharm, associate professor of psychology, director of undergraduate research, psychology department, Wheeling Jesuit University, Wheeling, West Virginia.

■ ■ ■ ■

Is Your Child's Car Seat Safe?

Most child car seats are too loose, and children are strapped too loosely into them. A car seat must be installed so that there is no more than one inch of side-to-side or front-to-back movement. The child should be strapped in so that only one finger fits between the strap and his/her collarbone. A child should be kept in a rear-facing seat until he weighs 30 to 35 pounds and as long as there is at least one inch of room between his head and the top of the car seat (though some groups recommend that a child should stay in a rear-facing seat until he is at least one year old and at least 20 pounds).

Children should start in booster seats when they weigh about 40 pounds and remain in them until they can wear a seat belt properly. This means that the lap portion rests firmly on the hip bone—low and snug on top of the thighs—when the child sits without slouching, with knees bending naturally over the edge of the seat. Children should not be out of booster seats until they are four feet nine inches tall, regardless of weight or age.

Alisa Baer, known as "The Car Seat Lady," based in New York City. www.thecarseatlady.com.

■ ■ ■ ■

Safety Seat Woes

Front seats of cars are not safe for children up to age 14—not age 12, as previously thought. Younger children are up to six times more likely to be injured than older kids when air bags deploy.

Reason: Bones and lean muscle protect the body, and age—not height or weight—determines their development.

Craig D. Newgard, MD, MPH, assistant professor, emergency medicine and public health and preventive medicine, Oregon Health and Sciences University, Portland, and author of a study of the effects of motor vehicle crashes on 3,790 children, published in Pediatrics.

What to Do When an Elderly "Someone" Won't Stop Driving

Helen Kerschner, PhD, president and CEO of the Beverly Foundation, a California-based nonprofit organization that advocates for senior transportation, www.beverly foundation.org, is the former president of the American Association for International Aging, Inc., and director of the University of New Mexico Center on Aging.

The comment, "I'm going to drive myself to the nursing home or the cemetery, whichever comes first" from an elderly driver shows what you might be up against when you try to persuade a parent, friend or other elderly person to stop driving.

But the effort can pay off. The US Department of Transportation reports that drivers over age 70 have higher rates of fatal accidents than do those in any other age group except teenagers.

While there are many individual exceptions, the chance of having an accident begins to increase around the age of 55, and the risk rises dramatically for people with diseases or who take medications that affect their motor skills, vision and/or judgment.

Still, many Americans think of driving as a fundamental right, and for older people, the car is often the last symbol of independence.

In trying to persuade a person to put away the car keys, you'll be attempting to influence a person who is probably accustomed to giving advice, not taking it. *Tactics that work...*

LAY THE GROUNDWORK

If possible, start your campaign before the danger of driving becomes immediate. Even if your loved one seems to be driving well, it's wise to suggest that he/she take a test to confirm the level of skill and/or take a refresher course for senior drivers. (AAA and many motor vehicle departments have information on the tests and courses.)

Advantage: These measures take some of the burden off you by letting drivers see their own shortcomings in a way that's difficult to deny.

Push your loved one to take a test or refresher course if you notice...

• **Friends no longer want to ride with him/her.**

• **Unexplained damage to the car,** such as scratches, dents or broken outside mirrors.

• **Incidents of confusion on well-known roads.**

• **An increase in accidents,** no matter who was at fault.

Reason: Accidents are often the result of a reduced ability to drive defensively.

AAA sells a compact disc, *Roadwise Review,* that lets people use a home computer to test themselves in such areas as physical flexibility, memory, visual acuity and leg strength.

For information on how to order the disc, phone a local AAA office, listed in the phone book. Prices vary from state to state but are usually in the $10 to $15 range.

The AARP's $10 Driver Safety Program is aimed at people age 50 and older and is usually taught in two four-hour sessions on different days.

Information: 888-227-7669, *www.aarp.org.*

OVERCOMING OBJECTIONS

It's very common that a senior driver will balk at the idea of taking a test or refresher course. *Countermeasures…*

• **Offer to join** the person and take the test or course together. (With AAA's *Roadwise Review,* it is mandatory to take the test with someone else present in order to verify results.) The offer doesn't always work, but it's often successful.

• **Point out** that most insurance companies give a discount to people who take the AARP course. The markdown is usually about 10%.

RELY ON INFLUENCERS

Despite a poor test and pleas from family members, some seniors still won't give up driving. When that's the case, it's wise to ask for help from the people in authority whom they do listen to. Doctors are at the top of the list.

Contact your family member's physicians and discuss the situation with them. Many doctors are willing to tell older patients how their diminished eyesight, loss of motor skills or effects of a disability can increase the risk of a serious accident.

Not every physician, however, is knowledgeable in this area.

Smart move: Give doctors a copy of *Physician's Guide to Assessing and Counseling Older Drivers.* The book, developed by the American Medical Association and the National Highway Traffic Safety Administration, gives doctors a checklist of conditions that impair driving ability.

Some of the conditions might not be obvious to doctors who haven't dealt with the issue before.

Examples: Insomnia, which can cause drowsiness during the day, and foot problems, which can prevent the proper use of the brake and accelerator pedals.

The book, which is free, can be downloaded from the Internet or ordered for delivery by mail.

Information: 800-621-8335, *www.ama-assn. org/ama/pub/category/10791.html.*

If doctors don't succeed in persuading your loved one not to drive, turn to friends, relatives or members of the clergy for whom he/she has a deep respect.

DRIVING ALTERNATIVES

Almost all elderly people—even those urged by doctors and confronted by evidence of diminished skill—use a powerful argument against turning over the car keys. They say that there's no other way to get to places they have to go. This is a reasonable concern that should be respected.

If arguments about safety won't overcome this concern, be prepared by knowing about alternative types of transportation that can make a car unnecessary.

My organization, the Beverly Foundation, lists more than 400 senior transportation programs. To download the list, go to *www.beverlyfoundation.org* and click on "The STP (supplemental transportation programs for seniors) Exchange."

Many elderly nondrivers require a combination of options…

• **Volunteer drivers.** Hundreds of volunteer driver programs have started up around the country, and more are being created each month. Typically sponsored by a charitable organization, these programs generally supply drivers to seniors free of charge. Many religious institutions also provide volunteer drivers.

The best way to locate a volunteer driver is through local departments of senior services, churches and interfaith volunteer groups. If there isn't an appropriate option in your community, consider the possibility of promoting one.

•**Paratransit.** That's a term coined by federal officials for transportation systems for the disabled operated by many cities and counties throughout the country.

Depending on the jurisdiction, many minor disabilities associated with advanced age may qualify a person for paratransit.

Examples: Poor vision in one eye or lack of full mobility in a foot. To find out if a loved one would qualify, contact your local department of transportation.

•**Regular taxis.** Taxicabs are an obvious option, especially in suburbs and other areas outside the city. Taxis can be a relaxing way to travel, almost like having a chauffeur. (That's particularly true once you develop a relationship with a taxi company.)

The strongest argument is that taxis are a bargain. AAA estimates that the average cost of owning and operating a car is about $7,000 a year, or nearly $135 a week—enough to pay for many taxi rides.

•**Assisted-living apartments.** If your loved one is contemplating a move, ask him to consider an assisted-living apartment complex. Many of them operate their own transportation system for regular trips to grocery stores, malls and medical centers.

Few people have quick success in persuading a senior to stop driving. But don't be discouraged. Before giving up, remember that if other friends and family members had been more persistent, some of the people cited in statistics on fatal accidents to seniors would still be alive.

■ ■ ■ ■

Road Travel Tips

Vehicle-related accidents are a major cause of accidental deaths of US citizens abroad. Especially in developing countries, taxi and bus drivers may take far more risks than in the US—overloading vehicles, ignoring stoplights, driving recklessly on mountain roads and failing to use headlights.

Self-defense: Avoid traveling at night, especially in rural areas. Sit in the backseat, and buckle up. Don't ride in taxis that don't have seat belts in the backseat.

Road safety information: Road reports for individual countries are available from the Association for Safe International Road Travel (*www.asirt.org*).

Stuart R. Rose, MD, president, Travel Medicine, Inc., Northampton, MA, and author of *International Travel Health Guide.* Mosby. *www.travmed.com.*

■ ■ ■ ■

Three Smart Supplements For Travelers

To stay healthy while traveling, take the right supplements, says Mark A. Stengler, ND. In addition to a multivitamin, take…

•*A probiotic* (follow label instructions) on an empty stomach, starting three days before leaving and during the trip, to prevent diarrhea and related problems.

•*Garlic*—preferably aged garlic—reduces risk of respiratory and digestive infections. Take two capsules a day for two days before you leave, during the trip and for two days after it.

•*Melatonin*—one to three milligrams—prevents jet lag and makes sleep easier. Take it the evening you arrive, at 9 pm in the time zone you are in, and for two or three more nights. Consult your physician before starting any supplements.

Mark A. Stengler, ND, naturopathic physician in private practice, La Jolla, California…adjunct associate clinical professor at the National College of Natural Medicine, Portland, Oregon…author of many books, including *The Natural Physician's Healing Therapies* and coauthor of *Prescription for Natural Cures* (both from Bottom Line Books)…and author of the *Bottom Line/Natural Healing* newsletter.

Danger in the Water: Drink Safely When You Travel

Connie Lohsl, RN, BSN, is a nurse manager and travel-health specialist with Passport Health, Inc., a nationwide chain of travel-health franchises that provide low-cost immunizations and other travel-related services, based in Baltimore. *www.passporthealthusa.com.*

Unprepared travelers who hope to enjoy exotic locales often spend their days in a hotel bathroom instead. About 40% of all travelers experience some form of stomach upset from mild to debilitating diarrhea. For those with underlying kidney or heart problems, the dehydration from diarrhea can be life-threatening.

Check the Centers for Disease Control and Prevention Web site (*www.cdc.gov*) to find out which countries have safe drinking water. *They're rated by risk—high, intermediate and low…*

High risk: Africa, Mexico and Central America, South America, most of Asia and the Middle East. Hepatitis A is a concern in Russia.

Intermediate risk: South Africa, Eastern Europe and some of the Caribbean islands.

Low risk: US, Canada, Japan, Northern and Western Europe, Australia and New Zealand.

To stay safe…

•**Drink bottled water, but inspect it first.** In some countries, a container of bottled water costs $4 or more. Unscrupulous vendors may refill empties with tap water. Always check that the factory seal is intact. Buy carbonated water, if available—it's harder to fake.

•**Wipe bottles and cans dry before drinking.** Bottled and canned beverages may be kept cold in tubs filled with ice water. Moisture on the outside may contain organisms that can get into your mouth when you drink. Of course, don't add ice cubes to beverages unless you are sure they are made from uncontaminated water.

•**Use bottled water for brushing teeth.** Stand your toothbrush upright between uses so it isn't contaminated with water from the sink.

•**Drink bottled water on cruise ships and airplanes.** Nonbottled water could be contaminated. Coffee and tea made with boiling water should be safe.

•**Sterilize your water.** *Two ways…*

•Boiling. Put the water in a clean pot, bring it to a rolling boil, then remove it from the heat and let it cool. Transfer to a sterilized container. Boiling is the most reliable way to kill most disease-causing organisms.

•Use a water-filtration bottle. This can protect against bacteria, protozoa and lead. Some also filter viruses, including hepatitis A. Check the product label. Available at my Web site, *www.passporthealthusa.com*, or at any local passport office or camping supply store.

Cost: $20 to $100 or more.

•**Beware of swimming.** Swimming in the ocean is usually safe—few bacteria and parasites can survive in salt water. But lakes and other bodies of freshwater can have high levels of contamination—and some organisms pass directly through the skin.

Showering and toweling off soon after swimming will assist in removing some kinds of parasites (but not all types) before they have a chance to burrow through the skin. Wearing swimming shoes can protect you from parasites and puncture wounds.

Well-maintained, chemically treated swimming pools generally are safe.

Best: Check the CDC site for high risk areas before swimming.

■ ■ ■ ■

Toxic Seafood Warning

Predatory tropical fish and subtropical reef fish, including amberjack, grouper, barracuda, hogfish, triggerfish, snapper, mullet and moray eels, can carry *ciguatoxin*, a seafood toxin that causes a food poisoning called ciguatera. The ciguatoxin does not affect the fish's taste, odor or color and is not eliminated by cooking. Those eating seafood in tropical areas such as Hawaii and the northern Caribbean are most at risk.

Victims experience cramping, diarrhea and nausea starting several hours after consumption.

Headache, muscle pain, dizziness and tingling or numbing of the lips may follow. In extreme cases, sufferers can experience cold-hot reversal —hot things feel cold and vice versa. Symptoms last one to four weeks but may recur for up to six months. See a doctor immediately if you think you might be infected. Treatment with intravenous mannitol has been shown to relieve symptoms effectively.

Ewen Todd, PhD, former director of the National Food Safety and Toxicology Center, Michigan State University, East Lansing. He was head of the Contaminated Foods Section of the Health Protection Branch of the Canadian government.

■■■■

Vaccinations Travelers Need Most

Every traveler, regardless of destination, should get vaccinated against tetanus and hepatitis A. Hepatitis A virus is found in food and water, even in the US. Get revaccinated for tetanus every ten years.

Also: Typhoid vaccination if going to Asia, Africa, the Caribbean, Central or South America. Yellow-fever immunization if visiting tropical South America or sub-Sahara Africa. Polio booster if you haven't been vaccinated since childhood and are going to Africa, South Asia, Southeast Asia and the Middle East. Influenza shot if visiting tropical areas in the southern hemisphere, where flu occurs year-round.

Carol DeRosa, RN, is senior vice president, clinical operations of Passport Health, Inc., provider of immunizations and travel consultations, Baltimore. 888-499-7277. *www.passporthealthusa.com.*

■■■■

Medical History in Any Language

Get your medical history in five languages. The Medistick carries your medical history —plus the medical histories of up to four more people—in a USB memory stick. Enter your information with the included software and the histories are recorded in German, English, French, Italian and Spanish. Update information whenever necessary. Prices start at $78.21 for one history.

For more information see Medistick GmbH, *www.medistick.ch.*

Beware: Hotels, Hospitals And Health Clubs Can Make You Sick

Jeffrey C. May, owner of May Indoor Air Investigations LLC, an air-quality assessment company based in Tyngsborough, MA, has conducted indoor environmental investigations in thousands of buildings. He is a nationally recognized authority and speaker on indoor air quality and author of *My Office Is Killing Me! The Sick Building Survival Guide.* Johns Hopkins University Press.

Mold in homes has been linked to asthma, headaches, fatigue, skin irritations and increased cancer risk.

Important: Mold and other health-threatening irritants can be everywhere, including hotels, hospitals, health clubs and libraries.

You should suspect that you're in a sick building if you experience respiratory symptoms (coughing, sneezing, etc.) that come on soon after you enter that space.

Places to watch out for and steps to take…

HOTEL ROOMS

Carpeting and heating/cooling systems pose the biggest risks because they may be contaminated with mold and/or cleaning residues. *Helpful…*

•**Ask for a room on the second floor or higher.** The carpeted ground floor of a two-story motel is typically the dampest and most likely to be moldy. Avoid rooms located directly off an atrium that has a waterfall or a fountain and rooms near an indoor pool.

•**Turn off the air conditioner/heater fan.** The fan coils may have mold.

Helpful: Before booking a room, ask if the windows can be opened. Keeping windows open can reduce exposure to indoor contaminants.

•**Ask for synthetic bedding.** The feathers in bedding shed millions of tiny particles that can trigger asthma attacks and other respiratory problems.

•**Cover the carpet with adhesive plastic,** such as Pro Tect (800-545-0826, *www.pro-tect. com*, $44 for a 2' x 200' roll). It traps mold spores and particulate allergens and irritants. For a short stay, just cover the most used areas—the walking path around the beds and to the bathroom and entry.

•**Avoid hotels and motels undergoing renovation,** which may result in irritating dust or chemical emissions from new furniture and carpeting.

LIBRARIES

Books can harbor significant amounts of allergen-containing dust, particularly if they aren't used often. *If you experience symptoms after being at a library or taking home library books…*

•**Open and close the books vigorously once you get outside.** The air currents help remove allergens.

•**Vacuum the tops and sides** of the books when you get home. Use a high-efficiency particulate arrestance (HEPA) vacuum.

•**Examine the bindings of older,** hardcover books for white, yellow or other discolorations, all of which can indicate mold. Airing books outdoors in bright sunlight for two or three hours may help. If not, get different copies.

PUBLIC BATHROOMS

The chemical air fresheners in public bathrooms are a common cause of respiratory symptoms. More than 10% of Americans have some degree of chemical sensitivity. Air fresheners—as well as scented candles—are a particular problem because they're designed to disperse chemicals into the air.

In offices and hotels, ask the cleaning staff to avoid using fragranced products and cleaners with chemical odors. If you're in a hotel, you could also ask the housekeeping staff to skip your room.

Breathe through a folded paper towel or T-shirt when entering an area with a strong fragrance. Or use an N95 mask (available at hardware and medical-supply stores for about $11 for a package of 20).

Be aware that the urinals in men's bathrooms often contain a block of *paradichlorobenzene* (the toxic substance that mothballs are made of), which can be extremely irritating to people with chemical sensitivities. If there is a window that vents to the outside, open it. A clean, well-ventilated restroom doesn't need chemicals to smell fresh.

ANTIQUES STORES

The backs and bottoms of old furniture often have mold. Even if an item has been kept in a dry place, it can harbor mold spores that are decades old. Consider wearing an N95 face mask when browsing in antiques stores.

After buying old furniture: If you notice a musty smell or are having symptoms, you may want to take the furniture outside and wipe unfinished surfaces with denatured alcohol. Apply a layer of clear finish to seal in mold spores and reduce mold growth. Mold growth on finished surfaces can be cleaned with any furniture cleaner (do this outdoors as well).

Caution: Don't do anything to an antique without consulting a dealer.

HEALTH CLUBS

Many fitness centers are warehouse-like structures that are built at or below ground level—an optimal environment for dampness and mold growth. If possible, join a health club that is above ground level—preferably one that can be ventilated with fresh air from open windows.

If there's a pool or hot tub, the smell of chlorine should not be so overpowering that it feels like your eyes or nose are burning. Chlorine and other pool disinfectants are a common cause of lung irritation. This problem can be worse in health clubs because people are exercising and breathing deeply.

HOSPITALS AND MEDICAL OFFICES

These often are modern, tightly sealed buildings, which, if the ventilation is inadequate, can result in high levels of indoor carbon dioxide. Medical and dental facilities also can trap large amounts of irritating chemical fumes—from anesthetics, disinfectants, etc.

If you notice strong smells: Wear a charcoal mask. (You can remove it during oral or nasal exams/treatments.) Unlike N95 masks, which trap only particles, charcoal masks also trap gases and chemical vapors. Reusable charcoal respirators with replaceable cartridges cost about $40 each, available at building-supply stores and some hardware stores.

Pilot Answers Top 10 Safety Questions

Meryl Getline, a pilot in Elizabeth, Colorado, with over 32 years of flying experience, including 15 as a captain with a major airline, is author of *The World at My Feet: The True (and Sometimes Hilarious) Adventures of a Lady Airline Captain.*

We trust our lives to airplanes and the pilots who fly them, but there is a lot that the average passenger doesn't know about modern aircraft. *We asked a veteran airline captain to answer some of the most common passenger questions...*

•**Where is the best place to sit on an airplane if you're prone to airsickness?**

The best spot is over the wing or a few rows in front of the wing. When a plane climbs or descends, it pivots on its center of gravity, which tends to be just in front of the wings. The closer you are to this point, the less you'll feel the movement, just as sitting in the middle of a seesaw subjects you to less movement than sitting at the end.

•**How do you prevent jet lag?**

I really don't suffer much from jet lag. I always observe local time, though many pilots keep their watches set to their hometown time and try to sleep accordingly. If you're traveling on business, this may be impractical.

The best advice is to stay well-hydrated and rest on the plane if you're traveling overnight and arriving in the morning. If you are traveling during the day, plan to read or watch a movie en route so that you're ready to sleep that night after you arrive.

•**Could the "autopilot" fly or land a plane without the pilots?**

Not really. Autopilot can't do much more than fly a programmed route or maintain the last heading or altitude entered by the pilots. Pilots are needed to manage the autopilot during the flight.

The autopilot sometimes plays a role in landings—it can keep the plane lined up with the centerline of the runway and even land the plane under certain conditions—but the pilot must control the air speed (even if autothrottles are used, they must be programmed and the speed monitored), flaps and landing gear. The autopilot plays no role at all in takeoffs, although some airplanes may employ autothrottles during takeoff.

•**How do I know that I can trust my pilot?**

Airline pilots are among the most thoroughly trained and tested professionals in the US. They also must go through rigorous retraining each year to remain certified. Any pilot at any airline in this country can be trusted to be a proficient flier.

The pilot certification process may not be as rigorous in some less-developed countries, however. Before you board a flight on a small airline in another country, consider checking the airline's safety record on the Web site *www.airsafe. com.* You can view accident reports and other statistics and reach your own conclusions.

•**Are air pockets dangerous?**

Not only are they not dangerous, they don't exist. The term "air pocket" was coined by a journalist during World War I, but he really just was referring to turbulence—irregular air currents that can shake aircraft around a bit.

When a plane "hits an air pocket" and seems to drop 1,000 feet, it really has just run into a little turbulence and probably dropped or climbed no more than 10 to 20 feet. Light turbulence is so common and inconsequential that experienced pilots scarcely notice it.

There is such a thing as "severe turbulence," which can be strong enough to injure passengers who aren't wearing their seat belts, but this is so rare that I have never encountered it in over 32 years of flying. Modern radar is advanced enough that pilots usually can steer clear of areas that have a high probability of moderate or severe turbulence.

Even when a plane does encounter severe turbulence, it won't crash because of it. When was the last time you read or heard of an airplane accident blamed on turbulence? If you're worried that a little turbulence will bring down your flight, watch one of those Discovery channel documentaries on "hurricane hunter" planes that fly right into the middle of huge storms and come out unscathed on the other side. A modern passenger jet is just as sturdy.

•**In the movies, when a plane hits severe turbulence, the baggage compartments open up and luggage tumbles out. Would that happen in a real plane?**

On occasion, if it gets really rough, an overhead compartment could open, especially if it isn't securely latched. I have never witnessed more than one compartment at a time come open due to turbulence, and I have only seen this once or twice.

•**How dangerous is it when a plane gets struck by lightning?**

My plane has been struck at least three times in my career. There's sometimes a bang, like a cannon going off, but it's not all that dangerous. The lightning charge simply travels around the plane's metal exterior, then off the "static wicks" (pencil-like protrusions) on the trailing edges and tips of the wings and tail.

It is true that lightning can cause problems for a plane's electrical systems. Once, on a flight from Oakland to Denver, a lightning strike knocked out my plane's power, but only for a few seconds. Even if the plane's main electrical system had been permanently disabled, we still had standby power. Some modern planes even are equipped with Ram Air Turbines (RATs), which use the airstream to power onboard electrical backup generators and hydraulic systems.

Between the emergency power systems and the extensive training that pilots receive, there's no reason to think that a plane would crash just because its main electrical system went out.

•**What advice do you have for people who are afraid to fly?**

I suggest that you consider the statistics regarding flying. It really is true that the drive to the airport is many, many times more dangerous than the flight. Personally, I feel far safer in a plane than I do in a car.

•**Are some airports safer than others?**

All US airports are safe, but some are more modern than others and thus probably a little safer.

Modern airports often have longer runways, easier-to-navigate approaches and more sophisticated electronics that allow pilots to land even with limited or no visibility.

Older airports, such as Chicago's Midway International Airport, Jackson Hole Airport, San Diego International Airport, New York City's LaGuardia Airport and Ronald Reagan Washington National Airport, are not this advanced, but I certainly wouldn't call them unsafe.

Ultramodern airports include Denver International Airport and Los Angeles International Airport.

•**Has air travel security improved since the tragedies of 9/11?**

Yes, mostly because the passengers themselves now are part of the security force. In the past, if a passenger started acting oddly, those seated near him/her would mind their own business. These days, if a passenger starts doing anything halfway suspicious, other passengers quickly alert a flight attendant.

■ ■ ■ ■

Beware of Ice!

Ice has more bacteria than the toilet water at some major fast-food restaurants?

Recent finding: Samples from served ice, self-serve ice machines and toilets at five fast-food restaurants were tested for bacteria and compared. Overall, toilet water fared better, although bacteria levels for all were in the acceptable range.

Jasmine Roberts, seventh-grade student, Tampa, whose project comparing bacteria in ice machines and public toilets won first place at the New Tampa School Science Fair.

■ ■ ■ ■

Less than Fresh Air

Some ionizing air cleaners could make your air unhealthy.

Recent study: Some ionizing air filters expose users to high levels of ozone. Experts agree that exposure to ozone in excess of 80 parts per billion for eight hours or longer can cause coughing, wheezing and chest pain and deaden the sense of smell. In one test, five ionizing room air cleaners performed poorly, and some emitted potentially harmful levels of ozone—Brookstone Pure-Ion V2, Sharper Image Professional Series Ionic Breeze Quadra S1737 SNX, Ionic Pro CL-369, Ioniz Air P4620 and Surround

Air XJ-2000 (these specific models are no longer sold by their manufacturers).

Best air cleaners: Freidrich C-90B and Whirlpool 45030—both effectively clean air and emit little ozone.

Mark Connelly, acting technical director of appliances and home-improvement department, Consumer Union, 101 Truman Ave., Yonkers, New York 10703, and leader of a test of five ionizing air cleaners, one electrostatic precipitator and one HEPA air cleaner. Consumers Union publishers *Consumer Reports.*

Best Ways to Prevent Food Poisoning

Ewen Todd, PhD, professor advertising, public relations and retailing, Michigan State University, East Lansing, previously headed the Contaminated Foods Section of the Health Protection Branch of the Canadian government.

There are an estimated 76 million cases of foodborne illness in the US each year. Many victims think they have contracted a "stomach flu" and never realize that food was to blame.

Most foodborne illnesses cause a day or two of nausea, diarrhea, abdominal cramping and, sometimes, vomiting. But in the US, 325,000 cases a year are severe enough to lead to hospitalization and about 5,200 are fatal, according to the Centers for Disease Control and Prevention. Foodborne illnesses are particularly dangerous for children under age five, adults over age 70, pregnant women and people with weakened immune systems. *Here, the foods most likely to cause problems...*

POULTRY

More than 60% of the raw poultry sold in the US is thought to contain disease-causing bacteria, including...

•**Campylobacter,** which can cause up to a week of diarrhea, abdominal pain and fever starting two to five days after the tainted food is consumed.

•**Salmonella,** which can cause four to seven days of diarrhea, fever and abdominal pain starting 12 to 72 hours after eating the contaminated food. Other sources of salmonella include undercooked eggs.

Note: Commercially prepared mayonnaise is made from pasteurized eggs, which are heat-treated to kill bacteria.

In 5% to 15% of cases, salmonella bacteria can lead to reactive arthritis, an inflammatory condition that develops in response to infection in another part of the body. This condition can last weeks, months, even years.

When poultry is cooked all the way through, the bacteria are killed.

Safest: Cook poultry until juices run clear and there is no sign of pink. Even then poultry can become contaminated if not handled properly—for example, if cooked poultry is placed on a cutting board that hasn't been washed after uncooked poultry rested on it.

It used to be common practice to wash raw poultry prior to cooking, but this has been identified as risky because splashes and drips can spread bacteria throughout the kitchen.

STEWS & SOUPS

Stews, soups, sauces and gravies containing red meat or poultry—or their juices—can be a perfect breeding ground for the *Clostridium perfringens* bacteria. When these dishes are cooked, allowed to cool slowly and then rewarmed, the bacteria thrive. It can cause an unpleasant day of nausea and diarrhea starting within 24 hours of consumption. To reduce the risk, refrigerate stews, soups, sauces and gravies in small containers, which cool faster, soon after cooking.

GROUND BEEF

The *E. coli* bacteria sickens about 70,000 Americans every year. Most victims experience about a week of cramping and bloody diarrhea starting four to eight days after the tainted food is consumed. Slightly less than one of every 1,000 victims dies.

E. coli bacteria live naturally in the intestines of many animals, including cattle. During the slaughter and processing of cattle, the meat can accidentally come in contact with fecal matter.

•**Ground beef is riskiest.** The E. coli bacteria can be present on the surface of any piece of raw beef, but steaks and roasts typically are sufficiently cooked to kill this surface bacteria—even when cooked rare. With ground beef, the surface of the meat gets ground up and can wind up in the middle of your burger. If the burger isn't cooked all the way through (to an internal temperature of 160°), bacteria can survive.

Important: If a steak has been punctured with a fork or knife prior to cooking, bacteria could find its way inside and survive. In that case, eat the meat only if it's cooked well-done.

Produce alert: E. coli also can be present in soil and has been found on lettuce, alfalfa sprouts and in unpasteurized apple juice and cider. Wash lettuce—even prewashed lettuce—carefully, and avoid sprouts (which are hard to clean) and unpasteurized juices.

DELI MEATS

Cold cuts, pâté and smoked fish are leading sources of the *Listeria* bacteria. Unpasteurized milk and milk products also can be contaminated. Listeria is found in soil and water. Animals also can carry the bacteria in their intestines. As a result, Listeria can spread to meat and dairy products. Ready-to-eat foods can become contaminated in the processing plant or en route from the plant.

There are about 2,500 cases of Listeria poisoning each year in the US, and about 20% of victims die, so it's important to be careful. Symptoms include fever, muscle aches and sometimes nausea or diarrhea.

Reduce your odds of infection by setting your refrigerator to just above freezing for storing deli meat, pâté and smoked fish. Consume or freeze these foods within four or five days of purchase.

LEFTOVERS

Discard leftovers that have been at room temperature for more than two hours or out in hot weather for more than an hour.

Use refrigerated leftovers within four days.

When reheating leftovers, bring them to an internal temperature of 165°. Reheat stews, soups, sauces and gravies to a boil.

If you think you have food poisoning: Drink lots of water and get plenty of rest. Don't use antidiarrheal medications—they may slow the elimination of bacteria from your system. Foodborne illness often improves within 48 hours. Call your doctor if you feel ill for longer than two or three days or if blood appears in your stool.

Water Can Explode In a Microwave

When water is quickly heated far above its boiling point, the bubbles that normally form in boiling water don't form.

When such superheated, non-bubbling water is removed from a microwave and jiggled or touched with a spoon, the bubbles may then form suddenly and spray the water up and out of the cup or container—potentially causing serious burns. *Safety...*

•**Don't overheat water**—microwave it on high for no more than one minute, then test it.

•**Put food contents (tea bag, soup mix, etc.) in the water before heating it.** This will prevent super-heating.

•**Let a cup of heated water sit for a minute after taking it out of the microwave—** and don't put your face over it.

Reassurance: Conventional ranges and stoves pose a much greater risk of fire and burns than microwave ovens do.

Scott Wolfson, spokesman, US Consumer Product Safety Commission, Bethesda, Maryland, *www.cpsc.gov.*

Beaches Are Full of Bacteria

Beach sand has five to 10 times more bacteria than adjacent water. Bacteria from bird droppings and human waste, such as E. coli, may survive longer in sand than in water because bacteria adhere to particles.

Self-defense: Wash hands after leaving the beach. Warn children not to put their hands in their mouths when digging in sand.

Walter McLeod, principal, EcoCapital, LLC (formerly Clean Beaches Council), Washington, DC.

Clean Veggies Safely

Remove pesticides and wax from fruits and vegetables. In a bowl or a basin, mix four tablespoons of table salt, four teaspoons of lemon juice and one quart of cool water. Soak fruits and vegetables for five to 10 minutes.

Exceptions: Soak leafy greens for two to three minutes...berries, one to two minutes. After soaking, rinse produce in plain cold water and dry.

Alternative: Veggie Wash. Made of 100% natural ingredients, it is available at supermarkets, health-food stores and on-line at *www.veggie-wash.com* (800-451-7096).

Joan Wilen and Lydia Wilen, authorities on folk remedies, New York City, and authors of *Bottom Line's Healing Remedies* and *Bottom Line's Household Magic, www.bottomlinesecrets.com.*

■ ■ ■ ■

Bug Off Naturally

New herbal insect repellent—*oil of lemon eucalyptus*—now is on the Centers for Disease Control and Prevention's recommended list. But it must be reapplied more often than DEET or Picaridin (frequency depends on the concentration).

Warning: Just one mosquito bite can transmit West Nile virus or other infections. Apply repellent to exposed skin whenever you are outdoors, especially between dusk and dawn.

Emily Zielinski-Gutierrez, DrPH, is a behavioral scientist, Division of Vector-Borne Diseases, Centers for Disease Control and Prevention, Fort Collins, Colorado.

■ ■ ■ ■

A New Blood Test for TB

The *T-Spot TB test* is as accurate as the skin test and requires only one doctor visit, but it is not offered by all providers, says Peter Barnes, MD.

Who needs regular TB tests: Hospital workers and others who might come in close contact with TB...residents of long-term-care facilities...and those receiving immune-suppressing treatment, such as chemotherapy.

Testing also may be required by schools, colleges and other places where disease can spread quickly.

Peter Barnes, MD, is professor of microbiology and immunology, Center for Pulmonary and Infectious Disease Control, University of Texas Health Center at Tyler. His study was published in *American Journal of Respiratory and Critical Care Medicine.*

■ ■ ■ ■

Air Freshener Warning

Room fresheners may cause headaches, depression and other maladies. A recent study finds that the "volatile organic compounds" found in aerosols such as air fresheners are associated with increased incidence of headache and depression among women, and higher levels of diarrhea, earache and other symptoms among young children. The study authors warn this may indicate heightened risk for other groups who are home a large percentage of their time, such as the elderly.

Safer: Use baking soda, lemons and other natural odor remedies. Don't use aerosols in confined spaces.

Alexandra Farrow, PhD, course director, School of Health Sciences & Social Care, Brunel University, Uxbridge, England.

Protect Against Killer Food Allergies

Steve L. Taylor, PhD, professor of food science and co-director of the Food Allergy Research Resources Program at the University of Nebraska, Lincoln, is a leading expert on food allergies.

Many people with food allergies have mild symptoms, such as a rash, runny nose or itchy eyes, when they eat small amounts of a problem food. But they may still be at risk for a potentially deadly reaction.

In the US, food allergies cause up to 125,000 emergency room visits and 3,000 resulting in hospitalization annually due to *anaphylaxis*, an acute reaction that can cause respiratory distress and/or a heart arrhythmia (irregular heartbeat).

Safer food: The Food Allergen Labeling and Consumer Protection Act, which went into effect in January 2006, requires food manufacturers to list eight major allergens on food labels to help people with food allergies identify and avoid problem foods.

IS IT REALLY AN ALLERGY?

Not all reactions to food are due to allergies. Tens of millions of Americans suffer from food *intolerance*. A food intolerance, such as a sensitivity to the lactose in milk, can begin in childhood. The most common symptom of lactose intolerance is gastrointestinal discomfort, including diarrhea, cramping and flatulence.

Food allergies affect about 12 million Americans. With a food allergy, the immune system mistakenly identifies as harmful the various proteins—or even a single kind of protein—within one or more foods. This triggers a cascade of events that causes immune cells to respond to the "threat" by releasing large amounts of histamine and other chemicals that produce the allergic symptoms.

The most common food allergen is shellfish. Up to 6.9 million Americans are allergic to shrimp and/or other shellfish, such as lobster, crab and crayfish. This type of allergy often is ignored—primarily because most people tend to eat shellfish far less often than other allergenic foods, such as eggs, peanuts and fish.

TESTING FOR ALLERGIES

A food allergy usually can be diagnosed with a thorough medical history taken by an allergist.

The doctor will want to know…

•**When do symptoms occur?** Food allergies typically cause symptoms within a few minutes to several hours after exposure. Symptoms include stomach cramping, hives, lip swelling, runny nose, congestion and asthma. With a food intolerance, symptoms may not occur until the next day.

•**How much did you eat?** With food allergies, any exposure can trigger symptoms. For some patients, 1 mg—an amount that's almost impossible to see—will provoke an allergic response. A reaction can even be triggered by kissing—or sharing utensils with—someone who has eaten a substance to which you are allergic. A skin reaction can occur from touching the substance.

With a food intolerance, symptoms usually are linked to the amount consumed. Someone who's sensitive to milk, for example, can often drink a small amount without a reaction.

Two tests can identify most food allergies. *They are…*

•**Skin prick.** Extracts of suspected foods are pricked into the skin with a needle. The appearance of a rash within a few hours—or even a few minutes—indicates a food allergy.

Caution: The skin-prick test isn't advisable for patients with severe allergies. The tiny amounts of food used in the test could trigger a life-threatening reaction.

•**Radioallergosorbent test (RAST).** This blood test detects antibodies to specific food proteins. The test occasionally produces false positives—indicating an allergy where none is present. It's often combined with the skin-prick test for more accurate results.

TREATMENT

People with a history of serious food reactions must carry an EpiPen. Available by prescription, it's a self-injector that delivers a dose of *epinephrine*. Epinephrine stimulates the heart and respiration and helps counteract deadly anaphylaxis.

Important: Use the EpiPen immediately if you experience difficulty breathing or throat constriction. Even if you take the shot promptly, get to an emergency room as soon as possible for follow-up treatments.

Also helpful: Take an antihistamine, such as Benadryl, according to label instructions. It can lessen the severity of symptoms while you get to an emergency room.

Also consider: Omalizumab (Xolair), a medication currently used for asthma, appears to significantly blunt reactions in food-allergy patients who receive a monthly injection of the drug. In an early study, patients who reacted to trace amounts of peanuts were able to eat eight to 10 nuts without experiencing problems. Further studies must be completed to determine whether the FDA deems it an effective—and safe—therapy for food allergies.

AVOIDING PROBLEM FOODS

Because there isn't a cure for food allergies—and even trace amounts of a protein can trigger reactions—strict avoidance is the best defense…

•**Always read food labels**—even if you've safely eaten that product in the past. Manufacturers frequently change or add ingredients.

•**Ask about "hidden" ingredients in medications.** Some prescription and over-the-counter (OTC) drugs, as well as vitamins and supplements, contain milk proteins or other common food allergens. This information should be on the label, but check with your doctor or pharmacist before taking any medication or supplement.

•**Talk to the chef or restaurant manager when eating out.** The waiter or waitress doesn't always have accurate information about food ingredients and preparation. Ask to speak to the chef or manager instead and tell him/her what you're allergic to. Explain that *any* contact with the offending food can be *life-threatening*.

If you're allergic to shellfish, for example, tell the chef or manager you can't eat a hamburger that was cooked on the same grill used to cook shrimp.

Other hidden sources of food allergens: Cooking oils that are used to cook different foods…knives and cutting boards that aren't washed clean between uses.

•**Wear a medical alert bracelet/necklace.** Anaphylaxis can potentially cause a loss of consciousness within minutes. A medical alert bracelet/necklace lets medical personnel know that you require urgent treatment for your allergy.

■ ■ ■ ■

Patch Warning

Wearing a pain patch may cause fatal breathing problems. The FDA has issued two warnings (in 2005 and in 2007) regarding overdose or improper use of *fentanyl*, which is administered via a transdermal patch and is used by people who suffer from severe chronic pain.

Self-defense: If you wear the fentanyl patch, often sold as the Duragesic patch, contact your doctor.

Crystal Rice, spokesperson, Center for Drug Evaluation and Research, US Food and Drug Administration, Rockville, Maryland.

■ ■ ■ ■

iPod Warning

If played too loudly, iPods can cause hearing loss and tinnitus (ringing in the ears), says hearing specialist Richard Tyler, PhD. To protect your hearing, these and other personal stereo devices using earphones should not be audible to anyone standing near you. No matter what sort of earpiece you use, set the volume at about the level of a conversation with someone near you—the music should never get so loud that it causes discomfort and you have to turn down the volume.

Richard Tyler, PhD, is an audiologist and professor of otolaryngology and speech pathology and audiology, University of Iowa, Iowa City.

■ ■ ■ ■

Unusual Drug Reaction

Some drugs can trigger a rare skin disease called *Stevens-Johnson Syndrome* (SJS). Symptoms include red blotches, welts and pimple-like bumps either in one area of the body or all over. Eyelids may swell and eyes may turn red. The patient can have persistent fever or flu-like symptoms. SJS usually appears within one week of starting a new medication. The most common medications that cause SJS include drugs containing *sulfa*, nonsteroidal anti-inflammatory medications, anticonvulsants and drugs to treat gout. SJS is treated with antibiotics and steroids. In rare instances, it can result in blindness or death. There are roughly 600 to 2,000 cases of SJS annually.

C. Stephen Foster, MD, founder and president, Ocular Immunology and Uveitis Foundation, and clinical professor of ophthalmology, Harvard Medical School, Boston.

■ ■ ■ ■

Deadly Heatstroke

People who become overheated—when spending hours in the sun—can lose their ability to sweat. This can cause heatstroke, in which body temperature soars to more than 104°F. Heatstroke can be lethal. It can cause brain damage and/or cardiac arrest if body temperature isn't lowered immediately.

Self-defense: Drink a lot of fluids—at least one-half ounce per pound of body weight daily.

Water and sports drinks are better than carbonated beverages. The carbonation makes it more difficult for the body to absorb fluids. Also, wear a hat and light-colored clothing.

Heatstroke warning signs: Dry mouth, dizziness, nausea, fatigue.

What to do: Find a cool, shaded area immediately. Get in front of an air conditioner or a fan, or get in your car and turn the air conditioner on high. If you don't feel better within a few minutes, have someone take you to a first-aid station or an emergency room.

Bottom Line/Personal newsletter, 281 Tresser Blvd., Stamford, Connecticut 06901.

■ ■ ■ ■

Pass the Tissues, Please

The best way to blow your nose is to use paper facial tissues, not handkerchiefs, in which bacteria can grow.

Also: Use a tissue once, then throw it away. Blow gently—too much pressure can push infectious fluid into ears and sinuses. Press a finger outside one nostril, then blow through the open one. Repeat on the other side. Always wash your hands after blowing. Wait 10 minutes after waking in the morning before blowing your nose—congestion decreases after you get up from a prone position.

Murray Grossan, MD, otolaryngologist, Cedars-Sinai Medical Towers, Los Angeles.

Are You Up-to-Date on Your Vaccinations?

William Schaffner, MD, professor and chair of the department of preventive medicine at Vanderbilt University Medical Center in Nashville. Dr. Schaffner has published more than 60 professional articles on vaccines.

If you are like most adults, the only time you think about vaccinations is during flu season or when you are planning an overseas vacation.

Problem: Only a very small percentage of American adults is receiving most vaccinations recommended by the Centers for Disease Control and Prevention (CDC). That's largely because few doctors are reminding their patients when they need to receive vaccinations.

Solution: Add vaccinations to the list of things you discuss with your doctor during your regular physical exam. Most of us know how crucial the flu vaccine can be, but there are other vaccinations that also are important. Vaccines, which generally are safe and effective, are usually covered by insurance when recommended by your doctor.

Most adults should receive vaccinations for the following infections...

TETANUS-DIPHTHERIA-PERTUSSIS

Vaccinations against tetanus (an acute disease that causes "lockjaw") and diphtheria (an infectious disease that causes difficulty breathing and swallowing) have long been given every 10 years. Now, adults are being advised to get a new combination vaccine that also protects against whooping cough, a disease caused by the bacterium *Bordetella pertussis*.

Nearly all infants are vaccinated against whooping cough, but there has been a dramatic increase in whooping cough among adults. At its worst, the cough can be strong enough to crack ribs. Adults can expose unimmunized infants and children to the disease, which can be fatal, especially in babies younger than six months.

Because the adult vaccine was introduced just three years ago, not all physicians think to recommend it. When it is time for your regular 10-year tetanus-diphtheria booster, ask for the "Tdap vaccine," which covers tetanus, diphtheria and whooping cough. The combination vaccine currently is approved for people up to age 65.

SHINGLES

If you've ever had chicken pox, you carry an inactive form of the varicella-zoster virus, which caused the infection. Years or decades later, the virus can become activated and develop into a disease known as shingles. (The reason for the reactivation is unknown, but it often occurs when immunity is weakened by another disorder or by the use of drugs that impair immunity.) Marked by a painful rash of fluid-filled blisters,

171

shingles usually appears on one side of the body. By age 80, half of all adults have had it.

With the shingles vaccine (administered once in adults age 60 and older), the chance of shingles and post-shingles pain, which can last for months or more in the area of the shingles outbreak, is cut by more than half.

Important: The shingles vaccine is generally covered by insurance for adults ages 60 to 65. After age 65, it is covered only under supplemental Medicare Part D insurance. If you are not covered for the shingles vaccine, the cost is typically $180 to $300. This vaccine should not be given to people whose immune systems are compromised, including those who take high-dose steroid medication and those who have received an organ transplant. Even if you've already had shingles, the vaccine may help prevent a recurrence.

PNEUMONIA

Pneumococcal pneumonia is a type of bacterial pneumonia that is a common complication of the flu. Each year, this type of pneumonia affects approximately 500,000 Americans and kills about 40,000.

The incidence of pneumococcal pneumonia starts to rise when people reach age 50—and increases even more after age 65. The reason: Older adults are more likely to have lung disease, diabetes or other illnesses that predispose them to pneumonia.

The pneumococcal pneumonia vaccine (administered at least once during a person's lifetime) is recommended for everyone age 65 and older...anyone ages 19 to 65 with a chronic illness (such as diabetes or heart or lung disease) or a compromised immune system (due to cancer treatment, for example, or an organ transplant).

HEPATITIS B

The hepatitis B virus attacks the liver. The virus is transmitted primarily through sexual intimacy and by infected blood. Mild cases may cause no symptoms, but severe cases can lead to cirrhosis, liver failure, liver cancer and even death.

The hepatitis B vaccine (given in a series of three shots) is recommended for adults whose occupation (such as health-care workers) or behavior (sexually active people who are not in a long-term, mutually monogamous relationship with an infection-free partner) puts them at increased risk of coming into contact with blood or body secretions infected with hepatitis B.

HUMAN PAPILLOMAVIRUS

The human papillomavirus (HPV) is sexually transmitted and consists of several dozen different strains. Some are relatively harmless, others cause genital warts and some cause cervical cancer. The HPV vaccine, currently recommended for all girls and women ages 11 to 26, protects women against two genital wart–causing strains and two cervical cancer–causing strains.

The vaccine (administered in three doses over a period of six months) was tested and approved for younger women to help protect them before they become sexually active. The more sexual partners a woman has, the greater the risk that she has become infected with one or more HPV strains.

The HPV vaccine is currently in clinical trials for use in women ages 26 to 45. Women over age 26 who are sexually active (and possibly infected with one or more strains of the virus) could potentially benefit from the vaccine because it protects against four strains of HPV.

Insurance covers the cost of the HPV vaccine for girls and women ages 11 to 26. Women over age 26 can ask their doctors about receiving the vaccine "off-label." This use may be covered by insurance. The cost is about $375 for the three doses.

■ **More from Dr. Schaffner...**

Precautions for Travelers

Ask your doctor about the following vaccinations at least six weeks, if possible, before leaving the US. This will give your body time to build maximum immunity. *Currently recommended by the Centers for Disease Control and Prevention (CDC)...*

•**Hepatitis A,** transmitted through food or water. Areas with high or intermediate risk include all parts of the world outside North America (except Mexico), Japan, Australia, New Zealand and developed European Countries.

•**Hepatitis B.** Areas with high risk include Africa, much of southeast Asia and the Middle East (excluding Israel). The vaccine is recommended for health-care workers and others who stay in these countries for long periods, as well as for travelers who have intimate relationships with residents of these countries.

•**Meningitis,** transmitted from person to person, especially in crowded conditions. The high-risk "meningitis belt" runs across central Africa, from Mali to Ethiopia.

•**Polio,** transmitted via contact with the feces of an infected person, is most common in areas where sanitation is poor. Risk is highest in Africa, South Asia, Southeast Asia and the Middle East.

Note: Even if you had a polio vaccination as a child, you should get a booster as an adult if you're traveling to these areas.

•**Rabies,** transmitted through contact with infected animals. Risk is highest in parts of Africa, Asia, and Central and South America.

•**Typhoid,** transmitted through food and water. Areas with the highest risk include all of South Asia…and developing countries elsewhere in Asia, Africa, the Caribbean and Central and South America.

Certain countries require a certificate of vaccination for such diseases as…

•**Meningitis and polio.** Saudi Arabia requires proof of these vaccinations during the annual pilgrimage to Mecca (due to the large numbers of visitors).

•**Yellow fever,** a mosquito-borne disease found predominantly in Central and South America, and sub-Saharan Africa.

For a more detailed summary, go to the CDC Web site, *www.cdc.gov/travel.*

■ ■ ■ ■

What You Need to Know About Bottled Water

Attracted by images of pristine springs and wary of dehydration, I guzzle bottled water, as many health-conscious Americans do. But is bottled water more healthful than tap—or am I needlessly squeamish about drinking from the same household water source I use to flush my toilets? *What I've learned…*

•**Emissions from manufacturing** and shipping plastic bottles add to global warming. An estimated 86% of water bottles wind up in landfills instead of recycling centers, and they will take centuries to biodegrade.

•**Repeatedly reusing bottles** meant for one-time use cuts down on pollution—but can promote bacterial growth as the plastic degrades.

•**Government standards for bottled water purity** often are less strict than for tap water. Bottled water packaged and sold within the same state is exempt from FDA oversight.

My plan for switching to tap…

•**Use a faucet-mounted or carafe-style carbon filter** ($20 to $60 at drugstores) to remove lead, chlorine and other contaminants from tap water…or install a reverse-osmosis filter ($300 to $600) on the main water line to the house.

•**Carry water in a stainless steel or enamel-lined thermos.** Avoid reusable bottles made with #7 polycarbonate plastic—potentially carcinogenic and/or hormone-disrupting chemicals may leach from the plastic into the water, especially when exposed to heat or sunlight.

Bottled water can cost up to 10,000 times more than tap. The money I save can pay my gym fees.

Tamara Eberlein, editor of the Bottom Line/Women's Health *newsletter. Boardroom, Inc., 281 Tresser Blvd., Stamford, Connecticut 06901.*

Protect Yourself from Killer Bacteria

Edward K. Chapnick, MD, director of the division of infectious diseases at Maimonides Medical Center in Brooklyn, New York, and associate professor of medicine at Mount Sinai School of Medicine in New York City. He has published more than 30 medical journal articles on infectious diseases.

Imagine entering a hospital for heart surgery, a joint replacement or some other procedure. The treatment is successful, but you contract an infection during your hospital stay.

Each year, this happens to 2 million Americans. The infection is usually minor—a simple rash and fever that can be cured with antibiotics. But about 10% of hospital-acquired infections are serious. Some bacteria are resistant to most—

if not all—antibiotics, and harmful organisms can quickly invade the bloodstream and damage skin, organs, muscles and/or bones. Nearly 100,000 Americans die of these hospital-acquired infections annually.

While most hospitals have stepped up their efforts to prevent infections, only recently have many patients become aware that they must be more assertive in protecting themselves.

HOW TO AVOID BACTERIA

Bacteria can live for hours—sometimes even days—on almost any surface and then transfer easily to skin. From there, bacteria can enter the body through breaks in the skin or via touching the eyes, nose or mouth. Hand-washing is the most effective way to help prevent the spread of bacteria and other infection-causing organisms.

Other ways to protect yourself—or someone you love…

•**Ask doctors and nurses to disinfect medical devices.** To prevent the spread of bacteria or other germs, stethoscopes, blood pressure cuffs and other such medical devices should be cleaned with a disinfectant alcohol wipe before they touch your skin.

•**Avoid touching surfaces touched by other people.** Some people do their best to avoid touching tabletops, chairs, elevator doors or any other surface. If this is impractical, use alcohol-based disinfectant gels and/or wipes. To prevent a possible infection, avoid rubbing bare skin from any part of your body against these surfaces. In a recent study, about three-quarters of hospital rooms tested were contaminated with bacteria.

•**Be aware that visitors can carry germs into your hospital room.** Ask visitors not to sit on your bed—they can transfer bacteria from their clothes to the sheets…or use the bathroom in your room—they can transfer germs to bathroom surfaces. Even doctors' neckties can carry bacteria or other germs, research shows.

Hospital patients typically are at greater risk of contracting an infectious disease due to their weakened immunity, but it's also wise for hospital visitors to follow hygienic practices to avoid getting sick.

PREP YOURSELF

Patients themselves often carry bacteria, such as *Staphylococcus aureus* (staph), on their bodies and/or clothes when they check into the hospital. These germs don't always cause symptoms—up to 30% of healthy adults carry staph on their skin. However, if your skin is colonized with bacteria when you go for surgery, it can enter your body at the surgical site. *To protect yourself…*

•**Wash your body.** Three to five days before surgery, start showering or bathing daily using a special 4% chlorhexidine soap. Chlorhexidine is a powerful antiseptic agent that will help remove bacteria from the skin's surface. Chlorhexidine soap (such as Hibiclens or Betasept) is available over the counter at most drugstores. If it is not in stock, ask the pharmacist to order it.

Caution: Because this soap can irritate the skin or cause an allergic reaction in some people, do not use the soap for more than five days…avoid the use of other skin products during that time…and be sure that your doctor gives his/her consent to use the soap.

•**Don't shave.** No matter how careful you are, shaving causes microscopic nicks in your skin. Any break in the skin can potentially create an entry point for bacteria. For 72 hours before surgery, do not shave the surgical site, even if the site is on your legs, underarms or face. If your surgery typically requires shaving, ask your doctor if clippers can be used instead of a razor by hospital personnel before your surgery.

•**Ask for a staph test.** A week to 10 days before surgery, ask your surgeon to test you for *methicillin-resistant Staphylococcus aureus* (MRSA) by taking a nasal swab. If this test shows that you are a carrier of the bacterium, specific infection-control procedures will be used in the hospital. A topical antibiotic also may be prescribed.

Helpful: Almost everyone will be given an oral antibiotic within 60 minutes of receiving surgery to help prevent an infection. However, it's common for busy hospital staff to forget this routine medication. Be sure to remind your doctor.

If you're scheduled for surgery: Call your state's health department and ask if hospitals in the state are required to report infection rates. If so, get the latest report for the hospital where you'll be treated. Discuss any findings with your doctor.

CATHETERS AND IVs

Having a catheter or intravenous (IV) line increases your risk for infection because bacteria from your own body or a health-care worker's hands can enter at the insertion site. Catheters are tubes that are used to drain liquids, such as urine, from the body. IV lines deliver fluids, such as medication and nutrients, directly into a vein. *You may not have a choice whether or not a catheter or IV is inserted, but always ask...*

•**Why is the catheter and/or IV there?** Often, a catheter or IV is used when a patient enters the emergency room, but is then forgotten for a time after it is no longer needed. If you don't know why you have a catheter or IV, ask.

•**How many days will I need the catheter and/or IV?** The answer largely depends on your condition, but it's important to let your doctor know that you want a catheter and/or IV removed as soon as possible. With urinary catheters, the risk for an infection increases by at least 5% each day it remains in place. That means that it should come out as soon as medically possible.

Helpful: Every day, ask your nurse or doctor whether the catheter can come out...don't wait for medical staff to think of removing it.

With peripheral IVs (the kind that are inserted into a vein in your hand or arm), the risk for infection is relatively low until the third or fourth day. If an IV has been in place for four days, ask when you are scheduled to have it replaced with a new one. (Central venous lines, which are inserted in large veins of the neck or chest, don't have the same risk and can stay in place almost indefinitely.)

■ **More from Dr. Chapnick...**

Hand-Washing Secrets

If you are hospitalized, everyone who enters your room should wash his/her hands. This includes family members, doctors, nurses and other hospital staff. If you feel embarrassed to remind your doctor or anyone else, raise the issue as a question: "Did you remember to wash your hands?"

Be sure that people who wash with soap and water dry their hands with a clean paper towel and not a cloth towel from the bathroom in your hospital room. The paper towel also should be used to turn off the faucet.

In most hospitals, alcohol-based hand-cleaning gel dispensers are mounted on the wall in or near each patient's room—these are for everyone to use, not just staff. These gels (which should contain at least 62% alcohol) are superior to hand-washing at killing germs. Alcohol dries out the skin less than soap and water does, so it is best for frequent cleanings. If hands are visibly soiled, soap and water must be used.

Important: Latex gloves are meant to protect the person wearing them, not the patient. If hands aren't washed before putting on gloves, bacteria will live on the gloves. If a hospital staff member enters your room already wearing gloves, ask him to remove the gloves, clean his hands and put on a fresh pair.

How NOT to Get a Deadly Infection

Susan Kellie, MD, associate professor of medicine in the division of infectious diseases at the University of New Mexico (UNM) Health Sciences Center.

More evidence emerged that the virulent strain of methicillin-resistant *Staphylococcus aureus* (MRSA) is causing dangerous infections in otherwise healthy adults and children.

In late 2007, MRSA made headlines when a Virginia high school student died after MRSA spread quickly through his internal organs. Local officials closed 21 schools for disinfection.

The Journal of the American Medical Association (JAMA) reported that MRSA infections may be twice as common as previously thought. Looking at data from 2005, government researchers estimated that there are more than 94,000 life-threatening MRSA infections in the US annually, contributing to the deaths of an estimated 19,000 Americans per year.

This could place MRSA in the top 20 causes of death. This so-called "superbug" kills more Americans than AIDS, Parkinson's disease or emphysema.

RISK IS SPREADING

The ordinary *Staphylococcus aureus* (staph) bacterium is among the most common causes of infection. Up to one-third of Americans have a relatively innocuous form of staph in the nose or on the skin. It usually causes nothing more serious than boils or a hair-follicle infection.

MRSA is a strain of this organism that is resistant to certain antibiotics and has long been a problem in hospitals. The *JAMA* study, conducted by researchers at the Centers for Disease Control and Prevention (CDC), found that about 85% of MRSA cases are connected with hospitals and other health-care settings—after surgery, in dialysis patients, etc.—but a new form of MRSA, known as *USA 300*, is increasingly found in healthy Americans. *Examples...*

•**The Veterans Administration** in Pittsburgh has reported a four-fold increase in emergency room treatments for skin and soft-tissue (tissue under the skin) infections caused by MRSA.

•**A study** in *The New England Journal of Medicine* found that nearly 60% of skin and soft-tissue infections at 11 university-affiliated emergency rooms were caused by MRSA.

•**In 2005, researchers investigated** an outbreak of skin infections among the St. Louis Rams and found that 9% of the football players had MRSA skin infections. In addition, 42% of nasal swabs taken from the players and staff members tested positive for MRSA. All carried the USA 300 form of MRSA, which was simultaneously being discovered throughout the country. This suggests rapid, widespread transmission.

•**Studies indicate that 1% of healthy Americans are colonized with MRSA**—bacteria are present but haven't caused infection. In group-living settings, such as prisons and military training camps, the colonization rate is as high as 2.5% to 3%. Among hospitalized patients, the rate of colonization is eight to 10 times higher than previously suspected.

WHAT TO LOOK FOR

MRSA—particularly the USA 300 variant—is a serious public health threat, but while MRSA is resistant to some antibiotics, it is still vulnerable to others, such as *Vancomycin*. Most patients, including those with systemic infection, can be treated successfully if they get an antibiotic promptly.

Infection with MRSA usually starts with the skin. Patients often notice what looks like a spider bite. There will be a small, swollen area with a halo of redness around it. The area will be tender...might become a larger abscess...and the middle area might turn black from tissue breakdown. Sometimes, the bacteria remain confined to the skin—but they also can burrow deep into the body, causing potentially life-threatening infections.

If you suspect that you have a staph infection, call your doctor. If he/she is not available, go to an emergency room.

PREVENTION

The CDC has identified five conditions, known as the *5 Cs*, that increase the risk for MRSA—crowding...contact (usually skin to skin)...compromised skin...contaminated surfaces...and cleanliness (or the lack of it).

Patients in health-care settings have the highest risk, followed by those who spend time in communal settings—team locker rooms, prisons, etc. But the emergence of the community-acquired USA 300 form of MRSA means that everyone is potentially at risk.

Important steps to protect yourself...

•**Wash your hands with friction.** Most people with MRSA carry it in the nose, and people tend to touch their noses frequently. Wash your hands at least four times a day, rubbing them together briskly for at least 15 seconds and applying friction to all surfaces. Be sure to do this before meals and after touching gym equipment, shaking hands, etc. Use regular soap —antibacterial soap isn't necessary.

If you are in the hospital or another health-care setting, insist that doctors, nurses and technicians wash their hands before touching you—even if they wear gloves while doing the procedure.

•**Dry your hands with an air blower or a disposable paper towel.** Don't share towels with others, even at home.

•**Use an alcohol-based hand-cleaning gel.** Look for a product that contains at least 62% alcohol. A thorough application of the sanitizer takes only a few seconds and is a highly effective alternative to hand washing.

•**Cover wounds.** Damaged, open skin is the main pathway to infection. Wash cuts and scratches carefully…and keep them covered until they're completely healed.

•**Stay safe in gyms and locker rooms.** Wipe down sweaty equipment (barbells, exercise benches and exercise machine handles) with disinfectant before using…shower after exercise…wear flip-flops to protect your feet in the shower and locker room…and sit on your own towel, rather than on a bare bench.

•**Get vaccinated.** People who have had the flu are vulnerable to post-influenza MRSA pneumonia, which is potentially deadly. In older adults, an annual flu vaccination can reduce mortality from all causes by 50%.

•**Don't take unnecessary antibiotics.** In hospitals and nursing homes, between 20% and 30% of MRSA infections are attributed to antibiotic use.

Reason: Antibiotics kill many of the normal, healthy bacteria in the body. Eradicating "good" bacteria can allow MRSA to proliferate.

Patients often ask their doctors for antibiotics when they have a cold or another viral illness —and doctors often give them to keep their patients happy. But antibiotics are useless for viral infections.

■ ■ ■ ■

Wear Your Slippers

Researchers asked 90 participants to place their bare feet in cold (50°F) water for 20 minutes, while 90 others kept their feet in an empty bowl. Thirteen people from the chilled group developed a cold within five days, compared with five people from the other group.

Theory: Chilling the body constricts blood vessels in the nose, reducing the supply of infection-fighting white blood cells to the nasal passages. This sets the stage for cold viruses to multiply and trigger cold symptoms.

Self-defense: Wear waterproof, insulated footwear during the winter to keep your feet warm and dry.

Ronald Eccles, PhD, director, Common Cold Centre, Cardiff School of Biosciences, Cardiff University, Cardiff, Wales.

Safe Ways to Kill Deadly Germs

Kimberly M. Thompson, ScD, adjunct associate professor of risk analysis and decision science at Harvard University School of Public Health in Boston. She is co-author of *Overkill: Repairing the Damage Caused by Our Unhealthy Obsessions with Germs, Antibiotics, and Bacterial Poducts.* Rodale.

The infectious diseases that make the headlines, such as severe acute respiratory syndrome (SARS), pose very little risk to most Americans. You're far more likely to get sick from microbes that already live in your own home.

Examples: A kitchen sponge can harbor 7 billion organisms…and a "clean" cutting board might have 62,000 bacteria per square inch.

The Centers for Disease Control and Prevention estimates that food-borne microbes *alone* cause 76 million illnesses a year. We can't even begin to estimate how many people get sick—or die— from bacteria and viruses found in the home.

Many families automatically reach for antibacterial products or heavy-duty cleaners. *But don't overdo it.* Antibacterial products can weaken your resistance to harmful bacteria, which may ultimately *increase* your risk of getting sick.

Smart idea: Use an antibacterial soap after handling raw meat—probably the most common source of household infection—or if someone in your home is sick or living with a compromised immune system due to chronic illness.

Otherwise, plain soap and water are fine for handwashing, and homemade natural cleaners can be just as effective as cleaning products that contain harmful chemicals.

KITCHEN

The sink is the most germ-ridden space in the house—and often contains more fecal matter (from washing meats) and *E. coli* bacteria than the average toilet.

Rinse the sink with hot water after every use. Clean it twice a week with a scouring powder, such as Ajax or Comet. Disinfect it weekly with a mild bleach solution—one tablespoon of bleach mixed with one cup of hot water. *Also…*

•**Replace sponges** once or twice a month—and run them through the dishwasher each time you use it. They're a perfect breeding ground for harmful germs.

•**Stock up on dishtowels**…and change them every other day to prevent germs from passing among members of the family. Washing them in hot water—and running them through the clothes drier—will kill bacteria as well as viruses.

•**Use separate cutting boards** for meats, poultry and seafood—and scrub them with dish detergent, such as Joy or Dawn, and hot water after each use. Clean plastic cutting boards in the dishwasher.

BATHROOM

Even if you wear gloves when cleaning the toilet or tub, it's a good idea to wash your hands afterward. This eliminates bacteria from water that may get on your hands as you take off the gloves. *Also…*

•**Clean the bathtub** at least once weekly with scouring powder or a solution made with one-half cup of bleach and one gallon of water.

•**Sweep the bathroom floor** at least once weekly and clean with a basic cleaner, such as Lysol, or a solution made with one gallon of hot water…two tablespoons of borax…one teaspoon of dish detergent…and five drops each of patchouli and lavender essential oils. These oils contain effective natural disinfectants.

•**Wipe the bathroom sink and counters after every use.** Once a week, use a disinfectant made with one-quarter cup distilled white vinegar and one-half teaspoon of dish detergent in two cups of warm water. The bathroom sink is a bacterial hot spot because germs on your hands can spread to faucets.

•**Disinfect the toilet bowl, seat and outer surfaces weekly** with a commercial cleaner or with a solution made with one-half cup of baking soda…one-half cup of borax…one-quarter cup of distilled white vinegar…one teaspoon of dish detergent…three drops of sweet orange essential oil…and two drops of patchouli essential oil. Let it soak for an hour, scrub then flush.

Wipe and disinfect the handle daily because it's frequently touched by unwashed hands.

•**Close the toilet lid when you flush.** During flushing, bacteria disperse into the air and can land on any surface within six feet—including toothbrushes.

WASHING MACHINE

If there are young children in your household, every time you wash dirty underwear, millions of fecal bacteria are deposited on the inner surfaces of the washing machine—and can spread to the next load. Every few weeks, disinfect the machine by running it empty, using hot water and adding one-half cup of bleach.

TELEPHONES

Many bacterial illnesses are transmitted by touching the telephone and then touching your eyes, nose or mouth. Wipe all phone surfaces every two weeks with a cotton ball moistened with rubbing alcohol or spray with a natural antibacterial.

To make: Combine one tablespoon of borax …one cup of hot water…one cup of distilled white vinegar…one-half teaspoon of dish detergent…one-half teaspoon of sweet orange essential oil…and one-quarter teaspoon each of rosemary and lavender essential oils.

DOORKNOBS

Disinfect them at least once a month with rubbing alcohol or the natural antibacterial spray described above. Wipe them daily if someone in your family is sick with a cold or flu. Doorknobs are great locations for bacteria to be transferred from the hands of a sick person to other members of the family.

Other spots to disinfect frequently: Refrigerator handles, light switches and bannisters.

Beware of Soaps And Moisturizers!

Marianne O'Donoghue, MD, associate professor of dermatology at Rush University Medical Center in Chicago, and past president of the Women's Dermatologic Society. She is a member of the *Bottom Line/Women's Health* advisory board.

Nasty surprise: Many common soaps—and even moisturizers—can make hands dry and itchy. Liquid soap is a common culprit because it is water-based and so must contain a preservative to prevent bacterial growth and boost shelf life. The preservative commonly used is a cousin of formaldehyde called *Quaternium-15*. It can trigger an allergic reaction that causes eczema—an inflammatory condition characterized by dry, cracked skin, redness and/or itching. As liquid soaps have become more popular, I've seen a marked increase in cases of hand eczema among my patients.

Better: In my experience, bar soaps—which contain little or no water and hence need fewer preservatives—are far less likely to irritate hands. I especially like moisturizing products, such as Aveeno, Cetaphil, Dove and Olay.

Also helpful: Gel cleaners are a good alternative. Alcohol-based gels with emollients are less irritating and allergy-provoking than soap, particularly for people who must clean their hands frequently (such as health-care providers and restaurant workers). Although rubbing alcohol can dry out skin when used alone, it is not drying when used in a gel with an emollient, such as aloe.

Moisturizer warning: Water-based liquid moisturizers also may contain preservatives that can dry and damage skin. Instead, use a waterless ointment, such as Vaseline or Aquaphor. Rub one-half teaspoon into hands before bed. Wearing cotton gloves over the ointment while you're sleeping isn't necessary if you use it sparingly, though doing so may help the moisturizer to soak in.

Infection control: If you do have eczema, proper cleansing and moisturizing is vital because germs can enter the bloodstream through cracks in the skin. Washing with bar soap or gel and applying ointment four times daily should smooth cracks within a few days. If eczema doesn't improve, consult a dermatologist—he/she can prescribe a topical steroid ointment, such as *triamcinolone*.

Shocking Places Germs Hide

Charles Peter Gerba, PhD, professor of environmental microbiology who specializes in virology, parasitology and risk assessment at the University of Arizona College of Agriculture and Life Sciences, Tucson. He is coauthor, with Allison Janse, of *The Germ Freak's Guide to Outwitting Colds and Flu*. HCI.

Bacteria and viruses are everywhere. The vast majority of germs don't make us sick—though some, of course, do. The average adult gets two to four colds or other respiratory infections annually…children may get up to 12 colds a year.

Surprisingly, the bathroom is not the main microbial hot spot. *Where the germs really are…*

CLEAN LAUNDRY

We know that dirty laundry is laden with germs. In fact, it has been associated with outbreaks of *salmonellosis* and *hepatitis A,* along with *rotavirus,* the most common cause of severe diarrhea.

But seemingly clean laundry also can be loaded with bacteria and viruses.

Fact: The average pair of used underwear contains 0.1 gram of fecal matter, one of the main sources of infectious organisms. Up to 99% of the organisms are killed during an average wash cycle, but that still leaves about one million infectious agents.

Self-defense: Wash undergarments in hot water (140°F or hotter)—about 95% of American households use cooler water. Add bleach to the wash cycle for whites—three-quarter cup per washer load. It will kill an additional 90% of the organisms. A 45-minute dry cycle can kill the majority of any remaining pathogens.

Also important: Wash your hands immediately after transferring damp clothes to the dryer. Damp clothes are more likely to harbor germs than dry ones.

RESTAURANT TABLETOPS

Every year in the US, there are about 76 million cases of food-borne gastroenteritis, with symptoms ranging from mild diarrhea to serious liver or kidney disease. Many of these cases originate in the home, but restaurants also can be bacterial hot spots.

When we swabbed restaurant tabletops, we found that 70% were contaminated with *coliform* (fecal) bacteria, such as E. coli, organisms that are commonly found on meats as well as on vegetables and in water and soil.

In the same study, we found that the bacterial load on tabletops was 45 times greater after the tables were wiped.

Reason: The damp cloths used in restaurants are supposed to be sanitized between uses, but this usually is not done. The cloths tend to stay damp for long periods, which encourages bacterial growth.

More than 89% of restaurant dishcloths were contaminated—and the bacterial level on bar dishcloths was even higher.

Self-defense: When you go to a restaurant, carry disposable disinfectant wipes and clean the table yourself. If you're at a bar, wipe the area in front of you with a disinfectant wipe—or spread a paper napkin to rest your elbows on.

Also: Clean your hands with a disinfectant wipe after touching restaurant menus and those gadgets that vibrate when your table is ready—both are very rarely cleaned.

KITCHEN SINKS

We tested 14 surfaces in each of 15 homes.

Result: The kitchen sink, including the faucet handles, had the highest bacterial load. There's more bacteria in the average kitchen sink than in the average toilet.

From a microbial perspective, the kitchen is the dirtiest room in the house. Many foods, particularly raw meats, transfer coliforms and other disease-causing organisms to sinks, counters and cutting boards. Some of these organisms can survive for up to 24 hours, providing ample opportunities to cause infection.

Self-defense: After preparing raw meats, clean the kitchen sink with a bleach solution (one-quarter cup of bleach per gallon of water) or a commercial cleaning solution with bleach.

Bonus: Use the same solution to sanitize countertops, refrigerator handles and other surfaces.

Also helpful: Pour one-quarter cup of bleach into the garbage disposal at least once a month.

Because a cutting board often is used for meats, merely wiping the board isn't enough. Use a generous amount of a bleach or cleaning solution, let it sit for five to 10 minutes, then rinse it off.

Also, sanitize sponges and dishcloths at least once a week. You can run them through the clothes washer and dryer. Or soak them in a bleach solution for about an hour. You also can sanitize sponges and dishcloths in the microwave—soak them with water, and microwave for 30 seconds.

TV REMOTE CONTROLS

Certain household gadgets are rarely cleaned, including TV remote controls. If someone in your house has the flu, more than 50% of household gadgets, including remote controls and telephones, can harbor the virus.

Self-defense: Wipe remote controls, telephones, your keyboard, mouse and other often-used devices with an alcohol sanitizer every two to three days—more often if someone who is using these devices is infected.

LIQUID HAND SOAPS

The refillable soap containers in public restrooms often are contaminated with fecal bacteria.

Reason: The antimicrobial preservatives used in liquid soaps can break down, allowing harmful organisms to proliferate. A single "pull" can dispense millions of bacteria.

Self-defense: Use only the soap from dispensers that contain bagged soap. This soap doesn't get contaminated. To play it safe, wipe your hands with a disposable wipe or alcohol-based gel.

If you use liquid soap dispensers at home, wash them carefully with hot water before you refill them.

GROCERY CARTS

About two-thirds of grocery store shopping-cart handles are contaminated with coliform bacteria. Many carts had a higher concentration of bacteria than public restrooms.

Self-defense: Some supermarkets offer sanitary wipes for cart handles or have installed systems to disinfect entire carts. Look for these supermarkets, or bring your own wipes.

Also: Place fresh produce (including melons), meat and poultry in plastic bags.

Tired? Gaining Weight? You May Have a Sluggish Thyroid

Ellen Kamhi, PhD, RN, a board-certified holistic nurse and a clinical instructor at Stony Brook University's School of Medicine and New York Chiropractic College, Seneca Falls. As "The Natural Nurse," Dr. Kamhi addresses millions of Americans through radio and television programs. She is author of *Definitive Guide to Weight Loss* and coauthor of *The Natural Medicine Chest* (both from Natural Nurse, *www.naturalnurse.com*).

Do you feel tired most of the time? Are you gaining weight for no apparent reason? A sluggish thyroid may be to blame.

Though approximately just 3% of all Americans suffer from an underactive thyroid, or *hypothyroidism* (sometimes referred to as a sluggish thyroid), as many as 10% to 15% of Americans have a subclinical (mild) hypothyroid condition. Because hypothyroidism often underlies other health conditions, the number of people who have the disorder may be even higher, perhaps as high as one in three.

Untreated hypothyroidism can lead to serious medical problems, including reduced immunity, high cholesterol and high blood pressure.

Finding: A study published in *Archives of Internal Medicine* reported that even mild changes in thyroid function are associated with an increased risk for mortality in patients with cardiac disease.

The good news is that a sluggish thyroid often can be corrected naturally.

WHAT IS A SLUGGISH THYROID?

The thyroid, a butterfly-shaped gland in the lower front of the neck, produces hormones that help your body regulate your metabolism and keep your heart, brain, muscles and organs functioning normally. Hypothyroidism has several causes that can trigger a shortage in formation or utilization of thyroid hormones.

RISKS

The risk for hypothyroidism grows with age, and being female puts you at even higher risk. According to the American Association of Clinical Endocrinologists, women are five to eight times more likely than men to have the condition. The risk for hypothyroidism increases if you have a family history of thyroid disease or if you have an autoimmune disorder, such as type 1 diabetes or rheumatoid arthritis.

SYMPTOMS

Symptoms of hypothyroidism include fatigue, depression, forgetfulness, weight gain, insomnia, intolerance to cold, constipation, dry skin, hair loss and/or chronic yeast infections.

For women, hypothyroid symptoms may include frequent and/or heavy menstrual periods. Also, symptoms commonly attributed to menopause, such as hot flashes and mood swings, can be signs of a sluggish thyroid.

If you regularly suffer from two or more hypothyroid symptoms over the course of several weeks or months, see your doctor. If your doctor suspects hypothyroidism, he/she will order a simple blood test that measures *thyroid stimulating hormone* (TSH) and "free" *thyroxine* (T4).

An abnormally high level of TSH means the thyroid gland is asked to make more T4 because there isn't enough available. A "free" T4 index can effectively measure how much T4 is circulating in the blood and available for your body to use.

If your doctor doesn't discover a thyroid problem but you have many of the symptoms, visit a holistic practitioner who may have a better understanding of hidden thyroid issues.

NATURAL REMEDIES

Lifestyle changes can go a long way toward correcting a sluggish thyroid…

•**Consume natural sources of iodine.** If you're low in iodine, it can lead to a thyroid deficiency. The best sources of iodine are iodized salt, sea vegetables, such as seaweed, as well as eggs and shellfish, including lobster, shrimp and crab.

You will need 100 micrograms (mcg) to 120 mcg of iodine a day. A three-ounce serving of shrimp—or one egg—contains about 30 mcg.

Also, to ensure a healthy metabolism, eat a balanced diet that includes adequate amounts of protein (beef, poultry, fish, eggs and milk products, such as yogurt and cottage cheese), whole grains and plenty of vegetables. Whenever possible, opt for organic foods—pesticides and herbicides have been linked to thyroid disorders.

•**Eat foods rich in vitamin E and selenium.** Studies reported in *BioFactors* and *European Journal of Endocrinology* show that vitamin E and selenium can revitalize an underactive thyroid.

Vitamin E is in various foods, including wheat germ, whole-grain cereals, nuts, avocados, green leafy vegetables and fish. Try to consume a total of 200 international units (IU) per day. One tablespoon of wheat germ oil has 30 IU...one ounce of almonds has 10 IU.

Selenium is in seafood, liver, poultry, red meat and grains—aim for 200 mcg a day. A four-ounce serving of most fish has 50 mcg to 75 mcg of selenium...four ounces of turkey breast has 33 mcg.

•**Exercise.** The research on hypothyroidism suggests that thyroid dysfunction may be linked to stress. A study in *Annals of the New York Academy of Sciences* found that exercise helps reestablish healthy thyroid function by decreasing the overall impact of stress.

Best: Aim for 30 minutes a day of any form of exercise.

7

Easy Pain Relief

How to Control Chinese Pain

One in 10 Americans suffers from moderate to severe chronic pain, most often due to osteoarthritis, back ailments or injury. Unfortunately, pain is often *undertreated.*

Pain control is not a luxury—it is a medical necessity. Chronic pain can cause muscle weakness due to inactivity, insomnia and fatigue. Chronic pain can even "rewire" the nervous system, increasing your sensitivity to pain signals and causing pain in areas that were previously pain-free.

PAIN INVENTORY

Your doctor's ability to prescribe the right treatment depends on knowing exactly where, when and how your body hurts. *Before your next appointment, create a personal pain inventory by answering the following questions…*

•**Where is the pain?** Is it shallow and near the surface of your skin, or deep below the surface? Is it worse in any particular location, or equally bad all over?

•**When do you feel pain?** Is it worse in the morning or at night? Does it hurt all the time, or only when you move? Which movements cause pain? Is your pain affected by stress, changes in weather, exercise or sleep?

•**How bad is the pain?** Rate your pain on a scale of 0 to 10 (0 represents no pain, and 10 is the worst pain you've ever had). These ratings might change during the day—for example, you may wake up with level 3 pain, but progress to level 7 by evening. Or you may have no pain most of the time, but level 8 pain with specific movements, such as sitting down, standing up or walking.

•**What does the pain feel like?** Is it sharp, stabbing, dull, burning or throbbing?

•**How has the pain interfered with your life?** Does the pain interfere with your sleep?

Jennifer P. Schneider, MD, PhD, a Tucson, Arizona–based physician, board certified in internal medicine, addiction medicine and pain management, is the author of *Living with Chronic Pain: The Complete Health Guide to the Causes and Treatment of Chronic Pain.* Hatherleigh.

What activities or aspects of your life are limited by pain? Physicians use this information to determine how aggressively to treat the pain, so be honest and thorough in describing how your life has changed.

• **What relieves the pain?** What have you tried, and what worked? Include all prescription and over-the-counter (OTC) medications, ice packs, rest, applied pressure, herbal remedies, etc.

WORKING WITH YOUR DOCTOR

Most primary care physicians can diagnose and treat common causes of pain, such as back pain, headaches and osteoarthritis. Depending on your problem, your doctor may refer you to a neurologist, orthopedic surgeon, rheumatologist or other specialist. These doctors may determine that you need surgery or other procedures to treat the underlying cause of your pain.

People in pain tend to minimize movement because it hurts. But the less you move, the weaker your muscles become, which worsens the pain when you do try to move. To end this vicious cycle, engage in as much physical activity, such as walking, as you can.

Your doctor may need to experiment with different drugs to see which works best for you. Often, a "cocktail" of medications, instead of just one type, offers the best pain relief. For each medication prescribed, ask the doctor how soon it will begin working and what side effects you can expect. For example, some pain relievers cause constipation.

Make a follow-up appointment before leaving the office. You may need frequent visits while your medications are being adjusted. Once your pain is controlled, you will probably need to see your doctor less often. Prepare a new pain inventory before each visit.

MEDICATIONS TO CONSIDER

Potent pain-fighting therapies, many of which are underused…

• **Anti-inflammatory drugs.** Because these medications both relieve pain and decrease inflammation, they are typically used to treat arthritis and other painful conditions that cause inflammation. The pain reliever *acetaminophen* (Tylenol) does not treat inflammation. First-generation nonsteroidal anti-inflammatory drugs (NSAIDs) include *ibuprofen* (Motrin, Advil) and *naproxen* (Naprosyn, Aleve). These medications have side effects that can limit their use, including gastrointestinal bleeding and elevated blood pressure. A second-generation NSAID, such as the prescription COX-2 inhibitor *celecoxib* (Celebrex), is much less likely to cause bleeding, but may increase risk for heart attack and stroke. Your doctor should weigh the risks against the benefits when recommending anti-inflammatory medication.

• **Opioids.** These medications are typically used to treat moderate to severe pain. Opioids include codeine, morphine, *hydrocodone* (Vicodin), *fentanyl* patches (Duragesic), *oxycodone* (OxyContin), and *oxycodone* combined with *acetaminophen* (Percocet). These drugs have been so stigmatized by illicit drug use that many doctors are afraid to use them to ease pain in patients who are truly suffering.

When used as directed, opioids are no more dangerous than any other drugs and can be taken indefinitely, if needed. Although most patients taking opioid analgesics for more than about three weeks become physically dependent on them, few become addicted. Physical dependency means the body has become used to the drug, and when it is stopped, withdrawal symptoms, such as muscle pain, vomiting and diarrhea, can occur. This can be avoided if your doctor tapers the drugs slowly. Addiction occurs when there is a loss of control over the drug use, continued use of the drug despite negative consequences and a mental focus on getting and using more than the prescribed amount.

• **Topical analgesics.** Some types of pain, especially pain on the surface of the skin—such as from shingles or joint pain due to osteoarthritis—respond well to drugs that are absorbed through the skin. Examples include the *lidocaine* (Lidoderm) patch and *capsaicin* (Zostrix) cream.

• **Antidepressants.** *Venlafaxine* (Effexor) and *duloxetine* (Cymbalta) have been shown to relieve nerve pain, such as that from shingles, and diabetic neuropathy (nerve pain in the extremities).

• **Anticonvulsants.** Typically used to control seizures, *topiramate* (Topamax) eases migraines, and *gabapentin* (Neurontin) is helpful for those suffering from diabetic neuropathy (an abnormal and typically degenerative state of the nervous system) or shingles pain.

■ ■ ■ ■

Cough Away Pain

In a new finding, coughing reduces the pain of a needle being inserted into the skin for local anesthetic, an intravenous (IV) line or when blood is drawn.

Reason: Coughing at the moment the needle is injected distracts a part of the brain that also perceives pain.

Important: Before trying this approach, ask the practitioner to observe whether you move your arm when you cough.

Taras I. Usichenko, MD, PhD, professor of anesthesiology, Ernst Moritz Arndt University, Greifswald, Germany.

What Relief! Natural Ways to Curb Your Pain

Mark A. Stengler, ND, naturopathic physician in private practice, La Jolla, California...adjunct associate clinical professor at the National College of Natural Medicine, Portland, Oregon...author of many books, including *The Natural Physician's Healing Therapies* and coauthor of *Prescription for Natural Cures* (both from Bottom Line Books)...and author of the *Bottom Line/Natural Healing* newsletter.

Not long ago, a 60-year-old woman came to my office suffering from severe arthritis pain in both hands. I gave her a bean-sized dab of a homeopathic gel that she applied directly to the skin on her hands. After a few applications in the span of 30 minutes, her pain was reduced by 90%. She did not need to apply the gel again for two weeks.

I witnessed a similar result with a retired National Football League player. He had severe chronic hip pain from past injuries. With one application of the gel, his pain was relieved by 70% for two full days.

The relief that these people experienced has given them each a new lease on life. *But here's the best news*—unlike pharmaceutical pain relievers, which often cause gastrointestinal upset or damage to internal organs, natural therapies can reduce pain without adverse effects.

WHAT ARE YOU TAKING FOR PAIN?

Most Americans take too many pharmaceutical pain relievers. An estimated 175 million American adults take over-the-counter (OTC) pain relievers regularly. About one-fifth of Americans in their 60s take at least one painkiller for chronic pain on a regular basis.

There has been a lot of news about the life-threatening risks of anti-inflammatory medications such as *rofecoxib* (Vioxx) and *celecoxib* (Celebrex), two pain relievers that had been heavily prescribed by conventional doctors to treat the chronic pain of arthritis and similar conditions. Vioxx was pulled off the market by its manufacturer, Merck, following research that linked it to increased risk of heart attack and stroke. Pfizer has revised all advertising for Celebrex to include warnings of increased risk, especially to those with heart disease and high blood pressure. Its safety is being scrutinized.

Of course, pain-relieving drugs can be a blessing in the event of injury, severe acute migraines or diseases, such as terminal cancer. A number of years ago, when I had a wisdom tooth extracted, I received a local anesthetic. Afterward, I went to an acupuncturist for pain relief so I wouldn't need any painkillers. For about one hour after the acupuncture, I was fine—but then the pain-relieving endorphins wore off. I tried a few natural remedies, but when the pain became excruciating, I resorted to the OTC pain reliever *acetaminophen* (Tylenol). That did the trick.

But many people use painkillers on a regular basis for several months or even years, which increases the risk of dangerous side effects. For instance, people who rely on acetaminophen increase their risk of developing stomach ulcers, liver disease and kidney disease. If you regularly take an OTC nonsteroidal anti-inflammatory drug (NSAID), such as aspirin or *naproxen* (Aleve), you run the risk of kidney and stomach damage. Regular use of NSAIDs also increases risk of heart attack, according to the FDA.

BETTER RESULTS, FEWER RISKS

Before you take any remedy, it's important for your doctor to identify what is causing your pain. Remember, pain is your body's distress signal that something is being irritated or damaged. Sometimes we protect ourselves by reacting instinctively. If you touch something hot, for example, you eliminate the pain by quickly pulling back your hand.

But what if your back hurts? You may need a pain reliever—but back pain also can be a signal that you're harming your body by bending or sitting the wrong way. You may need to address the underlying cause to prevent further injury. Pain receptors are found in the skin, around bones and joints—even in the walls of arteries. If a muscle is torn, for example, a pain signal is released from fibers in the shredded tissue.

In light of the dangers from prescription and OTC drugs, what safe alternatives are available to you? There are many natural supplements that I recommend.

NATURE'S PAIN RELIEVERS

If you take prescription or OTC pain medication, work with a naturopathic physician, holistic medical doctor or chiropractor who will incorporate natural pain fighters into your treatment regimen. With his/her help, you may be able to reduce your dosage of pain medication (natural pain relievers can be used safely with prescription or OTC painkillers)—or even eliminate the drugs altogether.

Natural pain-fighting supplements are even more effective when combined with physical therapies, such as acupuncture, chiropractic, magnet therapy or osteopathic manipulation (a technique in which an osteopathic physician uses his hands to move a patient's muscles and joints with stretching, gentle pressure and resistance). Physiotherapy (treatment that uses physical agents, such as exercise and massage, to develop, maintain and restore movement and functional ability) also is helpful.

Here are—in no special order—the best natural pain relievers, which can be taken alone or in combination...

•**White willow bark extract** is great for headaches, arthritis, muscle aches and fever. In Europe, doctors prescribe this herbal remedy for back pain, and recent research supports this use. One study conducted in Haifa, Israel, involved 191 patients with chronic low-back pain who took one of two doses of willow bark extract or a placebo daily for four weeks. Researchers found that 39% of patients taking the higher dose of willow bark extract had complete pain

relief, compared with only 6% of those who were taking a placebo. Those participants who benefited the most took willow bark extract that contained 240 mg of the compound *salicin*, the active constituent in this herbal remedy. (Aspirin is made from *acetylsalicylic acid*, which has many of the chemical properties of salicin.) However, aspirin can cause gastrointestinal ulceration and other side effects, including kidney damage. Willow bark extract is believed to work by inhibiting naturally occurring enzymes that cause inflammation and pain.

I recommend taking willow bark extract that contains 240 mg of salicin daily. In rare cases, willow bark extract can cause mild stomach upset. Don't take willow bark if you have a history of ulcers, gastritis or kidney disease. It also should not be taken by anyone who is allergic to aspirin. As with aspirin, willow bark extract should never be given to children under age 12 who have a fever—in rare instances, it can cause a fatal disease called Reye's syndrome. Willow bark extract has blood-thinning properties, so avoid it if you take a blood thinner, such as *warfarin* (Coumadin). For low-back pain, you may need to take willow bark extract for a week or more before you get results.

•**Methylsulfonylmethane (MSM)** is a popular nutritional supplement that relieves muscle and joint pain. According to Stanley Jacob, MD, a professor at Oregon Health & Science University who has conducted much of the original research on MSM, this supplement reduces inflammation by improving blood flow. Your cells have receptors that send out pain signals when they're deprived of blood. That's why increased blood flow diminishes pain.

MSM, a natural compound found in green vegetables, fruits and grains, reduces muscle spasms and softens painful scar tissue from previous injuries. A double-blind study of 50 people with osteoarthritis of the knee found that MSM helps relieve arthritis pain.

Start with a daily dose of 3,000 mg to 5,000 mg of MSM. If your pain and/or inflammation doesn't improve within five days, increase the dose up to 8,000 mg daily, taken in several doses throughout the day. If you develop digestive upset or loose stools, reduce the dosage. If you prefer, you can apply MSM cream (per the label instructions) to your skin at the painful area. This product is available at health-food stores and works well for localized pain. MSM has a mild blood-thinning effect, so check with your doctor if you take a blood thinner.

•**S-adenosylmethionine (SAMe)** is a natural compound found in the body. The supplement is an effective treatment for people who have osteoarthritis accompanied by cartilage degeneration. SAMe's ability to reduce pain, stiffness and swelling is similar to that of NSAIDs such as Advil (ibuprofen), Aleve (naproxen) and Celebrex (celecoxib). There's also evidence that SAMe stimulates cartilage repair, which helps prevent bones from rubbing against one another. A 16-week study conducted at the University of California, Irvine, compared two groups of people who were being treated for knee pain caused by osteoarthritis. Some took 1,200 mg of SAMe daily, while others took 200 mg of Celebrex. It took longer for people to get relief from SAMe, but by the second month, SAMe proved to be just as effective as Celebrex.

Most patients with osteoarthritis and fibromyalgia (a disorder characterized by widespread pain in muscles, tendons and ligaments) who take SAMe notice improvement within four to eight weeks. Many studies use 1,200 mg of SAMe daily in divided doses. In my experience, taking 400 mg twice daily works well. It's a good idea to take a multivitamin or 50-mg B-complex supplement daily while you're taking SAMe. The vitamin B-12 and folic acid contained in either supplement help your body metabolize SAMe, which means that the remedy goes to work faster.

•**Kaprex** is effective for mild pain caused by injury or osteoarthritis. It is a blend of hops, rosemary extract and *oleanic acid,* which is derived from olive leaf extract. These natural substances inhibit pain-causing chemicals called *prostaglandins,* which is the same way NSAIDS work.

I recommend taking one 350-mg tablet three times daily. Kaprex is manufactured by Metagenics (800-692-9400, *www.metagenics.com*). The product is sold only in doctors' offices. To find a practitioner in your area who sells Kaprex, call the toll-free number. Kaprex has no known side effects and does not interact with other medications.

•**Proteolytic enzymes,** including *bromelain, trypsin, chymotrypsin, pancreatin, papain* and a range of protein-digesting enzymes derived from the fermentation of fungus, reduce pain and inflammation by improving blood flow. You can find these natural pain fighters at health-food stores in products labeled "proteolytic enzymes." Take as directed on the label. Bromelain, a favorite of athletes, is available on its own. Extracted from pineapple stems, bromelain reduces swelling by breaking down blood clots that can form as a result of trauma and impede circulation. It works well for bruises, sprains and surgical recovery. If you use bromelain, take 500 mg three times daily between meals.

Repair is a high-potency formula of proteolytic enzymes that I often recommend. It is manufactured by Enzymedica (to find a retailer, call 888-918-1118 or go to *www.enzymedica.com*). Take two capsules two to three times daily between meals. Don't take Repair or any proteolytic enzyme formula if you have an active ulcer or gastritis. Any enzyme product can have a mild blood-thinning effect, so check with your doctor if you take a blood thinner.

•**Pain Med** is the homeopathic gel that gave such quick relief to the patients I described at the beginning of this article. It is remarkably effective for relieving the pain of arthritis, muscle soreness and spasms, sprains, strains, stiffness, headaches (especially due to tension) as well as injuries, including bruises.

Pain Med is a combination of nine highly diluted plant and flower materials, including arnica, bryonia, hypericum and ledum. Like other homeopathic remedies, it promotes the body's ability to heal itself. A bean-sized dab works well for anyone who has pain. It should be spread on the skin around the affected area. Following an injury, use it every 15 minutes, for a total of up to four applications. As the pain starts to diminish, apply less often. Do not reapply the gel once the pain is gone. Pain Med does not sting, burn or irritate the skin. It is clear, has no odor, does not stain and dries quickly. Because it has so many uses and works so rapidly, Pain Med is a good first-aid remedy to have on hand. To order, contact the manufacturer, GM International, Inc., at 800-228-9850.

■ ■ ■ ■

Exercise Reduces Pain

Many people know running is an excellent exercise for general health, but they worry that it causes strain on ankles, knees, hips and legs that may lead to arthritis or other medical problems.

Reality: Research shows the reverse is true. Running strengthens joints and bones, and reduces risk of arthritis and skeletal problems.

New study: In 1984, 492 exercisers over age 50 joined a long-term study in which those who exercised (including running) at least two hours a week were matched with non-exercisers. Today, the exercisers report experiencing 25% less musculoskeletal pain than the non-exercisers.

Bonnie Bruce, DrPH, MPH, RD, senior research scholar, department of medicine immunology & rheumatology, Stanford University, Palo Alto, California.

Heal Your Headache Without Drugs

David W. Buchholz, MD, associate professor of neurology at Johns Hopkins University School of Medicine and former director of the Neurological Consultation Clinic at Johns Hopkins, both in Baltimore. He is author of *Heal Your Headache: The 1-2-3 Program for Taking Charge of Your Pain.* Workman.

Most doctors traditionally distinguish minor "tension" headaches from migraine headaches. Until recently, it had been thought that tension in the head and neck muscles produced tension headaches.

New findings: Electromyograms—tests that record the electrical currents caused by muscle activity—of patients with so-called tension headaches reveal no abnormal muscle activity in the head or neck.

It now appears that the vast majority of headaches have the same underlying cause—and that they all should be considered forms of migraine.

Why it matters: Many of the medications for so-called tension headaches actually make the problem worse. Instead, the same steps that prevent migraine, such as avoiding "trigger foods," should be followed for virtually all headaches.

Headache expert David W. Buchholz, MD, of Johns Hopkins University School of Medicine explains that most patients can substantially decrease both the frequency and severity of headaches within one to two months. This often can be done without relying on drugs. *Here's how...*

TRIGGERS

The brain contains a headache-generating mechanism that causes swelling and inflammation of blood vessels in and around the head. When this mechanism is fully activated, patients experience the most severe symptoms—pain, as well as nausea, vomiting, sensitivity to light and other classic migraine symptoms.

The same mechanism also can be partially activated. When this happens, patients are likely to experience only mild-to-moderate discomfort. *Two factors determine whether—and how severely—the mechanism is activated...*

• **Triggers.** There are dozens of potential triggers—including hormones, foods, sleep deprivation and even weather changes—that can set off a headache. Each person responds individually to different triggers.

• **Trigger threshold.** Exposure to one or more triggers doesn't necessarily activate a headache. Patients first have to exceed their personal, built-in trigger threshold—a genetically determined level at which a headache is activated. People who get few headaches have high thresholds—whereas those who get frequent and severe headaches have lower thresholds.

Example: You might be sensitive to chocolate, along with changes in barometric pressure and high amounts of stress. A headache won't occur as long as the sum of the triggers doesn't push you past the threshold. But if you're exposed to all of these factors and the threshold is crossed, you might develop a splitting headache.

STEPS TO PREVENTION

One way to prevent headaches is to do aerobic exercise (biking, swimming, brisk walking, etc.) most days of the week. No matter what your particular triggers are, aerobic exercise raises the migraine threshold.

Also, take these measures to help control headaches...

***Step 1:* Avoid quick fixes.** It's understandable that people reach for analgesics (painkilling drugs) at the first hint of a headache—but beware. Many of these drugs cause rebound headaches by lowering the migraine threshold, which makes subsequent headaches more likely and eventually more frequent and severe.

What happens: Many headache drugs contain ingredients that relieve pain by temporarily constricting blood vessels. After the initial relief, the drugs lead to rebound vasodilation—the blood vessels tend to swell even more than they did before.

Drugs that cause rebound headaches include those that contain caffeine (Excedrin and Anacin)…as well as decongestants (Sudafed)…triptans (Imitrex, Relpax and others)…and narcotics, among others. Don't use these drugs more than twice a month.

Single-ingredient analgesics, such as ibuprofen, aspirin or acetaminophen, don't constrict blood vessels—but they aren't as effective for most patients. However, they're a better choice for occasional use—up to two days per week at the most—because they are less likely to cause the rebound effect.

The best way out of the rebound cycle is to stop taking rebound-causing analgesics altogether. Headaches may temporarily worsen for one to two weeks—the time it takes to recover from the rebound. You must escape from rebound in order for steps two and three to be effective.

***Step 2:* Reduce the trigger load.** There are dozens of migraine triggers. Foods and food additives are among the most common *and* the most avoidable. Some people react to inadequate sleep, strong smells (perfume, tobacco, etc.), humidity or high altitudes.

Some triggers cause a headache almost immediately. More often, there's a delay of hours or even a day or two. *The most common dietary triggers…*

• **Caffeinated beverages**—such as coffee, tea and colas. Caffeine is one of the most potent dietary triggers. Decaffeinated coffee and tea aren't completely safe, because they contain other chemicals besides caffeine that can act as triggers. Herbal teas are fine.

• **Processed meats,** such as bacon and salami, that contain nitrites.

• **Chocolate and cocoa.**

• **Monosodium glutamate (MSG),** a popular flavor enhancer.

• **Alcohol**—particularly red wine.

• **Citrus fruits and juices.**

• **Onions, sauerkraut, lentils and certain beans** (broad Italian, lima, fava and navy).

• **Soy foods,** particularly those that are fermented, such as tempeh and miso.

I advise my patients to avoid these foods as best they can for four months. After that, you can reintroduce individual items, no more than one item per week, to see if it leads to a headache. If it doesn't, it's probably safe, at least for the time being, and you can reintroduce the next item.

Other potentially avoidable triggers include medications, such as birth control pills, estrogen-replacement pills and proton pump inhibitors (Nexium, etc.) for reflux. Certain antidepressants are triggers, too, including selective serotonin reuptake inhibitors (SSRIs), such as Prozac…serotonin and norepinephrine reuptake inhibitors (SNRIs), such as Effexor and Cymbalta…and norepinephrine and dopamine reuptake inhibitors (NDRIs), such as Wellbutrin.

***Step 3:* Take preventive medicine.** Most people can control their headaches with steps one and two. If not, you may need to add preventive medication to raise your migraine threshold.

Some medications used for preventing headaches are not approved by the Food and Drug Administration (FDA) for this use, but they have been found to be safe and effective, including tricyclic antidepressants, calcium channel blockers and beta-blockers. FDA-approved medications include Topamax. Talk to your doctor about what might work best for you.

■ ■ ■ ■

How to Find Help for Your Migraines

Some migraines can be relieved with a dental device. Migraine pain usually stems from the trigeminal nerve, which also is involved in jaw clenching. When worn through the night, the *nociceptive trigeminal inhibition tension suppression system* (NTI-tss) dental mouthpiece reduces the intensity of clenching and frequency of migraines by 77%.

Cost: $600 and up. It may be covered by insurance, depending on your plan.

Find a dentist trained in NTI at *www.headache prevention.com* (click on "NTI Provider List").

Michael Steinberg, DDS, dentist in private practice, New York City.

∎∎∎∎

Migraine Relief

Migraines may be relieved when a minor heart defect is repaired. Research has found that when a hole in the heart called a patent foramen ovale was repaired in stroke patients, those who suffered migraines no longer had the headaches. If results of further studies are positive, this treatment may be available for migraine sufferers within several years.

Jonathan Tobis, MD, physician, medicine, cardiology, adult cardiac catheterization laboratory and interventional cardiology, UCLA Health System.

Breakthrough Treatments for Rheumatoid Arthritis

Harry D. Fischer, MD, chief of the division of rheumatology at Beth Israel Medical Center and associate professor of clinical medicine at Albert Einstein College of Medicine, both in New York City, is coauthor of *What to Do When the Doctor Says It's Rheumatoid Arthritis.* Fair Winds Press.

Rheumatoid, or inflammatory arthritis, which affects an estimated 2 million Americans, typically occurs in the hands and feet, resulting in swelling, pain and joint deformities. It is an autoimmune disease (a malfunction in the immune system that causes the body to attack cells), which affects the synovium (the thin membrane that surrounds the joints). But rheumatoid arthritis isn't just about achy joints. It also can affect other parts of the body.

In severe cases, rheumatoid arthritis can cause dangerous heart inflammation (pericarditis)... lung inflammation (pleurisy)...and eye inflammation that can damage sight (scleritis).

People with rheumatoid arthritis should be treated early not only to prevent permanent joint deformities but also to guard against the inflammation-related complications associated with the disorder. Most joint destruction caused by rheumatoid arthritis occurs in the first six to 12 months following diagnosis.

At one time, doctors mainly focused on relieving symptoms with pain medication.

Now: Drug therapies are aimed at curbing the progression of this debilitating disorder.

ARE YOU AT RISK?

Rheumatoid arthritis can occur at any age. About 75% of sufferers are women, which suggests that hormones may play a role in the disease. Some researchers believe that a viral or bacterial infection may trigger the disorder in some patients. Smoking and stress are thought to contribute to rheumatoid arthritis—but not cause it.

Rheumatoid arthritis is characterized by joint stiffness and swelling, often in symmetrical patterns on both sides of the body. Fatigue and a low-grade fever also may occur.

NEW TREATMENTS

Rheumatoid arthritis almost always requires drug therapy. Drugs can significantly reduce pain in more than half of patients and offer some relief to the others.

People who have rheumatoid arthritis should seek treatment from a rheumatologist (a medical doctor who specializes in the treatment of disease involving the joints, muscles and associated structures).*

Rheumatologists often prescribe nonsteroidal anti-inflammatory drugs (NSAIDs), such as *ibuprofen* (Advil) and *naproxen* (Aleve), or the corticosteroid *prednisone*, to control the pain and inflammation associated with the condition.

A majority of rheumatoid arthritis sufferers also are prescribed a medication known as a disease-modifying anti-rheumatic drug (DMARD),

*To find a qualified rheumatologist in your area, contact the American College of Rheumatology (404-633-3777, *www.rheumatology.org*).

which is designed to reduce pain and inflammation and slow progression of the disease.

•**Nonbiological DMARDs** are synthetic medications that have been available for many years. These drugs reduce joint damage. *Nonbiological DMARDs include…*

•*Methotrexate* (Rheumatrex). It suppresses the immune system and minimizes joint destruction. Most patients who take methotrexate experience reduced pain and joint swelling within weeks. It's among the best drugs for slowing the progression of rheumatoid arthritis.

Potential side effects include nausea, diarrhea and, in rare cases, liver scarring and/or inflammation. For this reason, periodic liver function tests are required.

•*Hydroxychloroquine* (Plaquenil). This antimalarial drug suppresses immune attacks on the joints. It's often combined with methotrexate for better results. This drug can cause nausea and decreased appetite and, in rare cases, retinopathy (a disorder of the retina, resulting in vision impairment). If you take this drug, you should have regular eye exams.

•*Sulfasalazine* (Azulfidine). This medication, often used for mild symptoms or in combination with other drugs for severe symptoms, can cause stomach upset, headache and, in some cases, a decrease in disease-fighting white blood cells.

Important: In addition to liver function tests, people who take nonbiological DMARDs require regular blood tests to monitor changes in blood counts.

•**Biological DMARDs** resemble substances that are naturally present in the body. Most patients who take these newer, more specifically targeted drugs experience improvements in a short time—and some even report a complete remission.

Three biologic agents are currently available that inhibit or block a cell protein known as *TNF-alpha*, which produces the inflammatory response.

•*Etanercept* (Enbrel). It is usually injected once or twice weekly.

•*Adalimumab* (Humira). It is given by injection once every two weeks, although it is sometimes given weekly.

•*Infliximab* (Remicade). This drug is taken in combination with methotrexate. It is given by intravenous (IV) infusion in a doctor's office, usually once every eight weeks. At times, it can be given as frequently as every four weeks.

These drugs may increase the risk for infection. They also can reactivate tuberculosis (TB) in patients who were previously exposed—even if they never had symptoms. A TB skin test is required prior to starting therapy.

Drawback: These drugs are extremely expensive, costing about $15,000 to $30,000 annually, depending on the dose.

NEW DRUG CHOICES

Several new drugs don't have the long-term data of the DMARDs, but they are an option for patients who don't respond to DMARDs.

•**Abatacept (Orencia).** Approved by the FDA in December 2005, abatacept inhibits the activity of *T-cells*, immune cells that play a central role in joint inflammation. It may increase risk for infection.

•**Rituximab (Rituxan).** Used for 10 years to treat lymphoma, this drug was recently approved to treat rheumatoid arthritis. It reduces *circulatory B-cells*, a type of white blood cell that has been shown to play a role in the development of rheumatoid arthritis. Rituximab is given by IV infusion every few months. It may increase infection risk.

Rheumatoid Arthritis May Cause Congestive Heart Failure

Paulo Nicola, MD, research fellow, Mayo Clinic, Rochester, Minnesota.
William Wilke, MD, rheumatologist, Cleveland Clinic.
John Klippel, MD, rheumatologist, and president and chief executive officer, Arthritis Foundation.
Arthritis & Rheumatism.

A study conducted at the Mayo Clinic confirms that there's a strong link between rheumatoid arthritis (RA) and congestive heart failure, a condition in which the heart progressively loses its ability to pump blood.

Previous studies have shown the same link. However, this latest study "followed patients from the beginning of the disease, describing how the increase in heart-failure risk was present in the early stages and throughout," says Dr. Paulo Nicola, a research fellow at the Mayo Clinic in Rochester, Minnesota.

THE STUDY

Nicola and other Mayo researchers looked at 165 Minnesota residents who had rheumatoid arthritis and found that they were twice as likely to develop heart failure over a 15-year period than 116 residents of similar age and gender who did not have this autoimmune disease.

While the study was not designed to address the reason for an increase in heart failure, "several studies in the general population suggest that inflammation may be a direct cause of heart failure," Nicola notes.

Rheumatoid arthritis is a disease in which the body mistakenly attacks its own healthy tissues, causing painful inflammation and loss of joint function.

The inflammation that attacks the joints in rheumatoid arthritis is believed to foster the process in which fatty plaques in the walls of arteries burst, leading to clots that can block the blood vessels.

IMPLICATIONS

The results of the study showed the need for the aggressive treatment of risk factors for heart disease and stroke, such as high blood pressure and diabetes, in people who have rheumatoid arthritis, Nicola says.

"The clinician should be aware of the higher risk of heart failure and look for the early symptoms of heart failure even in people without cardiovascular risk factors," Nicola advises. "Treatment should be focused not only on the rheumatoid condition, but also on control of those risk factors."

The severity of arthritis in individual patients must also be considered, explains Dr. William Wilke, a rheumatologist at the Cleveland Clinic.

"A more active rheumatoid disease is a sign of greater risk of heart disease," he says.

"If we treat people aggressively with medications, such as methotrexate and tumor necrosis factor inhibitors, we can significantly reduce the risk of heart disease," Wilke adds.

Nicola's research further stresses the importance of controlling RA quickly.

It also highlights rheumatoid arthritis "as a potentially life-threatening condition," says Dr. John H. Klippel, president and chief executive officer of the Arthritis Foundation.

"We've certainly become aware of cardiovascular disease as a risk factor for premature death in rheumatoid arthritis," Klippel says.

"People with rheumatoid arthritis have a life expectancy of roughly a decade less than those without the disease. At least one study has suggested that if one can get inflammation under control, there is increased survival," he says.

Faster Treatment For Rheumatoid Arthritis

Scott J. Zashin, MD, clinical assistant professor, division of rheumatology, University of Texas Southwestern Medical Center, Dallas, is author of *Arthritis Without Pain: The Miracle of TNF Blockers*. Sarah Allison.

Doctors used to recommend that patients "go slowly" in treating rheumatoid arthritis—start with nonsteroidal anti-inflammatory drugs (NSAIDs), such as *ibuprofen* (Advil, Motrin), followed by stronger drugs, as needed, over the years. This approach doesn't always work. In the past, up to 20% of patients with rheumatoid arthritis were disabled two years after diagnosis, and 50% were disabled 10 years after diagnosis.

Newer approach: Treatment with drugs called Tumor Necrosis Factor (TNF) blockers. People with rheumatoid arthritis have excessive amounts of the cell protein TNF-alpha. It mobilizes white blood cells, which travel to affected joints and cause inflammation, pain, stiffness and, eventually, joint damage. TNF blockers bind to *TNF-alpha*, rendering it inactive and relieving symptoms—sometimes in less than two weeks—and slowing down joint deterioration and deformity.

WHO SHOULD TAKE TNF BLOCKERS?

A newly diagnosed patient usually begins treatment with an NSAID, possibly combined with short-term steroid therapy. If that isn't effective within a few weeks, he/she might be given an antirheumatic drug, such as *hydroxychloroquine* (Plaquenil), *methotrexate* (Rheumatrex) or *sulfasalazine* (Azulfidine). If adequate results still aren't achieved in 12 to 24 weeks, the next step may be a TNF blocker. The FDA has approved three TNF blockers for rheumatoid arthritis. They appear to be equally effective. Your doctor can help you decide which is best for you.

•**Enbrel** (*etanercept*) is taken by self-injection, usually twice a week. It is not yet determined if a new once-a-week formula is as effective.

•**Humira** (*adalimumab*) also is taken by self-injection, usually once every two weeks.

•**Remicade** (*infliximab*) is given by intravenous infusion, usually in a doctor's office, once every six to eight weeks.

THE DOWNSIDE

TNF blockers are extremely expensive, costing at least $15,000 a year. You take them as long as the condition is active—often for life. The cost may be covered by insurance—check with your insurance company.

The drugs may cause itching, pain or swelling at the injection site. *More serious risks...*

•**Infection.** TNF blockers increase the risk of infection because they suppress the immune system. People who develop respiratory or other infections often are advised to discontinue the drugs until the infection is successfully treated. People who have insulin-dependent diabetes (type 1) have a high risk of infection and are not good candidates for TNF-blocker therapy.

Important: A tuberculosis (TB) skin test is required prior to starting a TNF blocker. TB can be activated in patients who have had any prior exposure, even if they never had symptoms of TB.

•**Cancer.** Some types of cancer, such as lymphoma, which affects the lymph system, have been associated with TNF blockers. But recent studies suggest that chronic inflammation, rather than the treatment, is responsible for the higher cancer risk.

Get Arthritis Relief Without Drugs

Vijay B. Vad, MD, a sports medicine physician and researcher specializing in minimally invasive arthritis therapies at the Hospital for Special Surgery in New York City, is an assistant professor of rehabilitation medicine at Weill Medical College of Cornell University, also in New York City, and the author of *Arthritis Rx*. Gotham.

Only about half of the people who suffer from osteoarthritis pain get significant relief from aspirin, *ibuprofen* (Advil) or other nonsteroidal anti-inflammatory drugs (NSAIDs)—and each year, an estimated 16,000 Americans die from gastrointestinal bleeding or other side effects from these medications.

New approach: Up to 80% of people who have osteoarthritis can experience significant improvement in pain and mobility—and reduce their need for medication and surgery—when they combine dietary changes, supplement use and the right kind of exercise. This program provides significant relief within six weeks.

DIET RX

Inflammation in the body has been implicated in heart disease, diabetes and kidney disease—and it also contributes to osteoarthritis.

The incidence of arthritis has steadily risen since the early 1900s, when processed foods, such as packaged crackers, cereals, bread and snack foods, began to dominate the American diet—and more people started becoming obese. Most of these foods actually promote inflammation, which can cause joint and cartilage damage and aggravate arthritis pain.

Studies suggest that adding more foods with anti-inflammatory effects to the average American diet—and reducing foods that promote inflammation—can curb inflammation by 20% to 40%.

Best anti-inflammatory foods...

•**Apricots and berries** contain large amounts of antioxidants, chemical compounds that reduce inflammation.

•**Almonds** contain fiber, vitamin E and mono-unsaturated fats, all of which curb inflammation.

Other important steps...

•**Increase omega-3s.** These inflammation-fighting essential fatty acids are mainly found in cold-water fish, such as salmon, tuna, mackerel and sardines. At least three three-ounce servings of fish per week provide adequate levels of omega-3s.

People who don't like fish, or don't eat it often, can take fish-oil supplements or flaxseed oil.

My advice: Take 2 g to 3 g daily of a fish-oil supplement that contains *eicosapentaenoic acid* (EPA) and *docosahexaenoic acid* (DHA)...or one to three tablespoons daily of flaxseed oil.

Caution: Because fish oil taken at this dosage can have a blood-thinning effect, check with your doctor if you take a blood-thinning medication, such as *warfarin* (Coumadin).

•**Reduce omega-6s.** Most Americans get far too many of these inflammation-promoting fatty acids in their diets. A century ago, the ratio of omega-6 to omega-3 fatty acids was about 2:1 for the typical American. Today, it's about 20:1. This imbalance boosts levels of a chemical by-product, arachidonic acid, that triggers inflammation.

My advice: Because omega-6s are found primarily in red meats, commercially processed foods (described earlier) and fast foods, anyone with arthritis should avoid these foods as much as possible.

•**Give up nightshades.** Although the reason is unknown, tomatoes, white potatoes, eggplant and other foods in the nightshade family have been found to increase arthritis pain. It has been estimated that up to 20% of arthritis patients get worse when they eat these foods.

My advice: If you eat these foods and have arthritis pain, give them up completely for six months to see if there's an improvement. For a complete list of nightshade foods, go to the Arthritis Foundation Web site at *www.arthritis.org*.

SUPPLEMENT Rx

Americans spend billions of dollars annually on supplements to ease arthritis pain, but many of them are ineffective. *Best choices...*

•**Ginger.** The biochemical structure of this herb (commonly used as a spice) is similar to that of NSAIDs, making it a powerful anti-inflammatory agent. A study of 250 patients at the University of Miami Miller School of Medicine found that ginger, taken twice daily, was as effective as prescription and over-the-counter drugs at controlling arthritis pain.

My advice: Add several teaspoons of fresh ginger to vegetables, salads, etc., daily or take a daily supplement containing 510 mg of ginger.

Caution: Ginger thins the blood, so consult your doctor if you take blood-thinning medication.

•**Glucosamine and chondroitin.** Taken in a combination supplement, such as Cosamine DS, these natural anti-inflammatories inhibit enzymes that break down cartilage and enhance the production of *glycosaminoglycans*, molecules that stimulate cartilage growth.

My advice: Take 1,500 mg of glucosamine and 1,200 mg of chondroitin daily. Or consider using a product called Zingerflex, which contains glucosamine and chondroitin as well as ginger.

Caution: If you have diabetes, consult your doctor before using glucosamine. It can raise blood sugar. Do not take glucosamine if you are allergic to shellfish.

EXERCISE Rx

Osteoarthritis pain weakens muscles, which diminishes joint support. The result is more inflammation and pain, and faster progression of the underlying disease.

Common exercises, including running and traditional forms of yoga, actually can *increase* pain by putting too much pressure on the joints. Patients benefit most from medical exercise, which includes modified versions of common strengthening and stretching exercises, supervised by a physical therapist.*

It's best to perform medical exercises under the guidance of a physical therapist for one to two months before beginning an exercise program at home. *Best choices...*

•**Medical yoga** improves joint strength and flexibility by strengthening muscles and moving

*To locate a physical therapist in your area, contact the American Physical Therapy Association at 800-999-2782 or *www.apta.org*.

joints through their full range of motion. Unlike conventional yoga, it does not require poses that put undue stress on the joints.

•**Pilates** combines yoga-like stretching and breathing control to strengthen the "core" muscles in the lower back and abdomen, as well as muscles in the hips. Like medical yoga, it puts very little pressure on the joints. A move called One-Leg Circle is typical of the Pilates exercises that are recommended for arthritis patients.

To perform One-Leg Circle…

•Lie on your back with your arms at your sides and your palms down. Tighten the abdominal muscles, press the lower back toward the floor and raise your right leg toward the ceiling. Point your toe.

•Rotate your right leg clockwise. Breathe in during half the rotation, then exhale during the other half. Then rotate the leg in the other direction. Repeat the sequence four times. Repeat with your left leg.

•**Healthy breathing.** Most of us take shallow breaths from the upper lungs—a breathing pattern that increases levels of stress hormones and heightens pain.

Better: Deep breathing, which promotes the release of pain-relieving chemicals called endorphins. Patients who breathe deeply for five minutes daily have less pain for several hours afterward. Practice deep breathing in addition to a regular exercise program.

Here's how…

•Sit in a chair with both feet flat on the floor. Close your mouth, place one hand on your stomach and breathe deeply through your nose until you can feel your stomach expanding. Hold your breath briefly, working up to 10 seconds. (If you experience any shortness of breath or gasping for air, you are holding your breath longer than you should.)

•Exhale through your nose, contracting your stomach until you've expelled as much air as possible. Hold the "emptiness" for a moment before inhaling again.

•Take 2 or 3 normal breaths until your breathing is smooth and regular.

•Repeat the cycle for at least five consecutive minutes daily.

Arthritis Treatments That Work Very Well

John D. Clough, MD, retired rheumatologist in the department of rheumatic and immunologic disease at the Cleveland Clinic, is author of *Arthritis: A Cleveland Clinic Guide*. The Cleveland Clinic Press.

More than 21 million Americans suffer from osteoarthritis, a degenerative joint disease. That's the bad news.

The good news—we know more about the disease now than ever before, including how to slow its progression.

CAUSES

There are many different forms of arthritis. Osteoarthritis is the most common form. When you have osteoarthritis, the cartilage that cushions the ends of the bones in your joints deteriorates. Over time, the cartilage may wear down completely, leaving bone rubbing on bone.

Osteoarthritis commonly affects the fingers, neck, lower back, hips and knees. *The exact cause of the disease isn't known, but the following are key risk factors…*

•**Advancing age.** People 45 years and older are at greater risk for the disease. In older people, the joint cartilage contains less fluid and may become brittle, which leads to deterioration.

•**Family history.** Heredity plays a role, especially in osteoarthritis of the hands. This particular type of osteoarthritis, which ultimately gives the fingers a gnarled appearance, is more common in women whose mothers also suffered from the condition.

•**Previous injury.** Not every joint injury causes a problem, but if you have had torn cartilage or a disruption of the ligaments in a major joint, then you are more likely to develop a problem in that area.

•**Obesity.** Being overweight puts unnecessary stress on weight-bearing joints—particularly hips and knees.

EARLY WARNINGS

Osteoarthritis often progresses slowly, but there can be early signs…

•**Joint pain during or after use,** after a period of inactivity or during a change in the weather.

•**Swelling and stiffness in a joint,** particularly after using it.

•**Joint instability,** especially noticeable in the knees, which can even take on a knock-kneed or bowlegged appearance as the cartilage deteriorates.

•**Bony lumps.** With osteoarthritis of the hands, these lumps (called Heberden's nodes and Bouchard's nodes) can appear on the middle or end joints of the fingers or at the base of your thumb.

PROTECT YOURSELF

There is no known cure for osteoarthritis, but lifestyle measures can help. *To prevent or slow progression of the disease…*

•**Lose weight.** While it's obvious that running and jumping can be hard on the joints, if you're overweight, even everyday tasks such as walking and climbing stairs can be problematic. Shed pounds, and you can ease the pressure on your weight-bearing joints.

•**Exercise.** Choose low-impact activities, such as walking, cycling and swimming, so that you don't put too much pressure on your joints.

If you've had a knee injury, it also pays to do quadricep-strengthening and hamstring-stretching exercises so that those muscles can better stabilize and operate the knee.

New finding: A study published in *Arthritis & Rheumatism* shows that people with knee osteoarthritis who exercised regularly for as long as 18 months had less disability and were able to walk much greater distances than people who dropped out of the program.

Check with your doctor before beginning a regular exercise program. He/she may recommend working with a physical therapist who can design an exercise program to meet your specific needs.

MEDICATIONS

Osteoarthritis sufferers have a range of treatment options…

•**Oral medications.** The most commonly used drugs for osteoarthritis are pain relievers, such as *acetaminophen* (Tylenol) and *non-steroidal anti-inflammatory drugs* (NSAIDs), which fall into two categories…

•Nonselective NSAIDs. Drugs such as aspirin, *ibuprofen* (Advil), *diclofenac* (Voltaren) and *naproxen* (Aleve) are commonly used to treat the symptoms caused by inflammation (pain, swelling, redness, etc.), and they work very well for some people. However, long-term use of NSAIDs can cause problems ranging from stomach upset to gastrointestinal bleeding.

•Selective Cox-2 inhibitors. These drugs were originally touted as being less likely to cause gastrointestinal problems than traditional NSAIDs, but most have been pulled from the shelves because of potentially devastating side effects. *Rofecoxib* (Vioxx), for example, was pulled in September 2004 after a study showed that the drug predisposed people to heart attacks. Currently, there's only one Cox-2 inhibitor, *celecoxib* (Celebrex), still in use.

Celebrex's manufacturer, Pfizer, has revised all advertising to include warnings of increased risk of heart attack and stroke, especially to those patients who are predisposed to heart disease or who have high blood pressure. Warnings also include increased chances of serious skin reactions or stomach and intestine problems, such as bleeding and ulcers. As of August 2008, the FDA has stated that for certain patients, benefits of Celebrex outweigh the risks. Patients should work closely with their doctor if taking Celebrex.

•**Injections.** In cases where a particular joint is acutely inflamed, a physician might opt to inject a corticosteroid preparation into the joint. This can provide rapid relief for up to several months, but long-term use of corticosteroids can be harmful to tissue and bones.

SUPPLEMENTS

Glucosamine and *chondroitin sulfate* play a role in the structure of cartilage and other connective tissue—and you can get them over-the-counter in supplement form. A massive study, known as the "Glucosamine/Chondroitin Arthritis Intervention Trial (GAIT)," coordinated by the University of Utah School of Medicine, found that in patients with moderate to severe pain, glucosamine and chondroitin provided statistically significant pain relief. However, the combination did not work any better than a placebo for the overall group of patients.

Also, a study suggests that glucosamine could potentially slow the progression of osteoarthritis of the knees, although not all studies of this supplement confirm this finding. More research is needed, but the supplements seem safe to use if you choose to try them.

Exception: People who are allergic to shellfish should steer clear of glucosamine, which is made from shellfish.

JOINT REPLACEMENT

In joint-replacement therapy (*arthroplasty*), the damaged joint is removed and replaced with a plastic or metal prosthesis. Joint replacement can be very effective, particularly for the major weight-bearing joints, such as the hips and knees, allowing you an active, pain-free life. Shoulder replacement also is effective, and the technology for smaller, more complex joints, such as the wrist and ankle, is improving.

■ ■ ■ ■

Pain in the Knee?

Acupuncture reduces pain from osteoarthritis of the knee.

Study: Patients who received acupuncture 12 times in eight weeks experienced less pain and more functionality eight weeks after the treatment than those who received "sham" acupuncture or none at all. One year after treatment, both groups fared the same.

Claudia Witt, MD, deputy administrative director, project coordinator, complementary medicine, Institute of Social Medicine, Epidemiology, and Health Economics, Charité University Medical Center, Berlin, Germany, and leader of a study of 294 people with knee osteoarthritis.

■ ■ ■ ■

Rose Hips for Arthritis

The anti-inflammatory properties of rosehips, found in wild dog rose (*Rose canina*), may help alleviate the pain and stiffness of arthritic joints. Rosehips are available at some health-food stores.

Best: Take 5 grams of rose hips daily.

Kaj Winther, MD, DMSc, head of research, department of clinical biochemistry, County Hospital, Gentofte, Denmark, and leader of a study of 94 osteoarthritis patients, published in *Scandinavian Journal of Rheumatology*.

Seven Ways to Ease the Pain of Fibromyalgia

Timothy McCall, MD, an internist, medical editor of *Yoga Journal* and author of *Examining Your Doctor* (Citadel Press) and *Yoga as Medicine* (Bantam). *www.drmccall.com.*

Fibromyalgia is a frustrating disease for doctors and patients alike. Because there is no definitive lab test to diagnose it, some physicians aren't sure it even exists. Many patients bounce from doctor to doctor, enduring a series of unrevealing lab tests and unhelpful drugs—and, too often, less than compassionate care—until finally someone hits on the diagnosis.

The typical symptoms of fibromyalgia syndrome (FMS) include widespread pain, fatigue and poor sleep. People with FMS often have other conditions, such as irritable bowel syndrome, depression and sleep apnea, a condition that temporarily interrupts breathing during sleep. Fibromyalgia is diagnosed by identifying characteristic symptoms as well as "tender points" that typically occur on the hips, shoulders and on either side of the spine. The condition affects seven times more women than men.

Although the cause of fibromyalgia is unknown, studies show that the condition is not "all in your head," as some patients are lead to believe. Researchers have found, for example, significantly elevated levels of a pain mediator, called substance P, and of nerve growth factor, in the spinal fluid of fibromyalgia patients, which suggests abnormalities in the way pain sensations are processed within the spinal cord and brain. Serotonin levels also tend to be low.

Because fibromyalgia is a chronic disease, it responds best to a holistic program of lifestyle changes, stress reduction, alternative measures (such as acupuncture, osteopathic manipulation, and gentle massage) and conventional medical interventions. *Here are some useful strategies...*

•**Get gentle exercise.** Exercise can help fibromyalgia, but be careful. Too much too soon can exacerbate symptoms. Gentle yoga is a good choice, because it is safe, easy and can be performed at home. Start slowly and gradually build up to 30 minutes daily, based on how you feel. Another good option is water aerobics.

- **Work to improve sleep.** Try getting up at the same time every day, winding down for an hour or two before bedtime, and taking a hot bath in the evening. Limit caffeine especially beyond the early afternoon.

- **Look into trigger point injections.** Doctors can treat pain by injecting a local anesthetic directly into tender points, then stretching the underlying muscles to relieve tension in them. The treatments usually need to be repeated a few times for optimal effect. Since the skill of the doctor doing the injections is key, if you don't get relief after a few treatments, try another doctor before giving up on this approach entirely.

- **Investigate supplements.** Two generally-safe ones that can improve mood, S-adenosyl-l-methionine (SAM-e) and 5-hydroxytryptophan (5-HTP), may also relieve tender point soreness.

- **Consider drug therapy.** Potentially helpful to some patients are tricyclic antidepressants, newer SSRI antidepressants and sleep mediations like *zolpidem* (Ambien). Topical capsaicin rubbed into sore muscles can lessen discomfort, and is very safe. For serious pain, a weak opiate called *tramadol* (Ultram) may bring significant relief.

- **Deal with psychological stress.** While stress and depression may not cause fibromyalgia, they can fan the flames. In addition to stress-reduction measures (such as yoga, meditation and walking in nature), you may benefit from cognitive-behavioral therapy, which helps you identify and counter negative thought patterns that contribute to psychological suffering.

- **Connect with others.** Consider joining a local or online support group. To learn more, check out the Fibromyalgia Network at *http://fm netnews.com* or call (800) 853-2929.

■ ■ ■ ■

Quick Relief for Jaw Pain

Waking up with a sore jaw or a headache may indicate that you grind your teeth in your sleep. This condition, called *bruxism*, is primarily caused by stress. Symptoms include tooth sensitivity to hot and cold food and drinks as well as pain while chewing. Sinus congestion can cause severe pressure on dental roots, leading sufferers to grind their teeth or clench the jaw.

Misaligned dental work can also trigger bruxism, leading to unconscious grinding. This grinding causes noticeable noise in only 30% of patients.

Your dentist can diagnose the problem by feeling muscle tension in the jaw and face...observing if teeth are worn or cracked...and viewing X-rays. Treatments include reshaping and polishing of tooth enamel to improve tooth alignment and/or the use of a mouth guard during periods of excessive grinding.

To ease jaw pain: Place your palm or fist under your chin and push up while barely opening your jaw against resistance. Hold for one to two seconds. Repeat 30 times, twice a day. This will stretch and strengthen jaw muscles, which helps alleviate pain.

Rob E. Sable, DDS, a restorative dentist in private practice in Alpharetta, Georgia.

Long-Lasting Relief for Neck Pain

Gerard P. Varlotta, DO, is a clinical associate professor of rehabilitation medicine and director of sports rehabilitation at the Rusk Institute of Rehabilitation Medicine at New York University Langone Medical Center in New York City.

There are very few upper-body movements that don't require use of the neck. That's why neck injury is one of the most common problems treated by orthopedists and physiatrists (doctors who specialize in rehabilitation medicine).

Most neck injuries are due to "onetime overload"—for example, putting too much strain on the neck by not keeping it in a neutral position while lifting a heavy object. Neck pain also can be caused by strain due to repetitive motions, such as twisting and turning the neck while exercising...muscle tension from stress...arthritic changes...or whiplash. Also, neck pain can be "referred" pain stemming from shoulder or elbow injuries or gallbladder disease.

Good news: Since neck pain usually includes muscle inflammation, it responds well to self-care. Even chronic pain usually can be relieved

—and prevented—with simple exercises. Surgery is recommended in rare cases, such as those in which neck pain is accompanied by radiating arm pain and compression of a nerve.

REASONS FOR NECK PAIN

Severe neck pain usually comes on suddenly, but often there's an underlying irritation and/or weakness in the muscles. In most cases, the sufferer reports that the neck feels a little weak or sore, then suddenly worsens—after turning the head abruptly, for example.

When to get help: Neck pain that doesn't begin improving within 48 hours or is accompanied by neurological symptoms—tingling in the arms, hand weakness, loss of muscle strength, etc.— indicates a more serious problem. *Examples...*

•**Disk damage.** A herniated disk (the gelatinous material inside a disk pushes through the outer coating and presses against nearby nerves) can be excruciatingly painful and, in severe cases, cause permanent spinal cord damage.

Red flag: A loss of bowel and/or bladder control or any of the above neurological symptoms. See a doctor immediately.

•**Arthritic changes.** The joints in the neck can deteriorate or stiffen due to osteoarthritis or rheumatoid arthritis.

•**Whiplash.** Injury results when the head is jerked violently forward and backward, as can occur during a car accident.

The above problems are diagnosed during a physical exam, often in conjunction with an X-ray and/or magnetic resonance imaging (MRI) scan. Treatment involves controlling inflammation and restoring strength and range of motion.

RAPID PAIN RELIEF

In the absence of neurological symptoms, arthritis or traumatic injury, patients can assume that neck pain is probably due to muscle strain. *To reduce muscle inflammation and pain...*

•**Apply ice immediately.** It's the quickest way to reduce inflammation as well as pain— but only if you apply it within the first 24 to 48 hours. Hold a cold pack or ice cubes wrapped in a towel or washcloth to the painful area for 20 minutes once an hour throughout the day.

Important: Do not apply heat during the first two days after an injury. It relieves stiffness but can increase inflammation and pain.

•**Take the proper anti-inflammatory drug.** Over-the-counter *ibuprofen* (Advil) and *naproxen* (Aleve) are equally effective at relieving muscle pain and inflammation.

Main difference: Ibuprofen is a relatively short-acting drug—generally lasting four to six hours. Naproxen lasts eight to 12 hours. *Acetaminophen* (Tylenol) may help, but it mainly eases pain, not inflammation.

Caution: Ibuprofen and naproxen can cause stomach upset...acetaminophen can cause liver damage when combined with alcohol. Don't take any of these drugs for more than a week without consulting your doctor.

•**Stretch muscles often.** Stretching lengthens muscle fibers and reduces the tension caused by neck-related ergonomic problems, such as how you sit at a computer or hold a telephone. *Helpful...*

While standing or sitting, slowly lower your ear toward your shoulder. Stop when pain significantly increases. Hold the stretch for a few seconds, then relax. Switch to the other side. Repeat eight to 12 times, five times a day.

Bring your chin toward your shoulder, following the directions above.

Although chiropractic treatment can help alleviate pain that emanates from the neck joints, its effects are not long-lasting. Acupuncture also may be helpful but needs to be repeated until the pain dissipates.

LONG-TERM NECK CARE

Most people with chronic neck pain need to perform strengthening exercises (consult your doctor first) and change their posture.

Important: Don't sleep on your stomach— and don't raise your head too high with pillows. Both put excessive pressure on the neck.

Better: Sleep on your side with your head level—propped just high enough to keep your nose in line with your navel. The pillow (when compressed) should be just thick enough to support the side of your head without elevating it.

If you spend a great deal of time on the telephone, use a headset. Cradling a phone between the neck and shoulder is one of the most common causes of neck pain. Choose a headset that is comfortable for you. Good ones, such as those made by Plantronics, are available for $130 and up at electronics stores.

If you spend time at a desk, adjust your workstation. The center of a standard computer monitor should be directly at eye level (a bit lower if it's a large monitor)...your knees should be slightly lower than your hips...and use your chair's armrests when possible to avoid hunching forward.

Strengthen your neck and shoulders—they share some of the same muscles. Keeping these muscles strong makes them more flexible and less prone to injury. Perform eight to 12 repetitions of each of the following exercises three times, two to three days a week. Once you can do 12 repetitions easily, gradually increase the weight lifted.

•**Shrugs.** While standing straight with your arms down at your sides, hold a two-pound dumbbell (or a household object, such as a can of soup) in each hand. With palms facing your thighs, shrug your shoulders as high as possible, keeping your head straight. Hold for five seconds, then return to the starting position.

•**Flies.** Lie on your back on an exercise bench, with a two-pound dumbbell in each hand. Hold your hands out to the sides so that the weights are about even with your chest. Keeping your back straight, raise your arms over your chest in a semicircular motion until the weights touch in the middle over your chest. Lower them back to chest level in the same semicircular motion.

•**Side deltoid raise.** While standing straight with your arms down at your sides, hold a two-pound dumbbell or other weight in each hand, with your palms facing your thighs. Keeping your elbows slightly bent, raise your arms up and out to your sides until they're shoulder level (your palms will be facing the floor in this position). Hold for five seconds, then slowly lower the weights.

Illustrations by Shawn Banner.

Better on Its Own

Sciatica pain often gets better on its own. There is no evidence that spinal decompression does any good. Anti-inflammatory drugs, cortisone shots and exercises that strengthen abdominal and back muscles may speed healing.

Also useful: Place a pillow behind your lower back while driving. Place a pillow under your knees when sleeping on your back—or between your knees when you sleep on your side.

Joel M. Press, MD, is medical director and chair in musculoskeletal rehabilitation, Spine & Sports Rehabilitation Center, Rehabilitation Institute of Chicago.

Relieve the Pain of a Pinched Nerve

David Borenstein, MD, clinical professor of medicine at George Washington University Medical Center, Washington, DC, is the author of *Back In Control: Your Complete Prescription for Preventing, Treating, and Eliminating Back Pain from Your Life*. M. Evans and Company.

Nerve pain is one of the worst kinds of pain. People with a pinched nerve (sometimes called a "stinger") may experience sharp, burning pain for anywhere from a few seconds to a few days or longer. The pain usually comes on suddenly and may disappear just as fast—only to return. There also might be temporary numbness or slight weakness.

A nerve gets "pinched" when surrounding tissue presses against it and causes inflammation of the nerve. Causes include repetitive motions, traumatic injuries and joint diseases, such as rheumatoid arthritis. The most common pinched nerves occur in the wrist, elbow, shoulder and foot. Nerve roots in the spinal canal also are vulnerable.

Red flag: Nerve pain that is accompanied by significant weakness or that doesn't improve within a few days needs to be checked by a physician. Excessive pressure on—or inflammation of—a nerve can result in loss of function and permanent damage.

SELF-HELP

To reduce the pain…

•**Stop repetitive movements.** A pinched nerve that's caused by performing the same movements over and over again usually will improve once the offending activity—leaning with your elbows on a counter, typing, working a cash register, etc.—is stopped for a few days. Avoiding these activities is also the best way to prevent a pinched nerve.

However, patients with job-related pain can't always afford to take time off. In that case, they should attempt to change their body position when doing the activity.

Example: Raising the back of a computer keyboard (most are adjustable) will enlarge the carpal tunnel in the wrist and reduce pressure on the nerve.

•**Ice the area.** Applying cold in the first 24 to 48 hours after nerve pain starts can reduce tissue swelling and nerve pressure. Use a cold pack or ice cubes wrapped in a towel. Hold cold against the affected area for about 15 minutes. Repeat every hour or two for a day or two.

•**Take an anti-inflammatory.** Over-the-counter analgesics that have anti-inflammatory properties, such as aspirin, *ibuprofen* and naproxen, reduce the body's production of chemicals that cause inflammation and swelling. Don't use *acetaminophen*. It will reduce pain but has little effect on inflammation.

•**Wear looser clothes.** It's fairly common for women to experience a pinched nerve in the outer thigh (*neuralgia paresthetica*) from too-tight jeans or skirts…or foot pain (*tarsal tunnel syndrome*) from tight shoes.

MEDICAL CARE

Nerve pain that's severe or keeps coming back—or that's accompanied by other symptoms, such as a loss of bowel or bladder control —requires immediate medical care. Customized splints or braces can be used to minimize pressure on a nerve from repetitive movements. *Also helpful…*

•**An injection of a corticosteroid** into the painful area—or a short course of oral steroid therapy. These drugs reduce inflammation very quickly and provide short-term relief. The pain may disappear after a single treatment, but most patients need repeated courses. Sometimes, if pain is not relieved, acupuncture may be used in addition to medication and physical therapy.

•**Surgery is recommended** when the pain is severe or keeps coming back. The procedures vary depending on the part of the body affected.

■ ■ ■ ■

Better Back Pain Relief

For 12 weeks, adults with persistent lower-back pain either took gentle yoga classes, performed conventional aerobic and strengthening exercises or followed advice from a back pain self-help book as part of a recent study.

Result: After 12 weeks, the participants who performed the gentle yoga poses showed the most improvement in back-related dysfunction, such as difficulty walking up stairs.

Caution: Vigorous styles of yoga could worsen chronic back pain.

To find a yoga instructor experienced in helping people with back pain, consult the International Association of Yoga Therapists, 928-541-0004, *www.iayt.org*.

Karen J. Sherman, PhD, MPH, senior investigator, Group Health Center for Health Studies, and affiliate assistant professor, epidemiology, School of Public Health and Community Medicine, University of Washington, Seattle.

A Simple 5-Step Plan to Get Rid of Back Pain… For Good

Miriam E. Nelson, PhD, associate professor at the Friedman School of Nutrition Science and Policy and director of the John Hancock Center for Physical Activity and Nutrition at Tufts University, Boston, is a fellow of the American College of Sports Medicine and author, with Lawrence Lindner, of *Strong Women, Strong Backs*. Putnam.

As many as 90% of all adults suffer back pain at some point in their lives. Back pain—lower-back pain, in particular—

ranks fifth among the most frequent reasons for hospitalizations.

Worse for women: Their musculoskeletal systems—ligaments, vertebrae, spinal disks, etc.—are more delicate than men's and more vulnerable to injury. Women also tend to be less active, on average, than men, and a sedentary lifestyle is a common cause of back pain.

Most back problems are caused by prolonged sitting or by lifting heavy objects the wrong way, but other factors contribute to back pain, including excess body weight, stress and depression. Even smoking is a factor for reasons that aren't exactly clear.

Simple lifestyle measures—maintaining a healthy weight, not smoking and controlling stress and depression—can prevent many cases of back pain. Most important, though, are exercises that strengthen muscles in the back, chest, abdomen, hips and sides. These are the core muscles—the scaffolding that supports the spine and enables the back to flex and twist without injury. Strengthening these muscles can relieve pain and also prevent it.

A FIVE-STEP PLAN

The following workout, which takes no more than 20 minutes, targets all of the core muscles. It can be done three to five times weekly (unlike most strength-training workouts, which should be done no more than three times a week, because muscles need time to recover between sessions). These exercises can be done more often because the intensity is lower—and they're less likely than traditional workouts to cause back pain or other injuries.

For each of the following exercises…

• **Complete 10 repetitions,** rest for one minute, then complete another 10 reps. If you can complete only five or six reps, the intensity is too high and you should do only what you can comfortably manage.

• **Work up to an advanced progression.** This is a way to increase the exercise intensity by making the movements more difficult.

• **Always warm up**—by taking a brisk walk around the block or stepping quickly in place—for five minutes before doing the exercises.

STEP 1: ABDOMINALS

Most people's abdominal muscles are weaker than they should be. Strengthening the abdominals is among the best ways to prevent back pain.

Starting position: Lie on your back on the floor with your knees bent and the soles of your feet flat on the floor. Lightly rest your hands on the lower part of the stomach.

The movement: Contract the abdominal muscles until you feel the small of the back pushing toward the floor. Imagine that you're pulling your belly button downward. Hold the "tense" position for three seconds, then relax.

Progression: Do almost the same exercise as above, with this difference. While the abdominal muscles are tight, raise the still-bent right leg a few inches off the floor and hold it up for three seconds, then place that leg down and raise the left leg for three seconds. The entire move will take 10 to 12 seconds.

STEP 2: CHEST MUSCLES

Along with abdominal exercises, chest workouts protect the back by strengthening the "front" of the core muscle groups.

Starting position: Stand facing a wall or a counter, about an arm's length away, with your feet hip-width apart and knees slightly bent. Put your palms on the wall (or lightly hold the edge of the counter).

The movement: Holding your body straight, bend at the elbows until you are leaning forward toward the wall or counter about 30 degrees. Pause in this position for a moment, then push with your arms until you're back in the starting position.

Progression: Work the same muscles with more intensity with a modified push-up. Lie facedown on the floor, with your palms directly next to your shoulders, elbows bent.

Keeping your knees on the floor, slowly push up only your chest. Keep your trunk in a straight line from your head to your knees. Push up until your shoulders are over your hands, but don't lock the elbows. Pause for a moment, then lower back down until your nose is about four inches from the floor. Keep your trunk in a straight line throughout the movements.

STEP 3: MIDBACK

Many exercises target the upper/lower back, but relatively few target the middle back—a common area for problems.

Starting position: Lie facedown on an exercise mat or carpet, with your arms straight out to the sides, perpendicular to the body.

The movement: Contract your shoulder blades to lift the arms up and slightly back. Hold the arms in the lifted position, and make four figure eights with the hands. Then lower your arms to the starting position.

Progression: Make the figure eights with the thumbs down or up…or while holding a balled-up sock in each hand…or with the little finger up or down. Varying the movement works different parts of the muscles.

STEP 4: UPPER BACK

This exercise increases shoulder strength as well as back strength.

Starting position: Tie a knot in the middle of an elastic exercise band (available at sporting-goods stores for $5 to $15). Place the knot over the top of a door, and then close the door to anchor the band in place. The two ends should be hanging down on the same side of the door. Sit in a chair facing the door, with your toes against the door. Hold one end of the band in each hand.

The movement: Slowly pull your hands down and in toward your chest. Keep your elbows pointed down and close to your body. Pause for a moment, then slowly let your arms extend back to the starting position.

Progression: When the exercise starts feeling easy, change to a higher-resistance band.

STEP 5: LOWER BACK

This is the area that gives most people problems.

Starting position: Lie facedown on an exercise mat or carpet. Reach your right hand in front of you, palm down. The left arm should be down alongside your body, with the palm up.

The movement: Slowly raise your right arm, chest and left leg about five inches off the floor. Keep your face down, so your spine is in a straight line. Keep your right leg and left hand on the ground. Pause for a moment, then return to the starting position.

Reverse the movement, raising your left arm, chest and right leg, and keeping the left leg and right hand on the floor.

Progression: Kneel on all fours. Raise your right arm straight in front of you while simultaneously raising the left leg straight behind. Keep the abdominal muscles contracted. Pause, return to the starting position. Then reverse the movement.

OPTIONAL EXERCISE: THIGHS, HIPS AND MORE

This optional exercise is a complex move that targets the upper legs as well as the trunk. It is good for improving stability and balance. The exercise requires the use of a stability ball, available at sporting-goods stores for about $20.

Starting position: Stand with your back to a wall, with the stability ball positioned between your back and the wall. Lean back against the ball, with your feet a bit more than hip-width apart. Hold your arms straight in front of you or crossed over your chest.

The movement: While keeping light pressure on the ball with your lower back, bend at the knees and slowly squat down—the ball will roll with the movement. Squat down as far as you comfortably can. The ball will then be positioned at about the midback.

Keeping pressure on the ball, contract the buttocks and slowly "roll" yourself up and back to the starting position.

Illustrations by Shawn Banner.

■ ■ ■ ■

Herbal Help for Back Pain

Back pain can be relieved with the herb devil's claw.

Recent study: A daily dose of 60 milligrams (mg) of *harpagosides*, found in devil's claw, is as effective in treating lower-back pain as a standard dose of the prescription drug Vioxx, which was linked to heart problems and removed from the market.

Caution: Do not take devil's claw if you are taking blood thinners or have any clotting disorders.

Joel J. Gagnier, ND, MSc, Institute for Evaluative Sciences, University of Toronto, and leader of a metastudy of 12 previous studies of harpagosides, published in *BMC Complementary and Alternative Medicine.*

■ ■ ■ ■

Knee Repair

Removing all or part of a damaged meniscus (a pad of cartilage in the knee joint), a common procedure to ease arthritis pain, may result in further wear and tear on the joint and loss of cartilage in the knee.

Better: Except in some cases such as a locked knee, nonsurgical strategies to alleviate knee pain may be more effective. These include weight loss…braces…shoes that prevent foot pronation, or flattening…and anti-inflammatory drugs such as *ibuprofen* (Advil).

David J. Hunter, MD, PhD, assistant professor of medicine, Boston University School of Medicine.

Foods That Trigger Headaches and the Foods That Relieve Them

Elaine Magee, MPH, RD, registered dietitian, Pleasant Hill, California, is the author of more than 25 books on nutrition, including *Tell Me What to Eat If I Have Headaches and Migraines.* New Page.

More than 45 million Americans annually seek medical treatment for frequent or severe headaches. Doctors have identified dozens of headache triggers, including stress, air pollution and weather changes, but one of the main triggers—especially for migraines—is diet.

At least 30% of migraine patients have one or more food triggers. In some cases, a single food may be responsible. Most patients have combination triggers—for example, red wine plus a high level of stress plus an extra cup of coffee in the morning.

Everyone who experiences migraines and other types of headaches should keep a food and lifestyle diary. Write down the foods and beverages you consume. Also note patterns that precede headaches—exercise activities, changes in sleep, stress level, menstrual cycle, etc. After a few weeks, review your diary and identify likely connections.

WHAT TO AVOID

•**Caffeine** is one of the main headache triggers. Some people get headaches when they consume any caffeine. Others get headaches when they consume less than they usually do and then need caffeine to relieve the headache.

If you drink coffee or other caffeinated beverages regularly, blood vessels in the brain become sensitized to the caffeine's effects. Eliminating or cutting back on caffeine causes rebound headaches in about half of patients.

People with chronic headaches often are advised to eliminate caffeine completely. Instead of quitting abruptly, gradually taper off. If you're used to drinking three cups of coffee a day, drink only two cups daily for a week. For several days after that, substitute decaf for one of your daily servings. Then dilute your regular coffee with decaf until you quit entirely.

•**High-fat foods.** Significantly reducing dietary fat decreases the frequency and intensity of headaches. Try to limit total fat intake to 20% of total calories. In particular, avoid saturated fats (mainly found in meats, fast food and full-fat dairy products) and trans fats (often called "partially hydrogenated oils" on labels and found in margarines, snack foods and packaged baked goods).

•**Tyramine** is a natural by-product of the amino acid tyrosine. Foods that are aged or fermented tend to be high in tyramine, which can cause vascular spasms that result in migraines.

Main offenders: Red wine, aged cheeses including blue and cheddar, deli meats and overripe bananas.

Stick with fresh meats and cheeses such as cottage cheese, ricotta and fresh mozzarella. White wine and beer have less tyramine than red wine—but any alcohol can trigger headaches.

•**Food additives,** including *monosodium glutamate* (MSG), nitrates and nitrites, dilate blood vessels and trigger migraines in people who are sensitive to these additives. Nitrates and nitrites are found mainly in processed meats, such as hot dogs, bacon and salami. MSG is added to literally thousands of processed foods. Check food labels, and avoid products that contain any of these additives.

FOODS THAT HELP

•**Omega-3 fatty acids.** The healthful fats in fish, flaxseeds and olive oil can reduce migraines by stimulating the production of body chemicals that inhibit inflammation in blood vessels in the brain.

Recommended: Two to three servings of fish weekly. Also, have one tablespoon daily of ground flaxseed (you can add it to cereal or smoothies or sprinkle on salads or yogurt). Cook with olive oil or canola oil, which contain more omega-3s than other vegetable oils.

•**Magnesium.** There is some evidence that adequate magnesium intake can help women prevent headaches (including migraines) associated with menstruation. The recommended daily intake for most women is 320 milligrams (mg). High-magnesium foods include whole grains, nuts, seeds, soy foods, legumes and dark green vegetables.

Examples: Almonds, two tablespoons (86 mg of magnesium)…artichoke, one medium (180 mg)…brown rice, two-thirds cup (57 mg)…peanut butter, two tablespoons (51 mg)…pumpkin seeds, two tablespoons (152 mg)…cooked spinach, one-half cup (78 mg)…tofu, one-half cup (118 mg).

•**Water** helps prevent dehydration—a common cause of headaches. Try to drink eight eight-ounce glasses every day.

The Best Pain-Relief Creams and Ointments

Beth E. Shubin Stein, MD, is assistant professor, Department of Orthopaedic Surgery, Weill Medical College of Cornell University, and assistant attending orthopaedic surgeon, Hospital for Special Surgery, both in New York City. Dr. Shubin Stein is a team physician for the U.S. Federation Cup Tennis Team.

If you suffer from chronic arthritis pain or have aching muscle strains or spasms after exercising, chances are you regularly take aspirin or another nonsteroidal anti-inflammatory drug (NSAID), such as *ibuprofen* (Advil) or *naproxen* (Aleve).

There is another option. Over-the-counter (OTC) topical pain relievers can be very effective without causing the stomach upset or gastrointestinal bleeding that may accompany oral pain medication.

Latest development: A topical form of the oral prescription NSAID *diclofenac* (Voltaren) has been approved by the FDA as the first topical prescription treatment that patients can apply directly to sites of joint pain associated with osteoarthritis. While Voltaren Gel has been shown to significantly reduce pain in the hand and knees and has a favorable safety profile, some adverse reactions have been documented. Ask your doctor if the prescription gel is right for you.

Meanwhile, a variety of OTC topical pain relievers are available to you directly. The products below relieve arthritis, backache and muscle strain. Most are used three to four times daily. Follow label instructions.

Helpful: If one type of topical pain reliever doesn't work for you, try one from another class until you find a product that provides relief.

Caution: Keep these products away from your eyes, nose and other mucous membranes.

SALICYLATES

These aspirin-based products dull pain and curb the inflammation that often accompanies and worsens pain.

How they work: Topical salicylates inhibit the production of *prostaglandins,* substances in the body that cause pain and swelling when they are released in response to strains, sprains and other injuries. *Salicylates include...*

• **BenGay Ultra Strength Pain Relieving Cream.**

• **Aspercreme Analgesic Creme Rub with Aloe.**

• **Sportscreme Deep Penetrating Pain Relieving Rub.**

• **Flexall Maximum Strength Pain Relieving Gel.**

Warning: Do not use salicylates if you are sensitive or allergic to aspirin or take blood-thinning medication that might interact with them. Consult a doctor before applying a salicylate to a large area several times a day.

COUNTERIRRITANTS

These pain relievers give the sensation of warmth or coolness to mask pain.

How they work: Creating a secondary stimulus to diminish the feeling of pain reduces physical discomfort. It's what you do instinctively when you stub your toe, then grab it to apply pressure. Both competing sensations travel to your brain at the same time—but because only a limited number of messages can be processed at one time, the initial feeling of pain is diminished. *Counterirritants include...*

• **Icy Hot Pain Relieving Balm, Extra Strength.**

• **Tiger Balm Extra Strength Pain Relieving Ointment.**

• **Therapeutic Mineral Ice.**

In most cases, coolness is beneficial for acute injuries, such as sprains, while warmth eases stiffness.

Caution: People sensitive to heat or cold should avoid counterirritants.

CAPSAICINS

These products, which are a type of counterirritant, contain capsaicin, an extract of hot peppers that causes a burning sensation.

How they work: Unlike most other counterirritants, capsaicin inhibits the production of substance P, a chemical that sends pain messages to the brain via the nervous system. *Capsaicins include...*

• **Zostrix Arthritis Pain Relief Cream.**

• **Capzasin HP Arthritis Pain Relief Creme.**

LIDOCAINE

Lidoderm is a prescription-only patch that contains *lidocaine*, a topical anesthetic similar to the novocaine that dentists often use to numb the gums.

How it works: Lidocaine blocks signals at the skin's nerve endings. The Lidoderm patch (lidocaine 5%) is worn for 12 hours a day over a period of days. It slowly releases medication, so it has longer-lasting effects than other pain relievers and helps with pain that emanates from nerves near the surface of your skin, such as that caused by shingles or diabetic neuropathy.

Caution: Side effects include drowsiness, dizziness and blurred vision. Allergic reactions are rare but may occur.

You Don't Need Drugs to Fight Arthritis

Harris H. McIlwain, MD, founder of the Tampa Medical Group and an adjunct professor of medicine at the University of South Florida College of Public Health in Tampa. A board-certified rheumatologist and former chair of the Florida Osteoporosis Board, Dr. McIlwain is coauthor of *Diet for a Pain-Free Life*. Da Capo.

Scientists have long known that inflammation is largely responsible for the pain associated with rheumatoid arthritis (an autoimmune disease that causes joint swelling and pain) and to a lesser degree osteoarthritis (age-related wear-and-tear arthritis).

That's why people with arthritis have relied heavily on nonsteroidal anti-inflammatory drugs (NSAIDs), including aspirin and *ibuprofen* (Advil)—even though only an estimated half of arthritis sufferers get adequate relief by taking such medication.

NSAIDs also can cause side effects, such as gastrointestinal bleeding. Prescription NSAIDs, may increase the risk for heart attack in high-risk individuals, especially if taken at maximum doses.

New thinking: Whether you have osteoarthritis or rheumatoid arthritis, you can dramatically reduce pain and/or stiffness by adopting an "anti-inflammatory lifestyle." This approach focuses not only on weight control and exercise, but also on strategies such as using certain spices and reducing stress, which are just now being recognized for their powerful effects on arthritis.

Even if you must take prescription medication for rheumatoid arthritis or occasionally use NSAIDs for acute flare-ups of osteoarthritis or rheumatoid arthritis, the following inflammation-fighting strategies may allow you to reduce—or even eliminate—your reliance on medication...

ELIMINATE "HIGH-TEMPERATURE" FOODS

Anything that's usually cooked at very high temperatures—mainly meats and fried foods—is likely to contain large amounts of compounds called *advanced glycation end* (AGE) products, which trigger inflammation in the body.

Scientific evidence: Several studies, including research conducted at Mount Sinai School of Medicine in New York City, have shown that consumption of AGE-containing foods is linked to increased risk for arthritis and other chronic diseases associated with inflammation.

What to do: I advise most of my patients to eliminate *all* red meat (poultry is acceptable) as well as processed foods and snacks, which are typically high in saturated fat and/or trans-fatty acids. Most people who eliminate these foods notice a significant reduction in arthritis pain within three weeks.

EAT MORE PLANT FOODS

Even though obesity is skyrocketing in the US, it affects no more than 6% of vegetarians—a fact that appears to have important implications for people with arthritis.

Scientific evidence: A study recently published in *Nutrition and Metabolism* found that arthritis sufferers who adopted a plant-based diet—particularly one rich in the so-called "super-antioxidants" (described below)—had significant reductions in pain.

The explanation? A plant-based diet is low in inflammatory chemicals and high in plant compounds that fight inflammation in the body. It also promotes weight loss.

What to do: Everyone with arthritis should eat little or no red meat...consume high-fiber foods, including legumes (such as black beans and lentils) and whole grains...and consume two to three daily servings of foods with the highest levels of anti-inflammatory compounds. *These include...*

• **Dark berries,** such as elderberries, black currants, blueberries, cranberries, cherries and blackberries (fresh or frozen). They are up to 50% higher in antioxidants than most fruits and vegetables. Consume one serving (for example, three-quarters of a cup of blueberries or 10 large cherries) daily.

• **Red grapes.** These contain *resveratrol,* a compound that inhibits the pain-causing COX-2 enzyme—the same mechanism that is used by the drug celecoxib. Red wine also contains resveratrol. Eat about 18 red grapes—and/or drink five ounces of red wine daily (purple grape juice can be substituted for red wine).

• **Citrus and other vitamin C–rich foods.** These greatly reduce inflammation and help the body repair damaged cartilage. A study in the *American Journal of Clinical Nutrition* found that people with high blood levels of vitamin C had a 45% reduced risk for inflammation. Eat one to two servings daily of vitamin C–rich foods, such as oranges and strawberries. Most daily multivitamins also provide sufficient vitamin C (60 mg daily).

• **Cold-water fish** (such as salmon, mackerel and sardines) and omega-3-containing nuts (such as walnuts, almonds and pecans). The omega-3 fatty acids found in these foods reduce levels of inflammatory chemicals in the body. Eat four ounces of cold-water fish daily and about one-half ounce (a small handful) of nuts daily. As alternatives, natural peanut butter without added fat or sugar (one tablespoon daily) and ground flaxseed (about three tablespoons daily) are good sources of omega-3s.

• **Green or black tea.** Both contain *polyphenols,* compounds that inhibit joint inflammation. Drink two to three cups daily.

USE ANTI-INFLAMMATORY SPICES

A number of kitchen spices and herbs, including turmeric and garlic, are powerful antioxidants that can relieve joint pain even when consumed in quantities used for cooking. Ginger is among the most potent and the best studied.

Scientific evidence: A study of 247 arthritis patients published in *Arthritis & Rheumatism* found that 63% who took an extract of ginger twice daily had less knee pain.

What to do: Use one teaspoon of fresh or dried ginger daily—the amount needed for noticeable anti-inflammatory effects. Also, add turmeric and garlic to dishes whenever possible.

TRY GLUCOSAMINE

Most studies indicate that glucosamine sulfate supplements don't help with acute pain, particularly when compared with anti-inflammatory drugs. However, glucosamine sulfate does appear to slow the breakdown of joint cartilage and can help prevent arthritis from worsening.

What to do: Ask your doctor about taking 1,500 mg of glucosamine sulfate daily. The addition of chondroitin, a compound often combined with glucosamine, doesn't seem to make a difference.

Caution: Because glucosamine is derived from the shells of shellfish, people with shellfish allergies should avoid it.

Also helpful: *S-adenosylmethionine* (SAM-e), a supplement that seems to lessen arthritis pain.

Recommended dose: 1,200 mg daily, taken with glucosamine sulfate or alone. Be sure to check with your doctor before taking SAM-e. It may interact with some drugs, including certain antidepressants.

MANAGE NEGATIVE EMOTIONS

Chronic stress increases levels of *cortisol*, a hormone that triggers the release of inflammatory compounds known as cytokines, and contributes to weight gain.

Scientific evidence: A recent Duke University study found that volunteers who were prone to anger and suffered from depression had levels of *C-reactive protein* (CRP), a protein associated with pain and inflammation, that were *two to three times* higher than levels in calmer volunteers.

What to do: Anything that relaxes you—meditation, yoga, walking in nature or visiting with friends. People who learn to set their stress aside, even for brief periods, have lower levels of pain-inducing chemicals.

Relief from Hip Pain Without Surgery

William Warren Brien, MD, an orthopedic surgeon and executive vice chairman, department of surgery, and chief of staff, Cedars-Sinai Medical Center, Los Angeles. He is also director of Cedars-Sinai Orthopaedic Center and Cedars-Sinai Institute for Joint Replacement.

Time isn't kind to aging hips. Every year, nearly 400,000 Americans, mostly seniors, undergo hip replacement surgery to relieve pain and improve mobility. Millions more have to curtail their normal activities because of hip pain and stiffness.

What happens: Most people with chronic hip pain suffer from osteoarthritis, a "wear and tear" disorder caused by decades of pressure and friction. The cartilage that cushions the ends of bones roughens and breaks down. The bones of the joint begin to "grab" sooner or later instead of sliding smoothly.

Result: Persistent inflammation and pain—and, often, disability.

Hip replacement procedures are effective, but they are major surgeries and carry risks, including infection, blood clots or dislocation/loosening of the prosthetic hip. Many people with hip pain—including those who think they need surgery—can often reduce discomfort with medications and lifestyle measures without the risks of surgery. *To reduce discomfort and protect the hips...*

MANAGE PAIN AGGRESSIVELY

Osteoarthritis sufferers typically experience flare-ups of heightened pain. This is usually due to joint inflammation. Take it seriously. Untreated inflammation accelerates joint damage and makes pain more difficult to manage.

Best approach: Ordinary, nonsteroidal anti-inflammatory drugs (NSAIDs), such as *ibuprofen* (Advil, Motrin), *naproxen* (Aleve) or even plain aspirin. These drugs block prostaglandins, inflammatory chemicals that cause pain as well as joint damage. Pain can persist for days when inflammation is allowed to "fester." Patients get the best results when they take an NSAID at the first hint of pain.

Helpful: Combine an NSAID with *acetaminophen* (such as Tylenol). The combination works at multiple pain sites and gives additional relief. *Also important…*

• **Start with a low dosing frequency.** Take the drugs twice daily—for example, in the morning and evening, when stiffness tends to be worse. If pain persists, increase the frequency to up to four times daily.

• **Take NSAIDs with food to reduce stomach upset.** Combining NSAIDs with an antacid can reduce this side effect. Follow the dosing instructions on the label and consult with your doctor about regular blood tests to assess kidney and liver functions.

• **Try different drugs as needed.** Most NSAIDs are chemically similar, but everyone responds to them differently. Try a drug for a week. If it doesn't seem to be helping, switch to something else—say, naproxen instead of ibuprofen, or aspirin instead of naproxen.

Caution: Many of the NSAIDs can prolong bleeding time (before blood starts to clot) in some patients. They may be dangerous for those with clotting disorders or who take blood-thinning medications, such as *warfarin* (Coumadin). Talk to your doctor before using NSAIDs on a regular basis.

HIP INJECTIONS

Oral pain relievers/anti-inflammatory drugs are often sufficient for mild to moderate hip pain, but they don't work for everyone—particularly for patients with more severe joint damage. *Two options…*

• **Hyaluronic acid,** a component of connective tissue, reduces inflammation, increases joint lubrication, inhibits cartilage breakdown and may stimulate cartilage growth.

How it's used: A doctor injects it into the joint once a week for three to five weeks. Many patients notice some improvement over a 10 to 12 week period after the last injection.

Some patients don't respond to hyaluronic acid. Those who do may be free of pain—or have reduced pain—for a few weeks to more than a year. The injections can be repeated every six to 12 months. It works best for patients with mild to moderate pain.

• **Corticosteroids.** Steroids decrease inflammation and reduce immune system response. Cortisone or other steroids can be injected into the joint for very rapid relief, within three to 14 days—important for patients with severe pain. In some cases, a single injection can relieve pain for many months.

Caution: The injections can increase cartilage degradation with repeated use. Most patients are advised to have no more than one or two steroid injections a year.

GLUCOSAMINE/CHONDROITIN

Glucosamine (a supplement derived from the exoskeletons of crustaceans) is thought to promote cartilage growth, and chondroitin (taken from cow and/or pig tissues) appears to inhibit cartilage breakdown. A number of studies have looked at the effects of these supplements— used alone or in combination—and the findings are mixed.

My experience: Many patients report that glucosamine/chondroitin provide lasting pain relief.

Recommended: A daily supplement that combines 1,500 mg glucosamine with 1,200 mg chondroitin. The supplements don't work quickly. Take them for two to three months to see how much they help.

Some patients experience stomach upset when taking these supplements, but that is rare. Most people who take them don't experience side effects.

WEIGHT CONTROL

Obesity substantially increases the risk of hip osteoarthritis and makes existing pain worse. The hips absorb three times our body weight when we walk. Someone who is 10 pounds overweight adds 30 pounds of force to the hip joints. And people who are overweight tend to be more sedentary, which decreases joint strength and flexibility.

Good news: People who lose as little as five to 10 pounds—with diet, exercise, etc.—often report a significant reduction in hip pain and stiffness.

KEEP MOVING

Exercise is among the best treatments for osteoarthritis. Increasing muscle strength and flexibility reduces joint stress…increases levels of pain-relieving body chemicals called endorphins…and increases the flow of synovial fluid, which lubricates the joints.

Recommended: Low-impact cardiovascular exercises, such as riding a stationary bike (set on low resistance) or using an elliptical machine (a treadmill-like device that also exercises the arms). Water exercises—swimming, water aerobics, etc.—are ideal because the water helps support the joints. Walking is also good for those with hip osteoarthritis, as long as you walk on a soft surface and avoid steep hills.

Most people with hip pain experience an increase in discomfort when they first start exercising. Stick with it—those who continue to exercise (working up to a minimum of 30 minutes, four or five days a week) report a long-term decrease in pain and an increase in flexibility and mobility.

LAST RESORT

Surgical hip replacement is a good choice for patients who can no longer do things they enjoy …have difficulty standing or sitting…get little relief from painkillers…or have trouble sleeping because of persistent pain. More than 90% of patients who have surgery experience significant improvement.

Important: Doctors often base their recommendations for surgery on imaging studies (such as X-ray evidence of joint damage) or on physical findings during an examination. But joint replacement is rarely an emergency procedure, so you can make your own decision. If hip pain is impairing your ability to enjoy life, and the "lifestyle" measures described in this article haven't worked, surgery might be a good choice.

Exercises for Pain-Free Joints

Harris H. McIlwain, MD, a rheumatologist and founder of the Tampa Medical Group and adjunct professor at University of South Florida College of Public Health, both in Tampa. He is coauthor, with Debra Fulghum Bruce, PhD, of *Diet for a Pain-Free Life* (Da Capo) and *Pain-Free Arthritis* (Holt).

I f you have joint problems, simply opening a jar or climbing stairs can cause pain. Easy tasks turn into daily chores.

Vicious cycle: When it hurts to move, you may stop exercising—yet moderate exercise eases joint aches and stiffness by increasing strength and flexibility and decreasing inflammation.

Solution: With your doctor's approval, try the exercises below.

• **Stretching** makes joints more limber, prevents muscles from becoming short and tight, and protects against injury. Stretch gently, moving each joint to the maximum range of motion possible without causing unusual discomfort. Do these moves daily, working up to 15 repetitions of each.

• Shoulder stretch. Sit with back straight and clasp hands behind your head. Move elbows forward as if trying to get them to touch in front of your face. Hold five seconds. Next, move elbows back until they point out to the side… hold five seconds. This increases shoulders' range of motion—making it easier, for instance, to style your hair.

• Bathtub stretch. Moist heat eases movement by increasing flow of blood, oxygen and nutrients to joints. During a warm bath or while seated on a shower stool, "circle" wrists by rotating hands, envisioning fingertips tracing the face of a clock. Next, circle ankles by rotating feet.

• Finger flexion. Bring the tips of your right thumb and forefinger together, making as round an "O" as possible…hold five seconds…repeat with other fingers. Switch hands.

• **Resistance training strengthens muscles that surround joints,** easing pain by providing muscular support. Try these exercises three times weekly, building up to 15 repetitions of each.

• Hand helper. Hold a tennis-ball–sized foam (Nerf) ball in one hand…squeeze, hold five seconds, release. Switch hands.

• Hip extension. Lie facedown on a mat or bed, legs extended. Bend arms and turn head to one side, resting your cheek on the backs of your hands. Knees straight, raise your right leg until your ankle is eight to 12 inches above the mat…hold five seconds…lower. Switch legs.

•Knee extension. Sit in a chair, feet flat on floor. Raise your left foot, straightening knee completely so the leg is parallel to the floor…tighten knee and thigh muscles…hold five seconds…lower foot to floor and relax. Switch sides.

•Foot and ankle strengthener. Sit in a chair. Place your bare foot on top of a tennis ball on the floor. Bearing down slightly, roll the ball underfoot, using the muscles of the toes, arch and ankle to move the ball back and forth and side to side. Continue for 30 seconds. Switch feet.

•**Aerobic activity,** such as walking, rowing and stair-climbing, burns calories and helps you lose excess weight that stresses joints. For sore shoulders: Swim in a heated pool. For problem knees and hips: Try biking or stationary cycling. Build up to five 30-minute sessions weekly.

Illustrations by Shawn Banner.

Put a Stop to Tingling And Numbness

Eva L. Feldman, MD, PhD, Russell N. DeJong Professor of Neurology and director of the Program for Understanding Neurologic Diseases at the University of Michigan in Ann Arbor.

Peripheral neuropathy is a nerve disorder that affects the arms, legs, face, hands or any other area not included in the central nervous system (the brain and spinal cord). The main symptom is numbness and/or tingling. Depending on the nerves affected, neuropathy also can cause pain, muscle weakness and/or a loss of muscle control.

Peripheral neuropathy is a nerve disorder that affects 15 million to 20 million Americans—and often it is one of the first signs of a serious medical condition. For example, 60% to 70% of patients with diabetes have peripheral nerve disease.

THE HIDDEN CULPRIT

The majority of people with neuropathy have an underlying disease that affects multiple nerves. *Main causes…*

•**Diabetes** (or prediabetes, a precursor to diabetes) is the most common cause of peripheral neuropathy. Although it is not known exactly how diabetes triggers neuropathy, it is thought that episodes of elevated blood sugar (glucose) can overwhelm *mitochondria* (the power plants inside cells that convert glucose to energy), resulting in accumulations of molecules (such as free radicals) that damage nerve cells.

Red flag: Persistent foot pain and/or numbness is often the first symptom of diabetes. If you experience these symptoms, see a doctor right away.

•**Autoimmune diseases** (such as lupus and rheumatoid arthritis) can lead to peripheral neuropathy. That's because the body's immune system attacks the layers of tissue, known as myelin sheath, that wrap around peripheral nerves.

•**Medications** can cause *toxic neuropathy* —particularly the chemotherapeutic drugs used to treat cancer. Other drugs that can cause peripheral neuropathy include certain antibiotics, such as *nitrofurantoin* (Macrodantin) and *metronidazole* (Flagyl). Exposure to workplace or environmental heavy metals, such as arsenic and mercury, also can cause neuropathy.

•**Vitamin deficiencies**—particularly a deficiency of vitamin B-12—can lead to a form of neuropathy most prevalent in older adults. These people are particularly at risk because they are more likely to have insufficient levels of *intrinsic factor*, a substance secreted in the stomach that's required for vitamin B-12 absorption.

GETTING THE RIGHT DIAGNOSIS

Neuropathy usually can be diagnosed in the doctor's office with a complete medical history, blood work and the following tests…

•**Pinprick.** The doctor will very lightly touch the patient's bare foot in several places with a pin. A patient with neuropathy—particularly when it's caused by diabetes—might not feel the pin.

•**Tuning fork.** Neuropathy patients may not feel the vibrations when the instrument is held against the big toe.

•**Reflex tests.** Rapping the ankle, knee or other affected body part with a small rubber hammer helps determine whether muscles are responding properly to nerve signals.

In addition, the doctor might perform an electromyography (a test of electrical activity in the muscles) and/or a nerve conduction study, in which electrodes are placed on the patient's skin and nerves are stimulated via an electrical pulse. The test measures the speed at which the nerves carry electrical signals.

BEST TREATMENT OPTIONS

Because neuropathy is almost always a symptom of another condition, the main goal is to identify and treat the underlying problem. Once that's achieved, the nerves will gradually start to heal—and the neuropathy will usually improve significantly—and even disappear.

For example, patients with prediabetes or diabetes who achieve good blood sugar control—with diet, regular exercise and/or the use of medication—often will have a complete reversal of neuropathy within one year.

Nerves that are severely damaged or entirely dead—as a result of chemotherapy, for example—may continue to cause pain or other symptoms indefinitely.

Most effective pain treatments…

•*Pregabalin* **(Lyrica) or** *gabapentin* **(Neurontin)** are used for treating diabetic neuropathy. Both drugs were originally developed for the prevention of epileptic seizures. Taken orally, the drugs are thought to work by affecting electrical activity in the brain and inhibiting pain sensations. Both drugs reduce pain by 20% to 30% in most patients.

Main side effects: Dizziness, sleepiness and/or peripheral edema (swollen ankles).

•*Duloxetine* **(Cymbalta),** an antidepressant, was approved by the FDA in 2004 for treating diabetic neuropathy—even in patients who aren't depressed. This medication increases levels of the brain chemicals *serotonin* and *norepinephrine*, which appear to work, in part, by increasing feelings of well-being. Like pregabalin and gabapentin, it reduces pain by 20% to 30% in most patients.

Main side effects: Nausea, dry mouth and/or constipation.

•**Opioid analgesics,** such as *oxycodone* (OxyContin) and codeine, are very effective painkillers. These drugs commonly cause sedation (and also pose a risk for addiction), so they're recommended only for patients with severe pain that does not respond to the therapies described above.

Main side effects: Nausea, sleepiness and/or dependency.

•**Nondrug therapies,** such as acupuncture and transcutaneous electrical nerve stimulation (TENS), are often used with or without medication. Many patients report that acupuncture helps relieve the pain related to neuropathy.

TENS, in which tiny electrical signals are transmitted through the skin, appears to block pain signals. In patients who respond to TENS treatment (typically performed by physical therapists), it can reduce pain by 50% to 70%.

For more information on peripheral neuropathy, contact the Neuropathy Association, 212-692-0662, *www.neuropathy.org*.

Stop Pain Without Drugs

Donna Finando, a Roslyn Heights, New York–based licensed acupuncturist (LAc) and massage therapist (LMT). She is the author of the *Trigger Point Self-Care Manual for Pain-Free Movement*. Healing Arts.

Most over-the-counter and prescription pain relievers temporarily ease aches and pains, but these medications do not address the root cause of the problem. In a surprising number of cases, muscular tightness is responsible for common types of pain.

Here's what happens: When any one of the more than 200 muscles in your body suffers from overuse or an injury, it can develop a *trigger point*—a tiny knot in which a strand of the muscle becomes constricted, making the muscle stiff and weak.

Left untreated, this condition can persist for years, causing pain to recur repeatedly. Fortunately, you can relieve this type of pain with a simple technique known as trigger-point therapy. It involves locating the associated trigger points and compressing them for 20 to 30 seconds several times a day. Press only hard enough to feel the tightness of the muscle and the soreness of the trigger point. Stretches for each condition (as illustrated on the following pages) also should be repeated several times daily.

Helpful: Whenever possible, also apply 20 minutes of moist heat once or twice a day to the affected muscle. Moist heat brings blood and body fluids to the muscle, increasing circulation. (Moist heating pads by Cara, Sunbeam or Thermophore can be purchased at most drugstores for $20 to $70.)

If you've worked on your muscles for several days and felt little or no relief, check with your doctor to make sure there is no other source of pain, such as arthritis.

Conditions often caused by trigger points—and how to treat them…

STIFF NECK

Stiff neck frequently occurs after sleeping with your head turned all the way to one side, or as a result of holding a phone between your ear and shoulder. The condition is often due to a trigger point in the *levator scapulae* muscle, which runs from the inner edge of the shoulder blade to the neck.

To find the trigger point: Reach the hand that is on your pain-free side over to touch your shoulder on the painful side. Locate the inside edge of the shoulder blade, then move your hand a bit closer to your spine, feeling for a hard band the size of a pencil running up toward your neck. While bending your neck toward your pain-free side, use your fingers to locate a tender spot along this band, then press it for 20 to 30 seconds.

Helpful stretch: Turn your chin 30 degrees away from the affected side, then drop your chin down slightly toward your chest. Hold for a slow count of 20.

HIP, BUTTOCK AND LEG PAIN

Pain in the hips, buttocks or legs is often diagnosed as sciatica (pain in your back that radiates into your buttocks and legs) when it actually may be caused by trigger points in the muscles of the back and buttocks. One of these muscles, the gluteus medius, lies midway between the top of your pelvis and the top of your thighbone.

To find the trigger point: Lie on the floor on your pain-free side with your knees slightly bent, and use your fingers to massage your hip under the top of your pelvis and down toward the top of your thighbone. If trigger points are present, you'll feel taut bands and tender spots. Once you've located a tender spot, roll onto your painful side and place a tennis ball between this spot and the floor. Then let your weight press the ball into the tender area for 20 to 30 seconds.

Helpful stretch: Stand facing a wall with your arms raised and the backs of your hands pressed against your forehead. Cross your pain-free leg in front of your other leg. Bend the knee of your rear leg into the back of your pain-free leg while shifting your weight onto your painful hip. This should create a stretch between your pelvis and the top of your thighbone. Hold for a slow count of 20.

CALF PAIN

If you're experiencing pain or soreness in your calf or the back of your knee, it may be caused by trigger points in the *gastrocnemius* muscle (the large muscle that gives the calf its characteristic shape).

To find the trigger point: Sit in a chair and place the sole of the foot of your affected leg on a footstool or coffee table in front of you. Place one hand on the outer side of this leg and the other on the inner side of this leg—in both cases, just above the ankle. Run your fingers along your Achilles tendon (the large tendon at the back of your heel) and work your way to the middle of the calf, feeling for tender spots. Continue upward, toward the back of the knee. When you find a tender spot, compress it with your fingers for 20 to 30 seconds.

Helpful stretch: While standing about 12 inches from a wall, facing the wall, place your hands on the wall at chest level. Keeping your feet hip-width apart and the toes of both feet facing the wall, move your painful leg 18 inches behind the other leg. Bend your front knee, keeping your rear leg straight. Your weight should remain on the front leg. Hold for a slow count of 20.

213

TENNIS ELBOW

Inflammation of the tendon on the outside of the elbow, known as "tennis elbow," can cause sharp pain down the back of the forearm into the wrist, making it hard to grip objects. However, sometimes the condition may not be an inflammation but a result of trigger points in the *extensor* muscles of the hand and fingers, which can be caused by repeated or forceful gripping, such as when holding a tennis racket—or even a coffee cup.

To find the trigger point: Rest the elbow and forearm of your sore arm on a table, with your palm facing up. Use your opposite hand to feel along the muscle on the outside (thumb side) of your elbow crease, then follow this muscle down toward your hand. When you find a tender spot, press down and hold for 20 to 30 seconds.

Helpful stretch: Sit on a chair, and keeping your elbow straight, place the back of the hand on the affected arm flat on the seat beside you, palm up, feeling a stretch in your forearm. Hold for a slow count of 20.

Illustrations by Shawn Banner.

in Bay Shore, New York, explains it this way: "The more you lean back, the more the weight of your body is supported by the chair, rather than putting pressure on the spine."

Standing puts less pressure on the lower back than sitting, but it isn't a practical solution for people who spend their days in seated positions, such as working at computers or watching television. What's the answer? *Dr. Weisberg advises...*

•**Sit in an adjustable chair** that allows you to lean back—and that also provides good lumbar support. Padding at the base of the spine creates a natural arch and reduces pressure.

Good brands: HealthyBack, 888-469-2225, *www.healthyback.com.*

Typical cost: $300 to $2,000.

•**Use a sliding keyboard tray if you work at a computer.** Adjust the keyboard/mouse so that you can work while leaning back. Or position a laptop so that you can work without sitting straight.

•**Take a break at least every 45 minutes.** Stand up...stretch your back...and walk around a little to keep the spinal ligaments loose.

Secrets to Pain-Free Sitting

Rebecca Shannonhouse, editor of the *Bottom Line/Health* newsletters, Boardroom Inc., 281 Tresser Blvd., Stamford, Connecticut 06901.

At one time or another, we've all heard the admonition to "sit up straight." Now, new research shows that this advice may not be sound.

Using magnetic resonance imaging (MRI) scans, researchers in Scotland found that spinal disks became more compressed—indicating increased pressure—when people sat straight up. When study participants leaned back, however, the disk compression was much less pronounced.

Joseph Weisberg, PhD, a physical therapist and dean of Touro College School of Health Sciences

Do You Really Need Back Surgery?

Eugene Carragee, MD, professor of orthopedic surgery and director of the Orthopedic Spine Center at Stanford University School of Medicine in Stanford, California. He is the author of an editorial discussing back surgery, published in *The Journal of the American Medical Association.*

For decades, doctors have recommended back surgery for people who have a damaged spinal disk that triggers sciatica (pain that radiates from the low back down the leg). Sciatica can cause shooting pains that some people describe as being as excruciating as childbirth.

The surgery, which involves the partial removal of the damaged disk, is the most common operation in the US for people who have back and leg pain due to sciatica. In at least 80%

of cases, the operation relieves symptoms and prevents nerve damage that could potentially cause permanent pain and disability, including paralysis and incontinence.

New finding: In a pair of recent studies comparing the results for back pain sufferers who received surgery versus those who waited, patients in both groups did equally well in the long run. Not one of the patients who delayed surgery—or didn't get it at all—experienced serious complications. Meanwhile, less than 5% of the patients in the surgery groups had complications, such as a tear in the membrane covering the spinal cord.

The studies, which included 1,244 patients and were published in *The Journal of the American Medical Association*, showed that the only major difference between the back patients who received surgery and those who did not was the speed with which they improved. In the surgery groups, a significant number of patients had regained all (or most) of their normal function within three months. A similar number of patients in the nonsurgical group also regained near-normal function, but it took much longer —up to two years, in some cases. Based on these findings, many doctors are now advising some sciatica sufferers to delay or even forgo surgery if their pain is not severe.

TO WAIT OR NOT

A herniated disk, which occurs when an injury or age-related spinal degeneration causes part of the cartilage between the vertebrae to bulge out, is not in itself an indication for surgery. Imaging studies indicate that up to 25% of adults have one or more herniated disks but don't have significant sciatica or related symptoms.

Even when sciatica causes severe pain initially, patients usually get better on their own within weeks or months as the body secretes *collagenases,* enzymes that break down disk collagen. Once the disk material breaks down—or when a disk protrusion retreats back into its normal space— pain and inflammation may gradually decrease.

Important: Prompt surgery may be needed when a large disk bulge or fragment compromises bowel or bladder control, or leads to leg paralysis. If you suffer from back pain that occurs suddenly, see your doctor—especially if you have fever and the chills, which could indicate an infection near the spine, or if you are taking a blood thinner (internal bleeding may be occurring).

When deciding whether to have surgery, points to consider...

• **Size of herniation.** Disk fragments/protrusions that are smaller than 5 mm (about one-fifth of an inch) are less likely than larger ones to cause serious sciatica—and even if they do, they're readily "mopped up" by the body. Herniations that are larger than 5 mm are more likely to cause severe, long-lasting symptoms.

• **Pain severity.** Some patients with sciatica are unable to sit or lie down—or even move—without excruciating pain. Others experience only minor discomfort, or are able to tolerate the pain for longer periods. Surgery is a reasonable choice for patients who are truly miserable and unable to function normally for a prolonged period.

• **Job/family requirements.** Some patients can't afford to wait six months—or two years— for their condition to improve on its own.

Example: A self-employed plumber or carpenter probably can't afford to wait months or years before going back to work. Patients with adequate personal/economic resources, on the other hand, may decide that it makes more sense to avoid surgery (and its risks, such as bleeding, infection and injury to the nerves or spinal cord).

NONSURGICAL ALTERNATIVES

Patients who decide not to have surgery can try to control pain/inflammation with a variety of nonsurgical treatments, including physical therapy.

Other important therapies...

• **Anti-inflammatory analgesics,** such as *ibuprofen* (Advil), *naproxen* (Aleve) and *indomethacin* (Indocin). These drugs can make a difference for patients with relatively mild sciatica, but they aren't very helpful for severe pain.

• **Daily exercise,** including walking, swimming and riding a bike, usually does not prolong episodes of sciatica. In fact, people with sciatica who exercise may recover more quickly than patients who are sedentary since exercise helps keep them physically fit.

• **Cold/heat applications** can help block pain signals as they travel to the brain.

215

What to do: Apply an ice pack to the painful area for about 20 minutes, followed by 20 minutes with a heating pad. Do this up to three times a day.

Caution: Do not use heat therapy within the first 48 hours of experiencing the pain, as this may increase the inflammation.

●**Steroid injections,** given into the open space that surrounds the spinal nerves, may reduce inflammation. Steroids used in this way are unlikely to cause the drug's typical side effects and can safely be given up to three times a year.

●**Oral steroids,** usually taken for a week, also reduce inflammation and may make the pain more tolerable. However, they are more likely to cause side effects (such as a worsening of diabetes or hypertension in patients with these conditions) than injections.

WHAT IS SCIATICA?

Sciatica is a common form of low back pain that radiates along one of the two sciatic nerves, each of which runs down the back of the thigh and calf and into the foot. Most cases of sciatica occur when one of the spinal disks—gel-filled pancakes of cartilage between the vertebrae—swells, tears (ruptures) or herniates (part of the interior of the disk bulges out), exerting painful pressure on a sciatic nerve. About 1 million Americans suffer from sciatica, and up to 300,000 a year have surgery to relieve the pain.

Make Back Pain Disappear Without Drugs or a Scalpel

Steven Shoshany, DC, a New York City–based chiropractor who specializes in spinal decompression. He can be reached through his Web site, *www.drshoshany.com.*

Most of us (80% by some estimates) will have back pain at some time or another—whether from over-exertion, injury or simply a result of the aging process. Chronic back pain is frustrating, not only because of how badly it hurts but also because it can be difficult to cure. It is one of the most common reasons for doctor visits.

A particularly common cause of such pain is a herniated disk, also referred to colloquially as a "slipped disk." For a long time, the usual mainstream medical solutions are surgery and pain medication, which do not work for everyone. An interesting approach is a non-surgical, non-invasive treatment for herniated disks called spinal decompression.

SPINAL DECOMPRESSION 101: A PRIMER

One of the first devices used for spinal decompression was approved by the FDA in 1995. Because spinal decompression requires special expertise and pricey equipment, few chiropractors have offered this treatment—but numbers are growing as training and better insurance reimbursement becomes more commonplace, said Steven Shoshany, DC, a New York City–based chiropractor who specializes in spinal decompression.

Here's how it works: The patient lies on a comfortable table made specifically for this purpose, comfortably strapped down with a pelvis and torso harness that resembles a girdle. Calling it a "high-tech traction device," Dr. Shoshany explained how it works. "Slowly and comfortably, almost imperceptibly, the machine creates traction by pulling and holding for one minute. Then, intermittently, it releases. It is believed that this creates a negative pressure, or a vacuum within the disk, which then draws back the herniated-disk material which was displaced." With less pressure inside the disk, and thus less on the spinal nerves, pain often decreases or might even disappear—sometimes instantaneously. For lasting treatment, numerous sessions may be required.

This technique also allows nutrient-rich fluid to go to the area where there is less pressure, stimulating the healing process. Most patients either sleep or watch a DVD during the treatment, Dr. Shoshany said. Each session takes about 30 minutes and a typical treatment program may take between 20 to 30 sessions.

Critics contend that there are no long-range, well-designed studies looking at efficacy over time, but there has been some research on the treatment and the results are promising. In one study published in *Neurological Research,* researchers reported that a spinal decompression therapy called VAX-D produced a success rate of 68.4% over a placebo therapy in treatment of chronic low back pain. Another study from a team of researchers at the University of Illinois at Chicago, and Coosa Medical Group, Rome, Georgia, found a 71% success rate for treatment of herniated disk and other causes of low back pain, with "success" defined as a reduction in pain to 0 or 1 on a scale of 0 to 5.

NOT FOR EVERYONE

Dr. Shoshany noted that some people get much more benefit from spinal decompression than others, and it is not an option for everyone. "It's not a good choice for a person who has metal implants in the spine," he warned. It's better for people with a single-disk herniation than those who have herniation in several or all of them. Also, people who are morbidly obese and/or who smoke likely won't find much relief from spinal decompression either.

The procedure is thought to be safe, though more research is needed to support its efficacy. If you do decide to seek out this somewhat unconventional form of treatment, it's safest and best to do so with the oversight of your orthopedic surgeon, who can help you ascertain whether it might work in your case. For more information on spinal decompression, go to *http://www.spinaldiscdecompression.com.*

Best Ways to Repair That Aching Hip

William Macaulay, MD, professor of clinical orthopedic surgery, director of the Center for Hip and Knee Replacement and advisory dean of students at the College of Physicians and Surgeons, New York-Presbyterian Hospital at Columbia University, all in New York City.

For decades, people whose severe hip pain did not improve with painkillers and/or physical therapy had only one option—a hip replacement.

Now: A procedure that "resurfaces" worn-out hip joints rather than replacing them is available in the US. Known as *hip resurfacing,* the technique can be as durable as hip replacement with less pain during recovery and greater long-term mobility. Originally introduced in England in 1997, the Birmingham Hip Resurfacing System (one of the products used for hip resurfacing) was approved by the FDA.

DO YOU NEED A BETTER HIP?

Osteoarthritis of the hip is the most common reason for hip pain. This disease occurs when the cartilage covering joint surfaces begins to wear out, causing pain and stiffness that can be so severe that sufferers limp and have difficulty climbing stairs, walking, standing and even sitting. Other causes of hip pain include rheumatoid arthritis and serious hip injury.

If you suffer from hip pain that does not improve with pain medication and physical therapy…interferes with activities that you enjoy, such as gardening or brisk walking…and/or disturbs your sleep, you may want to consider one of several surgical options.

A BREAKTHROUGH APPROACH

For several years, Americans who wanted to try an alternative to hip replacement have traveled to England, India or one of the other countries that have offered hip resurfacing. Now this procedure is available at approximately 100 medical centers throughout the US.

With hip resurfacing, the round head of the femur (thighbone) is reshaped and covered with a metal cap about the same size as the natural femoral head. The reshaped head moves within a smooth metal socket that is implanted into the pelvic bone. Enough bone is left in place to allow for a future hip replacement, if necessary.

Hip resurfacing is a good option for patients age 55 and younger…people of any age who have relatively healthy bones or who are highly active.

Hip resurfacing may take slightly longer than the hour to hour-and-a-half required for a standard hip replacement surgery. The incision is often two to three inches longer than the six- to 12-inch incision required for conventional hip replacement, due in part to the limited maneuverability the surgeon has with most of the thighbone left in place. As with traditional hip replacement, a two- to three-day hospital stay is usually required following hip resurfacing, and healing is more than 90% complete within six to eight weeks. The procedure typically costs about $48,000 and is usually covered by insurance.

HIP REPLACEMENT OPTIONS

If you are not a candidate for hip resurfacing (due to age, osteoporosis or bone weakness), *total hip replacement* is an option. During this procedure, the surgeon makes an incision, removes the femoral head and replaces the ball-and-socket mechanism with an artificial implant that functions much like a natural joint.

A significant amount of bone is removed with hip replacement in order to insert a metal stem that attaches the synthetic ball-and-socket mechanism to the femur. If any part of the implant loosens in the future, this loss of bone makes a follow-up surgery more difficult.

Traditional hip replacement (as described above) is usually recommended for patients who are obese or very muscular. Recovery time is the same as that for hip resurfacing.

With a newer minimally invasive approach, the surgeon uses specially designed surgical instruments to place the hip implant. Minimally invasive hip replacement generally takes one-and-a-half hours, uses one-and-a-half- to three-inch incisions and requires a one- to two-day hospital stay. It is usually recommended for people who are thin. The recovery period is comparable to that for hip resurfacing and a traditional hip replacement. However, the minimally invasive procedure is controversial, because it has been associated with significant complications in some studies.

The same type of artificial implant is used with both procedures. Each procedure costs about $25,000, which usually is covered by health insurance.

INSTALLING HIP IMPLANTS

More than 300 types of hip implants are now available, as well as dozens of different techniques for installing them. *Main choices...*

•**Cemented.** The implant is attached to bone of the thigh with an acrylic cement. The cement gives immediate strength and is extremely durable.

Recommended for: Patients with less-than-healthy bone, such as those with osteoporosis or osteoarthritis.

•**Uncemented.** The joint implants have a porous surface that allows the patient's natural bone to surround and grow into the implant.

Recommended for: Active patients with normal bone metabolism.

•**Metal/ceramic-on-plastic.** A metal or ceramic femoral ball (prosthetic head) is mated with a hard plastic (polyethylene) socket. It's one of the older configurations—proven to be durable and reliable.

Recommended for: Any patient.

RISKS AND RECOVERY

The main cause of hip-replacement failure is aseptic loosening (when normal bone loss occurs around the implant, causing the joint to separate). In this case, the hip replacement must be repeated. *Other risks...*

•**Deep vein thrombosis.** Blood clots can form in the leg veins—a life-threatening complication if a clot travels to the lungs. After the procedure, most patients are treated with blood thinners, such as *warfarin* (Coumadin), and advised to move their ankles up and down frequently (about 10 times at least three times daily), which helps prevent clots.

•**Uneven leg lengths.** In some cases, the leg on the side that was operated on will be slightly longer than the other leg. When this happens, a patient may need to wear a shoe with a slightly raised heel.

Important: Postsurgical exercise, including low-impact activities, such as walking or using an elliptical trainer, are among the best ways to stabilize the joint and maintain hip strength and/or flexibility.

■ ■ ■ ■

Arthritis Alert

Arthritis supplements often don't contain a key ingredient, warns Tod Cooperman, MD. The labels may say that they have glucosamine *and* chondroitin when they have little or no chondroitin, which is expensive.

Some that contain what they claim: Nutramax Laboratories Cosamin DS...Puritan's Pride Triple Strength Glucosamine Chondroitin...and

Walgreens Finest Natural Glucosamine Chondroitin Double Strength.

Tod Cooperman, MD, president of ConsumerLab.com, an independent evaluator of health products, White Plains, New York. *www.consumerlab.com*

Rhus Toxicodendron

Mark A. Stengler, ND, naturopathic physician in private practice, La Jolla, California…adjunct associate clinical professor at the National College of Natural Medicine, Portland, Oregon…author of many books, including *The Natural Physician's Healing Therapies* and coauthor of *Prescription for Natural Cures* (both from Bottom Line Books)…and author of the *Bottom Line/Natural Healing* newsletter.

Todd, a 60-year-old retired farmer, came to see me for his arthritis. He was already very interested in natural therapies. He pulled out a bag of supplements that he had tried for his osteoarthritis. They included glucosamine sulfate and about 12 other supplements as well.

"I hope you have something else that can help me," he said. "I'm taking all these supplements and even so, it's getting hard to walk."

He also complained of the expense of the supplements, which were costing him about $150 every month.

After asking Todd about all the symptoms he experienced, I recommended *rhus toxicodendron* (commonly called rhus tox, pronounced roos tox).

He asked me two questions: "Is this going to work?" and, "How much is the medicine going to cost me?"

"It should help reduce the joint pain and stiffness," I replied, "even in the first couple of weeks. As far as cost goes, you can buy a month's supply at the health food store for about seven dollars."

"Seven dollars, that's all it costs?" he questioned. "That's it," I replied.

I suggested that Todd stop taking all the other supplements, as he had not noticed any improvement in his condition. I advised him to take only the rhus tox. When he came to my office for a follow-up visit six weeks later, Todd reported a 70 percent improvement in his arthritic symptoms.

PALLIATIVE FROM A POISON

Rhus tox is the homeopathic dilution of poison oak. We know this as a plant that causes a nasty, blistering rash. However, this homeopathic is one of the best skin remedies for relieving symptoms in people who have touched poison ivy. It is also effective in treating eczema, where the skin is very itchy and feels better after the application of very hot water.

I have also used this for people with shingles. The itching, burning pain of the shingles blisters can be relieved in a few days with rhus tox.

Dosage: The typical dosage for rhus tox is 30C potency taken two to three times daily for a day or two for conditions such as stiffness from overexertion. For long-term use for eczema or arthritis, I generally start with a lower dose such as 6C taken two to three times daily.

What are the side effects? While rhus tox has few side effects, some people may experience skin irritation. People with chronic eczema or arthritis may experience a flare-up of their condition at the beginning of treatment. This is usually a sign that the remedy is working (known as a healing aggravation).

If you do have a flare-up and you begin taking the rhus tox less frequently, you'll probably notice that the flare-up subsides. Soon after, you'll probably notice an improvement in your condition.

If you are not sure whether you should use rhus tox, consult a homeopathic practitioner.

■ **More from Mark A. Stengler…**

Boswellia Herb—Better Than Arthritis Drug

Researchers compared *boswellia serrata extract* (BSE) to the anti-inflammatory drug *valdecoxib* (Bextra, Valdone). The study involved osteoarthritis patients who took either BSE (333 mg, three times daily) or valdecoxib (10 mg, once daily) for six months. Those taking BSE showed reductions in pain and inflammation after two months—and benefits lasted for one month after BSE use ended. Patients on valdecoxib improved after one month, but benefits disappeared when the drug was discontinued.

My view: Drugs like Valdecoxib do not slow the degradation of cartilage that arthritis causes—so over time, patients require higher doses to manage pain. Side effects include heartburn, stomach pain and gastrointestinal ulcers. Boswellia (sold at health-food stores) does slow cartilage damage and ease inflammation, so pain relief continues even if treatment is stopped. Side effects (mild digestive upset and/or skin rashes) are rare.

Note: Bextra has since been pulled from the market for safety reasons.

Speedy Healing—6 Steps To Faster Recovery From Illness or Injury

Julie K. Silver, MD, assistant professor in the department of physical medicine and rehabilitation at Harvard Medical School and a staff member of Dana-Farber Cancer Institute, both in Boston. She is author of *Super Healing: The Clinically Proven Plan to Maximize Recovery from Illness or Injury.* Rodale. She is a cancer survivor who perfected her healing techniques as she worked to speed her own recovery.

At any given time, about 90 million Americans are healing from an illness or injury. During this healing period, patients often experience declines in immune function and heart efficiency and a loss of bone and muscle strength.

Example: People assigned to bed rest—after surgery, for example—lose 1% to 3% of their muscle strength daily over the first two weeks. They may lose 50% after three weeks or more.

These and many other factors, including depression, can greatly slow recovery—*but you can take steps to stop this downward cycle and speed healing…*

1. SET SPECIFIC GOALS

Patients usually have an *idea* of what they want to achieve. Someone who has had back surgery might want to walk normally without pain. A patient recovering from a car accident wants to be able to get back to work.

But people often lack a plan—specific steps that can help them reach their long-term goals. The steps will be different for each person, depending on the underlying problem. For every

patient, however, setting goals helps him/her define what he wants…the steps needed to achieve each goal…and benchmarks to measure progress.

Short-term goals: I recommend that patients identify eight easy-to-achieve goals that they plan to accomplish within one month. At the end of the month, they check their progress and create eight new goals for the next month.

Examples: Using a pedometer to count the number of steps you take daily—and setting a goal of 1,000 more daily steps by the end of a month…meeting a friend for lunch at least once a week. Social interactions have been shown to reduce healing times (see step #6 for more).

Long-term goals: These represent where you want to be in the future for optimal health.

Examples: Walking at least 5,000 steps daily…meeting with a counselor/psychologist to cope with mood problems…eating five daily servings of produce for better immunity, etc.

2. REST TO RECOVER

Much of the body's recovery, including wound healing, occurs during sleep. Patients who sleep well have improved immunity and better blood sugar control. Sleep also improves mood.

Trap: Most patients who have experienced a significant injury or illness have difficulty sleeping. *What to do…*

• **Limit alcohol.** It's okay to have one drink with dinner but no more.

• **Ask your doctor about sleep aids.** Over-the-counter (OTC) and prescription drugs are safe for short-term use (seven to 10 days)—and are helpful for patients who need help establishing better sleep habits. OTC drugs include Nytol QuickCaps, Tylenol PM and Simply Sleep Nighttime Sleep Aid Caplets. Prescription sleep aids include Ambien, Lunesta and Sonata.

3. EXERCISE DAILY

Exercise increases muscle strength and accelerates every healing process, including the flow of nutrients to injured tissue…blood clotting and immune responses…and the synthesis of collagen for tissue healing.

In one study, researchers compared wound-healing rates in volunteers who exercised against volunteers who were sedentary. In the exercise group, the wounds took an average of 29 days to heal…in the sedentary group, the average healing time was about 40 days.

Almost everyone can exercise, regardless of the underlying condition. Someone with a broken leg might not be able to walk initially, but he/she can do upper-body exercises. Hospital patients often can use light hand weights…walk the halls…or do exercises to improve grip strength.

Ask your doctor to refer you to a physical therapist. He/she can design an exercise program that takes into account your physical limitations.

4. EAT TO HEAL

Studies have shown that people who don't get enough key nutrients have significant changes in blood chemistry, strength, physical performance, etc. Adequate protein is essential for tissue healing…vitamin C improves immune function…vitamin A supports skin and bone healing…and zinc is required for cell growth. *To get adequate nutrition, be sure to eat…*

• **Five or more servings of brightly colored produce daily**—broccoli, spinach, carrots, tomatoes and berries. These foods are high in antioxidants, which significantly improve immune function.

• **Foods rich in *serotonin*.** Many antidepressants work by increasing brain levels of serotonin, a neurochemical that affects both mood and appetite. People can naturally increase serotonin by eating bananas, kiwi, plums and pineapple.

5. COPE WITH PAIN

Patients who experience high levels of pain have impaired immunity and more stress. Pain also interferes with sleep, which can further delay healing.

Patients should never tolerate excessive pain. Most doctors aren't trained in sophisticated pain-management techniques, so you may want to see a pain-management specialist (ask your doctor for a referral)…or get a second opinion if you feel your complaints about pain aren't being addressed.

Don't get "behind" the pain. Pain-killing drugs, including mild analgesics such as ibuprofen, are far more effective when taken at the first signs of pain or even before pain starts. They're less effective once pain is under way.

Helpful: Take analgesics in the morning. Patients who treat their pain early in the day tend to get better relief—and often require less medication.

6. MIND YOUR EMOTIONS

Emotions play a large role in how quickly and how well you heal. A 2005 study in *Archives of General Psychiatry* evaluated wound healing among couples. The quality of the couples' relationships was rated as either "high hostile" or "low hostile," depending on how they got along with each other. Wounds in the low-hostile group healed almost twice as fast as wounds in the high-hostile group.

Thousands of studies have looked at the effects of stress and other negative emotions on health. People under stress tend to get more respiratory infections. They have an increase in *interleukin-6*, a type of protein produced by immune cells that is a sign of inflammation. They also have decreased immunity and an increase in blood pressure and heart rate. *What to do…*

• **Practice mind-body therapies**—meditation, progressive muscle relaxation, imagery, etc. For more information on these therapies, go to *www.nccam.nih.gov*, sponsored by the National Institutes of Health.

• **Reduce day-to-day stress** with regular exercise and pleasurable hobbies.

• **Foster nurturing relationships**—by getting together with friends, for example, and welcoming help from others.

8

Drugstore Remedies

Hidden OTC Dangers: Deciphering Labels

Over-the-counter (OTC) drugs can be purchased just as easily as a bottle of shampoo or a box of cereal —but that doesn't mean that they are harmless.

Few people realize that in some cases, OTC drugs contain the same amount of an active ingredient as that found in prescription medications. Using OTC drugs incorrectly—for example, taking them for too long or in excessive doses—can cause serious side effects.

Example 1: People with arthritis often treat their symptoms with OTC painkillers, such as *ibuprofen* (Advil) or *naproxen* (Aleve), for months or years—even though the label advises against taking these drugs for more than 10 consecutive days without consulting your doctor. The long-term use of such drugs greatly increases the risk for stomach bleeding as well as heart and/or kidney problems.

Example 2: If you have hypertension or heart disease, taking a cold remedy that contains *pseudoephedrine*, such as Sudafed, can cause a heart rhythm irregularity such as atrial fibrillation or even a heart attack.

All OTC medications include a standardized "Drug Facts" label (on the outside of the packaging and also in an insert) that details the approved uses of the drug…active ingredients… how to use it…and possible risks. Even though OTC drug labels were simplified in 2002, the information is often confusing and printed in such small type that it's almost impossible to read.

Note: The FDA recently has required drug manufacturers to redesign prescription drug labels so that they are easier to read.

Important: Bring your reading glasses or a small magnifying glass with you and read

Jack M. Rosenberg, PharmD, PhD, is director of the International Drug Information Center at the Arnold and Marie Schwartz College of Pharmacy Health Sciences at Long Island University in Brooklyn, New York.

the OTC drug label before leaving the store. If you're purchasing from a drugstore, ask a pharmacist to explain any instructions that you don't understand.

What to look for…

ACTIVE INGREDIENT

This term refers to the medication that relieves symptoms. There might be dozens of drugs in a pharmacy that have the same active ingredient.

Example: Advil Cold & Sinus Non-Drowsy coated caplets and Motrin Cold & Sinus caplets both contain 200 mg of ibuprofen and 30 mg of pseudoephedrine. Knowing the active ingredient makes it easy to comparison shop for the best price.

What you may not know: Manufacturers occasionally change the active ingredients in OTC products.

Example: The antidiarrheal drug Kaopectate once contained a type of clay called *attapulgite*. It was safe for patients who were taking blood-thinning medication. Kaopectate now contains *bismuth subsalicylate*, an aspirin-like ingredient that increases the risk for bleeding in patients taking blood thinners.

INACTIVE INGREDIENTS

This term refers to the chemicals that are used as preservatives, binders and colorants/flavors—but have no medical effects.

What you may not know: Some people are allergic to certain inactive (as well as active) ingredients.

Example 1: Hundreds of products, such as the OTC antihistamine *loratadine* (Alavert) and the OTC pain reliever Arthritis Strength BC Powder, contain the inactive ingredient lactose, a milk sugar that can trigger reactions in patients who are lactose intolerant.

Example 2: Gluten, a protein found in wheat, barley and rye, should be avoided by people with celiac disease, but starch, maltodextrin and other substances that could contain gluten are common inactive ingredients in both OTC and prescription medications, such as the OTC anti-gas drug Gas-X Regular Strength Chewable Tablets.

USES

Known as "indications" on some labels, this term refers to the list of symptoms that a drug is designed to treat.

The FDA allows drug manufacturers to list only uses for which the medication has been proven to be safe and effective.

Example: The label on an antihistamine such as *diphenhydramine* (Benadryl) says the drug treats sneezing, runny nose and other allergy symptoms.

What you may not know: It can be risky to take drugs "off-label"—that is, taking a medication for uses other than the indications and/or directions found on the label.

Example: Taking high doses of the OTC B-vitamin niacin to lower cholesterol is an off-label use. Prescription niacin is approved for lowering cholesterol, but taking it without being monitored by your doctor can lead to liver damage.

WARNINGS

Many patients ignore the warnings on OTC medications because they assume the drugs must be safe or they wouldn't be sold without a prescription. Not true.

OTC drugs can cause side effects that are just as serious as those caused by prescription drugs. Aspirin and related drugs, for example, cause about 100,000 hospitalizations annually in the US.

What you may not know: In addition to explaining the main risks of a medication, "warnings" may include information on who should not take the medication, when to consult your doctor if symptoms persist, when to take medications with foods (or when to avoid certain foods and beverages), whether it's safe to drive, etc.

Even if you've taken a particular OTC drug for years, check the warning label each time you purchase the medication. A drug that was safe when you first started taking it might cause problems if you've begun taking other medications or if the ingredients or your health needs have changed. Always check the expiration date.

FORMS AND FORMULATIONS

The label on an OTC drug lists the medication's form—tablet, capsule, caplet, etc. The form

can affect how quickly the product works…
what side effects occur…and how easy it is to
take.

Examples…

•**Buffered analgesics** (pain relievers) are
made slightly alkaline to protect the stomach.
Patients who experience stomach irritation,
pain or heartburn from aspirin or similar drugs
might do better with a buffered product.

•**Caplets** are ordinary tablets in the shape of
a capsule. They're easier to swallow than traditional tablets—an important point for patients
who have trouble swallowing. Gelcaps, geltabs
and capsules are coated with gelatin, making
them also easier to swallow.

•**Timed-release capsules or tablets.** These
drugs are designed with various types and layers of coatings around the active ingredients,
which allows the medication to be released
slowly, resulting in extended drug action.

An enteric-coated drug is treated so that it
passes through the stomach unaltered and dissolves in the intestines. Enteric-coated medications take longer to work, so if you have a
headache (and do not have a sensitive stomach),
it may be better to take regular aspirin than
enteric-coated aspirin.

•**Extra-strength drugs** contain a higher
dose of the active ingredient. These medications, such as Extra Strength Tylenol, are helpful if the regular dose isn't adequate to control
symptoms—and more convenient than taking
two or more doses of a lower-dose product.

•**PM** (or night formulas), including some antihistamines or pain relievers, such as Excedrin
PM, can cause drowsiness, so they're meant to
be taken at night.

•**Suspension formulas** are liquid medications in which the active ingredient isn't dissolved. They require shaking before use (and
typically indicate this on the label).

Example: The laxative Phillips Milk of
Magnesia is an oral suspension medication.

224

Everyday Painkillers May Block Memory Loss!

Lon Schneider, MD, professor of psychiatry, neurology and gerontology, Keck School of Medicine, University of Southern California, Los Angeles.

Theo Palmer, PhD, associate professor of neurosurgery,
Stanford University School of Medicine, California.

John C. Morris, MD, professor of pathology and immunology, and director, Alzheimer's Disease Research Center, Washington University School of Medicine, St. Louis,
Missouri.

Science.

Two studies indicate that nonsteroidal anti-
inflammatory drugs (NSAIDs), including
aspirin and other aspirin-like drugs such
as ibuprofen, can restore brain cell (neuron) production and decrease harmful levels of amyloid
beta proteins by reducing inflammation.

Amyloid beta proteins form clumps in the
brains of people who have Alzheimer's, and
those clumps are suspected to cause or at least
contribute to the disease. Amyloid beta-42 seems
to be the most harmful form of these proteins.

The results of these two studies suggest that
memory and learning problems in conditions
such as Alzheimer's and other types of dementia, stroke and traumatic brain injury might be
helped by a simple drug, a researcher says.

THE FIRST STUDY

In one study, Dr. Steven Paul and researchers from drugmaker Eli Lilly and Co. report
that anti-inflammatory drugs can reduce the
production of amyloid beta proteins, including
amyloid beta-42.

These results support the notion that
NSAIDs have a protective effect against future
neurodegeneration, says Dr. Lon Schneider, a
professor of psychiatry, neurology and gerontology at the University of Southern California.

Schneider believes trials are needed to see
which NSAIDs might prevent dementia and
treat head injury and stroke.

THE SECOND STUDY

In another study, a team led by Theo Palmer,
an associate professor of neurosurgery at Stanford University School of Medicine, experiment-
ed with rats to see if reducing brain inflammation
might have an effect on neuron production.

"The dogma for many decades has been that the brain doesn't replace neurons, but that is not true. There are regions of the brain that continue to make neurons throughout life. These new neurons are made by stem cells called precursors," Palmer says.

These new neurons may be important for memory and learning, he adds.

The team found that in rats with brain inflammation, the production of new neurons stopped. However, when they treated the rats with the anti-inflammatory drug indomethacin, the production of neurons was completely restored.

These results suggest that people who have Alzheimer's, stroke and brain injury might benefit from a simple drug such as indomethacin, Palmer says.

Dr. John Morris, director of the Alzheimer's Disease Research Center at Washington University School of Medicine, comments, "These reports suggest that commonly used anti-inflammatory drugs may lessen the toxic effects of brain inflammation believed to be important in Alzheimer's disease.

"However, neither study involved human subjects. Whether the positive effects shown in these experimental models translate to actual patients is far from clear," Morris says.

Get an explanation of how NSAIDs reduce inflammation at the American Academy of Orthopaedic Surgeons Web site, *www.aaos.org*.

■ ■ ■ ■

Aspirin vs. Stroke

Because aspirin can cause bleeding, it is typically avoided by people who have had a hemorrhagic stroke, which occurs when a blood vessel bursts in the brain.

New finding: In a study of 207 hemorrhagic stroke survivors, those who took an antiplatelet drug, such as aspirin, were not at increased risk for another hemorrhage.

Implication: Aspirin therapy may be appropriate for hemorrhagic stroke survivors who are at high risk for heart attack or ischemic stroke,

in which a blood clot blocks blood flow to the brain.

Anand Viswanathan, MD, PhD, assistant neurologist, neurology clinical trials unit, Massachusetts General Hospital, Boston.

The Dangerous Truth About Acetaminophen

Elham Rahme, PhD, assistant professor of medicine, McGill University, and medical scientist, Montreal General Hospital, Quebec, Canada.
John Klippel, MD, rheumatologist, and president and chief executive officer, Arthritis Foundation.
Arthritis and Rheumatism.

Acetaminophen is often a first line of treatment for arthritis because it is believed to have fewer side effects than other painkillers.

But Canadian researchers have shown that in high doses, acetaminophen is just as likely to cause gastrointestinal (GI) problems, such as upset stomach and ulcers, as *nonsteroidal anti-inflammatory drugs* (NSAIDs), such as *ibuprofen* or *naproxen*.

"Physicians need to know that if they are increasing the dose of acetaminophen rather than switching to another medication because they think they will see fewer GI events, they should look at other options," says one of the study's authors, Elham Rahme, an assistant professor of medicine at McGill University in Montreal.

Acetaminophen—the active ingredient in Tylenol, among other cold and headache products—is frequently recommended to manage the pain associated with arthritis.

HIGHER DOSE, GREATER RISK

After studying almost 50,000 arthritis patients, half of whom were taking acetaminophen, "we saw that there really is a difference," Rahme says.

"At the low dose of acetaminophen, GI events are much lower than in the NSAID group, but when you go to 2,600 milligrams [mg] a day and higher, there were similar rates of GI events," reports Rahme.

Rahme says the rate of stomach and intestinal troubles approximately doubled between the lowest dose (less than 650 mg per day) of acetaminophen and the highest dose (more than 3,250 mg daily).

The researchers started to see side effects at the equivalent of eight regular-strength or five extra-strength tablets a day.

Rahme says there are some limitations to the study. For example, there may have been a slight bias toward having GI problems because the patients included in the study were older and often on more than one medication. Many had already been on either acetaminophen or NSAID therapy. Rahme says the researchers tried to control for these variables and still saw more GI problems in patients on high doses of acetaminophen.

Dr. John Klippel, medical director of the Arthritis Foundation, wasn't surprised by the results of this study, but says that acetaminophen will probably remain the first line of treatment for many patients because it's cost-effective and still considered quite safe in low doses.

He cautions that consumers should check the label of any over-the-counter medication they are taking to be sure they're not getting extra doses of acetaminophen because it's contained in a lot of cold and headache preparations.

■ ■ ■ ■

Painkiller Risk

Combining painkillers can be dangerous. Patients regularly taking an over-the-counter nonsteroidal anti-inflammatory drug (NSAID), such as *ibuprofen* (Advil), and aspirin in the same day had two to three times the risk for ulcers and gastrointestinal (GI) bleeding as those who took either alone.

Theory: Acidity in the GI tract reaches more harmful levels when the common painkillers are combined.

If you must take multiple painkillers: Ask your physician about adding a proton pump inhibitor (PPI), such as *lansoprazole* (Prevacid), to reduce stomach acid.

Joseph Biskupiak, PhD, research associate professor, department of pharmacotherapy, University of Utah, Salt Lake City.

Aspirin Lowers Asthma Risk for Older Women

Tobias Kurth, MD, ScD, associate epidemiologist, Brigham and Women's Hospital, and assistant professor, medicine, Harvard Medical School, Boston.
Len Horovitz, MD, pulmonary specialist, Lenox Hill Hospital, New York City.
Thorax.

Taking a small dose of aspirin every other day seems to reduce the risk of developing asthma among older women, according to a recent study in an on-line issue of the *Thorax* journal. The findings essentially mirror a similar study in which men taking aspirin saw the same reduced risk.

BACKGROUND

The incidence of asthma is on the increase, possibly due to obesity, dietary factors, exposure to allergens and environmental factors. But the trend also coincides with a decreased use of aspirin as people have switched to other over-the-counter pain relievers.

That led some researchers to wonder whether the reduction in aspirin use was contributing to the rise of asthma.

THE STUDY

This premier randomized trial in women looked at nearly 40,000 healthy professionals, ages 45 and older, who were participating in the Women's Health Study. These women received either 100 milligrams (mg) of aspirin every other day or a placebo. This dose was much lower than that taken by men in a previous study (325 mg).

Over the next decade, there were 10% fewer new cases of asthma in the women who had been taking aspirin regularly. Yet aspirin had no effect in women who were obese, perhaps due to the low dose. Furthermore, the effect of the regular aspirin dose in non-obese women was smaller than that seen in men (they saw a 22% risk reduction), but that may be at least partly attributable to the lower dose as well.

IMPLICATIONS

Authors warned that the research was still not strong enough to recommend taking aspirin regularly for primary prevention of adult-onset asthma. Interestingly, aspirin can exacerbate symptoms in 4% to 11% of people who have already been diagnosed with the condition.

It's not clear exactly why aspirin has this effect. However, for the many older adults already taking aspirin for its salutary effects on heart health, this could be an added benefit.

The Secret Cause Of Asthma?

R. Graham Barr, MD, DrPH, assistant professor of medicine and epidemiology, Columbia University, New York City.

Susan Redline, MD, professor of pediatrics, University Hospitals, Rainbow Babies and Children's Hospital, Cleveland.

American Journal of Respiratory and Critical Care Medicine.

Frequent use of the popular painkiller *acetaminophen* may increase a person's risk for developing asthma, a study says. But experts caution that it's far too early to tell consumers to avoid it.

Women who were taking acetaminophen at least 15 days a month for six years had a 63% higher risk of developing asthma compared with women who didn't use the analgesic, according to researchers.

Individual reactions to pain relievers vary. "We are not trying to say that all asthmatics should stop using acetaminophen," says study author Dr. R. Graham Barr, assistant professor of medicine and epidemiology at Columbia University.

Soaring rates of asthma across the United States have alarmed public health officials and puzzled asthma experts.

Scientists estimate that in the past 30 years, asthma cases approximately doubled in younger children, says Dr. Susan Redline, an asthma expert at Rainbow Babies and Children's Hospital in Cleveland.

However, the exact cause of this steep climb remains unclear.

Rising rates of obesity—which can impair lung function—have been cited by experts as a possible culprit, as have indoor pollutants, such as dust mites and mold.

But the upswing in new asthma cases also coincided with the increasing popularity of over-the-counter acetaminophen, the researchers say. According to the American Medical Association, approximately 200 over-the-counter drugs contain acetaminophen.

THE STUDY

In their study, Barr and his colleagues examined data from the Nurses Health Study, which included nearly 122,000 adult women. As part of the study, each participant kept a record of her analgesic use, as well as the development of any new medical conditions, including asthma.

Among women who used acetaminophen for more than half of the days in a given month, "there was a significant increase—63%—in the risk of a new diagnosis of asthma," Barr says.

POSSIBLE EXPLANATION

Scientists know that acetaminophen lowers blood levels of a natural compound called *glutathione*. "Glutathione has an antioxidant effect in the body, particularly in the lungs," Barr explains. When glutathione levels plummet, "that may reduce the antioxidant defenses in the body and increase the possibility of developing asthma."

However, the study only demonstrates an association between acetaminophen and increased asthma—not a cause-and-effect relationship. And Barr notes that other analgesics such as aspirin, ibuprofen and nonsteroidal anti-inflammatory drugs (NSAIDs), such as *celexicob* (Celebrex), have also been shown to affect asthmatics in various ways.

"If individuals happen to notice that their asthma gets worse after they take aspirin or nonsteroidals or acetaminophen, it's worth reassessing that usage," Barr says. "But we're not making any blanket statements."

For information on controlling asthma symptoms, visit the Asthma and Allergy Foundation of America at *www.aafa.org*.

■ ■ ■ ■

OTC Risks

Acetaminophen may be a contributing cause of hypertension.

Recent finding: Women who take a daily dose of more than 500 milligrams of the aspirin-free painkiller—the equivalent of one extra-strength Tylenol—have double the risk of developing high blood pressure within three years. *Ibuprofen* (Advil and Motrin) and *naproxen* (Aleve) have been linked to hypertension, but until recently, acetaminophen was considered safe.

Best: Monitor blood pressure if you are taking these drugs.

Christie Ballantyne, MD, professor, department of medicine, and associate chief, atherosclerosis and lipoprotein section, Baylor College of Medicine, Houston.

Aromatherapy for Everyday Ailments

Jane Buckle, RN, PhD, director, RJ Buckle Associates LLC, Hunter, New York.

W hen you hear the word "aromatherapy," you probably think of a scented bath or a fragrant candle.

But medical practitioners in the United States and around the world are using distilled oils of aromatic plants medicinally. Essential oils activate the *parasympathetic nervous system*, causing relaxation, which speeds healing.

AROMATHERAPY IN ACTION

Plant oils can be used in a warm bath…in a "carrier oil"—such as almond or sesame oil—for massage…or in a lotion.

The oil aromas can also be sniffed from a bottle…a cotton ball…or a *diffuser*—a machine that emits the aroma into the air.

Clinical and scientific studies support the use of aromatherapy as an adjunct to medical care for treating…

•**Anxiety.** Essential oils that were inhaled for three minutes relieved anxiety in men and women, according to research published in the *International Journal of Neuroscience.* Use rosemary, Roman chamomile or patchouli.

Typical treatment: Sniff one to three drops when anxious.

Caution: Avoid using rosemary if you have high blood pressure.

•**Bronchitis.** Use spike lavender.

Typical treatment: One drop of spike lavender in a bowl of three cups of boiling water. Drape a towel over your head, close your eyes and inhale the steam. Do this for five minutes, four times a day.

•**Hair loss.** In people with patchy hair loss due to *alopecia areata*, essential oils helped restore hair growth, notes an *Archives of Dermatology* study that used a jojoba and grapeseed carrier oil (3 mL to 20 mL respectively) containing a mixture of thyme (two drops), rosemary (three drops), lavender (three drops) and cedarwood (two drops).

Typical treatment: Massage the mixture into the scalp for two minutes daily.

•**Headache.** Use peppermint. If pain isn't gone in five minutes, try Roman chamomile or true lavender.

Typical treatment: Five drops in one teaspoon of carrier oil. Apply to temples or sniff.

•**Hot flashes.** Use clary sage, fennel, geranium or rose.

Typical treatment: Ten drops in two cups of water in a spray bottle. Spray on face during hot flash.

•**Insomnia.** Use ylang ylang, neroli or rose.

Typical treatment: Five drops in a diffuser placed in the bedroom.

•**Lower-back pain.** Use lemongrass. If you feel no relief in 20 minutes, try rosemary or spike lavender.

Typical treatment: Five drops in one teaspoon of carrier oil. Apply to the painful area every three hours.

•**Menstrual cramps.** Use geranium.

Typical treatment: Five drops added to one teaspoon of carrier oil. Rub on the lower abdomen and lower back every three hours.

•**Muscle spasms.** Use clary sage, sage or try lavender.

Typical treatment: Five drops added to one teaspoon of carrier oil. Apply to the affected muscles at least every three hours.

•**Osteoarthritis.** Use frankincense, rosemary or true lavender.

Typical treatment: Five drops added to one teaspoon of carrier oil. Apply to the painful area every three hours.

WHAT TO BUY

Aromatherapy is most effective when the essential oils are prepared with no extraneous ingredients.

Good brands include Scents & Scentsibility (*www.scentsibility.com*). They are also available in health-food stores.

USING AROMATHERAPY SAFELY

Some essential oils can irritate or burn skin if applied undiluted. Always dilute oils before using topically. If skin stings or becomes red, dilute with a plain carrier oil and wash with unperfumed soap.

Essential oils are flammable. Store them away from candles, fires, cigarettes and stoves. Don't pour oil on lightbulbs to scent a room.

Caution: Essential oils can be lethal if they are ingested—even in tiny doses. Keep away from children and pets. People with asthma or epilepsy and pregnant women should consult their doctors before using aromatherapy.

Vitamin C May Help Block Ulcers

Joel A. Simon, MD, MPH, FACN, associate professor of clinical medicine and epidemiology, University of California, San Francisco, School of Medicine, and staff physician, San Francisco Veterans Affairs Medical Center.

James Everhart, MD, chief, epidemiology and clinical trials branch, division of digestive diseases and nutrition, National Institute of Diabetes & Digestive & Kidney Diseases, National Institutes of Health, Bethesda, Maryland.

Journal of the American College of Nutrition.

P eople who consume large amounts of vitamin C to try to protect themselves from colds might also be defending their stomach and intestines against ulcers.

The higher a person's blood levels of ascorbic acid, another name for vitamin C, the lower their risk of gastrointestinal trouble, according to a study.

"We are not the first to show this," admits Dr. Joel A. Simon, an associate professor of clinical medicine and epidemiology at the University of California, San Francisco, School of Medicine and a staff physician at the San Francisco Veterans Affairs Medical Center. "But it could be the largest study" so far.

THE STUDY

Simon and his team of researchers examined the Third National Health and Nutrition Examination Survey (NHANES III) and discovered that almost one-third of the 6,746 adults who were evaluated had antibodies against *Helicobacter pylori*. This strain of bacteria is now believed to cause most peptic ulcers.

Chronic infection with *H. pylori* is an important risk factor, Simon notes, for both peptic ulcer problems and gastric cancer.

Researchers found that higher blood levels of ascorbic acid in the people studied were associated with lower rates of H. pylori infection, Simon says.

After the researchers accounted for factors that might affect the relationship, including age and body mass index, they still found that the subjects with the highest blood levels of ascorbic acid had a 25% lower risk of having the infection.

When the researchers looked at infection with especially virulent strains of H. pylori, there was a 69% lower risk for those with higher blood levels of ascorbic acid.

NO CAUSE-EFFECT LINK DISCOVERED YET...

Simon does not know why vitamin C may work, although animal studies have found that ascorbic acid inhibits the growth of H. pylori.

If there is a true association, he says, higher intakes of vitamin C might help prevent infection and, in turn, ulcers. Simon's study was supported by a donation from Roche Vitamins Inc. and a Public Health Service grant.

"It's an interesting finding," says Dr. James Everhart, chief of the epidemiology and clinical trials branch of the division of digestive diseases and nutrition at the National Institute of Diabetes & Digestive & Kidney Diseases.

"But I think the results were not terribly strong." And it still doesn't prove cause and effect, he adds.

Every year, there are as many as 500,000 new cases of peptic ulcer disease in the United States, according to the American Gastroenterological Association.

In addition to infection, many ulcers are the result of irritation from nonsteroidal anti-inflammatory drugs (NSAIDs), such as aspirin and ibuprofen.

Contrary to popular belief, ulcers are not caused by eating spicy food.

For information on H. pylori and ulcers, visit the National Digestive Diseases Information Clearinghouse at *http://digestive.niddk.nih.gov.*

■■■■

Alarming Tylenol Danger

Accidental poisonings from *acetaminophen* (Tylenol) are rising. Acetaminophen is one of the safest painkillers when taken in the correct dose, but it can cause serious—even fatal—liver damage when dosing directions aren't followed. Adults should take no more than 4,000 milligrams (mg) of acetaminophen a day (the equivalent of eight extra-strength Tylenol pills). It's easy to exceed the maximum when you're feeling under the weather and perhaps using multiple products with acetaminophen without realizing it.

Example: 650 mg of acetaminophen every 4 hours from Tylenol Cold Multi-Symptom Severe, 250 mg per dose from Excedrin Extra Strength and another 500 mg from NyQuil Cold/Flu at bedtime can put you well above the 4,000 mg/day limit.

Caution: Some prescription drugs contain acetaminophen.

Examples: Percocet contains 325 mg per pill...Vicodin ES contains 750 mg.

Anne Larson, MD, associate professor of medicine and director, hepatology clinic, University of Washington Medical Center, Seattle.

Melatonin Reduces Blood Pressure

Mark A. Stengler, ND, naturopathic physician in private practice, La Jolla, California...adjunct associate clinical professor at the National College of Natural Medicine, Portland, Oregon...author of many books, including *The Natural Physician's Healing Therapies* and coauthor of *Prescription for Natural Cures* (both from Bottom Line Books)...and author of the *Bottom Line/Natural Healing* newsletter.

A study of melatonin involved 18 women, ages 47 to 63, half with hypertension being successfully controlled with ACE inhibitor medication and half who had normal blood pressure.

For three weeks, participants took either 3 mg of time-released melatonin (a supplement typically used to promote sleep) or a placebo one hour before bed. They were then switched to the other treatment for another three weeks. After taking melatonin for three weeks, 84% of the women had at least a 10 mm/Hg decrease in nocturnal (nighttime) systolic and diastolic blood pressure, while only 39% experienced a decrease in nocturnal blood pressure after taking the placebo. The reduction was the greatest in those with controlled hypertension. In both groups, no change was found in daytime blood pressure readings. Previous studies have found similar results when men with untreated hypertension took melatonin.

My view: Melatonin, a hormone produced by the pineal gland in the brain, is secreted in response to darkness and promotes a normal sleep cycle. A deficiency of melatonin may prevent relaxation of the cardiovascular and nervous systems, increasing blood pressure. (Normally, heart rate and blood vessel constriction decrease at night.) While people with hypertension often monitor their daytime blood pressure, they usually are unaware of their readings at night. This can be a mistake. High nighttime blood pressure is just as important as high daytime pressure.

For people with high blood pressure whose levels also tend to be elevated at night, I recommend taking 3 mg of time-released melatonin one hour before bed. To try to determine if you have elevated blood pressure at night, you can use a home blood pressure monitor to test levels several times during the day and twice a night (at midnight and 4:00 am) for three days.

Caution: Bear in mind that waking yourself might be enough to raise your reading. Consult your doctor before trying melatonin or making other decisions based on self-testing. Any new regimen may require an adjustment to your blood pressure medication. Women who are pregnant or breastfeeding, as well as those taking birth control pills, should not use melatonin.

■ **More from Mark A. Stengler...**

The Truth About Vitamin E

For more than 30 years, vitamin E has been one of the most widely used supplements. It's been touted as a key antioxidant, helping to prevent heart disease, certain cancers and other serious illnesses. But a few years ago, vitamin E became quite controversial, because some studies showed that it could be harmful. So it left many people wondering, *Is vitamin E safe? Is it effective? For what conditions? And what type of vitamin E should one use?*

Vitamin E is found naturally in wheat germ, nuts, seeds, whole grains, egg yolks and leafy, green vegetables. Animal products are a poor source of vitamin E. The recommended dietary allowance for vitamin E is 15 mg, or approximately 22 international units (IU), per day. Serious vitamin E deficiency is rare, although many Americans don't get enough of the vitamin. People on low-fat diets are susceptible to low vitamin E levels, because fat is needed for absorption of vitamin E. And people with the genetic condition cystic fibrosis have trouble absorbing vitamin E.

Vitamin E has been shown to be important as a supplement for people with specific diseases, such as Alzheimer's and diabetes, and those with a high susceptibility to certain conditions, such as bladder cancer and eye disease. Vitamin E prevents LDL "bad" cholesterol from becoming oxidized (damaged), thereby helping to guard against plaque formation in the arteries, known as atherosclerosis. Also, low vitamin E levels are associated with an increased risk of major depression, rheumatoid arthritis and preeclampsia

(a condition during pregnancy characterized by high blood pressure and swelling of the hands and face).

CONTROVERSIAL STUDIES

Two well-publicized studies have raised questions about vitamin E. The first was a meta-analysis (a study of other studies) led by researchers from the Johns Hopkins School of Medicine. The researchers reviewed 19 vitamin E studies that followed almost 136,000 patients. Most of these studies targeted populations at high risk for a chronic disease, usually coronary heart disease. The meta-analysis found that those taking 400 IU or more of vitamin E daily for at least one year were 10% more likely to die from all causes than those who took a smaller dose.

There are several problems with this analysis. First, researchers combined data that used both natural supplements (which provide the same type of vitamin E as that found in food) and synthetic forms of supplemental vitamin E. Previous research has shown that natural forms of vitamin E are better utilized by the body than cheaper, synthetic forms.

The biggest criticism of the meta-analysis was that most of the studies included elderly people who had existing health problems such as cancer, Alzheimer's disease, heart disease and other potentially fatal illnesses.

Another study, which was published in the *Journal of the American Medical Association*, focused on patients age 55 or older with vascular disease or diabetes. The study concluded that for people with vascular disease or diabetes, long-term supplementation with natural vitamin E does not prevent cancer or cardiovascular events and may increase risk for heart failure. This study provides no evidence that vitamin E is unsafe for people who are healthy.

POSITIVE FINDINGS

Many studies exist that demonstrate both the safety and effectiveness of vitamin E (in natural and synthetic forms). *A few examples...*

•**A Harvard study of more than 80,000 healthy, female nurses** ages 34 to 59 found a 41% reduction in the risk of heart disease in those who had taken daily vitamin E supplements of 100 IU or more for at least two years.

•**A study of almost 40,000 male health professionals** ages 40 to 75 found that those who took daily vitamin E supplements of at least 100 IU for more than two years experienced a 37% lower risk of heart disease.

•**A National Institute on Aging study** focusing on 11,000 people between the ages of 67 and 105 found that those who used vitamins C and E supplements in various dosages had a 53% reduction in mortality from heart disease and a 42% reduction in death from all causes, compared with nonusers.

•**One study of moderate-severity Alzheimer's patients** conducted at Columbia University in New York City showed that a very high daily dose of vitamin E (2,000 IU) delayed the progression of Alzheimer's disease.

DIFFERENT TYPES

Vitamin E really refers to a family of compounds. There are more than 12 vitamin E compounds found in nature (currently eight forms are available in supplement form). There are two main groups of compounds—*tocopherols* (found in foods such as corn, soy and peanuts) and *tocotrienols* (found in rice, barley, rye and wheat). Many foods contain a blend of these two groups. Both have subgroups called *alpha, beta, gamma* and *delta*.

The most commonly used natural supplement form is *alpha-tocopherol*, and most studies have researched this form. But taking just alpha-tocopherol can reduce blood levels of gamma- and delta-tocopherols, which is not beneficial. Studies indicate that higher blood gamma-tocopherol levels correspond to the reduction of prostate cancer and coronary heart disease. Also, delta- and gamma-tocotrienols reduce the liver's production of cholesterol.

Barrie Tan, PhD, president of American River Nutrition, Inc., and former adjunct professor of food science at the University of Massachusetts, Amherst, is a specialist in the production and supplementation of vitamin E. He explains that 70% of (dietary) vitamin E consumed by North Americans is the gamma-tocopherol form due to the abundance of soy and corn in our diets. He believes that vitamin E supplements used for disease prevention should be a blend of both tocopherols and tocotrienols. I agree with this

view, because these forms are more similar to what we find in food.

One example of a full-spectrum vitamin E product that has a good ratio of tocopherols and tocotrienols is Now Foods' Tru-E BioComplex. To find a health-food store that sells this product, call 888-669-3663 or go to *www.nowfoods.com*. A good dosage for anyone, healthy or not, is 200 IU daily. Consult with your doctor before using dosages above 400 IU, especially if you are taking a blood-thinning medication, such as *warfarin* (Coumadin)—vitamin E can have a blood-thinning effect.

■ **Also from Mark A. Stengler...**

Alpha-Lipoic Acid A True Cure-All?

The nutritional supplement *alpha-lipoic acid* (ALA) is touted as a treatment for cancer, chronic fatigue syndrome, diabetes, glaucoma, HIV/AIDS and liver disease.

ALA was identified as a vitamin-like substance more than 50 years ago. It is produced in the cells of the body and also is found in small amounts in certain foods, such as broccoli, spinach, tomatoes, peas, Brussels sprouts and liver.

ALA is a unique antioxidant that neutralizes free radicals (potentially harmful negatively charged molecules). ALA is absorbed into water-soluble and fat-soluble tissues, thereby providing antioxidant protection to all cells of the body.

Another important feature of ALA is that it facilitates the regeneration of antioxidants. This is helpful because antioxidants become inactivated after neutralizing free radicals. ALA reactivates these antioxidants, including vitamins E and C, coenzyme Q10 and *glutathione,* a group of nutrients considered to be the most powerful of the antioxidant network.

THE SCIENTIFIC EVIDENCE

There is reliable research supporting the use of ALA in the treatment of type 2 diabetes. Daily supplementation with ALA has been shown to improve blood sugar (glucose) uptake by cells and insulin resistance (allowing insulin to transport glucose into cells more effectively) and reduce nerve damage and pain associated with diabetic neuropathy.

A four-week, placebo-controlled multicenter study measured the effects of ALA on insulin sensitivity (the ability of the body's cells to recognize and respond to insulin). Seventy-four patients with type 2 diabetes were randomized to receive either a placebo or 600 mg of ALA once, twice or three times daily. Blood glucose and insulin levels were measured before and at the end of the study. Those receiving ALA had a 25% improvement in insulin sensitivity after the four weeks of treatment. All three doses of ALA had the same effect.

There is additional research showing that ALA at doses of 600 mg to 1,200 mg daily is helpful in alleviating diabetic neuropathy, a condition in which nerve damage causes pain, burning or numbness, especially in the lower legs and feet. Improvement with ALA can take three to five weeks.

In one Russian study, nearly half of glaucoma patients who took 150 mg of ALA daily for one month experienced improved vision. It is thought that the antioxidant properties of ALA improve the health of eye tissue and help the vision of people with glaucoma.

DOSAGE

For the treatment of type 2 diabetes and diabetic neuropathy, I recommend taking 600 mg to 1,200 mg of ALA daily. For glaucoma, cancer, chronic fatigue syndrome and liver disease, I recommend 300 mg to 1,200 mg of ALA daily. Its antioxidant and blood sugar–regulating properties support better immune function as well as energy production. ALA also can be taken at a dosage of 50 mg to 100 mg daily by anyone who wants to benefit from its immune-boosting property.

For optimal absorption, take supplemental ALA on an empty stomach. There are two main supplemental forms of ALA. The R form is found in plants and animals. The S form is a synthetic version. Recent data has found the R form to be more active in the body than the S form. I recommend taking the R form, which is commonly available in tablets at health-food stores. Side effects, including skin rash and digestive upset, are rare.

The Case Against Vitamins

Robert M. Russell, MD, director and senior scientist at Jean Mayer USDA Human Nutrition Research Center on Aging at Tufts University, Boston, is former chairman of the Institute of Medicine's Food and Nutrition Board.

At least half of American adults take vitamins and other supplements regularly, spending more than $23 billion a year on these nutritional aids in the belief that supplements can help prevent disease and improve health. However, evidence suggests that many supplements may be ineffective—and, in large doses, some may even do more harm than good.

Here's what you need to know now…

MULTIVITAMINS

According to a report by a panel of advisers at the National Institutes of Health, there is not enough evidence to recommend the use of multivitamin and mineral supplements to prevent chronic disease. And most people taking multivitamins don't really need them.

Reason: These individuals tend to be health conscious anyway, getting important nutrients from the food they eat.

There are, however, some people who do need supplements…

•**Anyone who eats fewer than 1,500 calories per day** should take a daily multivitamin that contains 100% of the Recommended Dietary Allowance (RDA) of all key nutrients.

•**Women who are trying to conceive** and those who are in the first trimester of pregnancy should take a daily prenatal multivitamin—which has 400 micrograms (mcg) of folic acid. Folic acid has been shown to reduce the risk of birth defects.

•**People over age 50** should take a B-12 supplement or a multivitamin containing at least the RDA of 2.4 mcg of B-12 if they don't get that amount in fortified foods, such as cereals. That's because as people age, the stomach produces less acid to digest food, making it difficult to absorb B-12 from food.

•**Those over age 70** have trouble getting enough calcium and vitamin D from food.

Example: To get the recommended amount of calcium, they would have to drink a quart of milk a day. People in this age group should have at least 600 international units (IUs) of vitamin D (15 mcg) and 1,200 milligrams (mg) of calcium a day.

MEGADOSES

The real concern is with the millions of Americans who consume nutrient-specific supplements in dosages that far exceed the RDAs.

Examples: Many people take vitamin C pills in hopes of boosting immunity and preventing colds...vitamins B and E to protect their hearts...beta-carotene and other antioxidants to help fight cancer.

Below are common supplements and the possible health problems that may result from taking high doses...

•**Vitamin E.** Although this antioxidant has been touted to improve heart health, recent "gold-standard" studies—randomized trials in which participants who are not aware of whether or not they are taking a supplement or a placebo are carefully tracked—show the opposite may be true. One meta-analysis, led by researchers from the Johns Hopkins School of Medicine, analyzed 19 previous trials involving almost 136,000 people and found that vitamin E supplements—especially in the often-sold daily dosage of 400 IUs—caused a slight increase in death from heart attack. In another study of 9,500 people, those who took vitamin E had a 13% higher risk of heart failure.

Another danger: Vitamin E supplements could interfere with chemotherapy or radiotherapy by suppressing free-radical production, which is necessary to kill cancer cells.

•**B vitamins.** Until recently, the belief was that vitamins B-6, B-12 and folic acid reduced the risk of heart attack and stroke by lowering the level of *homocysteine* in the blood, a well-documented risk factor for coronary artery disease. However, one study published in *The New England Journal of Medicine*, which followed people who had had a heart attack, found that the risk of a second attack increased after taking B-vitamin supplements.

Another danger: In animal studies, high doses of B vitamins seemed to stimulate cancer

growth. There is no proof of this effect in humans, but there is a theoretical risk.

•**Vitamin C.** Contrary to popular wisdom, there's no credible evidence that vitamin C supplements help prevent colds, although they may shorten the duration by a day or so. For people who eat healthfully, supplementing with vitamin C does not seem to boost immunity.

Dangers: Vitamin C supplements raise the risk of kidney stones. As with vitamin E, vitamin C supplements should be avoided by cancer patients who are undergoing chemotherapy or radiotherapy.

•**Vitamin A and beta-carotene.** Vitamin A comes in two forms—as preformed vitamin A or as one of several carotenoids, of which beta-carotene is the best known. Both forms of vitamin A supplements have proved risky.

Beta-carotene supplements have been found to speed the risk of death from lung cancer and heart disease in people who smoke. More recently, a study of 75,000 people found that supplements of preformed vitamin A—as well as diets rich in vitamin A—increased the risk of hip fractures by 48%. This was observed with dosages just slightly above the RDAs of 900 mcg for men and 700 mcg for women.

Other dangers: Unless you are deficient in vitamin A—rare in the US—taking supplements containing more than 3,000 mcg (10,000 IUs) can cause liver damage. In pregnant women, high-dose vitamin A supplements may cause birth defects.

•**Glucosamine and chondroitin sulfate.** In a federally sponsored clinical trial, the often-used combination of glucosamine and chondroitin sulfate, once believed to reduce osteoarthritis knee pain by rebuilding cartilage, proved no more effective than a placebo for most of the 1,583 participants. Only a small group of patients with severe arthritis experienced slight relief.

Dangers: Mild gastrointestinal upset is a possible side effect. Theoretically, people with seafood allergies may be allergic to glucosamine, which is derived from shellfish.

•**Saw palmetto.** Although taken by millions of men with an enlarged prostate, the herb saw palmetto didn't relieve symptoms any better than a placebo in a well-respected randomized trial published in *The New England Journal of Medicine.*

Dangers: Saw palmetto should not be taken with blood thinners, such as aspirin or *warfarin* (Coumadin). Possible side effects of saw palmetto include stomach pain, nausea, diarrhea and impotence.

•**Zinc.** Another antioxidant nutrient, zinc was once believed to help boost immunity and prevent colds. However, in most studies, supplements seem to benefit only those with zinc deficiency, which is rare among Americans eating a balanced diet.

Danger: Zinc supplements lower the body's copper levels, which in turn may increase the risk of cardiac arrhythmia.

•**Copper.** In adequate amounts—the RDA of 0.9 mg—copper helps in the formation of red blood cells, nerve fibers and collagen for healthy skin and bones. It also acts as an antioxidant. However, in higher amounts, copper may work as a pro-oxidant, promoting free-radical damage that could contribute to Alzheimer's disease—especially in people who eat a high-fat diet.

In a six-year study of 3,718 people whose average age was 75, published in *Archives of Neurology,* the rate of memory loss and other cognitive decline was equivalent to 19 years of aging in those who consumed 2.75 mg of copper per day—levels found in some multivitamins—and ate a diet rich in saturated and trans fats. However, copper intake wasn't associated with mental decline in people who ate low-fat diets.

Another danger: The risk of liver damage occurs with dosages above 10 mg a day.

THE BOTTOM LINE

Although high levels of certain nutrients help prevent disease and improve health, the benefit typically comes from diets rich in those vitamins and minerals. Foods also contain health-protecting *phytochemicals*—some of which have not yet been identified—and these substances are not in supplements.

The old advice still is best—eat a healthful, well-balanced diet to meet the RDAs of necessary nutrients.

■■■■

Smart Vitamin Buying

To get the most health benefit at the lowest cost from multivitamin supplements…

•**Avoid buying "mega-dose" supplements.** They provide far more than 100% of the recommended daily allowance (RDA) for vitamins, antioxidants and minerals. Such doses provide no benefit and might prove harmful.

•**Buy a basic multisupplement.** It should provide 100% of the RDA for a large number of vitamins and minerals—a "seniors' formula" containing an extra amount of vitamin B-12 and lesser amount of iron is fine.

•**Shop by price.** Generic and store brands are just as good as higher-priced name brands, and tablets are as good as capsules.

•**Look for "USP" on the label.** This indicates that the product meets United States Pharmacopeia quality standards.

•**Avoid vitamin combinations that contain herbs, enzymes and hormones.** The benefit of these is unproven and they could be harmful.

•**Don't pay more for unneeded features.**
Examples: All natural…timed release…stress formula…starch free…chelated (to promote absorption). They add no value.

Simeon Margolis, MD, PhD, medical editor, *The Johns Hopkins Medical Letter: Health After 50.* University Health Publishing.

What Supplement Makers Don't Want You to Know

James N. Dillard, MD, DC, former assistant clinical professor at Columbia University College of Physicians and Surgeons and past medical director of Columbia's Rosenthal Center for Complementary and Alternative Medicine, both in New York City. He is now in private practice in New York City and Stamford, Connecticut.

Samantha Heller, MS, RD, nutritionist, has appeared frequently on radio and TV and practices in Fairfield, Connecticut.

More is not better when it comes to the ingredients in your vitamin supplement. When a multivitamin pill is packed with extra nutrients or herbs along with vitamins and minerals, it's not the bargain you think it is, says Dr. James Dillard, a former clinical medical adviser at the Rosenthal Center for Complementary and Alternative Medicine at Columbia University.

Why? A tablet or capsule can only hold so much, and the more ingredients in a single pill, the less of each ingredient you can have; sometimes pills have so little of each nutrient, they are hardly worth taking, he says.

That can hurt if you think you're protecting yourself, especially if you're a woman who needs extra calcium, says registered dietician Samantha Heller.

"Calcium should always be taken as a separate supplement, as they simply can't fit all a woman's needs into one multivitamin pill," says Heller.

TOO MUCH OF A GOOD THING

Vitamin supplements with nutrient levels that soar above the recommended daily amounts (RDA) can also cause problems, increasing the risk of such side effects as diarrhea and nausea, Heller says.

Too much vitamin A and D, for example, can be toxic, she notes. A vitamin supplement can even make you feel ill.

According to Dillard, nuances in the way vitamins are made, or even the source of the nutrients themselves, can affect the way you react to any specific supplement. That can result in everything from dizziness to headaches, fatigue, hives or other allergic reactions.

"If you take a vitamin supplement and don't feel well, switch brands," Dillard says.

But which brand should you take? Many experts say that the bigger, more experienced companies are more likely to give you a higher-quality product.

Also important is a product with no sugars, starches, binders or fillers.

THE DISSOLVE FACTOR

Another key concern is getting the nutrients into your bloodstream, a goal that's often defeated when supplements are made with a hard-shell coating.

"If we X-ray someone's stomach, we can often see dark shadows indicating undissolved vitamin pills," Dillard says.

Look for products that carry the US Pharmacopeia seal of approval, usually noted as "USP Approved" on the label. This means the product was tested by a government agency and will dissolve in a minimum amount of time.

Here's a home test suggested by Dillard to see how well your vitamin dissolves—mix equal parts water and vinegar in a glass and drop in your vitamin pill. Within 40 minutes, it should be well on its way to being dissolved. If it's not, he says, it's probably going to pass through your body undigested.

Finally, always check the expiration date before buying a vitamin supplement. If you don't find one, don't buy the product.

■ ■ ■ ■

Vitamin K Cuts Arthritis Risk

In a study of 672 adults, those who had the highest vitamin K levels were less likely to have osteoarthritis of the hands and knees than people who had the lowest levels.

Theory: Insufficient vitamin K could affect proteins that build and maintain bone and cartilage.

Self-defense: Get the recommended daily intake of vitamin K—65 micrograms (mcg) for women and 80 mcg for men.

Good sources: Spinach, broccoli and olive oil.

Caution: If you take a blood thinner, vitamin K can reduce the drug's effectiveness.

Tuhina Neogi, MD, assistant professor of medicine, Boston University School of Medicine.

Avoid Dangerous Herb-Drug Interactions

Catherine Ulbricht, PharmD, adjunct assistant professor at Massachusetts College of Pharmacy and Health Sciences, Boston, is editor-in-chief of *Journal of Herbal Pharmacotherapy* and cofounder of Natural Standard (*www.natural standard.com*), a Web site dedicated to the scientific study of integrated medicine.

An increasing number of American adults now take herbs or nutritional supplements for a wide range of ailments, including arthritis, depression and nausea.

Problem: Unlike prescription drugs, herbal supplements are not regulated by the FDA, so there are no labeling requirements regarding potential interactions with prescription or over-the-counter (OTC) drugs.

Whether they are used in capsules, extracts, liquid, cream or tea, many herbal products can be harmful when combined with prescription or OTC medication.

What happens: Some herbs can interact with medications by affecting their absorption, metabolism or by other mechanisms. As a result, drug levels and their effects may become too high or too low.

Catherine Ulbricht, PharmD, a professor at Massachusetts College of Pharmacy and Health Services, is an expert on herb-drug interactions. *Her advice on commonly used herbs...*

CAYENNE

Cayenne is also known as chili or red pepper. Cayenne's active component, capsaicin, which is used as a spice in food, is commonly used as a pain reliever in prescription medicine, often for osteoarthritis, rheumatoid arthritis and diabetic neuropathy (nerve pain resulting from diabetes).

Possible interactions: When combined with aspirin, *ibuprofen* (Advil) or any other nonsteroidal anti-inflammatory drug (NSAID), cayenne may increase these drugs' side effects, especially gastrointestinal (GI) upset. In some people, cayenne also may enhance the pain-relieving action of NSAIDs.

*Check with your doctor or pharmacist before taking any herbal product.

Like NSAIDs, cayenne can have a blood-thinning effect, increasing the risk for bleeding. (When used topically, this risk is lessened because lower doses of cayenne are absorbed.) Do not use cayenne if you take a monoamine oxidase (MAO) inhibitor antidepressant, such as *phenelzine* (Nardil).

Caution: Avoid getting cayenne (in any form) in your eyes, nose, etc., where it can cause burning or stinging.

GINGER

Ginger is a popular antidote for nausea and/or vomiting. Research suggests that ginger also may help prevent blood clotting and reduce blood sugar levels.

Possible interactions: If you take an NSAID or antiplatelet drug, such as *clopidogrel* (Plavix), ginger may further increase bleeding risk.

Caution: Although there's strong evidence that it is particularly effective for nausea and/or vomiting in pregnant women, high-dose supplemental ginger (more than 1 g daily) is not recommended during pregnancy because of possible fetal damage and/or increased bleeding risk. Because of the lack of long-term studies on ginger, consult your doctor before taking it for an extended period of time.

GREEN TEA

As scientific evidence has revealed the disease-fighting benefits of antioxidant-rich green tea, an increasing number of Americans have begun drinking it—or, in some cases, taking it in capsules or extracts. Although new research questions the health benefits of green tea, some studies have found that it may help prevent cancer, especially malignancies of the GI tract, breast and lung. More investigation is needed to confirm these findings. To read more about clinical trials on green tea, go to the National Institutes of Health's Web site, *www.clinicaltrials.gov*.

Possible interactions: Most forms of green tea contain caffeine, which may intensify the effect of any medication that increases blood pressure and/or heart rate, such as the decongestant *pseudoephedrine* (Sudafed). Decaffeinated green tea is available, but this form still contains some caffeine and may not have the same health benefits.

Caution: People with arrhythmia (abnormal heart rhythm) should consume no more than moderate amounts of green tea, determined by their personal sensitivity to caffeine.

LICORICE

Licorice contains a compound known as *glycyrrhizin*, which has antiviral properties. For this reason, licorice is often used to treat the common cold and herpes infections (including cold sores). However, some studies have found that topical licorice cream did not help genital herpes.

Possible interactions: Licorice can interact with diuretics, such as *chlorothiazide* (Diuril) and *furosemide* (Lasix), and any medication that affects hormone levels, such as birth control pills.

Caution: It also may increase blood pressure and bleeding risk.

MILK THISTLE

This popular herb is used for liver problems, including cirrhosis and hepatitis. These benefits are well documented by research.

Possible interactions: Milk thistle may interfere with how the liver breaks down certain drugs, such as antibiotics and antifungals. Milk thistle also may interact with the anticonvulsant *phenytoin* (Dilantin). The herb may lower blood sugar and cause heartburn, nausea and vomiting or other GI upset.

Caution: If you take diabetes medication, do not use milk thistle unless you are supervised by a health-care professional.

ST. JOHN'S WORT

St. John's wort is commonly used for depression. Several studies show that it may work as well as a prescription antidepressant, such as *paroxetine* (Paxil), for mild to moderate depressive disorders. More research is needed before St. John's wort can be recommended for severe depression.

Possible interactions: St. John's wort may interact with drugs that are broken down by the liver, including birth control pills, the blood thinner *warfarin* (Coumadin) and migraine medications. People who take St. John's wort may experience stomach upset, fatigue, sexual dysfunction, dizziness or headaches.

Caution: St. John's wort should not be taken with prescription antidepressant medication.

Healing Herbs: What the Scientific Evidence Says About Herbal Therapies

Mark Blumenthal, founder and executive director of the American Botanical Council (ABC).

It was headline news when *The New England Journal of Medicine* published a study that cast doubt on the effectiveness of echinacea. The message to the countless consumers spending more than $300 million annually on the purported cold-fighting herb? *Save your money.*

University of Virginia School of Medicine researchers had found echinacea to be no more effective than a placebo at combating cold and flu symptoms. But don't clear out your herbal medicine chest just yet.

What went largely unreported was that study participants received only 900 mg of echinacea daily—less than one-third of the dose recommended by the World Health Organization for combating upper-respiratory infections. That's akin to expecting one-third of a dose of aspirin to relieve a headache.

What's the other side of the story? Dozens of clinical studies point to echinacea's effectiveness, including a Canadian trial in which volunteers who took echinacea at the onset of colds experienced 23% milder, shorter symptoms, such as sore throat, stuffy nose, chills and headache, than those taking a placebo—a benefit that researchers linked to a marked increase in circulating white blood cells and other cells of the immune system.

More work is needed to identify the optimal echinacea species (supplements are commonly derived from *E. purpurea*, *E. pallida* or *E. augustifolia*) and the most potent plant parts (roots, stems, leaves or flowers).

Meanwhile, best results have been achieved by taking 3,000 mg daily of an echinacea product that combines one of the above-mentioned species and parts at the first sign of cold or flu until symptoms resolve.

Caution: If you're allergic to ragweed, avoid echinacea supplements derived from stems, leaves or flowers—they may contain pollen and trigger a reaction. Use an echinacea root supplement.

Five other herbs with scientific evidence on their side…

GARLIC

What it does: Helps prevent and possibly reverse arterial plaque buildup (atherosclerosis), a major risk factor for heart attack and stroke…reduces risk for stomach and colorectal cancers…and acts as a blood thinner to reduce the risk for blood clots.

Scientific evidence: In a recent German study, 152 patients with advanced atherosclerosis who took 900 mg daily of garlic powder for four years experienced a 3% decrease in existing arterial plaques in their neck (carotid) and thigh (femoral) arteries. Those taking a placebo experienced more than a 15% *increase* in arterial plaques.

Potential side effects: Bad breath and indigestion. Because garlic has a blood-thinning effect, it should not be used if you take aspirin regularly or an anticoagulant drug, such as *warfarin* (Coumadin). To minimize bleeding risk, ask your doctor about discontinuing garlic supplements at least one week before undergoing elective surgery.

Typical dose: One clove of fresh, minced garlic daily, or 200 mg to 300 mg of standardized garlic powder, taken in pill or tablet form, three times daily.

GINKGO*

What it does: Improves memory and concentration in people with early-stage dementia or Alzheimer's disease, as well as in healthy adults, by increasing blood flow to the brain. May also relieve tinnitus (ringing in the ears), vertigo and altitude sickness, as well as vascular problems such as intermittent claudication, a painful calf condition caused by decreased circulation to the legs.

Scientific evidence: An overwhelming majority of ginkgo trials have shown positive results. At least 33 randomized, controlled trials have shown this herb to enhance mental functioning or slow cognitive deterioration in older patients with dementia, while another 13 controlled studies have shown ginkgo to boost memory and cognitive performance in healthy adults.

*Check with your doctor or pharmacist before taking any herbal product.

Potential side effects: Stomach upset, headache, rash and/or dizziness. Like garlic, ginkgo should not be taken with aspirin or a prescription blood thinner such as warfarin. The herb was previously believed to increase the effects of monoamine oxidase inhibitor (MAOI) antidepressants, such as *phenelzine* (Nardil), but this has been refuted.

Typical dose: 120 mg daily. Nearly all positive ginkgo trials have used one of three formulations that are produced in Germany and sold in health-food stores in the US under the brand names Ginkoba by Ginsana/Pharmaton Natural Health Products…Ginkgold by Nature's Way…and Ginkai by Abkit Inc.

MILK THISTLE

What it does: Because of its strong antioxidant activity, milk thistle detoxifies the liver and may help regenerate liver cells. It may be appropriate for patients with alcohol-related liver damage or infectious or drug-induced hepatitis, as well as anyone who is regularly exposed to industrial pollutants.

Scientific evidence: At least 19 out of 21 clinical studies (a total of 2,200 people out of 2,400) have shown milk thistle to protect the liver against invasive toxins and possibly even stimulate the generation of new liver cells.

Potential side effect: Loose stools.

Typical dose: Take 140 mg of milk thistle three times daily.

SAW PALMETTO

What it does: Relieves the symptoms of benign prostatic hyperplasia (BPH), a noncancerous swelling of the prostate gland, which causes frequent and/or weak urination and is common in men over age 50.

Scientific evidence: In nearly two dozen clinical trials, saw palmetto has proven almost equal to prescription drugs, such as *finasteride* (Proscar) and *terazosin* (Hytrin), for relieving the symptoms of BPH. Unlike prescription prostate medications, which can cause side effects, including diminished libido, saw palmetto causes only minor adverse effects. Saw palmetto does not inhibit the production of prostate specific antigen (PSA), a protein that, when elevated, serves as an early warning for prostate cancer.

239

(Conventional BPH drugs suppress PSA, complicating prostate cancer screening.)

Potential side effects: Stomach upset or nausea if taken on an empty stomach.

Typical dose: 320 mg daily. It requires four to six weeks to take effect.

VALERIAN

What it does: The root combats insomnia and acts as a mild sedative to relieve anxiety or restlessness.

Scientific evidence: All of the nearly 30 clinical studies to date have shown the herb to be effective against insomnia and anxiety. In a German trial, taking 600 mg of valerian root extract daily proved as effective as the prescription tranquilizer *oxazepam* (Serax) for improving sleep quality, but with fewer side effects. Unlike prescription sleep aids, valerian isn't habit-forming, won't leave you feeling groggy the next morning and doesn't diminish alertness, reaction time or concentration.

Potential side effects: None known. It is best to avoid combining valerian with conventional sedatives, such as *diazepam* (Valium), since the herb may heighten the drug's sedating effects.

Typical dose: 2 g to 3 g of the dried crushed root, infused as a tea…or 400 mg to 800 mg in supplement form, taken one-half hour before bedtime.

Fish Oil for Heart Health

Laurence S. Sperling, MD, associate professor of medicine and founder of the section of preventive cardiology at Emory University School of Medicine in Atlanta, coauthored the paper, "Understanding Omega-3s," published in *American Heart Journal*.

Ever since scientists observed 30 years ago that Greenland's Eskimos, who subsist largely on fish, have appreciably lower rates of cardiovascular disease than nonfish eaters, the bulk of evidence has demonstrated that the omega-3 fatty acids found in fish may significantly lower the risk of developing heart problems.

Landmark study: In an Italian study involving 11,324 heart attack survivors, patients who took about 1 g of fish oil daily for three and a half years had a 30% lower risk of dying from cardiovascular disease and a 45% lower risk of having a sudden fatal heart attack. In 2000, the American Heart Association (AHA) began recommending omega-3 fatty acids to prevent heart attack and stroke.

WHAT ARE OMEGA-3s?

Omega-3 fatty acids are a kind of polyunsaturated fat found chiefly in cold-water fish, such as salmon, mackerel, lake trout, herring and sardines. The two main omega-3 types are called *eicosapentaenoic acid* (EPA) and *docosahexaenoic acid* (DHA). Another type of omega-3, called *alpha-linolenic acid* (ALA), is found in walnuts, flaxseed, soybeans and canola oil.

Studies suggest that omega-3s may protect the heart by reducing systemic inflammation, which can damage arteries and leave them susceptible to plaque buildup. Omega-3s also are believed to decrease the "stickiness" of blood platelets, lowering the risk for clots that can cause heart attack and/or stroke.

Other research indicates that omega-3s may fight mild to severe depression, as well as autoimmune disorders such as rheumatoid arthritis, psoriasis and Crohn's disease. Unfortunately, most of us just don't eat enough omega-3–rich fish to reap the benefits.

How much is enough? The AHA recommends that healthy adults consume at least two fish meals weekly to help reduce the risk for cardiovascular disease—and it urges those with existing heart disease to get 1 g of fish oil daily to prevent future attacks, preferably from fatty fish.

I suggest that patients at increased risk for cardiovascular disease—including those with diabetes or peripheral arterial disease (a condition in which blockages restrict blood circulation, mainly in arteries to the kidneys, stomach, arms, legs and feet)—also consume 1 g of fish oil daily. You can do this by eating three to six ounces of fish every day, but it's more practical for most people to take a fish oil supplement.

The advantages of taking a fish oil supplement include…

•**Consistency.** With a supplement, you generally know the amount of omega-3s you're getting. Independent testing by both *Consumer Reports* and ConsumerLab.com has shown that fish oil supplements by and large contain the levels of EPA and DHA cited on their labels. Of the dozens of products tested by these two watchdog groups, only one failed to provide the promised amount of omega-3s. (For a partial list of brands approved by ConsumerLab.com, see *www.consumerlab.com/results/omega3.asp.*) Fish, on the other hand, vary greatly in their omega-3 content. While 3.5 ounces of salmon, mackerel or bluefin tuna supply more than 1 g of EPA and DHA in total, the same amount of catfish, cod or canned light tuna provides almost none.

•**Safety.** Virtually all fish contain mercury, PCBs and dioxins. And, unfortunately, some of the best sources of omega-3s—including bluefin tuna and swordfish—also are among the fish with the most potential toxins. Fortunately, fish oil supplements appear to be generally contaminant-free. Of the 16 brands recently tested by *Consumer Reports* and the 41 tested by ConsumerLab.com, not a single product contained more than negligible levels of mercury, PCBs or harmful dioxins.

THE RIGHT SUPPLEMENT

You don't have to buy the most expensive fish oil supplement to get a quality product. Low-price store or discount brands, such as CVS and Puritan's Pride, are comparable in both quality and content to higher-priced name brands. A month's supply can cost as little as $14.

So what should you look for? *When choosing a product, consider the following guidelines (as indicated on the label and/or package insert)…*

•**It contains both EPA and DHA** (most provide both at a 1.5-to-1 ratio favoring EPA).

•**It is "molecularly distilled,"** a process used to separate the oils from any metals or other pollutants.

•**It is encapsulated under nitrogen** rather than oxygen—oxygen can turn the oils rancid, giving them a "fishy" taste and smell.

•**It is highly concentrated** to minimize the number of pills you'll need daily. Over-the-counter omega-3 supplements may contain from 30% to 90% fish oil.

•**It is approved by the US Pharmacopeia (USP),** the independent authority that sets quality standards for all US-manufactured pharmaceuticals and dietary supplements.

USING FISH OIL SAFELY

The FDA considers up to 3 g of fish oil daily to be generally safe. At or below this level, fish oil supplements are typically well-tolerated, though some people do experience gastrointestinal (GI) upset or an unpleasant "fishy" aftertaste, particularly when they first start taking them.

To minimize GI distress and the fishy aftertaste, divide the dose and take it with food twice a day. Freezing or refrigerating your fish oil supplements may minimize any stomach or intestinal symptoms, as well as any fishy aftertaste, and reduce or slow decomposition of the supplements. Fish oils, like all fats, will eventually deteriorate and turn rancid at room temperature.

Always check with your physician before beginning a supplement, particularly if you're taking any medication. If you're allergic to seafood or iodine (found in some fish and shellfish), do not take fish oil supplements. Get your omega-3s through ALA-rich foods or supplements. *In addition, fish oil may not be advisable for people who…*

•**Take a daily aspirin** or another antiplatelet or anticoagulant drug. Because fish oil has a blood-thinning effect, it theoretically could increase your chances of bleeding, though in nearly 150 studies so far this has not emerged as a side effect.

•**Have type 2 diabetes.** Some studies suggest that high-dose omega-3s may trigger short-term increases in blood sugar in people with type 2 diabetes. However, I routinely advise my patients with diabetes to take up to 1 g of fish oil daily to stave off cardiovascular disease, and most do well on this modest dose. A person with diabetes should take omega-3 fish oil only under a doctor's supervision.

•**Have elevated LDL** ("bad") cholesterol (above 70 mg/dL). There's evidence that taking omega-3s may actually increase LDL—possibly because they decrease triglycerides. Studies have shown that lowering triglycerides may increase LDL in some patients.

If, on the other hand, you have low LDL levels (below 70 mg/dL) and very high triglycerides (above 500 mg/dL), your doctor may suggest Lovaza, a new prescription drug that is a highly concentrated form of omega-3. It was just approved by the FDA to treat high triglyceride levels.

Studies show that 4 g of Lovaza daily may lower triglycerides by as much as 45%. Just be sure that your doctor routinely monitors your cholesterol and triglyceride levels while you're taking this or any omega-3 fish oil at doses exceeding 3 g daily.

The Omega-3 Solution—Fatty Acids Fight Heart Disease, Arthritis, Obesity and More

Andrew L. Stoll, MD, director of the psychopharmacology research laboratory at McLean Hospital, Harvard Medical School, both in Boston. He is the author of *The Omega-3 Connection*. Free Press.

In Japan and other nations where fish is a dietary staple, many disease rates are significantly lower than in Western countries.

Omega-3 fatty acids—lipid compounds that are a major constituent of fish oil—receive much of the credit for this difference.

Many people now take omega-3 supplements to reduce their risk for heart disease, rheumatoid arthritis, obesity and other health problems. But do omega-3s really deliver all these salutary effects?

Researcher Andrew L. Stoll, MD shares some facts…

• **Why are omega-3 fatty acids important?** Essential fatty acids are dietary constituents that promote good health.

In addition to omega-3, there's another essential fatty acid known as omega-6. For optimum health, we need to consume roughly the same amount of omega-3s and omega-6s.

But Americans eat small quantities of fish and even less omega-3-containing plants, such as flax and the salad green purslane. Instead, our diets are loaded with omega-6-rich oils—corn, sunflower and most oils in processed foods. We eat 10 to 20 times more omega-6s than omega-3s.

• **Why is this unhealthful?** Omega-3s contain *eicosapentaenoic acid* (EPA). When we consume this beneficial fat, much of it gets converted into *eicosanoids*, hormone-like substances that direct the inflammatory response and other functions within the immune system, heart and brain.

Omega-6s contain the fatty acid *arachidonic acid*. This substance also turns into eicosanoids—but with a critical difference.

Omega-6 eicosanoids are strongly inflammatory, while omega-3 eicosanoids are only mildly inflammatory or, in some cases, anti-inflammatory.

That's why balance is so important. Without it, uncontrolled inflammatory responses can damage virtually any organ system in the body.

• **How do omega-3s protect the heart?** By offsetting omega-6s, omega-3s reduce *atherosclerosis* (hardening of the arteries). Without omega-3s, omega-6s can inflame and damage coronary arteries, allowing plaque buildup.

Omega-3s also raise levels of high-density lipoprotein (HDL), which transports plaque-causing cholesterol out of the body.

EPA prevents blood platelets from sticking together, reducing the risk for clotting.

Omega-3s also help inhibit *arrhythmia* (erratic heartbeat), the leading factor in fatal heart attacks. Research shows that at least 1 g daily of omega-3s reduces a heart patient's risk for sudden death by 30%.

• **How do omega-3s help prevent obesity and diabetes?** Obesity is a diabetes risk factor. Omega-3s are the only fats that may actually promote weight loss, since they cause the body to burn calories. Plus, people who eat omega-3-rich foods or take supplements often report fewer cravings for other more fattening foods, such as ice cream, butter and cookies.

Omega-3s fight diabetes by making the body's insulin receptors more responsive. In adult-onset (type 2) diabetes, the body's insulin receptors fail. This can lead to a dangerously high level of blood sugar.

•**What about diseases of the immune system?** The highly inflammatory eicosanoids produced by omega-6s are great infection fighters. But when left unchecked by omega-3s, they can damage healthy tissue.

In the digestive disorder known as Crohn's disease, the gut becomes inflamed…in rheumatoid arthritis, it's the joints…in asthma, the airways are inflamed.

In a remarkable Italian study published in *The New England Journal of Medicine*, 60% of Crohn's patients who took 2.7 g of fish oil supplements daily went into remission for more than one year. No medication has proven to be more effective in treating Crohn's disease.

Studies also indicate that omega-3s reduce the inflammation of rheumatoid arthritis and asthma.

•**Do omega-3s help fight other diseases?** Research conducted at Brigham and Women's Hospital in Boston showed that omega-3s block abnormal brain cell signaling in patients with bipolar disorder (manic depression). Therefore, omega-3s can be a powerful adjunct in treating this illness.

Many bipolar patients who take the antidepressant *lithium* (Lithonate) and other mood stabilizers, such as *divalproex* (Depakote) and *lamotrigine* (Lamictal), improve initially but later relapse. Omega-3s can enhance the drug's effectiveness and may allow some people to reduce their dosage.

If you're on a mood stabilizer: Do not alter the dose without your doctor's approval. Stopping these medicines abruptly can make the illness worse.

•**How much omega-3 does a healthy person need?** To maintain health, 1 g to 2 g a day. But it's hard to get that much in food alone. You'd have to eat, say, a large salmon steak daily.

You should certainly try to eat more omega-3-rich foods, such as salmon, tuna, mackerel, sardines…wild game meats, including elk, buffalo and venison…flax…purslane…and walnuts. Add one to two servings a day of these foods to your diet. Still, you may not get enough omega-3s in dietary sources. To ensure adequate intake, take a daily 1 g to 2 g supplement.

•**How do I choose the right supplement?** Look for distilled fish oil capsules with an omega-3 concentration of 50% or more.

Quality supplements cost more, but they allow you to take fewer and smaller pills, without the fishy aftertaste you often get with other brands.

•**What do you recommend for vegetarians?** Flaxseed oil is a good option for strict vegetarians or people allergic to fish. Consume one-half tablespoon daily of this plant-based omega-3.

Some people take flaxseed oil straight. Others can't tolerate the strong taste. However, it's virtually imperceptible when used in waffle batter and other recipes.

•**Do omega-3 supplements have any side effects?** Omega-3s may inhibit blood clotting. If you're taking a blood thinner, such as *warfarin* (Coumadin), or aspirin, check with your doctor before taking omega-3 supplements.

Some people experience stomach upset, but this usually goes away within seven days. You'll be less likely to have this problem if you use a quality supplement…take it with food…and divide your daily intake among two or three equal doses.

By the way, it's a good idea to take vitamins C and E with omega-3s. These antioxidant vitamins scavenge disease-causing molecules known as "free radicals." Once free radicals are eliminated, omega-3s can do their job.

In addition to other benefits of vitamin C, your colds might not last as long. Discuss the proper dosages of vitamins C and E with your physician.

■ ■ ■ ■

Cough Help

Allergy medications soothe coughs better than over-the-counter (OTC) cough remedies, such as *guaifenesin*. OTC allergy medications, such as those that contain *diphenhydramine, chlorpheniramine* and *brompheniramine*, help to quiet a cough due to the common cold by drying the secretions in the back of the throat.

Downside: These allergy medications may cause drowsiness as well.

Also helpful for a cough: Pain relievers, such as Advil and Aleve—they may lessen the severity and frequency of the cough by inhibiting chemicals that cause inflammation.

Richard Irwin, MD, professor of medicine, University of Massachusetts Medical School, Worcester, and editor-in-chief of the American College of Chest Physicians' journal, *Chest*.

■■■■

Cold Help

Zinc cold remedies should be used cautiously. There is evidence that zinc can lessen a cold's severity, but zinc products should be used only two or three times a day, primarily in the first 48 hours after symptom onset—not every three hours, as indicated on labels. Do not use zinc lozenges and nasal spray—choose one. High concentrations of zinc can cause nausea and diarrhea.

Neil Schachter, MD, is professor of pulmonary medicine and medical director of the COPD Program, Mount Sinai School of Medicine, New York City.

■■■■

Hemorrhoid Relief

There are no dietary treatments that have been shown to consistently help or heal hemorrhoidal symptoms. In most cases, if a food causes a flare-up of symptoms, it is best to avoid that food. If you want to use topical medication, first try petroleum jelly—an inexpensive but often effective treatment. Over-the-counter (OTC) hemorrhoid medications typically contain emollients designed to facilitate easier passage of stool and protect the anal area. The best prescription hemorrhoid creams, such as Analpram-HC (2.5%) with *hydrocortisone*, contain topical steroids that decrease inflammation of the tissue overlying the hemorrhoidal veins and may reduce discomfort.

Caution: Symptoms of diseases, such as colon cancer and inflammatory bowel disease, can mimic hemorrhoidal symptoms. Rectal bleeding demands immediate attention. Consult a physician for an evaluation before beginning self-treatment.

Gary H. Hoffman, MD, attending surgeon, department of surgery, Cedars-Sinai Medical Center, Los Angeles.

Vitamin K—The Forgotten Vitamin

Sarah Booth, PhD, director of the Vitamin K Laboratory at the Jean Mayer USDA Human Nutrition and Research Center on Aging and a professor at the Gerald J. and Dorothy R. Friedman School of Nutrition Science and Policy, both at Tufts University in Boston. She has led or participated in more than 50 scientific studies on vitamin K.

Vitamin K is the first nutritional supplement that most Americans ever receive. That's because newborns routinely get a shot of the nutrient—which is crucial for *coagulation* (blood clotting)—to help prevent a severe and sometimes fatal bleeding disorder.

Researchers are now discovering that vitamin K provides a wide variety of health benefits that extend well beyond blood clotting.

VITAMIN K FOR BETTER HEALTH

Vitamins C and E tend to get the most media attention, but recent findings on vitamin K's ability to help curb the development and/or progression of certain common medical ailments are worth noting.

Examples...

•**Arthritis.** Research shows that low dietary intake of vitamin K may play a role in the development of osteoarthritis.

Scientific evidence: In a study published in the journal *Arthritis & Rheumatism*, higher blood levels of dietary vitamin K were associated with a lower risk for osteoarthritis of the hand and knee.

•**Heart disease.** Vitamin K aids the function of the biochemical *matrix Gla-protein,* which helps prevent calcium buildup in plaque-filled arteries.

Scientific evidence: Researchers in the Netherlands studied more than 4,800 people over age 55. Compared with those with the lowest intake of vitamin K, those with the highest intake were 52% less likely to have severe calcification of the aorta, the major artery leading from the heart. The participants were 57% less likely to die of heart disease.

• **Liver cancer.** Cirrhosis of the liver, which occurs when alcoholism or infection with the hepatitis B or C virus results in scarred, abnormal liver tissue, can lead to liver cancer.

Scientific evidence: Studies of animal and human cells show that vitamin K may help control the progression of liver cancer. For example, in a study published in the *Journal of the American Medical Association,* Japanese researchers divided 40 women with viral cirrhosis of the liver into two groups. One group received vitamin K daily...the other did not. Two of the women in the vitamin K group developed liver cancer, compared with nine in the non-vitamin K group.

• **Osteoporosis.** Vitamin K aids in the formation of *osteocalcin* (a protein that helps calcium bind to bone). This bone-strengthening process may help prevent and/or treat osteoporosis, the brittle-bone disease that afflicts more than 10 million older Americans—80% of them women.

Scientific evidence: Scientists at Harvard Medical School analyzed data on vitamin K intake and bone health in more than 70,000 women. Those with the highest dietary intake of vitamin K had a 30% decreased risk for hip fracture compared with those who had the lowest intake. Other studies show similar results for men.

In England, researchers analyzed data from 13 Japanese clinical trials that used large, pharmacological doses of vitamin K to treat osteoporosis. Overall, the vitamin reduced the rate of spinal fractures by 40% and hip fractures by 13%.

Latest development: Scientists at the University of Toronto, Tufts University and the University of Wisconsin have completed three clinical trials to determine whether vitamin K can prevent bone loss in postmenopausal women.

ARE YOU GETTING ENOUGH?

The US government's recommended daily intake for vitamin K is 90 micrograms (mcg) for adult women...and 120 mcg for adult men. That level is high enough to prevent vitamin K deficiency, a rare condition that can lead to impaired blood clotting.

But is it high enough to keep your blood, bones and heart healthy? That's a question nutritional scientists are asking—but haven't yet answered.

However, scientists *do* know an easy, natural way to maximize your intake of vitamin K. It comes down to the classic maternal advice—eat your vegetables.

Green vegetables—leafy and otherwise—are among the best dietary sources of vitamin K.

One-half cup of broccoli sautéed in olive oil gives you plenty of vitamin K. Or try a lettuce salad (using any type except iceberg) with a teaspoon of salad dressing that contains vegetable oil (some fat is needed for absorption of vitamin K). And don't worry about cooking—it doesn't destroy the vitamin.

Among vegetable oils, the richest sources of vitamin K (per two-tablespoon serving) are soybean oil (50 mcg) and olive oil (13 mcg).

Another good source: Mayonnaise (23 mcg).

Should you take a vitamin K supplement? Scientists don't have enough data at this point to recommend a dietary supplement of this nutrient for healthy adults.

IF YOU TAKE WARFARIN

Warfarin (Coumadin and Jantoven) is a widely used blood-thinning medication given to people who have had or are likely to develop an artery-blocking blood clot. Warfarin is often prescribed following a heart attack, stroke, blood clot in the leg (deep vein thrombosis) or a clot that has traveled to the lung (pulmonary embolism). The drug is also used in people who have an irregular heart rhythm (atrial fibrillation) or an artificial heart valve.

Warfarin works by decreasing the activity of vitamin K.

If you take warfarin: Don't eat dark, leafy green vegetables. The amount of vitamin K in these foods can vary threefold, depending on where they're grown. For example, a serving of spinach could contain 200 mcg of vitamin K...or 600 mcg. That's a significant difference in vitamin K intake for someone taking warfarin, who should not have large fluctuations in intake of this vitamin.

Instead, eat three daily servings of vitamin K–rich foods with lower but predictable amounts of the nutrient. That could include one-half cup of broccoli, one-half cup of green peas or six ounces of tomato juice. Other good choices of foods that contain relatively low amounts of vitamin K include asparagus and green beans.

To help determine the dose of warfarin that prevents blood cots from forming, doctors test the coagulation time—a measurement known as the International Normalized Ratio and Prothrombin Time (INR/PT). INR/PT is checked monthly, and the patient is instructed to maintain a consistent dietary intake of vitamin K to avoid altering the effectiveness of warfarin.

VITAMIN K IN VEGETABLES
(estimated micrograms, per one-half cup, cooked)

	mcg
Kale	530
Collard greens	500
Spinach	440
Beet greens	350
Swiss chard	290
Turnip greens	260
Brussels sprouts	190
Dandelion greens	100
Broccoli	75
Asparagus	45
Cabbage	36
Green peas	20
Green beans	10

Source: US Department of Agriculture

Vitamin D Prevents Cancer

Michael F. Holick, MD, PhD, director of the General Clinical Research Center and professor of medicine, physiology and biophysics at Boston University School of Medicine, and director of the Bone Healthcare Clinic and the Heliotherapy, Light, and Skin Research Center at Boston University Medical Center.

Grade school was probably where you learned about vitamin D—the "sunshine vitamin" that helps grow strong teeth and bones. A lot more has been learned about the vitamin since then. *Breakthrough research shows that it can help prevent cancer, high blood pressure, diabetes, multiple sclerosis and more…*

CANCER

Compared with Northeasterners, people in the Southwest have lower rates of more than a dozen cancers, including bladder, breast, colon, esophageal, gastric, kidney, lung, ovarian, pancreatic, prostate, rectal, stomach and uterine cancers and non-Hodgkin's lymphoma. What does the Southwest have that the Northeast doesn't? A lot more sunlight.

A form of vitamin D is made in the skin after sun exposure. Then it travels to the liver and kidneys for biochemical "morphing," becoming what scientists call active vitamin D.

Active vitamin D fights cancer by…

•**Slowing or stopping unregulated cell growth.**

•**Increasing the death rate of cancer cells.**

•**Reducing blood supply to tumors.**

RECENT STUDIES

Recent research supports the cancer-preventing power of vitamin D…

•**Colon cancer.** Researchers at the University of California, San Diego, analyzed five studies on colon cancer and vitamin D. People with the highest blood levels of vitamin D (a form known as *25-hydroxyvitaminD*) had a 50% lower risk of colon cancer (*American Journal of Preventive Medicine*).

•**Breast cancer.** The same researchers analyzed vitamin D levels and breast cancer rates in 1,760 women. Again, those with the highest levels of vitamin D had a 50% lower risk (*Journal of Steroid Biochemistry and Molecular Biology*).

•**Prostate cancer.** Researchers at Harvard Medical School analyzed data from an 18-year study of nearly 15,000 men. Those with the lowest levels of vitamin D had twice the risk of developing "aggressive" prostate cancer—fast-growing and often fatal (*PLoS Medicine*).

GOOD NEWS

Statistical analysis shows that increasing blood levels of vitamin D among Americans could result in 185,000 fewer cases of cancer every year and 30,000 fewer deaths.

Vitamin D also *treats* cancer. In two recent studies, men with metastatic prostate cancer given pharmaceutical doses of active vitamin D had positive responses, including up to 50% reduction in prostate specific antigen (PSA), a measure of the disease's activity. The FDA may approve a high-dose active vitamin D drug soon.

HIGH BLOOD PRESSURE

The farther you live from the equator, the greater your risk of high blood pressure—probably because you're exposed to less sunlight. Vitamin D may help keep blood pressure low by regulating the kidneys' production of *renin,* an enzyme that controls the relaxation and constriction of arteries.

Landmark study: Dr. Holick led a study at Boston University School of Medicine that divided people with high blood pressure into two groups. One group was exposed to vitamin D–creating UVB radiation in a tanning bed three times a week for three months, while the other was exposed to UVA radiation, which doesn't boost vitamin D. The UVB group had a 180% increase in blood levels of vitamin D and an average six-point drop in diastolic and systolic blood pressure—the same drop typically produced by pressure-lowering medications. The UVA group had no change in either vitamin D levels or blood pressure.

OSTEOPOROSIS

Low levels of vitamin D can cause and worsen osteoporosis—the bone-eroding disease that often leads to hip fractures. A recent study shows that approximately one in three elderly men and one in five elderly women with hip fractures die within one year.

More than half of women receiving therapy to prevent or treat osteoporosis have low blood levels of vitamin D.

New studies: Researchers from Wake Forest University School of Medicine studied 976 people over age 65. Those with the lowest blood levels of vitamin D had the worst balance and least strength (*Journal of Gerontology: Medical Sciences*).

Researchers from the Institute of Aging Research in Boston gave either vitamin D or a placebo to elderly residents of nursing homes. During the next five months, those receiving 800 international units (IU) of vitamin D a day had 72% fewer falls than those taking the placebo (*Journal of the American Geriatrics Society*).

MULTIPLE SCLEROSIS

Multiple sclerosis (MS) is a slowly developing autoimmune disease in which the body's immune system attacks the myelin sheaths that surround nerve fibers in the brain and spinal cord. Common symptoms are fatigue, poor balance, memory problems and depression. Scientists speculate that vitamin D helps fight MS by strengthening the immune system.

Recent studies: Researchers at Harvard School of Public Health found that veterans with the highest blood levels of vitamin D had a 62% lower risk of developing MS than those with the lowest levels (*The Journal of the American Medical Association*).

Australian researchers found that MS patients with the highest blood levels of vitamin D had the lowest levels of disability (*Journal of Neurology*).

DIABETES

In type 1 (juvenile) diabetes, the body's immune system attacks the insulin-secreting cells of the pancreas. A study found that Finnish children who were given vitamin D–rich cod-liver oil during their first year of life were 78% less likely to develop type 1 diabetes.

Vitamin D deficiency also has been linked to type 2 (adult-onset) diabetes, in which the body is resistant to the effects of insulin or does not produce enough insulin. There is evidence that active vitamin D increases insulin production.

HOW TO GET ENOUGH

Taking a daily vitamin D supplement (1,000 IU) is the easiest way to maintain healthy blood levels of vitamin D.

Other ways to boost vitamin D…

• **Food.** Milk, some orange juices and a few other foods are fortified with vitamin D.

Beware: A study shows that many cartons of milk contain less than 50% of the vitamin D listed on the label. Vitamin D–fortified orange juice, breakfast cereals and bread are more likely to contain the labeled amount.

●**Oily fish,** such as salmon, are generally rich in vitamin D.

Beware: Scientists at Boston University Medical Center found that farm-bred salmon have 25% less vitamin D than wild salmon, so choose wild salmon whenever possible.

●**Sun.** Vitamin D from sun exposure is highly variable, depending on the time of the day, season, latitude and your skin pigmentation. However, the rule of thumb is to spend 10 to 15 minutes, three to four times a week, in the sun without sunscreen on your arms, legs and hands. Never sun to the point of burning, and always protect your face with sunscreen or a hat.

●**Tanning bed.** Researchers at Boston University School of Medicine found that people who regularly used a tanning bed had average blood levels of vitamin D that were 90% higher than those who didn't. A tanning bed can be helpful in winter, when it's more difficult to get adequate sun exposure.

Caution: Limit use to approximately three to eight minutes, three or four times a week. After a month or two, once a week should be enough.

■ ■ ■ ■

Potent Anticancer Agent: Vitamin D

Vitamin D can drive down the mortality rates from 16 types of cancer, including breast and ovarian, by up to 70%. As a possible cancer preventive, be sure to get at least 1,000 IU of vitamin D-3 (cholecalciferol—not D-2, ergocalciferol, which is less effective) in summer and 2,000 IU in winter. For most people, it is best to take 1,500 IU daily in supplement form.

William B. Grant, PhD, founding director, Sunlight, Nutrition and Health Research Center, *www.sunarc.org.*

Other Benefits of Vitamin D

Mark A. Stengler, ND, naturopathic physician in private practice, La Jolla, California…adjunct associate clinical professor at the National College of Natural Medicine, Portland, Oregon…author of many books, including *The Natural Physician's Healing Therapies* and coauthor of *Prescription for Natural Cures* (both from Bottom Line Books)…and author of the *Bottom Line/Natural Healing* newsletter.

Vitamin D has long been appreciated for its ability to improve bone density by boosting calcium absorption. But now we're hearing that this nutrient offers many additional health benefits—and should be taken at dosages that for decades have been considered toxic. Is vitamin D a potentially dangerous fad, or does it deserve superstar status? *The facts…*

Of the five known forms of vitamin D molecules, two types are of primary importance. *Ergocalciferol* (vitamin D-2) is found in plants, including shiitake mushrooms, yeast and some sea vegetables and in fortified milk. *Cholecalciferol* (vitamin D-3) comes from animal sources, such as fatty fish and eggs laid by hens fed vitamin D (as most are). Also, when the sun's ultraviolet-B (UVB) rays penetrate the skin, a chemical reaction converts a substance in the skin into D-3.

In the small intestine, vitamin D promotes absorption of calcium and phosphorous. It also has a hormonelike effect, working with parathyroid hormone to maintain normal blood calcium levels.

New evidence suggests that vitamin D reduces the risk of 17 types of cancer by normalizing cell replication and activating tumor-fighting white blood cells. It also may combat the recurrence of certain cancers and improve survival rates among people who do get cancer. For instance, a 2007 analysis of five studies found that people with a vitamin D intake of at least 1,000 international units (IU) daily, or with vitamin D blood levels of at least 33 nanograms per milliliter (ng/ml), experienced a 50% lower risk of colorectal cancer.

Vitamin D supplementation may decrease the risk of type 1 diabetes, multiple sclerosis and rheumatoid arthritis…lower blood pressure and the risk of stroke…and reduce asthma attacks, tooth loss and musculoskeletal pain.

Surprising: In a Swiss study, seniors who supplemented daily with 800 IU of vitamin D-3 and 1,200 mg of calcium reduced their number of falls by 49%, perhaps due to increased knee strength.

Formerly, doctors cautioned against vitamin D supplementation above 600 IU, fearing a rise in blood calcium levels that could provoke heart, lung and even bone problems. However, the Harvard School of Public Health now recommends 1,000 to 2,000 IU daily for the general adult population.

For adults who are likely to have low vitamin D levels, the optimal dosage is 3,000 IU to 4,000 IU daily. This includes people who spend little time outdoors…live in northern climes…have dark skin (which absorbs less UVB radiation)… are obese (because subcutaneous fat impedes UVB penetration of the skin's deeper layers)… have arthritis or fibromyalgia (since a deficiency may contribute to chronic pain)…or are over age 65 (because their skin produces less of the vitamin D-3 precursor and their kidneys are less able to convert vitamin D into its active hormone form).

I recommend 200 IU daily, or up to 600 IU (under a doctor's supervision) for children with asthma.

Your doctor can order a blood test called *25-hydroxy vitamin D*. Opinion varies as to the "normal" level, but I feel that the optimal level is 60 ng/ml to 100 ng/ml.

For supplementation, vitamin D-3 gets a grade of A+ because it is more effective than D-2 in increasing blood levels of vitamin D— so choose a product specifically labeled "D-3." Supplements are sold in health-food stores. Side effects include gastrointestinal upset. If you take medications that contain calcium, such as *atorvastatin* (Lipitor) or *rosuvastatin* (Crestor), wait two hours before taking vitamin D supplements to avoid interactions that could trigger inflammation.

Aspirin Update

Charles Campbell, MD, director of the Coronary Care Unit at the University of Kentucky's Gill Heart Institute and an assistant professor of medicine, both in Lexington. Dr. Campbell was lead author of an article on aspirin in the *Journal of the American Medical Association*.

Studies show that taking aspirin daily can lower your heart attack risk by 33% and reduce your combined risk for heart attack, stroke and cardiovascular death by 15%.

Despite these well-established cardiovascular benefits, doctors disagree on the optimal dose of aspirin—about 60% favor one 81-mg dose daily (often referred to as "low-dose" or baby aspirin), while about 35% recommend 325 mg daily (a standard-sized tablet).

What's new: At the University of Kentucky, researchers analyzed 11 major clinical trials comparing different aspirin doses in 10,000 patients with cardiovascular disease (CVD) and found that 75 mg to 81 mg daily prevents heart attacks and strokes as well as higher-dose (325 mg) aspirin does—in some cases, even better— with fewer reports of gastrointestinal bleeding.

HOW ASPIRIN WORKS

Aspirin helps guard against heart attack and stroke by inhibiting the effects of *cyclooxygenase-1* (COX-1), an enzyme that blood platelets require for coagulation (clotting). Aspirin's effect on this enzyme helps prevent the formation of clots that might choke off oxygen to the heart or brain.

Aspirin also inhibits *cyclooxygenase-2* (COX-2), a related enzyme that helps regulate pain and inflammation, such as that caused by arthritis. However, aspirin is a much more effective blood thinner than anti-inflammatory—it typically requires eight times as much of the drug to relieve pain and swelling as it does to reduce heart attack and stroke risk.

My advice: Enteric-coated aspirin should not be used to protect against heart attack or stroke. It has not been well studied for this purpose. The coating may allow aspirin to pass undigested through the stomach, possibly limiting its clot-inhibiting powers.

WHO SHOULD TAKE ASPIRIN?

The potential for gastrointestinal bleeding problems and other side effects means that aspirin should be used only by people who need it.

My advice: If you have a 10% or greater risk of having a heart attack within 10 years, consult your doctor about aspirin therapy. To learn your heart attack risk, ask your doctor or go to the Web site of the American Heart Association (*www.americanheart.org/riskassessment*).

If you're a man over age 40 or a woman over age 50 with atherosclerosis (fatty buildup in the arteries)...high cholesterol (total of 200 mg/dL or higher)...diabetes...or a first-degree relative (parent or sibling) with heart disease, you are among those who may benefit from aspirin therapy. Do not begin aspirin therapy without consulting your doctor. A previous heart attack or stroke also means you should discuss aspirin therapy with your doctor.

HEART ATTACK PROTECTION

Aspirin can be a lifesaver if taken during—and for up to 30 days following—a heart attack, reducing your risk of dying by up to 23%.

My advice: If you think you are having a heart attack, first call 911, then chew 325 mg of aspirin immediately to help prevent the worsening of blood clots.

Caution: Aspirin should be avoided by people who are allergic to it and by those who have a bleeding disorder or asthma that is exacerbated by aspirin.

Important: Chewing 325 mg of aspirin (or four baby aspirin) before swallowing it can cut the absorption time from 60 minutes for an aspirin swallowed whole to 15 to 20 minutes. Never use enteric-coated aspirin for heart attack symptoms—the coating prevents rapid absorption in the stomach.

Caution: Do not take aspirin if you think you are having a stroke. Testing is necessary to determine whether a suspected stroke is caused by a blood clot or bleeding, which could be worsened by aspirin.

ASPIRIN RESISTANCE

Not everyone who takes aspirin experiences a reduction in heart attack and stroke risk.

What's more, none of the dozen or so "aspirin-resistance" blood tests that measure a person's platelet response to aspirin is particularly reliable, according to research done to date.

My advice: Skip the aspirin-resistance tests, and ask your doctor about taking 81 mg of aspirin daily if you are at increased risk for heart attack or stroke.

IBUPROFEN AND ASPIRIN

A study by University of Pennsylvania researchers showed that *ibuprofen* (Advil) can block aspirin's blood clot–fighting activity—especially if the ibuprofen is taken before the aspirin and/or multiple times daily. Short-term use of ibuprofen (for a couple of days or less) is unlikely to interfere significantly with aspirin.

My advice: If you're relying on aspirin to prevent a heart attack or stroke, avoid long-term ibuprofen use. If you have arthritis or another chronic, painful condition, talk to your doctor about taking supplements of *glucosamine* (promotes cartilage formation) and *chondroitin sulfate* (promotes cartilage elasticity) using *acetaminophen* (Tylenol) at the dosage prescribed by your doctor...or receiving local steroid injections.

ASPIRIN'S OTHER BENEFITS

Research suggests that aspirin may also...

• **Prevent adult-onset asthma.** Among 22,000 men enrolled in the Physicians' Health Study, those who took 325 mg of aspirin daily for nearly five years were 22% less likely to develop asthma than those who took a placebo.

• **Reduce the risk for enlarged prostate** by up to 50%, possibly by fighting urinary tract inflammation, according to a recent Mayo Clinic study.

• **Curb cancer risks.** Of 22,507 postmenopausal women participating in the Iowa Women's Health Study, those who took aspirin once weekly were 16% less likely to develop cancer over a 12-year period than nonaspirin users. Other studies suggest that regular aspirin use may reduce the risks for skin, prostate, pancreatic and breast malignancies.

• **Improve longevity.** Aspirin may be a good preventive medicine overall. Cleveland Clinic researchers who tracked 6,174 adults for three years found that those taking aspirin daily were 33% less likely to die during that period, with the greatest benefits realized by people who are age 60 or older, unfit and/or diagnosed with pre-existing coronary artery disease.

Vitamins & Herbs That Don't Mix with Common Medications

George T. Grossberg, MD, faculty, department of neurology and psychiatry, Saint Louis University School of Medicine, St. Louis, Missouri. He is the author, with Barry Fox, PhD, of *The Essential Herb-Drug-Vitamin Interaction Guide*. Broadway.

Most doctors warn their patients about the potential dangers of combining some medications, but few doctors take the time—and some are not well-informed enough —to offer crucial guidance on the harmful effects of taking certain vitamins and/or herbs with common prescription drugs.

Recent study: Among 132 pharmacists surveyed, 47% had seen a patient with a suspected side effect from a vitamin-drug or herb-drug interaction, according to research published in *The Annals of Pharmacotherapy.*

Hidden danger: The problem is particularly common among Americans over age 65, who comprise about 14% of the US population but take approximately 40% of all drugs, vitamins and herbs. Older people also are more sensitive to the side effects of vitamin-drug or herb-drug interactions due to changes in metabolism and the brain.

HARMFUL INTERACTIONS

When some vitamins and/or herbs are taken with certain drugs, the supplement can…

• **Weaken** the effectiveness of the drug.

Example: The herb astragalus, which is used to boost immunity, may reduce the immunosuppressive effects of such drugs as *cortisone* (Cortone Acetate).

• **Strengthen** the effectiveness of the drug, causing a type of drug overdose.

Example: Black cohosh, an herb used to control the symptoms of menopause, can lower blood pressure. If taken with an antihypertensive medication, it can cause hypotension (severely low blood pressure) with symptoms such as dizziness and fatigue.

VITAMIN-DRUG INTERACTIONS

Vitamins that are among the most likely to cause dangerous interactions with drugs…*

• **Vitamin A** promotes immunity, proper bone growth and healthy skin. It also plays a role in night vision and the growth and maintenance of cells of the gastrointestinal tract.

Recommended Dietary Allowance (RDA): 2,300 international units (IU) for women…3,000 IU for men.

Supplemental vitamin A may interact with drugs including: The anticoagulant *warfarin*—vitamin A can increase the risk for bleeding and bruising.

• **Vitamin B-6** is involved in digestion, the production of red blood cells and the maintenance of a healthy brain and nervous system.

RDA: 1.3 mg for all adults ages 19 to 50…1.5 mg for women over age 50…1.7 mg for men over age 50.

Supplemental vitamin B-6 may interact with drugs including: *Amiodarone* (Cordarone), taken for heart arrhythmias—B-6 may increase skin sensitivity to sunlight…*carbidopa* and *levodopa* (Sinemet), taken for Parkinson's disease—B-6 may interfere with the medication's effectiveness…*theophylline* (Elixophyllin), taken for asthma—B-6 may increase the risk for seizures induced by theophylline.

• **Vitamin C** is important for immunity and helps the body manufacture and repair blood vessels, skin, muscles, teeth, bones, tendons, ligaments, hormones and neurotransmitters.

RDA: 75 mg for women…90 mg for men.

Supplemental vitamin C may interact with drugs including: The blood thinners *heparin* (Hepalean) and *warfarin* (Coumadin),

*Multivitamins or individual supplements containing nutrients that exceed the RDA may cause interactions.

taken for cardiovascular disease—vitamin C may reduce the effectiveness of these drugs.

•**Calcium** helps build strong bones and assists in wound healing, blood clotting, cellular metabolism and muscle contraction.

*Adequate intake (AI):** 1,000 mg for adults ages 19 to 50…1,200 mg for adults over age 50.

Supplemental calcium may interact with drugs including: *Digitalis* drugs, such as *digoxin* (Lanoxin), which improve the heart's strength and efficiency—calcium can decrease digitalis levels…*aminoglycoside* antibiotics, especially *gentamicin* (Garamycin)—calcium can increase the risk for kidney failure.

HERB-DRUG INTERACTIONS

Herbs that are among the most likely to cause dangerous interactions with drugs…

•**Valerian,** a mild sedative, is used to treat insomnia and anxiety.

Lowest effective dose: 400 mg, up to two hours before bedtime.

Valerian may interact with drugs including: A selective serotonin reuptake inhibitor (SSRI), such as *sertraline* (Zoloft), or tricyclic antidepressant, such as *desipramine* (Norpramin) —valerian can cause excessive sedation, depression and mental impairment.

•**Grapeseed extract** is rich in powerful antioxidants called *procyanidolic oligomers* (PCOs). It is used to treat high blood pressure, heart disease, varicose veins and macular degeneration.

Lowest effective dose: 75 mg daily.

Grapeseed extract may interact with drugs including: A blood-thinning medication, such as aspirin or *warfarin* (Coumadin)— grapeseed extract can increase the risk for bleeding and visible bruising.

•**Yohimbe** is an African herb that improves blood flow. It is sometimes prescribed for men who have erectile dysfunction.

Lowest effective dose: 5.4 mg daily.

Yohimbe may interact with drugs including: The allergy medication *phenylephrine*, found in over-the-counter products, such

*AI is sometimes used in place of RDA.

as Vicks Sinex Nasal Spray, or in prescription drugs, such as *promethazine hydrochloride* (Phenergan)…or the asthma medication *albuterol* (Proventil)—yohimbe can cause a potentially dangerous increase in heart rate and blood pressure.

•**Apple cider vinegar** is a popular folk remedy that has been used to treat arthritis, high blood pressure and leg cramps.

Lowest effective dose: One tablespoon daily.

Apple cider vinegar may interact with drugs including: Medication for congestive heart failure and/or high blood pressure, such as digoxin, *furosemide* (Lasix) and *hydrochlorothiazide* (Microzide)—apple cider vinegar can increase the risk for *hypokalemia* (lower-than-normal potassium levels in the blood), which can further complicate heart disease.

•**Evening primrose oil** is derived from the seed of the evening primrose plant. This herbal supplement delivers high levels of *gamma-linolenic acid* (GLA), an essential fatty acid. It is used to treat premenstrual syndrome, hot flashes, high blood pressure (during pregnancy) and rheumatoid arthritis.

Lowest effective dose: 540 mg daily.

Evening primrose oil may interact with drugs including: Antiseizure medications, such as *clonazepam* (Klonopin)—evening primrose oil can lower the effectiveness of such drugs, making a seizure more likely.

Natural Remedies That Work Like Drugs

Tod Cooperman, MD, founder and president of ConsumerLab.com, the leading independent evaluator of nutritional and vitamin/mineral supplements, White Plains, New York. Reports can be found at *www.consumerlab. com* (subscription required). He also is editor of ConsumerLab.com's *Guide to Buying Vitamins & Supplements*.

Most people assume that prescription medications are stronger and more effective than supplements. But some supplements can be just as effective—with fewer side effects than prescription drugs.

Also, people with chronic conditions who have no insurance or are under-insured or who have been hit with higher co-pays can save hundreds or even thousands of dollars a year by using supplements in place of drugs.

Caution: Always check with your doctor before stopping a prescription drug or taking a supplement.

Here, natural alternatives to commonly prescribed medications. If there are two alternatives, try one. If that doesn't work, try the other. Dosages are those typically prescribed, but always follow directions on the supplement label or from your health practitioner.

HIGH CHOLESTEROL

Statins, the most popular drugs for lowering cholesterol, can reduce LDL (bad) cholesterol by as much as 60%, depending on the drug and dose.

Drawback: Some of these drugs can cause liver problems and/or a type of muscle pain known as *myopathy.*

Alternative 1: **Red yeast rice.** It contains *monacolins,* chemical compounds that inhibit the body's production of cholesterol. One of these compounds, *lovastatin,* is chemically similar to the active ingredient in some statin drugs.

One study found that people taking red yeast rice supplements had reductions in LDL of 23%. When the supplements were combined with healthy lifestyle changes, LDL dropped by 42%.

Other benefits: Because red yeast rice contains a variety of cholesterol-lowering compounds, it may be effective in patients who don't respond to single-ingredient statins. It also appears to be less likely to cause liver problems and muscle pain.

Dose: 600 milligrams (mg) of red yeast rice extract, taken twice daily.

Alternative 2: **Phytosterols.** These are naturally occurring plant compounds that come in supplement form as well as in cholesterol-lowering margarines, such as Benecol. Plant sterols inhibit the absorption of cholesterol in the intestine and can lower LDL by between 10% and 14%.

Dose: 1.3 grams (g) of a plant sterol supplement daily, divided into two doses. Or two tablespoons of a cholesterol-lowering margarine.

OSTEOARTHRITIS

It's the most common form of arthritis, affecting up to 20 million American adults. Osteoarthritis occurs when cartilage in the joints wears and breaks down, causing pain and stiffness. People with frequent or severe symptoms often depend on prescription-strength anti-inflammatory drugs. These drugs reduce symptoms but don't change the outcome of the disease. They also can cause stomach upset or other gastrointestinal problems.

Alternative 1: **Glucosamine.** This supplement usually is derived from shellfish, though vegetable-based versions are starting to appear. It helps the body repair and rebuild damaged cartilage. It can help reduce pain as well as subsequent joint damage.

Dose: 1,500 mg, once daily.

Alternative 2: **Glucosamine plus chondroitin.** This supplement combination is more expensive than glucosamine alone, but it sometimes helps patients who don't respond to glucosamine. Chondroitin, the added ingredient that typically is made from cow or pig cartilage, promotes the absorption of fluids into connective tissue and aids in flexibility and repair.

Dose: 1,500 mg of glucosamine and 1,200 mg of chondroitin, once daily.

Important: Studies reveal that supplements protect joints better than they relieve pain. Most people who take them still need an occasional anti-inflammatory painkiller.

RHEUMATOID ARTHRITIS

This form of arthritis causes inflammation throughout the body that can damage joints as well as the eyes, lungs and/or heart. Most people with rheumatoid arthritis take prescription drugs, such as *methotrexate* (Rheumatrex) or *hydroxychloroquine* (Plaquenil). Most rheumatoid drugs are expensive, and many have a high risk for side effects, including suppressed immunity.

Supplementation can reduce inflammation and potentially reduce the dosage of prescription drugs.

Alternative: Fish and fish oil. The omega-3 fatty acids in cold-water fish, such as salmon and tuna, have potent anti-inflammatory effects. A study at the University of Pittsburgh School of Medicine found that 59% of patients given supplemental omega-3s had decreased joint pain.

Dose: A total of 1,200 mg to 2,400 mg of EPA and DHA (types of fish oil) daily, or eat three or more fish servings a week.

Caution: Fish oil may interact with blood-thinning drugs, such as *warfarin* (Coumadin).

DEPRESSION

Antidepressant medications, including selective serotonin reuptake inhibitors (SSRIs), such as *paroxetine* (Paxil), *escitalopram* (Lexapro) and *citalopram* (Celexa), have revolutionized the treatment of depression. Many people who take them, however, experience troublesome side effects, including heightened anxiety and reduced libido.

Alternative 1: St. John's wort. It appears to be as effective for mild-to-moderate depression as SSRIs but with milder side effects. It is not effective for patients with major depression and should not be taken with prescription antidepressants. It also may interact with other medications, including blood thinners, such as *warfarin* (Coumadin).

Dose: 300 mg, three times daily. Look for a product that contains 1% to 3% *hypericin,* the active ingredient.

Alternative 2: Fish oil. It improves a number of emotional and mental disorders, including depression and bipolar disorder. A study found that those who combined EPA with an antidepressant medication did better than those using either treatment alone.

Dose: 1 g of EPA, once daily, or eat three or more fish servings a week. (See fish oil caution above.)

ENLARGED PROSTATE

Starting in their 40s, many men experience a rapid growth of the prostate gland. If the inner part of the gland gets too large, it can press against the urethra. This condition, called *benign prostatic hyperplasia* (BPH), can cause irritation or difficulty urinating.

Some drugs, such as *finasteride* (Proscar), reduce the size of the prostate gland. Others, such as *terazosin* (Hytrin) and *doxazosin* (Cardura), relax the prostate and make it easier to urinate but also may cause dizziness.

Alternative: Saw palmetto. This herbal supplement helps prevent *testosterone* from fueling the growth of prostate cells. In some but not all studies, it has been shown to be as effective as finasteride for men with mild symptoms of BPH.

Dose: 160 mg, twice daily. It can take several months to a year before saw palmetto is fully effective.

■ **More from Tod Cooperman...**

The Best Multivitamins

There are problems with multivitamins. Half the brands recently tested had too little or too much of some nutrients...did not break down properly...or were contaminated with lead. There was no relationship between price and quality—some brands that cost $3 a day failed, while some costing five cents a day passed.

Among the multivitamins that passed the test: Centrum Silver...One-A-Day Women's ...and Puritan's Pride ABC Plus Senior.

9

Save on Your Prescriptions

Are You Taking Too Many Pills?

With our national pharmacy bill at $200 billion each year, and recent disclosures about harmful and ineffective drugs, more people are asking—*Are all those pills really necessary?*

John Abramson, MD, a Harvard Medical School clinical instructor who is widely recognized for his in-depth research of the drug industry, answers the tough questions...

•**Are most Americans overmedicated?** They sure are. Americans take many drugs unnecessarily, and when drugs *are* needed, people often take the wrong ones. For example, before *rofecoxib* (Vioxx) was withdrawn from the market because it was found to cause heart attacks and strokes (and was discovered to provide no better relief of arthritis symptoms than older, much less expensive anti-inflammatory

drugs), about 80% of the Vioxx that was prescribed worldwide was used in the US.

•**Are doctors to blame?** The vast majority of physicians prescribe medication because they think it's in their patients' best interest. But there have been radical changes in the way that our medical knowledge is provided. Prior to 1980, most clinical research was publicly funded, but now most is funded directly by the drug and other medical industries, whose primary mission is to maximize the return on investments for investors.

Ninety percent of clinical trials now are commercially funded—as well as 75% of published clinical research. When a pharmaceutical company sponsors a study, the odds are five times greater that the findings will favor its product.

Drug and medical industries fund 70% of continuing education lectures and seminars,

John Abramson, MD, clinical instructor in primary care at Harvard Medical School in Boston, is the author of *Overdosed America: The Broken Promise of American Medicine* (Harper Perennial) and coauthor of "The Effect of Conflict of Interest on Biomedical Research and Clinical Practice Guidelines: Can We Trust the Evidence in Evidence-Based Medicine?" in the *Journal of the American Board of Family Medicine*.

which are among the activities that doctors are required to attend to maintain their licenses to practice. Wherever doctors turn for sources of information, drug companies dominate.

•**Who should be monitoring doctors' relationships with drug companies?** The real failure is on the part of government agencies, such as the FDA and the Agency for Healthcare Research and Quality. Medical journals and academic researchers have become dependent on drug company money and/or are vulnerable to drug company lobbying. Doctors and the public still trust these institutions to independently oversee the integrity of the medical knowledge that informs our medical care, when they simply are not able to do this anymore.

•**We all know that cholesterol-lowering statins are widely prescribed.** Are they unnecessary? Despite being on the market for 18 years and becoming the best-selling class of drugs, statins have never been shown in randomized, controlled trials to provide a significant health benefit when used by women of any age without heart disease or diabetes. The same is true for men over age 65 without heart disease or diabetes. Even so, millions of people in both groups now are taking a statin drug.

•**Is it ever advisable to take a statin?** Yes, there is good evidence that statins are beneficial for people who already have heart disease and for at least some people who have diabetes. A good case also can be made for men who are at very high risk for heart disease (LDL "bad" cholesterol approaching 200 and other risk factors).

•**What other drugs do you think are being prescribed because of drug company influence?** Antihypertensives—drugs used to treat high blood pressure—are good examples. Newer medications, such as calcium channel blockers and angiotensin converting enzyme (ACE) inhibitors, are among the most popular. One of them, *amlodipine* (Norvasc), was the second most commonly prescribed drug for older adults in 2003. But a study funded by the National Heart, Lung, and Blood Institute found that diuretics, which have been around for decades, are as good or better than Norvasc in protecting against complications of hypertension, such as heart attack and stroke. A diuretic

might cost $29 per year, compared with $549 to $749 for Norvasc, depending on the dose. The patents for diuretics expired decades ago, so drug companies don't profit much from them.

•**Should everyone with high blood pressure just take a diuretic?** High blood pressure is a complex problem. Some people respond to one drug, some to another, and some need more than one. It would make sense, though, to start with a diuretic, and use expensive drugs such as Norvasc only when other alternatives haven't worked.

•**Are natural therapies a better alternative to some drugs?** If you look at the data rather than listen to the drug ads, you see that natural alternatives, such as improved diet and routine exercise, often are far more effective than drugs at achieving real health improvements, such as less heart disease and longer life.

Probably the most important test of a healthy diet's effect on heart disease is the Lyon Diet Heart Study conducted in Lyon, France. Heart attack patients were randomly counseled to eat a Mediterranean diet (high in unprocessed grains, fruits, vegetables and olive oil…very low in red meat, dairy fat and cholesterol) or a "prudent" post-heart attack diet (no more than 30% of calories from total fat and no more than 10% from saturated fat).

The people counseled to eat the Mediterranean diet developed 72% less heart disease than those in the prudent diet group over the next four years. There were 56% fewer deaths in the group counseled to eat the Mediterranean diet—that's two to three times the benefit achieved with statin drugs.

The same holds true for exercise. A study conducted at the Cooper Institute in Dallas followed 25,000 men who had undergone physical exams. Over the next 10 years, the men whose exercise endurance (as measured on a treadmill) was in the lowest 20% of the group were at a much higher risk of dying than those with high total cholesterol levels (above 240)—confirming that exercise is even more important than cholesterol control.

•**But many patients prefer pills because they're easier.** There is no question that many of us would rather take a pill than change our lifestyle. If the pills worked, it would simply be a question of how we want to spend our money. The problem is that the pills often are closer to folk medicine—empowered by our cultural beliefs but without a genuine scientific basis. About two-thirds of our health is determined by the way we live our lives, and—for better or worse—no pills can change that.

●**What's the solution?** Most doctors don't invest much time or energy helping patients to make healthy changes in diet and exercise or teaching stress reduction. If you are willing to consider these approaches before trying drug treatment, tell your doctor.

When medication is necessary, ask your doctor if a generic drug is just as effective as the expensive brand-name product. Remember, drug ads that tell you to "ask your doctor" about a particular drug have a single purpose—to sell more drugs, not to improve your health.

Prescription drug ads have become a normal part of our cultural landscape, but the US and New Zealand (with less than four million people) are the only two industrialized countries that allow them. The rest of the industrialized countries feel that assessment of the scientific information about prescription drug treatment should be left to doctors, who should work in a partnership with each patient to determine optimal medical care based on his/her individual situation.

Antibiotics: New Dangers, Latest Findings

Stuart Levy, MD, professor of medicine, molecular biology and microbiology, and director of the Center for Adaptation Genetics and Drug Resistance at Tufts University School of Medicine in Boston. He is founder and president of the nonprofit Alliance for the Prudent Use of Antibiotics (*www.apua.org*) and the author of *The Antibiotic Paradox*. Da Capo.

B y now, we've all heard about the growing threat of antibiotic-resistant bacteria. We know not to ask our doctors to prescribe an antibiotic unnecessarily, and we've been told that frequent handwashing cuts down on the transmission of bacterial infections. With such strong warnings, you might assume that antibiotic resistance is going away. It isn't.

Increasingly, bacteria that are responsible for sinusitis, ear and urinary tract infections and many types of pneumonia are resistant to one or more antibiotics. This means that many infections that were once easily cured by taking an antibiotic for a few days now can linger much longer—and even become life-threatening.

How antibiotic-resistance develops: Bacteria can become resistant to antibiotics by mutating to become insensitive to the drug. The surviving resistant organisms then multiply and create new strains of bacteria that don't respond to antibiotics that were previously effective. Emergence of resistance is enhanced when patients do not finish a full course of an antibiotic—or when antibiotics are overused or misused in general. *Latest developments…*

LAX HANDWASHING

What's new: Many people still aren't washing their hands. While about 91% of American adults claim to wash their hands after using the restroom, only approximately 83% actually do so, according to the American Society for Microbiology.

What this means for you: Since many viruses and bacteria are spread from hands to the mucous membranes of your mouth, nose or eyes, dirty hands are a prime means of transmitting infection.

Self-defense: In addition to washing your hands after using the restroom and before eating or preparing food, it's also important after handling garbage…playing with a pet…changing a diaper…blowing your nose, sneezing or coughing…and inserting or removing contact lenses.

What to do: Using soap and warm, running water, rub your hands together for at least 10 seconds. Don't forget the wrists and backs of your hands. Dry with a clean or disposable towel. Pocket-sized bottles of hand-sanitizing gels and disposable towelettes that contain alcohol are convenient ways to wash when water is not available.

MORE DRUG-RESISTANT STRAINS

What's new: The number of drug-resistant and multidrug-resistant strains of bacteria is up sharply from just a few years ago. About 70% of the bacteria that cause infections in hospitals are now resistant to at least one common antibiotic.

What this means for you: If you are hospitalized, you're now at increased risk of contracting an infection that can be difficult to treat and may even result in death. Recent studies show that 5% to 10% of hospital patients in the US get an infection during their stay, and nearly 100,000 die annually as a result. This compares with about 13,000 deaths from hospital-acquired infections in 1992.

Self-defense: Keep hospital stays as short as possible. Visitors and hospital staff should wash their hands before and after contact with you. With some infectious diseases, such as tuberculosis, visitors and staff may need to wear a mask, gown and gloves to prevent the spread of the infection.

ANTIBIOTIC BAN FOR POULTRY

What's new: The FDA has announced a ban on the use of the animal antibiotic *enrofloxacin* (Baytril) in poultry. Enrofloxacin is a *fluoroquinolone* antibiotic in the same class as *ciprofloxacin* (Cipro). The ban followed the finding that fluoroquinolone-resistant bacteria that infected poultry were becoming increasingly less responsive to Cipro in human infections caused by the same bacteria. This was the first time the FDA had banned an antibiotic used in animal health because of a potential harm posed to people by the emergence of drug-resistant bacteria.

What this means for you: Greater attention is being given to antibiotic use in agriculture, animals and people. Europe has instituted a ban on the use of all growth-promoting antibiotics. In the US, antibiotics are still given to poultry to increase growth. The FDA is currently reviewing the issue, and many experts believe the US should also ban growth-promoting antibiotics.

Self-defense: Although the FDA ban on enrofloxacin is in effect, poultry producers still can use growth-promoting antibiotics. To find poultry that is totally free of antibiotics, check with your local butcher or at a natural-food store.

NEW STAPH INFECTIONS

What's new: A drug-resistant strain of *staphylococcus* bacterium, community-acquired methicillin-resistant Staphylococcus aureus (CA-MRSA), formerly found only in hospitals, is now increasingly being detected within communities.

What this means for you: This particular staph bacterium appears to be more virulent and spreads from person-to-person, particularly through skin-to-skin contact sports, such as football and wrestling.

Self-defense: To prevent infection, wash well with soap and water immediately after any contact sports, being especially careful to clean any cuts. Never share towels or washcloths in a gym.

CIPRO RESISTANCE

What's new: *Ciprofloxacin* (Cipro), one of the first-line antibiotics to treat anthrax (a leading bioterror weapon), is becoming increasingly ineffective against other infections.

What this means for you: For now, other antibiotics can fill the gap for ear, sinus and urinary tract infections. Experts do not believe that Cipro's effectiveness against anthrax has been compromised—but this could change in the future if the antibiotic is overused.

Self-defense: Some experts believe that doctors are too quick to prescribe Cipro when another antibiotic would do. If your doctor prescribes Cipro, ask if another antibiotic could be used.

LATEST ANTIBIOTICS

What's new: *Tigecycline* (Tygacil), the first in a new class of antibiotics called glycylcyclines is available. It was approved by the FDA as a first-line treatment for hospital-based skin and soft tissue infections caused by bacteria that are resistant to other antibiotics. A new class of antibiotics called *diarylquinolones*, which treats drug-resistant tuberculosis, is now in clinical trials.

What this means for you: Despite these new drugs, antibiotic research is getting short shrift. That's because many major pharmaceutical companies have found that it is more profitable to fund research and development for new drugs that treat chronic illnesses, such as diabetes, arthritis and high cholesterol.

Self-defense: Write to your representatives in Congress and tell them that you support efforts to boost incentives (via tax credits and other means) for pharmaceutical companies to develop new antibiotics. To write to your congressional representatives on-line, go to *www.usa.gov*. This Web site also gives mailing addresses and phone numbers for your congressional representatives.

Troublesome Side Effects Of Common Drugs

Jack E. Fincham, PhD, RPh, A.W. Jowdy professor of pharmacy care, department of clinical and administrative pharmacy at the College of Pharmacy at the University of Georgia in Athens, is also editor of the *Journal of Public Health Pharmacy*.

Anyone who has ever waded through the fine print on the package insert of a prescription drug knows that the list of potential side effects can be long and alarming —and difficult to understand.

Latest development: The FDA has updated the design used for prescription drug package inserts to make them easier to read. The redesigned package inserts are required for prescription drugs approved on or after June 30, 2006. For drugs approved in the five-year period prior to that date, the new format will be gradually phased in. Inserts for drugs older than that will be revised by manufacturers on a voluntary basis.

However, this good news does not change the fact that all drugs can cause side effects. Depending on the medication, there are literally hundreds of side effects that can occur, potentially affecting every organ system and bodily function.

Gastrointestinal side effects are among the most common. Dozens of drugs, including the antibiotics *ciprofloxacin* (Cipro) and *erythromycin* (E-Mycin), commonly prescribed for urinary tract, respiratory and skin infections, can cause upset stomach, diarrhea and/or abdominal pain.

Other examples: The antibiotic *amoxicillin* (Amoxil) can cause nausea...*digoxin* (Lanoxin), a heart medication, can cause vomiting...narcotic pain medications can cause constipation.

Hives and/or rashes also are common side effects. These skin conditions, which often are the first sign of an allergic reaction to a medication, can occur with aspirin, antibiotics and *atorvastatin* (Lipitor), a cholesterol-lowering drug.

Anaphylactic shock, a potentially fatal type of allergic reaction in which the breathing passages are constricted and blood pressure drops precipitously, may not occur the first time a drug is taken but rather after a third or fourth dose. Swelling (especially around the face and throat) and/or difficulty swallowing are red flags that you may be suffering from a serious allergic reaction.

Important: Each person responds differently to medication—side effects may occur in some people but not in others. It's crucial to understand the potential side effects of the medications you are taking so that you can report any adverse reactions to your doctor and/or pharmacist.

Spend the 10 to 15 minutes it typically requires to carefully read the package insert. Use reading glasses or a magnifying glass, if necessary. Checking a drug reference book (preferably one with large print) also is helpful. When picking up a prescription, ask to speak to the pharmacist about potential side effects. And of course, discuss potential side effects with your doctor when medication is prescribed.

Once you're taking a prescription drug, it's not always easy to identify side effects, because they can mimic the condition that is being treated. Usually the only way to distinguish between the two possibilities is to stop taking the drug—with your doctor's approval—to see if the side effects stop.

Side effects that are often missed by patients —and doctors...

COGNITIVE PROBLEMS

Prescription drugs that affect the central nervous system can impair thinking, memory, alertness and judgment. These include barbiturates, such as *phenobarbital* (Bellatal), prescribed for epilepsy or migraines...anticholinergics, such as *atropine* (Sal-Tropine) and *scopolamine* (Scopace), prescribed to slow stomach motility (movement of food through the digestive system)...antispasmodics, such as *propantheline* (Pro-Banthine) and *dicyclomine* (Bentyl), for bowel spasms or cramping...muscle relaxants, such as *chlorzoxazone* (Paraflex) and *carisoprodol* (Soma), for muscle stiffness or back spasms...and antidepressants, such as *paroxetine* (Paxil) and *fluoxetine* (Prozac). Central nervous system stimulants, such as *methylphenidate* (Ritalin), also can affect cognition. Stimulant drugs are often used for attention deficit hyperactivity disorder (ADHD).

What you may not know: Certain blood pressure medications, such as *methyldopa* (Aldomet) and *clonidine* (Catapres), may affect heart rate and/or cardiac output (the pumping efficiency of the heart), leading to disorientation.

Cognitive symptoms to watch for: Cognitive changes, such as forgetting simple things that you normally remember, are worth noting. If family members and/or friends tell you that they see a change in your cognitive function, consult your doctor and/or pharmacist. Your doctor may be able to adjust the dosage, or it may help to take the drug at night. As an alternative, your doctor may prescribe an equally effective drug that won't trigger side effects in you.

SEXUAL DYSFUNCTION

Antidepressants, including the widely prescribed selective serotonin reuptake inhibitors (SSRIs), such as *fluoxetine* (Prozac) and *escitalopram* (Lexapro), are known to cause sexual dysfunction, including changes in libido, inability to reach orgasm and/or difficulty achieving an erection. Diuretics, such as *furosemide* (Lasix) and hydrochlorothiazide, can lead to male impotence. Some drugs that are used to treat benign prostatic hypertrophy (a condition in which the prostate gland is enlarged), such as *finasteride* (Proscar) or *dutasteride* (Avodart), also can affect sexual functioning, as can anti-anxiety agents, including *alprazolam* (Xanax), *lorazepam* (Ativan) and *diazepam* (Valium).

What you may not know: Older types of drugs used to treat acid reflux and ulcers, including H2 antagonist drugs, such as *cimetidine* (Tagamet), block androgen receptors, which are necessary for male sex hormone activity. These drugs also can decrease testosterone synthesis, leading to impotence and breast enlargement in some men. Newer H2 antagonist drugs, such as *famotidine* (Pepcid) and *nizatidine* (Axid), and some of the proton pump inhibitors, including *omeprazole* (Prilosec) and *esomeprazole* (Nexium), don't have this effect.

Symptoms to watch for: Report any changes in sexual function, including inability to have or maintain an erection, change in libido and inability to reach orgasm, to your doctor and/or pharmacist as soon as possible. Your doctor may adjust the drug dosage, prescribe an alternative medication in the same class or suggest alternative dosing schedules, such as taking the drug in the early morning.

WEIGHT GAIN

Some newer drugs, including the antipsychotic agents *olanzapine* (Zyprexa) and *quetiapine* (Seroquel), which are used to treat severe mental disorders, such as schizophrenia, may cause weight gain. The antidepressant *bupropion* (Wellbutrin), which is often used instead of an SSRI because it typically does not cause sexual side effects, also can trigger weight gain.

What you may not know: Some diabetes drugs, such as *glyburide* (DiaBeta) and *chlorpropamide* (Diabinese), can lead to weight gain.

Symptoms to watch for: If you gain more than five pounds in any four- to six-week period that you are taking a drug, speak to your pharmacist and/or doctor. Consider weighing yourself daily if you are prescribed a drug that can cause weight gain. Meanwhile, try reducing daily calories and/or exercising more to control any weight gain.

HOW TO AVOID SIDE EFFECTS

To help guard against potentially dangerous side effects, follow these steps when your doctor prescribes medication...

•**Review the dosage.** Drug dosages are usually determined by studies based on young, healthy volunteers or patients with uncomplicated diseases. People who have less body mass (under 120 pounds) don't need the same dose as someone who tops 200 pounds.

What to do: Ask your doctor if he/she is prescribing the lowest possible dose for a person your weight.

•**Mention your age.** As we age, our kidneys and liver are less efficient at metabolizing drugs.

What to do: Ask your doctor whether he is prescribing the lowest possible dose for a person your age.

Drugs That Are Dangerous to Stop Suddenly

Larry D. Sasich, PharmD, MPH, chair of the department of pharmacy practice at Lake Erie College of Osteopathic Medicine (LECOM) School of Pharmacy in Erie, Pennsylvania, and consumer representative on the Science Board of the Food and Drug Administration (FDA). Dr. Sasich is coauthor of *Worst Pills, Best Pills* (Pocket), which has sold more than 2.3 million copies. *www.worstpills.org*

Have you ever wanted to stop taking a medication because of an annoying side effect or some other reason? About 60% of people taking a prescription medication decide on their own, without talking with their doctors, to stop a medication, sometimes suddenly.

Warning: The consequences of suddenly stopping a medication can be deadly.

Some of the medications that you should never stop quickly…

BETA-BLOCKERS

Beta-blockers, which slow the heartbeat, are prescribed for high blood pressure, angina (chest pain) and even for stage fright.

Drowsiness is a common side effect. If you take the medication for high blood pressure, which has no symptoms, you may decide that you feel a whole lot better when you are not taking the drug than when you are taking it—and so you suddenly stop.

What can happen: Quickly stopping a beta-blocker can cause *arrhythmias* (heart rhythm disturbances), even in people without heart disease, and/or worsen angina, possibly even triggering a heart attack.

What to do: Stopping safely requires tapering the dosage—lowering the intake slowly and progressively over a period of one to two weeks. Do so only under the supervision of a physician or other health-care professional.

If you have any withdrawal reactions—for example, if angina worsens—talk to your doctor. You may need to return to the full dosage, at least temporarily.

Beta-blockers include: Acebutolol (Sectral)…*atenolol* (Tenormin)…*atenolol* with *chlorthalidone* (Tenoretic)…*betaxolol* (Kerlone)…*bisoprolol* (Zebeta)…*bisoprolol* with *hydrochlorothiazide* (Ziac)…*carvedilol* (Coreg) …*labetalol* (Normodyne, Trandate)…*metoprolol* (Lopressor, Toprol-XL)…*metoprolol* with *hydrochlorothiazide* (Lopressor HCT)…*nadolol* (Corgard)…*penbutolol* (Levatol)…*pindolol* (Visken)…*propranolol* (Inderal, Inderal LA)… *propranolol* with *hydrochlorothiazide* (Inderide LA)…*timolol* (Blocadren)…*timolol* with *hydrochlorothiazide* (Timolide).

DRUGS FOR DEPRESSION OR ANXIETY

Selective Serotonin Reuptake Inhibitors (SSRIs) and Serotonin-Norepinephrine Reuptake Inhibitors (SNRIs) work by increasing the level of neurotransmitters, brain chemicals that speed messages from neuron to neuron and play an important role in mood. SSRIs increase the neurotransmitter *serotonin*, while SNRIs increase both *serotonin* and the neurotransmitter *norepinephrine*.

SSRIs are prescribed for depression, anxiety disorders (such as panic attacks, general anxiety disorder, social anxiety disorder or posttraumatic stress disorder) and other types of intense and ongoing emotional distress. SNRIs also are prescribed for depression.

What can happen: If you suddenly stop taking an SSRI or SNRI, you may go through intense physical withdrawal. It usually starts one to three days after the drug is stopped, and symptoms can include dizziness, vertigo (a spinning or whirling sensation), poor coordination, nausea and diarrhea, and flulike symptoms, such as fatigue, headache, muscle pain and chills. You also might experience emotional symptoms, such as depression, irritability, agitation, anxiety, confusion or mood swings, along with insomnia. Withdrawal symptoms generally go away after one or two weeks.

What to do: If you and your doctor have decided that you should no longer take an SSRI or an SNRI—because of side effects (such as sexual dysfunction or weight gain) or cost, or because you feel that you are ready to go off the drug—create a plan to stop the drug gradually, by tapering the dosage.

If you begin to experience intolerable withdrawal symptoms while stopping the drug, return to the previous dose and decrease at a more gradual rate.

SSRIs include: Citalopram (Celexa)...*escitalopram* (Lexapro)...*fluoxetine* (Prozac, Sarafem)... *fluoxetine* with *olanzapine* (Symbyax)...*fluvoxamine* (Luvox)...*paroxetine* (Paxil)...*sertraline* (Zoloft).

SNRIs include: Duloxetine (Cymbalta)... *venlafaxine* (Effexor).

SLEEPING PILLS

The new generation of nonbenzodiazepine sleeping pills was formulated to replace *benzodiazepines*, such as Valium and Xanax (which also are prescribed for anxiety).

That's because benzodiazepines are highly addictive and work by sedating the body, which in turn adapts to the drug. As a result, higher and higher doses are needed to produce an effect. When a benzodiazepine drug is suddenly halted, you can experience symptoms similar to those experienced by an alcoholic who abruptly stops drinking—tremors, cramps, convulsions, sweating and vomiting. If you have been taking a benzodiazepine for insomnia and stop suddenly, you also may experience rebound insomnia, in which you have an even harder time falling asleep and more nighttime awakenings than before you started the drug.

What can happen: Even some doctors, don't realize that the nonbenzodiazepines—*eszopiclone* (Lunesta), *zaleplon* (Sonata) and *zolpidem* (Ambien), which are used mainly to help you fall asleep—work in almost the same way as benzodiazepines and, it turns out, also are addictive. Nonbenzodiazepines have a different chemical structure from benzodiazepines, but they act on the same area of the brain.

Sudden withdrawal from these sleeping pills can produce exactly the same type of physical withdrawal symptoms—such as nausea, sweating and shaking—and rebound insomnia as sudden withdrawal from a benzodiaz-epine. And those problems can develop after taking a nonbenzodiazepine every night for just a week or two.

What to do: As with all sleep medications, after a week or two of nightly use, work with your doctor to stop the drug gradually, tapering the dosage.

HOW TO WORK WITH YOUR PHYSICIAN

Some physicians might not know about the withdrawal reactions discussed here, particularly the reactions for nonbenzodiazepine sleeping pills. When you discuss stopping a drug with your doctor, bring a copy of the "professional product label" for the medication—the comprehensive printed descriptions and warnings that accompany each drug when you fill a prescription. With this information in hand, you can emphasize that caution is warranted and that the drug needs to be stopped gradually.

Resources: Print professional product labels for nearly 4,000 prescription drugs at *www.dailymed.nlm.nih.gov* or from select drug manufacturer's official Web sites. You can find detailed drug information in the *Physician's Desk Reference*, or *PDR* (Thomson Healthcare), available in libraries, bookstores or on-line at *www.pdrhealth.com*.

The Blood Pressure Pill That's Great for Your Bones

Bruno H.Ch. Stricker, PhD, professor, Erasmus University Medical Center, Rotterdam, the Netherlands.
Felicia Cosman, MD, clinical scientist and medical director, the Clinical Research Center, Helen Hayes Hospital, West Haverstraw, New York.
Annals of Internal Medicine.

Thiazide diuretics that control high blood pressure can also reduce age-related bone loss and the resulting fractures, but the protection vanishes once the drugs are stopped, researchers say.

Osteoporosis, which can sometimes lead to hip fractures, is a common problem in older men and women, as bones become thinner and weaker during the normal aging process.

Studies have shown that thiazides slow calcium loss and may be a factor in preventing age-related bone erosion.

Now, Dutch investigators have clearly shown that thiazides significantly reduce the risk of hip fractures.

In a large population of elderly patients, the use of a thiazide medication "offered a substantial protection from hip fracture," says lead researcher Bruno H.Ch. Stricker, PhD, a professor at Erasmus University Medical Center located in Rotterdam.

THE STUDY

In their study, the researchers collected data on hip fractures among 7,891 men and women older than age 55.

They classified patients as those who had never used a thiazide, those who had used a thiazide for a short time and those who had used a thiazide for a year or more.

They also looked at individuals who had stopped using a thiazide for a short period and those who had stopped the medication for six months or more.

RISK REDUCED BY HALF

During up to nine years of follow-up study, Stricker and his team found that compared with patients who had never taken a thiazide diuretic, those who had taken a thiazide for more than one year had about a 50% lower risk of hip fracture.

However, this lower risk disappeared within four months after the medication was stopped, the research team says.

WHAT THE RESEARCH IMPLICATIONS ARE

Because thiazide diuretics are relatively safe, Stricker believes that they might be useful for treating older patients who have high blood pressure and who are also at risk for hip fracture.

"But I do not advise using thiazides primarily to protect against hip fracture if you do not have hypertension—not until a clinical trial has demonstrated that it is truly effective and how big that effect is," he cautions.

According to Stricker, based on the current study's findings, "it is reasonable to treat an older woman with hypertension who is also [likely] to hip fracture with a thiazide as a first medication."

FINDINGS SUPPORT OTHER STUDIES

Dr. Felicia Cosman, clinical scientist and medical director of the Clinical Research Center, Helen Hayes Hospital, West Haverstraw, New York, comments that these findings are consistent with those of other studies.

According to Cosman, it is not surprising that the protective effect of thiazide medications wears off after use of the drug is discontinued. This is a common occurrence that can also be found with numerous other medications, she explains.

"We still need to follow the same preventive measures for osteoporosis. People need to maximize their calcium and vitamin D intake, exercise regularly and reduce any possible risk factors," she advises.

To learn more about how to prevent osteoporosis, visit the National Osteoporosis Foundation at *www.nof.org*.

Counterfeit Drug Watch

Rebecca Shannonhouse, editor of the *Bottom Line/Health* newsletters, Boardroom Inc., 281 Tresser Blvd., Stamford, Connecticut 06901.

Most people know there's a risk of buying counterfeit drugs on the Internet. *Problem:* Even drugs purchased from US pharmacies might be fake.

According to an FDA estimate, about 1% of the nation's drug supply—about 35 million prescriptions annually—is believed to be counterfeit.

What happens: Drugs are typically sold by manufacturers to wholesalers, who then sell them to pharmacies. However, some dishonest wholesalers tamper with drugs before selling them. Often, they buy cut-rate—sometimes phony—drugs from unlicensed or suspicious sources, explains Katherine Eban, an investigative journalist who has documented counterfeit drugs in her book *Dangerous Doses* (Harvest).

The drugs most vulnerable to counterfeiting are commonly used and/or expensive.

Examples: The cholesterol-lowering drug *atorvastatin* (Lipitor) and the anemia drug *epoetin* (Procrit). Even common antibiotics such as penicillin have been faked. *How to protect yourself...*

•**Sign up for free E-mail alerts on fake drugs** at *www.safemedicines.org*, the Web site of the nonprofit Partnership for Safe Medicines.

•**Become familiar with the shape, color and, if applicable, taste of the drugs that you take.** Some counterfeits appear and/or taste slightly different from the real medication.

•**Note if your medicine seems to stop working or causes new side effects.**

If you suspect that a drug is a counterfeit, tell your pharmacist and physician immediately—and report it on the FDA Web site at *www.fda.gov.*

Low-Cost Hypertension Drugs May Work Just as Well as Expensive Ones

Jackson T. Wright, Jr., MD, PhD, professor of medicine, Case Western Reserve University, Cleveland.

Lawrence J. Appel, MD, MPH, professor of medicine, Johns Hopkins University, Baltimore.

The Journal of the American Medical Association.

You might expect newer, more advanced and costlier medications for high blood pressure to be more effective than the older and less expensive *thiazide diuretics*. But a Cleveland study found that this is not necessarily the case.

In an eight-year trial, the incidence of heart failure was lower and the risk of fatal heart disease or heart attacks was no greater for people who took a diuretic than for those who took the newer *calcium channel blockers* or *angiotensin-converting enzyme (ACE) inhibitors.*

The study may be the most comprehensive effort ever made to compare the effectiveness of different blood pressure drugs. *Here's how each drug works…*

•**Diuretics** lower blood pressure by increasing the passing of water and sodium.

•**Calcium channel blockers** widen blood vessels by relaxing the muscles around them.

•**ACE inhibitors** block the activity of an enzyme that makes arteries constrict.

Diuretics, by far the oldest drugs, are generally available as relatively inexpensive generics, while the calcium channel blockers and ACE inhibitors often are higher-priced, brand-name products.

The approximately 50 to 60 million Americans who have been diagnosed with high blood pressure now spend an estimated $15.5 billion a year on drugs, the report says. A large proportion of patients need more than one drug, but the report says, "It is reasonable to infer that a diuretic be included in all multidrug regimens."

COST SAVINGS

A preliminary cost analysis showed that "if patients were switched from calcium channel blockers and ACE inhibitors to diuretics, the annual savings in direct costs would be between $250 and $600 per patient," says study leader Dr. Jackson T. Wright, Jr., a professor of medicine at Case Western Reserve University. There would be other savings from a reduced need for hospitalizations, Wright adds.

Diuretics have fallen out of favor with many doctors because they have potentially dangerous side effects, such as raising blood cholesterol and sugar levels, causing concern that they might actually be increasing the risk of heart disease, says Dr. Lawrence J. Appel, a professor of medicine at Johns Hopkins University.

However, the study "provides strong evidence that they should be first-line therapy," he says.

The National Heart, Lung, and Blood Institute at *www.nhlbi.nih.gov/hbp* provides information on managing your blood pressure.

What Are the Odds? Some Parkinson's Drugs May Cause Gambling

Mark Stacy, MD, associate professor of neurology and director, Movement Disorders Center, Duke University Medical Center, Durham, North Carolina.

Jay Van Gerpen, MD, assistant professor of neurology, Mayo Graduate School of Medicine, Mayo Clinic, Jacksonville, Florida.

Neurology.

A combination of some Parkinson's disease medications may produce a rare but potentially devastating side effect —addictive gambling behavior.

Researchers found nine pathological gamblers in a group of more than 1,000 people being treated for Parkinson's disease. These people said they hadn't had any gambling problems in the past.

THE STUDY

Dr. Mark Stacy, lead author of the study, says he began this study because he had two Parkinson's patients report huge gambling losses soon after Stacy had changed the doses of their medications. Stacy is associate professor of neurology and director of Movement Disorders Center at Duke University Medical Center in Durham, North Carolina, but was at the Muhammad Ali Parkinson Research Center in Phoenix at the time of the study.

He and his colleague reviewed the charts of 1,184 patients with Parkinson's disease, and found seven other cases of problem gambling.

In all of the cases, the gambling was severe enough to cause financial problems.

On average, the people who had gambling problems had been diagnosed with Parkinson's disease 11 years before the start of their addictive gambling behavior.

PARKINSON'S DRUGS MAY BE IMPLICATED

All nine people were taking *levodopa* and a *dopamine agonist* when their gambling problems began.

Levodopa is a drug that changes into dopamine in the brain, and dopamine agonists help the body use the created dopamine. People who have Parkinson's disease have low levels of dopamine, which is believed to help control smooth movement. Dopamine also appears to affect mood and personality.

Of those with a gambling problem, eight were taking a dopamine agonist called *pramipexole* and one was taking *pergolide*.

None of the people who were taking levodopa alone reported problem gambling, and none of those taking a different dopamine agonist, *ropinirole*, reported any gambling problems.

Stacy says he's not sure how the medications cause addictive gambling behavior, but seven of the patients reported that their problems started within a month of when their dosage was increased. This suggests, Stacy says, that the higher doses of the dopamine agonists act as a catalyst for problem gambling behavior.

When their medications were switched, or the doses were lowered, most of the patients were able to control or stop their gambling behavior, according to the study results. Some of the patients also attended Gamblers Anonymous meetings.

DON'T BE SURPRISED BY SIDE EFFECTS

Dr. Jay Van Gerpen, an assistant professor of neurology, Mayo Graduate School of Medicine, Mayo Clinic, Jacksonville, Florida, says he was not surprised by this study's findings.

"Medicines for Parkinson's disease may elicit unwanted side effects relating to mood and personality," says Van Gerpen. "Dopamine agonists can be associated with changes in personality, such as sexual inappropriateness, and changes in sleep cycles. Patients need to be aware of these possibilities," he adds.

Stacy says that although this side effect is rare, it's important for doctors and patients to know that higher doses of these medications may increase the risk of problem gambling.

If you think you or someone you love may have a gambling problem, find out for sure with a self-test from the National Council on Problem Gambling at *www.ncpgambling.org*.

■ ■ ■ ■

Steroid Warning

Corticosteroids can cause bone loss if taken for long periods and in high doses, warns Harris H. McIlwain, MD. High doses are used to treat lung disease, arthritis and other severe conditions. Patients taking corticosteroids daily for three months or longer also should take calcium and vitamin D supplements to prevent bone loss. Your doctor should arrange a bone-density test if you have been, or will be, taking high doses of these drugs or inhaled steroid drugs for asthma for longer than three months. Topical corticosteroids are usually safe.

Harris H. McIlwain, MD, is a lead investigator for clinical trials at the Tampa Medical Group and adjunct professor, University of Southern Florida College of Public Health, both in Tampa.

■ ■ ■ ■

Shingles Vaccine

The first shingles vaccine, *Zostavax*, has been approved by the FDA for adults 60 and older who previously had chickenpox. If you had chickenpox, you can develop shingles, which can cause itching, burning, tingling and a red rash that develops into painful pus-filled blisters. Pain can be intense and persists in some patients for months or years. The vaccine reduces shingles incidence by half. Ask your doctor if Zostavax is right for you.

Jesse Goodman, MD, MPH, director, US Food and Drug Administration's Center for Biologics Evaluation and Research, Rockville, Maryland.

■ ■ ■ ■

Drug Warning

People who take low-dose aspirin plus *clopidogrel* (Plavix) to prevent a first heart attack or stroke are 78% more likely to die from cardiovascular causes than people who take aspirin alone. Paradoxically, the aspirin/Plavix combination can help prevent a second heart attack or stroke.

Also: Patients who have had a stent should take the aspirin/Plavix combination.

Self-defense: If you use both drugs, consult your physician about the benefits of continuing. Do not stop either drug on your own.

Eric Topol, MD, is a heart researcher and professor of genetics, The Scripps Research Institute and chief academic officer at Scripps Health, both in La Jolla, California, and coauthor of a study of 15,603 people, published in The New England Journal of Medicine.

Time-Tested Drugs Are The Best Way to Go

Karen Elizabeth Lasser, MD, MPH, assistant professor of medicine, Massachusetts General Hospital, Boston, and Cambridge Health Alliance, Cambridge, Massachusetts. She is lead author of a study on the safety of new drugs published in The Journal of the American Medical Association.

A study published in *The Journal of the American Medical Association* examined all drugs approved by the US Food and Drug Administration (FDA) from 1975 to 1999. *One drug in five* was withdrawn from the market or required to have a "black-box" warning put on the package insert about serious risks.

During just one year of the study period, approximately 20 million Americans were given drugs that were later withdrawn.

The most common risks of the drugs were damage to the liver, heart and bone marrow and a variety of problems for pregnant women.

Self-defense: As long as other effective treatments are available, avoid any drug until it has been on the market for at least seven years. Approximately half of all problems with toxicity are discovered within that period.

Here is advice on common drugs to avoid —and better alternatives…

ALLERGY

Desloratadine (Clarinex). Introduced to the market in 2002, this antihistamine is essentially the same as the older drug *loratadine* (Claritin). When you take loratadine, the drug is broken down in the body into desloratadine. The manufacturer simply got a patent for the chemical by-product.

Drawbacks: Not only is there no evidence that desloratadine is clinically different from loratadine, neither drug is a particularly effective antihistamine.

In fact, when the manufacturer submitted four clinical trials to the FDA comparing doses of desloratadine with a placebo, only two of the studies found the drug to be effective.

Better choice: Over-the-counter (OTC) antihistamines, such as *chlorpheniramine* (Chlor-Trimeton) or *diphenhydramine* (Benadryl). Though many patients find them sedating, they are not only less expensive but they are usually more effective.

As an alternative to OTC drugs, ask your doctor about prescription nasal steroids, such as *flunisolide* (Nasalide) or *beclomethasone* (Vancenase AQ). They quickly ease congestion without the grogginess that is sometimes caused by antihistamines.

HEARTBURN

Esomeprazole (Nexium). Introduced in 2001, esomeprazole is the fifth member of the *proton pump inhibitor* class of drugs used for gastro-esophageal reflux disease (heartburn) and for duodenal ulcers that don't respond to antacids or H-2 blockers, such as *cimetidine* (Tagamet).

Drawbacks: An FDA evaluation suggests that esomeprazole is no better than *omeprazole* (Prilosec), an older OTC proton pump inhibitor that has a known safety record.

Better choice: People who have heartburn can choose among many drugs—Prilosec, Tagamet, antacids, etc.—that have been on the market for a long time and are known to be safe.

Non-drug treatments, such as not lying down after meals and avoiding chocolate or other foods known to cause heartburn, are often all that's needed.

INSOMNIA

Zaleplon (Sonata). Introduced in 1999, zaleplon was designed to help insomnia patients fall asleep without the residual grogginess that is so common with other sleeping pills. Zaleplon is quickly eliminated from the body, so you can potentially take it late at night or early in the morning and still be fully alert when you get up.

Drawbacks: It's less potent than the older *benzodiazepine* sleeping pills, such as *triazolam* (Halcion), *temazepam* (Restoril) and *flurazepam* (Dalmane).

Compared with a placebo, zaleplon decreases the time it takes to fall asleep by only eight to 20 minutes.

Zaleplon has a high risk for addiction when taken for more than several weeks.

It also has potentially serious interactions, such as excessive drowsiness, when it is taken with other drugs, including antihistamines and anti-ulcer medications.

Better choice: Behavioral and lifestyle adjustments, such as reducing caffeine intake and practicing yoga or other relaxation techniques, are much safer for treating insomnia.

For patients who need extra help for a few nights to two weeks, an older drug, such as *oxazepam* (Serax) or *zolpidem* (Ambien), can be effective.

Covered-Up Facts About Bone-Building Drugs

The New England Journal of Medicine.

Combining osteoporosis drugs may do more harm than good, according to two studies.

The studies sought to prove that combining *alendronate* and *parathyroid hormone* would work even better than using the drugs separately. Instead, it proved exactly the opposite, researchers say.

Alendronate, sold by Merck as Fosamax, helps stop any bone loss. Parathyroid hormone helps to build bone.

THE STUDIES

The first study looked at the drug combination in 238 women with untreated osteoporosis. Some got one drug, some got the other and some got both.

The study, which was conducted at several major hospitals nationwide for a year, found "no evidence of synergy" when both drugs were used. In fact, Fosamax reduced the effects of parathyroid hormone.

The second study, done at Massachusetts General Hospital, targeted 83 men with brittle bones. It, too, found that Fosamax canceled the effects of the parathyroid hormone.

Women should talk to their doctors about whether to take Fosamax alone.

BRISK WALKING BUILDS BONE MASS

According to Katarina T. Borer, professor of movement science at the Center for Exercise Research at the University of Michigan, postmenopausal women who walked three miles fast enough to become winded, five days a week for 15 weeks, increased their bone mineral density by 0.4%. This can be compared with a 1% bone-density loss in those who walked at a slower, less challenging pace.

Theory: Intense exercise triggers greater secretion of hormones that may increase bone mineralization.

Alzheimer's Drug Warning

Amy F.T. Arnsten, PhD, associate professor and director of graduate studies in neurobiology, Yale University School of Medicine, New Haven, Connecticut.

Paula Bickford, PhD, professor of psychology, University of South Florida Center for Aging-Neuroscience, Tampa, and past president, American Aging Association.

Neuron.

Experimental drugs designed to preserve memory function lost to age or brain disease may do so at the expense of other forms of recall.

Researchers believe that regional differences in the brain could undercut the effectiveness of drugs that are being developed to enhance memory in people with Alzheimer's disease and other age-related dementia.

UNDERSTANDING MEMORY

Two areas of the brain are associated with different types of memory. The hippocampus has been associated with long-term memory formation, while the prefrontal cortex has been associated with working or functional memory—such as remembering the phone number of your babysitter or remembering a phone number long enough to dial it.

In a healthy individual, the two brain systems work together. When a person gets older, however, both forms of memory can be adversely affected.

The prefrontal cortex—the working memory—naturally flags with normal aging, "so it's particularly important to see what this cortex loses, and give it back," says study author Amy F.T. Arnsten, an associate professor and director of graduate studies in neurobiology at Yale University School of Medicine.

"There's some deterioration in the hippocampus [the long-term memory function] with normal aging, but what really erodes the hippocampus is Alzheimer's."

Experts believe that increasing the activity of an enzyme called *protein kinase A* (PKA) in the hippocampus may improve memory and other cognitive deficits. There are drugs in development that may accomplish that.

THE PROBLEM WITH DRUGS

The problem, according to Arnsten and her colleagues at Yale, is that a particular drug can have vastly different effects on different parts of the brain.

Their study found that drugs that might benefit the hippocampus might have deleterious effects on the prefrontal cortex.

"Different regions of the brain that control various kinds of learning and memory may be affected differently by drugs that are targeted at improving cognition," explains Paula Bickford, a professor of psychology at the University of South Florida Center for Aging-Neuroscience in Tampa and a past president of the American Aging Association.

"They may improve one kind of cognition but impair a different type of cognition," according to Bickford.

THE STUDY

The researchers did a series of tests in rats and monkeys using drugs to increase or decrease PKA activity.

Inhibiting PKA in the hippocampus actually improved functioning in the prefrontal cortex. PKA activation in the hippocampus impaired functioning in the prefrontal cortex.

As people age, PKA activity declines in the hippocampus but increases in the prefrontal cortex, suggesting that different measures are needed to improve the situation in each area of the brain.

For more on memory and aging, visit the Memory and Aging Center of the University of California, Los Angeles, at *www.npi.ucla.edu/memory.*

■ ■ ■ ■

Pneumonia Vaccine

Adults who received the pneumococcal vaccine were 40% to 70% less likely to die from pneumonia when hospitalized for the condition than patients who were unvaccinated or had unknown vaccination status. Vaccination also reduces risk for respiratory failure, kidney failure and heart attack.

Theory: Vaccination prevents invasion into the bloodstream of pneumonia-causing bacteria, lowering risk for organ failure. The CDC recommends that adults age 65 and older and younger people with risk factors, such as diabetes or kidney disease, get the pneumonia vaccine.

David Fisman, MD, MPH, epidemiologist, Ontario Public Health Laboratory, Toronto.

■ ■ ■ ■

Infection-Fighter After Chemotherapy

Neutropenia—a low level of infection-fighting white blood cells—is a common complication of chemotherapy.

Study: More than 1,500 patients with breast, lung, testicular or other solid tumors or lymphoma took 500 mg of the antibiotic *levofloxacin* (Levaquin) or a placebo for seven days during each of six chemotherapy cycles.

Result: The patients taking levofloxacin experienced a 27% reduction in hospitalizations for infections during all six cycles. If you are undergoing chemotherapy: Ask your doctor about adding levofloxacin to your regimen.

Michael Cullen, MD, medical oncologist, Queen Elizabeth Hospital, University Hospital, Birmingham, England.

Simple Fixes for Medication Errors

Charles B. Inlander, a consumer advocate and healthcare consultant based in Fogelsville, Pennsylvania. He was founding president of People's Medical Society, a consumer health advocacy group active in the 1980s and 1990s. He is the author of more than 20 books, including *Take This Book to the Hospital with You.* St. Martin's.

Charles B. Inlander has been a member of a committee organized by the Institute of Medicine, a government advisory group in Washington, DC, to study and find solutions to the medication error problem in America.

Their report, based on the findings of several studies and the testimony of more than 100 experts, made front-page headlines across the country.

Among our findings: Each year, at least 1.5 million Americans are seriously harmed by medication errors (with at least 7,000 deaths). Statistically, every hospitalized patient can expect to be the victim of a medication error at least once a day for each day that he/she is hospitalized... tens of thousands of errors occur at local pharmacies each month....and more than 800,000 medication errors occur in nursing homes annually. Although the dangers of medication errors were widely reported in the media, the solutions were hardly discussed. *What you can do to help protect yourself—and your family...*

•**Keep a current list of all your medications.** One of the most dangerous medication errors involves a doctor prescribing a drug that causes a serious interaction with another drug or supplement. Most doctors do not know all the prescription and over-the-counter drugs, vitamins and other supplements their patients take, so keep a list of everything you take (and the dosage). Take the list with you to every doctor visit and hand it to the doctor before he writes a new prescription. For information on interactions, check the FDA Web site *(www.fda. gov/cder/consumerinfo/druginteractions.htm).*

•**Double-check drugs at the pharmacy.** Pharmacy errors can occur when the pharmacist is in a rush or can't read the doctor's handwriting.

Helpful: Ask your doctor to write the name of the drug on a piece of paper along with the dosage. Compare this information with what you are handed at the pharmacy or what is delivered to you from a mail-order pharmacy. If there is a discrepancy, do not accept the drug until you have checked with the pharmacist. If the prescription is a refill, make sure the pills match those you already have.

•**When hospitalized, bring an advocate.** Studies show that error rates drop dramatically if a family member or friend is with a hospitalized patient to help oversee medications. *Your advocate should...*

1. Create a list of the drugs you were taking before being hospitalized to share with every doctor and nurse who treats you.

2. Get a list of all the drugs you are taking in the hospital and the times they should be given.

3. Monitor the drugs themselves, looking for any differences, such as size, color or dosages, and keep a log of what medication was given when.

4. Refuse any new or different drugs that have not been discussed by a doctor or nurse with you or the advocate. If you have a loved one in a nursing home or assisted-living facility, having a family member or friend visit daily to monitor the medication log will reduce errors dramatically.

Drugs Work Differently In Men and Women

Marianne J. Legato, MD, founder and director of the Partnership for Gender-Specific Medicine at Columbia University and a professor emeritus of clinical medicine in New York City, is the author of *Eve's Rib: The New Science of Gender-Specific Medicine and How It Can Save Your Life*. Harmony.

Medical researchers have long known that men and women differ in their susceptibility to common diseases, such as diabetes, heart disease and cancer.

Now: Researchers are discovering that men and women often respond differently to the same medication.

Example: The allergy drug *terfenadine* (Seldane) was removed from the market in 1998 when it was discovered that women taking it had a higher risk for potentially deadly heartbeat irregularities (arrhythmias). Men taking the drug didn't experience the same risk.

THE GENDER FACTOR

Until recently, the pharmaceutical industry mainly tested new drugs on men. Women were not included in drug trials to protect them and any children they might conceive if pregnancy occurred during testing. Also, the hormone fluctuations experienced by women were thought to make them less desirable than men as study subjects.

In 1993, after researchers had discovered that men and women respond differently to drugs, the FDA began requiring that women be included in drug trials for medications that would be taken by them.

Among the most popular theories to explain gender-related differences in drugs...

•**Hormones.** The enzymes that metabolize drugs are affected by hormones, which differ greatly in men and women. For example, the "female" hormone progesterone, which increases just prior to menstruation, accelerates the breakdown of the steroid *prednisone* in the body. This means that a woman with asthma might require a higher dose of the drug just before her menstrual period to avoid an attack.

•**Fatty tissue.** Some drugs are stored in fatty tissue. Because women typically have a higher percentage of body fat than men, women might require a lower drug dose in some cases because the drug is stored in the fatty tissue and is available for a longer time after dosing.

Common drugs with sex-specific differences...

ANALGESICS

Women may be biologically more sensitive to pain than men—and they are known to experience more inflammation from infection and injury. Therefore, women may require higher doses of analgesics that have an anti-inflammatory component.

Women often do better with *ibuprofen* (Advil) or another nonsteroidal anti-inflammatory drug (NSAID), such as *naproxen* (Aleve), than with pain relievers, such as *acetaminophen* (Tylenol), that do not treat inflammation.

Best advice: For severe pain—following surgery, for example—women should ask their doctors for a "kappa opioid," such as *butorphanol tartrate* (Stadol), a morphine-like painkiller. This class of drugs is much more effective for women than other analgesics. In men, kappa opioids aren't as effective as other drugs.

ANESTHESIA

Women tend to wake up quicker than men following anesthesia—an average of six minutes faster—even when they're given the same dose relative to their body weight. Women experience more side effects from anesthesia than men do and are more likely than men to report some consciousness during surgical procedures.

Despite this, women tend to be given less pain-relieving medication in the recovery room following surgery.

Reason: A man's blood pressure rises when he's in pain. Doctors rely on this to indicate when to use drugs and how much to give.

Women in pain frequently have a drop in blood pressure—and a more rapid heart rate as a result, which is a better indicator of how much distress they are feeling.

Best advice: Before an operation, women should request that their heart rate be monitored as a pain indicator along with blood pressure. If the heart rate increases, their doctors should consider giving more pain medication.

ANTI-ARRHYTHMICS

This class of drugs is used to treat heart arrhythmias. One popular anti-arrhythmic, *sotalol* (Betapace), is more dangerous for women than for men. Due to differences in the characteristics of the cardiac cell membranes in men and women, sotalol, which acts on these cell membranes, can increase a woman's risk for *ventricular tachycardia*, a potentially life-threatening arrhythmia.

Best advice: A woman who needs an anti-arrhythmic drug can sometimes be treated with another drug in the same class. If she requires sotalol, she should be advised to stay in a hospital or other facility that can provide continuous heart monitoring—and cardiac resuscitation, if necessary.

ANTIDEPRESSANTS

These days, most people with depression are treated with a selective serotonin reuptake inhibitor (SSRI) antidepressant, such as *paroxetine* (Paxil) or *fluoxetine* (Prozac). These drugs increase brain concentrations of serotonin, a neurotransmitter that regulates mood.

However, a new study shows that men don't appear to benefit from SSRIs as much as women—perhaps because men are known to have about 50% more brain serotonin than women. Therefore, increasing the levels of this neurotransmitter through drug therapy has relatively modest effects in men.

Best advice: Tricyclic antidepressants, such as *amitriptyline* (Elavil) or *nortriptyline* (Pamelor), are often better choices for men. These older drugs have a higher risk for side effects, such as weight gain and dry mouth, than the SSRIs, but are more likely to be effective in men.

ASPIRIN

Millions of healthy Americans take aspirin daily or every other day to "thin" the blood and reduce the risk for clots, which can contribute to heart attack and/or stroke. However, doctors must weigh the potential benefits of aspirin therapy against the potential risks. In both sexes, regular use of aspirin has been shown to increase the risk for gastrointestinal bleeding.

New finding: In men, daily aspirin can lower heart attack risk by 32%, according to a recent analysis of aspirin therapy conducted by researchers at Duke University Medical Center in Durham, North Carolina. Aspirin does not have this effect in all women. However, women who take a daily or every-other-day aspirin were found to have a 17% reduction in the risk for stroke.

Best advice: For men who are at risk for heart attack (due to smoking, high blood pressure or family history), aspirin therapy is often a good choice.

Women under age 65 who are concerned about heart protection alone may want to forgo aspirin therapy and focus on other protective strategies, including weight control, not smoking, regular exercise, etc.

In women over age 65, the heart benefits of aspirin therapy may outweigh the risks for stomach problems.

Because women suffer strokes about as often as men—and their risk of dying from stroke is even higher—they should consider aspirin therapy if they have stroke risk factors, such as smoking, high blood pressure, etc.

Important: Consult your doctor before starting or discontinuing aspirin therapy.

Dangerous Medication Risks for Seniors

Robert N. Butler, MD, professor of geriatrics, Mount Sinai Medical Center, and president and CEO, International Longevity Center (*www.ilcusa.org*), both in New York City. He won the Pulitzer Prize for his book *Why Survive? Being Old in America* (Johns Hopkins University). He is also coauthor of *Aging and Mental Health* (Pro-Ed) and *The New Love and Sex After 60* (Ballantine).

Modern medications are so powerful that they both save lives and endanger them. After age 50, just when people are most likely to take several medications prescribed by multiple health professionals who often don't communicate with each other, they become increasingly vulnerable to adverse drug reactions.

Reasons: Aging slows recovery…diminished liver and kidney functions result in altered metabolism and excretion.

Also: Reapportionment of fat and lean body tissue changes drug distribution.

Surprising: The drugs most commonly implicated in adverse drug reactions are time-honored medications prescribed for chronic conditions.

Examples: Diuretics (water pills), such as *hydrochlorothiazide* (HydroDiuril) and *furosemide* (Lasix), to reduce fluid retention and blood pressure…oral anticoagulants (blood thinners), such as *warfarin* (Coumadin), to limit clotting after a heart attack or stroke.

DANGEROUS INTERACTIONS

An often-quoted study published in the *Journal of the American Medical Association* found that in the US, more than 2.2 million people a year have serious adverse reactions to prescribed drugs and 100,000 of them die, making drug interactions one of the leading causes of hospitalization and death. *Watch out for these…*

• **Drug-food interactions.** Some labels say, "Take with food." Which food? Grapefruit juice often triggers a drug-food interaction that may be good (helps the body absorb certain AIDS drugs) or bad (deactivates some blood pressure drugs and cholesterol-lowering drugs). Oat bran also can make blood pressure medication less effective.

Solution: Ask your doctor or pharmacist which foods might affect the actions of your medications and how.

Although taking drugs with a meal may reduce stomach upset, food may delay the drug's absorption, alter its characteristics or make its actions less predictable. Speak up—ask whether this applies to any medication you take.

Reduced body mass and increased fat make older people more sensitive to alcohol, which interacts with many commonly prescribed drugs and many commonly prescribed sleep aids, such as sedatives and hypnotics.

Danger: Alcohol is a major ingredient in many liquid medications, especially cough syrup.

• **Drug-drug interactions.** Prescription drugs known for interacting with other drugs include cholesterol-lowering statins, such as *atorvastatin* (Lipitor) and *pravastatin* (Pravachol), and blood pressure-lowering antihypertensives, such as *furosemide*, *propranolol* (Inderal) and *clonidine* (Catapres).

Self-defense: Find out which potential interactions apply to each medication you take now…and whenever a new one is prescribed, ask your doctor and/or pharmacist which drugs or foods not to take with it. Perhaps just separating the food and the drug by two or three hours would be safer.

Over-the-counter (OTC) drugs can wreak as much havoc as prescription drugs.

Examples: Antacids, antihistamines and heavy use of nonsteroidal anti-inflammatory drugs (NSAIDs), such as aspirin and *ibuprofen* (Advil, Motrin). According to an estimate by James Fries, MD, of the Stanford University School of Medicine, NSAID-induced gastrointestinal bleeding sends about 76,000 Americans to the hospital each year…and kills about 10% of them.

Antacids (Milk of Magnesia, Tums, Amphojel) can reduce the effectiveness of antibiotics, such as *tetracycline* and *ciprofloxacin* (Cipro)…antihypertensive drugs, such as *propranolol* and *captopril* (Capoten)…and heartburn drugs, such as *ranitidine* (Zantac) and *famotidine* (Pepcid AC). But antacids can also increase the potency of *valproic acid* (Depakote/Depakene), for seizures and bipolar disorder…*glipizide* (Glucotrol), for diabetes…*quinidine* (Quin-Release), for arrhythmias…and *levodopa* (Larodopa), for Parkinson's disease.

The older (first-generation) antihistamines, taken widely for allergies, colds and flu, can have dangerous interactions when taken with other drugs that cause drowsiness, such as antidepressants, alcohol, pain relievers, muscle relaxants and medications for seizures or anxiety.

Examples: *Brompheniramine* (in Robitussin Allergy & Cough) and *doxylamine* (in NyQuil).

The examples listed above are drops in the bucket. Check your own medications.

PERILOUS FALSE ALARM

Some drugs can drain certain vitamins from the body. If these vitamins aren't replaced, resulting symptoms may mimic those of dementia or other age-related conditions.

Examples: Tuberculosis drugs can deplete vitamin B-6, leading to amnesia, and vitamin-B complex, leading to apparent senility. Seizure drugs (anticonvulsants) can deplete vitamin D, leading to hearing and walking problems and general weakness. An older person displaying characteristics that are associated with dementia may just have an easily corrected vitamin deficiency.

MEDICATION ERRORS

More than 7,000 deaths in US hospitals were caused by medication errors in a single year, according to a major report published by the Institute of Medicine.

As it happens, the drugs found by the United States Pharmacopoeia* to be most frequently implicated in medication errors are commonly taken by seniors.

Examples: Insulin (for diabetes)...*warfarin* and *heparin* (to control clotting, such as in cardiovascular disease)...*albuterol* (Proventil, for asthma or bronchitis).

The Joint Commission asked hospitals to start providing every hospital patient with a list of all his/her prescribed medications and instructions for taking new ones. Patients, the Joint Commission said, should be encouraged to show the list to everyone providing care in the hospital, at any follow-up facility and after going home.

Have an advocate—a family member or friend—with you when you're in the hospital. Anyone hospitalized in my family is attended by a relative night and day.

Potentially fatal danger: Poor communication about meds when a patient is moved, such as from a critical-care unit to a general medical unit or from one health-care facility to another...or when nurses or other caregivers change shifts.

Self-defense: If you don't get a list from the hospital, maintain and hand out a list of your

*The nonprofit public standards–setting authority for prescription and OTC medicines, dietary supplements and other health-care products made and sold in the US.

own. A free form is available on-line from The Joint Commission at *www.jointcommission.org.* Also, question every drug you're given by anyone, anywhere, anytime.

For the most expert care, find a geriatrician—a physician specializing in seniors' medical needs. Medication needs differ as we age.

Example: A child's dose of *digoxin* (Digitek), used for congestive heart failure and other cardiac conditions, may be sufficient after age 65.

MEDICATION STRATEGIES

•**Brown-bag it.** You'll get your doctor's appreciation and attention by bringing in a bag containing every drug you currently take. Include prescription and over-the-counter drugs, vitamins, herbal supplements and nutritional supplements (such as chondroitin for joint pain). Go through the bag together.

Once you've agreed on which ones, if any, to change or drop, make a list of the ones remaining. Include the drug name, dose (amount and interval) and the name, specialty and phone number of the health professional who prescribed it. With every change, update the file.

•**Tell the world.** Post your master list on your refrigerator in case of a medical emergency at home. Keep a copy in your wallet near your driver's license. Give a copy to all your health-care providers, including surgeons, anesthesiologists and dentists. If you go to the hospital, take several copies and give them to all your health-care providers, including every nurse who hands you a pill or adds meds to your IV line. Ask to have a copy placed in your file or clipped to your chart.

•**Collaborate in your own care.** Our health system has no good mechanism for coordinating medical care. It's your job to give all your health-care providers the full picture.

Patients underestimate physicians' willingness to collaborate. Doctors are rushed, but they care. *Ways to help yourself...*

•If you suspect a possible interaction between drugs you're taking, either from symptoms or research, call the doctor immediately.

•Don't be afraid to raise concerns. You may be able to switch to a different drug that doesn't interact with your other meds.

•If you have trouble getting your doctor's attention, ask an office nurse to field medication-related questions.

•If your doctor is routinely unwilling to discuss your medications and to look up what he/she doesn't know, find one who will.

•Submit all prescriptions to the same pharmacy or chain. Typically, pharmacy computer systems automatically flag potential drug interactions. Ask your pharmacist.

EASY STEPS TO REMAIN SAFE

Prevention is far better than cure. *Keep medication crises at bay proactively…*

•**Use your eyes.** When you pick up a prescription, open and examine it on the spot.

Example: Coumadin, a brand-name product of the blood thinner warfarin, comes in nine doses. Is yours correct?

Before taking a new drug, read the side effects and interaction warnings in the patient information enclosure. Print too small? Type the drug name into Google or another search engine to find the manufacturer's Web site.

•**Don't take others' medications.** Doctors determine the best drug and dose according to age, weight, medical conditions and other drugs taken. What works well for someone else, even with the same condition, might be dangerous for you.

•**Drink lots of water.** Aspirin's tiny flakes can lodge in the esophagus, causing inflammation. *Acetaminophen* (Tylenol) in high doses can cause liver damage. Nonsteroidal anti-inflammatory drugs (NSAIDs), such as *naproxen* (Anaprox DS, Aleve), can cause ulcers. To reduce the risk, take pills with a large glass of water and drink several more glasses throughout the day.

•**Economize, but wisely.** Request a prescription for double the dose you need—a 10-milligram (mg) pill for a 5-mg dose, 20 mg for a 10-mg dose, etc. Cut each pill in half with an inexpensive pill cutter. You'll be taking the right amount at a lower cost per dose.

Warnings: Don't cut capsules or pills coated to prevent nausea or cut your prescription, taking half the prescribed dose, to save money. Ask an expert—your pharmacist will know whether your pills can safely be cut.

Popular Drugs That Steal Nutrients

Frederic Vagnini, MD, medical director of The Heart Diabetes & Weight Loss Centers of New York in New York City. Dr. Vagnini is coauthor of *The Side Effects Bible: The Dietary Solution to Unwanted Side Effects of Common Medications.* Broadway.

Depletion of nutrients is among the most common—and overlooked—side effects of both over-the-counter (OTC) and prescription drugs.

Here's what happens: Medications can cause improper absorption of vitamins and minerals—or they can accelerate the elimination of nutrients from the body. The consequences may range from bothersome symptoms, such as fatigue or stomach upset, to serious heart, muscle or nerve damage.

Most doctors are aware of some minerals that are depleted through the use of diuretics (water-excreting drugs). However, few doctors are aware of the dangers of nutrient depletion caused by many other types of medication, because the problem is not widely reported.

Popular drugs that deplete the body of nutrients…

ANTIBIOTICS

The most commonly prescribed antibiotics include *azithromycin* (Zithromax), *amoxicillin* (Amoxil), *ampicillin* (Omnipen), *ciprofloxacin* (Cipro), *ofloxacin* (Floxin) and *erythromycin* (Eryc).

Nutrients depleted…

•**B vitamins.** The B vitamins are essential for normal metabolism as well as immune and nervous system functioning.

•**Vitamin K.** This vitamin is critical for blood clotting and bone strength.

•**"Friendly" intestinal bacteria** known as *Bifidobacterium bifidum* and *Lactobacillus acidophilus.* Antibiotics kill not only harmful bacteria but also "good" bacteria that promote gastrointestinal health and help balance immune response.

If you are prescribed an antibiotic: Ask your doctor about also taking a B-complex vitamin—50 mg...vitamin K supplement—60 micrograms (mcg) to 80 mcg...and probiotic supplements providing 15 billion live B. bifidum and 15 billion live L. acidophilus organisms daily.*

In addition, eat more vitamin B–rich foods, such as beef, liver, chicken, pork, fortified breads and cereals, whole-grain pastas, legumes, nuts and dark, leafy greens.

To increase your intake of vitamin K, eat kale...collard, turnip or mustard greens...spinach...broccoli...and Swiss chard.

Caution: Do not take vitamin K supplements or eat excessive amounts of vitamin K–rich foods if you take *warfarin* (Coumadin) or another blood-thinning drug.

For additional B. bifidum, eat more asparagus, garlic and/or onions, which stimulate growth of this friendly bacteria. For L. acidophilus, yogurt containing live cultures is your best food source.

HIGH-CHOLESTEROL DRUGS

The most widely prescribed cholesterol-lowering "statins" include *atorvastatin* (Lipitor), *simvastatin* (Zocor), *fluvastatin* (Lescol), *lovastatin* (Mevacor) and *pravastatin* (Pravachol).

Nutrient depleted...

•**Coenzyme Q10 (CoQ10).** All cells require CoQ10 for the proper function of mitochondria (tiny energy-producing structures within the cells). The more energy a cell must produce, the more it depends on CoQ10. That's why cells of the heart, in particular—because it is constantly beating—require an abundance of CoQ10.

Unfortunately, statin drugs, which effectively block the production of harmful cholesterol, also prevent CoQ10 production.

Some doctors worry that long-term use of statins may worsen heart failure. Studies have found that patients with chronic heart failure have lower CoQ10 levels, and that CoQ10 supplements may improve their heart condition. Signs of CoQ10 deficiency include fatigue and muscle weakness.

If you are prescribed a statin: Ask your doctor about taking 30 mg to 100 mg of a CoQ10 supplement daily. This nutrient also is available

*If you're taking any medications, consult your doctor before changing your diet or beginning a supplement. In rare cases, increasing a nutrient may interfere with a drug's potency or worsen your condition.

in some foods, including beef, chicken, salmon, oranges and broccoli.

PAINKILLERS

Millions of Americans take a nonsteroidal anti-inflammatory drug (NSAID), such as *ibuprofen* (Motrin, Advil), *naproxen* (Aleve), *celecoxib* (Celebrex) and *nabumetone* (Relafen), to help relieve arthritis and other inflammatory pain.

Nutrient depleted...

•**Folic acid.** Your body needs this water-soluble B vitamin to produce new cells and DNA and to synthesize and utilize proteins.

Several large epidemiological studies have linked low folic acid levels to increased risk for colon, breast and pancreatic cancers.

Heart health is also affected by folic acid. As folic acid levels decline, levels of the amino acid homocysteine rise. Studies suggest that elevated homocysteine can raise the risks for blood clots, heart attack and stroke.

Low folic acid levels may cause loss of appetite, irritability, weakness, shortness of breath, diarrhea, anemia, headaches, heart palpitations and a sore tongue.

If you take an NSAID regularly (daily for at least one to two weeks): Talk to your physician about also taking 400 mcg to 800 mcg of folic acid daily.

You also can get more folic acid by consuming fortified breakfast cereals, orange juice, spinach and other leafy greens, peas and beans.

BETA-BLOCKERS

Beta-blockers, such as *propranolol* (Inderal), *atenolol* (Tenormin), *betaxolol* (Betoptic S), *carteolol* (Cartrol) and *labetalol* (Normodyne), are commonly prescribed for high blood pressure or glaucoma.

Nutrients depleted...

•**CoQ10.** Not only does CoQ10 appear to improve cardiac function in patients with chronic heart failure, studies suggest that it also may prevent second heart attacks and possibly protect against Parkinson's disease.

•**Melatonin.** The hormone melatonin is essential for healthy sleep-wake cycles, and there's some early evidence that it may slow aging.

If you take a beta-blocker: Ask your physician about taking 30 mg to 100 mg of CoQ10 daily…and 1 mg to 3 mg of melatonin nightly, just before bed, if you have trouble sleeping.

ACE INHIBITORS

Angiotensin-converting enzyme (ACE) inhibitors, such as *enalapril* (Vasotec), *benazepril* (Lotensin) and *ramipril* (Altace), as well as angiotensin II receptor blockers (ARBs), including *candesartan* (Atacand) and *irbesartan* (Avapro), are prescribed for high blood pressure and heart failure, and to help prevent heart attacks in high-risk patients.

Nutrient depleted…

•**Zinc.** Zinc boosts immunity, and some studies have shown that it reduces the duration of cold symptoms.

Zinc also is necessary for wound healing, strong bones and male potency, and it may help slow the progression of age-related macular degeneration (AMD).

In a recent six-year National Eye Institute study involving 3,600 people with AMD, zinc and antioxidant supplements reduced the risk of developing advanced AMD by 25%.

If you take an ACE inhibitor or ARB: Ask your doctor about taking 50 mg to 100 mg of zinc daily and eating more zinc-rich foods, such as oysters, beef, dark-meat chicken, pork tenderloin, yogurt, milk, peas, beans and nuts. If you continue to take zinc indefinitely, do not exceed 50 mg daily.

Important: Many medications combine an ACE inhibitor or ARB with a diuretic—for example, *enalapril* and *hydrochlorothiazide* (Vaseretic) is an ACE inhibitor plus a diuretic… *candesartan* and *hydrochlorothiazide* (Atacand HCT) is an ARB plus a diuretic.

If you're taking a combination drug, you'll need to compensate not only for zinc, but also for the electrolytes and nutrients excreted by the diuretic, including potassium, magnesium, thiamine (B-1) and calcium. Ask your doctor for advice.

DIABETES DRUGS

People with type 2 diabetes are often prescribed *tolazamide* (Tolinase), *acetohexamide* (Dymelor), *glimepiride* (Amaryl) or *glipizide* (Glucotrol)—all sulfonylurea drugs. These medications stimulate the pancreas to produce more insulin, which lowers blood sugar.

Nutrient depleted…

•**CoQ10.** Diabetes more than doubles your chances of dying from heart disease or stroke—and low CoQ10 levels increase those risks.

If you're taking a sulfonylurea drug: Ask your doctor about supplementing with 30 mg to 100 mg of CoQ10 daily.

REFLUX DRUGS

Proton pump inhibitors, such as *esomeprazole* (Nexium), *lansoprazole* (Prevacid), *omeprazole* (Prilosec) and *rabeprazole* (AcipHex), are prescribed for chronic heartburn—also known as gastroesophageal reflux disease (GERD)—and ulcers.

Nutrients depleted…

•**Vitamin B-12.** Vitamin B-12 is essential for producing red blood cells and maintaining a healthy nervous system. Deficits may cause fatigue, dizziness, shortness of breath, diarrhea, tingling in the hands or feet, unsteady gait, nervousness, cognitive changes and even dementia.

Vitamin B-12 is found in red meat, fish, eggs and dairy foods, but our bodies require stomach acid to release the vitamin from these foods. Proton pump inhibitors reduce the production of stomach acid, inhibiting the release and absorption of vitamin B-12.

•**Iron.** Low iron reduces the amount of oxygen your red blood cells can transport to body tissues, leaving you feeling weak and fatigued. A serious iron deficiency results in anemia.

If you take a proton pump inhibitor: Ask your doctor about taking 500 mcg to 1,000 mcg of vitamin B-12 daily and for advice on the best way to increase your iron intake.

Caution: Never take an iron supplement without consulting your physician—excess iron can accumulate in your major organs and cause severe damage. Most people, however, can safely eat more iron-rich foods, including liver, beef, dark-meat chicken or turkey, legumes and fortified cereals.

Risks of Acid Suppressants Like Prilosec

Andrew L. Rubman, ND, director, Southbury Clinic for Traditional Medicines, Southbury, Connecticut.

Andrew L. Rubman, ND, has long been concerned about the dangers associated with long-term use of drugs that suppress stomach acid, specifically the powerful proton pump inhibitors (PPIs) including *esomeprazole* (Nexium), *omeprazole* (Prilosec) and *lansoprazole* (Prevacid). A recent study adds to the alarm about the use of PPIs. This latest research shows an increased risk for hip fractures among older patients using PPIs. The risk is especially high for people taking higher doses or for those using PPIs for longer periods—and especially for people who do both.

THE STUDY

The study, from the University of Pennsylvania, reviewed 13,556 hip fractures from the United Kingdom General Practice Research Database, a collection of electronic medical records taken from 1987 to 2003. All of the data were from people older than age 50 at enrollment. The mean age at enrollment in the database was 77, and 79% were female. Researchers found that people who had used a PPI for more than a year had an associated increased fracture risk of 44%…long-term use of higher doses was even more startling, with 2.6 times elevated risk compared with non-users. Because 20% of the cases of hip fractures lead to death within a year, and older adults are increasingly being prescribed PPIs, these findings are especially scary.

WHAT'S THE CONNECTION?

Dr. Rubman notes that PPIs are effective medicine for people who have evidence of an ulcer. But use of a PPI for more than four weeks is always a risk, and a danger to those in the study who had used the medication for a year or more. Many people take a PPI not because of ulcers but to treat gastritis, an inflammation of the stomach lining that causes pain, belching, bloating and nausea.

When taken to quiet the stomach and used for more than three weeks, these drugs can end up significantly disabling the body's natural ability to produce digestive acids, says Dr. Rubman. This creates havoc in the digestive process and interferes with the body's ability to absorb calcium and magnesium. Both minerals are essential for strong bones, but they must be transformed in the stomach first in order to be absorbed and used in the body. This process requires a strong acidic environment, not one that has been suppressed. Without adequate levels of stomach acid, calcium and magnesium won't be absorbed properly.

Given the enormous popularity of PPIs, it's evident that there are many people who have compromised their stomach acid, and who may be in danger of fracture. One problem, notes Dr. Rubman, is that many older adults who have been long-term users of PPIs are likely to have become hypochlorhydric—meaning that they can no longer make enough hydrochloric acid to properly digest a meal. The solution, says Dr. Rubman, is to work with a naturopathic physician or other medical professional highly trained in enzyme use to begin rebuilding the body's ability to produce enzymes on its own. This will trigger the natural production of stomach acid. He considers this a necessity for anyone who has taken PPIs for longer than three weeks. It's possible that many people will have to take enzyme supplements with meals for the rest of their lives…but Dr. Rubman says that even in people with healthy stomachs, regular digestive enzyme use can be beneficial.

Are You Taking Too Much Lipitor?

Jay S. Cohen, MD, associate professor (voluntary) of family and preventive medicine, University of California, San Diego. Dr. Cohen is author of *What You Must Know About Statin Drugs and Their Natural Alternative* (Square One) and *Over Dose: The Case Against the Drug Companies* (Tarcher/Penguin). *www.medicationsense.com*.

The maker of *atorvastatin* (Lipitor) seems to be looking for even more new uses for its best-selling, cholesterol-lowering statin drug. The company, Pfizer, has significantly raised its profits by aggressively promoting the highest doses of Lipitor. (The 80-milligram dose costs over a third more than a 10-milligram dose.)

A Pfizer-sponsored study in *The New England Journal of Medicine* suggested that Lipitor should be taken not just by people with heart disease or by those at risk of a second heart attack, but also by people at risk of a second stroke, even if they don't have heart disease.

Jay S. Cohen, MD, author of *What You Must Know About Statin Drugs and Their Natural Alternatives*, says that while the results were positive in some respects, the real problem in this study, as in a previous trial involving high-dose Lipitor, is the overall mortality data. In this study, the risk of fatal stroke was reduced. But, when the total death rate was compared with the death rate of a group taking a placebo, there was very little difference. This raises safety concerns, since Lipitor—especially at high doses—is a powerful drug with potentially powerful side effects. Dr. Cohen also points out that study authors had financial ties to Pfizer, and several were Pfizer employees, which increases the potential for the authors to attach an agenda to the results of the study.

ABOUT THE STUDY

The study involved 4,731 individuals who had experienced a stroke or transient ischemic attack (a mini-stroke with symptoms such as numbness, confusion and dizziness, that may be a warning sign of a more serious stroke in the future) in the preceding one to six months, and had no known heart disease. Participants had LDL ("bad" cholesterol) levels of 100 to 190 mg/dL. Participants were randomly assigned to receive 80 mg of Lipitor a day, a high dose, or a placebo.

During the following 4.9 years, 265 people (11.2%) taking Lipitor and 311 people (13.1%) taking placebo had a stroke. The Lipitor group experienced 218 ischemic strokes (by far the most common strokes, caused by a clot in an artery in the brain) and 55 hemorrhagic strokes (strokes caused by the rupture of an artery or a blood vessel in the brain causing bleeding). The placebo group had 274 ischemic strokes and 33 hemorrhagic strokes. The researchers concluded that, in this risk group, 80 mg daily of Lipitor decreased the overall risk of stroke,

although it also resulted in what they called a "small increase" in hemorrhagic strokes. When comparing the two types of stroke that occurred in each group, hemorrhagic strokes accounted for 21% of the strokes in the Lipitor group, and only 11% of the strokes in the placebo group.

QUESTIONS RAISED

While these results are promising for stroke patients, the study also raises a number of questions. Of greatest concern to Dr. Cohen is the fact that the overall mortality rate was roughly the same in both groups. Elevated liver enzymes were also more common in those who took Lipitor, and he wonders why the study included no comparisons to lower doses of Lipitor.

Dr. Cohen also questions the use of statins—which have an anticlotting effect—in people who have had hemorrhagic strokes. Again, this raises safety concerns. Logically speaking, it seems that Lipitor and other statins would be safer for people who have had ischemic strokes. Additionally, while the study authors characterized the increase in risk as small, Dr. Cohen points out that there was in fact a 66% increase in risk of hemorrhagic stroke in those taking high-dose Lipitor, in comparison with those who were given a placebo.

Dr. Cohen's bottom line? "The improvement in ischemic strokes with maximum-dose Lipitor was tiny—1.9%. This is not a 'promising' finding. Instead, it shows a minimal effect. Another study should be done, preferably by independent researchers, to confirm the results before doctors start prescribing maximum-dose Lipitor to all stroke patients," explains Dr. Cohen.

There are many risks that must be weighed against potential rewards when it comes to Lipitor. This is no "slam dunk" for the drug company. If your doctor suggests you take it based on this study, question him/her and talk it through thoroughly.

■ ■ ■ ■

Can Antibiotics Cure Bronchitis?

After 640 bronchitis patients first saw their doctors, coughing lasted for 11 days whether they received antibiotics or not. Other symptoms, such as increased phlegm and shortness of breath, cleared up less than one day sooner in those who took antibiotics.

Bottom line: Most bronchitis is caused by viruses, not bacteria—and antibiotics are ineffective against viral infections.

Self-defense: Talk to your doctor about taking *acetaminophen* (Tylenol), which reduces fever and relieves sore throat and muscle pain. Inhaling steam for five minutes three times a day also may be effective.

Paul Little, MD, professor of medicine, health and life sciences, University of Southampton, England.

■ ■ ■ ■

Antidepressant and Dreams

Vivid dreams can be a side effect of some antidepressants, including *fluoxetine* (Prozac), *venlafaxine* (Effexor) or *bupropion* (Wellbutrin). The dreams are caused by chemical changes in the brain associated with these drugs. If the dreams are too disturbing, patients should ask their doctors about switching to a different antidepressant.

Jack M. Rosenberg, PharmD, PhD, director, International Drug Information Center, Long Island University, Brooklyn, New York.

■ ■ ■ ■

Medication Expiration Dates

Manufacturers guarantee product potency only until the expiration date. The medicine may be good later—but you can't be sure. Over-the-counter products in the original unopened manufacturers' packages kept under optimal conditions may last two years or more. Most prescription medicine is dispensed by pharmacists in patient-specific packaging and probably won't last as long.

Storage conditions also affect potency.

Example: If you keep medicine in a so-called medicine chest—a bathroom cabinet—it will degrade more quickly than if you store it away from bathroom heat and humidity.

Bottom line: After the expiration date, medicine should be discarded.

Susan Winckler, RPh, Esq., pharmacist, attorney and chief of staff, Department of Health and Human Services, US Food and Drug Administration, Rockville, Maryland.

■ ■ ■ ■

How Is Drug Dosage Calculated?

For certain medications with a narrow therapeutic effect (that is, the beneficial dose is just below the toxic dose), the dosage is calculated on a body-weight basis. Examples include some drugs used to treat cancer, many pediatric drugs and certain antibiotics, such as *gentamicin* (Garamycin) and *vancomycin* (Vancocin). In general, many factors other than weight are used to determine the dose of a drug, including kidney and liver function…the stage of a disease being treated…and other drugs the patient may be taking. For some medications, the dose is based on the actual level of the drug in the blood. But for many medications, the therapeutic dose is far below the toxic dose, and a fixed dose can be used for most patients.

Caution: In some cases, the lowest dose commercially available is still too high for older patients, due to reduced kidney and/or liver function and other physiological changes. In these cases, the drug is administered less often, or the dose is cut in half if the medication is suitable for splitting.

Jack M. Rosenberg, PharmD, PhD, director, International Drug Information Center, Long Island University, Brooklyn, New York.

■ ■ ■ ■

Rheumatoid Arthritis Medication Dangers

Many rheumatoid arthritis patients take *infliximab* (Remicade) or *adalimumab* (Humira), known as tumor necrosis factor (TNF)-blocking antibodies, usually after other treatments have failed to treat arthritis symptoms.

Finding: Scientists reviewed studies involving 3,493 patients who took one of these drugs and 1,512 patients who took a placebo.

Result: Those who took TNF-blocking antibodies had 3.3 times the risk of developing cancer, and 2.2 times the risk for serious infections, such as pneumonia, as those who took a placebo.

Theory: The drugs interfere with the body's infection-fighting mechanisms and its ability to defend itself against cancerous cells.

Self-defense: Patients who take these drugs should watch for symptoms of infection, such as fever and chills…get their vaccinations, such as those for influenza (flu) and pneumonia…and ask their doctors about appropriate cancer screenings.

Eric L. Matteson, MD, chair, division of rheumatology, professor of medicine, Mayo Clinic, Rochester, Minnesota.

■ ■ ■ ■

How Safe Are the Drugs from Canada?

Look for a pharmacy listed on the Web site of the Canadian International Pharmacy Association (CIPA), *www.ciparx.ca.* CIPA pharmacies must meet standards for handling drugs, licensing, business practices and more. They sell only medicines that have been tested and approved by Health Canada—the Canadian version of the US Food and Drug Administration (FDA). Health Canada and the FDA have equivalent safety standards.

Before ordering from a Canadian pharmacy site, be sure it is licensed as required by Canadian law. It should display its provincial license on-line. All pharmacies listed at the CIPA site have the necessary licenses.

Gary Passmore, spokesperson and executive assistant to the state president, Congress of California Seniors, nonprofit senior advocacy group, Sacramento.

■ ■ ■ ■

Vaccinations for Adults

You should get the Tdap vaccination every 10 years. It protects against tetanus, diphtheria and pertussis (whooping cough). This is especially important now because of recent outbreaks of whooping cough among adolescents and young adults.

If you are not in a monogamous long-term relationship, get the Hepatitis B vaccine to protect against this sexually transmitted liver disease.

Also, the new shingles vaccine has been approved by the FDA. Shingles is caused by the chickenpox virus. The vaccine is recommended for everyone age 60 and older—except those with weakened immune systems.

The pneumococcal vaccine prevents pneumococcal pneumonia. Everyone age 65 and older, as well as younger people with heart or lung disease or compromised immune systems, should get this vaccination.

An annual flu shot is recommended for people over age 50 and younger adults with diabetes, kidney disease, heart or lung disease, or a weakened immune system.

William Schaffner, MD, chairman, department of preventive medicine, Vanderbilt University Medical Center, Nashville.

Can Shipping Damage Mail-Order Drugs' Potency?

Gregory T. Chu, MD, staff intensivist, Banner Good Samaritan Medical Center, Phoenix.

Matthew Grissinger, RPh, medication safety analyst, Institute for Safe Medication Practices, Huntingdon Valley, Pennsylvania.

Ann Smith, spokeswoman, Medco Health Solutions, Franklin Lakes, New Jersey.

American College of Chest Physicians.

Mail-order drugs that are exposed to too much heat—in a car, transport truck or mailbox—may become less effective, say researchers.

THE STUDY

To test the effects of heat on medications delivered by mail, lead investigator, Dr. Gregory T. Chu, staff intensivist, Banner Good Samaritan Medical Center in Phoenix, and his colleagues recreated the conditions of a scorching Arizona mailbox in their lab. In the heat of an Arizona summer, a mailbox can reach a parching 158° Fahrenheit.

"The genesis of this study was our patients were actually calling us and telling us that that drug was being delivered to them in unsuitable conditions," says Chu.

In the study, capsules of the asthma drug *formoterol* (Foradil), still in their original blister packaging, were heated to 70° Celsius (or 158°F) for four hours.

When they were inspected, the heated capsules appeared grossly distorted and the formoterol formed clumps, according to Chu. His team also tested the effectiveness of the heat-exposed medication and found it delivered less than half of its intended dose.

CAUSE FOR CONCERN

With more Americans receiving prescriptions by mail, some medication-safety experts worry that exposing certain medications to extreme heat or cold could render them ineffective.

Their concern is not just limited to prescriptions that are received by mail or to formoterol, the focus of Chu's study.

"This is far more broad than what they present it to be," explains Matthew Grissinger, a medication-safety analyst at the Institute for Safe Medication Practices, a Pennsylvania-based drug safety organization.

Every prescription comes with information indicating the safe temperature for storing that medication, he notes. While some medications must be refrigerated, others should be kept at room temperature.

"Any time you exceed that temperature, there's no guarantee what you're going to get," Grissinger says.

Think about the heat and humidity in the bathroom—one of the worst places to keep prescription medications.

MAIL-ORDER PRECAUTIONS

However, Ann Smith, a spokeswoman for Medco Health Solutions, which dispenses approximately 78 million mail-order prescriptions a year, says the study fails to mention safe packaging requirements.

A mail-order pharmacy such as Medco has procedures in place for temperature-sensitive medications, including formoterol, she says. Such medications are shipped overnight in insulated packaging that includes ice or cold gel packs, depending on the type of medication and seasonal weather conditions.

For more tips on safe medication use, visit the Web site of the National Council on Patient Information and Education at *www.bemedwise.org.*

■ ■ ■ ■

Antibiotic Side Effects

A common antibiotic may cause high blood sugar levels (hyperglycemia) or low ones (hypoglycemia) in some patients, warns David N. Juurlink, MD, PhD. Tequin (*gatifloxacin*) is prescribed about two million times a year in the US, for pneumonia, sinus infections, urinary tract infections and some sexually transmitted diseases. If rapid heartbeat, sweatiness, nervousness, tremors, frequent urination or extreme thirst develop, contact your doctor to discuss alternatives. Tequin does not cause diabetes, as some recent reports suggested.

David N. Juurlink, MD, PhD, is a clinical pharmacologist at Sunnybrook and Women's College, Health Sciences Center, Toronto, and lead author of a study published in The New England Journal of Medicine.

Generic Drug Dangers

Joe Graedon, pharmacologist, and Teresa Graedon, PhD, consumer advocates who specialize in health issues related to drugs, herbs and vitamins. Their syndicated newspaper column "The People's Pharmacy" is widely distributed in the US and abroad, and they cohost an award-winning radio talk show. They are coauthors of 12 books, including the recently published Best Choices from The People's Pharmacy. NAL.

Generic drugs cost 30% to 80% less than their brand-name counterparts, but most people feel safe taking them because the FDA requires that both types of medications provide the same active ingredients and a comparable level of effectiveness.

Recent development: A survey found that about 25% of 300 doctors throughout the US don't believe that generics are chemically identical to brand-name drugs...nearly one in five believe that generics are less safe...and more than one in four believe that generics cause more side effects.

So what's the truth about generic drugs?

WHAT PATIENTS SAY

Since 1976, when our book *The People's Pharmacy* was originally published as a consumer guide to drug and health information, thousands of patients have contacted us about their experiences with medications.

In the last few years, we've received hundreds of letters and e-mails—most of them complaints—about generic drugs, including pain relievers, antidepressants and blood pressure medicines. The number of such complaints has increased dramatically in that time.

What we've learned: Some patients who switch from a brand-name to a generic drug report a decline in effectiveness—for example, blood pressure that isn't controlled as well or a worsening of depression. Others report having a rash or other types of allergic reactions, probably due to one of the inactive "filler" ingredients in generic drugs. There also seem to be problems with the timed-release mechanism of some generic drugs.

Example: We've heard more than 100 complaints about a generic version of the long-acting antidepressant Wellbutrin XL. At least one manufacturer's timed-release generic formulation appears to be different from the brand name—and may be releasing too much of the drug too quickly (known as "dose dumping"). This would explain many of the side effects, such as headaches and anxiety, that some people tell us they experience when they take the generic drug, but not the brand-name version.

We've contacted the FDA about the complaints regarding this generic drug, and we're also working with an independent laboratory to analyze this formulation.

IS THE FDA DOING ENOUGH?

Drug companies must apply to the FDA to sell generic versions of drugs. To gain FDA approval, a generic drug must contain the same active ingredients as brand-name medications and meet the same criteria for such factors as quality, strength and purity. *Possible problems with generic drugs…*

•**Periodic checks for impurities.** The FDA monitors generic drugs, testing for such things as proper dosing and active ingredients. But the agency only checks about 300 medication types, such as tablets and capsules, among brand-name and generic products a year—out of a total of more than *three billion* prescriptions.

•**Infrequent inspections.** The FDA is supposed to inspect each US drug manufacturing plant every two years—but lacks the resources to meet that requirement.

•**Overseas manufacturing.** An enormous percentage of drug ingredients and raw materials for drugs (primarily generic and over-the-counter) come from India, China and other countries where quality assurance is not as rigorous as in the US—and where drug counterfeiting has been a problem.

Trap: Overseas plants are inspected much less frequently than those in the US. Without testing, there's no way to tell whether drugs and drug ingredients derived from these plants have impurities—or come in "subtherapeutic" doses (for example, a drug labeled as 10 mg may be only 6 mg).

STAYING SAFE

Most of the evidence for problems with generic drugs is based on anecdotal reports. However, research published in *Neurology* reported that people with epilepsy who switched from the brand-name form of the antiseizure drug *phenytoin* (Dilantin) to the generic form of the drug began to have higher-than-expected rates of seizures. Investigators found that in many patients, blood levels of the active ingredient had dropped by 30%.

Even so, patients should not give up on generic drugs. The cost savings can be considerable…and there's no evidence so far that the majority of generic drugs will cause problems for most patients. Patients using generic drugs should simply take extra precautions…

•**Stick with one manufacturer.** This is particularly important if you're taking a drug with a *narrow therapeutic index* (NTI), such as the anticoagulant *warfarin*, the antipsychotic *lithium* or the anticonvulsant *carbamazepine*. NTI drugs, which typically require periodic blood tests to measure blood levels of the medications, have a very thin margin between an effective dose and a toxic dose. If you're taking a generic form, ask your pharmacist for the name of the manufacturer—and request that the pharmacy stick with that company, if possible, to avoid variations between products.

•**Track your numbers.** Many conditions, such as hypertension or high cholesterol, don't cause obvious symptoms. The best way to tell whether a drug is working is to monitor your numbers—by taking daily blood pressure readings, tracking blood-sugar levels and keeping track of cholesterol levels with frequent blood tests at your doctor's office.

Important: Ask your doctor to give you copies of your test results. Check them periodically to make sure that you're maintaining adequate control—particularly if you've recently switched from a brand name to a generic, or the reverse.

- **Trust your instincts.** Some medications affect the body in subtle ways. A patient taking a thyroid drug, for example, might feel slightly run-down if it isn't working exactly the way it should, even if test results appear to be normal. *Pay attention.* If you've switched to a generic and notice a difference—either in effectiveness or side effects—tell your doctor.

- **Do a "challenge, rechallenge" test.** If you suspect that a generic drug isn't working the way it should, write down changes in how long the drug works and side effects. Then, ask your doctor to switch you to the brand-name equivalent, and see if there's improvement—in most cases, it will be apparent in about two weeks. Under the close supervision of your doctor, repeat the test, going back and forth until you have a clear idea which drug is more effective for you.

- **Report problems to the FDA.*** The FDA can analyze generic drugs to determine if they contain the stated amount of active ingredient. When reporting a drug to the FDA, ask your pharmacist to provide the name of the manufacturer, the lot number and exactly when the drug was dispensed to you.

If you'd also like to report problems with generic drugs to us, go to The People's Pharmacy Web site, *www.peoplespharmacy.org.*

*Go to the FDA Web site, *www.fda.gov/medwatch*, or call 888-463-6332.

Boost Your Medication's Healing Powers

Leo Galland, MD, director of the Foundation for Integrated Medicine in New York City. His latest book is *The Fat Resistance Diet.* Broadway. *www.fatresistancediet.com.* Dr. Galland is a recipient of the Linus Pauling Award.

If you're among the millions of Americans taking medication for pain, asthma or allergies, hypertension, high cholesterol or depression, research shows that you may be able to maximize the benefits...curb the side effects...and maybe even lower the dosages of your drugs by combining them with the right supplements.

Important: Consult your doctor before adding a supplement to your drug regimen. Some supplements can interact adversely with medications—for example, some research shows that fish oil can reduce the time it takes for blood to clot and should be used with caution by people taking a blood thinner, such as *warfarin* (Coumadin).

Supplements (available at health-food stores) to consider using if you are taking any of the following...

ANTIDEPRESSANT

Supplement with: 1,000 mg to 2,000 mg daily of *eicosapentaenoic acid* (EPA), an omega-3 fatty acid found in fish oil. (Ask your doctor which dosage is right for you.)

What it does: Omega-3s are believed to enhance the ability of the brain chemical *serotonin* to act on the nervous system. In a recent British study, when depressed patients who were taking a prescription antidepressant, such as *fluoxetine* (Prozac) or *sertraline* (Zoloft), added 1,000 mg of EPA to their daily regimen for 12 weeks, they reported significantly less depression, anxiety and suicidal thoughts, as well as improved sleep, libido and energy.

Most standard fish oil supplements contain only 200 mg to 300 mg of EPA, so you'd need up to 10 capsules daily to get the recommended 1,000 mg to 2,000 mg of EPA. If you don't want to take that many capsules, take liquid fish oil—in an amount equal to 1,000 mg to 2,000 mg daily of EPA.

Helpful: To avoid "fishy-tasting" burping (the most frequent complaint), try taking the capsules on an empty stomach with a large glass of water. Some people also find that this unpleasant aftertaste is less likely to occur with liquid fish oil.

Also try: 500 micrograms (mcg) daily of folic acid, which promotes proper functioning of the nervous system. Low levels of folic acid have been linked to depression.

Harvard Medical School researchers report that depressed patients who had achieved remission

283

with fluoxetine were 13 times more likely to relapse during a six-month period if they had low blood levels of folic acid.

Caution: Supplemental folic acid may mask a vitamin B-12 deficiency, which can lead to nerve damage. Take a 500-mcg to 1,000-mcg B-12 supplement daily to prevent worsening of a B-12 deficiency.

NONSTEROIDAL ANTI-INFLAMMATORY DRUG

Supplement with: 350 mg of *deglycyrrhizinated licorice* (DGL), three times daily.

What it does: Studies show that DGL may reduce or prevent the gastrointestinal (GI) inflammation, bleeding and ulcerations caused by aspirin and other nonsteroidal anti-inflammatory drugs (NSAIDs)—prescription and over-the-counter.

Caution: Whole licorice extract also protects the stomach, but it contains *glycyrrhetinic acid*, which even in small doses may raise blood pressure. Stick with DGL.

Also try: 1,000 mg to 2,000 mg daily of vitamin C (in two divided doses) and 7 g of powdered glutamine (one heaping teaspoon dissolved in water, three times daily). Studies suggest that taking 1,000 mg of vitamin C twice daily may help prevent aspirin-induced inflammation of the small intestine.

Meanwhile, the amino acid glutamine, long used to help heal ulcers, may decrease the intestinal toxicity of other NSAIDs.

ASTHMA OR ALLERGY DRUG

Supplement with: 1,000 mg daily of *gammalinolenic acid* (GLA) and 500 mg daily of EPA.

What it does: GLA, an omega-6 fatty acid derived from evening primrose oil or borage oil, may inhibit production of *leukotrienes*, molecules that trigger inflammation and constriction of the bronchial airways. The asthma drug *montelukast* (Singulair) also works by inhibiting leukotrienes.

Important: Most omega-6 fatty acids (including those found in many processed foods) *increase* inflammation, unless they're balanced by sufficient amounts of anti-inflammatory omega-3s. GLA, however, is an anti-inflammatory, but at high doses—and in the absence of

omega-3s—it can become inflammatory. The recommended 500 mg of EPA daily creates an optimal balance of omega-6s and omega-3s.

Also try: Quercetin, a bioflavonoid derived from red onions, apples and other foods. In laboratory studies, quercetin has demonstrated antihistamine and anti-allergenic properties. Clinical trials are needed, but given its safety, I often recommend quercetin to my asthma and allergy patients. Try using 500 mg to 600 mg, twice daily, of quercetin—taken on an empty stomach for maximum benefit—as an adjunct to your antihistamine and/or GLA.

BLOOD PRESSURE DRUG

Supplement with: 1,000 mg of *arginine,* twice daily.

What it does: Arginine (also called L-arginine) is an amino acid used by the body to produce nitric oxide (NO), a molecule that helps keep blood vessels flexible and able to dilate—both of which stabilize blood pressure. Legumes (such as lentils, black beans and kidney beans) and whole grains (such as brown rice) contain some arginine, but you'll need a supplement to get the 2,000 mg daily that is recommended for blood vessel health.

Caution: Because some research has shown that arginine can be dangerous for people who have suffered a heart attack, it should not be used by these individuals. If you have the herpes simplex virus and want to take arginine, you may need to add 1,500 mg daily of *lysine*, another amino acid. The virus grows in the presence of arginine but is inhibited by lysine.

Also try: 100 mg daily of *Pycnogenol*. This plant extract appears to enhance NO synthesis in blood vessels. In a recent placebo-controlled trial, Chinese researchers found that hypertensive patients who took 100 mg of Pycnogenol daily for 12 weeks were able to significantly lower their dose of a calcium channel blocker, a popular hypertension drug.

STATIN

Supplement with: 100 mg daily of coenzyme Q10 (CoQ10).

What it does: Cholesterol-lowering statins deplete the naturally produced molecule coenzyme Q10—this depletion may lead to muscle damage.

Researchers at Stony Brook University in Stony Brook, New York, found that patients taking statins who added 100 mg of CoQ10 daily for one month reported a 40% reduction in severity of muscle pain, a common side effect of statins.

CoQ10 also may prevent oxidation of LDL "bad" cholesterol—an unfortunate side effect of statins that occurs to LDL cholesterol particles not eliminated by the drug.

Also try: Fish oil that contains 1,500 mg of EPA and 1,300 mg of docosahexaenoic acid (DHA) daily. Studies show that these essential fatty acids raise HDL "good" cholesterol and lower dangerous blood fats known as triglycerides—making EPA and DHA a valuable adjunct to statins, which mainly target elevated LDL cholesterol.

Timing Medications Helps You Recover Faster

Michael Smolensky, PhD, professor at the School of Public Health, and cofounder and former director of the Memorial-Hermann Center for Chronobiology, both at the University of Texas—Houston. He is coeditor of the medical journal *Chronobiology International* and coauthor of *Body Clock Guide to Better Health*. Henry Holt.

Most medical students are taught that the body is *homeostatic*—that is, having a "steady state" of biological functions. However, scientists now know that the body functions rhythmically.

The symptoms of chronic medical conditions, such as high blood pressure, arthritis and hay fever, vary greatly according to so-called *circadian* (24-hour) *rhythms*. By timing medications to your body's biological rhythms—a treatment approach known as chronotherapy—you can recover faster from a health problem or live better with a chronic illness.

HIGH BLOOD PRESSURE

One in every four American adults has high blood pressure. Most doctors agree that normal blood pressure is less than 120/80. (The top number is *systolic* pressure, when the heart beats...the bottom number is *diastolic*, when the heart relaxes between beats.)

Using a technique called *ambulatory blood pressure monitoring*, which measures pressure automatically 24 hours a day, doctors now know that blood pressure exhibits a circadian rhythm.

In most people, blood pressure is highest after awakening, rising by at least 25 systolic points. Blood pressure remains elevated during the day and declines in the evening, reaching its lowest level during nighttime sleep. It is important that prescription blood pressure medications control daytime highs without overcorrecting nighttime lows.

New advances: In the US, there are several medications specifically designed to keep drug levels in the body in sync with the circadian rhythms of blood pressure. These medications, called chronotherapies, include the calcium channel blockers *verapamil* (Verelan PM and Covera-HS) and graded-release *diltiazem* (Cardizem LA)...and the beta-blocker *propranolol* (InnoPran XL).

Intended to be taken at bedtime, their drug-delivery technology ensures that no medication is released until four hours after ingestion. Medication is then released so that peak levels of the drug are circulated during the day when blood pressure rises and the lowest levels of the drug are circulated at night when blood pressure is lowest.

Clinical studies show that these medications optimize the control of the morning blood pressure rise, which has been linked to stroke in at-risk patients. These drugs may also minimize risk for morning heart attack.

Caution: If you are taking a non-chronotherapy drug, do not change your dosing schedule. Studies show that taking certain medications at the wrong times can cause extreme lowering of blood pressure during nighttime sleep and may not control hypertension throughout the day.

New finding: Low-dose aspirin, when taken at the right time of day, may have a blood pressure–lowering effect. A study published in 2003 in the journal *Hypertension* found that taking low-dose aspirin before going to bed reduced systolic blood pressure by an average of five points but had no effect when taken first thing in the morning.

More research is needed, but the new finding suggests the importance of the body's circadian rhythm, even when taking non-prescription medications, such as aspirin.

ARTHRITIS

Osteoarthritis (OA) is an age-related disease of painful, stiff and swollen joints. Rheumatoid arthritis (RA) is an autoimmune disease that causes joint inflammation. These conditions are typically treated with nonsteroidal anti-inflammatory drugs (NSAIDs), such as *ibuprofen* (Advil), *ketoprofen* (Orudis) and *indomethacin* (Indocin).

New finding: Large clinical studies show that NSAIDs are more effective against symptoms of RA when taken at bedtime.

Moreover, NSAIDS produce fewer gastrointestinal (GI) complications, such as indigestion and stomach discomfort, when taken at bedtime than when taken in the morning.

Additional studies have found that patients with OA who experience their most severe symptoms in the afternoon and evening get the most relief from NSAIDs when they are taken at breakfast (even though there may be an increase in the risk for GI side effects at this time) or at midday with lunch.

If NSAIDs do not relieve RA symptoms, your doctor may prescribe anti-inflammatory corticosteroid medications, such as *prednisone* (Deltasone). These medications can cause side effects, such as insomnia, mood changes and appetite enhancement, especially when taken in high doses. Studies show that these medications are the most effective, and the least likely to cause side effects, when taken once a day, either in the morning or early afternoon.

HAY FEVER

Allergens, such as pollens, mold spores, dust mites or animal dander, cause this respiratory problem, also known as *allergic rhinitis*. Symptoms include sneezing, an itchy, stuffed or runny nose and swollen, puffy eyes.

One in 10 sufferers experience symptoms seasonally, while the remainder suffer year-round. As all hay fever sufferers know, symptoms typically are worst in the early morning, after waking up, although many sufferers complain that sleep is disrupted at night due to severe nasal congestion.

The circadian rhythm of hay fever symptoms is thought to be due to fluctuations in adrenaline and cortisol. That's because these hormones, which counter allergen-caused inflammation and swelling, are at their lowest during the night.

For better control of morning symptoms, such as sneezing and/or a stuffy, runny nose, take an antihistamine in the evening or at bedtime.

Save Money on Prescription Drugs

Timothy McCall, MD, internist, medical editor of *Yoga Journal* and author of *Examining Your Doctor* (Carol) and *Yoga as Medicine: The Yogic Prescription for Health and Healing*. Bantam. *www.drmccall.com*.

With some prescription drugs now costing hundreds of dollars per month—and many patients taking dozens of different pills—people wonder what they can do to keep their drug expenses down.

Some patients cut costs by skipping doses or by simply not filling prescriptions. Either approach can be dangerous. But there are many ways to lower costs without compromising your care. *Here are some suggestions...*

•**Ask your doctor the cost of each drug he/she prescribes.** Doctors often wildly underestimate the costs of the drugs they prescribe. By inquiring, you let your doctor know that price matters to you and you assess just how aware of costs your doctor really is.

If your doctor's estimate is way off, let him or her know. The doctor may then make another suggestion. At the very least, future patients may benefit from your inquiry.

•**Tell your doctor how you pay for drugs.** About 75% of Americans with health insurance are covered by a plan that pays for at least part of each prescription. If you're not one of the lucky ones, tell your doctor. Similarly, if meeting growing co-payments is a concern for you, let your doctor know.

•**Ask your doctor if there are any cheaper alternatives.** In general, generic drugs are just as safe and effective as name brands—sometimes at less than one-tenth the price. And most drug plans charge lower co-payments when patients use generics or other "preferred" medications. Ask, too, if there's an entirely different medication that might work just as well for your condition at lower cost.

Each time your doctor prescribes a drug for you, ask if there's any reason *not* to use the generic version. Occasionally, there are good reasons to stick with the name brand—for example, when you're taking a blood thinner, antiseizure medication or another drug that must be kept at precise levels in the bloodstream. If you choose a generic, some problems can be mitigated by being sure you always get a generic manufactured by the same company. Be wary of doctors who always oppose generic substitution.

•**Ask your doctor about nondrug alternatives.** For many illnesses, it's possible to forgo medication—or use lower dosages—if nondrug therapies are used.

Losing weight, for example, can reduce the need for medication in many cases of diabetes, arthritis and high blood pressure. Yoga has been shown to have similar effects. Acupuncture can lessen dependence on pain pills. Some herbs, such as saw palmetto for prostate enlargement, are effective but cost less than prescription drugs.

•**Ask your doctor to prescribe medication in large quantities.** Pharmacies often give discounts to patients who purchase more than 100 pills at a time. Similarly, a four-ounce tube of a salve may cost only a bit more than a one-ounce tube.

If you've never used the drug before, however, stick with a small quantity. That way, you won't wind up with lots of a drug that didn't work well for you—or that caused unacceptable side effects.

Another way to save money is to buy pills in a higher-than-needed dose and then divide the pills. If you take 20 mg per day, for example, ask your doctor if you could buy 40-mg tablets and cut them in half. Be careful, though. This strategy works only with "scored" pills, which have a groove down the middle, and some other

medications. Ask your pharmacist if you have any doubts.

•**Compare prices at several drugstores.** Drug prices vary enormously from store to store. A prescription that costs $30 at one store could easily run $50 at another.

It makes no sense to pick a drugstore solely on the basis of price. Service, location and the pharmacist's willingness to provide useful information also matter. But call at least three drugstores to find out what each charges for the medications you take regularly. Once you settle on a drugstore, it's best to use it for all your prescriptions.

•**Ask your pharmacist for a discount.** Drugstores give deep discounts to HMOs and insurance companies. You, too, may be able to get a price break—simply by asking for one. Your drugstore may have more room to cut the price on generics since the markups are higher than on brand names.

•**Consider mail order.** A mail-order drugstore cannot provide the personalized touch you get in a good neighborhood pharmacy. But sometimes the cost savings justifies the trade-off. Consider mail order only for drugs you take regularly, and order them a week or more before you run out. It can take several days to receive the drugs you order, and you don't want to be without needed medication.

•**Look into drug discount programs.** Many pharmaceutical manufacturers offer medications free of charge or at a steep discount to people with incomes below a certain threshold. To learn more, you can contact your drug's manufacturer directly or visit the Partnership for Prescription Assistance's Web site at *www.pparx.org* for listings of public and private patient assistance programs.

•**When evaluating a health plan, ask about its drug formulary.** A formulary is the list of drugs the plan agrees to pay for (minus any co-payment). If you take a particular drug on a regular basis, you will save lots of money if it's on the list. Plans with "closed" formularies make you pay the full cost of any unlisted medication. The only exception is if your doctor can convince the plan that you truly need a particular drug.

•**Don't store your pills in the bathroom medicine cabinet.** Humidity accelerates the rate at which drugs decompose, so bathrooms are just about the *worst* place to store pills. Instead, find a cool, dry place that's out of the reach of children. One good option is to keep your pills on a shelf in your office.

Properly stored, pills retain 70% to 80% of their original potency for a year or two after the expiration date. If the bottle was never opened, pills can remain potent for 10 years or more. The bottom line? You can safely use most drugs beyond their expiration dates. One dangerous exception is the antibiotic *tetracycline*. It becomes toxic as it decomposes.

•**Say no to drug samples.** Free samples are almost always of new drugs. These tend to be costly, and they have no long-term track record of safety. If you accept a sample for some new drug and buy more later, you may end up paying much more.

•**Think twice about drugs that are heavily advertised.** It costs millions to run the drug ads that have become ubiquitous on TV and in newspapers and magazines. As you might imagine, heavy promotion makes sense only for high-cost, high-profit medications, which because they are newer may have still unrecognized side effects. Those are the sorts of drugs you want to avoid, unless they offer real advantages. Remember—you want the best drug for your ailment, not the one with the cleverest ad campaign.

When Drugs and Juices Don't Mix

Beverly J. McCabe-Sellers, PhD, RD, professor of dietetics and nutrition at the University of Arkansas for Medical Sciences in Little Rock for more than 20 years. She is currently a research coordinator/nutritionist with the US Department of Agriculture, Agriculture Research Services and is a coeditor of the *Handbook of Food-Drug Interactions*. CRC.

If you take any kind of prescription or over-the-counter (OTC) medication, you may be unwittingly reducing its benefits and/or increasing its risks by drinking certain beverages when you swallow the drug. The potentially harmful interactions also may occur if you drink the beverage hours before or after taking the medication.

For example…

DANGERS OF GRAPEFRUIT JUICE

Grapefruit juice has long been known to interfere with the effectiveness of certain medications, but not all doctors warn their patients about these potential dangers.*

Grapefruit juice contains compounds that inhibit an important enzyme called *CYP3A4*, which is found in the liver and intestines. CYP3A4 is one of several enzymes that help metabolize up to 70% of all medications.

Grapefruit juice that is made from concentrate usually contains the entire fruit, including the rind—the primary source of the compound that affects drug metabolism. Grapefruit juice that is *not* made from concentrate contains less of this compound. However, to be safe, it's best to avoid grapefruit juice (and grapefruit itself) altogether if you take certain medications.

Among the drugs that can interact with grapefruit juice…

•**Anti-arrhythmic medications,** such as *amiodarone* (Cordarone), *quinidine* (Quinidex) and *disopyramide* (Norpace), which are taken for abnormal heart rhythms.

Risks: Heart arrhythmias as well as thyroid, pulmonary or liver damage.

•**Blood pressure–lowering calcium channel blockers,** such as *felodipine* (Plendil), *nifedipine* (Procardia) and *verapamil* (Calan).

Risks: A precipitous drop in blood pressure, as well as flushing, swelling of the extremities, headaches, irregular heartbeat and, in rare cases, heart attack.

•**Cholesterol-lowering drugs,** such as *atorvastatin* (Lipitor), *lovastatin* (Mevacor) and *simvastatin* (Zocor).

Risks: Headache, stomach upset, liver inflammation and muscle pain or weakness.

•**Sedatives such as *diazepam* (Valium) and *triazolam* (Halcion).**

Risks: Dizziness, confusion and drowsiness.

*As a general guideline, it is best not to drink any juice at the same time that you take medication. Instead, use water to swallow pills.

DANGERS OF APPLE JUICE AND ORANGE JUICE

New research shows that apple juice and orange juice can decrease the absorption of some drugs if the juice is swallowed at the same time as the pill. Grapefruit juice is also believed to have this effect.

Specifically, researchers found that apple, orange and grapefruit juice decrease the absorption of…

•**Allergy medication** *fexofenadine* (Allegra).

•**Antibiotics,** such as *ciprofloxacin* (Cipro) and *levofloxacin* (Levaquin).

•**Antifungal drug** *itraconazole* (Sporanox).

•**Blood pressure–lowering beta-blockers,** such as *atenolol* (Tenormin).

•**Chemotherapy drug** *etoposide* (Toposar).

If you are taking any of these drugs, it is probably safe to drink apple or orange juice (and eat whole fruits) at least two hours before or three hours after taking the medications. Check with your doctor first. Avoid grapefruit juice (and grapefruit itself) altogether.

DANGERS OF COFFEE

Coffee can interact with certain medications in a variety of ways. Do not drink coffee at the same time that you take any medication. *Limit daily consumption of coffee to one to two cups if you take…*

•**Antacids.** Because coffee contains acid, it counteracts the effectiveness of OTC antacids such as *calcium carbonate* (Tums) and *aluminium magnesium* Maalox.

•**Aspirin** or other nonsteroidal anti-inflammatory (NSAID) medications, such as *ibuprofen* (Advil) or *naproxen* (Aleve). Because coffee increases stomach acidity, combining it with these drugs may increase risk for gastrointestinal side effects, including stomach irritation and bleeding.

•**Bronchodilator** *theophylline* (Elixophyllin), used to treat asthma or emphysema. Consuming coffee with the bronchodilator can slow metabolism of the drug, leading to an increased risk for nausea, vomiting, palpitations and seizures.

•**Monoamine oxidase inhibitor (MAOI) antidepressants,** such as *phenelzine* (Nardil) and *selegiline* (Eldepryl). The combination may increase anxiety.

•**Osteoporosis drug** *alendronate* (Fosamax). Studies show that coffee (and orange juice) can inhibit absorption of Fosamax by 60%. If you take Fosamax or any other osteoporosis medication, ask your pharmacist about foods or other beverages that may interact with the drug.

DANGERS OF CRANBERRY JUICE

In the United Kingdom, there have been at least eight recent reports of bleeding in patients (one of whom died) after they drank cranberry juice with the blood-thinning medication *warfarin* (Coumadin).

Health officials were unable to definitively link the bleeding to the combination of cranberry juice and warfarin, but it's probably safest to avoid cranberry juice altogether if you're taking this medication. Cranberry juice has been shown to inhibit a key enzyme that is responsible for warfarin metabolism, but more research on this interaction is needed.

If you take another drug with blood-thinning effects, such as aspirin, you can probably drink cranberry juice occasionally (no more than four ounces—at least two hours before or three hours after taking the medication). Consult your doctor.

DANGERS OF MILK

The calcium in milk can interact with certain medications. *Drink milk at least two hours before or three hours after taking…*

•**Antacids,** such as calcium carbonate products (Rolaids) or *sodium bicarbonate* products (Alka-Seltzer and Brioschi). Drinking milk with these antacids can cause milk-alkali syndrome, a condition characterized by high blood calcium levels that can lead to kidney stones or even kidney failure.

•**Antibiotics,** such as *tetracyclines* and *ciprofloxacin* (Cipro). Calcium blocks absorption of these drugs, decreasing their effectiveness. Calcium-fortified juices are believed to have the same effect.

BETTER DRUG METABOLISM

Our bodies need nutrients to properly metabolize most medications. Chief among these nutrients is protein. Though we tend to eat less protein as we age—due to a variety of reasons, such as dental problems that make it harder to chew meat—we actually require *more* of this nutrient, since our bodies become less efficient at digesting and utilizing it.

Because the lining of the small and large intestines—where drugs are absorbed—regenerates every three to seven days, you need a continual supply of protein to maintain healthy levels of the enzymes that promote metabolism of medications.

To facilitate drug metabolism: Aim to eat about half a gram of protein daily for every pound of body weight.

Good sources: Fish, meats, eggs, peanut butter and soybeans.

B vitamins also play a key role in drug metabolism. Food sources rich in B vitamins include meats, fortified cereals, bananas and oatmeal.

Helpful: If you skip breakfast and aren't much of a meat eater, consider taking a multivitamin supplement containing the recommended daily intake of B vitamins.

To learn more about drug-beverage interactions, go to the FDA Web site (*www.fda.gov/ cder/consumerinfo/druginteractions.htm*).

■ ■ ■ ■

Dispose of Drugs Carefully

Don't toss unused prescriptions down the toilet. They could seep into drinking water and harm the environment.

To safely dispose of prescription medications: Remove the pills or liquid from the original container, and mix them with used coffee grounds, cat litter or another undesirable substance to prevent a child or pet from ingesting them. Put the combination in a nondescript, impermeable container, such as a jar or sealable bag, and seal it. Throw the container in the trash.

Alternative: Go to a pharmaceutical take-back site, which allows consumers to return drugs for safe disposal. Search for these locations at *http://earth911.org*.

Federal Guidelines for Proper Disposal of Prescription Drugs, Office of National Drug Control Policy, Washington, DC. *www.whitehousedrugpolicy.gov.*

10

Living Longer and Better

10 Easy Ways to Add Many Years To Your Life

How old are you really? We all have a "real age" that can be much lower—or higher—than our chronological years. A 50-year-old man, for example, could have the immune system of someone 20 years younger.

More than a decade ago, I introduced the RealAge concept—a scientific way of calculating a number that reflects the overall state of your health rather than your calendar age. We are constantly updating our data to reflect new research. The lower your RealAge, the longer you are likely to live.

We discovered that some changes can be hard to achieve—such as losing 25 pounds or quitting smoking—but others are relatively easy and can have a big impact on your life span.

Latest findings: Research pinpoints 10 simple changes that can lower your RealAge by almost 15 years…

TAKE ASPIRIN DAILY

RealAge benefit: 1.9 years.

In men over age 35 and women over age 40, 162 milligrams (mg) of aspirin daily (the equivalent of two baby aspirins) reduces the risk of heart attack by 36% and the risk of colon, esophageal, throat and stomach cancers by about 40%. We don't know how aspirin reduces cancer risk—we just know that it does.

Check with your doctor about taking aspirin. Some people can't take it because of stomach discomfort and/or bleeding. Ibuprofen may be an appropriate substitute.

Caution: Taking both aspirin and ibuprofen in the same 24-hour period blocks the protective

Michael F. Roizen, MD, chief wellness officer at the Cleveland Clinic, Ohio, is coauthor of *YOU: The Smart Patient* (Free Press). Dr. Roizen has cowritten *YOU: The Owner's Manual* (Collins), and served on the boards of five nonprofit foundations. He is former chair of a Food and Drug Administration advisory committee and has published over 160 peer-reviewed papers.

effects. Also, don't take aspirin in combination with blood-thinning drugs such as *warfarin* (Coumadin). It increases the risk of internal bleeding.

SUPPLEMENT WITH FOLATE

RealAge benefit: 1.2 years.

The B vitamin folate helps prevent errors in DNA duplication, an underlying cause of cancer. Taking 600 micrograms (mcg) to 800 mcg of folate daily could decrease breast cancer risk by 25% to 50%…colon cancer risk by 20% to 50%…and risk of childhood cancers by about 60% when taken by the mother during pregnancy. Folate also lowers levels of *homocysteine*, an amino acid linked to stroke, heart disease and other cardiovascular disorders.

Take a B-complex or multisupplement that includes 100% of the recommended daily amount of the vitamins B-6 and B-12…and add a folate supplement to get a total of 600 mcg to 800 mcg daily. You need all three to lower homocysteine—and the ability of the body to absorb B-12 declines with age.

DON'T SUPPLEMENT UNNECESSARILY

RealAge benefit: 1.7 years.

Millions of Americans take iron or vitamin A supplements daily. With the exception of some people who, for specific reasons, are advised by their doctors to take extra vitamin A or extra iron, the use of these nutrients (except in a multivitamin) can take years off your life.

The average vitamin A supplement contains more than 5,000 international units (IU), an amount that causes bone demineralization and increases the risk of liver and lung cancers.

Taking iron is dangerous because as many as one in 200 Americans has hemochromatosis, a condition that causes excess iron to accumulate in tissues, increasing the risk of heart or liver failure.

I advise taking a daily multivitamin that contains all the essential vitamins and minerals but no iron unless told to by your doctor. The multivitamin should contain less than 2,500 IU of vitamin A.

EAT SPAGHETTI SAUCE

RealAge benefit: 1.9 years for men, 0.8 years for women.

Tomatoes contain the carotenoid *lycopene*, which is believed to strengthen the immune system and reduce the risk of breast and prostate cancers by 30% to 50%. Try to get 10 tablespoons (a little more than one-half cup) of tomato sauce weekly. Processed tomatoes, such as those in spaghetti sauce, confer more benefits than fresh tomatoes because processing releases the lycopene. Eat canned tomatoes or tomato sauce with a little oil—for example, by cooking the sauce with olive oil—to improve absorption of lycopene.

CONSUME FAT FIRST AT MEALS

RealAge benefit: 1.8 years.

Starting meals with a little fat increases feelings of satiety and reduces overall calorie intake by about 7%. If you are overweight, you can lose about 10 pounds in a year if you do this at every meal.

Make sure that the fat is a healthy one—olive oil, nuts, etc. To get the benefits, you need about 70 calories of fat, which is about one-half tablespoon of olive oil, six walnuts or 12 almonds. One great way to start a meal is with a salad that has olive oil in the dressing and a few chopped nuts sprinkled on top.

WASH PRODUCE—AND YOUR HANDS

RealAge benefit: 0.4 years.

More than 40 million Americans suffer from food poisoning annually, and several thousand die from foodborne illness. Washing your hands frequently—and always before meals—is a key way to prevent this.

It's also crucial to wash produce thoroughly. Even organic fruits and vegetables require washing because they contain fertilizer residue that can cause illness. Wash produce twice in lukewarm water with a little dish soap, then rinse twice in regular water. You can put greens in a salad spinner and give them three cycles of rinsing/spinning.

DRINK MODERATELY

RealAge benefit: 1.9 years.

Alcohol reduces the tendency of blood platelets to clump together and form clots in the arteries, the cause of most heart attacks. It also inhibits the oxidation of fat that contributes to the development of plaque on artery walls.

The extensive Harvard Nurses' Health Study found that women who had three or more alcoholic drinks weekly had a 40% lower rate of heart attacks and arterial disease than those who did not. Studies in men show similar results.

Caution: Moderation is the key—no more than one drink daily for women, and no more than two drinks daily for men. Don't drink alcohol if you have a history of drug or alcohol abuse.

WEAR A HELMET

RealAge benefit: 1 year.

Wearing a helmet when riding a bike or a horse or when skiing can reduce your risk of head injury and related aging by as much as 80%. The RealAge benefit of one year assumes that you engage in the activity five times a month.

GET ENOUGH SUN

RealAge benefit: 1.7 years.

Vitamin D is essential for calcium absorption and bone strength. It also helps reduce the risk of breast, colon, prostate and lung cancers. Only a few foods (mainly fatty fish) contain vitamin D in a form that can be used by the body. Sunshine is required to convert fats in the body into a usable form of vitamin D.

I advise getting 10 to 20 minutes of sun exposure without sunscreen daily. Use sunscreen when you're in the sun longer than 20 minutes to prevent premature skin aging and skin cancer.

EAT FIBER EARLY IN THE DAY

RealAge benefit: 0.6 years.

Starting the day with a high-fiber cereal or fresh fruits or vegetables helps you feel full longer and reduces calorie intake. It prevents spikes in glucose that can damage arteries and increase the risk of heart disease.

Bonus: People who get at least 25 grams of fiber a day have a RealAge up to three years younger than those who get the national average of 12 grams.

Example: In a study at Northwestern University, a 10-gram-a-day increase in cereal fiber consumption decreased the risk of heart attack by 29%.

■ **More from Michael F. Roizen...**

Erase Years from Your Age in 30 Minutes a Day

Walking is the single best thing you can do for your health. I view it as the fountain of youth. In my first RealAge book, I showed how aging has little to do with calendar years. A 50-year-old man could have the arteries and immune system of a 75-year-old. Someone else might be 75 but have a RealAge—measured by the risk of disease, disability or death—of a 52-year-old. Exercise is a key factor in reducing your RealAge—and just 30 minutes of walking a day can make you healthier, more energetic and, in a real sense, younger.

HEALTH BENEFITS

Walking is easy to do, doesn't require any special equipment (except walking shoes) and conveys many of the same health benefits as more strenuous exercise.

Walking helps prevent fatty buildup in the arteries. When your arteries are clogged with fatty buildup, your cardiovascular system ages more quickly, and so does your entire body. Aging of the arteries brings on cardiovascular disease, the major cause of heart attacks and strokes. It also leads to loss of energy, memory loss and, in men, impotence. Walking can help keep arteries young and healthy.

Walking every day also decreases the risk of such conditions as macular degeneration (the leading cause of blindness in people over age 50) and arthritis. The long-running Framingham Heart Study found that people with arthritis who walked daily for 30 minutes and supplemented their diets with vitamins C and D and calcium were able to stop the progression of joint damage. Walking also prevented osteoarthritis in patients who didn't already have it.

Walking can even reduce the risk of some forms of cancer by as much as 50%.

GET READY

Studies show that people who walk as little as 10 minutes a day—or even just once a week—on a regular basis have less risk of dying prematurely than those who are sedentary. For optimal health gains, you should walk for at least

30 minutes daily. People who take three 10-minute walks each day have about the same health gains as those who walk for 30 minutes straight. *Helpful…*

•**Warm up before walking.** Walk more slowly than usual for the first several minutes. This warm-up heats the muscles and makes them more flexible and efficient and less prone to injury. It also increases circulation in the joints.

•**Wear a watch.** Measure time rather than distance. Time is easy to count, and you can walk for 30 minutes at a comfortable pace. You don't need to follow a track or a premeasured route—and you won't try to force yourself to go a certain distance.

•**Don't miss a day.** Make 30 minutes a day of walking a priority. Things like yard work and housecleaning help, too, but they can't take the place of your daily walks.

Malls are terrific places to walk if the weather is bad, and most YMCAs have walking tracks and treadmills. If your budget permits, buy a treadmill so you can walk any time of the day or night without leaving home.

POSTWALKING STRETCH

Once your routine becomes ingrained, set aside two to three minutes to stretch after you're done walking. Stretching improves joint range of motion. Without a normal range of motion in the joints, daily activities become more difficult and the risk of musculoskeletal injury increases. Some people find that stretching also reduces soreness, though I can't find hard evidence to support that claim.

To perform a stretch, move slowly into the stretch position until you feel a gentle pulling sensation, not pain. Hold the stretch for 10 to 30 seconds *without bouncing.* Repeat each stretch two or three times.

Here is a sample postwalking stretch for each key muscle group…

•**Hamstring.** Sit on the floor with both feet straight out in front of you. Keep your left leg extended, and bend the right so that the sole of your right foot is against the inner thigh of your left leg. Lean forward over the left leg until you feel a gentle stretch along the back of your extended thigh, keeping your back as straight as possible. Repeat with the right leg extended.

•**Quadricep.** Stand on your right leg, and bend the left so that your left knee is pointed toward the floor. Then reach your left hand behind you and take hold of your left ankle. Your hips should be pressed forward so that you feel a gentle stretch along the front of your left thigh. (You may need to stand near a wall for balance.) Repeat, standing on your left leg with the right leg bent.

•**Buttock.** Lie on your back, and bend both legs, keeping your feet flat on the floor. Cross the ankle of your right foot just above your left knee. Lift your left foot off the floor, and bring both legs toward your chest. Hold on to your left thigh to help pull your legs closer to your chest until you feel a gentle stretch near your right hip and buttock. Repeat with the other leg.

•**Adductor.** Lie on your back, and bend both knees. Open your knees out to the sides, and place the soles of your feet together. Pull your feet in toward you, allowing your knees to drop toward the floor until you feel a gentle stretch in the groin and inner-thigh area.

•**Hip flexor.** Stand with the left foot in front of the right, with your weight centered evenly between both feet. Keeping your back straight, bend your knees slightly, lowering yourself toward the floor and tucking your hips under. You should feel a gentle stretch along the front of your right hip. Repeat with the right foot in front of the left.

•**Calf.** Sit on the floor with both feet extended in front of you. Keeping your back as straight as possible, flex your toes toward you until you feel a gentle stretch in the back of both legs.

•**Lower back.** Sit on the floor cross-legged. Keeping your head in line with your spine, lean forward with your upper body and reach your arms out in front of you until you feel a gentle stretch in your lower back.

A Calorie-Restricted Diet May Slow Aging

Mark A. Stengler, ND, naturopathic physician in private practice, La Jolla, California…adjunct associate clinical professor at the National College of Natural Medicine, Portland, Oregon…author of many books, including *The Natural Physician's Healing Therapies* and coauthor of *Prescription for Natural Cures* (both from Bottom Line Books)…and author of the *Bottom Line/Natural Healing* newsletter.

A calorie-restricted diet could slow aging, according to new research. Investigators looked at lab reports and Doppler imaging of 25 people who had been practicing calorie restriction for about six years. The people, ages 41 to 65, consumed an average of 1,400 to 2,000 calories a day. Their blood pressure, heart function and inflammatory blood markers, including *C-reactive protein*—a measure of inflammation in blood vessels and elsewhere in the body—were compared to those of 25 people of similar age and gender with an intake of 2,000 to 3,000 calories per day, the amount in a typical Western diet. Researchers found that diastolic function of the heart in the calorie-restricted group resembled diastolic function in people about 15 years younger. (Diastolic, the bottom number in a blood pressure reading, measures the pressure when the heart is at rest, in between beats.) There was little difference in systolic function (the top number in a blood pressure reading, which measures the pressure inside blood vessels when the heart beats). Blood pressure overall and inflammatory markers were significantly lower as well in the low-calorie group.

My view: This was the first human study to show a correlation between calorie restriction and an anti-aging effect on heart function. Researchers theorize that chronic inflammation from a typical calorie-loaded Western diet, which is heavy in animal products and refined sugar but low in fruits and vegetables, causes damage to—and premature hardening of—heart muscle. More studies are needed. Keep in mind that the quality of your food choices is as important as calorie restriction. For best results, opt for fruits, vegetables, cold-water fish, lean poultry, whole grains and legumes, limited red meat—and watch your portion sizes.

■ **More from Mark A. Stengler…**

The Truth About Growth Hormone

For over 15 years, human growth hormone (HGH) has been touted as a miraculous anti-aging hormone. Some physicians prescribe it for obesity, sexual dysfunction, cognitive decline and fibromyalgia.

WHAT IS HUMAN GROWTH HORMONE?

HGH is secreted by the brain's pituitary gland. As its name implies, it stimulates the growth of tissues in the body. Most notably, it promotes growth in height during childhood. Most people have heard of a childhood deficiency of HGH, but in rare cases, adults can lack adequate amounts of the hormone. An HGH deficiency that occurs during adulthood can lead to a reduction in muscle mass, strength and bone density as well as sexual dysfunction and emotional problems, such as depression. If you have these symptoms, ask your doctor for a blood test. An HGH deficiency even can increase cardiovascular disease risk.

THE ANTI-AGING CRAZE

In 1990, *The New England Journal of Medicine* reported on a six-month study in which 12 healthy men, ages 61 to 81, who showed no signs of HGH deficiency were given twice the dose of HGH that an adult man with a deficiency would ordinarily receive. A control group of nine men did not receive HGH injections. The men receiving the injections experienced systolic (top number) blood pressure and fasting blood glucose concentrations that were significantly higher than when they started the study. On the positive side, they experienced an increase in lean body mass, a decrease in fat mass and an improvement in bone density, all of which led many people to believe that HGH could be used to effectively reverse some of these troubling signs of aging. However, there have been no studies of HGH's effect on longevity in humans.

SAFETY CONCERNS

I have tested many patients' blood levels of insulinlike growth factor (IGF-1)—a biomarker that is used to assess HGH levels. Only occasionally have I found a patient with a serious deficiency.

Typically, these patients suffer from fatigue. What concerns me is that some doctors routinely recommend HGH injections for virtually all of their patients who are over age 60 without testing for a deficiency. When these doctors do run blood tests, they often diagnose a deficiency by comparing their older patients' IGF-1 levels with those of a 20-year-old. I strongly disagree with this practice. HGH should not be used unnecessarily because of the side effects, which include swelling in the legs and arms, headache, arthritis-like symptoms, bloating, muscle pain, hardening of the arteries, high blood pressure, diabetes.

A rapid drop in HGH levels or an overt deficiency (a deficiency is characterized by IGF-1 readings below 90 µg/mL) can and should be treated, but a gradual decline over a period of years appears to be one of the body's ways of preventing cancer. Research now links elevated IGF-1 levels to increased risk for colon, pancreatic, endometrial, breast and prostate cancers.

MY RECOMMENDATION

HGH is a powerful hormone that should be used only by people who have been diagnosed with a deficiency. Even in these cases, HGH replacement should be monitored by a physician. To gain the benefits of extra HGH without the dangerous risks, there is a much more effective —and less costly—strategy. I recommend a combination of aerobic exercise (such as walking and cycling) and weight-lifting, each performed for 30 minutes three times a week. Sleep also is important for maintaining healthy HGH levels. There are a variety of supplements that claim to boost HGH levels, but no good data support their use. Save your money for the gym.

■ ■ ■ ■

Human Growth Hormone (HGH) Alert

Human growth hormone (HGH), sometimes touted as an anti-aging agent, has potentially dangerous side effects. Most mainstream doctors point to higher diabetes risk, carpal tunnel syndrome, muscle pain and possible tumor growth as reasons to avoid HGH. But some alternative medicine practitioners recommend using HGH under carefully controlled and supervised circumstances. They say that daily HGH injections have sometimes resulted in improvements in blood pressure, heart ailments and other conditions. HGH costs up to $20,000 a year and is not covered by insurance.

Robert N. Butler, MD, clinical professor of geriatrics and adult development, Mount Sinai School of Medicine, and president and CEO, International Longevity Center-USA (*www.ilcusa.org*), both in New York City. He won the Pulitzer Prize for his book *Why Survive? Being Old in America* (Johns Hopkins University). He is also coauthor of *Aging and Mental Health* (Pro-Ed) and *The New Love and Sex After 60* (Ballantine).

Amazing Health Protecting "Pill"

Bruce Ames, PhD, professor of biochemistry and molecular biology at the University of California at Berkeley, is best known for developing the Ames Test, a widely used procedure for identifying potential carcinogenic substances. He is the recipient of the National Medal of Science.

Wouldn't it be nice if you could take a pill that would help protect you against serious ailments, including cancer and heart disease?

You can. Dozens of studies have shown that taking a daily multivitamin/mineral supplement is one of the simplest and best ways to help fight age-related disease. But it has to be the *right* multi to get the job done. Unfortunately, only one in three American adults consistently takes a multivitamin.

To learn more, we spoke with Bruce Ames, PhD, a renowned biochemist who studies the effects of vitamin and mineral deficiencies on health...

ARE YOU GETTING ENOUGH?

There's no question that a balanced diet consisting of whole grains, vegetables, fruits, fish, dairy and lean meats is our best source of the nearly 40 vitamins, fatty acids, minerals and amino acids that are essential to human health.

While most Americans consume enough of these micronutrients to avoid acute deficiency diseases, such as scurvy (vitamin C deficiency) or anemia (iron deficiency), research shows that up to 10% of us consume less than half of the recommended levels of each key micronutrient —a dangerously low level. *Also...*

•**Up to 25%** of premenopausal American women consume less than half of the recommended intake of iron.

•**More than half of us** aren't getting enough magnesium or calcium.

•**Up to 80%** of American adults with darker skin (blacks, people from India and some Hispanics)—particularly those who live in northern states, where sun exposure tends to be limited—are deficient in vitamin D. Fair-skinned people who don't get much sun exposure and don't get vitamin D from a supplement also are at risk.

These nutritional deficiencies are serious threats to our health—on par with smoking or obesity. Even a marginal deficiency of only one key nutrient can significantly change our cells in a way that can lead to cancer and other serious diseases.

THE SCIENTIFIC EVIDENCE

At our laboratory at the Children's Hospital & Research Center in Oakland, California, we study nutritional deficiencies in human cells by limiting vitamins or minerals and examining how the cells respond.

Our findings: When cells are grown so that one of the vitamins (biotin or B-6) or minerals (iron, zinc, magnesium or copper) is limited, the cells' chromosomes undergo significant damage, changes that are linked to the development of cancer.

An abundance of research shows that inadequate levels of folic acid are linked to breast, pancreatic and colon cancers...low intakes of vitamin B-6 are implicated in colorectal cancer ...insufficient vitamin D increases the risk for colorectal cancer and may double the risk for prostate cancer...low zinc appears to heighten the risk for esophageal cancer...and low magnesium increases colorectal cancer risk.

If this isn't reason enough to get your daily vitamins and minerals, there's even more evidence. Nutrient deficiencies appear to disrupt the normal functioning of *mitochondria*, the tiny "engines" inside our cells that convert fuel (starches and fats) into energy. This process normally produces a small number of "free radicals," oxidized molecules that contribute to cellular aging.

However, when zinc, iron, copper, biotin or other key nutrients are in short supply, we've observed that mitochondria mass-produce free radicals. In the body, this may lead to premature aging and a raft of degenerative diseases, affecting everything from our hearts and brains to our bones.

Antioxidant nutrients may help stave off the damage, but supplying the missing nutrient is the key. In a recent Johns Hopkins University study, older people taking vitamins E and C were found to be less likely to develop Alzheimer's disease. In studies at The Cooper Institute in Dallas, patients who took multivitamins for six months had significantly lower blood levels of C-reactive protein, a marker for cardiovascular disease.

YOUR BEST DEFENSE

A multivitamin/mineral is a convenient way to fill in any nutritional gaps in your diet. An expensive brand-name supplement isn't necessary. I recently bought a year's supply for about $10 at one of the big national discount stores.

Just be sure to choose a multivitamin/mineral supplement that contains close to 100% of the Daily Value (recommended daily intake) of most vitamins and minerals.

Men and women age 50 and older who eat some red meat should choose an iron-free formulation, since most adults get sufficient amounts of this mineral in their food. Premenopausal women, who lose iron through menstruation, should choose a supplement with iron.

Be cautious about supplements providing "megadoses" (five to 10 times the recommended daily intake) of specific vitamins and/or minerals. In my opinion, there is little scientific evidence showing that the use of more than the recommended daily intake of any nutrient is beneficial for the general public (though future studies may change that). What's more, certain vitamins, especially vitamin A, and many of the minerals, including iron, manganese and selenium, are toxic at high doses.

Some manufacturers are now advertising multivitamins that offer a "bonus" ingredient—for example, the herb ginkgo to bolster memory... or the sugar-cane derivative policosanol to lower cholesterol. These combination products are generally safe, but most lack sufficient research showing that they're actually any better for you—or whether the added benefits are worth the additional costs. Talk to your doctor before starting a multivitamin with added ingredients, especially if you're taking medications.

297

Important: A multivitamin should be taken with food to help promote the body's absorption of fat-soluble vitamins, such as vitamins D and E.

OTHER IMPORTANT NUTRIENTS

In addition to a basic multivitamin, consider a calcium/magnesium supplement. Because calcium and magnesium are bulky, most multivitamin/mineral supplements contain no more than a small percentage of the recommended daily intake (otherwise the pills would be too big to swallow). Look for a product that offers a 2:1 ratio of calcium to magnesium—your body can't effectively use one without the other. And be sure your multivitamin contains 400 international units (IU) of vitamin D to aid absorption of these minerals.

Unless you eat three meals of cold-water fish (such as salmon, halibut, mackerel) weekly, I advise taking a fish-oil supplement with omega-3 fatty acids. These essential fatty acids promote brain and heart health.

If you feel your energy or cognition slumping, try taking two lesser-known nutrients—acetyl-L-carnitine (ALC) and alpha lipoic acid (ALA). In animal studies, these biochemicals lower oxidant levels caused by aging and improve physical and mental performance. Twenty-four clinical trials have shown ALC and ALA to be safe.

Good choice: The supplement Juvenon (*www.juvenon.com*) contains both ALC and ALA.

The Secret to Looking And Feeling Younger: Posture

Paul D'Arezzo, MD, a retired emergency physician and a posture-alignment specialist based in Colorado Springs, *www.posturealignment.com*, is the author of *Posture Alignment: The Missing Link in Health and Fitness*. Marcellina Mountain.

You can take years off your appearance and ease pain in your muscles and joints without expensive surgery, cosmetics or even highly demanding exercise routines.

All you need to do is spend a few minutes a day focusing on one of the most important—and neglected—aspects of a youthful appearance and an optimally functioning body…posture.

Think of your body as if it were a stack of building blocks. If the blocks are lined up unevenly, the structure is weak and is more likely to collapse. If they're carefully lined up one on top of the other, the structure is strong.

When the body is misaligned, it fails to function as efficiently as possible. Bad posture contributes to arthritis, muscle pain and injuries. These aches and pains cause us to avoid activities that we once enjoyed.

What went wrong? Modern society has evolved in such a way that we're no longer required to move as much during our day-to-day activities. And when we do move, we do so in the same repetitive ways, not utilizing all of our muscles or our full range of motion. Certain muscles get strong while others get weak—and we lose correct alignment.

BETTER ALIGNMENT

By performing the following simple exercises to correct and maintain posture, you can begin to achieve maximum physical function as you age. The following four exercises strengthen and stretch unique muscles in the body that hold us upright and stabilize us—muscles that usually aren't worked by standard aerobic and strength-training exercises.

Ideally, this alignment program should be practiced at least every other day as an adjunct to your usual aerobic, stretching and strength-training regimen.

Although it can take weeks to change posture, you will feel a difference in your alignment after doing the exercises only once.

GROIN STRETCH

Purpose: Stretches and aligns the groin muscles. Over time, it will align your hips and allow your shoulders and back to return to a more anatomically correct position.

What you need: A chair, coffee table or ottoman that is the right height so that when you lie on the floor on your back, one leg can rest on top of the object and form an approximate 90-degree angle.

What to do: Lie on your back, bend your right leg and place it on top of your "platform." Your right calf muscle should be resting on the platform. Stretch your left leg straight out on the floor, toes pointed toward the ceiling. Place your arms out to the sides, palms up. Rest in this pose for five minutes, allowing gravity to do the work, relaxing the body and letting the muscles stretch. Repeat with your left leg.

TABLE STRETCH

Purpose: Counteracts the tendency to hunch and roll shoulders forward.

What you need: A table, desk, counter or back of a chair.

What to do: Stand a few feet from the table, with feet hip-width apart and pointing straight ahead. Lean forward and rest your hands, palms down, on the table so that your legs and torso form a 90-degree angle. Relax. Let your head fall forward between your shoulders, and let gravity do the work. Hold for one to two minutes.

CATS AND DOGS

Purpose: Increases flexibility and movement in the pelvis and lower back.

What you need: A carpet, exercise mat or other comfortable floor surface.

What to do: Get on your hands and knees so that your back forms a small table. Place your hands directly below your shoulders, fingers pointing forward. Knees should be in line with your hips. Exhale and slowly arch your back upward like a cat, pressing your chin toward your chest. Hold for five seconds.

Then arch in the opposite direction (the way dogs do when they stretch), pulling your head and neck upward and your upper and lower back downward and lifting your buttocks into the air. Hold for five seconds. Smoothly transition from "cat" to "dog" for 10 complete cycles.

FACE THE WALL

Purpose: Stretches and aligns the muscles of the chest, shoulders and pelvis.

What you need: A wall.

What to do: Stand facing the wall with feet hip-width apart, toes turned inward and touching (pigeon-toed). Your chest and nose should almost touch the wall.

Lift your arms straight above your head, shoulder-width apart. Place the backs of your hands on the wall. Hold for one minute, eventually working up to three minutes. You will feel a stretch in your pelvis and shoulders.

At first you only may be able to reach the wall with the sides of your hands.

As your muscles align and stretch, you will be able to work up to reaching the wall with the backs of your hands.

Helpful: This may be uncomfortable at first, but after a minute your shoulders will begin to relax.

Illustrations by Shawn Banner.

10 Quick Energy Boosters

Jon Gordon, best-selling author of *Energy Addict: 101 Physical, Mental and Spiritual Ways to Energize Your Life* (Perigee), *The 10-Minute Energy Solution* (Putnam), and his latest book, *The Energy Bus: 10 Rules to Fuel Your Life, Work and Team with Positive Energy* (Wiley). His performance-energy consulting firm is based in Ponte Vedra Beach, FL. Clients include the PGA Tour, the Atlanta Falcons, Campbell Soup, and JPMorgan Chase. *www.jongordon.com.*

Three-quarters of the people I meet complain of tiredness during the day. This epidemic of exhaustion is brought about by mental and physical stress, including too much caffeine and sugar as well as too little sleep and exercise.

Here are easy ways to feel more alert and energetic...

•**Stop hitting the snooze button on your alarm clock in the morning.** Your brain goes through periods of light and heavy sleep. Falling back to sleep for just five more minutes can cut short a new sleep cycle, leaving you groggier when you do arise.

Better: Set your clock for when you really have to get up. Open your shades right away, and get as much light as possible—bright light wakes you up and invigorates you. Raise your heartbeat for at least five minutes in the morning by running in place or doing sit-ups, push-ups or jumping jacks.

•**Eat a power breakfast.** It will energize you as you start the day. My favorite power breakfast: Mix low-fat plain yogurt and one-half cup of old-fashioned raw oatmeal when you first get up. The yogurt will soften the oats while you shower and dress. Add a few chopped walnuts, one-half cup of pineapple or one-quarter cup of blueberries.

•**Sit up straight.** Bad posture can decrease your oxygen intake, and slouching exhausts your neck, shoulders and upper-back muscles.

Correct posture for sitting: Your back should be aligned against the back of the chair, so that you can work without leaning forward. Your knees should be a bit higher than your hips. Keep both feet flat on the floor and your arms flexed at a 75- to 90-degree angle.

•**Replace coffee with green tea.** The rich taste of coffee and the mental alertness it imparts make coffee drinking a tough habit to break. But coffee raises stress hormones, and just a few cups a day creates an energy roller coaster that increases overall fatigue. I have found that people who have the most success giving up coffee switch to green tea. It contains one-third the amount of caffeine (20 mg to 25 mg per six-ounce cup), so you get an energy boost without feeling irritable or experiencing a slump later on.

Bonus: Green tea is loaded with disease-fighting antioxidants.

If you have no intention of giving up your daily coffee, at least try cutting back to half regular/half decaf.

•**Consume protein with meals.** It helps your body absorb sugar at a slower rate, so your energy levels don't fluctuate so much during the day.

Examples: Fish, eggs, hummus, skinless poultry breast, lean red meat.

•**Go for a 10-minute walk after lunch.** It raises your metabolism and prevents you from falling into the familiar, post-meal "coma."

If it's inconvenient to go outside, try chair squats.

How to do that: With a chair behind you, stand with your feet positioned shoulder-width apart. Keep your back straight and your chin up. Squat down, and push out your rear as if you were going to sit in the chair behind you. Just as your rear touches the chair, return to your starting position. Repeat five to 30 times—or until you feel your muscles have had enough.

•**Take a short nap,** no more than 25 minutes. Longer than that and you move into a deeper phase of sleep, which, if interrupted, can leave you groggier than before your nap. The optimal time to take a nap is eight hours after you wake up.

•**Eat an energy snack,** such as a banana or a handful of walnuts or almonds. Avoid commercial energy drinks and energy bars—they often work by introducing caffeine and/or sugar into your system.

Helpful: I do recommend a caffeine-free, multivitamin energy powder that I use myself each day—Fatigued to Fantastic! from Enzymatic Therapy, available at health-food stores.

Cost: About $50 for a month's supply.

•**Try peppermint.** It boosts mood and motivation. Have a cup of peppermint tea, or dab peppermint oil (available at health-food stores) on your wrists.

•**Breathe.** We tend to hold our breath when we work intensely or are under stress—and this contributes to fatigue.

To practice energy-boosting breathing: Stand up straight with your arms at your sides. Inhale for two seconds as you raise your arms slowly over your head with your palms open. Continue lifting your arms until they are directly over your head with fingertips touching. Exhale for three seconds as you bring your arms down. Repeat 10 times.

The Anti-Aging Workout

Karl Knopf, EdD, an exercise physiologist and professor of adaptive/older adult fitness at Foothill College, Los Altos, California, and president of the Fitness Educators of Older Adults Association, is the author of five books, including his most recent, *Weights for 50+: Building Strength, Staying Healthy and Enjoying an Active Lifestyle.* Ulysses.

Most people know that cardiovascular exercise, such as walking and swimming, helps promote good health. Unfortunately, many neglect strength training.*

*Consult your doctor before beginning this or any new exercise routine.

People who do not perform regular strength exercises will lose 50% of their muscle mass and muscular strength by age 65. In fact, sarcopenia (age-related muscle loss) is one of the main reasons that many older adults become unable to live independently and must enter an assisted-living center or nursing home.

The following simple program, designed especially for those over age 50, is easily done at home using a stretchable rubber exercise band (about $15)...ankle weights ($13 per pair)...and dumbbells ($1 to $2 a pound). These products are available at sporting-goods stores.

Most of the following exercises recommend beginning with one- to two-pound dumbbells or ankle weights. Increase the weight when you can perform 15 repetitions easily. By performing this 30-minute full body workout two to three times a week, in addition to your regular cardiovascular exercise routine four to five times a week, you can enhance your energy, strength—and even your independence.

SIT TO STAND

Purpose: Strengthens the front leg muscles that are used to get up from a seated position.

What to do: Sit toward the front of a sturdy chair, with your feet flat on the floor. Lean slightly forward. Inhale. Exhale slowly as you stand up. If possible, do not use your hands. Cross your arms in front of your chest. Inhale and lower yourself slowly into the chair. Do six to 15 repetitions. When you can easily complete 15 repetitions, try holding a one- to two-pound dumbbell in each hand.

LUNGES

Purpose: Strengthens the legs and helps with balance.

What to do: Stand with your feet shoulder-width apart, arms at your sides, holding a one- to two-pound dumbbell in each hand. Inhale. Keeping your left leg in place, exhale and lunge forward with your right leg as far as you comfortably can while keeping your right knee in line with your right ankle. Inhale as you step back to the starting position. Do six to 15 repetitions. Repeat with your left leg.

Modification: If you find this exercise too difficult, do it without weights, and place your hands on your hips instead. If balance is an issue, hold on to a chair when lunging.

LATERAL ARM RAISES

Purpose: Strengthens the shoulders and upper back.

What to do: Stand straight, feet shoulder-width apart and knees relaxed. Place your arms at your sides and hold a one- to two-pound dumbbell in each hand. To protect your lower back, keep your torso firm by contracting your abdominal muscles and not arching your back. Inhale as you slowly lift your arms out to each side, no higher than shoulder level. Hold for one second. Exhale as you slowly return to the starting position. Do six to 15 repetitions.

Modification: If doing this exercise with straight arms is too difficult, bend your elbows and extend them out from your sides.

Caution: If this exercise causes pain and/or a clicking sound in the shoulder area, stop right away. Consult your doctor.

MODIFIED PUSH-UPS

Purpose: Strengthens the upper body.

What to do: While on your hands and knees, move your hands forward so your torso is slanted at a comfortable angle and your hands are shoulder-width apart. Keep your back straight and pull your abdominal muscles in. Inhale. Exhale as you bend your elbows to lower your chest toward the floor. Keep your elbows close to your body. Go only as far as you comfortably can. Inhale as you return to the starting position. Do six to 15 repetitions.

TRICEPS BAND EXTENSIONS

Purpose: Strengthens the backs of the arms.

What to do: Stand straight and drape an exercise band over your left shoulder, placing your right hand on the band to secure it (begin with the easiest resistance band and work up as you get stronger). Keeping your left elbow next to your body, grasp the band with your left hand to make a 90-degree angle with your arm, keeping the band taut at all times. Inhale. Then exhale as you slowly pull the band by extending your left arm downward. Inhale and slowly return to the starting position. Do 15 repetitions. Repeat with your right arm.

POSTURE STRENGTHENER

Purpose: Strengthens upper body muscles to improve posture.

What to do: Hold your exercise band out straight in front of your body at shoulder-height, one end in each hand. Extend your arms out to the sides, stretching the exercise band, squeezing your shoulder blades together and making a "T" with your body. Hold for two seconds. Slowly return to the arms-in-front position. Do 15 repetitions.

SEATED LEG EXTENSIONS

Purpose: Strengthens the front muscles of the legs.

Note: If you have long legs, roll up a towel and place it under your knees.

What to do: Strap a one- to two-pound ankle weight to each ankle and sit with your back against the back of a chair. Place your hands in a comfortable position. Inhale. Exhale and slowly extend your left leg until it is almost straight (but do not lock the knee). Hold for two seconds. Inhale and slowly return your leg to the starting position. Do 15 repetitions. Repeat with the right leg.

Modification: If you find this exercise too difficult, try it without weights.

Illustrations by Shawn Banner.

■ ■ ■ ■

Don't Act Your Age

Older adults who imagine themselves 20 years younger and think, act and speak as they did two decades earlier have better memory and manual dexterity than people of similar ages who act as old as they really are. The ones who act young look younger than their real ages, too, although not a full 20 years younger.

Bottom line: Positive expectations and beliefs about aging make people healthier and more vital.

Ellen J. Langer, PhD, professor, psychology department, Harvard University.

■ ■ ■ ■

Retirement Risks

Early retirement may lead to premature death. People who retire at age 55 are twice as likely to die by age 65 as those who keep working. Until recently, it was generally thought that retiring early increased longevity.

Shan P. Tsai, PhD, manager, department of epidemiology, Shell Health Services, Shell Oil Company, Houston, and leader of a study of 3,500 Shell Oil retirees, published in *British Medical Journal*.

Medical Breakthroughs For Aging Eyes

Neil F. Martin, MD, FACS, an ophthalmologist in private practice in Chevy Chase, Maryland, and a fellow of the American Academy of Ophthalmology.

As we age, our vision can be affected by a number of conditions, including cataracts, glaucoma, macular degeneration and diabetes-related eye damage as well as presbyopia (age-related farsightedness) and insufficient tear production (dry eyes). Catching and treating these problems early is the key to preventing long-term vision loss.

NEW EYE TREATMENTS

A number of new drugs and lens technologies are making it much easier to treat a variety of age-related eye ailments. The following treatments have become available just within the last several years...

•**Restasis eyedrops for dry eyes.** The drug *cyclosporine eye* (Restasis), used to prevent rejection in heart and kidney transplants, also relieves tear-deficiency syndrome (dry eyes) when used as eyedrops by decreasing inflammation in the tear glands. The drops are applied twice a day to increase tear production. Some people may experience slight stinging at first. Anyone with an active eye infection (such as conjunctivitis) shouldn't use the drops.

•**Improved glaucoma treatments.** A new eyedrop medication, *latanoprost eye* (Xalatan), reduces fluid buildup better than older eyedrops. (Glaucoma eyedrop treatments work by enhancing the eye's natural filtering process.) While very safe, latanoprost can cause occasional redness, tends to make eyelashes grow longer and may turn light-colored irises brown over time.

Other new treatments include selective laser trabeculoplasty (SLT), which uses a cool laser to enhance the eye's natural drainage canal and improve flow out of the eye without invasive surgery. SLT uses less energy than its predecessor, argon laser trabeculoplasty, lowering the risk of damaging surrounding tissue. SLT is so effective and safe that it may even become a first-line treatment for glaucoma, in place of eyedrops.

•**Eyeglasses with progressive lenses.** Progressive lenses are made by a computer to "morph" from one lens setting in the upper half of the eyeglasses (for far objects) into another in the lower half (for close objects). Progressive lenses have been around awhile, but the newest ones are a vast improvement over what was available just a few years ago.

Reason: Advanced computer designs allow a smoother transition from far to near.

•**Improved Lasik.** Lasik surgery uses an "excimer" laser that can be focused very precisely to reshape the cornea to correct nearsightedness or farsightedness.

The newest version, the Allegretto Wave, uses tiny pulses of laser light adjusted by computer to match your eye's specific curvature. It can be used to treat more severe cases of nearsightedness, farsightedness and astigmatism, previously untreatable by laser, and also causes fewer side effects (such as seeing halos around car headlights at night), with less need for corrective follow-up treatments.

•**New replacement lenses for cataract patients.** Cataract surgery, in which the cataract-clouded natural lens is removed and replaced with an artificial lens, has long been effective at restoring distance vision. Now, several new types of replacement lenses provide improved near and intermediate vision. Each has its own strengths and weaknesses. *Discuss with your doctor which is best for you...*

•The Crystalens from Eyeonics combines the distance vision of a traditional lens implant with an ability to flex slightly and turn into a lens for near vision when the eye muscles focus on closer objects. It's particularly good at providing clear intermediate vision.

•The ReZoom lens from Advanced Medical Optics employs alternating rings of near- and far-distance lenses.

•The AcrySof ReSTOR lens from Alcon Inc. has a series of tiny ridges that diffract light (instead of refracting it, like an ordinary lens), enhancing near and intermediate vision. This lens may be the best of the three for focusing on very close objects.

Note: Cataract surgery is extremely safe, with a success rate of more than 95% and a complication rate of less than 2%. Most complications, such as minor swelling of the cornea or retina, increased pressure in the eye or a droopy eyelid, generally resolve themselves with close doctor supervision and time. Rarely, cataract surgery can lead to severe visual loss as the result of surgery-related infection, bleeding in the eye or retinal detachment.

•**New intraocular contact lenses.** For those too nearsighted for Lasik, the FDA recently approved the first intraocular contact lens—High Definition VISIAN ICL from Staar Surgical. The lens is implanted directly in front of your own lens through a tiny incision. The procedure is safe, and the lens can be surgically removed if necessary. A similar lens for farsightedness and astigmatism is in clinical trials.

Here are some essentials for keeping your eyes healthy...

•**See an ophthalmologist for a checkup** at least every two years up to age 60, and annually after that. Be sure that the exam includes a careful check for cataracts, macular degeneration (a leaking of the blood vessels in the eyes) and glaucoma (a buildup of fluid inside the eye, which can damage the optic nerve).

•**Supplement your diet** with fish oil (2 to 3 grams daily) or flaxseed oil (one to two tablespoons daily) supplements containing omega-3 and omega-6 fatty acids. These supplements help reduce the inflammation in the tear glands that can lead to tear deficiency syndrome (dry eyes).

•**Eat dark, leafy greens,** such as spinach, collard greens and kale. These are good sources of lutein—a carotenoid (naturally occurring pigment) found in the eye's macula that absorbs dangerous blue light and may help prevent macular degeneration.

•**Eat plenty of oranges,** corn, nectarines and persimmons. These are good sources of zeaxanthin, another carotenoid.

•**Take supplements of antioxidants and zinc.** The Age-Related Eye Disease Study (AREDS), sponsored by the National Eye Institute, found that taking high levels of antioxidants and zinc reduces risk of developing advanced age-related macular degeneration by about 25% in certain at-risk patients.

The study used the following daily doses—500 milligrams (mg) vitamin C, 400 international units (IU) vitamin E, 15 mg beta-carotene, 80 mg zinc in the form of zinc oxide and 2 mg of copper in the form of cupric oxide (to prevent copper deficiency anemia, a condition linked to high levels of zinc consumption).

These antioxidant supplements should be taken in addition to a daily multivitamin. Products specifically formulated to meet AREDS levels include Ocuvite PreserVision (and an "advanced" formula that also contains lutein) and Viteyes Complete (which also contains lutein and zeaxanthin). Confirm dosage with your doctor.

•**Don't smoke.** Nicotine constricts the blood vessels in the eyes, increasing the risk of cataracts and macular degeneration.

Note: Smokers should not take beta-carotene supplements.

•**If you have diabetes,** work with your doctor to keep your blood sugar under control, and see an ophthalmologist at least annually, if not more often. Diabetes leads to damage of the eye capillaries, and ultimately to vision loss if untreated. By tightly controlling your blood sugar, you can largely prevent this damage. If capillary damage occurs, laser treatments can help mitigate the damage.

•**Wear UV-protective sunglasses outdoors.** To prevent cataracts, wear sunglasses that offer UVA and UVB protection. If you spend significant time outdoors in ordinary eyeglasses, get a transparent UV-protective coating applied at any eyeglass store.

•**Wear shatter-resistant polycarbonate goggles** whenever you use power tools, a weed whacker or a hammer or when playing sports like handball or squash.

•**Check with your eye doctor before using** the impotence drugs *sildenafil* (Viagra) or *vardenafil* (Levitra). In some cases, these drugs can attack the optic nerves, causing damage to vision or to the nerves.

Power of Attorney Traps You Need to Avoid

Adriane G. Berg, an elder law attorney in New York City, and a founder of the National Academy of Elder Law Attorneys, is author of 13 books on personal finance, most recently, *How Not to Go Broke at 102! Achieving Everlasting Wealth.* Wiley.

While most of us hope to age well, we all need specialized legal documents that ensure our wishes will be carried out with regard to our money and health care in the event we become mentally or physically incapacitated.

These documents include powers of attorney and several health-care directives, which appoint surrogates to carry out our financial and health-care wishes. The most comprehensive directives—living wills—set out our wishes for end-of-life planning and incapacity.

Other key directives: Health-care proxies, also called health-care powers of attorney, which delegate responsibility for carrying out these decisions to others…"Do not resuscitate orders," which cover care in emergencies.

If you should become incapacitated and don't have these documents, a court will appoint a conservator to take over your money and health-care decisions, potentially at considerable cost and heartache to you and your family.

Even worse: Strangers—doctors, medical institutions, etc.—will impose their decisions at critical times.

Careful—if these crucial documents are not drafted by an experienced elder law attorney, they can present a danger to your health and/or wealth. *Here are the pitfalls to avoid...*

Problem 1: A power of attorney is ineffective just when you need it. A power of attorney appoints an agent to spend your money...buy, sell or make gifts of investments and other property to people you have designated ...sign your name to other documents...cash checks...file your taxes...and engage in other financially related activities. Most people sign powers of attorney for use in the event that they become incapacitated, but a traditional power of attorney is void if you become incapacitated.

Solution: Create a "durable" power of attorney, which is effective unless specifically revoked by you. The document must specifically state that it is durable and goes into effect upon your incapacity. To prevent your agent from controlling your finances right away, make it a "springing" power of attorney. This means it "springs" to life when certain conditions are met.

Example: Two physicians certify that you have become incapacitated, whether temporarily or permanently.

Your surrogate can act for you only if you are incapacitated. You can take back control when you regain competency.

Entrepreneurs: Create a separate business power of attorney. A well-thought-out business power of attorney can be flexible enough to allow you to maintain control over your business for as long as possible, even if your competency waxes and wanes.

Problem 2: The directions on your power of attorney are incomplete or incorrect. Many powers of attorney are "one size fits all" forms that don't take into account individual needs or wishes. For example, giving your surrogate "the power to do everything I may have done under the law" may not give him/her the right to gift your property, making it difficult or impossible to plan for government assistance programs (see Problem 3).

Solution: Clearly establish your wishes. For example, a document might say, "It is understood that it is my wish to stay in my home in the event of incapacity. Therefore, I authorize my agent to make expenditures for home renovations, at-home medical equipment, mobility devices and services of a geriatric care manager and any other expenditure needed to create a state-of-the-art environment."

Problem 3: Your power of attorney fails to plan for long-term care.

Solution: If you don't have long-term-care insurance, give your agent the power to plan for government benefits that cover long-term health-care costs. Strategies include giving away assets or placing them in a trust so you can be eligible for government programs.

Caution: Most people name their closest heirs as surrogates, so there may be a conflict of interest in deciding who gets a gift if assets are transferred. Consider naming as surrogate a person who won't also be the recipient of the gift.

Problem 4: The wishes expressed in the health-care directives are too vague. Without clear health-care directives, decisions regarding your medical care, custodial care (for feeding, toileting, bathing and mobility) and even your end-of-life planning will be out of your hands. The quality of your final years may bear very little resemblance to what you wanted.

Solution: Make sure that your agent, usually a grown child or your spouse, understands and respects your desires. The American Bar Association (800-285-2221, *www.abanet.org*) and the National Academy of Elder Law Attorneys (520-881-4005, *www.naela.com*) offer information on holding a conversation with family members about your end-of-life preferences. *Specifically express your desires with regard to long-term care and pain treatment...*

•**Long-term care.** Make sure that the agent handling your money and arranging payment for your desired care is not at odds with your health-care agent. One easy fix is to make them the same person. If you have a clause in your durable power of attorney for "aging in place"

Bottom Line's Ultimate Healing

(in your home), make sure that a similar clause exists in your health-care power of attorney.

•**Pain treatment.** A typical clause gives your surrogate the power to arrange for various treatments.

Example: "The administration of pain-relieving drugs of any kind or other surgical or medical procedures to relieve my pain, including unconventional therapies that may be helpful, even though such drugs or procedures may lead to permanent physical damage, addiction or even hasten the moment of (but not intentionally cause) my death."

Problem 5: **Your surrogate reinterprets or disregards your wishes.** There are civil and criminal sanctions against surrogates who ignore your wishes deliberately or use your money for personal gain. But honest surrogates, even professional trustees, may decide to cut spending on health care because of concerns about objections from heirs.

Solution: One way to handle this is to specifically relieve your trustee or other surrogate of liability to your heirs if he spends too freely on your health care, so long as the decisions are in accordance with your expressed wishes. *Such a clause might read like this…*

"My trustee and my trustee's estate, heirs, successors and assigns are hereby released and forever discharged by me, my estate, my heirs, successors and assigns from all liability and from all claims or demands of all kinds arising out of the acts, except for willful misconduct or gross negligence, needed to carry out my wishes as expressed in clause X (*specify the relevant clause in your trust*) of this trust."

■ ■ ■ ■

Older and Nicer?

Older people get along better with others than younger people do. They also are more likely to avoid conflict by waiting for things to improve…younger people are more likely to engage in yelling and name-calling.

Kira S. Birditt, PhD, research assistant professor, Life Course Development Program, Institute for Social Research, University of Michigan, Ann Arbor, and leader of two studies of interpersonal relationships in different age groups, published in Journal of Gerontology: Psychological Sciences.

How to Keep an Eye on Elderly Family Members From Afar

Jim Miller, an advocate for senior citizens, writes "Savvy Senior," a weekly question-and-answer information column syndicated in more than 400 newspapers nationwide, and is a regular guest on the NBC *Today* show. *www.savvysenior.org.*

Many new technologies have been developed to help adults ensure that their older loved ones are safe…

HOME MONITORING

A basic form of this system—the personal emergency response system (PERS)—has been around for years. With a PERS, a person wears a device (panic button) that sends out a call for help if needed. The problem is that many who have such a device don't wear it or aren't alert enough to hit the button if they fall or become ill.

High-tech home-monitoring systems (which still offer the panic-button feature) require no input from the person being cared for. They work through wireless motion sensors placed throughout the senior's home and collect information on activities of daily living, such as getting out of bed, using the bathroom, eating and taking medicine. The system establishes the person's routines so it can detect when there are changes to those patterns, such as a person failing to leave the bedroom in the morning. Alerts are sent to the caregiver via phone or E-mail. Family members also can check on their loved one's patterns via the system's secure Web site. *Companies that offer this product…*

•**QuietCare.** A leader in the industry and the first to offer this service.

Cost: Less than $300, plus about $90 a month for monitoring (varies by area). 877-822-2468, *www.quietcare.com.*

•**Healthsense.** Offers a more comprehensive monitoring system that allows you to keep an eye on just about everything. With a variety of sensors, you can monitor such things as sleep patterns, shower and toilet use, whether the stove has been left on, when your loved one has left the house, etc.

Cost: $1,300, plus $60 for monthly monitoring, though prices vary depending on tier of service and size of the home. 800-576-1779, *www.healthsense.com*.

•**GrandCare.** In addition to monitoring, this system has a small computer that connects to the Internet and plugs into the TV, allowing family members to share pictures, E-mails, appointment reminders and more on a dedicated TV channel.

Cost: $2,000 to $2,500, plus a $30 to $50/month monitoring fee, depending on the service. 262-384-4903, *www.grandcare.com*.

MEDICATION MANAGEMENT

Remembering to take medications is a challenge for many seniors. The MD.2 system can help organize medications and dispense them on schedule. It also provides multiple reminders to take the medication. Caregivers are alerted if necessary. The system can be monitored via the Internet.

Cost: About $750, plus a $30 monthly monitoring fee, or it can be rented for less than $100 per month, but cost will vary by distributor. 877-563-2632, *www.imdsupportcenter.com*.

Helpful: *www.epill.com* offers a full line of medication-reminder products and services. 800-549-0095.

VIDEO CHAT SERVICE

An on-line video chat service allows you to speak to and see each other. It is easy to set up, though both parties need a computer, webcam and high-speed or broadband Internet connection. Two services are Windows Live Messenger (*get.live.com*) and SightSpeed (*www.sightspeed.com*).

All-in-one videophones (from such companies as *www.packet8.net*…and *www.ojoservices.com*) also can provide this service.

Cost: About $350 per phone, plus $15 to $20 per month.

■ ■ ■ ■

Best Osteoporosis Formulas

These products contain all the vitamins and minerals described in this article, in the therapeutic doses used for osteoporosis treatment…

•**Bone-Up by Jarrow.** To find an on-line retailer, call 800-726-0886 or go to *www.jarrow.com*.

•**Osteoprime by Enzymatic Therapy.** To find a retailer, call 800-783-2286 or go to *www.enzy.com*.

•**Pro Bone by Ortho Molecular Products** is available from health-care professionals, including naturopaths, holistic MDs, chiropractors, nutritionists and acupuncturists. If you cannot locate a health-care professional in your area who sells the formula, it is available from Dr. Stengler at *www.lajollawholehealth.com*.

Mark A. Stengler, ND, naturopathic physician in private practice, La Jolla, California…adjunct associate clinical professor at the National College of Natural Medicine, Portland, Oregon…author of many books, including *The Natural Physician's Healing Therapies* and coauthor of *Prescription for Natural Cures* (both from Bottom Line Books)…and author of the *Bottom Line/Natural Healing* newsletter.

Boost Your Brainpower To Keep Your Body Young

Gary Small, MD, professor of psychiatry, director of the UCLA Memory & Aging Research Center at the Semel Institute for Neuroscience & Human Behavior and one of the world's leading physician/scientists in the fields of memory and longevity. He is author of *The Memory Bible, The Memory Prescription* and *The Longevity Bible* (all from Hyperion).

Today's American expects to live a long life. Those who make it to age 65 are likely to survive another 17 or more years. But will they be good years? To a great extent, that's up to the individual.

It's easy to say that a genetic roll of the dice determines how rapidly and gracefully we age, but studies have shown that only one-third of the factors that predict how well we age are controlled by genetics.

I've spent more than 20 years researching the lifestyle practices that lead to quality longevity. We all know that a healthful diet is the first step, followed by regular exercise. But there are other

Living Longer and Better

307

commonly overlooked, yet simple, steps that also can make a real difference in the way you age.

A HEALTHY BRAIN

Your brain is the "operating system" of your body. When you protect it, a ripple effect is created. With a sharp memory and positive outlook, you're more likely to take the actions that contribute to overall health and longer life, such as watching what you eat…exercising…and staying attentive to other people, which strengthens your relationships.

How to keep your brain healthy…

•**Brighten your outlook.** Optimists live longer. A Mayo Clinic study found that people who scored high on optimism in a personality test had fewer physical and emotional problems and were 50% more likely to survive another 30 years.

What to do: Practice mental habits that promote positive thinking—focus on your strengths and achievable goals, rather than what's wrong or missing in your life.

•**Do more than crossword puzzles.** Although research is not conclusive, mental workouts, such as those provided by crossword puzzles, have been touted as a key to maintaining brain health. However, crossword puzzles and other brain teasers, such as the number-logic game Sudoku, are of little value unless you really challenge yourself with *difficult* versions of these and other brain exercises.

What to do: Spend at least 10 minutes each day performing some form of challenging "brain activity." If you like crossword puzzles or Sudoku, choose ones that give your brain a rigorous workout, gradually progressing to even more difficult puzzles. They should be challenging but possible to complete. If you enroll in a class to learn a foreign language, put in the study hours it demands. If you join a book club, make sure you go beyond the best-seller list.

•**Be mindful.** Staying in the moment—aware of your thoughts and bodily sensations, and what's going on around you—promotes the health of both your brain and your body. If you stay in the moment, you're less likely to do things like overeating, tripping and hurting yourself or multitasking, which studies show can be stressful.

What to do: Keep your mind in the present to avoid worrying about the future and/or dwelling on past mistakes—it's a proven stress and anxiety reducer. To achieve mindfulness, sit down and meditate for five to 10 minutes, or simply take a few slow, deep breaths and tell yourself to focus on the present.

Also helpful: If you practice mindful awareness at mealtime, portion control—the key to weight control—will come naturally to you. Notice how your body feels before, during and after each meal. Eat when you're hungry, and stop just before you feel full.

CULTIVATE STRONG RELATIONSHIPS

Spending pleasant time with other people can add years of good health. A Harvard study of about 3,000 men and women found that people who socialized most (attended sports events, played games, went to restaurants, etc.) had a 20% better chance of living long lives than loners. In addition, they had fewer disabilities and less cognitive decline.

Close, satisfying friendships and family connections are particularly helpful. The MacArthur Study of Successful Aging, conducted by researchers throughout the US, linked emotionally supportive relationships to lower levels of stress hormones. People with close relationships recover faster from surgery and need less pain medication.

Staying in the moment when talking with others—and being aware when your mind wanders—is the heart of true communication. The more attentive you are to another person's words, expressions and body language, the better you can feel what he/she is feeling. The capacity for empathy builds strong relationships.

What to do: Try this 15-minute exercise with a spouse, family member or friend: For three to five minutes, one partner talks about something that is going on in his life, such as a crisis, chronic issue or upcoming event. The listener should maintain eye contact and stay focused on what the other person is saying and should not interrupt. Switch roles for another three to five minutes, then discuss the experience.

COMBAT CLUTTER

If your environment is confusing and disorganized, you may feel constant stress. When you can't find what you need, you face a constant reminder that you're not in control of your life.

What to do: Schedule 15 minutes a day to put things where they belong. Declutter one room—or one corner of the room—at a time. Put away rarely used items, such as clothes or sports equipment not needed until the next season. Consider donating or throwing away anything you haven't used in the last 12 months. Sort mail, groceries—anything—as soon as it comes into the house. Organize and store similar items together so they will be easy to find later.

Apply the same principle to your personal life. We often maintain friendships even when they become unfulfilling. "Declutter" your social world by staying away from people who make you feel unappreciated, guilty or who simply irritate you. Or at least see them less often. This will create time for healthy relationships.

BRAIN EXERCISE

Starting with the word WARM,* change one letter at a time until you have the word FILE. Each change must result in a proper word.

WARM

——

——

——

FILE

*Solution: WARM, FARM, FIRM, FILM, FILE or WARM, FARM, FIRM, FIRE, FILE.

How to Keep Your Brain Sharp

Gene D. Cohen, MD, PhD, professor of health-care sciences and psychiatry, and director of The Center on Aging, Health & Humanities at The George Washington University in Washington, DC, is founding chief of the Center on Aging at the National Institute of Mental Health, past-president of the Gerontological Society of America and author of *The Mature Mind.* Basic.

Scientists used to assume that older adults don't learn as well as younger people and children...that creativity is strongest in youth...and that mental abilities in general go south after age 50. These long-standing myths prevailed even though there was virtually no science to back them up.

New findings: The brain has enormous plasticity—the ability to form new neurons (brain cells) and new connections between neurons. Brain plasticity doesn't decline with age. It can actually increase as people get older.

Example: The hippocampus is the part of the brain that processes information and integrates thinking and emotions. Nerve endings (dendrites) and connections between dendrites (synapses) increase in this area between the ages of 50 and 80.

The brain is not immune to age-related changes. Brain cells "wear out" and die with age. Older adults can't process math problems as quickly as younger people, and they experience declines in short-term memory storage.

However, other kinds of brain changes aren't caused by aging, but by underlying conditions, such as Alzheimer's, stroke and depression. *Assuming that you take care of yourself and stay healthy, you can improve mental function by doing the following...*

STIMULATE YOUR BRAIN

People who push themselves mentally can increase synaptic connections by at least 20%. They also experience increased neurogenesis, the formation of new neurons. The result is quicker thinking, better memory, etc. Mental challenges even can delay the onset of Alzheimer's disease. A study in the *New England Journal of Medicine* reported that patients at high risk for Alzheimer's who engaged in difficult mental activities, such as playing a musical instrument or word games, significantly delayed disease onset. Apparently, they built up a brain "reserve," which kept their minds robust longer.

Choose mental activities that really push your capacities.

Examples: Learning a language or instrument...doing challenging crossword puzzles... playing Scrabble or chess.

EXERCISE

People who exercise do better mentally and diminish the risk of Alzheimer's disease and other forms of dementia than those who are sedentary. Aerobic exercise in particular improves brain circulation and oxygenation. It appears to stimulate the release of chemicals in the body that increase synaptic connections as well as the formation of new neurons.

Example: A study of older women showed that those who increased their physical activity by walking had less cognitive decline and dementia over a period of six to eight years.

More is better. Just as vigorous exercise of the brain is good for cognition, vigorous physical activity is necessary for brain health.

Exercise for 30 to 45 minutes at least four days a week. Aerobic activities, such as brisk walking and swimming, are better for the brain than weight training. Aerobic workouts improve cardiovascular fitness, which is thought to increase networks of blood vessels in the frontal part of the brain and stimulate the release of chemicals that improve brain cell survival and plasticity.

ACHIEVE MASTERY

Older adults who work hard to get good at something experience feelings of empowerment and control. These feelings produce higher levels of T cells and natural killer cells—immune cells that battle disease and help keep brain tissue and blood vessels robust.

One study compared 150 older adults, average age of 80, who were involved in rigorous arts programs with a comparable group not enrolled in the programs. People in the arts group met weekly for a period of about nine months a year for two years and completed between-session assignments.

Many of those in the arts group showed no physical or mental health declines during the study—and some showed significant improvement. Those who didn't participate in the arts programs tended to have a reduction in overall mental health.

It's less important what you do—it could be embroidery, learning how to paint or understanding your computer—than learning to do it well.

STRENGTHEN BOTH SIDES OF THE BRAIN

It isn't true that some people are "right-brained" and others are "left-brained." We use both sides of our brain throughout life, but younger adults are more likely to use only one side at a time—for things such as reading, recognizing patterns,

etc. After middle age, however, people are more likely to use both sides simultaneously. This is probably a protective mechanism that allows the brain to overcome some degenerative changes associated with aging. Older adults who cultivate this capacity have quicker reaction times and improved cognitive abilities.

Best: Creative activities draw on both the right and left sides of the brain and improve the ability of both sides to work together. Take drawing classes. Join a book club. Write your autobiography.

STRENGTHEN SOCIAL NETWORKS

Close relationships are important throughout life, particularly for older adults. People who maintain active social schedules—going to church, getting together with friends and spending time with family—have lower blood pressure and less risk of stroke. They have lower levels of stress hormones, the chemicals that damage brain tissue and increase the risk of anxiety and depression.

New finding: Older adults experience negative emotions less often—including fear and anger, which interfere with relationships—than younger people. Imaging studies show that the amygdalae (the parts of the brain that generate some of our most intense emotions) get less active with age. We experience less intense negative emotions as we get older, but positive ones remain robust. We have an improved capacity to ride out emotional storms that often roil relationships.

Spend time with people you really care about. Volunteer and get involved in your community. Even people who describe themselves as wallflowers during their younger years often find that social connections get easier—and more rewarding—later in life. And they help keep your brain healthy.

■ ■ ■ ■

Keep Your Memory Strong

Keep your memory strong by using all five senses to help you remember tasks and learn new things. In addition to visualizing an object or event, imagine how it would smell, taste and feel.

Example: To remember to bring dessert to an event, imagine eating it—with all the sensations—earlier in the day.

Also: Relax—memory gets overwhelmed when the body is stressed.

And: If you cannot remember someone's name, try to recall where you were, or with whom, when you last saw the person, and the name may come to you.

Douglas Mason, PsyD, clinical neuropsychologist, Clermont, Florida, and author, *The Memory Doctor*. New Harbinger.

Raise Your IQ 9 Points In 10 Minutes

Arthur Winter, MD, neurosurgeon, and director, New Jersey Neurological Institute, Livingston. He is author of *Brain Workout* (Arbor House) and *Build Your Brain Power*. St. Martin's. *www.brainbody.com*.

Most people assume that everyone's mental capacities diminish with age. Fortunately, that's not true.

New studies show that cognitive decline doesn't occur in *healthy* older brains. With the right kind of physical and mental stimulation, most people can keep their cognitive abilities near maximum capacity as they age. Your brain continues to repair cell damage and form new neural networks throughout life. In fact, people who are active mentally can actually *improve* their performance on intelligence tests after age 60.

Activities that work…

EXERCISE YOUR BRAIN

As we age, reduced oxygen levels in our blood may contribute to memory impairment.

Example: A 75-year-old uses approximately two-thirds less oxygen per minute than an adult who is younger.

Recent study: Sedentary individuals ages 55 to 70 who enlisted in a four-month aerobic exercise program did significantly better on neuropsychological tests than subjects who didn't perform aerobic exercise. Researchers attributed improved cognitive performance to increased blood flow to the brain.

Any aerobic exercise—walking, swimming, biking, etc.—also increases oxygenation of the brain and can improve memory as well as mood and speed of decision-making. Brisk walking for 30 minutes daily is adequate.

USE ALL YOUR SENSES

We gather information with the senses—and we are more likely to remember information when we use multiple senses.

Example: It's common to forget the name of someone you just met, partly because you only use one sense (hearing) when you're introduced. The next time you meet someone, bring more of your senses into play. Shake hands. Notice his/her scent and appearance. The more sensory details you accumulate, the more likely you are to store the name in memory.

Exercise: Sniff a bar of sweet-smelling soap, and pay attention to how it looks and feels. Then read a paragraph from a book or magazine. Sniff the soap again. The next day, smell the soap again. You'll probably recall more details of the paragraph than you would if you did not sniff the soap.

MEMORIZE SOMETHING DAILY

Memory is like a muscle—the more you use it, the stronger it becomes.

The brain stimulation that occurs while you're learning new material triggers an increase in the number of *dendrites* (spider-like sensors on nerves) as well as *synapses* (gaps between the nerve cells).

Exercise: Learn one new word a day. Write it down on a notepad, and rehearse it in your mind a few times. The next day, write down a new word and review the one from the day before. Doing this daily will increase your vocabulary as well as your ability to retain new information of all kinds.

Smart idea: Use a free on-line service, such as A.Word.A.Day. To subscribe, go to their Web site at *http://wordsmith.org/awad*. Or, choose a word you don't know from your daily newspaper.

IMPROVE MEMORY WITH MUSIC

Music is a highly effective tool for improving brain function. The type of music is not important. Music of your choice reduces emotional and mental stress, both of which interfere with memory. Singing or playing a musical instrument stimulates the cerebellum and improves your ability to organize and recall new information that is presented to you.

A study of college students reported in *Nature* found that those who listened to Mozart for 10 minutes prior to a standardized intelligence test raised their scores to 119 (from 110 following silence).

Exercise: Practice a musical instrument or sing for 15 minutes several times daily. It doesn't matter if you can't carry a tune. Just the act of singing—accompanying words with rhythm—makes information easier to remember.

Helpful: If there's something specific you want to memorize—a phone number, address or shopping list—sing it out loud. This brings different parts of the brain into play and aids memorization.

MAKE ASSOCIATIONS

The brain is thought to store related information in discrete areas. When you recall a word from your long-term memory, there's a temporary increase in nerve activity in the locations of other nearby words. That's why the practice of association—linking certain words or concepts together—is an effective technique to practice to improve memory.

Exercise: Make a list of 20 simple words—dog, cat, bird, shovel, etc. Read the list of words once, then write as many of them as you can remember on a blank piece of paper. If you're good, you'll get about half of the words.

Then try the same thing while making associations for each word. The word "dog," for example, can be associated with a picture of a black Labrador or a pet you own. The more associations you make, the more words you'll remember.

PRACTICE SPEED

Using a timer or your watch, write down as many five-letter words as you can in two minutes. Repeat the exercise daily. If you want, practice with six-, seven- or eight-letter words. Your ability to recall all information—not just words—will improve.

■ ■ ■ ■

Memory Aid

To remember a word, get physical. If a word is on the tip of your tongue, but you just can't recall it, try gesturing. Physical movement can sometimes unlock a temporary memory block. If possible, move your hands in a shape related to the word.

Example: When trying to remember a type of bird, shape your hands like wings.

Elena Nicoladis, PhD, associate professor of psychology, University of Alberta, Edmonton, Canada.

Click Your Way to a Sharper Mind

Domenic Greco, PhD, a psychologist based in San Marcos, California, studies the effect of games on the people who play them. *Information:* SmartBrain Technologies, *www.smartbraingames.com.*

Don't scoff at the games kids play on computers. More and more adults are discovering that on-line games help keep their minds sharp and allow them to socialize via the Internet with people all over the world.

On-line games are by no means all fast-action electronic versions of what you once might have played at penny arcades. The Internet also gives you access to dozens of traditional games, including bridge, canasta, mahjong, hearts, dominoes, chess and backgammon.

Hundreds of Web sites let you play these and other games against a computer or real competitors.

GOOD FOR THE BRAIN

If you have any doubt that computer games are good for the brain, your skepticism might be allayed by the experience of James Rosser, Jr., MD. He's the director of the Advanced Medical Technology Institute at Beth Israel Medical Center in New York City—and he asked his staff of surgeons to periodically play video games.

Dr. Rosser recently reported that surgeons who played games three hours a week performed their medical tasks faster and more accurately than those who didn't. Rosser's findings aren't unique. Experiments at my own company, CyberLearning Technology, show that people who regularly play video games have an easier time learning new tasks.

For older people, on-line games have another benefit. They can introduce you to activities that you'll enjoy with younger members of your family.

GETTING STARTED

To best play games on-line, you need a computer with at least 128 megabytes of memory (preferably 256) and at least a 17-inch screen. A high-speed Internet connection isn't necessary, although it's helpful for some games.

In on-line games, the board or playing field is displayed on screen, often with stunning graphics and dramatic sound effects. Moves are made by manipulating the mouse or other types of controllers, such as joysticks or gamepads.

Depending on the game, winning usually requires a combination of coordination, memory and occasionally teamwork. Luck plays an important role, too.

For an overview of available on-line games, visit one of the major sites, called portals, that have links to hundreds of games. Some of the biggest game portals are *http://games.yahoo.com/games/front...http://games.aol.com...*and *http://zone.msn.com.* To find other game sites, enter "on-line games" into Google or another search engine.

At least one portal, *www.aboutseniors.com.au,* has links to games traditionally popular with seniors, including bingo, solitaire, cribbage and canasta.

Before you can play, you may have to register by submitting your E-mail address and choosing a password. Most sites are free, and those that charge usually have fees of less than $100 a year.

Caution: Don't register unless a site states that it won't share your e-mail address. Also, some on-line games require you to download software that enables you to play the game on your computer. Before you do, make sure your computer has a security program that screens downloads for viruses and other unwanted bits of computer code.

Game sites usually allow you to play with people you know, who must also register, or with anonymous opponents chosen by the site on the basis of the skill level that you select.

Though your identity won't be revealed when you play, many sites have chat rooms where players can exchange messages about game strategy and other topics. In chat rooms, players usually have the option of posting their real names and contact information.

CHOOSING A GAME

• **Backgammon.** "It's Your Turn" at *www.itsyourturn.com* has classic backgammon as well as several variations that you and a friend can sign up for and play for free. As in all backgammon games, winning requires you to remember complex numerical combinations and to vary your strategy as your opponent moves.

• **Battleships.** "Battleships-General Quarters II" at *www.battleships.f-active.com* has been a free site for young people and it's now attracting a multigenerational crowd. Each of two players is in command of a fleet of five ships, and the object is to "destroy" the opponent's fleet before the opponent destroys yours. The game is tricky, requiring physical coordination to work the computer's mouse as well as the ability to make quick decisions about the most likely location of the enemy.

• **Bridge.** "OKbridge" at *www.okbridge.com* has been sanctioned by the American Contract Bridge League. It is the oldest and largest on-line bridge club, with members from 100 countries.

Cost: $99 a year after a free seven-day trial. Unlike most other games, bridge is played with a partner, a feature that can hone your skill at communications and patience.

• **Chess.** "Free Internet Chess Server" at *www.freechess.org* allows you to play—free of charge—against its computer or a real person.

• **Crossword puzzles.** "Best Crosswords" at *www.bestcrosswords.com* has seven new puzzles a day. Solvers have the option of submitting their results so they can track their improvement and also compete against others. When competition results are posted, players are known only by their screen names. Like most other word puzzles, crosswords build vocabulary and remind you of words you may have forgotten.

•**Dominoes.** "GameDesire" at *www.game desire.com* has a classic domino game with 28 "bones," or pieces. Play is free.

•**Mahjong.** "GameHouse" at *www.game house.com/onlinegames* lets Internet users play a variety of solitaire mahjong games for free.

•**Zuma.** "PopCap" at *www.popcap.com* features Zuma, which has a reputation as one of the most addictive games in the "action puzzle" genre. To win this solitaire game, you must make your way through a visually perplexing temple in the mythical city of Zuma. It's not easy. You must use the mouse to fire magical orbs without letting them reach the golden skull in the middle of the temple. The game requires coordination and the ability to resist being distracted by the accompanying music (unless you turn off the sound).

The majority of portals let you download many types of games that you can play on your computer without actually being connected to the Internet. While some downloads are free, others require payment of a fee—usually under $25.

How Nuns Ward Off Alzheimer's

Guy McKhann, MD, professor of neurology and neuroscience and founding director of the Center for Mind-Body Research at Johns Hopkins University School of Medicine, Baltimore, is author of *Keep Your Brain Young*. Wiley. He is a fellow at The Royal College of Physicians.

Doctors still don't know what causes Alzheimer's disease. *Worse:* Today's treatments are far from ideal, but thanks to the ongoing Nun Study—a one-of-a-kind study of brain diseases in the elderly—scientists are beginning to identify some of the main risk factors, which could open the door to preventive strategies and more effective treatments.

Key finding: Scientists now believe that behaviors and personality traits established early in life are strongly linked to the development of Alzheimer's in later years. Some people have a genetic predisposition to getting the disease, but other factors—such as education, staying mentally active and a history of head trauma or stroke—are thought to play a bigger role.

MANY VARIABLES

Epidemiology is the field of medicine that deals with the differences between people who get sick and those who don't. The goal is to identify factors that cause or contribute to disease, such as genetics, diet, exercise and vitamin intake.

Over the years, Alzheimer's researchers have used epidemiology to identify risk factors. The difficulty in this approach is that populations are rarely static. Individuals within a group move away or come from different places… change their habits over time…or fail to accurately recollect their previous behavior. The greater the number of variables, the harder it is to determine which particular factors have positive or negative effects.

Example: It was once widely believed that people with the highest intake of vitamin E were less likely to get Alzheimer's. Yet these are also the people who tend to have healthier habits overall. This makes it difficult to determine if vitamin E itself is beneficial or if the lower disease rates are linked to different factors altogether.

What we have learned: A recent study of blood samples from the nuns showed that vitamin E did not protect against Alzheimer's.

A STABLE POPULATION

Starting in 1986, David A. Snowdon, PhD, now a professor of neurology at the University of Kentucky, Lexington, began studying nuns of the School Sisters of Notre Dame living in Mankato, Minnesota. The study was later expanded to include nuns living in the midwestern, eastern and southern US.

The researchers hoped to identify factors in early, mid- and late life that increase the risk of Alzheimer's and other brain diseases. The Nun Study, which initially included 678 participants ranging in age from 75 to 103, is providing answers.

Unlike most populations studied by epidemiologists, the School Sisters of Notre Dame live in small, relatively uniform communities. They get similar medical care and have similar lifestyles. And because convent archives contain detailed personal histories, researchers were able to collect accurate information spanning previous decades of the nuns' lives.

The Nun Study has revealed that even though symptoms of Alzheimer's typically appear in older adults, the underlying causes may be rooted much earlier in life. *Important findings…*

STROKE/HEAD TRAUMA RISK

When scientists examined the brains of nuns who had died, they found that nearly all of those with signs of Alzheimer's, such as brain deposits of a protein called *beta-amyloid*, showed evidence of a previous stroke or other forms of brain injury, such as head trauma from a car accident.

It's not yet certain that a history of stroke increases the risk of Alzheimer's, but it does seem likely that a stroke can accelerate the onset of symptoms and cause more rapid disease progression.

Reason: We all have brain reserves, "extra" neurons that give us the ability to maintain cognitive function after neurological damage. Those who lose some of their brain reserves early in life and then go on to develop Alzheimer's will experience mental impairment more rapidly than those without previous injuries and greater brain reserves.

What to do: Prevent strokes by keeping the cardiovascular system strong—don't smoke, manage blood pressure and cholesterol and get regular exercise. Protect against head injury—wear a helmet while biking, motorcycling and horseback riding, always wear seatbelts, etc.

FOLATE HELPS

A number of studies indicate that low levels of the B vitamin folate are linked to dementia and brain atrophy (shrinkage). The Nun Study indicates that a deficiency may be linked to Alzheimer's as well.

When researchers compared autopsy results with earlier blood samples, they found that nuns with higher blood levels of folate were less likely to show signs of brain atrophy associated with Alzheimer's.

Folate (the supplemental form is called folic acid) suppresses the amino acid *homocysteine*. Excessive homocysteine levels promote the development of atherosclerotic plaques in brain and heart arteries. These plaques increase the risk of stroke and heart attack. Homocysteine is also thought to damage neurons and increase brain atrophy in Alzheimer's patients.

What to do: Eat plenty of folate-rich foods—leafy green vegetables, legumes, fortified cereals and enriched grain products. Take a daily multisupplement that contains 400 micrograms (mcg) of folic acid for even more protection.

STAY MENTALLY ACTIVE

Scientists have learned from autopsies that people with brain changes characteristic of Alzheimer's don't necessarily exhibit impairments of cognitive function. Why do some Alzheimer's patients experience severe declines in mental abilities while others continue to function more or less normally?

When researchers analyzed biographies that the nuns wrote decades before taking holy orders, they found that those with a high "idea density"—a marker of education level and vocabulary—were less likely to develop Alzheimer's symptoms later in life, even when their brains showed signs of disease.

The brain continues to form neurons and connections between neurons throughout life. People who are mentally active form the most connections and develop brain reserves that can slow the onset of Alzheimer's symptoms.

What to do: Take classes at a local college. Read challenging books. Do crossword puzzles. Learn a new language. Mental activity increases the number of synaptic pathways, connections between neurons that enhance memory and cognitive function.

EXERCISE

Obesity and hypertension are among the leading causes of stroke. One of the best ways to reduce stroke risk—and protect brain reserves—is with daily physical activity. It's never too late to start. One of the sisters in the Nun Study, who was 91 years old when she was interviewed, attributed her longevity to an exercise program that she started when she was 70.

Exercise improves blood circulation in the brain and lowers blood pressure. It also lowers stress hormones and stimulates the release of trophic factors, brain proteins that repair neurons and keep them functioning at peak capacity.

What to do: Exercise daily. Even light physical activity, such as walking or yardwork, increases the release of trophic factors and promotes better cognitive function.

STRESS AND DEPRESSION

Depression, anger and stress increase the risk of cardiovascular disease as well as declines in cognitive function. A study of the nuns' biographies showed that those who expressed negative emotions died sooner and were more likely to have declines in mental function.

Stress and anxiety increase levels of *glucocorticoids*, hormones that damage the hippocampus, the part of the brain that controls memory. Depression saps motivation and self-esteem and can cause significant memory declines. In patients who already have Alzheimer's symptoms, depression and stress can accelerate mental declines.

Know the signs: Insomnia, changes in appetite, increasing irritability or a loss of interest in daily activities can indicate clinically significant stress/depression. See a doctor or therapist right away.

What to do: Reduce stress with activities you find relaxing, such as exercise, or even simply by taking deep breaths. Talk about your problems with friends and family. Sharing concerns with others can lower levels of stress hormones even when the source of the stress is ongoing.

■ ■ ■ ■

Slowing Alzheimer's

Alzheimer's is slowed by cholesterol-lowering drugs. In a three-year study of 300 Alzheimer's patients, the disease progressed more slowly (loss of 1.5 points in a 30-point mini mental status exam, or MMSE) in those who took a cholesterol-lowering drug than it did in those not taking the medication (loss of 2.5 points in MMSE).

Theory: High cholesterol levels increase the deposition of proteins that can impair brain function.

Florence Pasquier, MD, PhD, professor of neurology, University Hospital, Lille, France.

■ ■ ■ ■

Lung Capacity and Alzheimer's

Reduce Alzheimer's risk as easily as taking a single breath.

Recent finding: For 29 years, researchers monitored the lung capacities of 1,291 women with tests that measure exhalation rates.

Result: The better the lung function in middle age, the lower the risk of developing Alzheimer's later in life.

Theory: Poor lung function decreases the amount of oxygen that reaches the brain, raising the risk for Alzheimer's.

To maintain optimal lung function: Get at least 30 minutes of moderate-intensity exercise most days of the week—and don't smoke.

Xinxin Guo, MD, PhD, researcher, department of psychiatry and neuroscience, University of Göteborg, Sweden.

Smart Ways to Detect and Prevent Alzheimer's

Todd Feinberg, MD, chief of Division of Neurobehavior, Department of Psychiatry at Beth Israel Medical Center, and associate professor of psychiatry at Albert Einstein College of Medicine, both in New York City, is coauthor of What to Do When the Doctor Says It's Early-Stage Alzheimer's. *Fair Winds.*

Alzheimer's disease was first identified 100 years ago, but only recently have significant breakthroughs been made in recognizing the sometimes subtle mental deficits caused by the condition.

Important development: With sophisticated new brain scans and neurological tests, doctors are now able to identify telltale signs of this dreaded disease in its early stages, when treatment is potentially most helpful. *What you need to know...*

HOW IT STARTS

With normal aging, our brains begin to shrink a few cells at a time, which slows brain functioning. In patients with early-stage Alzheimer's, however, a much more insidious process occurs. For reasons that are not well understood, abnormal accumulations of protein fragments and cellular material (plaques) that contain an insoluble protein called *beta-amyloid* develop, as do brain-damaging bundles of neurofibers known as neurofibrillary tangles.

When memory lapses occur as a result of normal aging, the information can almost always be retrieved at some point later. With early-stage Alzheimer's, however, memories of recent events—those that have taken place in past weeks, days or even hours—completely disappear.

Lesser-known symptoms that also characterize Alzheimer's in its early stages…

•**Loss of initiative.** The person may lose interest in what had been favorite activities, such as gardening or taking walks. He/she may become passive and spend more time sleeping or watching television.

•**Loss of smell.** One study has linked Alzheimer's to an inability to identify certain smells—specifically, strawberry, smoke, soap, menthol, clove, pineapple, natural gas, lilac, lemon and leather.

•**Language problems.** Finding the right word or phrase becomes increasingly difficult, and vocabulary is diminished.

•**Difficulty reasoning.** This affects a person's ability to do things such as read and understand an instruction manual, balance a checkbook or follow a recipe.

People who have early-stage Alzheimer's also may have trouble making even simple decisions…take longer to perform routine tasks…or experience a change in personality (such as a person who is ordinarily very sociable becoming a recluse).

Important: Many early-stage Alzheimer's symptoms are similar to those caused by depression. Imaging tests, as well as a family history of either condition, can be used to distinguish the two.

During moderate-stage Alzheimer's disease, the patient may become less concerned with personal appearance…confuse the identities of family members (for example, thinking one's wife

is one's sister)…hear, see or smell things that are not there…and/or need help with basic hygiene.

Late-stage Alzheimer's is typically characterized by loss of bladder and bowel control…an inability to recognize close family members…difficulties chewing and swallowing…and a need for total assistance with activities of daily living, such as eating, using the toilet, bathing and dressing.

MAKING THE DIAGNOSIS

People who are concerned about memory loss —or experience two or more of the symptoms listed above for early-stage Alzheimer's—should be evaluated by a neurologist, psychiatrist and/or psychologist to rule out treatable conditions that can mimic Alzheimer's. These include nutritional deficiencies (especially those involving vitamin B-12 and folate)…metabolic or hormonal disorders caused by diseases of the liver, pancreas or kidneys…lung problems that reduce oxygen flow, such as emphysema or pneumonia…and alcohol abuse. Certain drugs, such as tranquilizers and antidepressants, also can cause Alzheimer's-like symptoms.

A brain autopsy is the only definitive way to diagnose Alzheimer's disease, but doctors can now make a "probable diagnosis" that is accurate about 90% of the time by using high-tech brain scans and behavior and memory tests.

A computed tomography (CT) or magnetic resonance imaging (MRI) scan is typically used to identify loss of brain tissue and/or decreased brain activity. If results are inconclusive, three-dimensional imaging techniques known as positron emission tomography (PET) or single photon emission computed tomography (SPECT) are used.

EARLY TREATMENT

If a person is diagnosed with Alzheimer's, medication is usually started right away to help slow the progression of the disease as well as curb or stabilize the symptoms. Alzheimer's drugs include *donepezil* (Aricept), *rivastigmine* (Exelon) and *galantamine* (Razadyne). Side effects, such as diarrhea, nausea, appetite loss and insomnia, usually are mild and often diminish within a few months. More recently, *memantine* (Namenda) has been approved for the treatment of moderate and severe Alzheimer's.

317

PREVENTION

Certain health habits are believed to help protect against Alzheimer's…

•**Control weight, blood pressure and cholesterol levels.** A recent study of nearly 1,500 people in Finland confirmed that risk factors for Alzheimer's and cardiovascular disease are strikingly similar. Researchers found that people who were obese and had high blood pressure and elevated cholesterol levels were six times more likely to develop Alzheimer's than people without those health problems.

•**Eat the right foods.** A nutritious diet rich in brightly colored, antioxidant-rich fruits (blueberries, plums, strawberries, oranges, cherries, raspberries and cranberries) and vegetables (kale, spinach, broccoli, brussels sprouts, red peppers, eggplant and onions) helps curb the damage that brain cells undergo in response to disease-promoting molecules known as free radicals.

•**Stay physically active.** Any kind of physical activity is valuable. But cardiovascular exercise, including walking, is particularly good for overall circulation—and blood circulation to the brain.

■ ■ ■ ■

Walk Away from Dementia

Abnormal walking may be an early sign of dementia. In a 21-year study of people over age 75, 43% of participants who had an abnormal gait, such as short-step shuffling or unsteady walking, developed non-Alzheimer's dementia over an average period of seven years. Only 26% of those with a normal gait developed dementia.

Theory: Vascular lesions, loss of nerve cells and other brain changes that alter movement patterns can also cause damage that may lead to dementia.

If you develop an abnormal gait: See your doctor for strategies to reduce your risk for dementia.

Joe Verghese, MD, associate professor of neurology, Albert Einstein College of Medicine, Bronx, New York.

Treating Varicose Veins Is Easier Than Most People Think

Neil M. Khilnani, MD, phlebologist at Weill Cornell Vascular and associate professor of interventional radiology at Weill Cornell Medical College and New York-Presbyterian Hospital/Weill Cornell Medical Center, all in New York City.

Up to 25% of all women in the US and about half of women age 55 and older have varicose veins. Men also get them but much less often.

What goes wrong: Veins, unlike arteries, are not simply hollow. They're lined with a series of one-way valves. Pressure—from the movement of muscles, for example—pushes blood upward through the valves. The valves intermittently open and close, allowing blood to move upward without being pulled back down by gravity.

In people with varicose veins, the vein walls dilate and lose elasticity, causing the valves to weaken.

Result: Blood flows backward, rather than circulating to the heart. The veins may appear blue from deoxygenated blood. If enough blood accumulates, the veins enlarge, causing unsightly bulges and twists. "Spider veins" are similar to varicose veins, but they are smaller and closer to the skin's surface.

Most varicose veins occur in the legs because gravity exerts more pressure on those rising columns of blood.

WHO GETS THEM?

People with a family history of varicose veins are more likely to get them. These veins often occur during pregnancy. The surge in *progesterone* that occurs during the first trimester causes blood vessels and valves to weaken. Obesity and prolonged standing also increase the risk.

For many people, varicose veins are primarily a cosmetic concern and unlikely to cause discomfort.

Exceptions: Large varicose veins are more likely than spider veins to cause leg fatigue, itching, sensations of heaviness and cramping. Even small veins, however, may cause symptoms.

Caution: In rare cases, pools of stagnant blood in varicose veins can damage the overlying skin and cause ulcers, usually on the ankles. There's also a small risk of *thrombophlebitis*, which causes a potentially dangerous blood clot.

People who aren't bothered by their varicose veins usually can manage them with exercise, weight loss and compression stockings, which are worn all day and steadily squeeze the legs, helping veins and leg muscles move blood more efficiently. Veins that cause symptoms, however, should be checked by a doctor.

EASY TO TREAT

Many varicose veins are caused by weakness or leaks in the *saphenous vein*, a blood vessel that runs through the leg and thigh. Blood from this vein can cause multiple varicose veins to form "downstream."

Most varicose veins can be treated with laser and/or chemical therapy. A vascular surgeon or a phlebologist, a physician who specializes in the treatment of veins, makes small nicks in the skin (about 3 millimeters long) to insert a tiny laser fiber into the saphenous vein. Heat from the laser seals the vein shut (*laser ablation*). That section of the saphenous vein eventually fades and disappears over six months to a year. The visible varicose veins may seem smaller almost right away.

The laser procedure takes about an hour and requires only a local anesthetic.

Any remaining varicose veins are then treated with a *sclerotherapy* or a *microphlebectomy*…

•**Sclerotherapy.** This procedure is usually done about one month after the laser procedure. The varicose veins are injected with *sodium tetradecyl sulfate* (Sotradecol), a chemical that shuts down the veins and causes blood to seek an alternate route. Injections of this chemical also are effective in patients who have only spider veins and don't require laser ablation.

•**Microphlebectomy.** During this procedure, small skin nicks are used to remove the vein. This often is done with larger varicose veins at the same time as the laser ablation.

Insurance doesn't usually cover the expense of elective cosmetic surgery for varicose veins. But if you have symptoms such as swelling and bleeding that are affecting your quality of life, insurance often will cover the procedures. The insurance company may require that you try other measures first, such as wearing compression stockings.

PREVENTION

Improving circulation and muscle tone can reduce your risk for developing varicose veins…

•**Exercise.** People who walk regularly or do other leg-strengthening exercises are less likely to get varicose veins.

Reason: Muscle contractions help move the blood upward.

•**Maintain a healthy weight.** Excess body weight exerts pressure on the leg veins and makes it harder for blood to circulate.

Myth: Doctors used to tell patients with varicose veins not to cross their legs. It was thought that this might constrict the veins and reduce circulation. Not true. There's no evidence that crossing the legs has any effect on varicose veins.

■ ■ ■ ■

Don't Forget: Wine and Coffee May Prevent Alzheimer's

Wine and coffee may help prevent Alzheimer's, reports Guilio Pasinetti, MD. Studies show that these slow the buildup of a damaging protein that kills brain cells.

Recommended: One to two four-ounce glasses of red wine a day (Cabernet Sauvignon was used in the study)…or three cups of coffee a day.

Another finding: People who drink fruit and vegetable juices more than three times a week have a 76% lower risk for developing Alzheimer's disease.

Giulio Pasinetti, MD, is professor of psychiatry and neuroscience Mount Sinai School of Medicine, New York City.

Secrets to Better Bone Health

Jamison Starbuck, ND, a naturopathic physician in family practice in Missoula, Montana. She is past president of the American Association of Naturopathic Physicians.

I f you are among the 44 million American women and men over age 50 who have or are at risk for osteoporosis, you've no doubt heard that it's important to boost your intake of calcium-rich foods. What most people do not realize is that other factors can have a significant impact on whether the nutrients in bone-building foods are actually absorbed so that they can provide the maximum benefit. Our bones are living parts of our anatomy, as vital and alive as the heart or the brain. What you eat—and how you assimilate what you eat—helps determine your bone health and whether or not you develop osteoporosis.

A recent study published in the *Journal of the American Medical Association* illustrates this point. Researchers examined data linking long-term use (more than one year) of heartburn and ulcer medications known as proton pump inhibitors (PPIs) and the risk for hip fracture in people over age 50.

The unequivocal results: Hip fracture risk increases with long-term PPI use. PPIs, such as *omeprazole* (Prilosec), *lansoprazole* (Prevacid) and *esomeprazole* (Nexium), reduce stomach acid. However, I've never recommended a PPI for a patient of mine, because I believe that a good supply of acid in the stomach improves the absorption of bone-building minerals, such as calcium and magnesium, and fat-soluble vitamins D and K, all of which are necessary for bone growth and maintenance.

For bone health, eat calcium-rich foods and/or take 600 mg of calcium citrate daily, which is readily absorbed, and perform weight-bearing exercise, such as walking, hiking, gardening or dancing. *Also…*

• **Limit mineral-robbing foods.** Eat plenty of mineral-rich whole foods, including whole grains, vegetables, fruits and nuts, but consume only small amounts of foods that steal minerals from your body. These include coffee, hard liquor and carbonated beverages.

• **Use vinegar or fresh lemon.** Add one teaspoon of vinegar or fresh lemon juice to your vegetables or salad at lunch and dinner. Substituting vinegar or lemon juice for fat-laden butter, ranch dressing or sour cream will enhance your body's absorption of essential nutrients.

Caution: Vinegar and lemon juice are not recommended for people with ulcers or gastritis.

• **Don't forget to take vitamin D.** Vitamin D, known as the sunshine vitamin, increases the absorption of calcium from the intestines, eventually increasing calcium deposition in bones. Get 800 international units (IU) of vitamin D through diet and supplementation.

• **Eat foods rich in vitamin K.** Good choices include broccoli, cabbage and spinach—and green tea. Recent studies show that vitamin K is very effective in maintaining and building bone.

Caution: If you take *warfarin* (Coumadin), consult your doctor before eating vitamin K–rich foods and do not take a vitamin K supplement. Vitamin K can interfere with blood-thinning medication.

■ ■ ■ ■

Memory Helper

B-12 shots can fight Alzheimer's disease, depression and panic disorders, reports Arthur Winter, MD. Vitamin B-12 inhibits a brain enzyme that breaks down chemicals involved in maintaining memory and mood.

But: One-fifth of Americans over age 40 do not produce enough stomach acid to absorb B-12 from protein in food, such as meat, eggs and dairy products, or from oral supplements, so they don't get a sufficient supply of the vitamin. Ask your doctor if monthly B-12 injections would be a good idea for you.

Arthur Winter, MD, director of New Jersey Neurological Institute, Livingston.

Chinese Herb Boosts Memory

Mark A. Stengler, ND, naturopathic physician in private practice, La Jolla, California…adjunct associate clinical professor at the National College of Natural Medicine, Portland, Oregon…author of many books, including *The Natural Physician's Healing Therapies* and coauthor of *Prescription for Natural Cures* (both from Bottom Line Books)…and author of the *Bottom Line/Natural Healing* newsletter.

Every so often, we learn that an ancient medicinal herb has new and astonishing health benefits. So it is with Chinese club moss. Perhaps you have heard of it by another name—*huperzia* or *Qian ceng ta*—but most people haven't heard of it at all. Yet as the baby boomer population ages, people will be talking a lot about Chinese club moss and its active ingredient, huperzine A (HupA).

New finding: HupA improves memory and slows age-related cognitive decline—even in early-stage Alzheimer's disease patients. (Neither HupA nor drugs help much in later stages of Alzheimer's.)

Chinese medicine practitioners have used club moss for centuries as a diuretic and an anti-inflammatory. Two decades ago, a Chinese scientist discovered that an *alkaloid* (an organic compound) in HupA could improve brain function. This sparked many studies, some ongoing, including a clinical trial at the National Institutes of Health.

I began prescribing HupA eight years ago for patients with memory problems—and many have been delighted with their improvement. HupA seems to work better than *ginkgo biloba*, an herb that increases blood flow to the brain. For ability to improve brain function, on a scale of one to 10, I rate ginkgo at six and HupA at nine. And unlike ginkgo, HupA is safe for people who take blood thinners, such as aspirin or *warfarin* (Coumadin).

For intermittent problems with short-term memory, I recommend that adults under age 55 take 50 micrograms (mcg) to 100 mcg of HupA daily…and that those age 55 and older take 100 mcg twice daily. For more severe memory problems, such as in early Alzheimer's, take 200 mcg twice daily.

HupA is generally safe and can be taken indefinitely. Occasional side effects include nausea, diarrhea, dizziness and/or loss of appetite. Before starting HupA, talk to your doctor. Do not take HupA if you have a cardiac condition that affects heart rate, such as *bradycardia* (slow resting heart rate) or congestive heart failure, because HupA can decrease heart rate and lead to fainting. If you take medication for Alzheimer's disease, do not use HupA, because it might worsen the drug's side effects (nausea, vomiting and sweating). If you are dissatisfied with the Alzheimer's drugs you are taking, ask your doctor about discontinuing them and trying HupA instead.

HupA brands I like include Source Naturals (800-815-2333, *www.sourcenaturals.com*), sold at health-food stores and on-line (for instance, at *www.iherb.com*)…and Ceriva by Metagenics (800-692-9400, *www.metagenics.com*), available from health-care practitioners. Cost runs about $20 for 120 200 mcg tablets. In my view, that's a small price to pay for improved memory and clearer thinking.

■ ■ ■ ■

Blood Pressure Meds That Help Your Memory Too!

In a six-year study of 1,074 patients who took blood pressure drugs, those using ACE inhibitors that cross the blood-brain barrier (a membrane that normally protects the brain) had 50% less cognitive decline, on average, than those using other blood pressure drugs, including ACE inhibitors that don't cross the blood-brain barrier.

Theory: ACE inhibitors that cross the blood-brain barrier, such as *captopril* (Capoten) or *fosinopril* (Monopril), may reduce cell damage in the brain.

If you take blood pressure medication: Ask your doctor if these potentially brain-protecting drugs are right for you.

Kaycee Sink, MD, assistant professor, gerontology and geriatric medicine, Wake Forest University Baptist Medical Center, Winston-Salem, North Carolina.

■ ■ ■ ■

Antacids May Cause Mental Decline

Stomach-acid medications can lead to mental decline. Mental decline can range from mild cognitive problems (such as confusion) to severe dementia.

Recent finding: People who used prescription and over-the-counter H2 blockers, such as Axid, Pepcid, Tagamet and Zantac, for more than two years were nearly two-and-a-half times more likely to develop cognitive difficulties than people who had not used them.

Self-defense: Talk to your doctor about safer alternatives.

Malaz Boustani, MD, MPH, assistant professor of medicine at Indiana University School of Medicine, Indianapolis, and leader of a study of 1,558 people, published in *Journal of the American Geriatrics Society.*

■ ■ ■ ■

Fight Free Radicals

Consuming foods with *epicatechin*, such as black or green tea, cocoa, blueberries and grapes, may improve memory. Epicatechin is an antioxidant, which reduces damage caused by harmful molecules called free radicals.

Recent finding: Epicatechin helps increase dilation of blood vessels in an area of the brain that is important for memory.

For a bigger boost: Exercise increases epicatechin's effect on memory.

Fred Gage, PhD, professor, laboratory of genetics, Salk Institute for Biological Studies, La Jolla, California, and leader of a study of the effects of epicatechin on mice, published in *The Journal of Neuroscience.*

■ ■ ■ ■

Seeds for Thought

Flaxseeds, sunflower seeds, sesame seeds and pumpkin seeds all contain high levels of polyunsaturated oils, as well as protein, vitamins and minerals—including magnesium, which is especially important for brain health.

Best: Nibble seeds instead of other snacks, or add them to salads. There is no need to measure them precisely—about three to four tablespoons a day is ideal.

Larry McCleary, MD, is a retired pediatric neurosurgeon in Incline Village, Nevada, and author of *The Brain Trust Program.* Perigee.

11

Healthy Mind

A Nobel Prize Winner Unravels Mysteries Of the Brain

The human brain, which weighs about three pounds and is composed of approximately 100 billion nerve cells (neurons), is the most complex organ in the body. The brain not only controls our heart rate, breathing, blood pressure and body temperature, but also allows us to walk and talk as well as see, hear, smell, think, remember and create.

Scientists have long sought to understand the inner workings of the human brain—and, more specifically, how we process learning and memory. Among the important discoveries in this field are those of Eric R. Kandel, MD, a winner of the Nobel Prize for his lifelong research into the biological basis of learning and memory.

Originally trained as a psychiatrist at New York University School of Medicine and Harvard Medical School, Dr. Kandel has written many scientific papers on brain function and is coauthor of *Principles of Neural Science*, generally considered to be the standard textbook in the field.

We interviewed Dr. Kandel to learn more about his research and its implications for a healthier brain and a happier life…

•**What is the essence of the research for which you were awarded the Nobel Prize?**
I was recognized for my work on the molecular biology of learning and memory. Throughout my career, I have been extremely interested in the biology of learning.

•**What changes in the brain as we learn?**
And, once something is learned, how is that information retained in the brain?

Eric R. Kandel, MD, cowinner of the 2000 Nobel Prize for Physiology or Medicine. Dr. Kandel is professor of physiology and cell biophysics, psychiatry, biochemistry and molecular biophysics as well as senior investigator, Howard Hughes Medical Institute, and director of the Kavli Institute for Brain Sciences at the Center for Neurobiology and Behavior, all at Columbia University in New York City. He is author of several books, including *In Search of Memory: The Emergence of a New Science of Mind.* W.W. Norton.

Our most basic finding was that the physical structure of the brain actually changes through the process of learning—whether it's learning to use a computer or speak a foreign language.

•**What does that finding mean in terms of memory in humans?** Over the past 50 years, my colleagues and I have delineated the biological—the molecular and cellular—basis of both short- and long-term memory in a simple experimental system, the marine snail aplysia.

Short-term memory (a memory that lasts for a few minutes) is controlled by a *functional change* in the brain—a change in the strength of communication from one nerve cell to another. This often is mediated by an intracellular "signaling" molecule, such as *cyclic adenosine monophosphate* (cAMP), that helps relay information from the synapse of a nerve cell to its nucleus.

Long-term memory (a stored memory that lasts days or even a lifetime) involves an *anatomical change*, with the growth and strengthening of synapses (connections between nerve cells). In this case, cAMP enters the nucleus of the nerve cell and stimulates memory-enhancer genes, which in turn activate the growth of these new connections. Short-term memory commonly is converted to long-term memory by repetition.

•**What are some of the implications of this research?** Based on these findings, several colleagues and I started the company Memory Pharmaceuticals in 1996 to develop drugs to treat memory loss. The company has created several families of compounds. One is for *benign senescent forgetfulness*—non-Alzheimer's age-related memory loss.

Age-related memory loss can begin in a person's 40s and worsen with time, and it affects the ability to convert short-term memory into long-term memory. For example, this could be remembering the next morning the name of a person you met at a dinner party the evening before. Another family of compounds is intended to reverse the early phases of Alzheimer's disease.

Currently, the compounds are being tested in the laboratory—some of them improve a rat's memory of a new task for months. Another few years of research and testing might lead to medications for humans that were scarcely imaginable just a few years ago.

•**What do these discoveries about short- and long-term memory tell us about human capability?** Obviously, there is a genetic predisposition for many capabilities, but superimposed upon that is a huge capability to modify predispositions through learning.

This capability allows you to change the very architecture of your brain. Since learning leads to anatomical changes, every single brain is different from every other brain—by virtue of learning.

•**What's the best way to keep one's brain healthy?** There are factors that are important for long-term mental functioning, such as not being overweight and not being physically inactive, both of which reduce blood flow to the brain.

It is also important to see life as an adventure—to see oneself not in a static state, but in a process of continual growth and a state of expanding knowledge. Otherwise, one can become intellectually lazy.

But most of all, you should stay intellectually active, through learning new things and facing new mental challenges, whether it is solving a crossword puzzle, or learning a new language.

Interacting with young people also is intellectually invigorating—they challenge your established thinking and help you think in new, fresh ways.

•**Dr. Kandel, you are one of the world's most successful scientists. What lessons have you learned that could be applied to any individual's professional life?** Three lessons have been most important to me throughout my career.

First, learn to trust your own judgment. When you reach a certain intellectual maturity—when you have developed a way of thinking that has not proven at least moderately effective—trust your instincts for new ideas.

I have often gone in directions that I felt were interesting but initially seemed to be quite "fuzzy"—yet they have turned out to be quite fruitful in the long run.

For example, I started my work on memory by studying marine snails, which seemed a wild idea to some scientists. However, I thought that the technical advantages of studying a particular species of snail were extraordinary, in part, because some of this snail's brain cells are the largest in the animal kingdom. That proved to be a sound judgment.

Second, don't be afraid to change directions, even if it involves learning a new discipline. At almost every phase of your life, you're fully capable of developing new intellectual skills. Don't be frightened of something because you're inexperienced. With time and effort, there's no reason why you can't master a new discipline.

Lastly, be willing to be bold. Within reason, take chances intellectually. If you tackle important problems in original ways—even if you fail—that's preferable to doing something everyone else can do as well as you can.

●**What will science reveal about the mind in the 21st century?** In the next 50 years, we will understand, through improvement in brain imaging and improvements in the use of animal models, many details of mental function. There will be a new "science of mind" that will revolutionize how we think about ourselves and our interactions with others.

We will begin to comprehend in biological terms the brain-based biology of behavior, social cognition, decision-making in business, our appreciation of the arts and much more.

We also will develop effective approaches, such as new medications, to treat brain diseases, including age-related memory loss, Alzheimer's disease and mental illnesses such as depression and schizophrenia.

The biology of mind—the science of mind—will enlighten all aspects of mental life, for the betterment of individuals and all of humankind.

Surprising Ways to Fight Fatigue! Boost Mood! Prevent Stroke!

Pierce J. Howard, PhD, a leading cognitive science researcher and cofounder and director of research at the Center for Applied Cognitive Studies in Charlotte, North Carolina, is adjunct professor of organizational psychology at University of North Carolina, Chapel Hill, and author of *The Owner's Manual for the Brain*. Bard.

Though many of the brain's inner workings remain a mystery, scientists make new discoveries about this powerful organ almost weekly. Recent brain research has revealed ways to significantly improve memory and mental ability along with practical ways to prevent stroke and other brain diseases, including Alzheimer's.

Highlights…

BOOST PERFORMANCE WITH STRESS

Scientists used to view stress as a detriment to mental performance. They advised people who were trying to improve learning and memory skills to minimize stress—with regular meditation, yoga, etc.

Recent finding: People learn more efficiently when they maintain an optimal level of stress. A principle called the Yerkes-Dodson Law has shown that a certain amount of stress (arousal) motivates people to try harder.

Balance is the key. People who experience very little stress—when taking a test or writing a paper, for example—tend to make errors of *omission*, such as forgetting to complete all the answers. People who experience too much stress make errors of *commission*, such as hitting the wrong computer keys.

What to do: If you find you're making more errors than usual in completing a task, you're probably experiencing too much stress. If you're bored, your stress levels are too low. For optimal mental performance, it is best to be in between these two extremes.

How to achieve stress balance: Too much stress is typically caused by one of two factors—having too few personal resources in a demanding situation or feeling that you have no options.

In the first case, increase your resources (practice, learn new skills, find helpers) or decrease the demands made on you (change to a less demanding task, simplify the task in some way).

In the second case, talk with your associates or with a counselor or doctor to identify ways to gain more control over the situation.

Too little stress is caused by having too many resources in a situation that is not very demanding—you are overqualified for the task at hand. Address this by handicapping or otherwise limiting yourself.

Example: When my daughter was younger and I played tennis with her, I would hit to her singles court, while she hit to my doubles lanes—so the tennis became more interesting for me. Or you can increase the level of difficulty or complexity of what you are doing. For example, if you are bored writing something, try doing it without using the verb "to be."

REDUCE STROKE RISK WITH CHOCOLATE

People who consume moderate amounts of chocolate have better brain circulation and can reduce their risk of stroke. Cocoa beans—the main ingredient in chocolate—contain natural antioxidants called cocoa flavonoids. The flavonoids in chocolate are more powerful than vitamin C at limiting fatty deposits (plaque) in arteries in the brain and heart. Buildups of plaque can impair mental performance and are the main cause of strokes.

Chemical compounds in chocolate also increase the levels of *nitric oxide,* a critical compound in the blood that relaxes the inner walls of blood vessels and promotes better blood flow and lower blood pressure. A study of 470 healthy men in the Netherlands found that those who ate the most cocoa beans—in the form of chocolate bars, pudding, hot cocoa, etc.—had lower blood pressure and half the risk of dying during the study period than those who ate the least.

What to do: Have one to two cups of cocoa or two small squares of a bar of chocolate daily. The darker the chocolate, the better. According to the ORAC scale—a measure of the antioxidant levels in foods—dark chocolate has double the amount of antioxidants of milk chocolate.

FIGHT AFTERNOON FATIGUE

Nearly everyone gets sleepy after lunch. You can prevent this afternoon slump by eating protein first during lunch, then carbohydrates. The protein triggers an energy-promoting amino acid in the brain.

Foods that are high in complex carbohydrates, such as whole-grain bread, fruits and vegetables, are good for you, but they contain an abundance of the amino acid *L-tryptophan*, which promotes relaxation and sleepiness. High-protein foods, such as meats and fish, contain *L-tyrosine*, which makes you more alert and less likely to feel tired.

Your energy level after lunch will depend on which of these amino acids reaches your brain first.

What to do: Start your meal with a bite or two of protein. This allows the L-tyrosine to reach the brain before the L-tryptophan. But don't just eat protein—carbohydrates are your body's main source of fuel.

GET HAPPY WITH OMEGA-3s

In countries such as Norway and Japan, where people eat the most fish—the best source of omega-3 fatty acids—the incidence of depression and suicide is much lower than in countries where people eat less. Omega-3s can help prevent and treat a variety of disorders, including bipolar disorder and attention deficit hyperactivity disorder (ADHD).

Unfortunately, Americans get excess amounts of another fatty acid group, the omega-6s, found mainly in meats, cooking oils and soybeans. In the last century, the ratio of omega-6s to omega-3s has soared, increasing the risk of mood disorders, including depression.

What to do: Eat three to four fish servings weekly to get more omega-3s. (Avoid fish high in mercury, such as shark, swordfish, tilefish and king mackerel, as well as large tuna, such as albacore, yellowfin, bigeye and bluefin.) Or you can eat nuts if you prefer. Ten to 15 walnut halves or 15 to 20 pecan halves provide the recommended daily amount of omega-3s.

REST—BUT DON'T NAP

The inventor Thomas Edison was famous for getting by on only two to four hours of sleep a night. When he was working on a particularly difficult problem, he would rest for five to 10 minutes. In the brief period between wakefulness and sleep, he often would experience an "A-ha!" moment and find the solution to his problem.

Scientists have found that when the brain goes into an "alpha state"—characterized by brain waves that are slower than the beta waves of wakefulness—people often develop insights, along with more focus and energy.

What to do: Shut your eyes and let your mind relax for five to 10 minutes. Resting in this fashion is not necessarily sleeping. People who slip into deep sleep may be groggy and less alert when they wake up.

PREVENT ALZHEIMER'S WITH "IDEA DENSITY"

The important Nun Study funded by the National Institute of Aging—a long-term study of 678 members of the School Sisters of Notre Dame, ages 75 to 106—revealed that cloistered nuns with brain changes characteristic of Alzheimer's disease didn't necessarily have cognitive impairments. Why do some people with these brain changes (apparent during autopsies) develop Alzheimer's, while others do not?

When researchers analyzed short biographies that the nuns had written upon taking their vows decades earlier, they found that those with a high "idea density" (many thoughts woven into a small number of words)—a marker of educational level and vocabulary—were less likely to develop Alzheimer's symptoms later in life, even when their brains showed signs of the disease.

The brain continues to form neurons and connections between neurons throughout life. People who are mentally active form the most connections and develop brain reserves that can slow the onset of Alzheimer's symptoms.

What to do: Stay mentally engaged. Take classes at a university or community college. Read challenging books and periodicals. Keep a diary or do crossword puzzles. Learn a new language.

TAKE LEARNING BREAKS

You'll learn most efficiently when you focus on one thing at a time, then take a break before moving on to new material.

Example: Someone learning a new golf swing needs about six hours for the new neural pathways to become established. If he/she tries to learn a second swing within that six-hour window, the new information will crowd out the previous learning.

What to do: If you're in school, studying for a professional exam or just trying to learn a new skill, save the beginning of each day for major new learning. Use the rest of the day for practice and repetition.

Suppose you're learning a new language, such as Spanish. You might spend the morning memorizing verbs with "–ir" endings. Practice this during the day or practice material learned on previous days, but don't introduce verbs with "–er" endings until the next day.

Stuck in the Same Old Routine? Don't Worry, It's Good for You!

Barbara Fiese, PhD, professor of psychology, Syracuse University, Syracuse, New York.
Irene Goldenberg, family therapist, University of California, Los Angeles.
Journal of Family Psychology.

Many Americans regularly engage in routines and rituals, and these practices improve their mental and physical health and sense of belonging, according to an analysis of 50 years of research.

Routine events, such as dinners together as a family, provide comfort simply by being events that people can count on, says study author Barbara Fiese, associate professor of psychology at Syracuse University in New York.

Children flourish when they can predict things in their life, such as family dinners or regular bedtimes, the study found. "Even a short period of time has a positive effect. It's related to physical health in infants and children, and academic performance in elementary [school] children," Fiese says.

Rituals, on the other hand, are symbolic practices people perform that help define who they are. The meaningful, symbolic parts of rituals seem to help emotional development and satisfaction with family relationships. When rituals are continued during times of stress, such as a death or divorce, they lessen the negative impact.

"It seems that at points of transition, such as [entering] school or [getting] married, rituals can increase one's sense of security," she says.

Irene Goldenberg, a family therapist at the University of California at Los Angeles, says that therapists routinely advise people to create rituals. "They represent an order and a sense of logic. They make the family more of a unit and tend to make it clear what the values are in the family."

To learn more about the importance of rituals to family life, visit ChildCareAware's Web site at *http://childcareaware.org* or read more from the Kansas State University Agricultural Experiment Station and Cooperative Extension Service at *www.oznet.ksu.edu.*

Dr. Bernie Siegel's Happiness Boosters

Bernie S. Siegel, MD, retired surgeon and well-known proponent of alternative approaches that heal the body, mind and soul, is author of several books, including *101 Exercises for the Soul: A Divine Workout Plan for Body, Mind, and Spirit* (New World Library) and the best-seller *Love, Medicine & Miracles* (HarperCollins).

In everyday life, it's easy to lose touch with your soul. I define "soul" as the authentic self that lies deep within you.

Your soul needs regular attention because it enables you to live with enthusiasm, vigor and joy. It also increases your ability to overcome difficulties that you encounter in your life. *Here's how to strengthen your soul...*

•**Access your creative side.** Take up painting, writing, sculpting or other creative endeavors. Expressing your creativity distracts you from emotional and physical pain. It also helps bring to the surface what is trapped within you so that you are able to heal emotionally and physically.

Example: More than 25 years ago, when I painted a self-portrait, I painted my face with a surgical mask. That helped me to realize that I was covering up my emotions even in the painting. Doctors aren't trained to deal with loss and pain—so we bury it. I knew I needed to uncover my feelings and express them.

•**Define your fears.** By specifically defining your fears, you can come up with solutions so you don't feel so powerless and frightened by them.

Example: If you're afraid of losing your job, dig deeper to find what that really means. Perhaps you fear that you'll end up homeless. If so, you can take steps to secure your home, such as setting aside enough savings to cover your mortgage for a year.

•**Get rid of the clutter in your life.** Release some of the negativity of the past, and make room for emotional growth by periodically cleaning your environment and letting go of belongings.

•**Get regular massages.** Being touched is therapeutic for your body and soul because it releases muscle tension, enhances the immune system and suppresses pain. Find a massage therapist, or exchange massages with your partner. Touch can be an effective tool to enhance your relationship.

•**Focus on the joyful.** All too often, we remember painful experiences—the annoying client, the traffic jam—rather than the happy moments. Carry a small journal to record happy moments in your life. Share funny stories at dinner. Watch funny movies and listen to comedy CDs while driving. My favorite is Mel Brooks's *2000 Year Old Man.*

Carry your baby picture in your wallet. Most likely, it will elicit feelings of joy when you look at it. Remind yourself that even though you're all grown up, there's still a happy, lovable child inside.

•**Find your chocolate—and eat it, too.** Chocolate, particularly the dark variety, stimulates the release of natural endorphins that boost mood. If you don't like chocolate, find "your chocolate"—whatever makes you feel good when you're feeling low. It could be music, gardening, reading or talking with a loved one.

■ ■ ■ ■

Live Longer by Meditating

Transcendental meditation (TM), a technique that produces a state of "restful alertness," has been shown to reduce stress levels and lower blood pressure. People with hypertension (average age 72) who regularly practiced TM for 20 minutes twice daily were 30% less likely to die from heart disease over an 18-year period than those who did not practice TM.

Theory: TM lowers levels of adrenaline and cortisol, stress-related hormones, in the body.

Helpful: Practice TM for 20 minutes twice daily.

Robert H. Schneider, MD, director, Institute for Natural Medicine and Prevention, Maharishi University of Management, Maharishi Vedic City, Iowa.

■ ■ ■ ■

Treating Depression

Depression in the elderly is best controlled by antidepressants, says Charles F. Reynolds III, MD. Over a two-year period, regular use of *paroxetine* (Paxil) was more effective at preventing a recurrence than psychotherapy. Doctors may want to keep depressed patients over age 70 on medication indefinitely—just as they would patients with diabetes or hypertension.

Also important: A depression care manager —a nurse, social worker or psychologist—to make sure the condition is kept under control.

Charles F. Reynolds III, MD, is a psychiatrist and professor of psychiatry, neurology and neuroscience at University of Pittsburgh School of Medicine and leader of the study, published in *The New England Journal of Medicine*.

■ ■ ■ ■

Botox Boosts Moods!

Botox may play a role in relieving depression. Two months after receiving Botox injections in their foreheads, nine out of 10 women previously diagnosed with depression were no longer depressed.

Theory: Injections prevented the patients from frowning. Researchers believe that there may be direct feedback between the facial frown muscles and the depression center of the brain.

Caution: Botox has risks. Ask your doctor.

Eric Finzi, MD, PhD, dermatologic surgeon and president, Chevy Chase Cosmetic Center, Chevy Chase, Maryland (*www.chevychasecosmeticcenter.com*), and lead author of a study of depressed patients, published in *Dermatologic Surgery*.

90% of Adults Don't Know They Suffer from ADD

Edward M. Hallowell, MD, instructor of psychiatry, Harvard Medical School, Boston, and director, Hallowell Center, Sudbury, Massachusetts.

Up to 10 million American adults have attention deficit disorder (ADD), but only about 10% know it. *Here are some of the myths about adult ADD that I want to dispel...*

Myth #1: People with ADD can't sit still or focus properly.

The Diagnostic and Statistical Manual of Mental Disorders, the "bible" of psychiatrists, refers to attention deficit hyperactivity disorder. The term isn't entirely accurate because hyperactivity (having trouble sitting through movies, for example, or frequently tapping your fingers or feet) may or may not be present.

The other important symptoms of ADD are *inattention* and *impulsivity.*

Examples of inattention include reading a book and spacing out or staring at someone's lips while they're talking to you but not taking in what they're saying.

Examples of impulsivity include taking unnecessary risks or having trouble waiting in line. Most adults suffer from only one or two of the three primary symptoms—hyperactivity, inattention and impulsivity.

Even the term *attention deficit* is misleading. Most people with ADD can focus intensely when necessary.

Myth #2: ADD is a learning disability.

Most adults who have ADD have normal IQs. They read and absorb new information as well as people who don't have the disorder—though they may have to make adjustments for their ADD symptoms.

Example: High-energy adults with ADD often avoid careers that are detail-oriented, such as accounting, bookkeeping and secretarial work. They like to work on multiple projects at the same time to stave off boredom. These individuals create systems (calendars, notes, etc.) to stay organized.

Myth #3: Poor parenting causes ADD.

This is totally false. People with ADD have a physical problem that they're born with, but it is often not diagnosed until adulthood. The exact cause still isn't known, but ADD is believed to be primarily due to genetics.

Most people with ADD have at least one relative with the disorder. Adults whose mothers smoked cigarettes, took illegal drugs or drank alcohol during pregnancy are at an increased risk for ADD, according to recent research. People who have been exposed to environmental toxins, such as dioxins and polychlorinated biphenyls (PCBs), are also at an increased risk.

Many people with ADD have more challenging careers than those without it.

Consider David Neeleman, founder and former CEO of JetBlue Airways. He found ways to compensate for his ADD. For example, he used to take a physical approach to his job, frequently going out onto the tarmac and checking up on his airplanes because he got bored sitting in the office. An assistant helped keep his schedule.

People who have ADD also tend to be creative, intuitive and highly energetic. In my own case, I have three kids, have written numerous books and do 60 lectures a year. I don't think I would have the energy for all that if I didn't have ADD.

Myth #4: ADD cannot be diagnosed with any degree of accuracy.

There isn't a single test for ADD, any more than there's a single test for anxiety or depression. But it can be diagnosed objectively by a psychiatrist, psychologist or neurologist.

First, a careful medical history is essential for an accurate diagnosis. Before ruling out ADD, doctors also should discuss the patient's symptoms with a family member. People with ADD are poor self-observers. A second point of view often reveals things that patients overlook.

To see if the patient exhibits the criteria representative of ADD, psychiatrists usually use a checklist—a sense of not meeting goals, trouble getting organized, frequent procrastination, etc.

A relatively new test known as *quantitative electroencephalography* (QEEG), which provides physical data by looking for slow brain waves in the frontal lobes, also should be administered. This test is 90% accurate in diagnosing ADD.

Myth #5: Stimulant drugs are really the only course of treatment.

Many patients do get better when they take stimulant drugs, such as *methylphenidate* (Ritalin) and *dextroamphetamine* (Dexedrine).

These drugs don't cure ADD, but they reduce many of the symptoms, such as hyperactivity, inattention and impulsivity.

The medications also stimulate the inhibitor neurons, which stop a great deal of the incoming and outgoing stimuli, allowing the patient to be more focused.

A relatively new drug, *atomoxetine* (Strattera), is the first nonstimulant medication approved by the US Food and Drug Administration (FDA) for adults with ADD. It works differently but just as effectively as stimulants, promoting higher brain levels of *norepinephrine*, a neurochemical that helps people focus and stay calm.

Nondrug treatments also are essential. *All ADD sufferers should…*

•**Exercise for at least 20 minutes every day.** Any exercise that you enjoy, that is convenient for you and can be added to your daily routine, will be beneficial. Physical activity increases brain levels of the neurotransmitter dopamine and helps people who have ADD release nervous energy.

•**Get a lifestyle coach.** Many psychiatrists refer ADD patients to professionals who are trained to help them make lifestyle adjustments. A coach will come to your home and suggest ways to improve everything from your work area and habits to your family dynamics.

•**Talk to a psychotherapist.** A directed, focused regimen of psychotherapy can be helpful in dealing with feelings that are often experienced by adults with ADD, such as low self-esteem and self-doubt.

To find a therapist, contact the Attention Deficit Disorder Association at 856-439-9099 or *www.add.org*.

Anxiety Relief—Without Prescription Drugs

Carolyn Chambers Clark, EdD, a board-certified advanced nurse practitioner, mental health specialist and faculty member in the health services doctoral program at Walden University in Minneapolis, is the author of *Living Well with Anxiety: What Your Doctor Doesn't Tell You…That You Need to Know.* Collins.

Anxiety is a normal reaction to the stresses of everyday living. For example, everyone feels insecure or worried at times. It's also common to feel anxious about job interviews, public speaking and meeting new people. But approximately 40 million American adults experience anxiety that is so persistent or excessive at some point during their lives that it interferes with their ability to function.

Anxiety disorders are among the most common mental health problems in men and women. Health effects associated with anxiety include tension headache, diarrhea and fatigue.

When people suffering persistent anxiety seek help, doctors typically prescribe anti-anxiety drugs, such as *alprazolam* (Xanax).

What many people don't realize: Drugs used to treat anxiety can be addictive and create severe withdrawal symptoms when patients try to stop using them.

ARE YOU AT RISK?

Anxiety is first learned by being around anxious parents or caregivers. If you have an excitable personality, which may be your temperament or genetic base, you are more prone to anxiety. Abuse victims and people who witness death, such as hospital workers, soldiers and firefighters, are prone to anxiety.

As a holistic nurse practitioner who has grappled personally with anxiety at different times during my lifetime, I've spent more than 30 years devising an effective nondrug approach to help myself and the people I treat. *Best strategies...*

REVIEW YOUR DIET

•**Caffeine** triggers the release of the brain chemical *norepinephrine*, which increases alertness. However, caffeine also causes your body to release adrenaline—just as if you're undergoing stress.

It's best to forgo caffeine altogether. Slowly withdraw over a few weeks. Try adding more decaffeinated coffee to your cup and less caffeinated coffee. Remember that coffee isn't the only source of caffeine. Tea, cola, cocoa and many over-the-counter medications, such as Anacin and Excedrin, may contain caffeine.

•**Sugar** is bad news for people with anxiety. It's well-known that simple sugars, found in candy, cakes, cookies and ice cream, cause your body to release too much of the blood sugar–reducing hormone insulin. If blood sugar drops too much as a result, some people feel light-headed and anxious. But all simple sugars —including corn syrup, fructose and honey— may have this effect.

What your body really needs is complex carbohydrates to burn as energy-producing fuel. Good sources include unrefined grains, found in cereal...vegetables, such as asparagus and avocados (both are rich sources of stress-reducing vitamin B)...and fresh fruit.

GET THE RIGHT MINERALS

•**Calcium** acts as a natural tranquilizer. People who are calcium deficient often suffer from heart palpitations, insomnia and nervousness. To increase your dietary intake of calcium, eat more sardines, tofu, broccoli, kale, Chinese cabbage, etc.

•**Magnesium** works with calcium to relieve anxiety. People who are magnesium deficient often experience nervousness, irritability and weakness. Magnesium-rich foods include halibut, avocados and almonds.

Eating a diet rich in the minerals potassium (salmon, cod and apricots)...zinc (whole grains, kidney beans and chickpeas)...and phosphorus (oat bran, chicken and sunflower seeds) is also important for alleviating anxiety. To ensure adequate mineral intake, take a multimineral supplement.

USE GENTLE HERBS

Because herbs can be as powerful as drugs and sometimes interact with prescription medication, I recommend those with the best safety records. Tell your health-care practitioner which herbs you are taking.

•**Chamomile** is a mild relaxant. Drink a cup of chamomile tea before bed or during a "coffee break." Start with one to two cups daily. Do not use this herb if you're allergic to plants of the daisy family.

•**Peppermint leaf** calms the nerves. Drink one cup of peppermint leaf tea after meals to help with digestion and promote relaxation.

•**Nutmeg** promotes sleep, which often is disrupted in people with anxiety. For best results, grind one whole nutmeg in a coffee grinder and place the powdered herb in empty capsules, which you can buy at health-food stores. Keep the capsules in the refrigerator and use within one week. As a sleep aid, take one nutmeg capsule four to five hours before bedtime. For daytime anxiety, take one capsule in the morning.

EXERCISE EVERY DAY

Exercise provides an ideal outlet for your body when you're exposed to excessive adrenaline due to stress. By triggering the release of "feel-good" chemicals known as endorphins, physical activity acts as a natural tranquilizer.

Everyone knows the benefits of exercise—but few people do it daily. Thirty minutes daily is ideal. If you have difficulty scheduling this, break your activity into three 10-minute sessions or two 15-minute workouts. You don't have to go to a gym—climb up and down some nearby stairs, garden or take a brisk walk at lunchtime.

To successfully integrate physical activity into your daily life, don't do the same thing all the time—instead, mix it up. For example, try swimming…yoga…weight-lifting…team sports…and dancing. The more variety, the more likely you are to stick to an exercise program.

CREATE NEW HABITS

Anxiety can encourage people to adopt bad habits, such as drinking too much alcohol and/or smoking. Do whatever you must to stop these behaviors—go to Alcoholics Anonymous, use a smoking-cessation program, etc. Subtle habits —ones that you might not realize are harmful—also contribute to anxiety.

•**Living with negative "self-talk."** Indoctrination from as far back as childhood can make for an anxious adult. Think back: Were you taught unhealthy beliefs, such as "Life is dangerous" or "I must be perfect"? Do your best to change these beliefs and replace them with affirmations.

Examples: "I am becoming more relaxed" …"I believe in myself"…"I can relax and breathe calmly." By replacing negative thoughts that cause tension with more positive ones that calm you, anxiety is reduced.

•**Not being assertive enough.** If you tend to do too much for family members and/or friends, learn to say "no." This may be easier said than done. That's why I often recommend taking a course in assertiveness training. Call your community college or look in your local newspaper to find a course near you.

Lack of assertiveness causes people to hold in feelings, which allows anxiety to mount. Assertiveness allows you to say what is on your mind in a constructive and respectful way, which reduces the tension associated with anxiety.

•**Accepting bad relationships.** Many times, family members and/or friends mean well but replicate old patterns that create anxiety. Speak to them about your anxiety. If they don't make changes that help relieve your discomfort, avoid these people whenever you can.

If they are binding relationships, it is important to seek out therapy or learn self-help skills, such as total body relaxation or imagery, to learn how to cope.

Diet and lifestyle changes should relieve some anxiety within a few days. Assertiveness skills may take longer. If you don't get adequate relief, seek counseling with a mental health professional or a counselor skilled in behavioral change.

How to Choose a Mental Healthcare Professional

Charles B. Inlander, a consumer advocate and healthcare consultant based in Fogelsville, PA. He was founding president of People's Medical Society, a consumer health advocacy group active in the 1980s and 1990s. He is the author of more than 20 books, including Take This Book to the Hospital with You. *St. Martin's.*

Choosing the right counselor, psychiatrist or other mental health professional can be confusing. But when you face a mental health issue, it is important to get appropriate care, because primary care doctors are not well trained in diagnosing and treating these problems.

•**Psychiatrist.** A psychiatrist is a medical doctor (MD) or doctor of osteopathy (DO)—two degrees with virtually the same training (four years of medical school, followed by four additional years of training in psychiatry)—who specializes in the prevention, diagnosis and treatment of mental and emotional disorders. Psychiatrists use both medication and counseling. Because of their medical training, they are the only mental health professionals allowed to write drug prescriptions. Before choosing a psychiatrist, check to see if he/she is board-certified by the American Board of Psychiatry and Neurology. Go to the American Board of Medical

Specialties Web site at *www.abms.org* and enter the practitioner's name, or call 866-275-2267.

Strengths: Good medical and psychological diagnosticians who can discover or rule out medical conditions that could be affecting your mental health.

•**Psychologist.** These professionals perform psychological testing and practice psychotherapy. Most psychologists hold an advanced degree, such as a doctor of philosophy (PhD) in psychology, a doctor of psychology (PsyD) or doctor of education (EdD) in psychology, all of which require the same minimum amount of schooling. Psychologists are licensed in the state where they practice. Some states also license psychologists holding master's degrees, but a certain level of work experience is required before a license can be granted. To determine if a psychologist is licensed, contact your state's health department.

Strengths: Best trained in a wide range of diagnosed mental health problems that require counseling.

•**Mental health social worker.** Social service agencies, hospitals and crisis centers employ mental health social workers, who usually hold a master's degree in social work with an emphasis in psychology. Licensing requirements for social workers vary widely from state to state. Contact your state's health department to find out if a specific practitioner is licensed.

Strengths: Skilled at helping people adjust to a new problem, such as a cancer diagnosis, and find resources and services.

•**Family, marriage or pastoral counselor.** These are general terms that are used by psychologists, social workers or even members of the clergy who specialize in particular areas of counseling. Some states require licensing for anyone calling himself/herself a "counselor," although no states require clergy to be licensed in order to offer counseling.

Strengths: Good general counselors for less serious mental health problems.

•**Psychiatric nurse.** Registered nurses with advanced training in psychiatry are called psychiatric nurses. They are found in general hospitals, psychiatric facilities and some nursing homes. They often administer and monitor medications and facilitate patient therapy sessions.

Depression: The Hidden Health Threat

Peter D. Kramer, MD, clinical professor of psychiatry and human behavior at Brown University in Providence, RI, is the author of *Listening to Prozac*, Penguin.

Depression is one of the most misunderstood health problems. Some people still stigmatize it as a "character flaw." Others romanticize it, claiming that it lends creativity, sensitivity—even wisdom.

However: Few people are aware that depression actually fuels the development of other serious medical conditions.

Unfortunately, the estimated 19 million Americans who suffer from depression—and their families—are paying the price for the misconceptions. Only one in eight depressed Americans gets treatment.

To learn more, we spoke with Peter Kramer, MD, a renowned psychiatrist…

•**As a health problem, how serious is depression?** In a very real sense, depression is the most devastating disease known to humankind—both in the developing world and industrialized nations. It is extremely widespread, it often strikes first in young adulthood or middle age and it frequently returns or becomes chronic. It robs more people of more years of active life than AIDS, heart disease or cancer. The disability that accompanies episodes of major depression is exceeded only in conditions such as dementia and quadriplegia.

And all this doesn't even take into account the effect that depression has on other diseases. Over the last 10 years, it's been firmly established that depression significantly raises the risk for heart attack and stroke. It also can accelerate bone loss and perhaps impair immune function. Even if depression didn't cause terrible emotional suffering, it would be important to treat it for these medical reasons.

There's also evidence that certain physical conditions and medical treatments can cause depression. In older adults, for example, tiny strokes that cause changes to the prefrontal cortex—a part of the brain that seems to be involved in depression—can lead to depression symptoms, such as altered sleep and appetite and impaired self-image. Some doctors call this "vascular depression." Thyroid disorders that affect hormone levels can be a direct cause of depression, while painful ailments, such as rheumatoid arthritis, can be an indirect cause. Fortunately, these types of depression are quite treatable with medication and other therapies. Drugs, such as the cancer medication *interferon*, steroids and some antihypertensives, can induce very severe depression.

•**Isn't depression a mental illness?** Research in the last decade has found that depression is associated with *physical* changes in the brain, similar to those that might occur with any neurological disease, such as epilepsy, Parkinson's or Alzheimer's disease. Depression causes atrophy—that is, brain cells die—and a loss of connections between brain cells. The longer the depression persists—or goes untreated—the greater the damage.

One study conducted by researchers at Washington University in St. Louis found that the hippocampus—a brain region linked to memory—was smaller in women who had a history of depression, and the longer they had suffered from the disease without treatment, the greater the shrinkage. Their loss of memory was proportional to the time they had spent depressed.

•**Can treating depression reduce the risk for heart attack, stroke and other related illnesses?** The evidence isn't as strong as we'd like, but some research does suggest that this is true. A recent study of 1,834 patients who had had a heart attack and were depressed found that the risk for death or a second heart attack over the next 29 months was approximately 40% lower in the 446 who were prescribed an antidepressant. Among stroke patients, one study conducted in Denmark showed that those who did not take an antidepressant were two to three times more likely to suffer a recurrent stroke over the next year.

•**How effective are current depression treatments?** The prescription antidepressants we have today are far from perfect, but they work pretty well. About 80% of patients who are treated properly get substantially better. But all researchers agree that depression is underdiagnosed and undertreated. Most people still don't get the treatment they deserve.

•**Aren't many people wary of antidepressants because of side effects?** Yes. However, although side effects do occur, they are usually well tolerated compared with the side effects of many other medications. For someone with major depression, minor side effects are tolerable. Although rare, antidepressants have been known to induce suicidal thoughts. When taking a new antidepressant, you should follow up with your doctor consistently.

•**How depressed do you need to be for treatment to make sense—and how do you gauge this?** Many more people should be evaluated for depression than currently are. Minor, or low-level, depression is just like major depression but with less intensity. There are many advantages to being assessed by a mental health professional to determine if you need treatment.

•**Does depression ever mimic other illnesses?** Yes. Some people may have a type of depression, often called pseudodementia, that has the pattern of a dementia illness. It resembles late-stage Parkinson's disease, resulting in problems in motivation, memory, concentration and word finding. Patients don't feel sad, but respond well to antidepressants.

•**What should a person with depression do to get help?** If you think that you—or someone close to you—might be depressed, act as you would for any serious disease and get professional help from a doctor or mental health professional. If you're under treatment for depression, expect to see some sign that it's working. With antidepressants and/or psychotherapy, you should start feeling at least somewhat better after four to six weeks. Don't settle for halfway—once you begin to improve, stay with the treatment until you and your doctor agree that you have achieved optimal results.

When Depression Won't Go Away: Bipolar Disorder Could Be to Blame

Jim Phelps, MD, a psychiatrist in private practice in Corvallis, Oregon, is the author of *Why Am I Still Depressed: Recognizing and Managing the Ups and Downs of Bipolar II and Soft Bipolar Disorder.* McGraw-Hill.

Until recently, bipolar disorder has been associated only with extreme mood swings—suicidal depressions alternating with manic periods of irrational and even dangerous behavior.

Now: A "soft" form of bipolar disorder has been identified and is estimated to affect 1% to 2% of the American population.

IS IT BIPOLAR DISORDER?

Depression associated with bipolar disorder has the same symptoms as common, or "unipolar," depression—sadness, lack of energy, sleep and appetite problems, loss of interest in life, etc. However, doctors can't always tell one disorder from the other. Psychiatrists are typically best suited to make the diagnosis, but they also can miss the telltale symptoms.

If you experience symptoms of depression in repeated, brief episodes, bipolar disorder should be suspected. Even though bipolar disorder is technically defined by "hypomania" (marked by phases of increased energy and activity), in the softer forms, hypomania can be accompanied by irritability and agitation—not just euphoria and grandiosity, the typical hallmarks.

Another red flag: People with bipolar disorder tend to eat and/or sleep more than usual, not less, when they're depressed.

THE RIGHT TREATMENT

For unipolar depression, standard antidepressants—such as *sertraline* (Zoloft), *fluoxetine* (Prozac), *bupropion* (Wellbutrin) or *venlafaxine* (Effexor)—usually reduce symptoms within several weeks. With bipolar disorder, an antidepressant alone can change a person's mood too dramatically—like flicking a switch from depression to mania.

The prescription drugs that work best for bipolar depression are designed to not only ease the depression but also even out the mood swings. These drugs often are combined with an antidepressant to increase the effectiveness of both medications.

Most effective mood-stabilizing drugs...

- **Lithium** is the oldest and, according to many doctors, the best mood-stabilizing drug. Side effects include tremor, diarrhea and confusion.

- **Lamotrigine** (Lamictal) is one of the newest mood-stabilizing drugs. In rare cases, it can cause a potentially fatal allergic reaction, marked by a rash.

- **Olanzapine** (Zyprexa) often reduces symptoms within hours. In some cases, it can cause major weight gain and even diabetes.

- **Valproate** (Depakote) is another tried-and-true mood-stabilizing drug. Side effects include sedation and weight gain.

A HEALTHFUL LIFESTYLE

To maximize the benefits of medication, it helps to adopt a healthful lifestyle. If your symptoms aren't too serious—for example, you're still able to work and maintain close relationships—this approach may stabilize your moods *without* the use of drugs. *Recommended...*

- **Exercise regularly.** Studies have shown that regular aerobic exercise can relieve depression as effectively as some prescription antidepressant medications.

To get started, try this simple strategy: Walk just seven-and-a-half minutes in one direction, then return. Do this every day. Gradually increase the duration if you can.

- **Consume omega-3 fatty acids.** Fish oil, the best source of these essential fatty acids, has been shown to improve depression and reduce mood swings. Try 1 g daily of *eicosapentaenoic acid* (EPA) from fish oil capsules or liquid. Right now, it's not known if the amount of *docosahexaenoic acid* (DHA) found in fish oil is significant for bipolar disorder.

Caution: Fish oil can have a blood-thinning effect, so check with your doctor if you use blood-thinning medication, such as *warfarin* (Coumadin).

- **Limit alcohol.** For many people, alcohol makes their moods more unstable. If you drink alcohol, abstain for several weeks and monitor your moods. Then slowly reintroduce it—begin with one or two drinks per week and track whether it affects you negatively.

LIGHT/DARK THERAPIES

Maintaining regular sleep habits and frequent light and dark exposure can help stabilize moods and reduce depression.

•**Light therapy** acts like an antidepressant, possibly by affecting levels of the neurotransmitter serotonin.

What to do: Expose yourself to light for 30 minutes or more per day.

Best approach: Use a light box, which can be purchased for about $175 to $300 at Costco or several Web sites, including *www.lightthera pyproducts.com.*

Warning: If you experience hypomania symptoms such as agitation, irritability or crowded thoughts, discontinue light therapy.

•**Dark therapy** acts like a mood stabilizer and is involved in regulating the biological clock.

What to do: Go to bed at the same time each night, keep your room as dark as possible and get up at the same time each morning. In addition, control your exposure to light. Even if you don't sit in complete darkness, keep lights low after 9 pm…don't watch TV or use the computer. Use a dawn simulator, a device that wakes you naturally by slowly turning up the lights each morning. For information about where to buy dawn simulators, check my Web site, *www.psycheducation.com.*

•**Blue light** is the wavelength that is believed to regulate the sleep-wake rhythm.

What to do: If it's past 9 pm and you want to use your computer or read without disrupting the cycle, wearing yellow-lensed sunglasses that block blue light may help, though this is still being researched. Yellow-lensed sunglasses are available at *www.lowbluelights.com.*

Eating and exercising at the same time each day also helps stabilize moods.

PSYCHOTHERAPY

Cognitive behavioral therapy (CBT), which helps identify and change thinking and behavior patterns that influence moods, has been shown to be as effective as antidepressants. When adapted for bipolar disorder, it may include strategies to help you maintain a healthful lifestyle, reduce stress and identify characteristic unhealthful thoughts.

To find a CBT practitioner near you, consult the Depression and Bipolar Support Alliance, 800-826-3632, *www.dbsalliance.org.*

■ ■ ■ ■

AA Alternatives

Alcoholism may be treated without intensive behavioral counseling.

Recent study: Alcoholics taking the oral medication *naltrexone* (Depade) who met for 20 minutes on nine occasions with a medical professional had clinical outcomes as good as those who had up to 20 psychotherapy sessions of 50 minutes each. Naltrexone costs up to $5 a day.

Mark Willenbring, MD, director of treatment and recovery research, National Institute on Alcohol Abuse and Alcoholism, Bethesda, Maryland, and a principal investigator of a study at 11 universities of 1,383 alcoholics, published in *The Journal of the American Medical Association.*

■ ■ ■ ■

Eating Disorder

Anorexia may be caused by dopamine overactivity in the brain.

Recent finding: Anorexia nervosa sufferers may have increased chemical activity in their dopamine receptors, which control reward and reinforcement. Dopamine affects how individuals respond to stimuli and how positive and negative reinforcement are viewed. This may explain why women with anorexia don't get any pleasure from losing weight. About 1% of American women have anorexia—it is the number-one cause of death from any psychiatric illness. Some medications that block dopamine receptors, such as antipsychotics, may benefit people with this illness, but more research is needed.

Walter H. Kaye, MD, professor of psychiatry and director of the eating disorders program at the University of California, San Diego. He was leader of a study of brain imaging, published in *Biological Psychiatry.*

Is Brain Stimulation The Best Treatment For OCD?

Ali R. Rezai, MD, head, section for stereotactic and functional restorative neurosurgery, director, Center for Neurological Restoration, and professor, department of neurosurgery, The Cleveland Clinic Foundation.

American Association of Neurological Surgeons annual meeting, San Diego, California.

People who have *obsessive-compulsive disorder*, or OCD, are tormented by their own repetitive, nagging thoughts, and for many, there's no treatment that offers relief.

But an experimental procedure may provide at least some improvement for patients who have severe OCD, letting them return to work and some semblance of routine.

However, the treatment, spearheaded by a Cleveland Clinic Foundation neurosurgeon, produces significant side effects, prompting some questions about the therapy's efficacy.

The study tested deep brain stimulation as a possible treatment for OCD. Because an estimated 20% of OCD patients don't respond to drug or behavioral therapies, the researchers hoped that they would be able to find a new way of treating the condition.

THE OCD LOOP

Those with OCD feel as though their brain gets snagged on a particular thought or impulse and it keeps playing the same message over and over again. For example, some people can't resist the nagging desire to wash their hands several times an hour, while others may constantly check the stove to make sure they haven't left it on. Patients who have OCD are unable to control their intrusive thoughts.

The researchers worked with 15 severely disabled OCD patients who had been on prolonged medication and behavioral therapy.

Each patient received deep brain stimulators —electronic devices that work like pacemakers—that were implanted into a fiber bundle located at the front of the brain.

A deep brain stimulator quiets activity in two regions of the brain where OCD patients appear to have abnormal activity, the researchers say.

After receiving the therapy, the patients experienced a 54% improvement in quality-of-life scores, and several were able to return to work.

PROS AND CONS

Some of the specific benefits of the treatment included mood elevation, anxiety reduction, decreased OCD symptoms and increased alertness. But some subjects also experienced depression, memory flashbacks, nausea, vomiting, visual blurring and abnormal heart rhythms, among other side effects.

But lead researcher Dr. Ali Rezai of The Cleveland Clinic Foundation says the side effects can be controlled by changing the dosage of electricity to the stimulator.

"Deep brain stimulation has the advantage of being reversible and adjustable. These [side effects] are not chronic and can be eliminated," Rezai explains.

Rezai agrees that a longer-term study is needed before his team embarks on a larger clinical trial. "The results are encouraging, but we need more follow-up before we enroll more patients."

For information on obsessive-compulsive disorder and other related disorders, visit *www.ocfoundation.org*, an educational and self-help group based in Connecticut.

■ ■ ■ ■

Contagious Yawning

The "contagious yawning effect" is due to our ability to empathize.

Recent finding: Many people yawn after someone near them yawns. Nearly every kind of animal yawns, but only primates, including gorillas and apes, mirror each other's yawns.

Steven M. Platek, PhD, nonclinical assistant professor of psychology, School of Biological Sciences, University of Liverpool, United Kingdom, and lead author of a study on yawning, published in *Cognitive Brain Research*.

A Good Night's Sleep Without Pills

Peter Hauri, PhD, consultant emeritus to the Sleep Disorders Center at the Mayo Clinic in Rochester, Minnesota, is coauthor of *No More Sleepless Nights* (Wiley), and one of the founders of the American Sleep Disorders Association, now the American Academy of Sleep Medicine, *www.aasmnet.org.*

More Americans than ever are taking sleeping pills. More than 42 million prescriptions for sleep medication are filled each year.

Insomnia is more than an annoyance. It can wreak havoc on the immune system, contributing to serious illnesses.

Newer sleep medications, such as *zolpidem* (Ambien), *zaleplon* (Sonata), *ramelteon* (Rozerem) and *eszopiclone* (Lunesta), are believed to be safe.

However: Even these medications can cause headaches, daytime drowsiness, dizziness and other adverse effects. Older adults, who are most likely to use sleeping pills, are particularly sensitive to them.

Is there a better option? Absolutely. New studies have found that natural treatments are just as effective as sleep medication for mild to moderate insomnia.

GETTING STARTED

Most people require eight hours of sleep a night to feel refreshed and stay healthy, but some of us need as many as 10 hours and others as little as four.

If you have trouble falling asleep, staying asleep or you regularly awaken earlier than you'd like, schedule an appointment with your primary care physician. Medical problems, such as thyroid disorders, pain and allergies, can compromise sleep. Treating such conditions can improve sleep.

Depression, anxiety, a panic disorder or even everyday stress also can disturb sleep. If you suspect that psychological issues may be causing sleeplessness, mention it to your doctor and consider consulting a mental health professional.

If your doctor can't find a medical problem, you can begin a natural self-help treatment plan. To determine whether natural approaches will be effective, you must try them for at least one or two weeks—one at a time.

Helpful: Keep a log of your sleep quality for at least a week, preferably two. Use a rating scale from one to 10, with 10 being optimal. Rate your sleep each night—preferably about a half hour after you get out of bed in the morning.

When you introduce one of the strategies described below, rate your nightly sleep again for about a week or two. If the ratings improve, you know that the technique you're trying works for you.

BEHAVIORAL APPROACHES

During my 40-year career, I've treated thousands of adults with sleep complaints. *Here are the simple strategies that I've found to be most successful...*

•**Create a sleep-inducing environment.** Keep your bedroom at a temperature that is comfortable for you (cooler is typically better)...turn out all the lights (darkness promotes the body's production of the sleep-promoting hormone melatonin)—some people, however, sleep better with a night-light...and, if necessary, adjust your sound level—some people like total quiet, while others prefer soft background noise, such as a radio or a "white noise" machine.

•**Go to bed at about the same time each night so that your body gets into a rhythm.** Some insomniacs are kept awake all night worrying what time it is, so putting a clock where you cannot see or reach it is often helpful. It is counterproductive to lie in bed desperately trying to fall asleep. Distract your mind by reading.

•**Get more physical activity.** Physically fit people tend to sleep more deeply. If you have been sedentary, start performing aerobic exercise, such as brisk walking or bicycling, three times a week.

Some sleep research indicates that it's best to exercise four to six hours before going to bed. If you exercise too close to bedtime, your body may be too stimulated for you to fall asleep.

•**Meditate.** Studies show that a period of meditation during the day or the early evening helps fight insomnia by promoting physical relaxation and/or slowing the mind.

SUPPLEMENTS

If the behavioral approaches described above don't work as well as desired, consider also trying a sleep-promoting supplement (available at health-food stores).*

Effective supplements…

•**Melatonin** has been shown to help restore a more normal sleep cycle—but it rarely lengthens the amount of time you sleep. If you have problems falling asleep, take it two hours before bedtime. If you wake up too early or in the middle of the night, take it when you awaken.

Recommended dose: Start with 3 mg once a day. If this does not work, gradually increase the dosage over a period of a month to a maximum of 9 mg daily.

Possible side effects: Headache, digestive upset and depression. Long-term use of melatonin has not been studied, so consult your doctor if you need to use this hormone for more than a few months or you develop side effects.

•**Valerian** is an herb that has been rigorously tested. It helps many people fall asleep faster and stay asleep longer.

Recommended dose: Take one-half to one teaspoon of liquid extract or 300 mg to 500 mg in powdered form or capsules about 20 minutes before bedtime.

Possible side effects: Stomach upset.

•**5-hydroxytryptophan (5-HTP)** is a compound derived from the seed of the African plant griffonia. 5-HTP is best known as a treatment for mild to moderate depression. The scientific evidence on 5-HTP's efficacy as a sleep aid is inconclusive at this time, but the compound may be worth trying if you don't get relief from the other supplements listed above. 5-HTP has helped some of my patients.

Recommended dose: Ask your doctor.

Possible side effects: Mild nausea.

•**Vitamin B-12 and/or calcium** can improve your sleep if you have a deficiency of either one. Both vitamin B-12 and calcium calm the nervous system and have a mild sedative effect in some people.

*The FDA does not regulate herbal and other natural supplements. Do not take these supplements if you are pregnant or nursing.

Recommended dose: Ask your doctor.

Possible side effects: None are known.

Important: If you are taking any medications, including prescription sleeping pills, consult your doctor before taking these supplements.

■ ■ ■ ■

New Help for Sleep Apnea

The FDA-approved Pillar Palatal Implant for sleep apnea—the sleep disorder that causes people to stop breathing intermittently—requires outpatient surgery, during which three pieces of polyester string are sewn into the soft palate. This procedure causes the tissue to stiffen, which reduces sleep apnea and snoring. The procedure is comparable to somnoplasty, in which microwaves directed at the back of the throat stiffen tissue. Either operation is simpler and less painful than the standard surgery to remove excess throat and soft palate tissue.

Bruce Corser, MD, is medical director, Sleep Management Institute, Cincinnati.

■ ■ ■ ■

Non-Drug Relief for Insomnia

In a study of 46 people with chronic insomnia, one group was trained in cognitive-behavior therapy (CBT) techniques, including relaxation practices and stimulus (noise, light) control. Two other groups took either the sleeping pill *zopiclone* (Imovane) or a placebo every night.

Result: After six weeks, time spent awake dropped 52% in the CBT group compared with 4% in the zopiclone group and 16% in those taking a placebo.

Theory: CBT helps patients identify and change negative thoughts, which can be an underlying cause of insomnia.

Borge Sivertsen, PhD, researcher and psychologist, University of Bergen, Norway.

Natural Remedies For Snoring

Jamison Starbuck, ND, a naturopathic physician in family practice in Missoula, Montana. She is past president of the American Association of Naturopathic Physicians.

Snoring is a problem that many of my patients suffer from but few admit to. For many of them, snoring is embarrassing. For example, Bill, a 44-year-old father of three, recently told me, "I'm just a heavy breather." However, based on the description from Bill's sleep-deprived wife, snoring was a definite problem in their household.

Snoring regularly affects 37 million Americans (about 25% female). It is defined as noisy breathing during sleep caused by air passing through a constricted airway. Mild snoring can be remedied by awakening the snorer or by changing his/her position…heavy snoring lasts most of the night, regardless of the person's position or how often he/she wakes. Snoring is not the same as sleep apnea. Sleep apnea is a breathing disorder. The sleeper (who may or may not be snoring) stops breathing and must awaken in order to start breathing again.

Chief causes of the airway constriction that triggers snoring are lack of fitness, being overweight, drinking alcohol before bed, smoking and nasal congestion. Men are more likely to snore than women, and if a first-degree relative (parent, sibling or child) snores, that also may make you more likely to suffer from snoring.

Food allergies are an often-overlooked cause of snoring. They lead to nasal congestion, allergic sinusitis and swelling in the upper respiratory tract. In Bill's case, a simple blood test revealed that eggs were a problem for him. Eliminating eggs from his diet cured his nighttime "heavy breathing" and brought peace to the household. For people who snore, dairy, wheat, eggs and soy are the most common food allergens. I've seen all of them trigger snoring in my patients. If you snore, try eliminating these foods for 10 days, one at a time, to see if your snoring is reduced.

For quicker answers, ask your doctor for an allergy test. Be sure to get a blood test, which checks for IgG-mediated antibodies to common foods. Skin scratch allergy testing will not adequately determine snore-inducing food allergens.

Other helpful steps for people who snore…

•**Get fit and lose weight.** Strengthening and tightening the muscles of the throat and losing weight will open airways and diminish snoring.

•**If you smoke, quit.** Smoke irritates the tissue of the upper respiratory tract, causing the congestion and swelling that can lead to snoring.

•**Don't drink alcohol within two hours of bedtime.** Drinking alcohol relaxes muscle tension. If you drink just before going to sleep, the muscles of your tongue and throat will be too lax and your airway will be narrowed—a perfect trigger for snoring.

•**Review your medications.** Drugs that relax the body—sleeping pills, antihistamines, tranquilizers and muscle relaxants—can cause snoring. Talk to your doctor about taking the smallest dose possible. Ask your pharmacist and/or doctor whether you can take the medication several hours before bedtime to help reduce the incidence of snoring.

■ ■ ■ ■

Snoring Stopper

Best treatment for snoring depends on the cause. Snoring occurs because of a blockage anywhere from the tip of the nose to the back of the throat.

Common cause: Being overweight. Losing weight should relieve the problem.

Other causes: Deviated septum, sinus infection, floppy uvula (the fleshy lobe that hangs from the back of the soft palate). These may require surgery or, when infection is present, treatment for the infection.

Best: A doctor who looks at the whole patient.

Example: An overweight smoker with allergies who complains of snoring may need to see an allergist, an acupuncturist to help stop smoking and a dietitian for weight loss. If snoring continues, the cause can be narrowed down

and treated directly—surgery for a deviated septum, for example.

Jordan S. Josephson, MD, scientist and snoring, ear, nose and throat-endoscopic sinus specialist in private practice, New York City. *www.drjjny.com.*

Use Your Dreams to Improve Your Health

Gillian Holloway, PhD, a psychologist and instructor at Marylhurst University in Marylhurst, Oregon, is the author of *The Complete Dream Book: Discover What Your Dreams Tell About You and Your Life.* Sourcebooks.

Dream interpretation has long been used to help people resolve troubling psychological issues.

But few people realize that dreams also can foretell health problems weeks to months before symptoms develop.

Landmark study: Vasily Kasatkin, a psychiatrist at the Leningrad Neurosurgical Institute, analyzed 10,240 dreams from 1,200 patients over a 40-year period. He concluded that illnesses, ranging from tooth infections to brain tumors, often caused distressing dreams that preceded the first symptoms.

Dreams related to health issues are typically recurring—and may include an intense physical sensation in the dream and/or pain or discomfort that lingers after awakening.

Most common health-related dreams and what they may mean...

VIOLENT INJURY

Dreams: In one version, a part of your body might get stabbed. On another night, that same body part might get branded with a hot iron. In yet a third dream, that part of your body may be shot. Although the method of injury may change, the body part you dream about remains the same.

What it means: You may be developing a health problem in that part of your body.

What to do: If the dream is a recurring one about a particular part of your body, ask your doctor for an exam.

EATING ROTTEN FOOD

Dreams: You eat food that is spoiled or has bugs all over it.

What it means: You may be overindulging in "junk food" or developing a problem involving digestion.

What to do: Ask yourself if you're under excessive stress. If so, try to change the stressful situation or take better care of yourself by getting more rest, eating a healthful diet and exercising.

SICK ANIMALS

Dreams: Your pet, former pet or a stray has become ill or suffered a violent injury.

What it means: Our pets are dream symbols of ourselves. This dream often means that some part of you is suffering. People who are in abusive relationships often have this dream. It also can mean that you have been abusing your own body by neglecting your health.

What to do: If you are in an abusive relationship, seek help from the authorities and/or a mental health professional. If you are not, take stock of your lifestyle and see if there is a way for you to improve your diet and/or get more exercise.

COLLAPSING HOUSE

Dreams: The floor in your house is collapsing, most commonly due to termites. Or perhaps the walls are crumbling. Or the stairs can't hold your weight.

What it means: Something is giving way or losing ground in your life, or you have a chronic health condition that might be worsening. For example, a woman with scoliosis (curvature of the spine) dreamed of a problem with a spiral staircase in her house at a time when her back was flaring up and needed adjustment.

What to do: Ask your doctor what therapies may be available for your condition. For example, people with chronic ailments often think that they must live with them. In some cases, there are treatments to relieve your symptoms.

CANCER DIAGNOSIS

Dreams: You go to the doctor and are told that you have cancer and have only a short time to live.

What it means: This is a very common dream, and it does not necessarily mean that you have cancer. It almost always means that you simply are overextending yourself and are anxious about it.

What to do: Reflect on what is causing anxiety in your life. If you're overloaded, delegate as much as you can to others. If you suspect cancer or have a family history of the disease, see your doctor.

■ ■ ■ ■

The Right Pillow

Your pillow should support your head in a way that lets your neck muscles relax. *Consider your primary sleeping position…*

•**Back sleepers** usually prefer medium- to low-density pillows (typically labeled as "medium" and "soft") because they provide the appropriate level of neck support.

•**Belly sleepers** are usually more comfortable with low-density pillows—they allow you to easily turn your head to one side to breathe.

•**Side sleepers** often prefer a medium- to full-density ("firm") pillow, depending on the distance from the head to the mattress (a person with broader shoulders, for example, would require a more supportive, thicker pillow). A contour pillow (with a recess for the head and support for the neck) may be a good choice if you sleep on your back and/or side.

Roger Herr, PT, a Seattle-based physical therapist, past president of the American Physical Therapy Association's Home Health section and member of the board of the Physical Therapy Association of Washington.

■ ■ ■ ■

"Sleeping Sickness"

Patients with sleep apnea may stop breathing after surgery, warns Kevin Finkel, MD. People with obstructive sleep apnea (OSA) temporarily stop breathing during sleep. Sedatives and pain medicines used during surgery can suppress the mechanism that causes arousal and may prevent these patients from waking up during the postoperative period, resulting in respiratory arrest.

Best: Tell your doctor if you snore, have daytime headaches, fall asleep during the day or have other signs of OSA.

If OSA is suspected: After surgery, fewer sedating drugs may be used…you may be positioned on your side…and you should be monitored for apnea or low blood-oxygen levels.

Kevin Finkel, MD, is a Washington University anesthesiology resident at Barnes-Jewish Hospital, St. Louis, and lead author of a paper on handling apnea patients during surgery, published in *Sleep Review*.

■ ■ ■ ■

Help for Sleep Apnea

Heart failure patients with central sleep apnea (in which breathing repeatedly stops and starts during sleep due to a brain malfunction) took either *acetazolamide* (Diamox), a mild diuretic and respiratory stimulant, or a placebo for six nights in a new study.

Result: Those who took acetazolamide slept better, had improved blood oxygen levels and were less fatigued during the day compared with those in a placebo group. Over time, treatment of sleep apnea is believed to aid cardiac function through improved oxygenation.

Shahrokh Javaheri, MD, medical director, Sleepcare Diagnostics, Mason, Ohio. *www.snorenomore.com*.

Stress-Proof Your Personality

Redford Williams, MD, director of the Duke University Behavioral Medicine Research Center in Durham, North Carolina, is coauthor of *In Control: No More Snapping at Your Family, Sulking at Work, Steaming in the Grocery Line, Seething in Meetings, Stuffing Your Frustrations.* Rodale.

Nobody escapes stress, but some fortunate people seem to be able to negotiate the shallows of life with apparent ease. They take setbacks in stride and don't waste their time or inflame their arteries by flaring up unnecessarily. They enjoy loving relationships and supportive friendships.

While their talent for living may seem mysterious, it's actually a matter of skill. Like the musician who knows how to draw lovely music from a violin, they know how to bring happiness and harmony to themselves and others.

These people have skills that put them in control of their emotions and relationships. Fortunately, these skills can be learned—at any age.

THE ADVANTAGE OF BEING IN CONTROL

Research conducted over the past three decades has shown that psychological stress increases the risk for heart disease and other major illnesses, such as depression and anxiety. Higher mortality rates are particularly linked to hostility, which can manifest as a cynical mistrust of others, a low threshold for anger and/or a high level of aggression.

New finding: A study recently published in the *American Heart Journal* found that coronary-bypass patients who underwent a training program to increase control of their emotions showed significantly less depression, anger and stress, along with more social support and satisfaction, compared with healthy people who received no training.

The trained participants' pulses slowed, and their blood pressure reacted less to stress after the training—clear signs that they were taking strain off their hearts. These factors remained unchanged or worsened in the other group.

SHORT-CIRCUIT STRESS

You can't deal with stress properly unless you recognize it. *How to cope when a negative situation arises...*

Step 1: **Ask yourself, how important is it?** The goal is to know how to separate trivial situations that are outside your control from those that are worth getting worked up over.

Helpful: Step back and decide whether you should allow yourself to react to a setback, annoyance or obstacle. Is there anything you actually can do about it? Is it important enough to go to the mat over?

Step 2: **Change your reaction.** If your evaluation of the stressful situation tells you that it's not that important, practice turning off the negative thoughts and calming the bad feelings.

Helpful: When you're alone and feel irritated, tell yourself to STOP! in a sharp voice. Repeat the command silently when stressful situations arise in public.

During a calm time, write a list of topics that make you feel good when you think about them—a beloved relative...a pleasant vacation spot. When you're stressed or upset, close your eyes and picture items from your list.

Step 3: **Take action.** If your analysis leads you to conclude that the stressful situation is worth acting on, take positive steps.

Helpful: Problem-solve in a systematic way. Define the problem...list possible solutions...make a decision...and implement it.

Example: Max was not comfortable driving at night. When he found out he had a book club meeting scheduled for 8 pm in a neighboring town, he at first became anxious. After considering his options (having a friend pick him up and drive him home...not going at all), he settled on calling a taxi.

IMPROVE RELATIONSHIPS

Intimate relationships, friendships and pleasant encounters with coworkers and acquaintances provide social support—a buffer against life's difficulties.

You can improve your relationships by being considerate, treating others with respect, offering help when needed, etc. One of the best strategies is to become a good listener. People appreciate you and like you when they feel heard and understood.

To improve your relationships, practice these skills...

•**Keep quiet while others are talking.** Suppress your desire to add information, ask questions, give advice or steer the conversation to yourself. Limit your input to the occasional nod or "Uh-huh." If your mind wanders, refocus on the other person's words. Your turn will come...wait for it.

•**Use appropriate body language.** To show interest, maintain a relaxed but attentive facial expression. Relax your shoulders, uncross your arms and lean slightly forward.

•**Repeat what the other person says.** Before you comment, summarize what you think you heard, focusing on facts or feelings.

Example: "It sounds like you had a great time with your grandkids last weekend."

•**Be open.** This doesn't mean you must change your mind, only that you're receptive to the possibility. When your mental attitude is open rather than rigid, it shows. You may even learn something useful.

ACCENTUATE THE POSITIVE

Several years ago, a University of Washington study found that marriages last longer when positive communications (compliments, affectionate touching, smiling, sharing enthusiasm) outnumbered negative ones (criticism, nasty looks, withdrawal) by a ratio of five to one.

Use the same principle in all your relationships—make a conscious effort to distribute five times as many compliments as criticisms.

Most important, apply the five-to-one ratio to yourself. Overwhelm negative self-talk ("I'm unprepared…my nose is too big…their house is nicer than mine") with positive messages.

Helpful: List your five best traits and count five of your blessings. Also, become aware of your five biggest self-criticisms and pledge to stop them.

■ ■ ■ ■

Stay Alert with DIY Acupressure

Stay alert with self-applied acupressure. Use your index and middle fingers to massage stimulation points in a circular motion—90 seconds in one direction, then 90 seconds the other way. Use a very firm touch—slight discomfort is normal.

Best places to massage: Back of the head at the hairline, on left and right sides at the same time…area between thumb and forefinger, just beyond the webbing on each hand…front of the leg, between kneecap and knee bone…just below the ball of the foot, toward the arch.

Richard Harris, PhD, division of rheumatology, University of Michigan Medical School, Ann Arbor.

Winning Strategies to Stop Smoking

Patrick Reynolds, founder and president of the non-profit Foundation for a Smokefree America, Box 492028, Los Angeles 90049. The organization provides resources and information for smokers who want to stop. *www.tobaccofree.org* and *www.anti-smoking.org.*

For Patrick Reynolds, it was natural to start smoking cigarettes. He's the grandson of R. J. Reynolds, founder of the tobacco company that bears his name. But he made the decision to stop smoking after his father, a brother and other family members died of smoking-induced emphysema and lung cancer. Today, Reynolds heads the Foundation for a Smokefree America, an organization that is dedicated to motivating youth to stay tobacco free and to empowering smokers to quit. He knows firsthand how difficult that can be. Reynolds tried to stop smoking 11 times before he succeeded in April 1985.

After just 20 minutes of not smoking, blood pressure and pulse rate decrease, says the American Lung Association.

After 24 hours, the risk of a heart attack decreases. After 48 hours, there's improvement in the ability to smell and taste.

Between two weeks and three months after quitting, circulation improves, walking becomes easier and lung function improves. A few months later, there's less coughing, sinus congestion, fatigue and shortness of breath.

After one year, quitters run less risk of coronary heart disease, and after five to 15 years, former smokers have the same risk of a stroke as people who never smoked.

After 10 years of not smoking, the risk of lung cancer drops by as much as 50%, and there's less chance of developing cancer of the mouth, throat, esophagus, bladder, kidney and pancreas.

After 15 years, the risk of coronary heart disease is about the same as it is for people who never smoked.

Just because you've tried unsuccessfully to stop smoking, don't give up. Becoming a nonsmoker will increase your chance of living a longer and healthier life.

Problem: Each time you try to stop smoking and fail, you believe more and more that quitting is impossible. In fact, the majority of former smokers made several attempts before they succeeded.

Instead of looking at failures as evidence that you can't quit, think of them as normal steps on the road to becoming a nonsmoker.

TOUGH REALITIES

The nicotine in tobacco is addictive. Giving it up can be as difficult as turning away from other powerful drugs. The biggest mistake smokers make when they decide to stop is believing that they can do it on their own. Most statistics show that chances of success double or triple for people who follow a structured stop-smoking program.

Because addiction affects people differently, a stop-smoking program that's effective for one person may not be helpful for another. But the good news is that today smokers have more ways to get help than ever before. Some of the most effective programs are listed below.

Pick a program based on your personality. If you enjoy meeting with other smokers who are trying to quit, consider a program with support meetings. If you prefer to work alone, try an on-line program or one based on written materials.

If a particular stop-smoking program doesn't work, try it again or look for another one.

KEYS TO SUCCESS

Stop-smoking methods that are proven to work…

•**Nicotine replacement.** Accessing nicotine by a skin patch, lozenge or gum satisfies the craving without exposing you to dozens of harmful substances in tobacco.

Once the craving for nicotine is satisfied, smokers have an easier time giving up tobacco products. After about one month, reformed smokers can usually reduce their use of nicotine replacement devices.

Nicotine patches, lozenges and chewing gum are now available over the counter at pharmacies.

Typical prices per day: $4 for patches, $6 to $12 for lozenges and $5 for chewing gum.

Important: Consult your doctor about this and any other type of medication or therapy.

•**Zyban (bupropion hydrochloride).** This prescription drug contains the same active ingredient as the antidepressant Wellbutrin and has been successful in reducing the craving for tobacco products, especially in combination with nicotine replacement.

Typical price: About $3 a day for a generic form, or less with insurance coverage.

Caution: The FDA has issued a warning for this drug. Consult your doctor.

•**Hospital programs.** Many hospitals throughout the country offer smoking-cessation programs that usually include counseling plus nicotine replacement therapy.

Typical price: Less than $200 for counseling.

A few hospitals treat smokers on an inpatient basis, including the St. Helena Center for Health in Deer Park, California (800-358-9195 and 707-963-6475, *www.sthelenahospital.org*) and the Mayo Clinic in Rochester, Minnesota (800-344-5984, *www.mayoclinic.org*).

Week-long programs include psychological services, lectures, nutritional instruction, exercise, medical assessment and a lung screening.

Price: Roughly $4,000 at the St. Helena Center, $5,500 at the Mayo Clinic.

Though inpatient programs are expensive, for people who enjoy being pampered, treatment is effective because it can reduce the stress that comes in the first days after giving up tobacco.

Some insurance plans, including Medicare, cover all or part of the cost of both inpatient and outpatient treatments.

To find convenient outpatient and inpatient programs, contact your physician, local hospitals or your state health department.

•**Nicotine Anonymous.** The organization's 12-step program—modeled to some extent on the Alcoholics Anonymous regimen—is taught at free meetings in many cities. Smokers get support from former smokers who have quit as well as from fellow smokers who are trying to quit.

Information: 415-750-0328, *www.nicotineanonymous.org*.

•**National cessation programs.** Popular programs are run by the American Cancer Society (800-227-2345, *www.cancer.org*) and the

American Lung Association (800-586-4872 and 212-315-8700, *www.lungusa.org*).

The programs offer a combination of written materials, help in avoiding triggers that stimulate the urge to smoke, advice on using medication and support by telephone hotline and/or the Internet.

Whether or not the program you choose includes the following steps, we at the Foundation for a Smokefree America have found them especially helpful…

•Deep breathing. Every time you want a cigarette, take three deep breaths, each time exhaling slowly. As you exhale, visualize the tension leaving your body.

•Drink lots of water and other nonalcoholic liquids. They help flush nicotine from your body.

•Stay away from alcohol, sugar and coffee. They can stimulate the desire for a cigarette.

•Nibble on low-calorie foods, such as celery, apples and carrots. They help satisfy the need for oral stimulation.

•Get more exercise.

•Write down 10 good things about being a nonsmoker and 10 bad things about smoking. The effort can reinforce your self-image as a person who is a permanent nonsmoker.

•Ask for support from coworkers, friends and family members. Request that they don't smoke in your presence.

Very helpful: The National Cancer Institute's toll-free Smoking Quitline. By phoning 877-448-7848, smokers can talk to professional counselors trained to help smokers quit.

Most valuable secret: Even after the urge to smoke has diminished, overwhelming surprise nicotine attacks can—and will—happen. For instance, you may be at a party and someone will light up, and you'll be tempted to have "just one." This is where most would-be quitters fail. Knowing it will happen and being prepared for it will help ensure that you succeed.

Best plan of action: Try to wait five minutes after the onset of an urge. It will pass. Deep breathing while you wait also helps.

12

Heart and Stroke Help

Five Common Misconceptions About Heart Disease Risks

One out of every five Americans has some form of heart disease. Literally millions of cases could be prevented if people had better information about the best prevention and treatment strategies.

Despite the abundance of health information reported in the media, many people are endangering their health because they are still ill-informed about key aspects of heart disease. Barry L. Zaret, MD, one of the country's leading specialists in cardiovascular health clarifies the most common misconceptions regarding heart disease.

Misconception 1: High cholesterol is the main risk factor for heart attack.

Fact: While high cholesterol does increase risk, recent studies show that elevated levels (3 mg per liter or higher) of *C-reactive protein*

(CRP), a protein that circulates in the bloodstream, may have an even stronger link than high cholesterol to heart attack and stroke.

Everyone has at least a small amount of CRP in the bloodstream. At higher levels, it indicates the presence of inflammation—possibly caused by an underlying bacterial or viral infection that may damage the linings of blood vessels and promote the development of atherosclerosis.

Every patient with a high risk for cardiovascular disease—smokers and/or those with a family history of heart disease, for example—should have a high-sensitivity CRP blood test. This test, unlike the standard CRP test, distinguishes between inflammation due to cardiovascular disease and other inflammatory conditions, such as arthritis. The high-sensitivity CRP test is particularly important for patients who have had a previous heart attack or who have unstable angina (chest pain caused by lack of blood to the heart). An elevated CRP level in these patients

Barry L. Zaret, MD, Robert W. Berliner Professor of Medicine and professor of radiology at Yale University School of Medicine in New Haven, Connecticut, is coauthor of *Heart Care for Life*. Yale University Press.

indicates a very high risk for heart attack—even if cholesterol levels are normal.

Misconception 2: All adults should take a daily aspirin.

Fact: Daily aspirin therapy is often recommended for patients who have an elevated heart disease risk due to family history, smoking, obesity, diabetes and atherosclerosis. Studies show that it can curb heart attack risk in men by more than 40%.

For women, the evidence is less clear. New research indicates that women who take aspirin are more likely to experience gastrointestinal upset or bleeding problems than men. Although research shows that in women age 46 or older aspirin protects against stroke, it does not reduce heart attack risk in all of these women. Aspirin has been shown to lower heart attack risk only in women age 65 or older, whether or not they have risk factors for the disease. Women of any age who smoke or have a family history of heart disease or other risk factors may benefit from aspirin therapy. The standard recommendation for women is 81 mg daily.

There's no evidence to suggest that aspirin helps prevent a heart attack in healthy women who are under age 65. For these women, not smoking, controlling body weight, getting regular exercise and maintaining a healthful diet are the best ways to guard against the development of heart disease.

This also is true for men age 64 and younger who are healthy and have no risk factors for heart disease. However, men age 65 or older, even if healthy, should take 81 mg of aspirin daily to protect against heart disease.

Misconception 3: The greatest danger of smoking is lung cancer.

Fact: Lung cancer is obviously a concern for smokers, but the risk for cardiovascular disease is actually higher. Of the approximately 440,000 premature deaths caused annually by smoking, the majority are due to cardiovascular disease, according to the Centers for Disease Control and Prevention.

Smoking increases levels of carbon monoxide in the blood, which damages artery linings and promotes atherosclerosis. It appears to lower HDL "good" cholesterol and increase

blood levels of fibrinogen, a substance in the blood that promotes clotting.

Good news: One year after quitting, the risk for heart disease drops to one-half that of current smokers—and within 15 years becomes about the same as for someone who never smoked.

Misconception 4: Exercise is dangerous if you've already had a heart attack.

Fact: Heart attack patients especially benefit from regular exercise. An analysis of 22 different studies that followed more than 4,000 patients for three years found that the death rate among patients who participated in a cardiac rehabilitation program that included exercise was 20% to 25% lower than among those who didn't exercise.

Heart patients who exercise have increased endurance, fewer chest or leg pains and improved heart function. Regular exercise also lowers blood pressure, raises HDL cholesterol and lowers resting heart rate.

Patients who have heart disease or have had a heart attack, or those who have been sedentary, should get a thorough checkup before starting an exercise program. This should include a treadmill stress test, which evaluates blood flow to the heart. Once your doctor determines that it's safe to exercise, aim for 30 minutes at least three to five days a week. Aerobic exercise—fast walking, swimming, etc.—provides the most benefits for heart patients. If you've had a heart attack or other cardiac event, start your exercise routine at a rehabilitation center, if possible. Ask your cardiologist to recommend one near you.

Misconception 5: Reports saying that chocolate is good for the heart are mostly hype.

Fact: The cocoa beans used to make chocolate are extremely rich in flavonoids, plant compounds that appear to relax small blood vessels and lower blood pressure. Some of the flavonoids in cocoa also appear to inhibit the ability of platelets to form clots in the arteries.

Harvard researchers recently studied residents of Kuna (an island off Panama), who drink an average of three to four cups of cocoa a day. (They consume even more cocoa in other foods.) Hypertension among these people is almost nonexistent—until they leave the island and forgo their cocoa-rich diet. At that point, their rates of hypertension and heart disease rise.

Of course, there is a downside. The high levels of fat and sugar in chocolate can lead to obesity and elevated blood sugar. But one to two small squares daily of dark chocolate that's at least 70% cocoa and low in added sugar does appear to be good for the heart.

Surprising Symptoms of Heart Attack

Joseph Ornato, MD, professor and chairman of the department of emergency medicine at Virginia Commonwealth University in Richmond. He has authored numerous scientific papers on cardiopulmonary resuscitation.

Chest discomfort in the center of the chest—the most common heart attack symptom—occurs only in about two-thirds of all heart attack sufferers. Roughly one-quarter of heart attacks produce atypical symptoms, and the rest produce no noticeable symptoms. These so-called "silent" heart attacks are detected only later on, if the person happens to undergo an electrocardiogram (EKG), a test that involves placing electrodes on the patient's chest to map the heart's electrical activity.

Recent finding: In an international study involving nearly 21,000 patients from 14 countries, including the US, researchers found that people who experience symptoms other than chest pain—for example, sweating, fainting, breathlessness, nausea or vomiting—are more likely to be misdiagnosed…are significantly less likely to receive appropriate treatments…and are three times more likely to die in the hospital than people suffering telltale chest pain symptoms.

People over age 75, anyone with high blood pressure, women and diabetics are more likely to experience atypical heart attack symptoms that elude diagnosis—but they can happen to anyone. People with heart failure (a disorder in which the heart pumps blood inadequately due to narrowed arteries, heart valve disease, etc.) also are at increased risk for heart attack accompanied by atypical symptoms.

Problem: Failure to recognize atypical symptoms results in an estimated 20,000 to 50,000 heart attacks that are *not* diagnosed in US emergency rooms and doctors' offices, leading to potentially thousands of preventable deaths annually.

RECOGNIZING THE SYMPTOMS

A heart attack, also called *myocardial infarction* (MI), usually occurs when a blood clot (often the result of fatty buildup in the arteries) blocks a vessel to the heart, depriving the heart muscle of oxygen and nutrients. In a matter of minutes or over the course of hours, the starved heart cells begin to die, typically causing a feeling of deep pressure or tightness just beneath the breastbone.

Unfortunately, most people experiencing heart attack symptoms delay seeking treatment for two to three hours or even longer—often because they don't recognize the symptoms or they fear that they'll be embarrassed if it turns out to be nothing serious.

CALL 911

About half of heart attack patients are driven to the hospital by someone they know—or, even worse, they drive themselves—instead of arriving by ambulance. But studies have consistently shown that heart attack victims who arrive by ambulance are diagnosed and treated more quickly and have better outcomes than those who arrive on their own.

If your heart suddenly stops, which happens during about 5% of heart attacks, emergency medical technicians (EMTs) can use a defibrillator (a device that delivers an electric shock to the heart) to try to get it beating again. In addition, EMTs usually know which emergency facilities in the area are best equipped to handle cardiac emergencies. And, arriving at the hospital by ambulance usually means you'll be seen immediately by a nurse or physician.

In some areas of the country, EMTs are able to perform an EKG on the way to the hospital, substantially speeding diagnosis and treatment. It sometimes takes at least two EKGs, taken 20 to 30 minutes apart, to reveal a heart attack.

A PROPER DIAGNOSIS

The EKG is an invaluable, noninvasive diagnostic tool, but it's far from perfect. The EKG is very good at detecting damage to parts of the heart that lie closest to the chest wall, but it can miss heart attacks that cause damage to the back or far left or far right portions of the heart.

If your EKG is normal—and if you don't fit the profile of the typical heart attack patient and/or you are experiencing less common symptoms, such as shortness of breath without chest pain—it's wise to ask for a more thorough workup.

A blood test, known as a troponin test, screens for cardiac markers (proteins that increase after a heart attack).

Depending on your symptoms and blood test results, other diagnostic tests may include…

•**Coronary angiography.** This common procedure involves threading a catheter through an artery in the groin or an arm and into the heart. A contrast dye is injected through the catheter and traced via X-rays to detect narrowing and blockages in the cardiac arteries.

If a significant blockage is found, coronary angiography can immediately be followed by angioplasty, a procedure in which a tiny balloon is inflated at the tip of the catheter to open the artery, and a stent may be placed to keep it open. These catheter procedures do pose a small risk for stroke, heart attack, cardiac arrest or a punctured blood vessel. But angiography and angioplasty remain the gold standard for diagnosis and treatment of many patients with blocked arteries.

Caution: People with shellfish allergies may be allergic to the contrast dye. Medication is available to prevent an allergic reaction.

•**Computed tomographic angiography (CTA).** This noninvasive test involves the injection of a contrast dye, which is then traced by a high-resolution rapid computed tomography (CT) scanner to create a three-dimensional image of the heart and blood vessels. CTA provides information similar to that obtained by angiography without the risks associated with an invasive procedure, but it is not widely available.

•**Nuclear heart scan.** This noninvasive procedure involves injecting a radioactive material into your arm and tracking the material as it moves through the heart with a special camera that performs single photon emission computed

tomography (SPECT). The image that is generated often allows doctors to identify a blockage that may lead to a heart attack or a heart attack itself that is not detected with an EKG. If nuclear scanning is available, patients often undergo this test to decide whether a more invasive test, such as angiography, is necessary.

•**Cardiac magnetic resonance angiography (MRA).** This cutting-edge technology produces three-dimensional images of the heart and surrounding vessels, revealing both structural and functional damage. Unlike CTA and nuclear scanning, which use radiation, MRA relies on electromagnetic energy, which cannot be used in patients with pacemakers or defibrillators because it may pull on iron-containing objects in the body.

As nuclear scanning as well as CTA and MRA techniques become more widely available, physicians are likely to miss even fewer heart attacks.

■ **More from Joseph Ornato, MD…**

Red Flags for Heart Attack

Any chest discomfort or pain that lasts for more than a few minutes requires immediate medical attention. *Less common heart attack symptoms…*

•**Pain or discomfort in the back,** between the shoulder blades, in the neck, the jaw, the left shoulder and/or one or both arms.

•**Shortness of breath.**

•**Cold sweats.**

•**Nausea and/or vomiting.**

•**A feeling of indigestion.**

•**Sudden fatigue or weakness.**

•**Dizziness, light-headedness or fainting.**

•**Sense of impending doom (especially in women).**

If you experience any of the above symptoms for more than five minutes—and think you may be having a heart attack—immediately call 911.

Silent Heart Disease: Every Year 500,000 Americans Have a First Heart Attack—Often Without Warning

Prediman K. Shah, MD, director of the division of cardiology and the Atherosclerosis Research Center at Cedars-Sinai Heart Center in Los Angeles, is a professor of medicine at the David Geffen School of Medicine at the University of California, Los Angeles, and was the leader of the Screening for Heart Attack Prevention and Education (SHAPE) Task Force editorial committee.

U p to 50% of people who have a first heart attack—which often results in sudden death—don't experience prior chest pain, shortness of breath or other red flags for cardiovascular disease. A heart attack is their first and only symptom.

In the past, cardiologists relied solely on the presence of risk factors—a family history of heart disease, smoking, diabetes, etc.—to identify "silent" heart disease.

New approach: An international task force of leading cardiologists has issued new guidelines that could prevent more than 90,000 deaths from cardiovascular disease each year in the US. Most of these patients have no prior symptoms.

RISK FACTORS AREN'T ENOUGH

Most heart attacks and many strokes are caused by atherosclerosis, buildup of cholesterol and other substances (plaque) within artery walls.

Over time, increasing accumulations of plaque can compromise circulation—or result in blood clots that block circulation to the heart (heart attack) or brain (stroke).

Plaque can accumulate for decades within artery walls without causing the arterial narrowing that results in angina (chest pain) or other symptoms. Even patients with massive amounts of plaque may be unaware that they have heart disease until they suffer a heart attack or sudden death.

RECOMMENDED TESTS

Guidelines created by the Screening for Heart Attack Prevention and Education (SHAPE) Task Force call for noninvasive screening of virtually all asymptomatic men ages 45 to 75 and women ages 55 to 75.* The tests can detect arterial changes that are present in the vast majority of heart attack patients. The SHAPE Task Force identified two tests—a computed tomography (CT) scan of the coronary arteries and an ultrasound of the carotid arteries in the neck—that are more accurate than traditional risk-factor assessments in identifying high-risk patients.

Most patients require only one of these tests. Which test is recommended will depend on insurance coverage and/or other underlying health conditions and risk factors. Although these tests are widely available, health insurers do not always cover the cost, which ranges from about $200 to $400 each.

● **Coronary artery screening.** Calcium within the coronary arteries always indicates that a patient has atherosclerosis (whether or not blockages are present). Calcium is a marker of actual disease, not just the risk of disease.

What's involved: The patient is given a CT scan of the heart and three coronary arteries. Undressing isn't required—the test is noninvasive and takes about five to 10 minutes.

Dozens of images are taken during the test and then analyzed with computer software. If calcium is present, it's given a score based on severity. A score of 0 is ideal...less than 100 indicates moderate atherosclerosis...100 to 400 represents a significant problem...and more than 400 is severe.

In patients with a score of 0 (no calcium is present), the risk of having a heart attack or stroke over the next 10 years is 0.1%. Patients with a score of 400 or higher are 20 to 30 times more likely to have a heart attack or stroke than those with a score of 0.

● **Carotid ultrasound.** This test measures the intima media thickness (the gap between the inside of the blood vessel wall and a layer called the media) of the carotid arteries. It also measures the amount of plaque that may be present.

A thickening of the intima media (the values are adjusted for age and sex) is a predictor of stroke as well as heart attack. The presence of any

*Screening for adults age 75 or older is not recommended because they are considered at high risk for cardiovascular disease based on their age alone.

plaque is a red flag—patients who have plaque in the carotid arteries generally will also show evidence of plaque in the coronary arteries.

What's involved: The patient lies on an examination table while a technician moves a *transducer* (a device that emits and receives ultrasound signals) over the carotid arteries on both sides of the neck. Like the CT scan, the test is noninvasive. It takes about 45 to 90 minutes to complete.

TREATING SILENT HEART DISEASE

With screening tests, doctors can target high-risk patients more precisely—and recommend appropriate treatment. The aggressiveness of treatment should be proportionate to the risk level.

It's possible that drugs to reduce levels of existing plaque will be on the market within the next five years. *Until then, patients diagnosed with asymptomatic cardiovascular disease (based on one of the above tests) should...*

•**Get a stress test.** Patients who test positive for calcium or plaque in the coronary or carotid arteries should undergo a cardiac stress test. The test, which uses an electrocardiogram, involves walking on a treadmill or riding a bicycle. The test detects impediments in circulation through the coronary arteries and identifies abnormal heart rhythms (arrhythmias) that can occur during exercise in patients with heart disease. Nuclear stress tests (which involve the use of radioactive dye) or echocardiogram (a type of ultrasound) stress tests generally are more reliable than simple electrocardiogram tests.

Patients with significant blockages in the coronary arteries may require invasive procedures, such as angioplasty or bypass surgery, to restore normal circulation to the heart.

•**Control cholesterol and blood pressure.** They're two important risk factors for heart attack and stroke—and both are modifiable with medication and/or lifestyle changes. A patient who tests positive for asymptomatic cardiovascular disease needs to treat these conditions much more aggressively than someone without it. For cardiovascular health, aim for a blood pressure of no more than 110 mmHg to 120 mmHg systolic (top number) and 70 mmHg to 80 mmHg diastolic (bottom number). An ideal LDL "bad" cholesterol level is no more than 70.

Most patients can significantly lower blood pressure and cholesterol with lifestyle changes —exercising for 30 minutes at least three to four times a week...losing weight, if necessary...eating less saturated fat and/or trans fat...and increasing consumption of fruits, vegetables, whole grains and fish.

Other risk factors to control: Smoking, obesity, diabetes, as well as emotional stress/anger, which may lead to a heart attack or angina. It's important to control all of these risk factors because they can amplify each other—for example, a sedentary lifestyle promotes obesity, which can lead to diabetes—or have a cumulative effect that's much more dangerous than an individual risk factor.

For more on silent heart disease, consult the Society for Heart Attack Prevention and Eradication, a nonprofit group that promotes heart disease education, early detection and research, 877-742-7311, *www.shapesociety.org.*

■ ■ ■ ■

Heart Risk Predictor

A blood test that measures levels of NT-proBNP, a protein produced when the heart is under stress, helps diagnose heart failure.

Finding: In people seeking emergency care for shortness of breath, a common symptom of heart failure and heart attack, those with high levels of NT-proBNP were three times more likely to die within one year than those without.

If you suffer from shortness of breath: Ask about getting this test to help determine your long-term prognosis. A clinical trial is underway to evaluate more aggressive drug therapy for patients with high levels of NT-proBNP.

James L. Januzzi, Jr., MD, associate medical director, coronary care unit, Massachusetts General Hospital, Boston.

■ ■ ■ ■

Breath Warning

Shortness of breath may indicate heart disease—especially if it is a new symptom in someone 50 or older.

New study: People with unexplained breathing problems have more than twice the risk of dying from cardiac causes as people who report chest pain.

Reason: Patients with chest pain are more likely to be treated.

Self-defense: If you experience shortness of breath, call your doctor.

Daniel S. Berman, MD, is director of cardiac imaging/nuclear cardiology, Cedars-Sinai Heart Center, Los Angeles, and leader of a study of 17,991 patients, published in *New England Journal of Medicine*.

■■■■

Aspirin and Surgery

Heart and stroke patients should not stop daily aspirin therapy prior to surgery unless directed by a physician.

Reasons: Patients who stop taking aspirin have triple the risk of suffering a stroke within a month. Studies also suggest that when patients stop taking aspirin, blood becomes even stickier for a few weeks than it would have been if they had never taken aspirin in the first place. These findings raise doubts about the practice of halting aspirin therapy for the weeks prior to surgery.

Self-defense: Talk to your doctor about the risks of discontinuing aspirin therapy before surgery.

Patrik Michel, MD, director, acute stroke unit, Lausanne University, Switzerland, and leader of a study of 309 stroke patients, published in *Archives of Neurology*.

■■■■

Aspirin, Stat!

If you think you may be having a heart attack, take an aspirin immediately and be sure to chew it. This gets the aspirin into your system quicker.

When taking an aspirin as a preventive: Do not chew it. There is no hurry in getting it into your system, and chewed aspirin can erode tooth enamel and cause other damage to teeth.

Jack M. Rosenberg, PharmD, PhD, is director of the International Drug Information Center at the Arnold and Marie Schwartz College of Pharmacy Health Sciences at Long Island University in Brooklyn, New York.

■■■■

Speak Up

To protect your body from coronary heart disease, speak up for yourself. People who feel they are typically treated fairly at work, with their ideas recognized, are less likely to have heart disease later in life than ones who feel they are not fairly treated.

Mika Kivimaki, PhD, professor, Finnish Institute of Occupational Health and University of Helsinki, Finland.

Detecting Heart Attacks Before They Happen

W. Gregory Hundley, MD, associate professor of internal medicine and radiology, Wake Forest University School of Medicine, Winston-Salem, North Carolina. *Circulation.*

Magnetic resonance imaging (MRI) has been used for peering at the body's organs, but scientists say it can also tell whether chest pain is a harbinger of a future heart attack.

An MRI scan creates three-dimensional images and can predict the odds of a heart attack or heart-related death in people with chest symptoms, even after accounting for risk factors such as high blood pressure, smoking and diabetes. Intriguingly, the authors of a recent study say, the device can even pinpoint reduced blood flow to the apex of the heart, a particular signal of trouble.

The MRI pictures are clearer than conventional noninvasive heart imaging, says Dr. W. Gregory Hundley, a radiologist at Wake Forest University School of Medicine in Winston-Salem, North Carolina, and leader of the research team.

Doctors generally create an image of the heart using ultrasound technology. That test is cheap and portable, but it doesn't work very well on obese people or smokers. In fact, up to 20% of patients have pictures that are difficult to read.

TESTING THE MRI

Hundley's group gave MRI "stress tests" to 279 people who had cardiovascular disease and poor sound wave images. To simulate the effects of exercise, doctors gave the patients drugs that make the heart beat faster.

People whose blood flow was reduced by 40% or more had four times the risk of a heart attack or heart-related death over the next two years than those with normal results.

Hundley's group was the first to take pictures of damage to the apex—near the lower left portion of the heart. People who had such damage were six times more likely than those without injury to experience more heart attacks or to die of cardiovascular illness.

Unfortunately, MRI is not for everyone. The machines don't function properly in the presence of metal plates, pacemakers or defibrillators, so some people can't undergo the test.

■ ■ ■ ■

Defibrillator Warnings: Keep Cell Phones Away

Don't place a cell phone within six inches of your implanted defibrillator when the phone is on. The defibrillator could misinterpret the cell phone's signal as a heartbeat and withhold pacing. You can talk safely on the cell phone as long as it is at least six inches from the defibrillator. The defibrillator may set off airport and other types of security systems, so be sure to carry the card that identifies you as a defibrillator patient to show security personnel. Handheld metal detectors contain magnets that may interfere with defibrillators—ask security personnel to scan you for less than 30 seconds or, better yet, search you by hand. Some medical equipment also may interfere with a defibrillator—be sure your doctor and the technician know about the unit if you need an MRI or other procedure involving electromagnetic energy.

Mayo Clinic Health Letter, 200 First St. SW, Rochester, Minnesota 55905.

■ ■ ■ ■

An Unexpected Link to Heart Attack and Stroke

Researchers reviewed the medical records of 69,493 adults admitted to hospitals for vascular events—strokes, heart attacks and transient ischemic attacks (ministrokes)—over a two-year period.

Result: Vascular events were 27% more likely to occur on patients' birthdays than on other days—and 88% more likely if the patient had a history of high blood pressure.

Theory: Birthdays can trigger emotions that can lead to higher blood pressure, a spike in adrenaline or other reactions that may cause vascular events in at-risk individuals.

Gustavo Saposnik, MD, director, stroke research program, St. Michael's Hospital, Toronto.

'Open-Heart' Surgery Without Opening Your Chest

Michael Argenziano, MD, director of robotic cardiac surgery, NewYork-Presbyterian Hospital/Columbia University Medical Center, New York City.
American Heart Association scientific sessions, Chicago.

Your next heart surgeon may be a robot. Well, not exactly; but instead of standing over you wielding a scalpel, the surgeon will be sitting at a console, manipulating controls to manage robotic arms that repair a damaged portion of your heart.

And the surgery will be done in a less invasive way. Instead of making a foot-long incision in the chest, as is often required for heart surgery, the surgeon will work through four small holes that keep the damage to your body to a minimum.

"This is open-heart surgery without opening the chest," says Dr. Michael Argenziano, director of robotic cardiac surgery at NewYork-Presbyterian Hospital/Columbia Medical Center in New York City.

Argenziano has used Intuitive Surgical's da Vinci System, which is increasingly available at medical centers in the United States and around the world.

The system costs $1 million, but Argenziano says it is clearly worth it. "We were able to perform the operation with all the benefits we expected," he says. "There was minimum pain postoperatively and the patients went home a few days earlier than expected."

European surgeons are ahead of Americans in use of the system because the US Food and Drug Administration (FDA) has stricter requirements for approval, Argenziano says.

The FDA has approved the use of the da Vinci System for repair of the mitral valve, which controls the flow of blood between the two left chambers of the heart, and its use in bypass surgery could be next.

BENEFITS OF ROBOTIC SURGERY

The robotic procedures did take longer than conventional surgery; the heart had to be stopped for an average of 34 minutes, compared with 20 minutes. The reason might be the need for the surgeon to learn how to use the new system, Argenziano says. The average stay in the intensive care unit after surgery was 18 hours, the same as for traditional surgery, but patients did get to go home much sooner.

The benefits of the robotic cardiac surgery include…

•**Instruments can be manipulated with more accuracy than fingers.**

•**Magnified images of the surgery site** are finer than the view available to the surgeon's own eye.

•**Pencil-sized instruments are minimally invasive,** and they allow for a shorter recovery time for the patient.

"Instead of being in the hospital for seven to 10 days, the patient is there for three days," Argenziano says. "Instead of a recovery time of six to 12 weeks, it is two to four weeks. This is definitely part of the future."

More information about minimally invasive robotic surgery can be found at the Columbia University Department of Surgery Web site at *www.columbiasurgery.org*.

■■■■

Go to the ER!

If you think you are having a heart attack, don't rely solely on the new dial-up EKG service. Get to an emergency room immediately. The *EKGuard* transmits information to the service's on-call doctor by phone so that he/she can try to decide if you really are having a heart attack.

But: The transmitting device takes time to set up, and heart attack diagnosis is not always simple. Some attacks are easy to spot, but a small one may not be, and some people have atypical symptoms.

Bottom line: Call 911 for an ambulance or have someone drive you to the nearest emergency room.

Edward Berman, MD, cardiologist in private practice, Gardena, California.

■■■■

Winter Danger

Rapid decreases in barometric pressure (usually associated with precipitation, especially during winter) are linked to heart attack.

In a review of 1,300 hospital admissions of heart attack patients over a three-year period, when the pressure dropped one unit on the barometer, heart attack risk was 10% greater during the next 24 hours…a two-unit drop per hour resulted in a 20% increase in risk.

Theory: A rapid drop in barometric pressure causes inflamed atherosclerotic plaque to break off and trigger a heart attack.

Philip D. Houck, MD, associate professor of internal medicine, Texas A&M University, Temple, Texas.

How to Get Your Life Back After A Heart Attack

Paul Kligfield, MD, medical director of the Cardiac Health Center at NewYork-Presbyterian Hospital, and professor of medicine at Weill-Cornell Medical College, both in New York City, is author of *The Cardiac Recovery Handbook: The Complete Guide to Life After Heart Attack or Heart Surgery*. Hatherleigh.

Every year, about 650,000 Americans have their first heart attack—a temporary interruption in blood flow to the heart that causes permanent damage. Thanks to improvements in emergency and hospital care, more people than ever survive. But what comes next?

Paul Kligfield, MD, medical director of the Cardiac Health Center at NewYork-Presbyterian Hospital answers the questions cardiologists hear most often.

DRUGS

•What medications should I take to prevent another heart attack?

The American Heart Association and American College of Cardiology recommend that nearly everyone who has had a heart attack take all four of the following types of drugs...

•**Blood thinners.** These important drugs reduce platelet adhesion, the first step in the formation of blood clots that can block arteries. Low-dose aspirin (81 mg) often is used, but some patients may need a higher dose (325 mg) each day. If you're at higher risk of clotting (after certain kinds of heart attack, for example), your doctor also might prescribe *clopidogrel* (Plavix).

If your heart attack caused enough damage to continue to reduce heart action or disturb its rhythm, your risk of clots may require a different blood thinner, *warfarin* (Coumadin), to prevent the kind of blood clots that form within the chambers of the heart.

•**Beta-blockers,** such as *propranolol* (Inderal) and *atenolol* (Tenormin), also are routinely prescribed after heart attacks. These drugs lighten the load on the heart by slowing the pulse and lowering blood pressure.

•**Angiotensin-converting enzyme (ACE) inhibitors** and *angiotensin receptor blockers* (ARBs) lower blood pressure and seem to have a stabilizing effect on the arteries, allowing blood to flow from the heart more easily.

•**Statins,** such as *lovastatin* (Mevacor) and *atorvastatin* (Lipitor), are powerful cholesterol-lowering drugs.

After a heart attack, the acceptable level of LDL cholesterol is lower than before the attack (100 mg/dl, compared to 130 mg/dl), and it appears that bringing it down still lower (to 80 mg/dl or even lower) can cut heart attack risk further. Statin drugs also help keep arteries healthy, perhaps by blocking inflammation.

EXERCISE

•Will I be able to be as active as I was before my heart attack?

It depends on how bad the heart attack was, but most people can safely return to their pre-attack activities.

One key factor is *cardiac rehabilitation*—a program of gradually increasing exercise. By helping the heart work more efficiently, this regimen can reduce the risk of future heart attacks, too. I usually start patients on a cardiac rehabilitation program two to four weeks after they leave the hospital.

•What does a cardiac rehabilitation program consist of?

A post–heart attack program usually requires that you exercise three times a week for 12 weeks, following a plan tailored by a cardiologist to your needs and capacities and under the supervision of a nurse. Your heart function will be tracked by electrocardiography to ensure exercise is at a safe level and to spot abnormalities quickly.

With this program, you can increase the level of exercise while keeping it safe. An analysis of 48 clinical trials involving nearly 9,000 patients found that cardiac rehabilitation programs significantly reduce the rate of death from all causes, including heart disease.

•Can I do the program on my own?

After most heart attacks, you can—as long as it's not entirely on your own. Before starting to exercise, have a full examination by your cardiologist, including a stress test, to confirm that it is safe to exercise and to determine the right level. Regular check-ins should guide you in increasing the amount and intensity of exercise as your capacity improves.

Aerobic exercise is best—brisk walking, swimming, riding a stationary exercise bike.

Rule of thumb: A good level of intensity is one that you can sustain comfortably for 30 minutes while being able to talk but not sing. Work out at least three times a week.

You may want to track your pulse rate to make sure it remains at a level your doctor says is safe, possibly with the help of a watchlike heart monitor, available in drugstores and online for between $50 and $80.

•What danger signs should I look for when exercising?

Chest pain or shortness of breath disproportionate to the level of exertion are signals that your heart isn't getting enough oxygen and that you should stop. If these recur or you have unusual fatigue, consult your doctor.

•When is it safe to have sex?

There's no one timetable that is appropriate for every heart patient. Sex makes demands on the heart that are at least as strenuous as walking up stairs, so it's usually okay to have sex once you can climb a flight or two without difficulty.

DIET

•What foods should I eat?

Aim for 25% to 30% of calories from fat (no more than 7% of that from saturated fat, found in meat, butter, etc.), lots of fruits, vegetables and whole grains and other complex carbohydrates. Alcohol in moderation is okay.

Even if you're taking a statin to reduce cholesterol, diet still counts. It will help the medication work better and even may enable you to cut the dose.

Perhaps the most important thing is to keep calories down enough to maintain a healthy weight. Obesity is associated with worsening heart disease.

OTHER PROBLEMS

•Are there any diseases I should watch out for?

The big two are diabetes and high blood pressure—each substantially increases your risk of having another heart attack. Work with your doctor to keep blood pressure below 130/80. If you have diabetes, use diet and medication, if necessary, to control it.

•Is there anything else I should be concerned about?

Depression, which is fairly common after a heart attack, increases the risk of dying from heart disease. Although it hasn't been proven that treating depression reduces this risk, relieving it with medication and/or therapy certainly improves life and makes you better able to take care of your heart.

Signs and symptoms of depression may include irritability, loss of interest in activities that used to interest you and excessive tiredness.

Drug-Free Ways to Reduce Artery Plaque

Mark A. Stengler, ND, naturopathic physician in private practice, La Jolla, California…adjunct associate clinical professor at the National College of Natural Medicine, Portland, Oregon…author of many books, including *The Natural Physician's Healing Therapies* and coauthor of *Prescription for Natural Cures* (both from Bottom Line Books)…and author of the *Bottom Line/Natural Healing* newsletter.

Amid the clamor created by pharmaceutical companies hyping cholesterol-lowering statin drugs, important information is going unheard.

You need to know: Four natural therapies can protect, and even restore, the health of your arteries—without the dangerous side effects of statin drugs.

Michael, a 60-year-old executive, is living proof. A computed tomography (CT) scan showed a buildup of plaque—a mix of fat, cholesterol, cellular waste products, calcium and other substances—in Michael's arteries.

Diagnosis: Atherosclerosis, a condition that affects one in four Americans and is a major contributor to cardiac disease, the number-one killer of both men and women in the US. Michael's medical doctor recommended statin medication, commonly used in an attempt to slow the progression of arterial disease by lowering cholesterol and reducing inflammation. Then the doctor recited a litany of side effects from the drug, including muscle pain, fatigue, weakness and potentially fatal liver damage.

That's when Michael came to me, saying, "I want to get rid of the gunk, not just keep it from increasing. And I want to do it with safe, natural therapies." He succeeded—and so can you—by using the four substances described below.

These natural substances help to *reverse* the process of plaque buildup—to dissolve plaque, eliminating the danger it presents. They are available over-the-counter from health-food stores, on-line and/or from holistic physicians. Unless otherwise noted, they have no side effects, can be taken indefinitely and are safe for everyone, including people who take statin drugs. *Important…*

• **If you have atherosclerosis or any other cardiovascular condition,** you need to be under a cardiologist's care.

• **If you take blood-thinning medication,** such as aspirin or *warfarin* (Coumadin)—typically given to improve blood flow and prevent blood clots—talk to your doctor before using the natural therapies below, because they could affect your medication dosage.

• **If you are pregnant,** speak to your doctor before taking these or any other supplements or drugs.

• **Discontinue use of these substances 10 to 14 days prior to scheduled surgery to reduce the risk of excess bleeding.** Resume use according to your doctor's instructions (typically 10 days after the procedure).

• **To determine which substance or combination of substances to use,** see "The Right Regimen for You" to follow on page 359.

1. TOCOTRIENOLS

Vitamin E is not just one vitamin, but rather a family of eight slightly different molecular structures that function differently in the body. There are two principal categories of vitamin E, called *tocopherols* and *tocotrienols*. Each of these has four subcategories—alpha, beta, gamma and delta.

Some vitamin E supplements contain synthetic alpha-tocopherol. If that's what is in your cupboard—indicated on the label as "dl-alpha-tocopherol"—throw it out! Synthetic alpha-tocopherol hogs the space on cells' vitamin E receptors (slots into which molecules must fit in order to be used by the body), leaving less room for the more healthful tocopherols you ingest from food or natural supplements (labeled "d-alpha-tocopherol"). Natural tocopherols reduce free radicals, helping to prevent new plaque, but they have not been shown to reduce plaque that is already present. For that, you need tocotrienols.

Tocotrienols are found in rice bran, coconut, barley and wheat germ—but only in small amounts. Supplements with mixed tocopherols/tocotrienols are sold in health-food stores—but they are not the best for reducing plaque.

Better: A tocotrienol-only supplement. I like Allergy Research Group Delta-Fraction Tocotrienols hypoallergenic soft gels (800-545-9960,

www.allergyresearchgroup.com), available from holistic doctors. The dosage is 300 mg per day.

2. VITAMIN K

Vitamin K is a key player in *bone calcification*, whereby calcium is transported from the blood into the bones to keep them strong. To do this, the body requires the aid of the protein *osteocalcin*, which cannot do its job without vitamin K. When vitamin K is insufficient, calcium that is stranded in the blood heads for the walls of the arteries, which in turn become stiffer and more prone to forming dangerous blood clots. In other words, vitamin K promotes beneficial bone calcification and protects against harmful arterial calcification.

Forms of vitamin K include *phylloquinone* (K1) and *menaquinone* (K2). Vitamin K1 is abundant in dark green leafy vegetables, such as lettuce, spinach and broccoli. However, vitamin K2 is better absorbed and remains active in the body longer than vitamin K1. Good food sources of vitamin K2 include natto (fermented soybeans) and, to a lesser degree, fermented cheeses (the type with holes, such as Swiss and Jarlsberg), beef liver, chicken and egg yolks.

People taking warfarin are at higher risk for atherosclerosis and osteoporosis (brittle bones) due to the drug's effects on calcification. A study in *Pharmacotherapy* demonstrated the safety and benefit of low-dose vitamin K supplementation in patients taking warfarin. (This study did not distinguish between vitamins K1 and K2.)

Note: It is vital that a person who takes blood thinners use vitamin K only under the close supervision of a doctor, because the medication dosage may need to be adjusted.

I think daily supplementation with 150 mcg to 200 mcg of vitamin K2 is appropriate for all adults—and especially important for those with atherosclerosis. If you take warfarin, the daily dose may be modified, depending on blood tests that indicate how your clotting mechanism interacts with vitamin K. A brand I like is Jarrow Formulas' MK-7 (800-726-0886, *www.jarrow.com*).

3. GARLIC EXTRACT

Legend tells us that garlic protects against vampires—but its true power lies in its ability to protect arteries. Most beneficial is aged garlic extract (AGE), available in capsule or liquid form.

A study from the University of California, Los Angeles, involved 19 cardiac patients who were taking statin drugs and aspirin daily. Participants took either a placebo or 4 milliliters (ml) of a liquid brand called Kyolic AGE for one year.

Findings: Participants who took AGE had about a 66% reduction in new plaque formation compared with those who took a placebo.

Research demonstrates that AGE also can…

• **Reduce LDL cholesterol by up to 12%…** total cholesterol by up to 31%…and triglycerides by up to 19%.

• **Protect against the LDL oxidation** that can trigger arterial plaque formation.

• **Thin the blood.**

• **Lower blood pressure.**

• **Reduce blood levels of *homocysteine*—** the amino acid that, when elevated, raises cardiovascular disease risk.

• **Reduce *C-reactive protein*,** a blood marker of inflammation and a risk factor for atherosclerosis.

• **Combat carotid plaque.**

I think it is wise to supplement daily with aged garlic extract.

Dosage: 4 ml to 6 ml of liquid AGE or 400 mg to 600 mg in tablet or capsule form.

4. POMEGRANATE JUICE

Once considered exotic, pomegranate juice now is sold in supermarkets and is a proven boon to arterial health. Israeli researchers verified this in a three-year study of 19 men and women, ages 65 to 75, with severe carotid artery blockage. Ten participants drank 50 ml (about two ounces) per day of 100% pomegranate juice, and nine participants drank a placebo.

Results: Among juice drinkers, plaque thickness decreased by an average of 13% after three months and 35% after one year. This is phenomenal—no drug can come close to reducing plaque like this! Placebo drinkers had a 9% *increase* in plaque after one year.

Pomegranate juice is loaded with antioxidants called *polyphenols*, which prevent cholesterol oxidation and improve blood flow.

Note: Choose 100% juice with no added sugar. Pomegranate juice contains a lot of naturally occurring sugar, so dilute two to four ounces of juice with an equal amount of water. Drink it with meals to slow the absorption of sugar into the bloodstream and help to maintain stable blood glucose levels. Use twice daily.

THE RIGHT REGIMEN FOR YOU

Arterial plaque buildup can be detected and its severity gauged using imaging tests, such as computed tomography (CT), magnetic resonance imaging (MRI) scan and/or ultrasound. Results help to determine the appropriate therapy for you. Tests may be repeated periodically to see if your regimen needs to be modified.

The four natural substances described in this article, used alone or in combination (following the dosage guidelines in the main article), can improve the health of your arteries. Here's how to tell which ones are right for you.

Note: If you take blood-thinning medication, talk to your doctor before using these substances.

If you do not have atherosclerosis, take one or more of these…

• **Vitamin K**

• **Aged garlic extract (AGE)**

• **Pomegranate juice**

For mild atherosclerosis, take all of these…

• **Vitamin K**

• **AGE**

• **Pomegranate juice**

For moderate or severe atherosclerosis, take all of these…

• **Tocotrienols**

• **Vitamin K**

• **AGE**

• **Pomegranate juice**

• **Statin medication**—but only if you and your doctor are not satisfied with your level of improvement after 12 months of daily use of all four natural substances.

How to Survive a Heart Attack

Marjory Abrams, publisher, *Bottom Line* newsletters, Boardroom Inc., 281 Tresser Blvd., Stamford, Connecticut 06901.

Choosing the right hospital can be the key to surviving a heart attack, says cardiologist Richard Stein, MD, director of the Vascular Biology and Disease Program at New York City's New York University Medical Center and author of the book *Outliving Heart Disease*.

To find the best hospital in your area, he advises checking the Hospital Compare heart attack statistics at *www.hospitalcompare.hhs.gov*. Do it now before an emergency. Call hospital cardiology departments to find out which perform emergency angioplasty to open blocked arteries and if it is done less than 90 minutes after arrival at the hospital. (Medication can be used instead, but angioplasty generally is more effective if done soon after arrival.) If possible, pick a hospital where your doctor has admitting privileges.

HEART ATTACK SURVIVAL CHECKLIST

1. Know the symptoms. The classic heart attack symptoms are chest pain or discomfort that may also be felt in the neck or left arm and may be accompanied by nausea. Women are more likely than men to have atypical symptoms—shortness of breath, profound fatigue, sweating, racing heart, burning stomach.

2. Call 911 for an ambulance to take you to the hospital immediately if you experience symptoms. Don't let embarrassment or concern that it is something minor prevent you from getting checked.

3. Chew two full-strength aspirin.

4. Tell ambulance and hospital staff that you think you are having a heart attack. Don't minimize your symptoms.

5. Have the appropriate tests, including an electrocardiogram (EKG) and blood tests to measure certain cardiac enzymes. Dr. Stein notes that women with the atypical symptoms cited above (or their health advocates) may need to be assertive to get these tests.

According to Dr. Stein, accurate diagnosis may require several EKGs and/or blood tests within the first few hours. In 2000, former vice president Dick Cheney experienced chest and shoulder pain. The initial EKG and blood tests showed no evidence of a heart attack. Several hours later, the second set of tests revealed that he had indeed suffered a minor heart attack.

6. Get the proper treatment. Treatment should begin even before all test results are in…

•Aspirin right away if you didn't take it at home.

•A beta-blocker, such as *metoprolol* (Lopressor) or *propranolol* (Inderal) should be given to most patients to decrease the heart's need for oxygen-rich blood and minimize heart damage.

•Nitroglycerin, prescribed for chest pain or if the heart is short of blood, dilates blood vessels.

•ACE inhibitor to decrease blood pressure and the heart's workload.

•Clot-busting treatments, such as the drug tPA, and/or angioplasty.

Photocopy this page so that you can take it with you to the ER. I hope that you will never need it, but if you do, it may save your life.

Deadly Blood Clots: Deep Vein Thrombosis Kills 200,000 Americans

Geno J. Merli, MD, a leading vascular expert, is director of the Jefferson Center for Vascular Diseases at Thomas Jefferson University Hospital, and Ludwig A. Kind Professor of Medicine at Jefferson Medical College, both in Philadelphia.

Blood clots that form in the coronary arteries cause heart attacks. However, many people don't realize that clots also can form in other parts of the vascular system—particularly in the deep veins of the legs, causing *deep vein thrombosis* (DVT). These clots can be even more dangerous than clots in the coronary arteries because they are more likely to go undiagnosed.

Of the more than 200,000 Americans who die each year from clots due to DVT, about 80% of them experience no symptoms. The worst danger of DVT is *pulmonary embolism*, in which one or more clots travel from the legs to the lungs. One in five people who experience a pulmonary embolism dies from it.

Clots that form in veins near the surface of the skin (superficial thrombosis) are rarely serious. But those that form in the deep veins in the legs—particularly in the *femoral* (thigh), *iliac* (groin) or *popliteal* (behind the knee) veins—are often life-threatening. They rarely dissolve on their own. If anything, they're likely to keep growing—and eventually break free and travel to the lungs.

Even for patients who survive a pulmonary embolism, the risk for complications is high. About 4% to 5% will go on to develop pulmonary hypertension (high blood pressure in the lungs). Others are at risk for *venous* insufficiency, in which the leg veins are damaged, resulting in chronic leg swelling, skin thickening and skin ulceration.

MAJOR RISK FACTORS

About 10% of patients with DVT have a genetic tendency to form blood clots. *Other risk factors...*

•**Prolonged periods of inactivity** can allow dangerous blood clots to form. This can occur during lengthy (more than five hours) plane flights or car trips. Long-distance air or car travelers who have other risk factors, such as congestive heart failure, previous heart attack, obesity or a history of previous blood clots, are at even greater risk than healthy people of developing DVT.

Orthopedic surgery, particularly hip or knee replacement, causes immobilization, often for days to weeks. Anticlotting drugs are given to prevent clots from forming.

•**Lung, pancreatic or ovarian cancer.** Patients with these cancers have increased levels of procoagulants, substances in the blood that promote clotting.

•**Pregnancy and childbirth.** Pulmonary embolism is a cause of death in women during childbirth. Many women who die from pulmonary embolism during or soon after childbirth may have an underlying genetic disorder that increases the risk for clots.

Women who take the breast cancer drug *tamoxifen* (Nolvadex) or supplemental estrogen in birth control pills or hormone therapy also are at increased risk for DVT and pulmonary embolism.

DIAGNOSIS AND TREATMENT

Although patients with DVT frequently do not have symptoms, when clots completely block a vein, persistent symptoms of leg swelling, redness, increased warmth and pain develop.

Red flag: A pulmonary embolism from DVT typically causes sudden shortness of breath, chest pain or a cough that produces blood-tinged mucus. If you experience these symptoms, get to an emergency room *immediately*. About 10% of patients with pulmonary embolism die within one hour.

DVT usually can be diagnosed with ultrasound, a painless, 30-minute test that uses high-frequency sound waves to view the veins.

If your doctor suspects that you have a pulmonary embolism, he/she may recommend a pulmonary computed tomography (CT) scan, in which a dye is injected into an arm vein and computerized images are taken as the dye passes through the blood vessels in the lungs.

Most patients require medication to prevent the clot from growing—and to prevent additional clots from forming.

Typical treatment approaches...

•**DVT patients with a pulmonary embolism who are hemodynamically stable**—that is, their blood pressure and level of oxygen in the blood are close to normal—are hospitalized for five to seven days and treated with intravenous heparin, an anticoagulant medication.

Recent development: A new formulation known as low-molecular-weight heparin, which is better absorbed and lasts longer than intravenous heparin, can be given as a subcutaneous shot at home for five to seven days.

After one of these initial treatments, *warfarin* (Coumadin) is given for three to six months.

•**DVT patients with a pulmonary embolism who are hemodynamically unstable** are at the greatest risk for death—they have low blood pressure and poor oxygen saturation. These patients are typically given *tissue plasminogen activator* (tPA), an intravenous, clot-dissolving drug that is often used to treat stroke patients. This therapy is followed by intravenous or subcutaneous heparin for five to seven days. Warfarin is then given for three to six months to prevent recurrent clots.

In rare cases, when a patient can not receive anticoagulant therapy because of bleeding, recent surgery or an allergy to the medication, doctors may use a vein filter, a small metal trap that's inserted into the *inferior vena cava* (the large vein that carries blood from the lower part of the body to the heart). The filter prevents pulmonary embolism by catching clots before they can be carried to the lungs.

PREVENTING DVT

Patients at risk for DVT who are hospitalized and bedridden are usually treated with subcutaneous heparin.

If they cannot take heparin, they may be fitted with graduated compression stockings or external pneumatic compression sleeves (which inflate and deflate every 30 seconds by air compression). Both exert varying amounts of pressure along the legs to keep blood from pooling in the legs and forming clots.

Other ways to prevent DVT...

• **Rotate your ankles and flex your toes** at least every 20 minutes when traveling by plane or car. On airplanes, periodically stand and rise up on your tip-toes repeatedly. These exercises flex the calf muscles, which pushes blood out of the legs and helps prevent DVT.

• **Walk daily.** Walking, like other forms of leg exercise, keeps blood moving upward out of the leg veins. The more that blood moves, the less likely it is to form unwanted clots. It's particularly important for hospitalized patients to attempt to walk with appropriate supervision or at least move their legs while they're in bed.

Recent studies indicate that about 15% of hospitalized patients get DVT. Bedridden patients also should flex their feet, ankles and calves every 20 to 30 minutes when awake for clot prevention.

• **Drink water.** Airplane and car travelers on trips of five hours or more should drink two to four eight-ounce glasses of water during the flight or car ride. This increases blood volume, which may help prevent blood clotting.

■ ■ ■ ■

Clot Buster

Dangerous blood clots can be eliminated with a new ultrasound device. The device consists of a hair-thin wire with transducers attached. After it is positioned near a clot, the transducers emit a high-frequency sound to loosen blood fibers and force an anticlotting drug through the clot. The device is in limited use for people who have deep-vein thrombosis or arterial-bypass grafts in the leg or acute blood clots in leg arteries. It is being studied for more uses, including dissolving stroke-causing clots in the brain.

James F. Benenati, MD, is medical director, Peripheral Vascular Laboratory, Baptist Cardiac and Vascular Institute, Miami, Florida.

Abdominal Aortic Aneurysms Kill 15,000 Americans Each Year

David Tilson, MD, Ailsa Mellon Bruce Professor of Surgery at Columbia University and director emeritus of the department of surgery at St. Luke's-Roosevelt Hospital Center, both in New York City, was chairman of a recent international conference on abdominal aortic aneurysm in New York City.

Until recently, hypertension, diabetes and other chronic conditions have been identified as America's biggest health threats.

Now: As the baby boomer population ages, abdominal aortic aneurysm (AAA), a potentially fast-acting condition that can be fatal, appears to be on the rise.

An aneurysm is a bulge in a blood vessel wall. Some aneurysms affect blood vessels in the brain. Others occur in the aorta, the main artery of the body. About the diameter of a garden hose, the aorta travels from the heart through the chest and abdomen, then forms separate branches that enter the legs. Aortic aneurysms usually form in the abdominal cavity—the artery walls may be weaker in this area.

Surgeons can repair AAAs before they rupture—if they are identified. An AAA can be discovered during tests, such as X-rays or computed tomography (CT) scans, for other conditions. But what makes an AAA so deadly is that it usually is not identified and typically causes no symptoms prior to rupturing.

Caution: If you have symptoms of an AAA—abdominal or back pain, along with a pulsating mass in the abdomen—seek immediate medical attention.

A SILENT THREAT

Most AAAs grow slowly—about 3 millimeters (mm) to 4 mm (about one-eighth inch) per year. A person can have an AAA for decades before it becomes large enough to rupture—if it ever does. Even when doctors detect an AAA, they're unlikely to recommend surgery if the aneurysm is smaller than 5 centimeters (cm)—about two inches—in diameter.

Warning: AAA patients must be closely monitored with imaging tests for the rest of their lives because the risk of dying from a rupture is so high. An AAA that's 5 cm or larger—or that's growing more than 1 cm a year—has a significant risk of rupturing and needs to be surgically repaired.

CAUSES OF AAA

AAAs have some of the same risk factors as those for atherosclerosis, the accumulation of fatty deposits (plaque) that weaken artery walls. The same measures that doctors recommend to prevent heart attacks—not smoking, controlling hypertension and cholesterol, for example—also can help prevent AAAs.

Some patients, particularly those with Marfan's syndrome (a genetic condition that's characterized by extreme height), are born with a weakness in the aorta wall. In rare cases, infection or inflammation (vasculitis) in a blood vessel can predispose patients to AAA.

For small or slow-growing AAAs, "watchful waiting" is usually best. Patients are advised to have ultrasound screenings every six months to determine whether the AAA is getting large enough or expanding fast enough to rupture.

Caution: Patients with high-risk AAAs should avoid heavy lifting and intense aerobic exercises.

These activities can cause surges in blood pressure that can increase the risk for a rupture.

Researchers have investigated the use of medications—for example, beta-blockers, such as *propranolol* (Inderal), and tetracycline antibiotics—to slow the growth of AAAs. The results have been disappointing. New drugs are being investigated, but surgery is currently the best option.

NEW TREATMENT STRATEGIES

Surgery to repair an AAA involves opening the abdomen, removing the damaged section of artery and replacing it with a synthetic graft.

Newer approach: A procedure known as endovascular surgery involves the insertion of a catheter into an artery in the leg. The surgeon threads the catheter upward into the damaged section of artery. Once the catheter is in place, it's used to insert and fasten a metal-covered mesh tube (stent) that reinforces the blood vessel.

The initial success rate of both procedures—open surgery and endovascular repair—has been determined to be about 96% to 98%, respectively. However, patients who undergo an endovascular procedure spend less time in the hospital and recover more quickly.

Recent finding: A study of 28,000 Medicare patients, published in the *Journal of Vascular Surgery*, found that the risk for death with endovascular procedures was 1.9%, compared with 5.2% for conventional surgery. It's still not known, however, whether the stent-grafts used in endovascular repair are as durable as the repairs performed in conventional surgery.

Guidelines…

•**Relatively young,** healthy AAA patients are generally advised to have conventional surgery. These patients are typically better able to withstand the operation, and the hand-sewn repair might last longer than an endovascular graft.

•**Older patients** who may not be healthy enough to withstand conventional surgery—and who have a shorter life expectancy—will probably benefit more from an endovascular procedure.

REGULAR SCREENING

Because an AAA rarely causes symptoms but is so deadly, anyone with risk factors—men who are current or former smokers or are age 65 or older…and men and women who are age 65 or older and have a first-degree relative (parent, sibling or child) with an AAA—should undergo an ultrasound test to detect changes in the artery wall. If you have a family history of AAA in one or more relatives who was diagnosed with an AAA under the age of 65, then you should be screened at a younger age.

An initial ultrasound at age 65 for people with any of the above risk factors is recommended. Cardiovascular risk factors, such as elevated blood pressure and/or cholesterol, also may be considered. Patients with no signs of disease at this age don't require additional tests. Exception: Patients with a family history of AAAs should be retested every five years. Their risk is at least three times higher than that of someone without a family history.

Medicare and most other health insurers will pay for ultrasound screening in patients age 65 and older who have AAA risk factors.

■ ■ ■ ■

Bad Noise

An excessively noisy environment can cause a heart attack.

Recent findings: Men who live in noisy areas are 50% more likely to suffer a heart attack than men who live in quiet areas. Women living in noisy areas are 300% more likely to have a heart attack than women who live in quiet areas.

Probable reason: Prolonged exposure to noise in the 65- to 75-decibel range (such as that in a city street-level apartment) causes your body to release *adrenaline*, which drives up blood pressure. Normal conversation levels are at about 60 decibels, so if you have to repeatedly raise your voice to be heard, you're in an unhealthy noise environment.

Mehmet C. Oz, MD, medical director of the Integrated Medicine Center and director of the Cardiovascular Institute at NewYork-Presbyterian Medical Center and professor of cardiac surgery at Columbia University, both in New York City, is coauthor of *You: The Smart Patient: An Insider's Handbook for Getting the Best Treatment.* Free Press.

■ ■ ■ ■

Early Warnings

Women may experience heart attack warning symptoms more than a month before the attack. The most common symptom is overwhelming fatigue, reported by 71% of women. Other reported symptoms are sleep disturbance (48%), shortness of breath (42%), indigestion (39%) and anxiety (35%). Only 30% experience chest discomfort.

Self-defense: If you are experiencing these or any suspicious symptoms, contact your doctor.

Jean McSweeney, PhD, RN, professor, University of Arkansas for Medical Sciences, Little Rock, and lead researcher of a survey of 515 female heart attack survivors, published in *Circulation.*

The Upside to Being Overweight: Heart Attack Survival

Kristin Newby, MD, associate professor of medicine, Duke University Medical Center, Durham, North Carolina.

Terrence J. Sacchi, MD, chief of cardiology, Long Island College Hospital, Brooklyn, New York.

Eric Eisenstein, assistant research professor of medicine, Duke Clinical Research Institute, Durham, North Carolina.

American College of Cardiology scientific sessions.

You know that being obese is bad for you. And no one should misconstrue the following information as an excuse for being fat. But there may be a short-term silver lining to all the fat that Americans typically accumulate.

Much to their surprise, scientists at Duke University Medical Center found that overweight and obese individuals actually have better one-year survival rates following a heart attack than people whose weight is within a healthier range.

Not so surprisingly, the researchers also determined that the United States had the highest combined rate of obese and very obese people, while Asia had the highest percentage of healthy-weight people.

One of the ironies in these findings is that being heavy is a risk factor for coronary artery disease, and may have been what helped land these patients in the hospital in the first place.

THE STUDY

Dr. Kristin Newby, coauthor of the study, had initially hypothesized with her colleagues that overweight and obese people would have higher mortality rates in the first year following a heart attack. But the results of the study showed that the opposite was true.

To test the hypothesis, the researchers looked at data already collected for two related international trials and divided the 15,904 participants into four groups according to their body mass index (BMI)—normal (18.5–24.9), overweight (25–29.9), obese (30–34.9) and very obese (35 and higher).

One year after a heart attack, individuals in the obese group had the lowest death rate (2.2%), followed by those classified as very obese (2.6%), overweight (2.7%) and, finally, normal bringing up the rear (4.3%). Normal-weight participants also had the highest death rate after 90 days, and a similar pattern was evident even at 30 days.

AGE vs. GIRTH

The results may have more to do with the age of the people studied than their girth, says Dr. Terrence J. Sacchi, chief of cardiology at Long Island College Hospital in Brooklyn Heights, New York. "It seems that the patients in the overweight and obese group were younger, and also they were treated more aggressively," he says.

"When adjusted for confounders, the findings still held up in overweight and obese people, but not in the very obese group," says Eric Eisenstein, Newby's coauthor and an assistant research professor at the Duke Clinical Research Institute. "Even after adjusting for all those factors, we still found that at one year, the overweight and obese groups had a lower hazard of death than the normal people and the very obese people," he says.

RESULTS NOT AN INDICATOR OF LONG-TERM SURVIVAL

One thing to keep in mind is that this study looked only at intermediate-term survival, not long-term survival. "I don't think anyone is advocating remaining obese," Sacchi says. "It is associated with multiple risk factors."

For a handy online calculator that quickly computes your BMI, visit the National Heart, Lung, and Blood Institute's Web site at *http://nhlbisupport.com/bmi/bmicalc.htm.*

What Your Doctor Won't Tell You About High Blood Pressure

Aggie Casey, RN, associate in medicine at Harvard Medical School, and Herbert Benson, MD, associate professor of medicine at Harvard Medical School, are coauthors of *The Harvard Medical School Guide to Lowering Your Blood Pressure.* McGraw-Hill.

High blood pressure (hypertension) has long been termed "the silent killer." That's because it usually causes no symptoms, but it sets the stage for stroke, heart attack and serious kidney damage.

Hypertension is defined as a blood pressure reading of 140/90 millimeters of mercury (mm/Hg) or higher.

Now: Data compiled from several studies indicates that risk for death from heart disease and stroke starts to increase with a blood pressure above 115/75 mm/Hg.

After reviewing more than 30 clinical trials, the National Heart, Lung, and Blood Institute recently created a new category of hypertension called "prehypertension"—a systolic (top number) blood pressure of 120 to 139 mm/Hg and/or a diastolic (bottom number) blood pressure of 80 to 89 mm/Hg.

Result: An estimated 90 million Americans —including 40 million who previously were considered not to be at risk—are now said to have prehypertension or hypertension. *Medication is the most common treatment, but you can avoid medication or reduce the dosage by following these important but often-overlooked strategies...*

TAKE STRESS SERIOUSLY

When treating hypertension, doctors rarely pay attention to stress—but that's a mistake. Stress hormones, such as *epinephrine* and *norepinephrine*, make the heart beat faster and blood vessels constrict, significantly raising blood pressure.

The stress response can be triggered by driving in traffic...waiting in long lines...or arguing with a family member, friend or colleague. Many studies have demonstrated that emotional stress can contribute to high blood pressure.

Solution: Allocate time each day to elicit the relaxation response. This is a quiet state that can be brought forth by meditation or breathing exercises. Start with five or 10 minutes several days a week, and gradually increase it to 20 minutes daily.

For optimal benefit, add a "minirelaxation" exercise whenever you feel stress building.

Examples: Count slowly from 10 to zero, inhaling and exhaling slowly with each number. Or sit quietly and focus on your breathing for one minute. With every inhalation, repeat "I am" to yourself. With each exhalation, repeat "at peace."

Important: Activities that people often perceive as "relaxing," such as watching TV, do not have a quieting effect on the mind and body.

LOW-PRESSURE EATING

Most people know the basics of a healthful diet—unsaturated fats, whole grains, low-fat dairy and at least five servings of fruits and vegetables daily. But there's more.

In the landmark Dietary Approaches to Stop Hypertension (DASH) study, 459 men and women with high blood pressure were divided into three groups—one group followed the typical American diet...one added more fruits and vegetables...and the third followed a diet designed specifically for the program.

The DASH diet contained four daily servings of fruits, four servings of vegetables, two to three servings of low-fat dairy foods and a moderate intake of fish, poultry and nuts, along with a decreased intake of saturated and total fats. Blood pressure dropped most significantly in the DASH group—by an average of 11.4 mm/Hg systolic and 5.5 mm/Hg diastolic.

Researchers are unsure why the DASH diet helps control blood pressure so effectively, but they speculate that it may be the potassium, calcium and magnesium that it contains...the antioxidant compounds...and/or the fiber.

Also, most people still are consuming too much salt. The usual recommendation for daily sodium intake is 2,400 mg (approximately one-half teaspoon of salt) or less, but most Americans consume 3,300 mg or more daily.

For the 50% of people who are salt sensitive (they experience an increase in their blood pressure after eating salty foods), even 2,400 mg daily is too high.

A later DASH study found that cutting sodium intake back to 1,500 mg daily reduced blood pressure by 12 mm/Hg systolic and 6 mm/Hg diastolic.

Surprisingly, only 15% of an average person's sodium intake comes from the salt shaker. Processed foods are the biggest source.

To detect sources of hidden sodium, it's crucial to read food labels. A snack should have no more than 200 mg per serving and a meal entrée no more than 500 mg. Less is even better.

Unexpected sodium sources...

•**Processed foods** labeled "healthy" or "lean." A serving may be low in calories, cholesterol and saturated fat but include up to half your daily sodium quota.

•**Packaged meats** and some soy-based meat substitutes.

•**Canned foods,** including beans, tomatoes and other vegetables as well as tuna (even if it's packed in water).

•**Breakfast cereals,** including some "heart-healthy," high-fiber or whole-grain varieties.

■ ■ ■ ■

Cola, Not Coffee, Raises Blood Pressure in Women

The association between hypertension and caffeine had been attributed to coffee, but a new study shows that caffeinated colas increase women's risk of hypertension. Researchers speculate that some other compound in soda is responsible for increased risk.

Wolfgang Winkelmayer, MD, department of pharmacoepidemiology and pharmacoeconomics, Brigham and Women's Hospital, Boston, and leader of an analysis of 12 years of data from 155,594 women, published in *The Journal of the American Medical Association.*

■ ■ ■ ■

Prehypertension Alert

Prehypertension—blood pressure of 120 to 139 mmHg/80 to 89 mmHg—usually is treated with lifestyle measures, such as weight loss, salt restriction and exercise.

Finding: In a study of 800 prehypertension patients, those who took the blood pressure medication *candesartan* (Atacand) for two years while making lifestyle changes had a

15.6% lower risk of developing hypertension than those who didn't take medication.

If your blood pressure is in the upper range of prehypertension: Ask your doctor about medication in addition to lifestyle changes.

Shawna D. Nesbitt, MD, associate professor of internal medicine, University of Texas Southwestern Medical Center, Dallas.

■ ■ ■ ■

Better Blood Pressure Reading

Systolic (the top number) blood pressure averaged 14 points higher when taken shortly after a patient arrived in the exam room and sat on an exam table than when he/she sat in a chair for five minutes.

Theory: Foot and back support induce a relaxed state, which helps allow for accurate blood pressure readings.

Self-defense: The next time you have your blood pressure taken, ask if you can sit in a chair with your back supported and feet flat on the floor for five minutes. Remain in this position (instead of sitting on an exam table) while the reading is taken.

Melanie F. Turner, RN, cardiology clinic practice nurse, University of Virginia Health System, Charlottesville.

■ ■ ■ ■

Skim Milk Helps

Skim milk lowers hypertension risk, according to Alvaro Alonso, MD, PhD.

Recent finding: A two-year study of 5,880 people found that those who consumed more than two to three servings of skim milk and other low-fat dairy products daily had half the risk of developing high blood pressure of those who rarely or never consumed such foods. Whole milk products were not found to reduce hypertension risk.

Theory: The calcium, which is highly absorbable in skim dairy products, may decrease blood pressure.

Alvaro Alonso, MD, PhD, assistant professor, division of epidemiology and community health, School of Public Health, University of Minnesota, Minneapolis.

Nobel Prize Winner's Secrets for a Healthy Heart

Louis J. Ignarro, PhD, the winner of the 1998 Nobel Prize in Physiology or Medicine, distinguished professor of pharmacology at the University of California, Los Angeles, David Geffen School of Medicine, and author of *NO More Heart Disease*. St. Martin's Press.

The 1998 Nobel Prize in Physiology or Medicine was awarded to Louis J. Ignarro, PhD, for ground-breaking research into nitric oxide (NO), a naturally occurring molecule in the body that may be the key to cardiovascular health. Dr. Ignarro's discovery has prompted every major pharmaceutical company to conduct research into the benefit of NO on heart and circulatory systems. *The results include...*

DRUGS FOR ERECTILE DYSFUNCTION

Viagra (*sildenafil citrate*) was the first drug to utilize the NO pathway. In the late 1980s, researchers at Pfizer who were testing a new angina (chest pain due to heart disease) drug realized that about 75 percent of male patients who took it reported more frequent and firmer erections. Pfizer quickly decided to market the drug for erectile dysfunction instead of angina.

TREATMENT FOR INFANTS' LUNGS

NO is now used in hospitals to treat persistent pulmonary hypertension—a form of hypertension that only affects blood vessels in the lungs—in newborns. In the past, newborns with this condition were unlikely to survive. NO gas, given via inhalation for one to five days, can *completely* reverse this condition.

A BETTER BETA-BLOCKER

A new drug Bystolic (*nebivolol*) developed in Europe—and first marketed in the US in late 2007—is the *first* beta-blocker that also elevates NO. Millions of Americans take beta-blockers (also called beta-adrenergic blocking agents), drugs for treating heart disease, hypertension and many other conditions. They cause the heart to beat more slowly and with less force, reducing blood pressure and improving circulation.

The drug is mainly used for hypertension and treating elderly patients with heart failure. Because it raises NO, it also reduces blood clots and arterial buildups that can lead to heart disease/heart attack. It's the *only* beta-blocker that produces these benefits.

HOW TO INCREASE YOUR NITRIC OXIDE LEVELS

Nitric oxide (NO) causes blood vessels to dilate, prevents blood clots, regulates blood pressure and may inhibit the accumulation of arterial plaque—the underlying cause of most heart attacks. It's possible that *most* cases of heart disease could be eliminated by elevating NO.

It isn't yet known how much NO is normally present in the body, or what levels are optimal. NO is difficult to measure because it's a gas that breaks down almost instantly with air exposure. Simpler tests will be needed before doctors can measure NO as a standard part of patient care.

It's thought that NO levels remain at normal levels until early adulthood, and then gradually decline.

Reason: Damage to the endothelial cells from factors such as lifetime exposure to high blood pressure, a high-fat diet, a sedentary lifestyle, arterial inflammation and oxidation from free radicals. Damage to the cells causes a reduction in NO.

Increasing NO is a critical component of heart-disease prevention.

The difficulty: Developing ways to administer it. Because it's an unstable gas that's destroyed by hemoglobin in the blood, it can't be taken as a drug/supplement. However, patients can take other supplements that increase production of NO in the blood vessels. Lifestyle changes, including not smoking, can cause levels to rise.

Important steps…

•**Take L-arginine.** It's an amino acid found in nuts, meats, grains, fish, etc. It passes through the intestine into the blood. From the blood it enters endothelial cells, where it's converted to NO. A Mayo Clinic study found that patients taking L-arginine had significant improvements in endothelial function and blood flow, compared to those taking placebos.

Recommended: 5,000 to 6,000 milligrams (mg) of arginine daily.

Eat nuts: A cup of peanuts contains about 5,000 milligrams of arginine. Fish and soy milk are also good sources. Or take arginine supplements—2,000 to 3,000 mg, twice daily.

•**Combine L-arginine with L-citrulline.** Supplemental arginine doesn't enter cells readily unless it's combined with L-citrulline, another amino acid. Melons are the richest food sources of L-citrulline, but don't provide high enough levels to significantly increase NO. Supplemental amounts are probably required.

Recommended dose: 200 to 1,000 mg, taken once daily.

•**Get more antioxidants.** We now believe that vitamin E and other antioxidant nutrients may *protect* NO by reducing its breakdown by free radicals. This might be the *main* reason that antioxidants promote cardiovascular health. *Helpful…*

•A daily multi that includes vitamin E. Don't take high-dose vitamin E supplements; recent studies suggest that patients taking daily doses of 400 IU or more may have *more* disease than those who don't supplement at these levels. The amount of vitamin E in most multi-vitamin-mineral supplements, usually about 50 IU, is well within the safety zone—and can promote NO production.

•500–1,000 mg vitamin C daily. Like vitamin E, it reduces oxidation in the blood vessels and may cause a rise in NO. A study in the journal *Circulation* that looked at 11,000 patients found that those who consumed high levels of vitamin C experienced less thickening of the carotid arteries. A reduction in arterial plaque is associated with higher NO levels.

•**Exercise at least 20 minutes three days a week.** It stimulates endothelial cells to *continuously* produce more NO, even on days you don't exercise.

•**Minimize saturated fat.** It contributes to the accumulation of arterial plaque and impairs NO production.

Better: Olive, canola or other vegetables oils, along with the omega-3 fatty acids found in fish and flaxseed. These fats help protect the endothelium by elevating levels of beneficial HDL cholesterol and lowering the harmful, LDL form.

•**Get more fiber.** The dietary fiber in grains, fruits and other plant foods lowers blood pressure and LDL cholesterol and raises HDL, thereby protecting endothelial cells.

Bonus: Many of the foods that contain fiber are also rich in antioxidants, which can protect NO.

Recommended amount: At least 25 g fiber daily. Patients who follow the government's dietary recommendations get at least this much.

•**Enjoy a glass of red wine.** It contains resveratrol, a powerful antioxidant that can delay the breakdown of NO. It's about *1,000 times* more potent than vitamin C.

If you don't drink wine: Have a daily glass of pomegranate or grape juice. They contain many of the same antioxidants as red wine.

■ ■ ■ ■

Better Treatment for Low Blood Pressure

Orthostatic hypotension occurs when blood pressure drops rapidly upon standing. It can result in dizziness, light-headedness or fainting.

Finding: Patients with orthostatic hypotension who took *pyridostigmine* (Mestinon), either alone or with *midodrine* (ProAmatine), another medication used to treat low blood pressure, had a smaller drop in standing blood pressure than when they took a placebo.

Bonus: Unlike midodrine, pyridostigmine did not increase blood pressure when patients were lying down. In rare cases, pyridostigmine can cause digestive upset and diarrhea.

Wolfgang Singer, MD, senior resident, department of neurology, Mayo Medical Center, Rochester, Minnesota.

■ ■ ■ ■

Achilles Warning

Pain in the Achilles tendon could indicate cholesterol problems. People with hereditary high cholesterol are seven times more likely to report Achilles tendon pain lasting three days or more than people without the condition.

Self-defense: If Achilles tendon pain persists, have your cholesterol tested.

Paul N. Durrington, PhD, professor, University of Manchester division of cardiovascular and endocrine science, Manchester, England.

You Don't Need Drugs to Control Your Cholesterol

Allan Magaziner, DO, a clinical instructor in the department of family practice at the Robert Wood Johnson University of Medicine and Dentistry in New Brunswick, New Jersey, and the medical director of the Magaziner Center for Wellness and Anti-Aging Medicine in Cherry Hill, New Jersey (*www.drmagaziner.com*). A past president of the American College for Advancement in Medicine, he is the author of *The All-Natural Cardio Cure.* Avery.

It's widely known that low cholesterol levels help prevent heart attack and stroke. But that's only part of the story. Levels of HDL "good" cholesterol must be high enough to carry harmful forms of cholesterol to the liver to be excreted.

Recent finding: Research has shown that decreasing LDL "bad" cholesterol by 40% and increasing HDL by 30% lowers the risk for heart attack or stroke by 70%—a much greater reduction of risk than occurs from lowering either total cholesterol or LDL levels.

The pharmaceutical industry has worked feverishly to develop a prescription medication that significantly increases HDL levels, to be used as a complement to cholesterol-lowering statins that focus primarily on lowering LDL levels.

Recent development: The new drug *torcetrapib* was pegged as a blockbuster that increases HDL levels by 60%—that is, until late-stage clinical trials showed that torcetrapib actually increased heart problems and death rates.

What you may not know: Therapeutic doses of niacin (vitamin B-3) effectively boost HDL levels—and lower LDL and total cholesterol.

THE "CHOLESTEROL VITAMIN"

Fifty years ago, Canadian scientists discovered that high doses of nicotinic acid—a form of niacin—could lower total cholesterol. In a 1975 study of men with heart disease, niacin was shown to reduce the rate of second heart attacks. Later, niacin was found to boost heart-protective HDL levels.

Although niacin alone cannot help everyone with abnormal cholesterol levels—often it is best used in combination with a statin—the vitamin is one of the most effective nondrug therapies available.

Ask your doctor about taking niacin if after trying cholesterol-lowering medication you have suffered side effects or your cholesterol levels have not improved within three months of getting a cholesterol test. Or consider trying niacin with the nondrug therapies described below.

How to use: Start with 100 mg of niacin daily and build up over one week to 500 mg a day. Every week, increase the dose by 500 mg until you reach 2,000 mg a day, taken in three divided doses, with meals. Be certain to use nicotinic acid, not niacinamide, a form of B vitamin that does not improve cholesterol levels. Consult your doctor before taking niacin.

The most common side effect of niacin is flushing—a warm, itchy, rash-like reddening of the face, neck and chest, which lasts about 10 minutes. Flushing is caused by niacin's ability to trigger vasodilation (widening of blood vessels).

To lessen this side effect, choose a form of niacin known as inositol hexanicotinate. It helps prevent the flush without reducing niacin's effectiveness.

Caution: Niacin should be avoided by people with a history of liver disease or stomach ulcers and used with caution by patients with diabetes and/or gallbladder disease. In addition, high-dose niacin (2,000 mg or more) may interact with certain medications, including alpha-blockers, such as *doxazosin* (Cardura), and the diabetes drug *metformin* (Glucophage).

OTHER NONDRUG THERAPIES

A diet that keeps sugar and processed food to an absolute minimum and emphasizes fruits and vegetables…whole grains…beans…fish…lean meats…and nuts and seeds can help lower LDL cholesterol and raise HDL levels. So can regular exercise, such as brisk walking, and losing excess weight.

Other nondrug approaches can lower total and LDL cholesterol and boost HDL. Combine the following nondrug therapies with niacin for maximum effectiveness…

•**Red yeast rice.** This Chinese medicine—a yeast that is grown on white rice, then fermented—contains monacolins, substances that act as naturally occurring statins. Research in China shows that red yeast rice can lower total cholesterol by 11% to 30%.

Typical use: Take 1,200 to 2,400 mg a day of red yeast rice, in two to four doses, with meals.

Not recommended: Policosanol—a supplement derived from cane sugar that also contains natural statins—has been widely promoted as effective for lowering cholesterol. However, several recent studies show that policosanol has no significant effect on cholesterol.

•**Fish oil and flaxseed.** Fish oil and flaxseed supply omega-3 fatty acids, which lower total cholesterol and LDL levels and raise HDL levels.

Typical dose: For fish oil, take supplements containing a total of 3 g daily of eicosapentaenoic acid (EPA) and docosahexaenoic acid (DHA). If you take a blood-thinning drug, such as aspirin or *warfarin* (Coumadin), check with your doctor before taking this dose of fish oil. Or use one to three teaspoons of ground flaxseed a day, sprinkled on food or mixed with water or juice. Flaxseed also can help relieve constipation and ease arthritis pain.

•**Soy.** Many studies show that soy can help lower total and LDL cholesterol.

Typical use: Try to get 20 g of soy protein a day—the equivalent of eight ounces of tofu…or one cup of edamame (soy) beans.

Important: Soy ice cream and other processed soy foods don't deliver enough soy to help reduce cholesterol.

Caution: If you have been diagnosed with a hormone-dependent cancer, such as some breast malignancies, or are at risk for such a condition, check with your doctor before adding soy to your diet.

•**Plant sterols.** These natural substances, which block the absorption of cholesterol in the intestines, are found in fruits, vegetables, beans, grains and other plants. Regular intake can reduce total cholesterol by 10% and LDL by 14%. Products with plant sterols (or a similar form, plant stanols) include spreads, salad dressings, snack bars and dietary supplements.

Typical use: Aim for 1 to 2 grams daily of plant sterols.

•**Walnuts.** A study published in the medical journal *Angiology* showed that people who ate a handful of walnuts daily for eight weeks had a 9% increase in HDL. Walnuts contain polyphenol antioxidants, which also inhibit oxidation of LDL cholesterol.

■ ■ ■ ■

Red Grapefruit Lowers Cholesterol

Red grapefruit lowers LDL (bad) cholesterol even in people who don't respond to statin drugs, such as Lescol and Lipitor.

Recent study: After eating one red grapefruit a day for four weeks, people whose cholesterol levels had failed to respond to statins lowered their LDL by 20%. People who ate white grapefruit did not benefit as much.

Caution: Chemicals in grapefruit can interfere with enzymes that break down certain drugs in your digestive system, such as Celebrex and Mevacor. Ask your doctor before changing your diet.

Shela Gorinstein, PhD, is chief scientist of medicinal chemistry and natural products, The Hebrew University of Jerusalem, Israel, and leader of a study of antioxidants, published in *Journal of Agricultural and Food Chemistry.*

Important! Do You Have This Leading Cause of Stroke?

Jonathan Halperin, MD, director of clinical cardiology at Mount Sinai Medical Center and a professor of medicine at Mount Sinai School of Medicine, both in New York City, is also a spokesman for the American Heart Association, *www.americanheart.org.*

Atrial fibrillation (AF) is a common type of arrhythmia (irregular heartbeat) affecting more than two million Americans. This figure includes up to 5% of people over age 65, many of whom may not know they have the disease. If untreated, AF significantly increases risk of stroke and other blood-clot-related ailments. Fifteen percent of all strokes occur in people with AF, and it's the leading cause of stroke in women over age 75.

Some good news: In recent years, doctors have learned a great deal about AF. If it's detected and treated promptly, AF-related strokes can usually be prevented.

WHAT IS ATRIAL FIBRILLATION?

The job of the two upper chambers of the heart (*atria*) is to pump blood into the lower chambers (*ventricles*), which in turn pump blood to the rest of the body. Normally, a regular electric pulse courses through the heart around 60 times per minute, triggering each heartbeat. But in AF, the atria beat several hundred times a minute, causing them to wiggle, or *fibrillate*, instead of contract in a regular heartbeat.

Unlike *ventricular fibrillation*—which can cause sudden death if not treated within minutes—atrial fibrillation is not immediately life threatening. But because it causes blood to stagnate in the atria, it sharply increases the risk that a blood clot could form there, then break off and lodge in the brain, causing a stroke, or in another organ or limb, blocking circulation.

With AF, increased electrical signals also reach the ventricles, causing them to beat more rapidly and less efficiently. This can lead to increased heart rate as well as reduced blood flow—which, in turn, may cause heart palpitations, dizziness, shortness of breath, fatigue or angina (chest pain).

These symptoms aren't always present, however, and when they are, they can vary from person to person. In some older individuals, for example, overall heart rate may not increase. Some people with AF have no symptoms at all.

Trap: Many other disorders, including other types of arrhythmias, can mimic the signs of AF.

DIAGNOSIS

While signs of AF may sometimes be detected by feeling the pulse or listening to the heart through a stethoscope, the only sure way to accurately diagnose AF is with an electrocardiogram (EKG), which will clearly show if any abnormal heart rhythm exists. In an EKG, electrodes are placed on the chest and body to record the heart's electrical impulses while the patient lies on an examination table. The test is quick and painless.

If someone has persistent AF (meaning the arrhythmia is occurring constantly), it can be uncovered by having an EKG. In the case of episodic AF (meaning the AF lasts for minutes or hours, then stops for a while before recurring), it may be necessary to wear a Holter monitor, which makes an EKG recording of the heartbeat for 24 hours, or use another type of heart monitor.

If an EKG reveals AF, then an echocardiogram (which uses sound waves, like a sonogram, to take a picture of the heart chambers) may also be done, either at the chest wall or, for more revealing pictures, via a tube inserted into the esophagus, to check for abnormalities of the valves as well as for blood clots.

TREATMENT

Treatment of AF involves several priorities…

•**Controlling the heart rate**—which can race up to 200 beats per minute during a bout of AF—is a doctor's first priority. This is done by administering one of several types of blocking agents that slow the transmission of electrical signals across the *A-V node* (connecting the atria and the ventricles), thus preventing too many signals from reaching the ventricles. Blocking agents include beta blockers, such as *propranolol* (Inderal), *metoprolol* (Toprol) and *atenolol* (Tenormin)…and calcium channel blockers, such as *verapamil* (Verelan) and *diltiazem* (Cardizem), which are preferred. If these are not effective enough or cause side effects, then the blocking agents *digoxin* (Lanoxin) or *amiodarone* (Cordarone) are used.

A Holter monitor—a portable device which continually records the EKG—is often employed to see how well a given medication works throughout the day. A patient may need to try several medications before finding the one that works best.

•**Administering blood-thinning medication** to reduce risk of a dangerous blood clot forming and to allow clots that have formed to dissolve. The standard medication in this case is *warfarin* (Coumadin), although patients deemed to be at low risk of dangerous blood clots (younger patients without heart disease) may be given aspirin instead. This treatment is the most important aspect of stroke prevention.

The anticoagulant may continue to be prescribed for months or years, if necessary.

•**Identifying and eliminating the underlying causes of AF.**

These might include: Excessive intake of alcohol and/or caffeine on a regular basis…use of a stimulant, such as a decongestant containing *pseudoephedrine*, or an illicit drug, such as cocaine…coronary artery disease…high blood pressure…a leaky mitral valve in the heart…hyperthyroidism…pericarditis…lung disease, such as emphysema or chronic obstructive pulmonary disease (COPD)…or congestive heart failure.

If the AF persists after such causes are addressed, as is the case in about 30% of patients, then an *antiarrhythmic drug*, such as *sotalol* (Betapace), *flecainide* (Tambocor) or *amiodarone* (Cordarone), may be prescribed. These drugs work by blocking ionic channels in the walls of the heart cells. (All heart cells have channels in their walls, through which ions travel back and forth, altering the electrical charge of the cell—including sodium channels, potassium channels and calcium channels.)

These drugs have a number of side effects, such as thyroid disturbances and lung damage.

Note: These drugs can interact dangerously with a number of other drugs, including warfarin (in which case the combo can cause excessive bleeding), tricyclic antidepressants and antipsychotic medications.

If the AF still isn't corrected, then more aggressive treatments may be tried…

•**Cardioversion,** in which an electrical shock is applied to the heart using paddles externally placed on the chest and back (similar to those used for ventricular fibrillation) to "reset" the heartbeat. This restores normal heart rhythms in many patients, but the success may not last. Anesthesia is administered before the procedure to minimize discomfort. The patient "jerks," but just for a moment.

•**Ablation therapy,** in which a catheter electrode is inserted into a vein and threaded into the heart, where a hole is poked in the wall connecting the right and left atria. Radio waves are then used to create a small burn in the heart lining. In many patients, this can eliminate AF altogether.

Newest ablation techniques have yielded success rates of more than 70% (keeping in mind that this procedure is done on carefully selected patients), though the long-term recurrence rate isn't yet clear.

■ ■ ■ ■

Bacteria Linked to Dangerous Heart Rhythm

Patients who have *atrial fibrillation* (AF)—rapid, irregular rhythm in the heart's upper chambers—are 20 times more likely than others to test positive for *Helicobacter pylori* bacteria.

Scientists now believe that H. pylori is the primary cause of most stomach and duodenal ulcers.

Self-defense: If you are diagnosed with AF, you should be checked for H. pylori. Controlling the infection using antibiotics reduces—or eliminates—the heart problem.

Annibale Sandro Montenero, MD, director, arrhythmia center, and chair of cardiology, MultiMedica General Hospital, Milan, Italy.

■ ■ ■ ■

Looking on the Bright Side May Save Lives

Pessimistic heart patients are almost twice as likely to die within six to 10 years as heart patients with an optimistic outlook.

Possible reason: Patients with positive expectations about the future may be more likely to make lifestyle changes and follow their doctors' treatment recommendations. Also, positive thoughts may lessen the damaging effects of stress on the body.

John C. Barefoot, PhD, professor of psychiatry, Duke University Medical Center, Durham, North Carolina, and leader of a study of 2,825 heart disease patients, presented at a recent meeting of the American Psychosomatic Society.

Latest Research: Half Of Angioplasties May Not Be Needed

Richard A. Stein, MD, director of preventive cardiology at Beth Israel Medical Center and professor of clinical medicine at the Albert Einstein College of Medicine, both in New York City. He is the author of *Outliving Heart Disease* (Newmarket) and a recipient of the National Institutes of Health's Preventive Cardiology Academic Award.

Most Americans who die each year from heart disease have *atherosclerosis*, fatty deposits (plaques) in the arteries that limit blood flow to the heart. Many cardiologists routinely recommend angioplasty (inflating a small balloon inside an artery), usually with stenting (inserting a wire mesh tube), to remove or flatten the plaques.

Recent research: *The New England Journal of Medicine* published a study that found that at the end of five years, angioplasty with stenting was no better than medication (such as cholesterol-lowering statins and beta-blockers to control heart rate), plus lifestyle modifications, for non-emergency heart patients. Based on these findings, some experts estimate that at least half of the 1.2 million angioplasties performed in the US each year may be unnecessary.

Surprising: The clots that cause most heart attacks usually form in areas with only minor plaques—not in the severely clogged areas that look so threatening on imaging tests. That's why preventing clots (by treating plaques) is actually preferable to restoring "normal" circulation to diseased arteries with an invasive procedure.

A BETTER APPROACH

Angioplasty with stenting as well as bypass surgery (grafting healthy veins from other parts of the body) can curb symptoms and prolong life when used appropriately (see "Surgical Options" below).

However, researchers have found that the incidence of heart attacks in some non-emergency patients could be reduced by as much as 70% by combining nonsurgical "medical management," such as that used to lower cholesterol and blood pressure, with changes in diet and other life-style factors. The steps required to achieve this level of risk reduction are easy to follow—the key is simply to do *all* of them.

People who smoke should most certainly give up cigarettes. It's also important to address stress and depression—taking care of how you feel is critical to taking care of your heart. Most people know by now to eat salmon or other cold-water fish. The Harvard Physicians' Health Study found that people who eat fish once or twice weekly have a significant reduction in the number of cardiovascular events, including heart attacks.

Anyone who is at risk for heart disease (due to family history, high blood pressure or diabetes, for example) or has a history of heart disease also should be aware that...

• **Statins do more than lower cholesterol.** This family of cholesterol-lowering drugs—*lovastatin* (Mevacor) and *simvastatin* (Zocor)—has revolutionized both the prevention and treatment of heart disease. These drugs can reduce heart attack risk by up to one-third...and they're just as effective for primary prevention (preventing a first heart attack) as for secondary prevention (preventing a heart attack in patients who already have had one).

Finding: Statins may reduce the size of arterial plaques. When LDL "bad" cholesterol is reduced to extremely low levels (below 70 mg/dL), plaques stop growing or even shrink. But this isn't the only benefit. Statins also prevent plaques from getting larger...convert plaques from *vulnerable* (likely to rupture and cause clots) to *stable* (less likely to rupture and cause clots)...and reduce damaging inflammation in the blood vessels.

Suggested: An LDL reading below 100 mg/dL in patients with heart disease...or 130 mg/dL or lower in patients without heart disease. Every patient with elevated LDL should ask his/her doctor if he should take a statin. (Red yeast rice, a dietary supplement that has the same active ingredient as statins, can be taken as an alternative.)

• **Not paying attention to HDL "good" cholesterol is dangerous.** Doctors tend to focus on reducing their patients' LDL levels because there are many treatment options—and each point reduction can reduce the heart attack risk by 1%. However, HDL cholesterol may be even more important. For every point *increase* in HDL, heart attack risk drops by 2% to 3%. HDL should be 40 mg/dL or higher in men...or 50 mg/dL or higher in women.

Suggested: Taken in high doses (more than 1.5 g daily), the B vitamin niacin can increase HDL levels by 50% or more. Unfortunately, niacin at these doses frequently causes side effects, mainly itching and/or facial flushing. A slow-release form, such as Niaspan, taken at bedtime, makes side effects less troublesome. Taking a baby aspirin one hour before taking niacin also reduces side effects.

Also helpful: Regular exercise can raise HDL by about 10%. People who stop smoking also will experience a slight increase in HDL.

• **The definition of high blood pressure has changed.** High blood pressure is one of the major risk factors for heart disease. Your blood pressure should be checked by your doctor at least once a year. If it is elevated—now defined as 120/80 mmHg or above, rather than 140/90 mmHg or above—a category now called prehypertension, work with your doctor to lower it through diet, exercise and/or medication.

• **Low-dose aspirin is all that is needed.** Aspirin reduces the risk for a first heart attack by about 20%, and the risk for a second by about 25%. In patients who also have high blood pressure, it can reduce the risk for a stroke by about 35%.

Suggested: A low-dose (81-mg) aspirin daily. Higher doses are no more effective in most patients and are more likely to cause stomach upset and/or bleeding. Aspirin therapy is not recommended for women age 65 or younger who don't have heart-disease symptoms, such as chest pain (angina) during exertion. In this group, the risk for bleeding outweighs the heart-protective benefits. Talk to your doctor before beginning daily aspirin therapy.

• **Fruits and vegetables are more powerful than most people realize.** Eating nine daily servings (one-half cup each) can reduce the risk for a heart attack by as much as 30%. Fruits and vegetables contain antioxidants, which curb inflammation, and fiber, which lowers cholesterol.

Best: A Mediterranean-style diet, which consists mainly of plant foods…moderate amounts of fish and poultry…and olive oil instead of butter or other saturated fats. People who follow this diet can reduce heart disease risk by 50% or more. For more information on the Mediterranean diet, go to *www.oldwayspt.org*, the Web site of the Oldways Preservation Trust, a non-profit food issues advocacy group.

•**Drinking wine really does help.** There's been so much talk about the heart-protective benefits of wine (red or white) that some people think it's hype. But it is true that small amounts of wine (five to 10 ounces daily for men…and five ounces daily for women) are good for the heart. Beer and spirits, in small amounts, also can be beneficial. People who drink moderately can reduce their risk for a first or second heart attack by 7% to 10%.

•**Burning calories is more important than the type of exercise you do.** Exercise increases blood flow through the coronary arteries. The rushing blood stimulates cells lining the blood vessels (endothelial cells) and makes them more resistant to plaque buildups.

The Harvard Alumni Study looked at exercise in terms of calories burned, rather than the type or duration of exercise. Men who burned 3,000 calories a week by performing moderate-intensity exercise had the lowest incidence of heart disease. (Women should aim to burn 2,500 calories weekly.) This can be achieved by walking briskly for about 45 to 60 minutes most days of the week.

SURGICAL OPTIONS

There are instances when angioplasty with stenting or bypass surgery is usually necessary. These include when a patient has severe blockages in all three coronary arteries…when the heart muscle is damaged (often due to a previous heart attack) and there are blockages in two coronary arteries…or when there's a blockage of more than 50% in the left main coronary artery.

In addition, these procedures can be lifesaving if a patient is in the early stages of a heart attack or has pre-heart attack symptoms, such as worsening chest pain and/or elevated levels of certain blood enzymes.

Are You Headed For a Stroke?

James F. Toole, MD, Walter C. Teagle Professor of Neurology and director of the Stroke Research Center at Wake Forest University Baptist Medical Center in Winston-Salem, North Carolina. He is past president of the International Stroke Society (now the World Stroke Organization).

What if people received warnings about coming strokes a week or even a month before they occurred? You might assume that such an alert would cause people to seek medical attention so that the patient and his/her doctor could take measures to prevent a stroke. Usually, that's not the case.

Each year, an estimated quarter-million Americans receive a warning in the form of a transient ischemic attack (TIA), commonly known as a "ministroke." Unfortunately, the majority of patients who experience a TIA don't recognize its importance—and fail to get prompt medical care that likely could prevent a full-blown stroke. About 11% to 20% of patients who experience a TIA go on to suffer a stroke within three months.

Good news: Patients who experience a TIA and then take preventive steps can greatly reduce their risk for further problems.

Important: A TIA is an *emergency*, and everyone should know the symptoms. If you experience one of the symptoms described below for at least five minutes, see a doctor the same day—go to the emergency room, if necessary.

KNOW THE SYMPTOMS

Like the majority of strokes, a TIA is usually caused by a blood clot and/or material that breaks free from artery walls and temporarily blocks blood flow to parts of the brain. The blockage of the artery lasts long enough to stop blood flow and cause stroke-like symptoms, but not long enough to kill brain cells.

What to watch for…

•**A dizzy spell that occurs for no obvious reason,** such as standing too quickly or dizziness from a middle ear disease.

•**Weakness and/or numbness on one side of the body**—usually in the face or an arm or leg.

•**The sensation that there's something in the eye,** causing blurriness, double vision or even temporary blindness.

•**Difficulty speaking or difficulty understanding what others are saying.**

People should *not* panic if they experience one or more of these symptoms—they aren't always caused by a TIA. Dizzy spells can be caused by something as simple as a plug of earwax. The only way to know for sure whether you've suffered a TIA is to see a doctor.

DIAGNOSING TIAs

Researchers are in the process of identifying brain enzymes that are released during a TIA. Blood tests that diagnose TIAs based on the presence of these enzymes are being developed.

In the meantime, doctors diagnose most TIAs by taking a medical history of the event—what the patient felt, how long the symptoms lasted and whether the person has stroke risk factors, such as high blood pressure, family history, diabetes or smoking.

Physical findings: Atherosclerosis (hardening of the arteries) is the underlying cause of most TIAs (and the majority of strokes). Patients who have atherosclerosis elsewhere in the body, such as in the arteries leading to the legs, kidneys, heart, etc., are very likely to also have damaged carotid arteries—blood vessels in the neck that carry blood to the brain.

In some cases, a doctor can detect problems in the carotid artery by listening carefully with a stethoscope. There are characteristic sounds (bruits) that indicate atherosclerosis.

In other cases, additional tests are required...

•**Carotid ultrasonography** uses sound waves to detect blood-vessel narrowing and/or clots in the carotid arteries. This is a good screening test for people with stroke risk factors or a family history of strokes or TIAs.

•**Magnetic resonance imaging (MRI)** also measures blockages in the carotid arteries.

If atherosclerotic blockages of 50% to 70% are found from either test, further evaluation and treatment is necessary.

TREATMENT APPROACHES

Patients with carotid artery blockages of 50% or more are usually advised to take strict steps, including the use of medication, to reduce risk.

If their disease progresses to 70% blockage, surgery is typically recommended...

Carotid endarterectomy is an in-patient procedure in which an incision is made to expose the carotid artery, and plaques are removed from the artery. When performed by a skilled surgeon, the risk for stroke or death is less than 1%, and the patient recovers within a week.

Stenting is an inpatient procedure in which an expandable metal net is threaded into the carotid artery. The net presses against the artery walls...dilates the opening for better circulation...and helps prevent the artery from "shedding" more clots.

Stenting, however, has not been performed long enough for its long-term effectiveness and durability to be known. One possible risk is that a dislodged blood clot could get carried in the bloodstream to the brain.

TIA patients who don't require surgery are almost always treated with drugs to prevent blood from clotting. *Main drug therapies...*

Aspirin is most often used. Taking a regular aspirin (three times weekly) or baby aspirin (daily), depending on the patient, can reduce stroke risk by up to 20%.

Adding other active anticlotting ingredients to aspirin can reduce stroke risk by an additional 3% to 5%.

Example: Aspirin plus the antiplatelet drug *dipyridamole* (Aggrenox) may be beneficial.

Aspirin alternatives, such as *clopidogrel* (Plavix) and *ticlopidine* (Ticlid), can prevent excessively sticky platelets from clumping together and forming clots. These drugs are a good choice for patients who are allergic to aspirin or who have an ulcer or acid reflux disease, which can be aggravated by aspirin.

■ **More from James F. Toole, MD...**

Stroke Prevention

Most stroke risk factors can be reduced with lifestyle modifications. *Most important...*

•**Not smoking.**
•**Limiting dietary fat.**
•**Eating fruits and vegetables.**
•**Exercising regularly.**

Patients who maintain healthy blood pressure readings (less than 120/80) and total cholesterol levels (less than 200)...avoid (or reverse) obesity...and control underlying diseases, such as diabetes, are far less likely to develop hardening of the arteries, thereby reducing their risk for TIAs and stroke.

Yes, You Can Bounce Back After a Stroke

Cathy Sila, MD, is associate medical director of the cerebrovascular center at The Cleveland Clinic in Cleveland.

If you suffer a stroke, one of the most common—and devastating—mistakes is failing to seek treatment fast enough. When blood supply to the brain is cut off by a clot (ischemic stroke) or there is bleeding in or around the brain (hemorrhagic stroke), damage starts within minutes. Getting help right away could save your life—or profoundly improve your recovery.

IS IT A STROKE?

The onset of stroke symptoms is sudden and consists of episodes of neurological dysfunction. Transient ischemic attacks, or TIAs, are stroke warning symptoms that usually last 15 minutes to several hours and are not associated with permanent damage. About 10% of patients who suffer a TIA go on to have a stroke within the next three months. If you think that you may be having a stroke, call 911. Studies have shown that treatment may be delayed if you first call your doctor or hospital. While waiting for emergency help, lie down in a comfortable position that allows you to breathe freely.

Caution: It is not recommended that you take aspirin for a suspected stroke. While its clot-fighting ability may help if you are having an ischemic stroke (or heart attack), it could make things worse if you are having a hemorrhagic stroke.

THE RIGHT DIAGNOSIS

At the hospital, brain imaging is one of the first tests performed to help diagnose a stroke and determine its type. Usually, this is done with a standard computed tomography (CT) scan. This painless, noninvasive test takes multiple detailed images of the brain.

A hemorrhagic stroke is easy to identify on a CT scan. That's because blood, which pools in or around the brain during a hemorrhagic stroke, appears different from brain tissue. With an ischemic stroke, the brain can appear normal on a CT scan if swelling or damage has not yet occurred. In this case, the scan rules out other causes, and ischemic stroke is diagnosed by a clinical history and exam. A follow-up CT scan is performed a few days later to confirm the diagnosis.

ISCHEMIC STROKE

During the period immediately following an ischemic stroke, medication may be needed to stabilize blood pressure and heart rate. If the stroke sufferer has a fever, it is treated with acetaminophen (Tylenol) or a cooling blanket—even a slight fever can worsen brain damage. *Other treatments...*

•**Medication.** The clot-dissolving drug *alteplase* (Activase) is the most effective emergency treatment for ischemic stroke. Also known as a *tissue plasminogen activator*, or tPA, the drug works with the body's own chemicals to dissolve the clot that is blocking circulation to the brain. To be effective, tPA must be given within three hours of the first stroke symptoms. TPA also has risks. As a potent "clot buster," it can cause bleeding. About 6% of patients who receive it develop bleeding into the stroke-damaged area of the brain, which can be fatal.

Latest development: Administering clot-busting drugs via an intra-arterial route through a catheter threaded up to the blocked artery itself may extend the treatment window to six hours. This approach requires special imaging, such as angiography, to pinpoint the blockage and can be performed only at centers with such equipment and personnel trained in the technique. Although studies have shown this technique to be effective for some patients, the bleeding risk is higher (10% to 12%) than standard tPA.

•**Surgery.** After a TIA or minor stroke due to blockage of the carotid (neck) artery, other options include clearing the carotid artery to prevent another stroke. This can be performed with *carotid endarterectomy* (cutting open a blocked artery and removing the clot to restore circulation) or with *angioplasty* and *stenting* (inserting a balloon via a catheter, expanding it at the site of the clot to widen the blood vessel, and inserting a wire mesh framework to keep the artery open).

Latest development: Another new approach uses a corkscrew-shaped device called the MERCI (*mechanical embolus removal in cerebral ischemia*) Retriever. It is approved by the FDA for removing clots from brain arteries, which are causing an acute stroke. The device looks promising, but it has not been definitively shown to improve the outcomes of patients and also carries a risk of bleeding into the brain.

HEMORRHAGIC STROKE

Hemorrhagic stroke treatment first focuses on stabilizing the patient—using a ventilator, if necessary, to restore breathing and treating life-threatening heart problems caused by the stroke, such as disturbances in heart rhythm (fibrillation). *Other treatments...*

•**Medication.** Blood pressure must be brought down quickly to prevent additional bleeding in other parts of the brain. Blood pressure medications often are administered intravenously for rapid effect.

Bleeding in the space between the inner layer and the middle layer of the tissue covering the brain (subarachnoid hemorrhage) is usually caused by a ruptured aneurysm—a burst bubble in a brain artery. Your doctor may prescribe *nimodipine* (Nimotop), a calcium channel blocker that prevents arteries from going into spasm and causing more damage. After the first hemorrhage, rebleeding can occur unless corrective steps are taken.

•**Surgery.** The standard treatment for brain aneurysm is *clipping*—a surgical procedure that involves opening the skull and placing a small clip at the base of the aneurysm to close it off from blood flow. It is the preferred form of treatment for aneurysms in certain areas of the brain, particularly in medically stable patients.

Latest development: For aneurysm patients who are not medically stable, a new technique known as coiling may be the best form of treatment. With coiling, a catheter is guided up through a blood vessel to place a collection of tiny platinum coils in the aneurysm, which causes

a clot to form within the aneurysm. The procedure is less invasive and safer than clipping, but some aneurysms cannot be completely treated with this technique. The risks of both procedures include rebleeding from the aneurysm.

ONGOING CARE

Perhaps the most frustrating aspect of stroke recovery is waiting to determine the extent of brain damage. During this time, an antidepressant may be needed if there are signs of depression.

For most stroke survivors, physical and/or occupational therapy over a period of months—or indefinitely—is essential to optimize functions, such as speech and the physical capacities that were impaired by brain damage.

Latest development: Nutrition has only recently been fully recognized for stroke sufferers. In a 2005 update, the American Stroke Association recommends assessing and correcting nutritional problems, such as malnutrition, in stroke sufferers.

Turn Around Carotid Artery Disease Before It Causes a Stroke

Claudette Brooks, MD, a neurologist at the West Virginia University Medical Center, Morgantown, is a spokesperson for the American Stroke Association.

Most people know about coronary artery disease, in which plaque builds up in the arteries feeding the heart, reducing blood flow and increasing heart attack risk. But plaque can also build up in the carotid arteries—the large arteries on both sides of the neck that carry blood to the front and middle part of the brain. This carotid artery disease significantly increases stroke risk if not treated.

Carotid artery disease has the same causes as coronary artery disease—blood cholesterol adheres to the walls of the artery over time, forming plaque deposits. These deposits can cause a stroke if a piece of plaque breaks off and gets lodged in a smaller brain artery, blocking blood flow...or the plaque cracks or becomes roughened, triggering a blood clot that blocks blood flow to the brain…or the carotid artery becomes so narrowed by plaque that the blockage itself prevents sufficient blood from getting to the brain.

WHO IS AT RISK?

Risk factors for carotid artery disease include smoking, high cholesterol, high blood pressure, diabetes, obesity, physical inactivity, previously diagnosed coronary artery disease and a family history of coronary or carotid artery disease. Age is also a risk factor. Only one out of every 200 people between age 50 and 59 has significantly narrowed carotid arteries, but this rate climbs exponentially in each decade after 65. Of those age 60 to 79, one out of 100 people has blockage. Among those age 80 to 89, one out of 10 has significant carotid artery blockage of 50% or greater.

EARLY WARNING SIGN

Most people with early-stage carotid artery disease don't realize it.

Reason: Arteries with blockages of 60% or less usually produce no symptoms. For many, the first sign that they have carotid artery disease is a transient ischemic attack (TIA). TIAs may occur when a small piece of plaque breaks off or a small plaque-related blood clot forms, temporarily reducing blood flow to the brain. These attacks typically last only a few minutes and cause no permanent damage.

Symptoms include loss of sight in one or both eyes…weakness, numbness or tingling on one side of the body…loss of coordination…dizziness or confusion…slurred speech…difficulty swallowing.

If you experience any of these TIA symptoms, seek medical attention immediately. Someone who has had a TIA is 10 times more likely to have a stroke than someone who hasn't. Even if you haven't experienced symptoms, you should be examined for possible carotid artery blockage if you have any of the above risk factors—particularly if you're older than age 45.

DIAGNOSIS

•**Stethoscope exam.** The first step in this examination, which your internist can perform, is to listen with a stethoscope to the flow of blood through each carotid artery. If the doctor hears a *bruit*—a rushing sound that indicates turbulent blood flow through the artery—then it's possible that you have carotid artery blockage. The absence of bruit does not rule out carotid artery blockage, however.

•**Carotid duplex ultrasound.** If your doctor suspects carotid artery blockage because you have heart disease, high cholesterol, high blood pressure and/or diabetes, the next step is a carotid ultrasound exam. In this test, an ultrasound image of the blood flow through the carotid artery is examined to determine whether there are blockages or other structural abnormalities. The exam is noninvasive and painless.

•**Catheter angiography and CT/MRI angiography.** If an ultrasound indicates carotid artery blockage, one of several follow-up tests is typically done to get a still-better picture of the blockage. In a *catheter angiogram*, a special dye is injected into the blood vessels of the head and neck through a catheter, and the carotid arteries are then X-rayed. In a *CT angiogram* or an *MRI angiogram*, the carotid arteries are studied using a CT or MRI scan. In all three tests, both carotid arteries are typically scanned, along with the two vertebral arteries in the back of the head that supply the rear brain.

Reason: 20% of people with carotid artery disease also have blockages in the vertebral arteries. While these tests are more invasive than ultrasound and therefore carry some risk, they give a more in-depth picture of the blockages.

Note: Catheter angiogram is considered the gold standard for accuracy and gives the clearest picture—it also has the most risk.

TREATMENT

If the carotid artery disease is asymptomatic —which is usually the case when the artery blockage is 60% or less—the first line of treatment involves controlling the underlying risk factors, including…

•**Bringing LDL cholesterol down** through a low-fat diet and cholesterol-lowering medications.

•**Controlling high blood pressure** with a low-sodium diet and antihypertensive medications.

•**Keeping blood sugar under tight control,** if you have diabetes.

•**Quitting smoking.**

•**Losing weight,** if you are overweight.

•**Getting 30 minutes or more of daily physical activity** such as walking, cycling and swimming.

Also, one or more antiplatelet medications may be prescribed to reduce the risk of dangerous blood clots—including aspirin, *dipyridamole* (Persantine), *clopidogrel* (Plavix) and *ticlopidine* (Ticlid).

SURGERY

Surgery to reduce asymptomatic carotid artery blockage is usually only recommended if the blockage exceeds 70%.

Reason: Studies have shown that for lesser blockages, risks of surgical complications (reaction to anesthesia or mid-operation stroke or heart attack) outweigh stroke prevention benefits. The main causes of mid-operation stroke or heart attack are emboli (air bubbles or particles of plaque or blood clot in the blood). The risk of serious complications is 2.3%.

The most common operation is a carotid endarterectomy, in which an incision is made in the neck at the point of the blockage—the plaque and, if necessary, the diseased artery walls are surgically removed. A shunt (tube) is used to route blood around the area being worked on. If artery tissue is removed, a length of artery is taken from the leg and grafted onto the carotid artery (similar to what's done in coronary bypass surgery). It usually involves a hospital stay of two to four days. After carotid surgery for patients with asymptomatic blockage of greater than 70%, there is a 40% reduction in risk of stroke over five years. However, other risk factors must still be treated since atherosclerosis and narrowing can return.

How to Prevent a Stroke

Patrick Lyden, MD, professor of neurosciences and director of the Stroke Center at University of California, San Diego, is chief of the Stroke Clinic at the San Diego VA Medical Center.

A stroke occurs when blood supply to a part of the brain is interrupted. Without oxygen and nutrients, brain cells die within minutes, damaging areas that control movement, speech—and even involuntary activities, such as breathing.

Stroke is the most *preventable* cause of death and disability in the US. Yet more than 750,000 Americans suffer strokes each year…about 160,000 of these people die…and 200,000 live with lasting disability. What are we doing wrong?

You can't change some risk factors, such as family history. If you have a parent or sibling who has suffered a stroke, you are at greater risk yourself.

Your age also plays a role. While strokes can occur even in young children, overall risk steadily increases as we grow older. That's why more than two-thirds of strokes occur in people over age 65.

Beyond these factors, whether we suffer a stroke is largely up to us.

STROKE PREVENTION

What most affects stroke risk…

•**Smoking.** Everyone knows that smoking increases heart disease risk, but did you know that smoking is actually more likely to cause a stroke than a heart attack? Not only does smoking promote the development of fatty deposits that narrow arteries (atherosclerosis), but the nicotine in tobacco causes blood vessels in the brain to constrict.

Result: Smokers have up to four times the stroke risk of nonsmokers.

What you can do: Quit smoking. If you've tried but can't kick the habit, consider using nicotine-replacement patches or gum.

•**Blood pressure.** High blood pressure gradually damages blood vessels and substantially increases the risk for both ischemic and hemorrhagic strokes. The risk is greater because high blood pressure rarely causes symptoms, so the problem goes unrecognized in 30% of sufferers.

What you can do: If your blood pressure exceeds 120/80, take steps to reduce it. Weight loss and exercise may be enough, but you also may need medication, such as diuretics or beta blockers.

•**Cholesterol.** For stroke prevention, maintain the same cholesterol levels that are recommended to reduce heart disease risk—total cholesterol under 200...LDL "bad" cholesterol under 100...HDL "good" cholesterol above 40.

What you can do: Weight loss and exercise help control cholesterol levels. If these strategies are insufficient, cholesterol-lowering medication may be needed.

•**Diabetes.** Maintaining tight control of blood sugar (glucose) will minimize small blood vessel damage that can lead to stroke.

What you can do: Work with your doctor to create a treatment plan that keeps your hemoglobin A1C (blood sugar over time) level at less than seven.

•**Diet.** Stroke risk, like heart disease risk, can be related to diet.

What you can do: Maintain a diet that's low in saturated fats (no more than 30% of total fats per day) and high in fruits and vegetables (five to nine one-half cup servings per day).

Research shows that people who are deficient in potassium are 1.5 to 2.5 times more likely to suffer a stroke. Aim for the government's recommended potassium intake of 4,700 mg daily. Although bananas are a popular source of potassium (one medium banana contains 457 mg of potassium), cantaloupe can be an even richer source (one cup of cantaloupe balls contains about 547 mg).

If you determine that sodium raises your blood pressure, limit your daily sodium intake to 2.4 g (slightly more than one teaspoon of salt).

•**Exercise.** Physical activity reduces risk for heart disease, diabetes and hypertension—and may offer stroke protection as well.

What you can do: Work with your doctor to create an exercise program based on your history of heart disease, smoking, etc.

•**Daily aspirin.** Aspirin reduces the tendency of platelets to clump, which helps prevent blood clots that can lead to ischemic stroke.

What you can do: If you're over age 55 and have diabetes, high cholesterol or other stroke risk factors, ask your doctor about starting daily low-dose (81-mg) aspirin therapy.

In patients who have never had a stroke or heart attack, and who do not have hypertension, diabetes or elevated cholesterol, the risk of hemorrhage may outweigh the potential benefits of aspirin.

•**Alcohol.** Moderate drinking has been shown to benefit the heart, but it does not curb stroke risk.

What you can do: Men should limit alcohol intake to two drinks per day...one drink per day for women. A drink is defined as 1.5 ounces of hard liquor, 4 ounces of wine or 12 ounces of beer. Risk for hemorrhagic stroke jumps substantially if you exceed this amount.

OTHER RISK FACTORS

Some medical conditions significantly raise your stroke risk...

•**Atrial fibrillation.** About 2.2 million Americans are affected by atrial fibrillation (AF), a heart rhythm disturbance that increases stroke risk five- to sixfold.

AF can cause dizziness, shortness of breath and constriction or other uncomfortable sensations in the chest. Or it may cause no symptoms and be found during a routine examination or when you have an electrocardiogram.

What you can do: Taking a blood-thinning drug, such as *warfarin* (Coumadin), can virtually eliminate AF's added stroke risk by preventing the formation of blood clots. Aspirin may be nearly as effective.

•**Transient ischemic attack (TIA).** If you have had one or more of these brief stroke-like episodes, your risk for a full-blown stroke increases dramatically. A TIA can cause dizziness, numbness or paralysis on one side of the body, difficulty speaking, double vision or other stroke symptoms that disappear after minutes or hours.

What you can do: After a TIA, ask your doctor about taking antiplatelet medication, such as aspirin, *clopidogrel* (Plavix) or *dipyridamole* and aspirin (Aggrenox).

•**Carotid stenosis.** When fatty deposits accumulate in the carotid artery, which carries blood up through the neck, they can impede brain circulation enough to cause a stroke. Up to half of all ischemic strokes are associated with carotid stenosis.

What you can do: If you have had a stroke or TIA, get an ultrasound of your carotid artery. If blockage is 70% or more, ask your doctor about surgery.

■ ■ ■ ■

Stroke Signs ER Doctors Miss

Strokes affecting the right side of the brain are not always accurately diagnosed by emergency room doctors soon enough—even though these strokes are as common as those that affect the left side of the brain.

Reason: Right-sided stroke symptoms—such as vision problems, memory loss, skipping food on the left side of the plate—often are overlooked by the patient and don't appear critical to family members and doctors.

Result: Patients get to the hospital later and often don't get the treatment they need.

Self-defense: If you or a loved one experiences any stroke symptoms, seek immediate care.

Vladimir Hachinski, MD, Hon. Dr. Med, University of Western Canada, London, Ontario, and part of a study of emergency care given to more than 750 right-brain stroke victims, published in *Neurology.*

Leg Pain: A Risk for Stroke and Heart Attack

Jonathan L. Halperin, MD, professor of medicine and director of clinical cardiology services at Mount Sinai School of Medicine in New York City, was a member of the writing committee that produced the American College of Cardiology/American Heart Association *Guidelines for the Management of Patients with Peripheral Arterial Disease.*

When most people hear about the condition atherosclerosis, they think of heart attack and stroke. But the same disease process (plaque buildup in the arteries) also can impair circulation in internal organs, such as the brain, heart and kidneys. When it happens in the legs, the result is a potentially life-threatening condition known as peripheral arterial disease (PAD). Unfortunately, it often goes undiagnosed and untreated, largely because symptoms seldom occur until the affected artery is more than 70% narrowed.

New development: The American College of Cardiology and the American Heart Association

have just released guidelines to help doctors identify PAD and treat it effectively.

Here's what you need to know about this often overlooked condition...

ARE YOU AT RISK?

More than 8 million Americans have symptomatic PAD, and it is estimated that 16 million have PAD with no symptoms. The most common form of PAD affects the legs. Known as lower extremity PAD, the risk factors for this condition are the same as those for coronary heart disease—high cholesterol (over 200 mg/dL)...high blood pressure (over 140/90)...and advancing age (over age 50). Smoking and diabetes significantly increase risk for the disorder.

You should be screened for lower extremity PAD during your regular physical if you are...

•**Over age 70.**

•**Over age 50 and have a history of diabetes or smoking.**

•**Under age 50 and have diabetes and one other atherosclerosis risk factor,** such as high cholesterol or hypertension.

The *ankle-brachial index* (ABI) is used to identify the disorder. To determine your ABI, your doctor takes your blood pressure on your upper arm—and at your ankle. The second systolic (top) reading should be divided by the first systolic reading. A ratio of less than 0.9 or greater than 1.65 is abnormal and is associated with a higher risk for PAD.

A less accurate way to test for lower extremity PAD is to use a stethoscope to listen to the pulse at various points on the legs—for example, the thigh, the knee and the back of the foot—to see whether the pulse is weak at any of those places or there are unusual sounds, such as a *bruit* (a murmur), that suggest blood flow is disrupted. If your doctor performs this test only, ask for the ABI.

SYMPTOMS TO WATCH FOR

The classic symptom of lower extremity PAD is *intermittent claudication.* This condition causes aching pain and/or fatigue, and sometimes burning, in the calf of one or both legs when you walk. The pain subsides when you stop.

The pain also may be in the thigh or the front of the foot. Some people say, "It doesn't exactly hurt. I just need to stop walking." In all these cases, it's crucial to see a doctor.

If you are suffering from this type of leg pain and your doctor determines that your ABI is normal, you'll need additional tests that are often performed at a vascular lab. In these tests, blood pressure in the toe is measured and/or the arteries in the abdomen are examined using an ultrasound.

If either test result is abnormal, an aggressive program to reduce risk factors for heart attack and stroke, including cholesterol-lowering medication, diet and exercise, is recommended. Your doctor also may suggest a cardiovascular evaluation, perhaps with stress testing and/or an ultrasound examination of the neck (carotid) arteries that feed the brain.

TREATING YOUR ARTERIES

If blockage is beginning to occur in your leg arteries, chances are the same thing is happening elsewhere in your body. This means that your risk for heart attack and stroke is high, and you need to act promptly to curb it—by stopping smoking, treating diabetes and/or controlling blood pressure and cholesterol levels.

Important: If you have lower extremity PAD, you should follow the same guidelines for cholesterol, blood pressure, etc., as those for people with coronary heart disease.

Example: Maintain LDL "bad" cholesterol at no more than 100 mg/dL (or 70 mg/dL if your doctor feels you are at particularly high risk), using a cholesterol-lowering statin drug to do so, if necessary.

Like someone with coronary heart disease, you may need an antiplatelet drug, such as a daily low-dose (81-mg) aspirin, to prevent tiny clots from blocking circulation.

Your doctor also may recommend an ACE inhibitor, such as *enalapril* (Vasotec) or *ramipril* (Altace). These drugs are commonly prescribed for high blood pressure but have been shown to reduce heart attack risk as well.

If you also have diabetes, good foot care—including thorough cleansing and daily inspection for cuts and infections—is especially important because poor circulation impairs healing.

REDUCING THE PAIN

When leg pain due to intermittent claudication is severe enough to cause you distress or interfere with your activities, there are ways to ease the pain.

Best options include...

•**Exercise.** A supervised exercise program (usually in a rehabilitation center) is the first step. Potential benefits of this approach, such as increasing the distance you can walk without pain, are greater than those offered by any medication. Exercise improves circulation and trains muscles to use oxygen more efficiently.

The best strategy is to walk until pain becomes moderately severe, rest until symptoms go away, then walk some more. For maximum improvement, sessions should be three times a week and last longer than 30 minutes each. The supervised program should last for six months. Afterward, exercise should be continued from home.

•**Medication.** If exercise alone isn't enough, or if you'd prefer another approach, the prescription drug *cilostazol* (Pletal) has been shown to improve circulation in the legs and can increase walking distance by 40% to 60% after three to six months of treatment. Don't use cilostazol if you have congestive heart failure—a class of drugs chemically related to cilostazol was found to increase mortality in heart failure patients. The drug *pentoxifylline* (Trental) can be taken instead, though it is much less effective.

SURGICAL OPTIONS

Arterial blockage in the legs also can be treated with procedures similar to those that are used to improve coronary circulation.

Your doctor is likely to suggest one of these procedures when exercise and medication haven't relieved symptoms sufficiently, or when tests show that the blockage occurs in a location where bypass or angioplasty is likely to be particularly effective—for example, in the abdominal artery that feeds the leg.

•**Angioplasty.** During this procedure, a catheter is inserted into the affected artery, and a balloon is inflated to open the artery. A wire mesh tube called a stent may then be inserted to keep the artery open.

•**Bypass surgery.** This operation involves reconstruction of blocked arteries with grafts taken from blood vessels elsewhere in the body or made from artificial materials, such as Gortex or Dacron.

Angioplasty or bypass is almost always necessary when the blockage has advanced enough to threaten the loss of part or all of the leg—a condition known as *critical limb ischemia* (CLI).

Important: CLI requires urgent care. See your doctor immediately if you start having leg pain even when at rest—or if you develop ulcers on your leg or foot.

The Only Aspirin Dose That Actually Prevents Stroke

Mark Alberts, MD, director, stroke program, Northwestern Memorial Hospital, Chicago.
Marshall Keilson, MD, director of neurology, Maimonides Medical Center, Brooklyn, New York.
American Stroke Association conference, Phoenix.

Baby aspirin and coated aspirin might not be sufficient to prevent strokes, according to research performed at several major stroke centers.

People at risk for a stroke who take baby aspirin (81 milligrams [mg]) were less likely to reap its blood-thinning benefits than those taking an adult-sized pill. The same was true of those who took coated aspirin compared with the uncoated kind, say researchers.

This research could have major implications because it could lead to aspirin as a dose-adjusted medication, says Dr. Mark Alberts, lead author of the study and director of the stroke program at Northwestern Memorial Hospital in Chicago. Instead of a one-size-fits-all approach, he says, doctors would measure the effect of the dose and see if the patient needs a different dose.

THE ACCEPTED DOSE

Right now, doctors believe that 50 to 325 mg of aspirin may help prevent ischemic stroke, says Dr. Marshall Keilson, director of neurology

at Maimonides Medical Center in Brooklyn, New York. *Ischemic* strokes are the most common type of stroke and occur when blood flow in an artery to the brain is pinched off, usually because of clotting. Aspirin thins the blood and prevents clots from forming.

Keilson says doctors use low doses of aspirin because they feel it reduces such complications as gastrointestinal upset and bleeding.

Many patients taking aspirin are still having strokes and, for that matter, heart attacks (aspirin is also thought to prevent some heart attacks). "Those episodes are indicating that the low doses that are commonly being used—around 81 mg—may not be adequate for stroke prevention," Keilson says.

In his study, Alberts and his coauthors measured how effective different doses and formulations of aspirin were at thinning blood in patients who had cerebrovascular disease.

WHAT WORKS BEST

More than half of the patients taking 81 mg a day did not have an anticlotting effect. Of those taking coated aspirin, more than 60% did not have an anticlotting effect. But only 28% of the people taking 325 mg of uncoated aspirin did not have an anticlotting effect. In other words, higher doses and uncoated formulations seemed to work better. But, there's a long way to go before these early results become routinely recommended.

The study measured only thinning of the blood, and not whether a person had another stroke. "We want to see if this is predictive of clinical results, which is the holy grail of research," Alberts says.

Keilson agrees. "Sometimes things that are done in a laboratory don't carry over in people," he says, adding that a large trial with thousands of patients is needed.

For more on the different types of stroke, visit the National Stroke Association at *www.stroke. org*. The association also has information on current guidelines for the use of aspirin in preventing strokes and heart attack.

How to Tell If Someone Is Having a Stroke

Amy Hurwitz, University of North Carolina at Chapel Hill School of Medicine.

Robert Felberg, MD, medical director, Stroke Center, Ochsner Clinic Foundation Hospital, New Orleans.

American Stroke Association conference, Phoenix.

Can you tell if someone is having a stroke? Yes, say researchers. The odds are good that you can, even for a complete stranger, if you know how to spot the symptoms.

Even though treating stroke patients requires extensive training, people without training can easily learn to detect stroke symptoms, says study author Amy Hurwitz, then a medical student at the University of North Carolina at Chapel Hill School of Medicine.

SPEED IS ESSENTIAL

A quick diagnosis is vital because a treatment is available for strokes caused by blood clots, but it only works if it's given within three hours of the onset of symptoms.

"Even a delay of 20 minutes can make a huge difference," says Dr. Robert Felberg, medical director of the stroke program at Ochsner Clinic Foundation Hospital in New Orleans.

He says that, ideally, you should get to the hospital within the first hour after symptoms appear, because doctors need time to make the diagnosis and run a computed tomography (CT) scan to confirm it before they can safely give the clot-busting stroke medication.

TESTING THE THEORY

For this study, the researchers chose 100 random visitors to the hospital and put them in a room in the emergency department where a stroke survivor and one of the researchers were waiting for him/her.

The stroke survivors still had visible symptoms, such as arm weakness, facial weakness or slurred speech.

The visitor learned how to give a three-item exam used by doctors to assess stroke victims.

1. See if the patient's smile is symmetrical.

2. Can the patient keep both arms raised?

3. Ask the patient to speak a standard phrase.

The volunteers were then asked to decide if the patient had performed normally or abnormally on the tests.

The visitors correctly gave the test nearly all of the time.

In patients with facial weakness, they correctly identified that symptom approximately 70% of the time, arm weakness was correct in nearly all of the patients and speech problems were found nearly 90% of the time.

"The biggest problem we have is that 75% of the American population doesn't know what a stroke is," Felberg says.

■ ■ ■ ■

Stroke Patients Recover Faster With Hot/Cold Therapy

Thermal stimulation applies hot and cold packs alternately to a stroke patient's impaired hand and wrist for 20-to-30-minute sessions. In addition to standard physical therapy, it appears to significantly improve wrist extension and sensation and grasping strength more than physical therapy alone. Thermal stimulation is suggested five times a week for six weeks.

Fu-Zen Shaw, PhD, associate professor, Institute of Cognitive Science, National Cheng Kung University, Taiwan, and leader of a study published in *Stroke*.

■ ■ ■ ■

Better Stroke Survival

Patients treated within 90 minutes of the onset of an ischemic stroke (caused by a blood clot) are almost three times more likely to have a favorable outcome than those who wait longer for care. The longer the wait, the worse the outcome. Compared with those who received a placebo, stroke patients treated in 91 to 180 minutes had only a 50% better chance of a favorable outcome...and a 40% better chance if treated in 181 to 270 minutes. (Consent was obtained from all patients.) If you experience paralysis in the arm, face or leg, slurred speech, vision loss, dizziness and/or headache, call 911 immediately.

Thomas G. Brott, MD, professor of neurology, Mayo Clinic, Jacksonville, Florida.

13

Diabetes and Other Diseases

The Diabetes Epidemic: You May Have It—And Not Know It

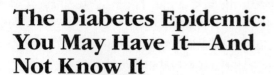

The US is in the midst of a diabetes epidemic. More than twenty million Americans currently have type 2 (adult-onset) diabetes, putting them at risk for such serious complications as blindness, kidney failure, heart disease, nerve damage and circulatory failure leading to amputation.

Another 41 million have prediabetes, which can turn into full-blown diabetes. The problem is that people with high blood sugar levels often don't feel any different—which is why one out of three Americans with diabetes don't even know they have the disease.

Main reason for this epidemic: More Americans are overweight and physically inactive—both of which make the body less responsive to insulin, the chemical that transports sugar from the bloodstream into the body's

various cells. This condition, known as insulin resistance, forces the body to produce more and more insulin in an effort to keep blood sugar within normal limits. Among those with genetic vulnerability (including many people who aren't overweight), this eventually causes the insulin-producing cells of the pancreas to "burn out," leaving the body unable to produce enough insulin to control blood sugar.

The result: Soaring blood sugar levels.

The good news: Complications can be avoided by catching insulin resistance early and then taking basic steps to bring your blood sugar levels within normal limits.

GET A FASTING BLOOD SUGAR TEST

The best way to learn whether you have insulin resistance is a fasting blood sugar test—a simple blood draw, taken 10 to 12 hours after you've last eaten. It should be included in your annual

Anne Peters, MD, professor of clinical medicine, Keck School of Medicine of the University of Southern California in Los Angeles, and director of the USC clinical diabetes program, is author of *Conquering Diabetes—A Cutting-Edge, Comprehensive Program for Prevention and Treatment.* Hudson Street Press.

physical. If you haven't had a fasting blood sugar test within the past year, call your primary care physician and schedule one—*especially* if you have a family history of diabetes.

A fasting blood sugar level of 126 milligrams per deciliter (mg/dl) or higher indicates diabetes, while a result between 100 and 125 mg/dl indicates prediabetes.

I always recommend a second test to confirm a high reading. If your test result is below 100, your blood sugar is within normal range, but you still may have early-stage insulin resistance—particularly if you are overweight or have close relatives with diabetes. If you and your doctor suspect this may be the case, you should follow the steps outlined below.

TEST FOR RISK FACTORS

Since insulin resistance is associated with significantly increased risk of heart disease, it's important that your doctor order a cholesterol (lipid) panel and check your blood pressure and body mass index (BMI). Body mass index is a measurement indicating how your weight/height ratio stacks up against the general population.

Triglyceride (a type of blood lipid) levels above 150 mg/dl and HDL (good) cholesterol levels below 50 (for women) or 40 (men), blood pressure of more than 130/80, and a BMI over 25 are all signs that you may be at risk for both heart disease and prediabetes/diabetes.

DEVELOP A TREATMENT PLAN

Some doctors still believe that there's nothing to worry about as long as your fasting blood sugar is less than 126. However, if one of my patients has a fasting blood sugar above 100 (or less than 100, but with other risk factors for insulin resistance or a family history of diabetes), I generally treat that patient as if he/she already has diabetes.

Reason: Damage from insulin resistance starts before blood sugar reaches "diabetic" levels.

This is why I urge everybody to ask their doctors for copies of their blood test results, rather than take a doctor's word that everything is OK. If your blood sugar is above 100, you need to discuss setting up a treatment plan with your doctor, or find another doctor if yours isn't responsive. *This plan should include five elements...*

•**Lose weight and exercise.**

•**Reduce cardiac risk associated with diabetes.** This includes taking a baby aspirin daily to reduce risk of heart attack and stroke, and, if your test results warrant, a statin drug to lower high cholesterol (Lipitor, Zocor, Crestor), fibric acid derivatives (Lopid, Tricor) to lower triglycerides and ACE inhibitors (Lotensin, Vasotec, Zestril, Altace) or angiotensin receptor blockers (Avapro, Cozaar, Hyzaar, Diovan) to treat high blood pressure.

•**Test blood sugar regularly.** If your fasting blood sugar test is above 100, I recommend getting another fasting blood sugar test every three months. If your blood sugar test is above 125, you'll need to test more often. My diabetic patients do home blood tests every day, including first thing in the morning and two hours after each meal, and also get an A1C blood test every three months. This test shows what your average blood sugar level was for the previous several months. The goal is to keep your A1C below 7, and preferably between 4 and 6.

•**Consider diabetes medication.** If your blood sugar levels continue to be high despite weight loss and exercise, you and your doctor might consider *glitazone* medication—either *pioglitazone* (Actos) or *rosiglitazone* (Avandia*) —to increase your body's sensitivity to insulin.

Your doctor may also prescribe *metformin* (which reduces the liver's glucose production and can be used with glitazones) and/or alpha-glucosidase inhibitors, such as *acarbose* (Precose) or *miglitol* (Glyset), which decrease the amount of carbohydrates absorbed by the intestines. (Unfortunately, they also tend to produce large amounts of intestinal gas.) Also, the new injected drug *exenatide* (Byetta) can help lower blood sugar level and weight at the same time.

If all else fails, your doctor can prescribe daily insulin doses to supplement your body's natural insulin production.

•**Test for complications of insulin resistance.** Since cell damage from diabetes begins early, I also recommend regular tests for

*Recent evidence suggests that Avandia may increase the risk of myocardial ischemia, a condition in which the heart muscle does not receive enough oxygen-rich blood, causing symptoms like angina. In 2007, the FDA required the manufacturers to add a severe warning label that Avandia may increase the risks of heart failure.

complications, even if your blood sugar is only slightly elevated.

Reason: Diabetes-related complications may be treatable early on, but once damage becomes serious, treatment becomes difficult or impossible.

Tests include: An annual dilated eye exam by an ophthalmologist...a yearly urine test for microalbuminuria (an early sign of kidney damage)...yearly cholesterol and triglyceride tests...a check for normal foot sensation at every doctor's visit, and if numbness is detected, twice daily home foot exams for cuts or sores that you can't feel.

Losing weight is the single most effective way to prevent type 2 diabetes.

Reason: Putting on even as little as 10 pounds—especially around your middle—automatically increases insulin resistance. Losing just 15 pounds reduces your risk of developing diabetes by more than half.

A simple, proven way to lose weight: Eat smaller portions. Use small (10-inch) plates at home—and therefore serve smaller portions—since studies show that people tend to finish whatever is on their plates. Also, avoid fruit juices and soft drinks as well as "white" foods (white bread, baked potatoes and French fries, pasta, white rice), all of which cause sharp rises in blood sugar. Finally, make sure that every meal contains a mix of high-fiber fruits and vegetables and high-quality protein (fish or lean meat).

Another key: Do an hour of exercise at least five times a week. A good program for most people is 45 minutes of aerobic exercise—such as walking, biking or swimming—and 15 minutes of light weight lifting.

Reason: Regular exercise encourages weight loss and increases your body's sensitivity to insulin. This effect only lasts a short time, however, which is why it's important to exercise often.

For many, these steps will be enough to prevent diabetes. If your body's ability to respond to insulin is 75% of normal and you can lower your insulin resistance by 25% through diet and exercise—a typical response—then your blood-sugar regulation will be brought back in balance.

■ ■ ■ ■

Diabetes—Tests and Symptoms to Look for

You have diabetes if any one of the following test results occurs on at least two different days...

•**A fasting blood glucose level** of 126 mg/dL or higher.

•**A two-hour oral glucose tolerance test result** of 200 mg/dL or higher.

•**Symptoms of diabetes** combined with a random (nonfasting) blood glucose test of 200 mg/dL or higher.

Symptoms of diabetes are...

- •Increased thirst.
- •Frequent urination (especially at night).
- •Unexplained increase in appetite.
- •Fatigue.
- •Erection problems.
- •Blurred vision.
- •Tingling or numbness in the hands and/or feet.

American Diabetes Association, *www.diabetes.org.*

■ ■ ■ ■

Antidepressants and Diabetes Risk

Antidepressants may increase diabetes risk, warns Richard Rubin, PhD. In a recent study, people at high risk for type 2 diabetes who did not take diabetes medications were two to three times more likely to develop diabetes if they were taking antidepressants than similar people who were not taking antidepressants. High-risk patients who were given the diabetes drug *metformin* (Glucophage) did not have a higher risk of diabetes. If you are taking an antidepressant and are at risk for diabetes–for example, because you are overweight or have a family history of diabetes—talk to your doctor.

Richard Rubin, PhD, is a coinvestigator with the Diabetes Prevention Program Research Group, Baltimore, and leader of a study of 3,187 people with elevated blood glucose levels, presented at the annual scientific session of the American Diabetes Association.

How Not to Get Diabetes

Robert A. Rizza, MD, professor of medicine and director for research at Mayo Clinic College of Medicine in Rochester, MN, is past president of the American Diabetes Association, *www.diabetes.org*. Winner of prestigious Banting Medal for Service.

The epidemic of type 2 diabetes is alarming —and more dangerous than many people ever imagine. The disease, which affects more than 20 million Americans, increases the risk for heart attack and stroke. Complications include blindness, kidney failure, impotence and poor wound healing that can lead to amputation.

Until recently, doctors diagnosed diabetes only when a patient had full-blown symptoms, which typically develop gradually over a period of years.

Now: You can stop diabetes in its tracks if you recognize and take action against "prediabetes," which affects more than 41 million people ages 40 to 74. *Here's how...*

WHEN SUGAR ISN'T SWEET

Glucose, a simple sugar molecule that is metabolized from the food you eat, is basic fuel for your body. It's broken down in cells of all kinds to produce energy that powers your muscles, lets you think and keeps your heart pumping and your lungs breathing.

The hormone insulin, which is produced by your pancreas, plays a key role, escorting glucose from the bloodstream into the cells. When there isn't enough insulin to do the job or the insulin is not effective, sugar builds up in the blood. That's when the trouble begins.

To diagnose diabetes, doctors order blood tests that measure the amount of glucose in your bloodstream. One test, fasting plasma glucose (FPG), checks the level first thing in the morning, before you've eaten anything. A normal glucose level is less than 100 milligrams per deciliter (mg/dl).

The oral glucose tolerance test (OGTT) is a bit more complicated—after fasting all night, you're asked to drink a sugary liquid, and your glucose level is tested two hours later (normal is less than 140 mg/dl).

If your FPG is 126 mg/dl or higher...or the two-hour OGTT is above 200 mg/dl, you likely have diabetes. Either your pancreas no longer secretes enough insulin for proper glucose metabolism or you have become resistant to its effects. This means that your chance of developing complications, such as heart disease, kidney failure or vision loss, has more than doubled.

AN EARLIER DIAGNOSIS

There's also an intermediate condition. Fasting blood sugar of 100 mg/dl to 125 mg/dl is called impaired fasting glucose. If the two-hour OGTT is 140 mg/dl to 200 mg/dl, it is known as *impaired glucose tolerance.*

Nowadays, these conditions are called prediabetes. With prediabetes, your insulin activity has already started to fall short of the amount your body needs. And if something isn't done, there's a good chance you'll go on to develop full-blown diabetes.

What are the odds? Fasting blood sugar between 100 mg/dl and 110 mg/dl means you have a 20% chance of developing diabetes within five to 10 years. If it's above 110, it's a 40% chance. If both the fasting blood sugar and two-hour glucose tolerance tests are elevated, the odds increase even more.

At the prediabetes level, excess blood sugar already has started to take its toll, researchers have discovered. For example, the risk for heart disease is one-and-one-half times higher than that of people with normal blood sugar.

DO YOU HAVE PREDIABETES?

To determine whether you have prediabetes, ask your doctor for a fasting glucose test—especially if you are at increased risk due to...

•**Excess body weight.**

•**Family history of diabetes** (parent, brother or sister).

•**Diabetes during pregnancy** (gestational diabetes).

•**Asian, African-American or Hispanic ethnicity.**

If any of these risk factors applies to you, have your blood sugar checked at your next physical —after age 45, do it at least every three years. Given the high rates of diabetes today, *everyone* over age 45 should consider getting tested.

TREATMENT FOR PREDIABETES

Slightly elevated blood sugar doesn't mean you're destined to get diabetes. With fairly moderate lifestyle changes, you can reduce that risk by more than 50%.

Obesity increases diabetes risk. If you are overweight, bring your weight down by 5% to 10% (an achievable goal for most people). Ideally, your weight should be brought down to the normal range, which means a body mass index (a ratio of weight to height), or BMI, of 18.5 to 24.9. To find your BMI, use the free calculator at the National Heart, Lung, and Blood Institute Web site at *http://nhlbisupport.com/bmi.* Or use the formula (weight in pounds × 703) ÷ height in inches squared.

Important finding: A Finnish study of 522 middle-aged, overweight people with prediabetes found that diabetes risk among those who participated in a diet and exercise program for three years was reduced by 58% compared with a control group, who experienced no reduction.

How to stop prediabetes…

•**Diet wisely.** Consuming fewer calories than you burn is the key to weight loss. Some research also suggests that reducing saturated fat (most beef and some dairy products), and the resulting weight loss that can occur, helps reverse prediabetes, allowing your body to use insulin more efficiently. A diet rich in complex carbohydrates, such as fruits, vegetables and whole grains, will meet these goals—and is best for general health.

•**Exercise regularly.** Physical activity helps control your weight and improves your body's ability to use insulin. Aim for at least 30 minutes five or more days a week. The type of exercise doesn't seem to matter, as long as it requires modest exertion—brisk walking, swimming, riding a bike, etc.

•**Forgo medication.** Blood sugar in people with prediabetes can be reduced with prescription diabetes medication such as *metformin* (Glucophage). However, research on prediabetes suggests that this drug is not as effective as diet and exercise in preventing diabetes.

Important finding: In a *New England Journal of Medicine* study, 3,234 men and women with prediabetes were randomly assigned to a healthy lifestyle program or the drug metformin.

Weight loss and exercise reduced diabetes incidence nearly twice as much as drug treatment over the next three years (a reduction of 58% versus 31%).

■ ■ ■ ■

Diabetes Pain Reduced

Twenty-four percent of 716 people with diabetes who took an alpha-lipoic acid supplement daily for three weeks felt an improvement in pain, burning and numbness in their feet due to diabetic neuropathy (nerve damage caused by high blood sugar) compared with 16% of 542 diabetics taking a placebo.

Theory: Alpha-lipoic acid neutralizes the damage caused by small molecules that accumulate when blood sugar is elevated.

If you suffer from diabetic neuropathy: Ask your doctor about taking 1,200 mg to 1,800 mg daily of controlled-release alpha-lipoic acid, available at most health-food stores. Taking alpha-lipoic acid may alter insulin or drug requirements.

Ira Goldfine, MD, professor of endocrinology, University of California, San Francisco.

Diabetes Reversed Forever

Annals of Surgery.
University of Pittsburgh Medical Center.

The weight-loss procedure called gastric bypass surgery, which has been gaining popularity recently, can improve or eliminate type 2 diabetes in people who are obese, according to Pennsylvania researchers.

Laparoscopic gastric bypass surgery makes the stomach smaller. Patients lose weight because their smaller stomach can't take in as many calories as before.

THE STUDY

A study by scientists at the University of Pittsburgh Medical Center found that 83% of obese patients with type 2 diabetes who underwent the operation saw improvement in, and even total reversal of, their disease.

"Most patients in the study with type 2 diabetes who underwent bypass surgery achieved excellent biochemical [blood sugar] control and were able to reap the clinical benefits of withdrawing from most, if not all, antidiabetes medications, including insulin," says principal investigator Dr. Philip Schauer, director of bariatric surgery.

"Younger diabetes patients with less severe disease stand to gain more from the surgery by circumventing years of progressive, debilitating disease," Schauer adds.

THE PROCEDURE

Gastric bypass surgery is intended for the estimated 8 million Americans who are considered morbidly obese—100 pounds or more above their ideal weight.

Morbid obesity is believed to cut between 15 and 20 years off a person's life, according to the University of Arkansas for Medical Sciences.

Most people who have gastric bypass surgery lose approximately two-thirds of their excess body weight during the first year after the procedure. Most are able to keep that weight off for years.

SYMPTOMS

Type 2 diabetes has some symptoms similar to type 1, including frequent urination, excessive thirst and hunger, dramatic weight loss (without dieting), irritability, weakness and fatigue and nausea and vomiting.

But there are also symptoms more likely to occur in type 2 diabetes, such as recurring or hard-to-heal skin lesions, gum or bladder infections, blurred vision, tingling or numbness in hands or feet and itchy skin.

Symptoms for type 2 diabetes usually occur gradually over a period of months or perhaps even years, and some people who have type 2 diabetes have symptoms that are so mild, they go undiagnosed.

TREATMENTS

There are a number of different treatments for people who have type 2 diabetes, including drugs other than insulin.

Very often patients can control their sugar and glucose levels through a diet that is recommended by a physician, as well as an exercise plan and careful daily monitoring of their blood sugar levels.

The US National Diabetes Education Program lists four steps to control diabetes on their Web site at *www.ndep.nih.gov/diabetes/control/4Steps.htm.*

Living Donors Help People with Diabetes

David E.R. Sutherland, MD, PhD, head, division of transplantation, and director, Diabetes Institute for Immunology and Transplantation at the University of Minnesota Medical Center department of surgery, Minneapolis.

If at first you don't succeed, try, try again. Such is the lesson learned from a recent experimental surgery in Japan in which doctors implanted pancreatic islet cells, which produce insulin, from a living donor into a woman with severe diabetes. Results so far are encouraging—the woman with diabetes is no longer insulin-dependent.

According to David E.R. Sutherland, MD, PhD, head, division of transplantation, and director, Diabetes Institute for Immunology and Transplantation at the University of Minnesota Medical Center department of surgery, a similar surgery was tried in the 1970s at the University of Minnesota Medical Center, though with unsuccessful results. The recent attempt by the Japanese team, led by Dr. Shinichi Matsumoto, of Kyoto University Hospital, and who trained at the University of Minnesota, is very encouraging for the possibility of using living donor pancreas tissue donations to aid cases of severe diabetes. To date, most pancreas replacement surgery has involved taking the pancreas from a cadaver, but results have been poor. With live tissue donation, the quality of the islets isolated is better and there is less chance of rejection.

ABOUT PANCREAS TRANSPLANTS

One function of the pancreas is to make digestive enzymes to secrete into the intestine. The other is to make insulin, which is done by little groups of cells called islets of Langerhans that are scattered throughout the gland. Dr. Sutherland describes the islets as being like BBs scattered throughout the pancreas. Fortuitously, the pancreas is shaped like a dumbbell and each half has a separate blood supply. Thus, it is possible to divide the pancreas and take one half for transplantation from a living donor, much as surgeons do routinely by removing one kidney for transplantation.

Pancreas transplants from living donors have been done successfully at the University of Minnesota since the 1970s. Using islets from living donors sounds like the future, and perhaps it will be, says Dr. Sutherland—not to make the surgery easier for the donor, but to make it minimally invasive for the recipient. We know that people can survive with half a pancreas (or for that matter, no pancreas at all—though they become instantly diabetic and must take digestive enzymes as well as insulin for life). However, even with the less invasive islet surgery, the recipient requires immunosuppressive medications similar to that of other transplant recipients.

ABOUT THE JAPANESE SUCCESS

The Japanese team removed half the pancreas of a woman, harvested the islet cells and transplanted them to the woman's 27-year-old diabetic daughter, who was suffering severe attacks of hypoglycemia from reactions to insulin injections. (Most diabetics are able to anticipate and prevent such extreme blood sugar drops, but some are not and they often pass out as a consequence—a condition called hypoglycemic unawareness.) The newsworthy aspect is that the donor is doing well and her diabetic daughter remains insulin-independent. Part of this latest success may be the fact that improved islets isolation techniques combined with the extreme freshness of tissue from a live donor enhance function, and the genetic match of the donor and recipient help prevent rejection. Dr. Sutherland says he salutes this effort for its early success but longer follow-up is needed to see if rejection is less than with cadaver tissue.

Transplant surgery is not useful for pancreatic cancer because the cancer is virtually never detected until it has already metastasized. However, for people with diabetes or whose pancreas has been removed because of severe pancreatitis, Dr. Sutherland says doctors hope that someday beta cell islet transplantation from living donors will be routine. In this country, the procedure is still considered investigational and needs approval from the Institutional Review Board and the FDA before doctors can move forward with it. We'll keep watching.

■ ■ ■ ■

The Diabetes–Cancer Link

Diabetes and pancreatic cancer may be linked, says recent research.

Recent finding: About 1% of patients ages 50 and older were diagnosed with pancreatic cancer within three years of being diagnosed with type 2 diabetes. This rate is eight times higher than in the general population.

Self-defense: Consult your physician if you are newly diagnosed with diabetes.

Suresh T. Chari, MD, Mayo Clinic College of Medicine, Rochester, Minnesota, and leader of a study of 2,122 people ages 50 and older, reported in *Gastroenterology*.

Developments in Glucose Monitoring

Richard Bergenstal, MD, endocrinologist, executive director, International Diabetes Center at Park Nicollet, Minneapolis.
American Diabetes Association annual meeting, Orlando, Florida.

New devices that monitor blood sugar levels may one day help ease the painful daily management of diabetes.

GLUCOSE MONITORING

Keeping a close eye on the body's blood sugar levels is critical to staying healthy. Right now, patients with type 1 diabetes (and many with type 2) draw blood up to four times each day to gauge their blood sugar levels.

"Good glucose control prevents eye, kidney and nerve problems, and seems to be associated with a lower risk of heart disease," says Dr. Richard Bergenstal, an endocrinologist and executive director of the International Diabetes Center at Park Nicollet in Minneapolis. Still, he adds, only 57% of people test even once a day.

One group of researchers is working on a device that measures levels of volatile organic compounds in human breath, eliminating the need for diabetics to prick their finger to test their blood sugar levels.

Another group of researchers described the HypoMon, a chest-belt transmitter that serves to continuously take glucose measurements on the surface of the skin.

One advantage of this system is that it would be able to monitor glucose levels even during sleep. The downside is that movement and sweat could affect the readings.

Bergenstal stresses that short-term monitoring of blood glucose levels should not replace long-term monitoring with the *hemoglobin A1c test*, which reflects an average of blood sugar readings for a two- to three-month period. In fact, the two should work together. "A1c has been best correlated to long-term complications," Bergenstal says.

■ ■ ■ ■

Diabetes Supplement Warning

The mineral *selenium* may increase diabetes risk. It had been thought to help protect against certain illnesses, including type 2 diabetes. According to recent research, people who took selenium supplements long-term—for an average of 7.7 years—were 50% more likely to develop diabetes during the study period than people who did not take selenium.

Self-defense: Talk to your doctor before taking selenium.

Saverio Stranges, MD, PhD, associate professor of cardiovascular epidemiology, Warwick Medical School, Coventry, England, and lead author of a study of the selenium/diabetes link in 1,202 patients, published in *Annals of Internal Medicine*.

Keep Down the Cost of Diabetes

Judith H. McQuown is a writer and editor in New York City who was diagnosed with diabetes in 1987. She is author of *1001 Tips for Living Well with Diabetes: Firsthand Advice That Really Works*. Marlowe & Company.

People with diabetes not only have a life-long, life-threatening ailment they have to manage on a day-to-day basis, they also bear the burden of enormous costs associated with it. Even if you have a good insurance plan, insulin and other medications can cost hundreds of dollars a year. Then there's the cost of testing strips…glucose monitors…and frequent doctor visits. It's estimated that more than 10 cents of every health-care dollar is spent on diabetes. For patients who have limited or no insurance coverage, individual costs can be staggering.

However, according to Judith McQuown, author of *1001 Tips for Living Well with Diabetes: Firsthand Advice That Really Works*, there are a number of ways that people with diabetes can save money without compromising care.

JUDITH'S SUGGESTIONS

•**Buy supplies on eBay.** There usually are hundreds of listings for test kits, glucose-monitoring devices, test strips, etc. You'll pay considerably less than retail prices.

Important: Check expiration dates on items you're buying. Also check the seller's customer feedback to make sure he/she is reputable.

•**Buy mail order.** There are a number of large, reputable mail-order pharmacies, such as Liberty Medical (*www.libertymedical.com*). Because they deal in large volumes, they typically charge less than local pharmacies.

•**Buy generics.** The Food and Drug Administration requires generic drugs to be identical to the original brand-name drugs in dosage, quality, safety and strength—and the savings can be tremendous.

Example: A newer brand-name prescription drug can cost up to 10 times more than older drugs that are available as generics. That said, there have been incidents of generic drugs not being as effective as the brand-name version. Talk to your doctor to be sure the generic versions are acceptable. Then double-check that the generic version is identical to the brand-name drug.

•**Split pill doses.** Ask your doctor to prescribe pills that are double your usual dosage, and then cut them in half. Most drugs come in several doses. The cost of higher-dose pills is usually the same or only slightly higher than the lower doses. Cutting pills in half can turn one month's supply into two.

Caution: Some drugs—those with enteric coatings or timed-release ingredients, for example—must be taken whole. Ask your doctor if pill splitting is appropriate for any of the drugs you're currently taking. And, be sure to use a "pill splitter" to ensure equal distribution.

•**Participate in clinical trials.** Patients who enroll in studies to test new drugs and/or treatments usually get free checkups, tests, consultations with specialists, etc. Many clinical trials compare active drugs with a placebo. Talk to your doctor about whether a given trial would be appropriate for you—and the potential risks if you happen to be in the placebo group. The upside of being in a trial is that your overall care will be state-of-the-art and you will be very well monitored. The downside is that there is risk involved with new medications. Depending on what's being tested, it may be worth considering.

•**Know the formulary.** Most health-insurance plans have a list of brand-name and generic drugs that they'll cover. This list is known as the formulary. If your doctor prescribes a drug that's not in the formulary, you will have to pay full price.

Example: Cipro antibiotic eardrops, which weren't in McQuown's medical group's formulary, would have cost her $134. A prescription of Cortisporin, a similar, brand-name antibiotic that was in the formulary, was going to cost $10 for the co-pay. Since people with diabetes are prone to an array of health challenges, having the full formulary can be very helpful.

Although these strategies won't make the diabetes go away, they can help ease some of the burden of it.

■ ■ ■ ■

Coffee and Green Tea Cut Diabetes Risk

In a study of 17,413 adults, those who reported drinking six or more cups of green tea or at least three cups of caffeinated coffee daily were one-third less likely to develop type 2 diabetes than those who drank less than one cup of green tea or coffee a week.

Theory: Caffeine stimulates oxidation (burning) of fat.

Caution: A high caffeine intake—more than 500 mg per day—has been linked to benign arrhythmias (irregular heart rhythms).

One eight-ounce cup of coffee contains about 100 mg of caffeine…green tea, about 35 mg. Ask your doctor how much caffeine is appropriate for you.

Hiroyasu Iso, MD, PhD, MPH, a professor of public health at Osaka University Graduate School of Medicine, Osaka, Japan.

Drink More Coffee, Lower Diabetes Risk

Rob M. van Dam, PhD, assistant professor of medicine, Harvard Medical School, and associate epidemiologist, department of medicine, Brigham and Women's Hospital, Boston.

More good news for latte lovers comes from researchers at the Harvard School of Public Health (HSPH). They found that people who drink coffee on a regular basis experience a substantially lower risk for type 2 diabetes.

ABOUT THE STUDY

In a retrospective review of nine studies of coffee consumption and type 2 diabetes risk, Harvard researcher Rob M. van Dam, PhD, and his colleagues looked at 193,473 regular coffee drinkers who experienced 8,394 cases of type 2 diabetes. They excluded studies of people with type 1 diabetes and studies of short-term exposure to coffee or caffeine.

Researchers calculated the risk of type 2 diabetes relative to how many daily cups of coffee the participants consumed. *It turned out that the more coffee, the better…*

•**The incidence of diabetes was lowest** for people who consumed the most coffee each day (six or more cups). They were 35% less likely to develop diabetes

•**Those who drank four to six cups daily** had a 28% reduction in expected incidence of diabetes.

•**People who drank the least coffee** (which was no consumption in US studies, and two or fewer daily cups for Europeans) had only a 6% reduction in their risk of diabetes.

These numbers did not differ significantly according to sex, obesity or geographic region (which in this case meant the US and Europe).

However, Dr. van Dam adds that the results were rather diverse in the lowest consumption category. He would not be surprised if future studies that are able to measure coffee consumption more precisely find a lower diabetes incidence for any amount of coffee.

MORE COFFEE, LESS DIABETES

These findings serve to underscore the results of an earlier HSPH study, in which men who drank more than six cups of coffee a day reduced their risk of type 2 diabetes by more than 50% in comparison with men who did not drink coffee…and women by 30% in comparison with women who were not coffee drinkers. This beneficial effect was observed independent of lifestyle choices such as smoking, exercise and obesity.

Scientists don't know exactly how coffee cuts diabetes risk. Paradoxically, caffeine reduces insulin sensitivity and raises blood sugar—both no-nos for diabetes. However, Dr. van Dam emphasizes that coffee is a complex beverage that contains numerous chemical compounds and minerals, which may have both helpful and harmful impacts on the body. Components other than caffeine—such as the antioxidants chlorogenic acid and magnesium—actually improve sensitivity to insulin and thus help lower diabetes risk. In animal studies, trigonelline and lignans improved glucose levels. Dr. van Dam adds that additional studies on effects of coffee components in humans are clearly needed.

WHAT ABOUT DECAF?

For those who prefer decaf, coffee still packs some protection against type 2 diabetes. Although the effect appears to be more modest, some of this discrepancy may be attributed to study limitations. Decaffeinated coffee consumption was substantially lower than caffeinated coffee consumption, and this may have affected the estimates, explains Dr. van Dam. He points out that it is easier to detect larger contrasts in consumption than smaller differences. In addition, one can expect some misclassification when you ask for the amount of coffee people consume (change over time, differences in strength and cup size, etc.).

Dr. van Dam notes that in a study on coffee consumption and C-peptide concentrations (a marker for insulin resistance), the association was actually similar for decaffeinated and caffeinated coffee consumption. He adds that it is currently unclear whether caffeine has detrimental effects on insulin sensitivity over the long term, because only short-term studies have been conducted. Nor is it clear if non-coffee sources of caffeine would have similar effects.

THE JOLT OF JAVA

Other trials have already lined up in coffee's favor, demonstrating that it can lower the risk of liver problems, gallstones, colon cancer and Parkinson's disease. Of course, there's also a downside to coffee (which pregnant women, children and people with colitis, hepatitis and other dietary challenges should not drink), such as jitteriness, insomnia and a rapid heartbeat. (Coffee stimulates liver function, which in healthy people is fine in moderation, but those with active liver disease may have symptoms worsen when they consume coffee.)

Promising as it seems, Dr. van Dam and his colleagues do not go so far as to recommend drinking coffee to prevent type 2 diabetes. They emphasize that while coffee consumption may provide greater control over diabetes and possibly reduce the need for pharmaceuticals, it cannot replace the myriad health benefits of diet, exercise and weight management.

Many people stop drinking coffee because they think this is good for their health. Now coffee drinkers can take comfort in knowing that their daily jolt of java not only gets them up and moving, it may also provide health benefits.

The Amazing Healing Power of Coffee

Joe A. Vinson, PhD, a professor of chemistry at the University of Scranton in Pennsylvania. A specialist in food-based chemical compounds, he was the lead author of an article on antioxidants published in *Journal of Agricultural and Food Chemistry.*

When most people think of a healthful diet, fresh fruits and vegetables typically top the list.

Surprising: An eight-ounce cup of caffeinated or decaffeinated coffee contains *more* disease-fighting antioxidants than a typical serving of fresh blueberries or oranges.

Although coffee does not contain some of the other nutrients found in healthful foods, it is the main source of antioxidants in the American diet (followed by tea and chocolate, respectively). Of course, the stimulating effects of coffee's caffeine are not always desirable—some people experience nervousness, insomnia or even spikes in blood pressure.

But most people who drink moderate amounts of coffee (typically defined as one to three cups daily) seem to have a lower risk for a number of chronic conditions, including heart disease, diabetes and age-related cognitive declines.

WHAT'S IN A CUP?

The amount of caffeine that is found in coffee varies, depending on how the coffee is prepared.

Examples: One ounce of espresso contains about 50 mg...an eight-ounce cup of instant coffee has 95 mg...and eight ounces of plain, brewed coffee has 150 mg.

A serving of espresso, instant or brewed coffee each contains roughly the same amount of antioxidants. In fact, coffee contains hundreds of antioxidants, particularly *polyphenols*—plant compounds that can inhibit cell damage or inflammation, two of the main causes of many chronic diseases. The addition of milk and/or sugar does not appear to affect the antioxidant levels.

Important: Most of the research linking coffee to reduced disease rates is based on epidemiological studies, in which scientists have analyzed the past dietary habits of large groups of people.

This type of research helps to develop hypotheses that deserve further study, but definitive answers won't be possible until scientists conduct more large-scale clinical studies, in which factors such as coffee consumption are tightly controlled (rather than merely self-reported by test subjects).

What the newest research on coffee consumption tells us...

GOOD FOR THE ARTERIES

Recent finding: In a study published in the *American Journal of Clinical Nutrition*, Norwegian researchers found that postmenopausal women who drink one to three cups of coffee daily are 24% less likely to develop cardiovascular disease than non-coffee drinkers.

Theory: The antioxidants in coffee—like those in fruits and vegetables—are thought to inhibit the damaging effects of free radicals on cells lining the arteries.

Result: A decrease in inflammation, now thought to be the underlying cause of heart disease.

Caution: Because of the stimulating effects of caffeine, blood pressure rises temporarily (for about one hour) when regular coffee is consumed. People who drink several cups in a row may keep their blood pressure elevated, thus increasing the risk for heart disease or a heart attack.

Helpful: Space out coffee consumption. For example, have one cup in the morning and another at lunch or in the afternoon. Or switch to decaf, which doesn't cause the blood-pressure spikes of regular coffee—but offers the same health benefits, except for those that improve cognitive function.

BLOOD PRESSURE STABILIZER

Recent finding: An analysis published in the *American Journal of Clinical Nutrition* found that older adults (age 65 and over) who have four or more daily servings of caffeine—in the form of coffee, soft drinks, etc.—have less than half the risk of dying of heart disease than those who consume smaller amounts.

Theory: Older adults are prone to occasional *hypotension* (low blood pressure). They are especially vulnerable to drops in blood pressure after meals, which can increase the risk for heart attack. Caffeine, by quickly raising blood pressure, appears to reduce the risk for such coronary events.

Caution: The oils found in *steeped* coffee, such as that made in a French press (a glass beaker to which hot water and ground coffee are added...then a plunger is depressed, filtering out all the grounds and sediment), can significantly raise cholesterol and increase the risk for elevated blood pressure.

Better for health: Coffee that is drip brewed (water is poured over ground coffee and seeps through a filter into a pot). The filter traps most of the oils.

LESS DIABETES

Recent finding: Research published in the *Archives of Internal Medicine* found that among 28,812 postmenopausal women studied, those who drank four to five cups of coffee (especially decaffeinated) per day were 16% less likely to develop type 2 diabetes than women who didn't drink any coffee.

Theory: The antioxidants in coffee may protect the pancreas's insulin-producing *beta cells* from oxidative damage.

BETTER BRAIN HEALTH

Recent finding: Coffee appears to slow the rate of cognitive decline in elderly adults. In a study published in the *European Journal of Clinical Nutrition* researchers gave memory tests to 676 healthy men in Finland, Italy and the Netherlands, then repeated the tests 10 years later. Non-coffee drinkers had four times more cognitive decline than men who drank three cups of coffee a day.

Theory: The antioxidants in coffee reduce age-related damage to brain cells (neurons) and/or cause beneficial changes in the hormones/neurotransmitters that are involved in cognitive function.

Scientific studies also suggest that moderate consumption of coffee reduces the risk for Parkinson's disease as well as Alzheimer's disease. Researchers have yet to explain why coffee reduces risk for these two diseases, but the mechanism is thought to be similar to that associated with reduced cognitive decline.

A HEALTHIER LIVER

Recent finding: According to research published in the *Archives of Internal Medicine*, coffee may reduce the risk for cirrhosis (irreversible liver scarring that, in severe cases, can be life-threatening without a transplant), especially in alcoholics. This link may be due to the anti-inflammatory effects of the antioxidants in coffee.

In addition, coffee may help protect against gallstones. Specifically, data from the ongoing Harvard Nurses' Health Study found that women who drank four or more cups of coffee daily required fewer operations for gallstones than women who didn't drink coffee.

Theory: Caffeine stimulates gallbladder contractions, which cause the gallbladder to empty more often and may reduce the risk for gallstone formation.

Caution: Caffeine interacts with certain medications, causing some to become more potent or increasing the amount of time caffeine remains in the body. These drugs include certain selective serotonin reuptake inhibitors (SSRIs), such as *fluvoxamine* (Luvox)...antiarrhythmics, such as *mexiletine* (Mexitil)...and bronchodilators, such as *theophylline* (Theo-Dur). Caffeine also may interact with the herbal dietary supplement ephedra. In addition, consumption of more than five cups of coffee daily has been linked to higher risk for bone fractures in postmenopausal women.

Power Supplement Fights Diabetes Problems

Bruce N. Ames, PhD, professor of biochemistry and molecular biology, University of California, Berkeley; senior scientist, Children's Hospital Oakland Research Institute, Oakland. He was appointed member, President's Committee, National Medal of Science.

One of the more popular supplements to come along is alpha-lipoic acid (ALA). Although studies are ongoing, this is one of the better-researched supplements, with demonstrated benefits as a disease-fighting antioxidant and as a treatment for diabetes.

Bruce N. Ames, PhD, a professor of biochemistry and molecular biology at the University of California in Berkeley, has conducted a number of studies of alpha-lipoic acid. *His thoughts about its many health benefits...*

A VERSATILE ANTIOXIDANT

As you probably already know, antioxidants protect our bodies from the cellular damage caused by unstable oxygen molecules called free radicals. Left unchecked, this damage can lead to ailments including cardiovascular disease, diabetes, arthritis, cataracts and Alzheimer's disease.

Because it is soluble in both fat and water, alpha-lipoic acid is an especially valuable antioxidant. It can reach both tissues composed primarily of fat (including the brain and nervous system) and those of water (such as the heart). ALA also enhances the action of other well-known antioxidants—vitamins E and C.

A BRAIN FUNCTION BOOSTER

As we grow older, there is a drop in mitochondrial function in the body's cells. According to Dr. Ames, mitochondria—the power plants of cells—provide energy for basic cell processes, and their decay with age impairs cellular metabolism and leads to performance decline. At UC Berkeley, scientists have demonstrated that ALA can help reverse this type of age-associated decline as it relates to brain function. In laboratory experiments, old rats that were given high doses of ALA along with another supplement—N-acetyl-L-carnitine, typically used as an anti-aging supplement to enhance mental functions such as memory and improve the symptoms of Alzheimer's disease—experienced improved cellular function, which in practical terms translated into better performance on memory tasks.

AN AID TO THE LIVER

In hospitals, ALA is administered intravenously to treat cases of mushroom poisoning and heavy metal poisoning. With its antioxidant abilities, ALA assists the liver in flushing toxins from the body. This supplement helps to shield the liver from harmful cell changes and offers protection against disorders such as hepatitis and cirrhosis.

WEAPON AGAINST DIABETES AND ITS COMPLICATIONS

Many studies of ALA have taken place in Germany, where this compound is commonly prescribed to treat diabetic neuropathy (a frequently agonizing complication of diabetes that begins with pain and numbness in the feet). ALA has been shown to increase blood flow to nerves and fine-tune the transmission of nerve impulses. Even more important, it improves insulin function and thus blood sugar regulation by expediting the more efficient removal of glucose from the blood. Poorly regulated, chronically high levels of blood sugar contribute to complications of diabetes including diabetic neuropathy and heart disease.

A FAT FIGHTER?

A recent study at the University of Ulsan College of Medicine in Korea suggests that ALA may even play a role in combating obesity. When ALA was added to the food of rats, it reduced their food intake and body weight. This research is still in its infancy, with clinical studies in humans not yet planned.

HOW TO USE ALPHA-LIPOIC ACID

Tiny amounts of ALA are present in foods such as spinach, liver and yeast...however, only supplements provide substantial benefits such as antioxidant effects. Suggested dosages of ALA vary. As an antioxidant, a typical range is 10 mg to 50 mg daily. Therapeutic doses for problems such as diabetes can be as high as 600 mg daily. But be careful. While very promising, doctors do not yet have full information on side effects or long-term effects of ALA usage at "normal" and at "high" doses. While you should work closely with your doctor to monitor usage, be aware that few conventional doctors are experienced in ALA's usage at this point in time. According to Dr. Ames, side effects are very rare—mainly a mild rash in one in 300 people. The most important interaction is with the dosage of diabetes medications. It's not contraindicated for anyone, but you should, of course, consult your doctor about taking it (especially if you have diabetes).

■ ■ ■ ■

New Diabetes Drug

Diabetes drug spurs insulin production after a meal. *Exenatide* (Byetta) is the synthetic version of a protein in the saliva of the Gila monster, a lizard. People with type 2 diabetes inject the drug twice daily to supplement the action of *metformin* (Glucophage) or other oral medications.

Most common side effect: Nausea. Dosages of older drugs may need to be reduced to avoid low blood-sugar levels (hypoglycemia).

David M. Nathan, MD, is director of Massachusetts General Hospital Diabetes Center and professor of medicine, Harvard Medical School, both in Boston.

■ ■ ■ ■

Important Little-Known Diabetes Test

The A1C test shows average blood sugar levels over the past 180 days. It is done by a lab or in your doctor's office in addition to home monitoring of blood sugar. The A1C test tells whether diabetes treatment is working effectively—but 61% of diabetics recently surveyed did not know what it was. The A1C test can help diabetics adjust diet, activity and medication to avoid possible complications of the disease. Ask your doctor how often you should have an A1C test.

Robert A. Rizza, MD, professor of medicine and director for research at Mayo Clinic College of Medicine in Rochester, Minnesota, is past president of the American Diabetes Association, www.diabetes.org. Winner of prestigious Banting Medal for Service.

Are You at Risk for Hidden Bone Loss?

Harris H. McIlwain, MD, chair of the Florida Osteoporosis Board and adjunct professor, University of South Florida College of Public Health in Tampa, is coauthor of Reversing Osteopenia: The Definitive Guide to Recognizing and Treating Early Bone Loss in Women of All Ages. Henry Holt.

Calcium alone won't protect you from *osteopenia*—early osteoporosis. Most women —as well as men—who are past age 50 know that they are at risk for osteoporosis, the leading cause of bone fractures in older adults. But few older adults realize that they may already have a precursor to osteoporosis known as *osteopenia*.

Recent finding: Estimates suggest that half of all women over age 45 and about 30% of men of the same age group have the mild bone loss that characterizes osteopenia.

Painful bone fractures, which are commonly associated with osteoporosis, also can occur in people who have osteopenia. These fractures can cause spinal deformities…hand or wrist disability…and severe hip injury.

SAY GOODBYE TO BONE

In women and men, new bone is constantly being produced and old bone broken down in a process called remodeling.

Until recently, doctors believed that a woman's peak bone-building years began in her childhood and extended to her 20s or 30s.

Recent finding: Bone growth slows significantly about 10 years earlier than previously thought.

For women, when estrogen levels decline at menopause, bone loss accelerates greatly. In the first five years after menopause, some women lose up to 25% of bone density.

Typically, men start to lose bone 10 years later than women. Testosterone deficiency and the use of certain steroid medications, such as *prednisone* (Deltasone), are some of the most common causes.

RISK FACTORS

A sedentary lifestyle, not getting enough bone-building calcium and vitamin D, and low body weight in women (less than 127 pounds) are the main causes of osteopenia.

Other key risk factors…

•**Very low-calorie diets.** Men and women who severely restrict calories—for example, consuming fewer than 1,000 to 1,200 calories daily—may not get enough dietary protein to ensure healthy bone growth.

•**Cola consumption.** Research has shown that drinking more than one 12-ounce cola daily significantly lowers bone density. That may be because cola contains phosphoric acid, which blocks calcium absorption.

•**Smoking.** It doubles the risk for osteopenia in women and men.

EARLY DETECTION

All menopausal and postmenopausal women as well as women and men of any age with two or more of the risk factors listed above should get a bone density test.

The most accurate test is dual-energy X-ray *absorptiometry* (DEXA). It is painless and takes only about 10 minutes and exposes patients to less radiation than that used for a chest X-ray. It usually costs about $200 and is covered by most insurance plans.

DEXA measures bone mineral density and converts the measurement into a standardized value called a T-score. The result shows how a patient's bone density compares with that of a typical 25-year-old woman. A higher T-score means stronger bones. A normal T-score is above -1.0...osteopenia, -1.0 to -2.5...and full-fledged osteoporosis, less than -2.5. If your results are abnormal, the test should be repeated every one to two years.

MAINTAINING BONE STRENGTH

Patients can stop further bone loss—or, in some cases, reverse osteopenia—with lifestyle steps...

•**Get adequate calcium.** You've heard it before—but there's no way around the importance of calcium. From age 25 to menopause, women need 1,200 mg daily, and 1,500 mg daily thereafter. Men need 1,000 mg daily from age 30 to 65, and 1,500 mg daily thereafter.

Dairy foods, including milk, have long been the most popular sources of calcium. An eight-ounce glass of milk provides about 300 mg—but only 25% to 30% of the mineral is actually absorbed.

What most people don't know: Juice can be a better calcium source than milk. An eight-ounce glass of calcium-fortified orange juice contains 350 mg (36% absorption).

Absorption rates are useful to know, so you can choose your calcium sources wisely. However, total daily calcium intake is based on the food product's available calcium rather than its absorption rate.

Supplements are acceptable if you don't get enough calcium in your diet. Calcium citrate and calcium carbonate supplements are equally effective. Calcium citrate can be taken at any time...calcium carbonate should be taken with meals. You can only absorb 500 mg to 600 mg of supplemental calcium at one time. If you're taking more, divide it into several daily doses.

•**Don't skip vitamin D.** Most younger adults synthesize adequate vitamin D from the sun, but older adults are less efficient at converting vitamin D into calcitriol, the hormone that stimulates calcium absorption.

What most people don't know: If vitamin D levels are low, bone building can be compromised.

Because it can be difficult to get enough of this vitamin, I recommend taking a 400-international unit (IU) supplement of vitamin D daily up to age 65...and 800 IU daily thereafter.

•**Eat vitamin K-rich foods.** Vitamin K aids calcium absorption.

Good sources: Red meat, eggs, cereals, fruit (prunes and blueberries) and vegetables (kale and spinach).

Caution: Sudden increases in vitamin K intake may decrease the effect of *warfarin* (Coumadin).

What most people don't know: Eating a single daily serving of vitamin K-rich green, leafy vegetables cuts the risk for hip fracture by 50%, compared with eating one serving weekly, according to the landmark Nurses' Health Study.

•**Perform strength training.** In addition to performing weight-bearing exercises, such as walking, running or using the stairs, back-strengthening exercises performed two to three times weekly can significantly increase bone strength.

What most people don't know: Bone responds better to heavier loads than frequent repetitions when weight-lifting.

Example: It's better to lift 25 pounds 10 times than to lift five pounds 50 times.

Important: If lifestyle measures are not adequate, medications, such as *alendronate* (Fosamax), *raloxifene* (Evista) or *calcitonin* (Miacalcin), may be needed.

Good News About Multiple Sclerosis

Moses Rodriguez, MD, division chair of neurology and professor of neurology and immunology at Mayo Clinic College of Medicine in Rochester, Minnesota, is the author of over 300 scientific papers on multiple sclerosis.

Multiple sclerosis occurs when immune cells target and destroy the myelin sheath that covers nerve cells in the brain and spinal cord, causing scarring that interferes with normal nerve-signal transmission. Depending on the location of the scarring, patients may suffer muscle spasms, vision loss, slurred speech, bladder, bowel or sexual dysfunction, dizziness, depression, numbness or tingling, cognitive problems and/or extreme fatigue.

Until recently, multiple sclerosis (MS) has been viewed as a debilitating disease that can condemn sufferers to wheelchairs and nursing homes.

Now: New studies at the renowned Mayo Clinic in Rochester, Minnesota, offer reason for optimism.

Background: Each year, more than 10,000 Americans are diagnosed with MS, an inflammatory disorder of the central nervous system. About 90% of MS patients have the "relapsing-remitting" form, suffering intermittent attacks of symptoms such as difficulty walking, visual disturbances, numbness, tingling and memory loss. Flare-ups are sometimes separated by years, followed by full or partial recovery.

The remaining 10% of patients have "primary-progressive" MS, which causes more continuous symptoms and a steady deterioration over a period of 10 to 20 years.

Researchers at Mayo Clinic have studied MS in Olmsted County, Minnesota (population 100,000), for 100 years. We've literally gone door to door to identify every person in the county with MS—and for the past 25 years we have tracked the progression of the disease in more than 170 confirmed patients. This method allows us to study patients with absent or mild MS symptoms, who are often missing from clinic-based studies that use only patients whose disease is active.

Our findings for the 90% of patients with the relapsing-remitting form of MS…

•**MS is benign in up to one-third of these patients,** causing minimal or no disability even after decades. For reasons that are still under investigation, these patients seem to have an intrinsic ability to repair themselves following acute MS flare-ups.

Although there is no way to predict at the onset whether MS will prove benign or progressive, we do know that people who do not suffer disability, including deficits in fine motor skills and coordination and bowel and bladder problems during the first five years, have a less than 10% chance of seeing their condition worsen over the next 10 to 30 years.

•**Another 50% of patients develop mild to moderate disabilities,** such as arm and/or leg weakness, tingling and/or numbness and mild incoordination, but are still able to walk unassisted after 10 or more years with MS.

•**Less than one-quarter of the patients with relapsing-remitting MS** ultimately suffer significant declines in their ability to function. Even for these patients, medications can alleviate symptoms.

IS MEDICATION NECESSARY?

In 2005, a new medication that had shown significant promise in early clinical trials—reducing the incidence of MS flare-ups by as much as 67%—was linked to two deaths. As a result, the drug *natalizumab* (Tysabri) was abruptly recalled just three months after receiving FDA approval.

National Multiple Sclerosis Society (NMSS) guidelines call for all patients with relapsing-remitting MS to begin treatment with older drugs to slow the disease's progression when a diagnosis is made. Patients are diagnosed after suffering two isolated attacks at least one month apart that damage more than one area of the central nervous system myelin—the sheath that surrounds and protects nerve fibers.

Recall, however, that our studies show that for one-third of MS patients who have the relapsing-remitting form, there will be minimal or no disease progression, even without treatment. This is no small consideration. The disease-modifying drugs prescribed for MS, including *glatiramer* (Copaxone), can reduce the frequency of MS attacks by 30% but can cost more than $20,000 annually and may not be covered by insurance. They must be injected as often as every other day and can produce serious side effects, including nausea, vomiting, fatigue, muscle aches and liver damage.

DR. RODRIGUEZ'S VIEW

The NMSS and many experts in the MS field believe that MS demands early intervention with these powerful drugs because the disease is so unpredictable. Based on our new research, however, I recommend that newly diagnosed patients take a wait-and-see approach when considering medication. If the patient experiences more than two attacks a year or shows signs of neurological deterioration, such as deficits in coordination and fine motor skills, we will initiate drug therapy.

For patients who go years between flare-ups, recover fully from attacks and experience minimal or no disability, the cost and side effects of drug treatment may be more damaging than the disease itself. For patients with this type of benign or mild MS, self-care measures can help keep the disease in check. *Key strategies...*

•**Reduce stress.** Studies have shown that stress can compromise healthy immune functioning, increasing your risk for MS flare-ups. Get plenty of rest and adequate sleep, and practice daily relaxation exercises, such as deep breathing or meditation.

•**Keep cool.** Many MS patients are heat-sensitive. Increases in body temperature brought on by warm weather or physical activity exacerbate their symptoms. Studies suggest that lowering body temperature by a degree or two can help bolster nerve-signal transmission. This may help relieve fatigue and improve mental functioning and muscle strength in MS patients. Cooling can be achieved with special garments (vests, hats, scarfs, etc.) designed for people who work in high-heat conditions. For more information, contact the Multiple Sclerosis Cooling Foundation, *www.mscooling.org*.

•**Take aspirin.** In a Mayo Clinic trial, we showed that taking 650 milligrams of aspirin twice daily significantly improves MS symptoms.

Researchers are unsure of aspirin's mechanism but believe it may work by reducing body temperature.

•**Exercise.** While heat-sensitive patients may need to limit vigorous aerobic activity, research confirms that moderate exercise greatly improves mobility and mood in people with MS. Swimming is an ideal choice, because the water prevents overheating.

•**Take vitamin D.** Studies suggest that not getting enough vitamin D through sun exposure or diet—in foods such as milk or sardines—is a significant risk factor for MS. Aim to get 15 or 20 minutes of sun exposure daily, before applying sunblock. Or take a daily supplement that provides 400 international units (IU) of vitamin D.

Ample evidence supports the use of these lifestyle changes, combined with a healthy diet (and avoiding smoking and alcohol), to help slow or halt the progression of mild to moderate MS.

Others with more serious symptoms or emerging disabilities should practice these measures and take a disease-modifying drug, such as *glatiramer, interferon beta-1a* (Avonex, Rebif) or *interferon beta-1b* (Betaseron).

The immune-suppressing drug *mitoxantrone* (Novantrone) also has recently been approved for treating steadily worsening relapsing-remitting MS. But this drug should be used with caution, due to serious potential side effects, including aggressive leukemia or lymphoma. There is still no approved treatment for primary-progressive MS.

ON THE HORIZON

New research suggests that estrogen and cholesterol-lowering drugs may prove useful in treating MS. In one small but promising study, the Alzheimer's drug *donepezil* (Aricept) improved memory in MS patients.

Kidney Stones: New Prevention Strategies

Glenn M. Preminger, MD, is professor of urologic surgery and director of the Comprehensive Kidney Stone Center at Duke University Medical Center in Durham, North Carolina.

A kidney stone is a hard mass that forms when certain minerals—calcium, oxalate and uric acid—fail to dissolve in the urine and then accumulate into solid crystals. Normally, urine contains chemicals, such as citrate, that inhibit stone formation. But some people are prone to stones due to diet, lifestyle and certain medical conditions, such as inflammatory bowel disease. Kidney stones can trigger sudden, searing pain in the back and side, often accompanied by blood in the urine, nausea and/or vomiting.

When a kidney stone creates a blockage in a ureter (one of the tubes that connect the kidney to the bladder), it can be excruciatingly painful. Each year, kidney stones affect more than one million Americans. Fortunately, new research is identifying highly effective prevention and treatment options.

Recent findings…

• **Lemonade fights kidney stones.** Researchers recently tracked stone-prone patients for up to four years and found that those who drank two quarts of lemonade daily had fewer new stones…and little or no growth of existing ones.

Why it works: Lemon juice contains high amounts of *citrate*, a substance that inhibits kidney stones by reducing urine acidity and binding with urinary calcium. Potassium citrate, in pill or liquid form, is routinely prescribed for stone prevention. Lemonade isn't as potent as potassium citrate, but it does appear to be a viable alternative for patients who can't take or tolerate the drug (people with impaired kidney function, for example), or for those who wish to avoid another medication.

To reap the study-proven benefits, you need to drink two quarts of homemade lemonade daily. The lemonade should be made by mixing two quarts of water with four ounces of reconstituted lemon juice. To reduce or eliminate sugar and/ or calories, consider using artificial sweeteners. Since stone formers are advised to drink three quarts of fluid daily as a preventative, you'll benefit even more if two of those quarts are lemonade.

• **Alpha blockers can speed stone passage.** For years, researchers have searched for ways to facilitate spontaneous passage of kidney stones that are stuck in a ureter so that patients would be spared stone removal via a procedure such as an endoscopic technique, using a thin, telescopic tube.

Good news: In multiple trials conducted over the last five years, alpha blockers—prescription drugs traditionally used to treat an enlarged prostate—have proven to be remarkably effective for speeding and easing the elimination of small stones (less than six millimeters in diameter) from a ureter. These drugs increase the likelihood of spontaneous passage of small stones by about 90%.

Alpha blockers work by relaxing smooth muscle cells lining the ureter, improving urine flow and preventing the painful contractions that can slow or block stone movement. It's now become the standard of care to start most ureteral stone patients on a trial of alpha blockers. In a majority of cases, the drugs allow the stones to pass spontaneously. A small percentage of patients who take alpha blockers experience orthostatic hypotension—light-headedness when quickly standing up.

• **Obesity and weight gain elevate kidney stone risk.** Several recent studies confirm that being overweight and/or gaining weight significantly increases kidney stone risk. A large-scale, long-term study shows that obese men are 44% more likely, and obese women 90% more likely, to develop stones than are their leaner counterparts. Gaining more than 35 pounds during adulthood also heightens risk (by 39% for men and up to 82% for women), compared with maintaining a stable weight.

What's the connection between kidney stones and weight gain? As recent studies show, many adults who are significantly overweight also have type 2 diabetes (often undiagnosed) or are insulin resistant—that is, their bodies have a reduced ability to respond to insulin, which causes the pancreas to secrete excessive amounts of insulin. Insulin resistance and diabetes raise the acid levels in urine—a primary risk factor for stones. Losing weight is the ideal antidote. But if that's not possible, alkali therapy, in the form of potassium citrate, may be prescribed to reduce the acid load in urine to prevent stones.

DIETARY MEASURES

For prevention, people with a personal or family history of kidney stones should…

• **Drink three quarts of fluid daily,** mostly noncaffeinated. Coffee and tea are fine in moderation.

• **Get enough calcium.** Though stone formers had long been advised to limit calcium intake, recent studies link insufficient calcium to increased risk for stones.

That's because calcium can bind with stone-producing oxalates in the digestive tract, preventing these minerals from concentrating in the urine. Aim for two to three servings daily of low-fat milk, cheese, yogurt or calcium-fortified juice or cereal.

Caution: Calcium supplements may not be the best source. Studies show that they may raise urinary calcium excretion, a risk factor for stones. If you have a personal or family history of kidney stones and wish to take calcium supplements, have your urine tested after three months to check for elevated calcium levels.

•**Limit salt.** Excess sodium steals calcium from your bones and causes it to accumulate in your urine, increasing your risk for kidney stones. Don't add salt to your food…and avoid highly processed, prepackaged foods.

•**Avoid high-oxalate foods,** such as spinach, tea, chocolate, nuts, asparagus and rhubarb. Our bodies also convert some vitamin C into oxalates, and studies suggest that too much can raise urinary oxalate levels. Stone formers should not exceed 2,000 mg (2 g) of vitamin C daily.

•**Cut back on meat.** Animal protein, particularly from red meat, raises acid levels in the urine, increasing kidney stone risk. Aim for three or fewer red meat servings weekly.

The Disease Doctors Misdiagnose

L. Ebony Boulware, MD, MPH, an internist and assistant professor of medicine and epidemiology at the Welch Center for Prevention, Epidemiology and Clinical Research at Johns Hopkins University School of Medicine in Baltimore, was lead author of a study on physicians' recognition of the signs and symptoms of kidney disease. Dr. Boulware won a Clinician Investigator Award from the Society of General Internal Medicine.

It's widely known that diseases such as high blood pressure (hypertension) and diabetes can go undetected for quite some time. But few patients—and a relatively small percentage of doctors—realize that chronic kidney disease (CKD) is equally threatening and often remains hidden.

Danger: CKD—and subsequent kidney damage—can be markedly slowed with medications and also by controlling the underlying causes. Yet many primary care physicians don't fully understand how to diagnose this condition or how to assess the main risk factors.

Result: Many of the estimated 20 million Americans with CKD aren't diagnosed as early as they could be. By the time symptoms appear, the kidneys could have lost more than 75% of their normal function. At that point, the damage may be so extensive that patients will eventually require dialysis or a kidney transplant—or they die waiting.

Simple blood and urine tests can detect most cases of early CKD. Patients who are diagnosed and referred to a nephrologist (kidney specialist) early are often able to delay dialysis or transplant, or even avoid them altogether.

WHAT'S GETTING MISSED?

One of the main functions of the kidneys is to eliminate wastes, such as urea, from the body. In CKD, damage to the filtering units (nephrons) in the kidneys is typically caused by hypertension or diabetes, usually over a period of decades. About 45% of CKD cases are caused by diabetes, while 27% are caused by hypertension. Because CKD causes no symptoms, laboratory tests are the only way to detect it early.

That's why patients with hypertension, diabetes or other risk factors for CKD should have tests for kidney function during annual exams. But even that might not be enough. A new study reports that many doctors miss the signs of early CKD even when those signs should be apparent to them.

The study: Researchers at Johns Hopkins University School of Medicine asked 304 randomly selected US doctors, including kidney specialists, internists and family physicians, to evaluate the medical files of a fictitious patient.

The doctors also were given the raw data needed to calculate the glomerular filtration rate, an important measure of kidney function. They were asked to calculate this number themselves using accepted equations.

Result: Of the kidney specialists surveyed, 97% accurately diagnosed CKD, and 99% of those said they would have recommended that a primary care physician refer the patient to a kidney specialist. Among the internists, only 78% made the proper diagnosis of CKD, and 81% of those recommended a referral to a kidney specialist. Even worse, only 59% of the family physicians made an accurate diagnosis of CKD, and only 76% of those recommended a specialist referral.

The implications of this study are troublesome. Delays in diagnosing CKD greatly increase the risk for complications, including heart disease.

Recent finding: CKD promotes atherosclerosis and is an independent risk factor (like smoking, diabetes or hypertension) for cardiovascular disease.

SELF-PROTECTION

Blood and/or urine tests, when interpreted properly, can easily detect early CKD, but doctors don't order these tests as often as they should. Patients who have been diagnosed with diabetes or hypertension should insist on getting tested for CKD. This is particularly important for African-Americans. They are six times more likely than Caucasians to develop hypertension-related kidney failure. People age 60 or older—even if they don't have diabetes or hypertension—also may want to be tested, because they are at higher risk for CKD. The testing can be done by a primary care physician. *Main tests...*

•**Serum creatinine.** CKD curbs the ability of the kidneys to remove wastes from the body. One such waste is creatinine (a substance derived from protein metabolized in muscle). Elevated levels in the blood indicate kidney disease.

Trap: Creatinine alone is not a good marker of kidney function. An older adult, or someone with a small frame, could have a normal level of creatinine and still have CKD. An additional step (below) is needed for accurate results.

•**Modification of Diet in Renal Disease equation.** Many physicians aren't aware of this equation. It's considered the gold standard for calculating glomerular filtration rate, the best measure of kidney function. The equation, which is available to physicians on the National Kidney Foundation Web site (*www.kidney.org*), takes into account the creatinine level as well as the patient's age, gender, race and other factors.

•**Albumin.** This is a protein that's often present in the urine of patients with CKD. It's detected by dipping a test strip in a urine sample. The presence of albumin usually indicates kidney damage caused by diabetes. This test is mainly recommended for patients with diabetes or other risk factors for CKD.

•**Cystatin C.** This is a relatively new test—and might be more accurate than creatinine for diagnosing CKD. Cystatin C is a protein that's normally filtered out of the blood by the kidneys. Elevated levels indicate that the kidneys aren't working at optimal levels.

TREATING CKD

Apart from a transplant operation, there isn't a cure for CKD. The most important strategy is to control (or prevent) hypertension and diabetes through medication and lifestyle changes, such as following a low-fat, low-salt diet. These conditions can double or triple the risk of CKD—and accelerate the damage in patients who already have it.

Because many patients with CKD also have hypertension, doctors often prescribe blood pressure medication. Lowering blood pressure to below 120/80 mmHg can significantly slow the progression of CKD. These drugs also are helpful for patients with CKD caused by diabetes.

Important: Studies have shown that using an angiotensin converting enzyme (ACE) inhibitor, such as *captopril* (Capoten) or *ramipril (*Altace), or angiotensin II receptor blocker, such as *irbesartan* (Avapro) or *candesartan* (Atacand), can slow the progression of CKD by as much as 30%. These drugs are effective even in CKD patients who don't have hypertension or diabetes.

What Most Doctors Don't Know About Heartburn

Lauren Gerson, MD, an associate professor of medicine at Stanford University School of Medicine and the director of the school's Esophageal and Small Bowel Disorders Center, both in Stanford, California. Dr. Gerson is the recipient of the Gastroenterology Research Group Young Investigator Clinical Research Award.

Most doctors tell patients who suffer from the searing, shooting pain of heartburn to avoid spicy foods, alcohol and chocolate. But new research has shown that for the majority of heartburn sufferers, switching to a bland diet doesn't eliminate pain-causing acid reflux.

SURPRISING NEW RESEARCH

Heartburn occurs when acid from the stomach backs up into the esophagus through a relaxed lower esophageal sphincter (the valve that prevents stomach acid from entering the esophagus). For decades, physicians have told heartburn patients to stop eating foods that can cause the sphincter to exert less pressure—namely, spicy, fried or fatty foods, as well as citrus, caffeinated or alcoholic beverages.

However, in my own practice, most of my patients who severely limited their diets for heartburn relief still had reflux. With this in mind, my colleagues and I set out to determine whether food avoidance actually has any benefit.

In an analysis recently published in *Archives of Internal Medicine*, we reviewed more than 2,000 studies published between 1975 and 2004 and found no evidence that removing specific foods or beverages from the diet would eliminate heartburn in most people.

A small percentage of heartburn sufferers do have triggers.

Example: Red wine causes immediate heartburn in sensitive patients, possibly because of its acid content. Such people should avoid red wine and/or take preventive medication.

Some so-called heartburn triggers, such as caffeine-rich coffee and chocolate, as well as tea and cola, have been linked to relaxation of the esophageal sphincter. However, our findings suggest that the sphincter would relax regardless of the types of food eaten. Therefore, avoiding caffeinated foods won't eliminate heartburn.

We found the same to be true for spicy foods, citrus, alcoholic beverages and even smoking —no studies have shown that eliminating these "triggers" caused an actual reduction in heartburn symptoms. More research is needed to determine systematically if food avoidance can benefit heartburn sufferers, since very few published studies have been designed to examine this question.

LIFESTYLE CHANGES

Although diet had no effect on reflux relief, our research found that there are two factors that could reduce the incidence of heartburn—weight loss and elevating the head of the bed. Try these approaches—and other proven strategies—for four to six weeks before taking heartburn medication, which can cause headache, diarrhea and other side effects.

•**Weight loss.** Excess body weight places additional pressure on the abdomen, which may cause the lower esophageal sphincter to relax.

Researchers have found that normal-weight adults in the Nurses' Health Study who gained 20 pounds developed acid reflux or worsened existing symptoms. Risk increased with greater weight gain.

Fortunately, studies have shown that weight loss brings relief. Portion control is more important than the foods you select.

•**Raise your head at night.** Elevating the head of the bed at least six inches by putting blocks or bricks under the frame guards against heartburn by helping keep acid out of the esophagus. If you don't feel comfortable raising the bed frame, buy a foam wedge pillow six to eight inches thick to place under your pillow. Wedges can be found in pharmacies or on-line at sites such as *www.medslant.com* (800-346-1850)…or *www.foamcenter.com.*

Typical cost: $20 to $90.

•**Avoid large meals.** Overeating can aggravate heartburn, since the stomach produces more acid for digestion. Additionally, fatty foods can delay emptying of the stomach, and that can lead to reflux.

•**Stop eating three hours before going to bed.** Late-night eating may cause problems for some people. A few studies have shown that heartburn didn't disappear when patients skipped late-night meals, but the pH level of acid in the esophagus improved, indicating that less acid was present.

•**Exercise.** Staying active can help you lose weight, which can offer relief. Some people find that vigorous physical activity worsens heartburn—exercise can slow stomach emptying and interfere with gastrointestinal absorption, but low-impact exercise, such as walking, typically does not have that effect.

HEARTBURN MEDICATIONS

If the above steps don't work within several weeks (or longer if you're trying to lose weight), consider...

•**Antacids.** Start with fast-acting over-the-counter (OTC) antacids, such as Tums or Mylanta. Use them for intermittent reflux, not for long-term treatment (six weeks or more).

Warning: The calcium in Tums can cause constipation, and the magnesium in Mylanta can cause diarrhea. Check with your pharmacist if you're taking other medications—antacids can interfere with the absorption of some drugs.

•**H2 blockers.** When antacids aren't strong enough, consider an H2 blocker, such as *famotidine* (Pepcid) or *ranitidine* (Zantac), both of which are available OTC. Side effects, such as headache and diarrhea, are uncommon.

•**Proton pump inhibitors.** If heartburn isn't squelched by other medications, try a proton pump inhibitor, such as *omeprazole* (Prilosec) or *lansoprazole* (Prevacid). Side effects, including headache and diarrhea, are rare.

A recent study examined whether the use of proton pump inhibitors was linked to infection with *Clostridium difficile*, a bacterium that can cause diarrhea, fever and abdominal pain. These drugs reduce the amount of stomach acid, so researchers thought some C. difficile bacteria that would normally be killed in the stomach could survive, causing intestinal problems. Additional research is needed.

DRUG-FREE ALTERNATIVES

Some people who want to relieve heartburn without medication try consuming papaya juice or ginger. No studies have examined the relationship between these products and heartburn, but ingesting them shouldn't cause health problems.

SCREEN FOR CANCER

Long-term heartburn sufferers are at increased risk of developing Barrett's esophagus, a precancerous condition caused by years of acid being regurgitated into the esophagus. Barrett's can lead to esophageal cancer. People with chronic reflux lasting more than six to 12 months should get an endoscopy (in which a flexible, lighted tube is used to examine the digestive system) to screen for Barrett's and esophageal cancer.

Natural Heartburn Relief

Ara DerMarderosian, PhD, is professor of pharmacognosy (the study of natural products used in medicine) and is director of the Complementary and Alternative Medicine Institute at the University of the Sciences in Philadelphia.

Many people who suffer from heartburn take over-the-counter antacids or expensive prescription medication, such as *esomeprazole* (Nexium) and *lansoprazole* (Prevacid). These treatments can help but often cause side effects, such as diarrhea and dry mouth.

Heartburn, a sharp, burning pain under the rib cage, occurs when stomach contents "back up" (reflux) into the esophagus.

Chamomile, ginger and deglycyrrhizinated licorice have long been used (in tea, extract and tincture) to relieve heartburn as well as indigestion and intestinal irritation. Their effectiveness is supported by anecdotal evidence.

For relief proven in clinical studies, try pectin, a substance found in the outer skin and rind of fruits and vegetables. Apples and bananas are among the best sources of pectin. If you suffer from heartburn, try eating an apple (do not choose green or other tart varieties) or a banana to see if it relieves your symptoms.

Pectin supplements, which are available at most health-food stores, are another option. Take at the onset of heartburn until it subsides. For dosage, follow label instructions. Pectin supplements are generally safe but may interfere with the absorption of some medications, so check with your doctor before trying this supplement.

Caution: Chronic heartburn (more than twice a week) may indicate gastroesophageal reflux disease (GERD), a condition that should be treated by a gastroenterologist.

■ ■ ■ ■

Heartburn Drug Warning

Drugs for heartburn and reflux disease increase risk of intestinal infections. Medications such as *esomeprazole* (Nexium), *lansoprazole* (Prevacid), *cimetidine* (Tagamet) and *ranitidine* (Zantac) suppress the stomach acid that fights bacteria.

Side effect: A two- to threefold increase in risk of a *Clostridium difficile* bacterial infection, which can cause diarrhea, colitis and other intestinal problems.

Self-defense: If you use a heartburn or reflux drug, be vigilant about washing your hands, which will kill C. difficile bacteria. Consult your physician if you have frequent diarrhea containing mucus or blood. C. difficile infections are treated with antibiotics.

Sandra Dial, MD, is assistant professor of medicine and director of respiratory medicine, McGill University, Montreal, Quebec, Canada, and leader of a study, published in *Journal of the American Medical Association*.

■ ■ ■ ■

Fatty Foods Lead to Heartburn

High-fiber, low-fat diet may prevent heartburn, according to research.

Recent finding: People who ate four servings of fat were twice as likely to have heartburn than those who ate one serving. Heartburn, which affects about one in five Americans, is caused when stomach acids enter the esophagus. Fat may increase reflux by filling the lower end of the esophagus, thus making it easier to reflux. It also promotes obesity, which is a risk factor for reflux. Fiber may bind to some of the fat, making reflux less harmful. If left untreated, heartburn can lead to ulcers, bleeding in the esophagus and esophageal cancer.

Hashem B. El-Serag, MD, MPH, associate professor of medicine, Baylor College of Medicine, Houston, and leader of a study of 371 people with and without heartburn symptoms, published in *Gut*.

Nausea? Heartburn? Stomach Pain? You Might Have a Hernia

Robert Kozol, MD, FACS, is professor and chair, department of surgery, University of Connecticut Health Center, Farmington, and is part of the colon cancer prevention program team. He has been a member of the European Union Hernia Research Cooperative and participated in the Veterans Administration Cooperative Hernia study, published in *The New England Journal of Medicine*.

Most hernias cause no symptoms or only mild discomfort. Many people don't even know that they have one until it is discovered during tests for other problems. Some hernias, however, cause nausea, heartburn or abdominal or testicular pain. Some can be life-threatening.

A hernia is the protrusion of an internal organ into an area where it's not supposed to be. For example, part of the intestine can poke through the diaphragm or protrude into the groin or through the abdominal wall.

The most common types of hernia and best treatments…

HIATAL HERNIA

A hiatal hernia occurs at the opening in the diaphragm (the hiatus), where the esophagus passes through to join the stomach. If the opening is larger than it should be or the surrounding tissue is weak, the upper portion of the stomach can bulge through the diaphragm into the chest cavity.

One-quarter to one-half of Americans have hiatal hernias. They are four times more common in women than men. Most cause no symptoms. In a minority of cases, they result in gastroesophageal reflux disease (GERD), which causes heartburn and occasionally nausea or cramping. *Two main types…*

Sliding hiatal hernias, which account for at least 90% of cases, occur when the hiatal junction—the area where the esophagus meets the stomach—slides into the chest cavity. These require treatment only when they cause severe or persistent GERD.

Paraesophageal hiatal hernias account for less than 10% of cases, but they are more dangerous. Part of the stomach protrudes into the chest, but the hiatal junction remains in the abdomen. There's a risk that the stomach and junction will twist and block circulation, causing stomach or esophageal tissues to die.

Warning: See your doctor immediately if you have severe pain in the upper abdominal or lower chest areas…suddenly have trouble swallowing…or can't eat more than a few bites at a time. These are signs that the stomach has twisted. You may need emergency surgery.

SELF-CARE

Patients without symptoms don't need treatment. If you're experiencing GERD, lifestyle approaches, such as eating smaller meals, avoiding fatty foods and not lying down within three hours of eating, can help relieve it. *If these steps don't work, try...*

•**Over-the-counter antacids,** which neutralize acidity in the esophagus and reduce heartburn in most patients. *If they don't work, your doctor may prescribe...*

•H2 blockers, such as *famotidine* (Pepcid), *cimetidine* (Tagamet) and *ranitidine* (Zantac), which reduce stomach acid and usually are taken before meals. These are available over-the-counter and in stronger prescription strengths.

•Prescription and over-the-counter proton pump inhibitors, such as *lansoprazole* (Prevacid) and *omeprazole* (Prilosec), which reduce stomach acid secretion and are taken once a day.

SURGERY

You may need surgery if medications and lifestyle changes don't control GERD...or if the stomach has twisted...or there's pressure on the esophagus that is causing bleeding or obstruction.

The surgery, *Nissen fundoplication*, usually is done laparoscopically through small incisions in the abdomen.

The top of the stomach is wrapped around the esophagus, and the opening in the diaphragm is sutured or stapled to make it smaller so the stomach can't protrude.

Most patients who have this procedure spend one or two nights in the hospital and recover fully within a month. GERD symptoms disappear in more than 90% of cases.

INGUINAL HERNIA

This type of hernia occurs when an organ pokes through a weak point in the groin. It can be painful, especially when you cough or lift a heavy object.

In men, the weak spot often occurs along the inguinal canal. This is where the spermatic cord enters the scrotum. Men are almost 10 times more likely to develop these hernias than women.

In women, the inguinal canal carries a ligament that helps hold the uterus in place. Hernias may occur where connective tissue from the uterus attaches to tissue surrounding the pubic bone.

Most inguinal hernias get larger over time. Though they can be excruciatingly painful, they aren't dangerous. However, a loop of intestine may get trapped in the weak point in the groin and obstruct the bowel or block circulation to the intestine. This condition—strangulation—can kill bowel tissue and is a life-threatening emergency. Warning signs include severe pain at the hernia site, skin redness and vomiting.

SELF-CARE

You may notice a bulge in the groin or the scrotum from the protruding intestine. You also may experience groin or scrotal pain when bending over, coughing or lifting. *You can temporarily relieve mild discomfort by...*

•**Lying on your back** and gently pushing the bulge into the abdominal cavity.

•**Sleeping with your hips higher than your abdomen** to make the intestine less likely to protrude.

SURGERY

If the hernia is painful or growing larger, your doctor may recommend surgery. *There are two main types...*

•**Herniorrhaphy.** The surgeon makes an incision in your groin and pushes the protruding intestine back into your abdomen, then repairs the weakened area by sewing it together. It may take as long as six weeks before you're able to resume normal activities.

•**Hernioplasty.** This is like patching a tire—a piece of synthetic mesh is sutured or stapled over the weak area. It closes the opening and prevents the intestine from protruding. It can be performed conventionally with a single long incision or laparoscopically with several small incisions. With laparoscopic repair, most people are back to work within a few days. Laparoscopy might not be an option if you have a very large hernia or if your intestine is pushed down into the scrotum.

PREVENTION

Some hernias are caused by congenital (inborn) weakness in the tissue walls. Other hernias are caused by "wear and tear." *To reduce your risk...*

•**Maintain a healthy weight.** Obesity puts extra pressure on weakened tissue.

•**Treat a cough.** A chronic cough increases abdominal pressure. This is another reason to quit smoking.

• **Avoid heavy lifting** to reduce pressure on the abdomen.

• **Eat a high-fiber diet** and drink water to avoid constipation. Straining can worsen hernias.

Is Your Heartburn Really A Hidden Hernia?

J. Scott Roth, MD, assistant professor of surgery at the University of Maryland School of Medicine, director of the University of Maryland Hernia Center and head of surgical endoscopy at the University of Maryland Medical Center, all in Baltimore.

Most people are familiar with the type of hernia that appears as a bulge in the groin. Much more common in men than in women, this type of hernia (known as an *inguinal* hernia) occurs when part of the intestine protrudes into the groin, possibly as a result of pressure caused by lifting heavy objects and/or straining during a bowel movement.

WHAT IS A HERNIA?

A hernia is a protrusion of an organ or tissue into a part of the body where it does not belong. Some types of hernias appear as bulges on the outside of the body—in the groin, for example —while other hernias can be detected only with medical tests, such as a barium X-ray.

What you may not know: There is another type of hernia, called a *hiatal* hernia, that far fewer people are aware of, even though estimates show that it occurs in up to six out of 10 people over age 60. A hiatal hernia, in which a portion of the stomach protrudes into the chest cavity, usually causes no symptoms. When symptoms do occur, however, they are often misdiagnosed as ordinary heartburn and/or nausea.

WHEN THE STOMACH MOVES

The *diaphragm* (a dome-shaped muscle that helps with breathing) separates the abdominal and chest cavities. The esophagus passes from the throat through an opening in the diaphragm (*hiatus*) to the stomach. The diaphragm opening is normally less than one inch across.

In patients with hiatal hernias, the opening is larger—sometimes up to 4.7 inches.

Result: The upper portion of the stomach can poke through the enlarged hole into the chest cavity. As the hernia enlarges, an increasing amount of the stomach may enter the chest. Large hiatal hernias may cause swallowing difficulties, nausea and vomiting.

Very large hiatal hernias, in which a significant portion of the stomach has entered the chest, can sometimes be detected during a physical exam. A doctor may be able to detect bowel sounds inside the chest cavity. In most cases, hiatal hernias can be diagnosed only with a barium X-ray (the patient drinks a chalky liquid that coats—and illuminates—the upper digestive tract) or an endoscopic procedure, in which a doctor uses a lighted tube to view the esophagus and stomach.

RISK FACTORS FOR HERNIAS

Some people have a genetic susceptibility to hernias—they're born with an unusually large hiatus or the opening enlarges due to weakness in the surrounding muscles.

As with inguinal hernias, repeated abdominal pressure—from lifting heavy objects, straining to have bowel movements, being overweight, and/or severe coughing, sneezing or vomiting —may increase risk for hiatal hernias.

Two types of hiatal hernias…

• **Sliding hernias** are the most common. They occur when a small portion of the stomach (typically about an inch) "slides" into the chest cavity, then returns to its normal position. This movement reduces pressure on the lower esophageal sphincter (LES), a circular band of muscle at the base of the esophagus, allowing reflux (backing up) of stomach acid.

• **Paraesophageal hernias,** though quite rare, are potentially more serious. The upper part of the stomach rises until it's next to the LES. This can restrict (strangulate) blood flow in the stomach, which if untreated, can result in necrosis (death) of the stomach. If the necrosis is not treated, it can be fatal.

If a paraesophageal hernia causes symptoms, such as chest pain, it should be surgically repaired.

CONTROLLING HEARTBURN

Without treatment, the chronic surge of stomach acid that occurs in patients with symptomatic hiatal hernias can cause inflammation of the esophagus…iron-deficiency anemia from esophageal bleeding…or premalignant changes (Barrett's esophagus) that can lead to esophageal cancer. Some patients experience difficulty breathing or even severe chest pain that resembles a heart attack.

Most people with hiatal hernias don't require surgical repair as long as they can minimize discomfort and damage caused by the reflux of stomach acid. *My advice…*

•**Make lifestyle changes.** Most patients with hernia-related heartburn require medication, but some improve significantly with lifestyle adjustments…

•Avoid eating within four to five hours of bedtime. Eating stimulates the production of stomach acid, which is more likely to cause heartburn when patients lie down soon afterward.

•Avoid peppermint and caffeine. Both reduce muscle tension in the LES, the muscular band that helps prevent reflux.

•Raise the head of the bed about six inches. Gravity can prevent stomach acid from moving into your esophagus while you sleep. Use bricks, wood or plastic risers designed to elevate the head of the bed.

•**Consider taking medication.** For most medical conditions, doctors usually prefer to start treatment with the mildest drugs first. In my experience, the opposite approach—starting strong, then tapering off, if possible—seems to work better for hernia-related heartburn…

•Proton-pump inhibitors (PPIs) are considered the strongest heartburn medication, so your doctor may advise you to start with one of these drugs. PPIs, such as *omeprazole* (Prilosec) and *esomeprazole* (Nexium), inhibit acid production in the stomach and allow damaged tissues to heal. If a PPI taken twice daily improves symptoms within about six weeks, your doctor may suggest that you cut back to one dose a day.

•Antacids and H2-blockers. If heartburn symptoms continue to improve over roughly a six-week period, you can probably switch to a milder (and less expensive) drug, such as an over-the-counter antacid or H2-blocker, including *famotidine* (Pepcid) or *cimetidine* (Tagamet), for occasional relief.

WHEN TO CONSIDER SURGERY

Most people with hiatal hernias can control heartburn with drugs alone. Therefore, surgery is recommended only if you have a twisted stomach that endangers your stomach's blood supply…complications, such as scarring or bleeding due to reflux…or severe discomfort or reflux of stomach contents (such as bile or digestive enzymes) that isn't relieved by medications. Surgery also is recommended for patients who no longer wish to take reflux medications.

Most hernias, including hiatal hernias, are repaired with laparoscopic "keyhole" surgery, in which the surgeon inserts a camera and instruments through four or five small (less than half an inch) incisions in the abdomen.

About 95% of patients who receive surgery for hiatal hernias will no longer need medication to control symptoms.

Herbal Remedies For Flatulence

Anil Minocha, MD, professor of medicine and director of the division of digestive diseases at the University of Mississippi Medical Center in Jackson, is the author of *Natural Stomach Care*. Avery.

Eating certain foods, such as beans and some fruits and vegetables, can lead to flatulence (gas or air in the stomach or intestine that is expelled through the anus). Fortunately, dozens of carminative (gas-reducing) herbs can help relieve flatulence. Use them one at a time or in combination. *Best choices…*

•**Chamomile** relaxes the bowel, which reduces intestinal spasms. Steep a tea bag in hot water for about 10 minutes. Drink one cup before bedtime.

•**Ginger** is an antispasmodic that reduces the force and frequency of intestinal contractions. It's good for most digestive complaints, including gas. Peel and slice one inch of ginger root and boil in three cups of water for 20 minutes. Drink one to three cups daily. Or take 500 mg of ginger capsules or powder three times a day.

•**Fennel seeds** calm an upset stomach and reduce gas. Munch on a handful of seeds to ease or prevent gas. They're available at health-food stores. *For additional relief...*

•**Massage your abdomen** when you have painful gas. With moderate pressure, use your palms to massage your abdomen clockwise— the direction that food moves through the gastro-intestinal tract—for five to 10 minutes. Massage pushes out gas and relieves discomfort.

•**Try a simple yoga posture** to help purge gas from your intestine.

What to do: Lie on your back, pull your knees to your chest and rock in a circular motion.

•**Perform daily exercise** to help move gas out of the intestine and reduce painful pressure.

Best: Walking, tai chi and bicycling.

The Covered-Up Cause of IBS

Nancy Kraft, RD, clinical dietitian, University of Iowa, Iowa City.
Theodore M. Bayless, MD, professor of medicine, Johns Hopkins University, Baltimore.
American College of Gastroenterology annual meeting, Baltimore.

Cutting back on sugar and fat makes sense for people trying to control their weight, but there may be another health benefit. Two studies suggest that fat and fructose, the sugar in fruits and honey, also can contribute to gastrointestinal discomfort.

Irritable bowel syndrome (IBS) is a common disorder of the intestines that leads to pain, gassiness, bloating and changes in bowel habits, according to the American Gastroenterological Association. The disorder can lead to constipation in some and diarrhea in others. Some people experience both. Another common symptom may be a crampy urge to move the bowels.

In the first report, Nancy Kraft, a clinical dietitian from the University of Iowa, and her colleagues say some patients who have IBS are fructose-intolerant, and restricting that type of sugar can improve their symptoms.

Kraft says fructose intolerance often is an overlooked component of IBS.

Her colleague Dr. Young Choi says that, "a fructose-restricted diet significantly improved symptoms in patients with IBS and fructose intolerance. Fructose intolerance is yet another piece of the IBS puzzle."

THE STUDY

In the study, the 14 patients with IBS who followed a fructose-free diet for one year experienced a significant reduction in abdominal pain, bloating and diarrhea.

However, IBS symptoms remained the same for the 12 patients who did not stick with the diet, the researchers report.

Kraft believes these results are encouraging, because "people who limit their intake of fructose see their symptoms improve or disappear," but that further study is needed.

SECOND STUDY

Researchers from the Mayo Clinic in Rochester, Minnesota, led by Dr. Yuri Saito, collected data on the diets of 221 adults, aged 20 to 50 years. Of these patients, 102 had gastrointestinal disorders and 119 were healthy.

The research team found that patients with IBS or dyspepsia (indigestion) reported eating more monounsaturated fats compared with healthy patients. These patients also ate fewer carbohydrates than their healthy counterparts.

The Mayo investigators concluded that "future studies are needed to determine whether fat intake causes gastrointestinal symptoms."

Dr. Theodore M. Bayless, a professor of medicine at Johns Hopkins University, is not surprised that fat and fructose are linked with IBS and dyspepsia.

He notes that both fat and fructose are hard to digest and can aggravate both conditions. But Bayless does not believe that restricting fructose cures IBS; it may only relieve symptoms.

He advises his patients to avoid fatty foods and foods that contain high levels of fructose, such as grapes, dates, nuts, honey and apple and pear juice. Another common source of fructose is high fructose corn syrup, a sweetener in many processed foods. He also advises patients to increase fiber intake.

Understanding IBS and How to Control It

Elizabeth Lipski, PhD, CCN, who has been working in the field of holistic and complementary medicine for more than 25 years. She is director of doctoral studies at Hawthorn University in Whitethorn, California and author of *Digestive Wellness* (McGraw-Hill) and *Leaky Gut Syndrome* (McGraw-Hill). *www.lizlipski.com.*

Your abdomen bloats and cramps. You pass so much gas that you think you might be contributing to global warming. You have diarrhea or constipation or an alternating assault of both.

Your problem: Irritable Bowel Syndrome (IBS), the most common gastrointestinal complaint, accounting for 10% of doctor's visits and about 50% of referrals to gastroenterologists. But the fact that doctors see a lot of IBS doesn't mean that they understand the condition or treat it effectively.

IBS is a well-recognized but unexplained set of symptoms—medical science knows *what* is happening but not exactly *why*. A diagnosis isn't made by detecting telltale biochemical or structural changes unique to IBS—it's made after other digestive disorders, such as colorectal cancer and inflammatory bowel disease, have been ruled out.

At that point, the typical doctor offers a predictable prescription—eat more fiber, drink more water, get more exercise, reduce stress.

While that regimen may work for some, it fails many because it overlooks a common but often ignored trigger of IBS—*food hypersensitivity.*

TRIGGER FOODS

To understand food hypersensitivity, you first need to understand what it is not—a food allergy. Food allergies are relatively rare, affecting 1% to 2% of the adult population. The ingested food attracts the immune system's *immunoglobulin E* (IgE) antibodies, which identify the food as "foreign" and attack it, sparking the release of *histamine* and *cytokines,* inflammatory chemicals that cause tissue to swell, eyes to tear, skin to itch and other allergic symptoms. Eggs, milk, nuts, shellfish, soy and wheat are common allergy-causing foods.

Food hypersensitivity involves other antibodies, such as IgA, IgG and IgM. Their attack isn't immediate—it can occur hours or days after eating an offending food and cause bloating, cramping, constipation and/or diarrhea.

What to do: For one week, eat an "elimination diet" consisting solely of foods that almost never cause hypersensitivity—fruits (except citrus), vegetables (except tomatoes, eggplant, white potatoes and peppers), white rice, fish and chicken. You can use olive and safflower oils. If after seven days you are symptom-free, food hypersensitivity is triggering your IBS. *Follow these steps...*

Step 1: Reintroduce one category of food every two to three days. Start with one of the foods that together account for 80% of food hypersensitivity—beef, citrus, dairy products, eggs, pork and wheat. For two days, stay on the elimination diet and eat as much of the reintroduced food as you like.

If IBS symptoms return, you have detected a hypersensitivity. Stop eating the offending food, and wait until symptoms disappear to reintroduce another food.

If you don't get symptoms, try the next food after the two days of eating the previous one. Repeat this process, reintroducing foods one by one.

Step 2: For the next six months, avoid all foods that caused IBS during the elimination testing. This will help your bowel heal.

Step 3: After the six months, you can try a "rotation diet"—reintroduce the offending foods (as long as they don't cause symptoms), but eat any offending food no more than once every four days. Now that your digestive tract is healed, you may be able to handle small amounts of the offending foods.

Also helpful: Digestive enzyme supplements can help reduce gas and bloating. Effective products include Tyler Enterogenics...Transformation Enzymes DigestZyme and TPP Digest...Enzymedica Digest and Digest Gold...and Enzymatic Therapy Mega-Zyme. These products are available at most health-food stores and many drugstores.

INFECTIONS

Food hypersensitivity triggers 50% to 75% of all cases of IBS. Another 25% or so is caused by infections.

Research: Israeli doctors studied 564 travelers. While traveling, people are more likely to be exposed to new microbes that can cause diarrhea. Those who developed traveler's diarrhea were five times more likely to later develop IBS. In reviewing eight studies, American scientists found a seven times higher risk of IBS among those who had infections in the gastrointestinal tract.

What to do: See your doctor—he/she can perform tests to detect abnormal bacteria, fungi and parasites, and prescribe the appropriate treatment.

NATURAL REMEDIES

Supplements to help relieve IBS symptoms…

•**For diarrhea.** Probiotic supplements provide friendly intestinal bacteria that can help restore normal bowel function. *Saccharomyces boulardii* is an unusual probiotic—it's yeast, not bacteria—but doctors have used it for decades to control diarrhea effectively.

Look for a product called Florastor or other probiotic brands containing the yeast. Take 250 milligrams (mg), three times a day. If that works, try twice a day and then once a day, finding the lowest dosage that works for you.

•**For constipation.** You've probably tried fiber supplements—and found that they didn't work. Instead, take a magnesium supplement, which naturally loosens bowels.

Use magnesium glycinate, starting with 300 mg a day. If that dosage doesn't work, increase the dose by 100 mg per day, until you develop diarrhea. Then cut back by 100 mg—to produce regular bowel movements.

Probiotic supplements can help as well (see above).

THE PROBLEM WITH MEDICATIONS

Doctors have tried a range of drugs for IBS—bulking agents for constipation, antidepressants to affect brain chemicals that play a role in digestion, spasmolytics to decrease cramping. In 2005, a review by Dutch doctors of 40 studies on medications for IBS concluded, "The evidence of efficacy of drug therapies for IBS is weak."

The drugs also can be dangerous. In March 2007, the FDA pulled the IBS drug Zelnorm (*tegaserod maleate*) from the market when studies showed that it increased the risk for heart attack and stroke 10-fold.

Keep Your Liver Healthy

Howard J. Worman, MD, associate professor of medicine, anatomy and cell biology at Columbia University and assistant attending physician at NewYork-Presbyterian Hospital/Columbia, both in New York City, is the author of *The Liver Disorders Sourcebook*. McGraw-Hill.

The liver, which weighs about three pounds, is the body's second largest organ (after the skin). It purifies the blood by breaking down and/or filtering out toxins and pollutants. The liver also breaks down nutrients for absorption by cells…creates proteins that transport nutrients and hormones through the bloodstream…stores vitamins and minerals…and helps regulate insulin and other hormones.

The liver is capable of performing most of its functions—including regenerating damaged cells—even when it's harmed by infection or inflammation.

Caution: Popular medications are one cause of potential liver problems.

Examples: Cholesterol-lowering statins…anticonvulsants such as Dilantin…birth control pills…and anabolic steroids used to treat such conditions as anemia or weight loss associated with a severe illness. Overdoses of *acetaminophen* (Tylenol)—the recommended maximum daily dose is 4 g, or eight extra-strength tablets—also can harm the liver.

Other facts you should know…

SUBTLE SYMPTOMS

People with liver disease usually have only mild symptoms, such as fatigue or abdominal pain (often in the upper-right abdomen, where the liver is located)—or none at all.

Red flag: Jaundice (yellowing of the skin and whites of the eyes) and/or dark urine often are the first signs of acute liver disease. With chronic liver disease, jaundice may not appear until the liver is severely damaged—often decades later.

Often-overlooked symptoms: Unexplained itching or bruising…and red dots on the skin above the waist with "legs" radiating from the center (spider angioma). If you have any of the above symptoms, consult your primary care physician, who can refer you to a liver specialist, if necessary.*

FATTY LIVER DISEASE

Nonalcoholic fatty liver disease is a silent disorder that is estimated to affect up to one-third of American adults. It often occurs in people with hypertension and obesity, particularly abdominal fat.

Over a period of years, high levels of fat accumulate in the liver and cause severe inflammation that can lead to cirrhosis (irreversible scarring) or liver failure. The deposits usually can be detected with an ultrasound or computed tomography (CT) scan.

What you may not know: For many people, losing weight (about one to two pounds a week) reduces the amount of fat in their livers. For other people, it requires less weight loss.

CARDIAC CIRRHOSIS

Some people with congestive heart failure (CHF) are misdiagnosed with cirrhosis of the liver.

What you may not know: Because the heart is unable to pump blood effectively in people who have CHF, blood can back up (congest) in the liver, possibly resulting in scarring or "cardiac cirrhosis." Treating the heart disease with medication or surgery is the only way to prevent subsequent liver damage.

VIRAL HEPATITIS

Hepatitis A, B and C are the most common viruses known to infect the liver.

•**Hepatitis A** is usually transmitted by food and/or water contaminated by infected fecal matter. In rare cases, it also can be passed during sexual activity with an infected partner. Hepatitis A can cause extreme fatigue and muscle and/or joint pain but usually clears up on its own in a few months.

*The American Liver Foundation, 800-465-4837, *www. liverfoundation.org*, can give you a list of local chapters that can provide the names of liver specialists in your area.

Self-defense: Wash your hands often if you live with someone with hepatitis A…use a condom during sex…avoid undercooked shellfish (which may be contaminated by water that harbors the virus)…and in countries where sanitation is questionable, drink bottled water and avoid raw, unpeeled produce.

•**Hepatitis B** is more serious than hepatitis A—5% of adults infected with the hepatitis B virus go on to develop the chronic form of the disease, which can result in permanent liver damage or liver cancer. Hepatitis B also causes extreme fatigue and muscle and/or joint pain. It is mainly transmitted by unprotected sex with an infected partner or via blood-contaminated needles.

Self-defense: Use a condom during sex… use sterile needles…and don't share razors or toothbrushes.

•**Hepatitis C** often causes no symptoms for 20 to 30 years, at which point permanent liver damage and/or liver cancer may have developed. Many of the 4 million Americans infected with the hepatitis C virus contracted it from blood transfusions prior to 1990 (when screening became routinely available) or via contaminated needles. Body piercing and tattoos given with unsterilized instruments also may transmit the hepatitis C virus.

Most doctors choose to use drugs to fight the hepatitis C virus because there's no way to predict which people will go on to develop severe liver problems later in life. Injections of *pegylated interferon*, a cancer drug, often combined with oral doses of the antiviral drug *ribavirin* (Rebetol), can eliminate the virus in about half the cases. Side effects of interferon include muscle aches, fatigue and depression, while ribavirin can cause anemia, birth defects and nausea.

What you may not know: A relatively new vaccine, Twinrix, protects against both hepatitis A and B. Health-care workers and people who travel to areas where sanitation is not regulated are among those who should consider receiving the vaccine. There is no vaccine to prevent hepatitis C.

ALCOHOLIC LIVER DISEASE

Alcohol is more dangerous for women than men because women produce less *alcohol dehydrogenase*, an enzyme that breaks down alcohol.

Studies indicate that men who average two drinks or fewer a day and women who average one drink or less daily are unlikely to develop alcohol-related liver problems.

What you may not know: Some drinks poured in bars, such as martinis, can contain the equivalent of three servings of alcohol. Two of these drinks may contain six servings of alcohol—the level at which the risk for liver disease sharply rises.

Natural Therapies For Ulcers

James N. Dillard, MD, DC, is a former assistant clinical professor at Columbia University College of Physicians and Surgeons and past medical director of Columbia's Rosenthal Center for Complementary and Alternative Medicine, both in New York City. He is now in private practice in New York City and Stamford, Connecticut.

I f you've got an ulcer, chances are you're taking antacids and/or an over-the-counter (OTC) or prescription medication to neutralize gastric acid or inhibit its production. These medications include proton pump inhibitors (PPIs), such as *esomeprazole* (Nexium) and *lansoprazole* (Prevacid), and H2-blocking drugs, such as *cimetidine* (Tagamet) and *ranitidine* (Zantac).

What most people don't realize: There are several natural, complementary remedies that help reduce ulcer symptoms and promote healing while conventional treatment is under way. Some of these treatments also can help prevent ulcers in some patients.

WHAT CAUSES ULCERS

It's been more than 20 years since doctors learned that an infectious disease—rather than emotional stress—was the primary cause of most ulcers.

A screw-shaped bacterium, *Helicobacter pylori*, or *H. pylori*, burrows through the protective mucous lining in the small intestine and/or stomach, allowing harsh digestive fluids to accumulate and ulcerate the lining. About 50% of Americans over age 60 are infected with H. pylori. The bacterium doesn't always cause ulcers—but about 60% of patients with ulcers harbor H. pylori.

The remainder of ulcers are caused by regular use of stomach-damaging nonsteroidal anti-inflammatory drugs (NSAIDs), such as aspirin, *ibuprofen* (Advil) and *naproxen* (Aleve)...alcohol...and/or smoking. Excessive alcohol wears down the lining of the stomach and intestines. Nicotine causes the stomach to produce more acid.

Best complementary treatments...*

NONDRUG THERAPIES

•**Probiotics.** The intestine contains up to four pounds of "friendly" bacteria, which aid digestion. There's some evidence that maintaining adequate levels of beneficial bacteria helps create an inhospitable environment for H. pylori and makes it harder for this ulcer-causing bacterium to thrive.

Self-defense: Take a probiotic supplement that contains *Lactobacillus acidophilus* and *Bifidobacterium bifidus*. These organisms create a healthful mix of bacteria and can inhibit the growth of harmful organisms. Probiotics are helpful if you've taken antibiotics, which can kill off some beneficial bacteria.

The optimal dose for probiotics hasn't been determined. Preliminary research cites a daily dose of up to 10 billion organisms—the amount usually included in one to two capsules. Probiotics are available at health-food stores.

•**Cabbage juice.** This folk remedy has some evidence to support it. Cabbage is high in vitamin C, which seems to inhibit growth of H. pylori. It also contains *glutamine*, an amino acid that may strengthen the protective lining in the stomach.

A small Stanford University School of Medicine study found that ulcer patients who drank about a quart of cabbage juice daily healed significantly faster than those who didn't drink it.

Self-defense: If you have an active ulcer, consider drinking a quart of cabbage juice (about the amount in half a head of cabbage) once daily for up to two weeks.

•**Deglycyrrhizinated licorice (DGL).** Herbalists often recommend fresh licorice root to heal ulcers. Licorice contains *mucin*, a substance that protects the stomach lining, and antioxidants that may inhibit H. pylori growth.

*Check with your doctor before taking supplements. They can interact with prescription medications.

However, natural licorice can increase the effects of *aldosterone*, a hormone that promotes water retention and can increase blood pressure in some people. DGL supplements (available at health-food stores) are a better option, because the substances that increase blood pressure have been removed.

Self-defense: Take one DGL tablet before meals, and another before bed. DGL may be effective for people with ulcers whose H. pylori has been successfully treated with antibiotics but who still have some stomach irritation.

•**Vitamin A.** Vitamin A helps repair damaged mucous membranes. A report in the British medical journal *The Lancet* suggests that ulcers heal more quickly in patients given supplemental vitamin A.

Caution: High-dose vitamin A therapy can be toxic, so get your vitamin A from dietary sources along with a daily multivitamin—*not* from a separate vitamin A supplement.

Self-defense: Get 10,000 international units (IU) of vitamin A daily if you're undergoing ulcer treatment. (A multivitamin typically contains 3,500 IU to 5,000 IU of vitamin A.)

Good food sources: Beef liver (one-and-one-half ounces contains 13,593 IU)…carrots (one raw carrot contains 8,666 IU)…and spinach (one cup of raw spinach contains 2,813 IU).

•**Zinc.** Like vitamin A, zinc is involved in tissue healing. In Europe, a drug compound made with zinc plus an anti-inflammatory is often used for treating ulcers. Early studies indicate that zinc alone can speed ulcer healing and possibly even help prevent some ulcers.

Self-defense: Don't exceed the recommended daily intake (15 mg) of zinc. Take a daily multivitamin that includes zinc…and get adequate intake from dietary sources (five medium fried oysters, 13 mg…¾ cup fortified breakfast cereal, 15 mg…three ounces lean beef tenderloin, 5 mg).

ANOTHER WAY TO FIGHT ULCERS

NSAIDs alleviate pain by inhibiting the production of pain-causing chemicals called prostaglandins. However, the body produces several kinds of *prostaglandins*, including some that protect the stomach lining. That's why NSAIDs, which block the production of pain-causing *and* stomach-protecting prostaglandins, make people who regularly use the drugs more susceptible to ulcers.

Self-defense: If you require regular pain relief, start with *acetaminophen* (Tylenol). It relieves pain without depleting stomach-protecting prostaglandins.

Caution: Taking more than the recommended dosage or drinking alcohol with acetaminophen can cause liver damage.

Also helpful: Ask your doctor about taking Arthrotec, a prescription drug combination that includes the NSAID *diclofenac* along with *misoprostol*, which protects the stomach and intestinal lining. One study found that patients taking Arthrotec experienced up to 80% fewer ulcers than those taking an NSAID alone.

How to Treat Overactive Bladder

Rebecca G. Rogers, MD, director of the division of urogynecology at the University of New Mexico Health Sciences Center, and associate professor of obstetrics/gynecology at the University of New Mexico School of Medicine, both in Albuquerque, is the coauthor of *Regaining Bladder Control*. Prometheus Books.

People with bladder problems are often too embarrassed to report their symptoms to their doctors—and feel that it is just a problem they must learn to live with. Not true.

Bladder problems aren't life-threatening, but they can be *life-altering*. Patients with overactive bladder (OAB)—increased urinary urgency and/or frequency with or without incontinence—often are ashamed…and they're *always* uncomfortable.

An estimated 34 million American adults have OAB (it affects men and women equally), yet only one in 25 sufferers seeks medical treatment.

Good news: Up to 85% of patients who undergo OAB treatment experience significant improvement or are cured.

BRAIN-BLADDER DISCONNECT

The bladder normally holds approximately eight to 12 ounces of urine before it sends the "have to go" message to the brain. In patients with OAB, as little as a few ounces can trigger the urge to urinate.

Patients with OAB have one or more of the following symptoms…

•**Frequency**—the need to urinate more than eight to 10 times in a 24-hour period.

•**Urgency**—an extremely strong need to urinate immediately.

•**Nocturia**—the complaint that one has to wake more than one time at night to urinate.

About 90% of cases of OAB are idiopathic, meaning the cause is unknown. The remaining cases may be due to spinal cord injuries, neurological diseases (such as Parkinson's), interstitial cystitis (irritation of the bladder wall), a urinary tract infection or a prolapsed (dropped) uterus in women or an enlarged prostate gland in men.

DIAGNOSING OAB

Most cases of OAB can be diagnosed with a medical history. The doctor will ask questions about the frequency of urination, the urgency of sensations, etc. In addition, he/she will diagnose or rule out any identifiable underlying causes for the symptoms.

Tests may include…

•**Urinalysis** to identify a urinary tract infection.

•**Abdominal and/or vaginal or rectal exam** to identify possible obstructions, such as uterine prolapse (descent of the uterus into the vagina) or an enlarged prostate gland.

•**Postvoid residual volume measurement** to determine how completely a patient's bladder empties. Incomplete emptying can result in excessive urinary frequency/urgency. For this outpatient test, the doctor uses a catheter or ultrasound to measure the volume of residual urine in the bladder after the patient urinates. A large volume of residual urine could indicate an obstruction or problems with the nerves/muscles in the spine or bladder.

TREATMENTS

Most patients with OAB improve with a combination of behavioral and physical therapies, plus medication in some cases.

Important: Patients with OAB symptoms should keep a voiding diary for at least three days. The diary should include how much you drink…how much and when you urinate (your

doctor can provide a plastic "hat," which attaches under the toilet seat, or a urinal, to measure urine output)…whether you've had incontinence episodes, etc. This diary can aid your doctor in making an accurate diagnosis. Also, many patients naturally improve once they become more aware of their urinary habits and may modify the volume and timing of fluid intake and other behaviors.

Best treatment choices for men and women who suffer from OAB…

•**Dietary changes.** Alcohol as well as caffeine, including that found in chocolate, tea and cola, can trigger symptoms in some people. Eliminate these offenders one by one to see if symptoms improve.

•**Pelvic-floor exercises.** Known as Kegels, these simple exercises reduce OAB by strengthening the urinary sphincter (a circular muscle that constricts to retain urine or relaxes to allow urine to pass from the urethra to outside the body) as well as the muscles of the pelvic floor. Contracting pelvic-floor muscles prompts the spinal column to send a message to the bladder to stop contracting.

What to do: Imagine that you're trying to stop the urine flow in midstream. Tightly squeeze the muscles that control urine flow…hold for a count of three…relax for a count of 10…repeat. Do the exercise for five minutes twice daily.

Helpful: Perform Kegels when you feel a sudden sense of urgency. They can help prevent urine leakage on your way to a bathroom.

•**Timed voiding.** Urinate "by the clock" instead of in response to internal signals. Your doctor might advise you to urinate every hour for several days…then every two hours…working up to every two and a half to three hours during the day. Timed voiding trains the bladder to hold more urine for longer periods of time.

•**Medications.** They're often used when behavioral techniques do not work or as an adjunct to these therapies to help patients gain better control—and may be the first choice for some patients with nocturia (since behavioral therapies cannot be used while sleeping). *OAB medications include…*

Anticholinergic and antispasmotic drugs, such as *tolterodine* (Detrol), *oxybutynin* (Ditropan), *solifenacin* (Vesicare), *trospium* (Sanctura) and *hyoscyamine* (Levsin). These medications relax the bladder and reduce sensations of urgency. Some studies have found tolterodine to be slightly more effective than the other drugs.

Main side effects: Dry mouth and constipation. Some older patients may suffer temporary cognitive impairment. Newer drugs in this class, such as solifenacin and trospium, may be less likely to cause cognitive difficulties.

•***Imipramine* (Tofranil).** This anti-depressant reduces bladder contractions and also increases the "holding power" of the urethra. Imipramine is typically used to treat nocturia.

Main side effects: Extreme sedation. When used by older patients, it may increase the risk for low blood pressure and falls.

TREATMENTS ON THE HORIZON

Preliminary studies indicate that inserting a cystoscope into the bladder to inject Botox (normally used to treat wrinkles) in the bladder wall blocks the release of chemicals that cause the bladder to contract. The procedure involves 20 to 30 injection sites and may require anesthesia. Risks include urinary retention.

•**Electrical stimulation.** Electrodes temporarily placed in the vagina or rectum deliver electrical impulses that inhibit nerves in the bladder wall from firing inappropriately. Most patients receive the treatments in a doctor's office once weekly for six to eight weeks. I recommend electrical stimulation, but it has not been well studied and the long-term effects are not known. It's mainly used as a last resort for patients who don't respond to other methods.

Urinary Incontinence: Treatments That Work

Jonathan M. Vapnek, MD, urologist, associate clinical professor of urology and director of neurourology at Mount Sinai School of Medicine in New York City, is a member of the American Urological Association.

For the more than 13 million Americans with urinary incontinence, poor bladder control can severely disrupt daily life. Some people don't always make it to the bathroom in time or they can't hold it in when they cough or sneeze. Some even curtail social activities because they don't have reliable bladder control.

Yet the majority of people with this condition never see a doctor—either because they're too embarrassed to discuss it or because they assume that it's a normal part of getting older.

Not true. About 80% of patients can regain nearly normal bladder control with lifestyle changes or, if necessary, medication or surgery.

TYPES OF INCONTINENCE

As the bladder fills with urine, it eventually sends signals to the brain that tell the person "it's time to go." Before that happens, the bladder walls relax to permit urine to accumulate. This gradual process is what allows most people to wait hours before going to the bathroom. Urinary control also is achieved by a ring of muscle called the urinary sphincter. It contracts to keep urine in, then relaxes to let it out.

Incontinence occurs when there's a problem with either muscular or nervous system control—or a combination of both. Women are about twice as likely as men to have incontinence, although men who have prostate enlargement or have had prostate surgery have an increased risk of incontinence.

The main types…

•**Stress incontinence** is most common, affecting at least 50% of the women who have urinary incontinence. It occurs when the urinary sphincter isn't strong enough to hold in urine, particularly during activities that cause an increase in abdominal pressure, including laughing, coughing, sneezing and exercise.

Stress incontinence frequently occurs during pregnancy and can persist in women who have had several vaginal births. Large babies and long labors can stretch and weaken the pelvic floor muscles and/or damage some of the bladder nerves. The drop in estrogen that occurs after menopause can weaken the urethra, inhibiting its ability to hold back the flow of urine.

•**Urge incontinence** often is caused by inflammation or irritation of the bladder or urethra —due to infection, urinary stones or, in men, irritation of the prostate gland. This causes frequent (and sudden) urges to urinate. This type

of incontinence also may be caused by bowel problems and neurological problems, such as stroke or Parkinson's disease.

•**Overflow incontinence.** Patients with nerve damage (from diabetes, for example) or damage to the bladder may constantly dribble urine because they're unable to empty the bladder completely when they urinate.

•**Other potential causes** of incontinence are an enlarged prostate gland, a tumor in the urinary tract or bladder cancer. The majority of patients have either stress or urge incontinence—or a combination of both, known as mixed incontinence.

DIAGNOSIS

Most cases and types of incontinence can be diagnosed with a medical history alone. Keep a bladder diary for a week or two before you see your doctor. Write down how often you urinate… when you leak…and if you have trouble emptying your bladder. The answers to these questions usually are sufficient to allow a definitive diagnosis.

Tests may be required to provide additional information. *Most common…*

•**Stress test.** The doctor examines the urethra while the patient coughs or bears down. A leakage of urine indicates that the patient has stress incontinence.

•**Urodynamic testing.** There are a variety of tests that measure pressure in the bladder and how much fluid it can hold.

Example: The doctor might insert a catheter into the bladder, inject small amounts of fluid and measure changes in bladder pressure. Sudden increases in bladder pressure and/or spasms could indicate urge incontinence.

Patients may require an ultrasound to check how well the bladder empties. Your doctor also should perform urinalysis to check for blood or signs of infection in the urine.

TREATMENT

Some forms of incontinence are transitory and will go away when the underlying problem (an infection or inflammation, for example) improves. Most incontinence requires one or more of the following treatments, which can bring about significant improvement for most patients.

•**Behavioral techniques.** These techniques are used to help patients achieve better bladder control and are considered the mainstay of treatment. *Examples…*

•*Bladder training* requires patients to avoid going to the bathroom for longer and longer periods. A person might try to wait an extra 10 minutes when he/she has the urge to urinate. The goal is to lengthen the waiting time over a period of days or weeks. With practice, most patients are able to wait several hours. This is for patients with bladder overactivity and frequent urination.

•*Timed urination* means going to the bathroom at specific intervals—say, once every hour, even if you don't feel as though you have to go. This might be used for frail, elderly people who tend to wet themselves because they can't hold it once the urge hits. The idea is to void before the bladder hits that point of no return.

•*Kegel exercises.* Patients are advised to tightly squeeze the same muscles that they would use to stop the flow of urine. Contract the muscles for three to five seconds, relax, then repeat again. Do the cycle several times daily, working up to more repetitions each time. Kegels are helpful for men and women and for both stress and urge incontinence cases.

•**Medications.** Antispasmodic drugs reduce bladder contractions that contribute to urge incontinence. These drugs often cause dry mouth as a side effect. They're usually used in combination with behavioral treatments.

•**Surgery.** If behavioral changes and medications don't adequately control incontinence, patients may require surgery. *Main approaches…*

•*Tension-free vaginal tape (TVT) procedure.* This is standard for women with stress incontinence. A mesh-like tape is slung under the urethra like a hammock. It compresses the urethra to prevent leaks.

•*Bulking injections.* Collagen or synthetic bulking agents are injected into tissue surrounding the urethra or urinary sphincter. The extra bulk causes surrounding tissue to tighten the seal of the sphincter. The procedure usually needs to be repeated every six to 18 months because collagen is absorbed by the body over time.

•*Sphincter replacement.* An artificial, doughnut-shaped device is implanted around the urethra. When patients are ready to urinate, they press a valve that causes the device to deflate and let out urine. This procedure is mainly used for men who have had prostate surgery.

Drugs That Cause Severe Diarrhea

Douglas L. Seidner, MD, is director of nutrition in the department of gastroenterology and hepatology at the Cleveland Clinic, Ohio. Dr. Seidner has contributed to *The American Journal of Gastroenterology* and the *Journal of Parenteral and Enteral Nutrition*, among others.

Diarrhea—bowel movements that are looser and more frequent than usual—is the second most common medical complaint (after respiratory infections) in the US.

Most people associate a bout of diarrhea with a viral infection or food poisoning.

Now: Researchers are identifying new—and sometimes surprising—triggers, including the use of some medications.

Latest development: The *Journal of the American Medical Association* recently published a study that links the use of acid-lowering heartburn drugs, such as *omeprazole* (Prilosec), *lansoprazole* (Prevacid) and *ranitidine* (Zantac), to increased infection with the bacterium *Clostridium difficile*—a cause of severe and persistent diarrhea.

In an unexpected finding, the same researchers identified an association between diarrhea and regular use of nonsteroidal anti-inflammatory drugs (NSAIDs). More study is needed to confirm this NSAID-diarrhea link.

HOW DIARRHEA DEVELOPS

What's left of food after most of it has been digested reaches the large intestine as a sort of slurry. There, the body absorbs water from this material, creating a solid mass to be excreted. Normal stool is 60% to 90% water. Diarrhea occurs when stool is more than 90% water.

When stool does not remain in the large intestine long enough, it is excreted in a watery form. This "rapid transit" diarrhea can be caused by stress, overactive thyroid (hyperthy-roidism) and certain drugs, such as antacids and laxatives that contain magnesium, and chemotherapy for cancer.

Other types of diarrhea...

•**Osmotic diarrhea** occurs when too much food remains undigested or unabsorbed. Water is drawn into the colon to dilute unabsorbed chemicals, which makes the stool looser.

Large amounts of certain fruits and beans as well as sugar substitutes (sorbitol and xylitol) that are used in some brands of fruit juice, chewing gum and candy are common causes of osmotic diarrhea. When the diarrhea sufferer stops eating the offending food, the condition stops.

Lactase deficiency—a lack of the enzyme needed to break down milk sugar (lactose)—is another cause of osmotic diarrhea. Most people know if they have this deficiency and avoid milk products.

Osmotic diarrhea also may develop in people taking antibiotics. That's because the drug eliminates beneficial bacteria that live in the intestinal tract, allowing harmful bacteria to proliferate. These microorganisms normally help the body process and absorb the small amount of food that hasn't been digested yet. Diarrhea usually develops within a few days of treatment. If it's bothersome enough, your doctor may prescribe a different antibiotic.

More rarely, diarrhea develops toward the end of antibiotic treatment—or even up to a month later. This may be caused by C. difficile or another bacterium that can flourish and cause inflammation of the large intestine when beneficial bacteria are eliminated.

Helpful: This infection is usually treated with the antibiotics *vancomycin* (Vancocin) or *metronidazole* (Flagyl).

•**Secretory diarrhea** occurs when an excessive amount of water, salt and digestive fluids are secreted into the stool. Viral infections, bacterial toxins that cause some types of food poisoning and rare tumors of the small intestine and pancreas can trigger the secretions that lead to secretory diarrhea.

With food poisoning, excess secretions are stimulated by chemicals produced by bacteria that have contaminated something you ate. This diarrhea usually lasts for 12 to 24 hours and stops without treatment. If it persists, your doctor may order tests, such as stool cultures, to determine whether a virulent bacterium, such as *Salmonella*, *Shigella* or *Campylobacter*, is involved and will require medication.

Travelers' diarrhea has a similar cause. The culprit is generally a mild strain of a toxin-producing bacterium, such as *Escherichia coli*, that is present in food and/or water. Natives of the region you're visiting have been exposed to the microorganism for years and usually are immune to it. You're not. Traveler's diarrhea typically goes away within one to two days.

•**Exudative diarrhea** occurs when the large intestine's lining becomes inflamed. This triggers the release of blood, mucus, proteins and other fluids. Infection with the bacterium Shigella can cause this type of diarrhea. Crohn's disease (chronic inflammation of the small bowel or colon) and ulcerative colitis (chronic inflammation and ulceration of the colon) can also cause exudative diarrhea.

An antibiotic is sometimes used to treat a bacterial infection. Medication, such as the corticosteroid *prednisone* (Deltasone), and sometimes surgery are used to treat the inflammatory conditions.

Seek medical attention if any of these danger signs appear...

•**The diarrhea is severe** (six or more stools a day), especially if there are signs of dehydration (parched lips, sunken eyes).

•**The diarrhea is bloody or includes mucus,** rather than just water.

•**It has lasted more than two days**—if mild, two weeks.

•**You have a fever over 101.5°F.**

•**Diarrhea is accompanied by severe abdominal pain** (anything more than moderate cramping).

BEST RELIEF STRATEGIES

In some cases, diarrhea can be a sign of a serious infection and should be treated by a doctor. *Even though most types of diarrhea run their course within a few days, the following steps can hasten the process and ease your discomfort...*

•**Eat right.** If food poisoning is the problem, you should abstain from all food until symptoms resolve, usually one to two days.

For other acute diarrhea, follow the "BRAT" diet: bananas, rice, applesauce and toast. Bananas and applesauce contain *pectin*, a water-soluble substance that helps firm up the stool...the carbohydrates in white rice and white toast are easy to digest. If you eat other foods, stick to small portions and avoid dairy products.

Yogurt is an exception. If it's made from live and active cultures, such as *Lactobacillus bulgaricus* and *Streptococcus thermophilus*, yogurt may replace beneficial bacteria in the colon, helping to relieve antibiotic-related diarrhea.

When the diarrhea subsides, return to your normal diet cautiously. For the first few days, avoid fatty foods (they're harder to digest).

Important: Drink 64 ounces of fluids daily to replace what you're losing. Choose weak tea, water and/or small amounts of clear juice or soda, such as apple juice or ginger ale.

If diarrhea is severe: Drink "replacement fluids," such as CeraLyte, Pedialyte or Enfalyte. These contain salt and simple sugars that help the body retain water. Diarrhea-related dehydration isn't a danger for most adults, but it is a danger for children and many adults over age 65. Young children do not have as large a reserve of water in the body as healthy adults. Older adults may have heart or kidney disease, which can be exacerbated by dehydration.

•**Medication.** Several over-the-counter preparations can help relieve diarrhea...

•*Loperamide* (**Imodium**) is a semi-synthetic narcotic that slows food as it passes through the bowel, allowing more time for water to be absorbed. Try loperamide if diarrhea is mild and hasn't been resolved in one to two days. It should not be taken if you have a fever or the stools are bloody.

•*Bismuth subsalicylate* (**Pepto-Bismol, Kaopectate**) absorbs toxins—it's quite effective for traveler's diarrhea. It should not be taken with aspirin. Do not take it if you have a fever or bloody stools. Children should not take this product.

Natural Remedies For Constipation

Mark A. Stengler, ND, naturopathic physician in private practice, La Jolla, California…adjunct associate clinical professor at the National College of Natural Medicine, Portland, Oregon…author of many books, including *The Natural Physician's Healing Therapies* and coauthor of *Prescription for Natural Cures* (both from Bottom Line Books)…and author of the *Bottom Line/Natural Healing* newsletter.

Constipation is one of the most common digestive complaints, accounting for about 2 million doctor visits every year. But it occurs much more frequently than this number indicates because the majority of people with constipation treat it at home with over-the-counter laxatives.

Big mistake: Regular use of certain laxatives can make constipation worse by damaging the large intestine, making it "lazier" and even less efficient.

Most patients who experience constipation can prevent it permanently with dietary changes and other natural approaches. Even patients who have had constipation for years often can restore normal bowel function within two weeks.

WHAT'S NORMAL?

In a healthy body, waste travels through the digestive tract in a predictable, regular cycle, over a period of six to 24 hours. Most people have one to three bowel movements daily. Others have as few as three bowel movements a week. There's a lot of individual variability—what's normal for you might not be normal for someone else.

Red flag: Any change in your normal bowel habits. See a doctor if the frequency of bowel movements changes…you have blood in your stool…or you are experiencing intense abdominal pain. Constipation by itself is rarely dangerous, but it may be a sign of other problems, including colon cancer.

Stool in the intestine contains bacteria, fungi and metabolic by-products of digestion. If it remains in the colon for too long, these harmful substances cause a number of uncomfortable symptoms, such as bloating, painfully hard stools and a general sense of fatigue.

SUPPLEMENTS & FOODS

The right diet and supplements can relieve constipation. *Best choices…*

•**High-fiber foods,** including brown rice, whole-wheat bread, oatmeal, fruits, vegetables and legumes, such as beans and lentils. Fiber absorbs water in the intestine, which makes the stool bulkier. This triggers the intestinal contractions that cause bowel movements. Fiber also makes the stool softer, so it is easier to pass.

If you don't eat a lot of plant foods, you can supplement with an over-the-counter product containing psyllium (such as Metamucil), following the directions on the label. Or take one teaspoon of ground psyllium seed husks twice daily. Psyllium acts as a bulking agent and increases the frequency—and comfort—of bowel movements. Be sure to drink plenty of water or juice to avoid making constipation worse.

Ground flaxseed also works. It's a highly concentrated source of fiber, with the added benefit of supplying healthful omega-3 fatty acids. Have one to two tablespoons of ground flaxseed daily. You can sprinkle it on yogurt or cereal or just eat it plain. Be sure to drink at least 10 ounces of water with it. Don't eat whole flaxseed. It has a tough outer coating that is not broken down during digestion.

Some people take stool softeners. Common ones, such as *docusate* (Colace), are not laxatives and not habit forming, but you can get similar results with flaxseed oil. Take one to two tablespoons daily. The oil can go in a shake or on a salad.

•**Magnesium.** People with constipation often are deficient in this mineral. Magnesium helps in three ways—it increases the strength and regularity of the intestine's muscular contractions…it relaxes the nervous system…and at higher doses, it promotes the accumulation of water in the intestine, which boosts bowel function.

Foods high in magnesium: Green, leafy vegetables (such as spinach), brown rice, avocado, berries, cabbage, broccoli and bananas.

If you have acute constipation, take 250 mg of magnesium two to four times daily. Don't take supplemental magnesium for more than about a week. It can lead to dependence—reducing the colon's natural ability to contract—and can interfere with the normal absorption of nutrients.

Don't take supplemental magnesium if you are pregnant unless authorized by your doctor.

•**Fermented foods.** People who eat sauerkraut, live-culture yogurt and/or kefir (a fermented milk) are less likely to experience constipation because fermented foods contain probiotics. These beneficial organisms crowd out harmful microbes that may impair digestion and elimination.

Eat fermented foods daily, or take a probiotic supplement. Look for a product that provides at least four billion active organisms, preferably a combination of *Lactobacillus acidophilus* and *bifidus bacteria.*

•**Milk thistle (*Silybum marianum*).** A traditional remedy for hepatitis, milk thistle improves the flow of bile, a digestive juice that breaks down fats in the intestinal tract. Bile improves the colon's motility (the ability of the colon to contract and eliminate wastes).

Dose: 200 mg to 250 mg of a product standardized to 80% *silymarin* (the active ingredient) with meals twice daily for six to eight weeks. Don't take it if you are pregnant or breastfeeding.

HOMEOPATHY

In homeopathy, individuals are given very small amounts of substances that would produce the same or similar symptoms of an illness in a healthy person if given in larger doses. These remedies stimulate the body's defenses to prevent or treat an illness.

It can be a challenge to find the right homeopathic remedy for constipation—but when it works, the results can be impressive. It's safe to self-medicate with homeopathy, but people tend to have better results when they work with a trained practitioner who can match specific remedies with symptoms. *Remedies to try...*

•**Alumina** is recommended for patients who typically go several days without having a bowel movement.

•**Calcarea Carbonica** is for patients with chronic constipation who often feel cold, have clammy hands and/or feet and experience a lot of stress.

•**Lycopodium** can be helpful for patients who experience gas and bloating along with constipation.

For each remedy, take two pellets of 30C potency twice daily for two weeks (or follow directions on the label).

GIVE UP DAIRY

A *New England Journal of Medicine* study of 65 children with chronic constipation reported that cow's milk was the cause in two-thirds of cases. It contains the protein casein, which has been shown to cause constipation.

Also, reduce the amount of saturated fats in your diet. A diet high in saturated fat slows motility—and the longer the stool stays in the intestine, the more likely it is to harden and interfere with normal bowel movements.

DAILY EXERCISE

Mild-to-moderate aerobic exercise—a 30-minute brisk walk, for example—helps stimulate intestinal contractions. It also reduces stress and relaxes the nervous system, which improves muscle movements in the intestine and helps prevent or treat constipation.

STRESS CONTROL

Yoga, Pilates, meditation and other stress-reducing activities can reduce constipation. Studies show that people who experience high levels of stress often have reduced intestinal efficiency. In addition, people with high stress levels often have hectic lifestyles and don't take the time for regular bowel movements. Every day, set aside time for mental and physical relaxation.

Tired All the Time?

James L. Wilson, ND, PhD, cofounder of the Canadian College of Naturopathic Medicine in Toronto and is the author of *Adrenal Fatigue: The 21st Century Stress Syndrome.* Smart Publications.

Most people know very little about their adrenal glands, but their proper functioning can have a profound effect on health.

The adrenal glands, located on top of the kidneys, are only about the size of walnuts but produce more than 40 different hormones, including the stress hormones *cortisol* and *adrenaline*. Cortisol is involved in a variety of functions, including adapting your body to—and protecting it from—stress, while adrenaline is a short-acting hormone involved in the "fight-or-flight" response.

People who experience high levels of chronic stress can develop "adrenal fatigue." With this condition, the hormone-producing cells of the adrenal glands are unable to keep up with the unremitting demand of chronic stress, which can be due to serious health problems, for example, or a high-pressure job.

People with adrenal fatigue may experience unusual tiredness, difficulty waking or getting up in the morning along with an afternoon lull, low blood sugar, lack of concentration and, in some cases, mild depression.

Some of these symptoms can be related to a variety of conditions, including general fatigue and thyroid disorders, so it is common for these patients to be misdiagnosed or go undiagnosed. But when these symptoms appear as a group—especially consistent morning fatigue—adrenal fatigue should be suspected.

A CONTROVERSIAL DIAGNOSIS

Most conventional doctors have never heard of adrenal fatigue—or deny that it's a legitimate medical problem. Unlike Addison's disease, a recognized condition in which cortisol levels drop precipitously due mainly to autoimmune problems, adrenal fatigue causes relatively modest declines in cortisol. It isn't life threatening, and conventional doctors rarely test for it.

Research has confirmed the link between low cortisol levels and fatigue. Researchers have noted that patients with low cortisol also have less resistance to disease. They are even less likely to survive a heart attack than those with normal levels.

WHAT CAUSES ADRENAL FATIGUE?

Levels of cortisol fluctuate in the body throughout the day. Levels typically are highest in the morning, drop in midafternoon, rise slightly about 6 pm, then gradually decrease until the next morning. People with adrenal fatigue may have unusually low cortisol levels at night, which prevents them from getting the deep, restorative sleep they need.

Result: Because a good night's sleep is important for the adrenal glands' recovery, the hormone-producing cells in these glands don't get a chance to recoup their ability to respond to the body's needs. Without adequate rest periods, the cells get overwhelmed and stop producing efficiently.

TESTING AND TREATMENT

The blood and urine tests that are used to diagnose Addison's disease aren't sensitive enough to detect adrenal fatigue. Saliva hormone testing is more useful because it measures the amount of cortisol that's actually available to cells.

The test requires saliva samples that are collected by the patient four times throughout the day—usually at 8 am, noon, 4 pm and 11 pm. (Cortisol levels for people who work night shifts would be measured at different times during the 24-hour period.) The samples are placed in test tubes and analyzed in a laboratory. It's a good idea to repeat the saliva hormone testing every six months after you have begun treatment.

Based on my experience with adrenal fatigue patients, approximately 80% to 90% will improve significantly in six months to two years after starting a program that includes lifestyle changes and the use of dietary supplements that promote a more normal output of adrenal hormones.

My recommendations…

•**Sleep in at least one day a week.** Adrenal cells undergo repair and recovery during sleep. Sleeping in between 7 am and 9 am—even for only one day a week—allows the adrenal glands to rest during a time when high demands are ordinarily placed on these glands.

•**Use herbs.** A number of herbs help the body normalize the production of cortisol. Follow label instructions. *Try the following herbs until symptoms subside…* *

•Licorice root stimulates the adrenal glands to produce more cortisol.

Caution: Because licorice root can raise blood pressure, check with your doctor about blood pressure monitoring.

•Ashwagandha root, from a plant found in India, is an adaptogen, a substance that helps the body return to a normal state. It's helpful for adrenal fatigue because it can stimulate the adrenal glands to produce normal levels of cortisol.

•Siberian ginseng, a popular medicinal plant grown in Siberia, Japan, Korea and China, normalizes adrenal function and increases the body's resistance to stress.

*The FDA does not regulate herbal supplements. Check with your doctor before taking any of these products. They can interact with prescription medications. Pregnant women should avoid most herbal supplements.

•**Take vitamins.** Even though most health-conscious adults take multivitamins, certain vitamins are needed in higher doses to fight adrenal fatigue. Best choices…

•Vitamin C is used by the adrenal glands to help manufacture stress hormones. Vitamin C is also an antioxidant that helps prevent and repair damage to hormone-producing cells.

Recommended daily dose: 2,000 mg of time-released vitamin C.

Helpful: If your bowel movements become loose while taking high-dose vitamin C, reduce the amount of vitamin C you take daily by 500 mg until your stool is normal. Take a vitamin C supplement that includes 250 mg of bioflavonoids per 500 mg of vitamin C. The combination makes vitamin C more active.

•B vitamins affect the ability of the adrenal glands to function at peak capacity—this includes, for example, the formulation of coenzymes and other substances required for the production of cortisol.

Recommended daily dose: A B-complex supplement with 50 mg to 100 mg of vitamin B-6…and 75 mg to 125 mg of vitamin B-3.

•Combine protein, fat and carbohydrates with every meal. Each of these provides energy to cells at different rates. Combining them at each meal ensures that your blood sugar will be stabilized. Good combinations include peanut butter and whole-grain bread…cheese and rice crackers…and a chicken sandwich topped with vegetables.

Also helpful: Be sure to chew food slowly—at least 30 times per mouthful—to aid digestion and metabolize nutrients more efficiently.

■ ■ ■ ■

Bloat Buster

Natural remedy for bloating: Boil two tablespoons of fennel seeds in two cups of water for at least three minutes. Strain the seeds, add honey to taste and drink. Bloating should be relieved in one to two hours. Fennel promotes gastrointestinal motility and acts as an antispasmodic. Fennel seeds are available at health-food stores.

Birgit Rakel, MD, integrative physician, Jefferson-Myrna Brind Center for Integrative Medicine, Thomas Jefferson University Hospital, Philadelphia.

Soothe Your Stomach Without Drugs

Leo Galland, MD, director, Foundation for Integrated Medicine, New York City. He is author of *The Fat Resistance Diet.* Broadway. *www.fatresistancediet.com.* Dr. Galland is a recipient of the Linus Pauling Award.

Millions of Americans take drugs to relieve excess stomach acid. In fact, acid-suppressing drugs are among the most frequently prescribed medications in the US. Although these drugs can relieve symptoms, such as heartburn and abdominal pain, they can have serious long-term side effects. The good news is that there are natural remedies that work even better than drugs, without the side effects.

THE DRUGS

Acid-suppressing drugs fall into two basic categories…

•**Proton-pump inhibitors** (PPIs), such as Prilosec, Prevacid, Nexium, Aciphex and Protonix, inhibit the enzymes that transport acid from acid-secreting cells into the stomach cavity.

•**Histamine-2 (H2) blockers,** such as Zantac, Pepcid, Axid and Tagamet, inhibit the activity of *histamine* in the stomach. Histamine stimulates stomach cells to secrete more acid.

THE DANGERS

Regular use of acid-suppressing drugs is associated with increased risk of hip fractures, probably because these drugs hinder calcium absorption.

Taking acid suppressors also increases your risk of acquiring a foodborne intestinal infection or experiencing the overgrowth of bacteria in the stomach and small intestine. Bacteria overgrowth in the stomach probably explains some other risks associated with regular use of acid suppressors, including pneumonia, stomach cancer and vitamin B-12 deficiency.

Acid-suppressing therapy is primarily used to treat two kinds of problems—gastroesophageal reflux disease (GERD) and gastritis (inflammation of the stomach lining). *Here are the natural remedies…*

GERD

In GERD, the contents of the stomach flow backward up the esophagus and may reach all the way to the mouth. Symptoms include heartburn, chest pain, regurgitation of food, sore throat, hoarse voice and cough.

Although acid suppressors are commonly prescribed, GERD isn't caused by excess production of acid. It is caused by failure of the muscle (called the lower esophageal sphincter, or LES) that acts like a valve and separates the esophagus from the stomach. This muscle valve usually is closed and opens only for swallowing so that it keeps the stomach contents out of the esophagus. Because acid is among the most irritating components of stomach juice, reducing acid may reduce irritation. But acid suppression doesn't prevent reflux—it merely converts acid reflux into nonacid reflux. *To prevent reflux itself...*

• **Don't stuff yourself.** Eating a lot at one time causes stomach distension, which triggers relaxation of the LES.

• **Avoid high-fat foods,** including fried foods and creamy sauces. These weaken the LES.

• **Don't smoke.** It weakens the LES.

• **Don't eat for three hours before lying down.** When you're upright, gravity helps to keep food down.

• **Maintain a normal weight.** Being overweight increases your risk of GERD. Excess pounds put pressure on the abdomen, pushing up the stomach and causing acid to back up.

• **Don't eat immediately before strenuous exercise.** Strenuous activity increases the likelihood of GERD.

• **Avoid foods that cause discomfort until you're better.** So-called "acidic" foods, such as oranges and tomatoes, may irritate an already inflamed esophagus.

• **Try supplements.** The simple steps above prevent symptoms of GERD in the majority of people and may allow you to avoid the use of acid-suppressing drugs. *If not, try the following...*

• Calcium. Calcium tightens the LES. This is not an antacid effect. In fact, the best type of calcium—because it is the most soluble—is *calcium citrate,* which is itself mildly acidic. The most effective preparation is calcium citrate powder. Take 250 milligrams (mg), dissolved in water, after every meal and at bedtime (for a total daily dose of 1,000 mg). Nutricology (800-545-9960, *www.nutricology.com*) makes calcium citrate capsules

that can be opened and mixed in water. Swallowing calcium pills does not prevent reflux, because the calcium is not instantly dissolved.

• Digestive enzymes. These appear to work by decreasing distension of the stomach. The enzymes should be acid-resistant so that they work in the stomach itself, not in the small intestine. A powdered enzyme preparation (one-half teaspoon) can be mixed together with the calcium powder above and taken after each meal. Digestive enzymes are available in health-food stores and pharmacies. I use Absorbaid powder from Nature's Source (866-502-6789, *www.natures-source.com*).

GASTRITIS

The leading cause of gastritis (inflamed stomach lining) in the US is the regular use of aspirin and nonsteroidal anti-inflammatory drugs (NSAIDs), such as ibuprofen (Advil, Motrin) and naproxen (Aleve). Other causes include other medications, especially antibiotics...cigarette smoking...and regular use of alcohol.

For some people, infection of the stomach is the underlying cause of gastritis. Anyone with gastritis should be tested for *Helicobacter pylori,* the most common cause of bacterial gastritis. If *H. pylori* is found, treatment with antibiotics is necessary.

Whatever the cause of the gastritis, when the stomach is inflamed, it becomes sensitive to its own acid. The usual symptom is burning pain in the middle part of the upper abdomen, above the belly button. This pain is often affected by food (food can ease the pain or make it worse) and may be associated with nausea and changes in appetite. Antacids, such as Maalox and Mylanta, and acid-suppressing drugs may relieve symptoms by buffering or decreasing acidity, but they do not address the underlying cause of gastritis. *To prevent gastritis...*

• **Eat anti-inflammatory foods.** The diet I developed, called the Fat Resistance Diet is helpful in preventing or relieving gastritis. The diet is rich in anti-inflammatory fruits, vegetables and spices.

• **Try supplements.** Scientific studies have shown benefits from the following. If your symptoms are severe, you might want to try them all. If not, use one at a time in the order listed until you get relief. If you want to use only one, choose the deglycyrrhizinated licorice (DGL).

• Carrot juice and/or cabbage juice, one cup per day. The addition of aloe vera liquid, up to four ounces a day, also can help, although aloe has a laxative effect. If you can't find cabbage juice, sauerkraut juice is a suitable substitute.

• DGL. This herbal extract—600 mg taken twice a day with meals—helps the stomach lining to heal and can be combined with other soothing herbs, such as slippery elm (200 mg twice a day) and marshmallow root (400 mg twice a day).

• L-glutamine powder. L-glutamine is an amino acid. One teaspoon of L-glutamine powder in four ounces of water taken with each meal can help heal gastritis and even stomach ulcers.

• Mastic gum. The sap of the Mediterranean plant *Pistacia lentiscus,* mastic gum has been used to treat stomach problems for centuries and now is available in capsule form. Take 500 mg of mastic gum twice a day after meals (for a total of 1,000 mg a day).

GO SLOWLY

People who have been taking acid-suppressing drugs daily for several weeks or more may have difficulty discontinuing them. When the stomach is deprived of acid, it compensates by producing more acid-secreting cells. The result is that even though the initial symptoms are not due to hyperacidity, attempting to stop the drug creates hyperacidity. The solution is to taper off the drug slowly, under a doctor's supervision, while taking steps to remedy the underlying cause, as described above.

■ ■ ■ ■

Cranberry Update

Take cranberry extract daily to prevent bacteria from adhering to bladder walls and triggering infection. Avoid cranberry juice—its acidity irritates bladder tissues.

Amy E. Rosenman, MD, assistant clinical professor of obstetrics and gynecology, David Geffen School of Medicine, University of California, Los Angeles. She is founder of the Pacific Continence Center in Santa Monica, and co-author of *The Incontinence Solution: Answers for Women of All Ages.* Fireside.

14

Cancer Fighters

The 7 Big Cancer Myths

Despite all the medical information in the media, many people are misinformed about the realities of cancer. These misconceptions can prevent people from getting appropriate treatment. *Here, the truth behind common myths about cancer...*

Myth 1: **Cancer usually is fatal.** In a recent American Cancer Society (ACS) survey, 68% of respondents said that they believe the risk of dying of cancer is increasing. Not true. Though the number of Americans diagnosed with cancer has increased (because the US population is increasing and getting older), the risk of dying of cancer has decreased due to early detection and improved treatment. More than half of people diagnosed with cancer survive the disease—and for some cancers, such as lymphoma and leukemia, the cure rate is between 70% and 80%.

Cancer isn't a single disease. It includes many types of tumors, all of which behave differently.

Some tumors, such as those in the breast, are very responsive to chemotherapy and other treatments. Lung tumors are more resistant to treatment. The likelihood of a cure depends not only on the type of tumor but how far advanced it is at the time of diagnosis.

Myth 2: **Cancer runs in families.** Only about 8% of cancers are genetically linked. These usually are cancers that occur in younger patients, such as sarcoma or early-onset colon cancer. The vast majority of cancers occur without a known cause or are related to lifestyle.

A family history does increase risk for certain cancers. For example, if a woman has a first-degree relative (such as a mother or sister) who developed the BRCA1 form of breast cancer at an early age, her risk for getting that cancer is increased.

However, only about 10% to 20% of women diagnosed with breast cancer have a family history of the disease. That's why it's important for

---

Gregory Pennock, MD, a medical oncologist, is medical director of clinical research at M.D. Anderson Cancer Center, Orlando, Florida.

429

every woman to undergo regular mammograms and do breast self-exams on a regular basis.

Myth 3: **Stress causes cancer.** There's a long-standing belief that people who experience a lot of stress or lack a positive attitude are more prone to cancer. A survey of long-term breast cancer survivors in Canada found that 42% attributed cancer to stress. This causes many people with cancer to blame themselves or feel that they always have to be upbeat to prevent a recurrence.

There's surprisingly little evidence that stress or a negative attitude causes cancer. In a study reported in the journal *Cancer*, 8,500 people were scored on factors such as fatigue, irritability, etc. After following the participants for almost nine years on average, researchers found no link between emotional distress and cancer risk.

However, positive thinking may play a role in recovery. Patients with a positive attitude are more likely to do things that improve outcomes, such as following medical instructions and maintaining a healthy lifestyle.

Myth 4: **Surgery causes cancer to spread.** In the ACS survey, 41% of respondents said they believe that cancer spreads through the body during surgery. In reality, the risk of cancer spreading during surgery is close to zero. This myth probably started in the days before early detection of cancer. It was common for doctors to find advanced cancers during surgery—even in patients who may have had only mild symptoms. Patients and their families concluded that the surgery itself made the disease worse.

Some cancers in the abdomen or ovaries produce large amounts of malignant fluid. In those cases, it's theoretically possible for cancer cells to spread if the fluid leaks into the abdomen during surgery, but there is no actual evidence of that happening.

Myth 5: **Injuries cause cancer.** More than one-third of respondents in the ACS survey thought that injuries such as a bruised breast or a hard fall could cause cancer later in life.

These types of injuries don't cause cancer. What may happen is that people hurt a part of the body, see a doctor about the injury and then learn that they have a tumor—but the tumor was already there. The injury just triggered the discovery.

That said, a few cancers are caused by certain types of injuries. A serious sunburn during childhood, for example, increases the risk of skin cancer later in life. Chronic reflux disease (heartburn) can burn the esophagus and increase the risk of esophageal cancer.

Myth 6: **It's okay to keep smoking after a lung cancer diagnosis.** Some people believe that because the damage is done, they don't have to quit smoking—but those who continue to smoke after a lung cancer diagnosis have significantly poorer outcomes than those who quit. There's also evidence that the chemicals in cigarette smoke interfere with radiation and chemotherapy. People with lung cancer who quit smoking respond better to the treatments.

Important: Lung cancer is the leading cause of cancer deaths in men and women. Lung tissue gradually returns to normal when people quit smoking. Ten years after quitting, lung cancer risk is reduced to one-third of what it was.

Myth 7: **Cell phones cause brain cancer.** Large population studies have shown no evidence that cell phones cause any kind of cancer, including brain cancer.

Cell-phone use today is vastly higher than it was a decade ago. If there were any truth to the cancer/cell-phone link, we would be seeing an increased incidence of brain cancers by now, but that hasn't happened.

Supporting Someone With Cancer

Lori Hope, a lung cancer survivor in Oakland, California, and author of *Help Me Live: 20 Things People with Cancer Want You to Know.* Celestial Arts.

One in two men and one in three women will get cancer during their lifetimes, according to the American Cancer Society. The advent of new treatments has allowed many cancer patients to live relatively normal lives, and about nine million Americans are cancer survivors.

When someone has cancer, friends and family members want to help and give support, but sometimes they unknowingly say things that may be disturbing. There are many ways to express concern and love when someone is faced with cancer or any serious illness…and just as many ways to make someone cringe. *Here's what cancer survivors wish people would do…*

BE PRESENT

People may disappear or withdraw when a loved one gets sick. Some are afraid of saying or doing the wrong thing. Others are geared toward fixing problems and get frustrated when they can't help. Still others have experienced their own tragedies with cancer and don't feel strong enough to face the emotional turmoil again.

Though it's uncomfortable to confront a person's outpourings of fear and grief, make the effort. Cancer patients need to cry and release their pain. One of the greatest acts of love is to be with him/her, to listen as he shares his fears.

If you live far away, call or write. Let him know that he's loved…that he matters…and that your heart is with him.

If you simply can't be there, at least try to explain why the situation is too difficult for you to handle.

GIVE HOPE

People often talk about their own experiences when they meet a person who has cancer. Their intention may be to show empathy or unload their own burdens, but the stories can hurt more than help.

Example: When people heard about my diagnosis, many said things like, "Lung cancer—that's really bad." A waiter at an Italian restaurant even told me that his wife died of the same cancer. He shared all the gruesome details—about the surgery, how the cancer returned and how she died. It brought back all of my own terror.

People who have cancer don't need to be reminded that they could die—they live with that fear every day. They would rather hear stories of hope and success.

Better: When I told my cousin about my diagnosis, she told me about one of her professors who had had the same cancer 20 years before—and who is still alive and healthy.

When I told my best friend, with whom I have always taken an annual vacation, she said that we would still be vacationing together when we're old ladies. That's the type of encouragement people with cancer need to hear.

ASK PERMISSION

Few of us ask permission before sharing our feelings or advice, but asking permission is important when you are dealing with someone who has a life-threatening illness. That's when people are at their weakest and most vulnerable.

People say things like, "You really should try this immune-boosting herb" or "You should ask your doctor about this new treatment I read about." The word "should" suggests that the person with cancer would be remiss not to take your advice.

Instead, ask him if he is interested in your advice or information or wants to hear your stories. Back off if he says no. *Possible ways to test the water…*

"I have been looking into this type of cancer. Would you like to hear some of the treatment options I've read about?"

"A friend told me about an herb that might help. Would you like to hear about it?"

LAUGH

We all tend to be overly serious when we're with people who have serious illnesses. That's appropriate some of the time, but not all the time. People with cancer may want to forget the pain and just laugh and be happy.

I interviewed a woman who received a cancer diagnosis on a Friday. She had all weekend to worry before she saw her doctor again on Monday, so to make herself feel better, she went to a video store and rented a bunch of comedies.

Going through cancer is not all about fear. There's always room for humor and joy.

DON'T HARP ON POSITIVE THINKING

It's normal to be angry, depressed or sad when you have cancer. No one feels positive all the time. Nevertheless, friends and family members often nag cancer patients about the importance of positive thinking and tune them out when they express worries, pessimism or fear.

The implication is that the cancer is somehow the patient's fault or that he can control the outcome. There's a myth that some people have a "cancer personality." There's no truth to it—and it implicitly blames the patient for causing the disease.

It is important to understand that people who have cancer need to allow themselves to feel everything. They shouldn't have to hide their true emotions. It's okay to feel rotten sometimes.

SPARE THE PLATITUDES

Platitudes are reassuring words that are said without much thought or understanding.

Everyone with cancer has heard things like, "You never know how much time any of us has —you could go outside tomorrow and get hit by a truck."

One woman I talked to had heard this cliché at least 10 times from people she knew—even from her doctor. Her comment? "Okay, so then in addition to the fact that I could die from cancer, I might also get hit by a truck." That isn't comforting.

Few who have had cancer see it as "a gift." Cancer patients don't want to hear how lucky they are or what they can learn from the experience. They just want to get better.

Silence and compassion are more helpful than empty words.

The New Integrative Cancer Prevention Plan

D. Barry Boyd, MD, director of the Integrative Medicine Program at Greenwich Hospital-Yale New Haven Health System, and the Boyd Center for Integrative Health, both in Greenwich, Connecticut, is the author of *The Cancer Recovery Plan: Maximize Your Cancer Treatment with This Proven Nutrition, Exercise and Stress-Reduction Program.* Avery.

The best surgery, chemotherapy and radiation therapy are not always enough to prevent a cancer recurrence. In an estimated four out of every 10 cancer cases, the malignancy comes back despite state-of-the-art medicine.

To maximize the effectiveness of standard cancer treatment, seek an *integrative* program that includes a healthful diet, emotional support and regular exercise. This type of approach may give the approximately 10 million

Americans who are cancer survivors the best possible chance of avoiding a recurrence—and help protect people who have never had cancer and want to do all they can to prevent it.

THE MYSTERY OF METABOLISM

Conventional oncologists usually advise patients to avoid weight loss, a significant side effect of chemotherapy and radiation. But for most people with cancer, avoiding weight gain is just as important. Research shows that excess weight increases the risk for the development and recurrence of many cancers as well as associated mortality.

What's the link between weight and cancer? Insulin resistance is one theory that is being extensively studied. Insulin, a hormone produced by the pancreas, is vital for glucose (blood sugar) metabolism—it brings this simple sugar into the cells to be broken down for energy. Trouble develops when the cells become less sensitive to insulin, usually as a result of a person being overweight and/or underactive. The pancreas responds by producing more insulin, and higher levels of the hormone remain in the bloodstream.

Excessive insulin levels have been linked to persistent, low-grade inflammation, which releases chemicals that stimulate the growth of cells. Many experts believe that inflammation also stimulates the growth of cancer cells. Cancer and some cancer treatments, such as hormone therapy, may increase insulin resistance as a result of decreased metabolism, reduced activity levels and changes in nutritional intake.

People diagnosed with cancer, especially if they are overweight, should be tested for insulin resistance by checking levels of fasting blood sugar, insulin and lipids, and seek treatment with medication if necessary.

A CANCER-FIGHTING DIET

Weight control is one of the most important ways to help your body fight cancer and promote recovery. Unfortunately, many cancer patients seek fattening comfort food, or their doctors tell them to eat whatever they want.

The ideal cancer-fighting diet consists of 45% complex carbohydrates, 25% protein and no more than 30% fat. Strong evidence has shown that this kind of balanced diet is associated with lower rates of cancer and cancer recurrence.

The Mediterranean diet—including ample amounts of fruits and vegetables, whole-grain cereals and olive oil—is a wise choice. Small meals eaten four to six times a day also are recommended. That's because people who consume their food over the course of the day—rather than in one to three big meals—tend to take in fewer calories and stay healthier.

The same guidelines are important if your appetite is diminished by nausea caused by chemotherapy or the cancer itself. In these cases, a balanced diet is important because it helps prevent nutritional deficiencies that can result from appetite loss.

To create a cancer-fighting diet...

•**Choose the right carbs.** The amount of carbohydrates you consume isn't as critical as the kind. Sharply limit pastries, candies, beverages containing high-fructose corn syrup, such as soft drinks and some fruit-juice drinks and refined grain products, such as white rice and bread made from white flour. The carbohydrates in these foods are broken down immediately and deposited into the bloodstream, triggering an insulin surge. With repeated exposure to insulin peaks, cells become less sensitive to the hormone.

Complex carbohydrates, such as fruits and vegetables, beans, brown rice, whole-grain cereals and whole-grain baked goods, are digested and absorbed gradually. Insulin is produced at a steady, moderate rate, fueling the body's cells with maximum efficiency. What's more, the fiber in complex carbs fills you up, so you can satisfy your hunger with fewer calories.

•**Eat a variety of vegetables and fruits.** Specific "superfoods," such as beans and blueberries, have received a great deal of attention for their healing properties, but it's crucial to get a broad selection of healthful foods.

Fruits and vegetables should be a mainstay of your diet—the American Cancer Society recommends five or more daily servings. Nine daily servings are even better. One-half cup is the standard serving size. In addition to fiber and complex carbohydrates, fruits and vegetables contain chemicals known as phytonutrients that protect against carcinogens and enhance the body's own healing powers.

Broccoli, cauliflower and cabbage have different phytonutrients than garlic and onion. Berries, citrus fruits and leafy, green vegetables each have their own nutrients. Eating a variety of fruits and vegetables ensures that you get them all.

•**Avoid dangerous fats.** Saturated fats, found mostly in meats and high-fat dairy products, promote insulin resistance, so limit your meat intake to two servings (three ounces per serving) of lean red meat per week and consume only low-fat or nonfat dairy products (one to three servings daily). Good protein sources include poultry, fish, nuts and legumes.

Trans fat, found in many baked goods and processed foods, also causes inflammation.

Beware: Even in food products that claim "0" trans fat on the food labels, small amounts may be present and listed as "partially hydrogenated oil."

On the other hand, omega-3 fatty acids, found in cold-water fish, such as salmon, sardines and herring, have been shown to reduce inflammation and provide a range of other anticancer benefits. Other sources of omega-3s include walnuts and flaxseed.

Important: Food is the best way to get vitamins, minerals and other nutrients. High-dose supplements should be taken only under the supervision of a health-care professional who is knowledgeable about nutrition and cancer care.

EMOTIONAL SUPPORT

Serious illness, such as cancer, can trigger the release of stress hormones that increase your risk of developing excessive insulin levels.

My advice...

•**Get emotional support.** In a Yale study that followed more than 300 women with breast cancer for 10 years, those who felt free to talk about their illness with others were significantly more likely to survive. Don't be reluctant to ask friends and family for help in performing difficult chores and for company during doctor visits.

•**Choose a doctor who gives you hope.** Hopelessness and helplessness are the worst stressors for people with cancer. Make sure your care is directed by a medical professional who focuses on the most positive possible outcome, even if the disease is severe.

EXERCISE IS ESSENTIAL

Exercise reduces insulin resistance by building up lean, metabolically active tissue—which is better than fat tissue for cancer prevention.

In a study of 2,987 breast cancer patients, women who walked three to four hours a week had a 50% lower risk of dying from breast cancer than women who did little or no exercise. Researchers believe that physical activity also helps fight other types of malignancies.

For cancer prevention, strive for 30 minutes of brisk walking per day—or its equivalent in comparably strenuous activities, such as swimming or cycling.

Cancer-Free in a Week

Mark Kaminski, MD, professor of internal medicine, division of hematology and oncology, University of Michigan Cancer Center, Ann Arbor.

Marshall Lichtman, MD, retired executive vice president, research and medical programs, The Leukemia & Lymphoma Society, White Plains, New York.

The New England Journal of Medicine.

Just one week of radioactive-based therapy put 75% of people who had advanced follicular lymphoma into complete remission.

BACKGROUND

The radioactive-based therapy, known as *131 I-tositumomab*, is currently approved for people who have relapsed after having chemotherapy. Of the patients who use the therapy after chemotherapy, 20% to 38% go on to have a complete remission, and 47% to 68% have some kind of response to the treatment. Approximately 30% of these patients have remissions that last between one and 10 years.

THE STUDY

Given the success of 131 I-tositumomab as a follow-up treatment, Mark Kaminski, lead author of the study, and his team decided to test it as an initial treatment on 76 patients who had stage III or stage IV follicular lymphoma. Each participant got two infusions, one week apart.

RESULTS

Overall, 95% of the patients showed some response, and 75% went into complete remission. Of those who had a complete remission, 77% remained disease-free after five years. The percentage of people who relapsed decreased each year.

"Instead of a 30% complete response rate, we're now up to 75%, and the complete response is very much key in getting a long remission," says Kaminski, professor of internal medicine in the division of hematology and oncology at the University of Michigan Cancer Center in Ann Arbor.

The duration and ease of the treatment is almost unknown in cancer treatment. Kaminski notes that he knows of only one other instance where a quick treatment induced a remission—and that was for hairy cell leukemia, a rare form of cancer.

The 131 I-tositumomab contains an antibody tagged with a radioisotope that emits radiation. Scientists believe that when the compound is injected into the bloodstream, the antibody binds to a certain protein on the tumor cells, so the radiation from the radioisotope can kill those cells. The antibody itself can also kill tumor cells, resulting in a lethal one–two punch to the cancer.

While the results achieved with this treatment were similar to those achieved with other therapies, there has been no head-to-head comparison with other treatments.

The results of this trial may push the treatment, currently approved for use after chemotherapy, towards being a first-line treatment, says Kaminski.

"It hasn't been compared to the best current therapy, so we still don't know what role this agent would play," says Dr. Marshall Lichtman, retired executive vice president of research and medical programs at The Leukemia & Lymphoma Society. "Would it be used alone, used initially, used with chemo? It had pretty substantial activity, so one could begin thinking about using it earlier."

The patients in this trial were also younger than the average population, which could skew results. "This may be the very best therapy for a subset of patients and may be a very useful addition to other therapies for other subsets. All of these details have to be worked out," Lichtman explains.

IMPLICATIONS

Kaminski is optimistic. "I think this is going to open the door to people feeling more comfortable…and treating patients with this earlier."

"I think it's an important incremental step," Lichtman says.

STATS

Follicular lymphoma, the second most common form of non-Hodgkin's lymphoma, is diagnosed in approximately 15,000 adults in North America each year, with more than 90% of those diagnoses made when the disease is already in an advanced stage.

The Lymphoma Information Network has more on follicular lymphoma at *www.lymphoma info.net/nhl/follicular.html.*

■ ■ ■ ■

Bladder Cancer Test

The BladderChek test screens urine for high levels of the protein NMP22, which is associated with bladder cancer. The test costs about $30. It can be done in a doctor's office, and results are available within 50 minutes. It is good for detecting a recurrence of bladder cancer and useful as a supplement to other tests for diagnosing it initially. Bladder cancer is the fourth most common cancer in American men and the tenth most common in women—about one American in 600 has had it. BladderChek is appropriate for people over age 40 who have hematuria—blood in urine—one of the first signs of bladder cancer. Smokers with hematuria should have the test at any age.

H. Barton Grossman, MD, is professor of urology and cancer biology, University of Texas M.D. Anderson Cancer Center, Houston, and leader of a study of 668 bladder cancer patients, published in *Journal of the American Medical Association.*

■ ■ ■ ■

Cancer Care Varies by State

The cancer care you receive often varies depending on where you live.

Example: More than twice as many patients with stomach cancer survive for five years in Hawaii—where doctors remove an average of 15 lymph nodes when treating the disease—as in Utah, where the average removed is six. Cancer researchers are developing standard care recommendations in hopes of getting all patients the best available care, no matter where they happen to live.

Ezekiel J. Emanuel, MD, PhD, chair, department of clinical bioethics, Magnuson Clinical Center, National Institutes of Health, Bethesda, Maryland, and liaison between the American Society of Clinical Oncologists and a Rand Corporation–Harvard team that studied US cancer care by geographic area.

Doctors Destroy 'Inoperable' Tumors

Thomas Jefferson University Hospital.

A new kind of radiation technology called *shaped beam surgery* allows doctors to destroy brain and spinal tumors that cannot be treated using conventional surgery.

BETTER APPROACH

Shaped beam surgery, available at only a few US medical centers, including Thomas Jefferson University Hospital in Philadelphia, can mold radiation beams to match the exact size and shape of a tumor.

"Shaped beam surgery is a major advance in treating both benign and malignant tumors in the brain and the spinal cord regions," says Dr. David Andrews, a professor of neurosurgery at Jefferson Medical College and director of the division of Neurooncologic Neurosurgery and Stereotactic Radiosurgery at Thomas Jefferson University Hospital.

So far, this new technology has been used mostly to destroy benign brain tumors that couldn't be treated before.

"Shaped beam surgery gives us infinite flexibility to deal with lesions from the top of the head to the bottom of the spine," Andrews says. "We can wrap doses around structures, such as the spinal cord, and can create a very high dose of radiation and leave the cord untouched. There's no other technology out there that can do this."

■ ■ ■ ■

Proton-Beam Promise

A relatively new cancer treatment is much more effective for some types of cancer. It's called *Proton-beam therapy* and is best for

435

tumors that can't be controlled with low doses of radiation and that are in or near sensitive areas, such as the prostate, chest, lungs and brain. There are proton-beam facilities in California, Florida, Indiana, Massachusetts and Texas. Treatment costs more than standard radiation but is covered by most insurers.

James D. Cox, MD, is professor and head of the division of radiation oncology, M.D. Anderson Cancer Center, Houston, Texas.

■ ■ ■ ■

Better Colon Cancer Screening

The fecal occult blood test (FOBT) detects blood in feces and often is used as a preliminary screening test for colon cancer.

However: False-positive results can result from eating red meat or such vegetables as radishes, turnips, beets or broccoli. Aspirin and other nonsteroidal anti-inflammatory drugs (NSAIDs), such as *ibuprofen* (Advil), also may cause a false-positive result. A diet high in vitamin C can cause false negatives.

Self-defense: Avoid these foods and medications within three days of the FOBT.

David Lieberman, MD, professor of medicine, chief, division of gastroenterology, Oregon Health & Science University, Portland.

New Technique Studied For Inoperable Liver and Lung Cancers

Riccardo Lencioni, MD, professor of diagnostic and interventional radiology, University of Pisa, Italy.

Jeff Geschwind, MD, associate professor and director, department of vascular and interventional radiology, Johns Hopkins University School of Medicine, Baltimore.

Society of Interventional Radiology annual scientific meeting, New Orleans.

For the many Americans diagnosed with inoperable lung or liver cancer each year, two new techniques may offer hope for longer survival, according to a pair of studies.

THE FIRST STUDY: LUNG CANCER

An Italian research team used *radiofrequency ablation*, in which a heated needle is inserted through the chest wall directly into the tumor site, to effectively "cook" the malignancy. The technique was performed on 106 patients who had a total of 186 malignant, inoperable tumors measuring 3.5 centimeters in diameter or smaller.

Researchers report the minimally invasive heated probe was successful in eradicating inoperable tumors in 93% of the cases.

Of the patients enrolled in the study, 91% were still alive two years after the intervention, the researchers report.

Further, complications linked to the procedure were minimal and easily managed.

IMPLICATIONS

That technique "is creating a new chapter in oncology," says Dr. Riccardo Lencioni, lead researcher and professor of diagnostic and interventional radiology at the University of Pisa located in Italy.

He stresses that surgery must still be the first option for people who have lung cancer whenever it is feasible.

However, because of late detection and/or poor cardiovascular health, surgery is often out of the question for many patients, he says.

According to Lencioni, the best candidates for radiofrequency ablation are "patients with early-stage, limited disease. Whether radiofrequency ablation could be used to also treat patients with more advanced tumors is not defined yet."

Lencioni says the value of radiofrequency ablation against other cancers was less known, but he did say "the treatment has been shown to be successful in treating tumors in the liver."

The treatment is catching on in the United States, Lencioni adds, especially at large teaching hospitals, but "many more doctors need to be trained to have the procedure widely available."

THE SECOND STUDY: LIVER CANCER

According to the American Cancer Society, approximately 22,000 cases of *primary* liver cancer originate within the organ itself.

However, up to 100,000 Americans each year develop secondary, metastatic tumors in their livers after battling cancer in other parts of their bodies.

More often than not, detection comes too late for surgery, says Dr. Jeff Geschwind, a researcher at Johns Hopkins University School of Medicine.

For these patients, systemic chemotherapy—with its often painful side effects—is the only treatment available.

"A lot of these patients present with far-advanced disease and they have no other options," Geschwind says.

His team of researchers hopes to change that scenario, however.

Geschwind's study looked at 149 liver cancer patients who had inoperable tumors. They were treated with a new technique called *chemoembolization*.

"This involves the delivery of highly concentrated chemotherapy suspended in an oily medium," Geschwind explains.

At the same time, doctors used tiny microspheres, which served as obstructing agents to temporarily prevent the tumor from getting its full blood supply.

"In our data, we've shown an extended mean survival of about six years, when otherwise, patients usually only survive without treatment for maybe one year, at most," according to Geschwind.

Because it is so localized, chemoembolization is also much easier on patients than systemic chemotherapy, which affects tissues throughout the body.

"We really have the ability to target the tumor while preserving healthy tissue," he says.

TECHNIQUE AVAILABLE, BUT NOT USUAL TREATMENT

The technology is currently available at most academic medical centers throughout the United States.

"Unfortunately, many patients and many primary-care physicians don't yet know about the success of this therapy," Geschwind says.

"I'm not saying it's a cure for liver cancer, but when you see the results in terms of prolongation of life, it's quite significant," he adds.

"I think we're on the cusp of something even bigger," he adds, "because now we have at our disposal new drugs that can be even more cancer-specific."

For more on these and other non-surgical breakthroughs in cancer care, visit the Society of Interventional Radiology at *www.sirweb.org*. Click on "patients."

■ ■ ■ ■

Fever Signals

Fever of unknown origin may signal cancer, according to Henrik Toft Sorensen, MD.

Recent finding: Patients hospitalized with fever of 101.5°F or more for which a cause never was determined were twice as likely to be diagnosed with cancer within the next year as the general population. The increased risk was high for cancers of the liver, brain, kidney, colon and/or pancreas as well as sarcoma (cancer of soft tissue).

Reason: Cancer can cause fever through inflammation and infection.

Self-defense: If you are hospitalized due to a fever of unknown origin, ask your doctor whether cancer could be a cause.

Henrik Toft Sorensen, MD, professor, department of clinical epidemiology, Aarhus University Hospital, Denmark.

■ ■ ■ ■

Cancer Vaccine

A cervical cancer vaccine helps protect girls and young women ages nine to 26.

Recent finding: In two large-scale, placebo-controlled studies, the vaccine was 100% effective after a 17-month follow-up when three doses were given over six months (as recommended by the vaccine maker) and 97% effective after an average two-year follow-up when one dose was given. The vaccine, called Gardasil, blocks infection caused by both *human papilloma virus* (HPV) 16 and 18, the two types of HPV that together cause 70% of all cervical cancers. The vaccine is not intended to replace regular Pap smears to screen for cervical cancer. The FDA approved Gardasil in 2006.

Kevin Ault, MD, associate professor of obstetrics and gynecology, Emory University School of Medicine, Atlanta.

Deadly Skin Cancer

Perry Robins, MD, professor emeritus of dermatology at New York University Medical Center, New York City, and founder and president of the Skin Cancer Foundation, is author of *Sun Sense: A Complete Guide to the Prevention, Early Detection and Treatment of Skin Cancer*. Skin Cancer Foundation.

Melanoma is the deadliest type of skin cancer. The incidence of melanoma is increasing so fast that it has been called one of the nation's most serious epidemics.

Since 1986, the diagnosis rates of melanoma have more than doubled. This is partly due to an increased awareness of skin cancer. More people are being tested, so more cases are detected. But the real numbers also are rising. The population is aging, and half of adults diagnosed are in their 50s.

Melanoma is more likely than other cancers to spread (metastasize) to other parts of the body. About 12% of patients with melanoma die from the cancer.

Important: No one needs to die from skin cancer. With regular screenings, melanoma can be detected and removed before it has a chance to spread.

KNOW THE SIGNS

Telltale signs of melanoma and other skin cancers...

A. Asymmetrical shape. Normal moles have a uniform appearance. Moles with irregular shapes are more likely to be cancerous.

B. Border that is irregular. The edges of the mole might be notched or scalloped.

C. Color changes. Moles should have a uniform color. If a mole has different colors, it could be melanoma.

D. Diameter. A mole larger than about one-quarter-inch (six millimeters) across should be checked.

The Skin Cancer Foundation recommends annual skin exams for people age 40 and over. An exam every three years is enough for younger people. The doctor should examine every inch of skin and note or diagram suspicious moles or skin changes for future evaluation and/or treatment.

CAUSES

Melanoma occurs in cells (melanocytes) that produce melanin, the "tanning" skin pigment. When you spend time in the sun, these cells produce more melanin as a protective mechanism against sun damage. However, excessive sun exposure (along with other, still unknown factors) can damage the DNA in melanocytes and result in cancer.

The sun produces three types of UV radiation. Both UV-A and UV-B rays have been linked to melanocyte damage and melanoma. The third type of radiation, UV-C, is absorbed in the atmosphere and doesn't reach Earth.

Melanomas usually form on parts of the body that aren't regularly exposed to sun. Low levels of melanin in these areas make cells more sensitive to damage. Men tend to develop melanomas on the back. Women are more likely to get them on the legs. Less often, melanomas may occur under a finger- or toenail or in the eye or in mucous membranes that line the nose, mouth, esophagus, anus, urinary tract and vagina.

Heredity also plays a role in melanoma risk. About one out of every 10 patients diagnosed has a family member who has had the disease.

PREVENTION

Most melanomas can be prevented with simple precautions...

•**Apply sunscreen before going outdoors year-round.** Use it on all exposed skin, including the face, ears, backs of the hands, etc. Apply it a half-hour before going outdoors so that it penetrates the skin and provides maximal protection. Use a product that filters out both UV-A and UV-B rays.

Certain sunscreens may cause a reaction in some people.

Self-test: Apply a small amount to the inside of your arm at night. In the morning, check for a rash, itching or other signs of sensitivity. If there are no changes, the sunscreen should be safe for you.

• **Use a product with an SPF (sun-protection factor) of 30.** Don't pay extra for products with higher SPF numbers—they provide little or no additional protection. Apply a thin layer of sunscreen every two or three hours. Apply it more often if you're swimming or perspiring heavily.

• **Wear protective clothing.** Sunscreens don't completely block UV radiation. Wear a cap or broad-brimmed hat…tightly woven clothing…and sunglasses that block both UV-A and UV-B rays.

• **Stay away from tanning beds.** Some tanning salons advertise that they are safe, but that is not true.

• **Perform monthly self-exams.** Stand in front of a full-length mirror, and examine your skin. Use a hand mirror to check hard-to-see areas. Check the soles of your feet and the spaces between your toes, as well as the scalp, groin, etc. New growths…moles that have changed…and sores that don't heal should be checked by a doctor.

TREATMENT

Nearly everyone with melanoma survives when it's detected at an early stage, before it has spread.

The only effective treatment for melanoma that hasn't spread is surgical removal. This usually can be done in a doctor's office and with a local anesthetic.

Very small melanomas may be entirely removed during the biopsy. For larger ones, the doctor will remove the cancer, and an additional amount of healthy tissue may be removed.

If melanoma has spread: Patients may require chemotherapy, radiation therapy or other treatments, along with surgical removal of the original cancer.

There are a number of new vaccines that can extend life by several years in patients who have melanoma that has spread. However, they don't eliminate the cancer and are not a cure.

New Hope for Brain Tumor Patients

Michael Vogelbaum, MD, PhD, associate director of neurosurgical oncology and vice chairman of the Brain Tumor Institute at The Cleveland Clinic in Ohio, is also director of the institute's Center for Translational Therapeutics, which conducts studies to evaluate the ability of new drugs to reach their targets in brain tumors.

Primary brain tumors—those that originate in the brain rather than metastasizing from other parts of the body—are among the most virulent of cancers. The most common type, glioma, tends to strike otherwise healthy adults with seeming randomness and is often fatal.* An estimated 17,000 to 20,000 Americans will be diagnosed with a primary brain tumor this year.

Good news: Recent research is giving these patients reason for hope. *If you or a loved one has been diagnosed with a brain tumor, here's what you need to know…*

TREATMENT ADVANCES

The most aggressive of all gliomas, *Glioblastoma multiforme* (GBM), is also the most common, with about 10,000 to 12,000 diagnosed in the US annually, most after age 50. The median survival time for someone with GBM is about one year.

These tumors rapidly spread and infiltrate normal parts of the brain, so it's impossible to excise them completely. The traditional approach to treating GBMs has been to surgically remove as much of the tumor as possible and then administer radiation therapy. When the tumor regenerates, as GBMs often do, doctors have prescribed chemotherapy to slow the growth.

Breakthrough: In a recent trial by Canadian and European researchers, GBM patients who were given radiation therapy and the chemotherapy drug *temozolomide* (Temodar) following surgery did significantly better than those who received radiation alone. A full 26.5% of the patients who received combination therapy were living two years after their diagnoses, versus only 10.4% of the control group. These results

*Meningioma, a type of brain tumor that is usually benign, is about twice as common as glioma.

were so positive that this approach is now the standard of care for all GBM patients in North America and Europe. More studies are needed to determine its long-term efficacy and safety.

On the horizon: It may soon be possible to identify which GBM tumors will respond optimally to the new protocol. In reviewing their trial data, Canadian and European researchers noticed that patients whose tumors had an inactivated gene, known as 06-methyl-guanine-DNA methyltransferase (MGMT), did markedly better on the combination therapy than those whose tumors had an active MGMT gene. The median survival among patients with inactive MGMT was nearly 22 months, and an astounding 46% of them were alive at two years. Those who had an active MGMT gene survived for a median of nearly 13 months. The gene enables cancer cells to repair themselves after being damaged by certain chemotherapy drugs, rendering the chemotherapy ineffective. We're exploring ways to safely "turn off" the gene in patients for whom it remains active.

OTHER RESEARCH ADVANCES

All cancers are in part genetic, since genes play a role in the development and progression of the disease. Genetic variations also appear to affect whether and to what extent another type of tumor, called an *oligodendroglioma*, will respond to chemotherapy. This slow-growing tumor is rare and typically occurs in middle-aged adults.

We've long known that an estimated two-thirds of these tumors are sensitive to chemotherapy drugs, while the remaining one-third are largely impervious. Researchers at Massachusetts General Hospital, in collaboration with Canadian colleagues, discovered in 1998 that responsive oligodendrogliomas had one thing in common—loss of parts of chromosomes (cell structures that carry genetic information), specifically chromosomes 1p and 19q. For reasons that are not yet clear, parts of these chromosomes "disappear" in some of these tumors. About 50% of patients with oligodendrogliomas lack these chromosomes. Virtually all oligodendrogliomas lacking both of these chromosomes will have a prolonged response to treatment, while those that retain them, particularly the 1p chromosome, are unlikely to have durable responses to treatment.

While patients with oligodendrogliomas are now routinely screened for loss of 1p and 19q chromosomes, doctors have yet to reach a consensus on how best to treat tumors lacking them. Some still recommend aggressive surgery to remove the bulk of the tumor, followed by radiation and chemotherapy. Others suggest starting with chemotherapy, hoping that patients may be able to avoid surgery and radiation. Both approaches are meeting with success. The median survival rate for these patients now exceeds seven years. Clinical trials are under way to study these treatment approaches.

CLINICAL TRIALS MATTER

All new therapies—surgical, radiological, pharmacological—must prove safe and effective in clinical trials before being prescribed to the general patient population.

One big challenge we face in advancing brain cancer therapies is making patients aware of the clinical trials that may benefit them personally…or lead to lifesaving treatments for future generations. For patients whose brain tumors do not respond to traditional treatment, an investigational therapy may be their best hope.

To learn more about clinical cancer trials, or to find a trial that may be right for you or a loved one, consult the National Cancer Institute, 800-422-6237, *www.cancer.gov*, or the American Cancer Society, 800-227-2345, *www.cancer.org*.

■■■■

Cancer Warning

Hiccups are a surprising sign of cancer, according to Thomas Noel Walsh, MD.

Recent finding: 27% of esophageal cancer patients had experienced persistent hiccups prior to diagnosis. People who have hiccups for more than 48 hours—especially if accompanied by swallowing problems and/or weight loss—should see their physicians. The incidence of this very serious cancer is on the rise.

Thomas Noel Walsh, MD, is associate professor of surgery, Royal College of Surgeons in Ireland (RCSI), Dublin, and leader of a study of 99 esophageal cancer patients.

The Fastest-Growing Cancer Threat

Herman Kattlove, MD, is a medical oncologist and medical editor with the American Cancer Society.

Cancer rates are generally declining in the US, but the incidence of adenocarcinoma, the most common type of esophageal cancer, has increased more rapidly since the 1970s than any other cancer.

Until recently, cancer of the esophagus—the foot-long muscular tube that carries food from the mouth to the stomach—has been considered deadly, though relatively rare. Now both of these beliefs are being challenged.

At one time, people diagnosed with esophageal cancer who underwent surgery had a low chance of surviving for five years. That survival rate is now as high as 50%, most likely due to earlier screening and diagnosis.

Fortunately, healthy lifestyle changes can reduce your risk of developing esophageal cancer.

WHO IS AT RISK?

As with many cancers, the risk for esophageal cancer increases with age—nearly 80% of new cases are diagnosed in people ages 55 to 85.

There are two main types of esophageal cancer—*squamous cell carcinoma*, which develops in the cells that line the entire esophagus, and *adenocarcinoma*, which occurs in the part of the esophagus closest to the stomach.

More than half of all squamous cell carcinomas are linked to smoking. Risk of adenocarcinoma is doubled in people who smoke a pack of cigarettes or more per day. Carcinogens in tobacco are believed to enter the bloodstream and contribute to the development of esophageal cancer. Excessive alcohol consumption—more than two drinks daily—also increases the risk for the squamous cell type of cancer, although it is not known why.

Tobacco *and* alcohol are a potentially deadly combination. A person who drinks excessively and smokes one to two packs of cigarettes a day has a 44 times higher risk of getting esophageal cancer than someone who does neither.

A diet low in fruits and vegetables accounts for approximately 15% of esophageal cancer risk. To help avoid the disease, eat at least five daily servings. Some scientific evidence suggests that berries, particularly black raspberries, which are rich in cancer-fighting antioxidants, protect against esophageal cancer.

Body weight also is a factor. Obese men are twice as likely to die from adenocarcinoma of the esophagus as men of normal weight.

THE HEARTBURN CONNECTION

Frequent heartburn, known as gastroesophageal reflux disease (GERD), is caused by stomach acid backing up into the esophagus. Up to 14% of Americans experience heartburn at least weekly, while 44% suffer from it monthly. GERD is linked to nearly one-third of esophageal cancer cases.

An additional factor for esophageal adenocarcinoma is a condition called *Barrett's esophagus*, in which cells of the esophagus begin to resemble those that line the stomach. People with Barrett's esophagus are about 50 times more likely to develop esophageal cancer than those without the condition.

People who suffer from chronic heartburn (three or more times per week for more than three months) should be screened for Barrett's esophagus. If they are found to have the condition, screenings every year may be recommended to detect esophageal cancer.

Screening involves the use of *endoscopy,* an invasive procedure that requires sedation. During the test, the doctor passes a thin, flexible tube (endoscope) through the mouth to view the entire length of the esophagus.

Prompt and effective treatment of GERD might reduce the risk for esophageal cancer, although this has never been proven. A number of effective prescription and over-the-counter GERD remedies, which block the production of stomach acid, are available. These include H2 blockers, such as *ranitidine* (Zantac) and *famotidine* (Pepcid), and proton pump inhibitors, such as *omeprazole* (Prilosec).

SYMPTOMS AND DIAGNOSIS

Difficulty swallowing is the most common symptom of esophageal cancer. If you notice that swallowing has become even slightly harder—you must swallow more firmly or food doesn't go down properly—see your doctor immediately. It could save your life.

Weight loss commonly occurs because of difficulty swallowing and loss of appetite. Frequent bouts of hiccups, another sign of esophageal cancer, may result when cancer irritates the nerves leading to the diaphragm. More advanced cancer may compress the nerves that control the vocal cords, which can lead to hoarseness.

If your doctor suspects cancer, endoscopy will be performed and a biopsy taken. Additional tests may be necessary—endoscopic ultrasound, a procedure that involves the use of high-frequency sound waves, to pinpoint the tumor thickness...and a computed tomography (CT) scan and a positron emission tomography (PET) scan to determine whether the tumor has spread to nearby lymph nodes.

TREATMENT

Surgery is the main treatment for esophageal cancer. Most often, the surgeon will perform *esophagectomy*, in which the cancerous part of the esophagus and nearby lymph nodes are removed, or *esophagogastrectomy*, in which the lower part of the esophagus and upper part of the stomach are removed. With both procedures, the remaining part of the esophagus is reconnected to the stomach, often with a segment of the large intestine.

These procedures are extremely complex and demand a high degree of surgical expertise, as well as a skilled team of nurses and other personnel to provide after-care. Choose a major cancer center that performs more than 10 esophageal cancer surgeries a year.

Chemotherapy and radiation before surgery have been shown to improve the outcome, possibly because they destroy microscopic tumor tissue before it can spread.

In one study of 802 patients, 42% of those who had two rounds of chemotherapy before surgery were still alive two years later, compared with 34% of those who had surgery alone.

New finding: A long-term clinical trial showed that esophageal cancer patients who received so-called "triple therapy"—treatment with two cancer drugs (*5-fluorouracil* and *cisplatin*) and daily radiation for five weeks before surgery—had a 39% chance of surviving for five years, compared with 16% of patients who received only surgery.

■ ■ ■ ■

Bladder Cancer Danger

Of 214 patients who had their bladders removed within 93 days of being diagnosed with cancer that had invaded the bladder wall muscle, 39% died, and the rest had a 51% chance of living for three years. When surgery was performed after 93 days, 54% died, and the rest had a 38% chance of living for three years.

Self-defense: Bladder removal for this type of cancer should be done within three months.

Cheryl Lee, MD, director, bladder cancer program, University of Michigan Comprehensive Cancer Center, Ann Arbor.

The #2 Cause of Cancer

Julie Parsonnet, MD, professor of infectious diseases at Stanford University School of Medicine in Stanford, CA, is the editor of *Microbes and Malignancy: Infection as a Cause of Human Cancers*. Oxford University.

People tend to think that cancer is caused only by unhealthful habits, such as smoking, or environmental factors, including exposure to asbestos or excessive sunlight. They don't realize that cancer often is triggered by an infectious disease.

The shocker: At least 25% of malignancies are caused by viruses, bacteria and parasites. After smoking, infection is the leading cause of cancer.

Although millions of Americans are infected with cancer-causing organisms at some time during their lives, most of these people don't develop cancer as a result. There are additional risk factors that work in tandem with infectious microbes to trigger the biological changes that lead to cancer.

THE INFECTION LINK

Viruses are the main cancer-causing organisms, followed by bacteria and parasites.

Primary ways that these organisms cause cancer...

•**Genetic changes.** Viruses can't replicate on their own. When viruses enter your body, they inject their own genetic material into your cells and take over the cells' inner workings.

Some viral genes, known as *oncogenes*, cause cells to divide much more rapidly than usual. Rapid cell division increases the odds of genetic "mistakes" that can lead to cancer. Viruses also inhibit our body's natural ability to destroy damaged cells, which may otherwise continue to grow and divide in ways that make us more vulnerable to cancer.

•**Chronic inflammation.** Some organisms, such as those that cause stomach and liver cancer, irritate tissues and trigger persistent inflammation. Inflammation causes cells to divide at a faster rate than normal, increasing the likelihood that they will mutate and undergo changes that lead to cancer.

CANCER-CAUSING INFECTIONS

Numerous cancers are believed to be caused, in part, by infectious organisms. *The most common cancer-causing infections—and steps you can take to protect yourself...*

•**Helicobacter pylori.** Between 30% and 40% of Americans are infected with *Helicobacter pylori*, a screw-shaped bacterium that burrows into the stomach lining and causes chronic inflammation. About 20% of these people will eventually develop ulcers—another 5% will develop stomach cancer.

Infection with H. pylori is a very strong risk factor for cancer, presumably because the bacterium causes inflammation and cell proliferation. More than 80% of stomach cancer cases are caused by H. pylori. Infection with this bacterium increases your risk of developing stomach cancer by at least eightfold.

Self-defense: Ulcer patients are routinely tested for H. pylori and treated with antibiotics if infection is present. Once the bacterium is eliminated, the risk for ulcers drops significantly. It is not yet known if treating bacteria will help prevent stomach cancer. Patients with a family history of stomach cancer should talk to their doctors about getting tested for H. pylori.

Also helpful: Eat a nutritious diet that is rich in fruits and vegetables and low in salt and food preservatives known as nitrates. Such a diet may reduce cancer risk.

•**Epstein-Barr virus.** The Epstein-Barr virus (EBV) causes infectious mononucleosis, which leads to extreme fatigue and other flu-like symptoms. EBV is found in the tumors of a significant number of patients with Hodgkin's disease (a form of lymphoma that strikes most often between the ages of 15 to 35 and after age 55).

The risk that an individual patient who has had mononucleosis will go on to develop Hodgkin's disease—or non-Hodgkin's lymphoma, which also is associated with the EBV virus—is still very low.

The main risk for non-Hodgkin's lymphoma in people with EBV appears to be in those who have severely compromised immune systems —for example, those who have undergone transplant surgery and/or are taking immune-suppressing drugs.

Self-defense: Transmission of EBV is impossible to prevent because many healthy people can carry and spread the virus for life. People who receive transplants and immune-suppressing drugs should ask their doctors about symptoms of EBV-related malignancies. Decreasing immunosuppression can often reverse lymphoma when caught early.

•**Hepatitis B.** The hepatitis B virus (HBV) is spread by contact with body fluids of an infected person, including blood, saliva, vaginal secretions and semen.

At greatest risk: People who have sex with infected partners...and drug users who share needles.

Most cases of HBV are acute, lasting six months or less. This form of hepatitis is not linked to cancer. However, the *chronic* form of HBV, which is almost always acquired in childhood and lasts for more than six months, greatly increases the risk for cirrhosis (destruction of normal liver tissue) as well as liver cancer.

Self-defense: All newborns are now given the HBV vaccine. It's also recommended for children ages 18 years or younger who weren't previously vaccinated. Adults don't require the vaccine for cancer prevention—but it is recommended for those in high-risk groups because it can reduce the risk for long-term liver disease.

Among those who should get the vaccine: Health-care workers...those who are sexually active with people who may have HBV and/or have household contact with them...and dialysis patients.

•**Hepatitis C.** Most people with the hepatitis C virus (HCV) were infected by tainted blood transfusions prior to 1992, when blood-screening tests first became available. HCV also can be transmitted by having sex with someone who is infected…sharing contaminated hypodermic needles…and receiving nonsterile tattoo or body-piercing procedures.

About 5% of patients with HCV will develop liver cancer. A much higher percentage will develop cirrhosis or other chronic liver diseases—usually decades after the initial exposure.

Self-defense: In addition to the high-risk practices mentioned above, do not share razors, toothbrushes or nail clippers in households with an HCV-infected person. Patients who received a blood transfusion prior to 1992, or who engage in high-risk practices, should be tested for HCV.

Treatment depends on the type and extent of the HCV infection. For example, a combination of *interferon* (such as PEG-Intron) and an antiviral drug called *ribavirin* (Rebetol) can eliminate infection in 50% to 80% of cases.

•**Human papilloma virus.** A majority of sexually active American women will be exposed to one of the many strains of human papilloma virus (HPV) at some time during their lives. HPV is a sexually transmitted infection that may cause no symptoms itself but increases the risk for cervical cancer.

Fortunately, only a small percentage of women with HPV go on to develop cervical cancer. There also are relatively harmless forms of HPV, such as those that cause genital warts—these do not increase cancer risk.

A new HPV vaccine appears to be extremely effective. It is now available.

The use of condoms and other safe-sex practices aren't very effective at preventing the spread of HPV. That's because condoms may not cover enough of the penis to prevent exposure. The virus also can be transmitted by hand-to-genital contact.

Self-defense: Women should get regular Pap tests to look for precancerous changes in the cervix. The American Cancer Society recommends an HPV test in addition to a Pap smear for women ages 30 and older. The cure rate for cervical cancer is about 90% when it's detected at an early stage.

Vitamin A vs. Cancer

John Erdman, PhD, professor of food science and human nutrition in the division of nutritional sciences at the University of Illinois at Urbana-Champaign, has participated in more than 100 scientific studies and authored 140 scientific publications on vitamin A and other areas of nutrition.

Vitamin A has traditionally been known for its role in helping to prevent night blindness (a condition in which you cannot see well in dim light).

In fact, that's why carrots, which are rich in beta-carotene (a vitamin A precursor), are said to be so good for your eyes.

Now, scientists are identifying new health benefits of the vitamin.

Recent finding: Researchers at the Harvard School of Public Health analyzed the diets of 450 men without prostate cancer. Among those under age 65, the men with the highest dietary intake of beta-carotene were 36% less likely to develop prostate cancer than those with the lowest intake.

How vitamin A could potentially help you…

WHAT VITAMIN A DOES

Vitamin A was discovered in 1920. As one of the first known vitamins, it was designated by the first letter of the alphabet.

Vitamin A helps prevent night blindness because it is a crucial component of *rhodopsin*, a light-sensitive molecule in the eye. It also helps maintain the health of the cornea (the front of the eye), guarding against the development of blindness, especially in children.

In addition to its beneficial effects on vision, vitamin A helps keep almost all the surfaces of the body healthy—the skin, the mucous membranes and the linings of the respiratory, urinary and intestinal tracts.

Vitamin A also improves the function of the immune system by supporting the action of various infection-fighting immune cells, such as neutrophils, macrophages and natural killer cells. In addition, it helps with reproduction, aiding the production of sperm and the development of eggs.

WHERE VITAMIN A IS FOUND

Foods of animal origin (egg yolks, liver and milk products) contain a preformed version of vitamin A known as *retinol*. Some fortified foods, such as low-fat milk and breakfast cereals, are supplemented with this highly usable form of vitamin A.

Vitamin A also can be produced in the body when you consume foods that contain *beta-carotene*, including sweet potatoes, pumpkin, mangoes, cantaloupe, apricots, tomatoes, red peppers, peas, peaches, papayas, winter squash, spinach and kale.

HOW MUCH DO YOU NEED?

The federal government sets a daily recommended dietary allowance (RDA) for vitamin A. This amount includes vitamin A derived from retinols (found in foods of animal origin) and carotenoids, such as beta-carotene (derived from brightly colored fruits and vegetables).

For women age 19 and older, the RDA is 2,310 international units (IU). For men age 19 and older, it is 3,000 IU. The RDA for pregnant women is 2,565 IU…for lactating women, it's 4,300 IU.

Approximately 56% of Americans do not meet the RDA for vitamin A, according to the US Department of Agriculture. This segment of the population is believed to have a generally poor diet that includes significant amounts of fast foods and other low-nutrient food products.

Because vitamin A is *fat-soluble* (that is, it is stored in the liver and does not dissolve in water), it takes longer for a deficiency to develop than it would with a water-soluble vitamin, such as vitamin C.

Many Americans may suffer from a *subclinical* deficiency, a low level of vitamin A that has no observable symptoms. This type of deficiency could diminish a person's ability to recover from significant stress, such as a major illness or operation.

People who have illnesses that inhibit the absorption of nutrients, such as Crohn's disease (an inflammatory bowel disorder) and celiac disease (an intolerance to gluten, a protein found in barley, wheat and rye), should ask their doctors whether they would benefit from a vitamin A supplement. Vegans, who consume no foods derived from animals, including eggs and dairy products, also may need a vitamin A supplement. A multivitamin typically is a good choice.

CAN YOU GET TOO MUCH?

Vitamin A toxicity has been well studied by scientists.

Most important findings…

•**Vitamin A and bones.** A handful of studies over the past five years have shown that postmenopausal women who got approximately twice the RDA of vitamin A were at greater risk for osteoporosis and had an increased rate of hip fractures compared with women who received the RDA. A study from Sweden showed the same result in men.

It's important to remember, however, that while these studies show an association between increased intake of vitamin A and bone problems, they do not prove that the nutrient causes bone loss.

Best advice: Postmenopausal women who are concerned about vitamin A-related bone loss should make sure that the nutritional supplements they take do not contain a total amount of vitamin A that exceeds the RDA.

•**Vitamin A and lung cancer.** By the 1990s, 24 out of 25 epidemiological studies of various populations had shown that smokers who consumed the most beta-carotene-rich fruits and vegetables had the lowest levels of lung cancer. Researchers theorized that the nutrient functioned as an antioxidant, protecting lungs from cellular damage.

To test the theory, in two studies conducted a decade ago, men at high risk for lung cancer (those who smoked a pack a day or more for decades…and/or were exposed to lung-damaging asbestos) were given 20 mg to 30 mg daily of supplemental beta-carotene for approximately six years. More of these men got lung cancer than a similar group who did not receive beta-carotene supplements.

Researchers explain this increased lung cancer risk by noting that the high-risk men who were studied had received 80 times more of a highly absorbable form of supplemental beta-carotene than the amount usually consumed from fruits and vegetables in a typical diet found in the epidemiological studies. As the study participants' bodies attempted to break down and eliminate this high dose of beta-carotene, harmful by-products were created that promoted the development of cancer in the lung.

Best advice: Get your beta-carotene from food.

VITAMIN A AS MEDICINE

•**Acne and psoriasis.** Retinoids (synthetic derivatives of vitamin A) are used to treat acne, psoriasis and other skin disorders.

Caution: The acne drug isotretinoin (Accutane) can cause severe side effects, including birth defects, and should be used only under close medical supervision.

•**Breast cancer.** Another synthetic derivative of vitamin A—4-hydroxyphenylretinamide (4-HPR)—is being used experimentally to prevent the recurrence of breast cancer.

■ ■ ■ ■

Another Reason Not to Smoke

Nicotine prevents the most common lung cancer drugs from working, laboratory tests show. This raises the possibility that nicotine gum and patches might have a similar effect.

Better for lung cancer patients: Use a smoking-cessation program that focuses on behavioral modification rather than nicotine replacement.

Srikumar Chellappan, PhD, associate professor, department of oncology, H. Lee Moffitt Cancer Center and Research Institute, Tampa, and leader of a study, published in *Proceedings of the National Academy of Sciences.*

■ ■ ■ ■

Curry Fights Cancer

In a lab study of human cells, curcumin (the compound that makes curry yellow) was shown to interfere with the development of melanoma cells. Past studies have shown that people who eat curry in abundance have lower rates of lung, colon, prostate and breast cancers.

Theory: Curcumin curbs inflammation, a risk factor for cancer.

Self-defense: Eat a half tablespoon of curry every day.

Bharat B. Aggarwal, PhD, professor of cancer medicine, University of Texas M.D. Anderson Cancer Center, Houston.

■ ■ ■ ■

Customized Chemo

Customized chemotherapy is just around the corner, reports Anil Potti, MD. A recent study shows that genomic tests, which analyze a cancer's molecular traits, are 80% accurate in predicting which drugs will be most effective in destroying tumors from breast, lung and ovarian cancers.

Advantages: In many cases, physicians won't have to try out drugs one by one to see what works. Treatment should progress faster—and patients will be exposed to fewer toxic drugs.

Anil Potti, MD, is assistant professor, Institute for Genome Sciences and Policy, Duke University Medical Center, Durham, North Carolina, and leader of a study of more than 350 tumors, published in *Nature Medicine.*

■ ■ ■ ■

This Exam Prevents Oral Cancer

In a recent study, when dentists and other health-care workers visually examined patients for signs of oral cancer, they uncovered numerous otherwise hidden cases, reducing risk for death by 79% compared with an unscreened control group. Researchers estimate that regular screening of the oral cavity by visual inspection once every three years could prevent at least 37,000 oral cancer deaths annually.

Self-defense: Make sure your dentist or general practitioner carefully examines the inside of your mouth at least once every three years.

Rengaswamy Sankaranarayanan, MD, head, screening group, International Agency for Research on Cancer, Lyon, France.

■ ■ ■ ■

Better Radiation Therapy

Radiation therapy for breast cancer no longer damages women's hearts. In the past, women with breast cancer on the left side who received radiation treatment risked heart attacks. Recent improvements now allow radiation to be delivered more accurately. Nearly 40%

of women with breast cancer are treated with radiation therapy following surgery.

Sharon Giordano, MD, MPH, assistant professor, University of Texas MD Anderson Center, Houston, and lead researcher of a study of the records of more than 26,000 women with breast cancer, published in *Journal of the National Cancer Institute*.

■ ■ ■ ■

Ineffective Cancer Test

New lung cancer test may lead to unnecessary invasive procedures. The spiral, or helical, CT scan can detect tumors that are small enough to be treated successfully.

Problem: The baseline test yields false-positives as much as 60% of the time—although physicians experienced in interpreting CT scans can reduce the number of postscan invasive procedures. Cancer researchers are studying ways to make spiral CT scans more accurate.

Thomas J. Glynn, PhD, director of cancer science and trends, American Cancer Society, Washington, DC.

■ ■ ■ ■

Missed Diagnosis

Sigmoidoscopies miss advanced precancerous colon growths in almost two-thirds of women—a failure rate twice as high as that in men. Sigmoidoscopies evaluate only one-quarter or one-half the colon and do not allow for removal of precancerous growths.

Self-defense: Everyone age 50 and over—and women, in particular—should have regular colonoscopies to screen for colon cancer. Many insurers will cover only sigmoidoscopies —colonoscopy is more expensive ($500 or more, depending on location) and requires use of a sedative.

Philip Schoenfeld, MD, associate professor of internal medicine, University of Michigan, Ann Arbor, and chief, division of gastroenterology, Ann Arbor Veterans Affairs Health System. He is leader of a study of 1,463 women, published in *The New England Journal of Medicine*.

■ ■ ■ ■

Chicken Lowers Colon Cancer Risk

In a study of 1,520 people, those who ate the most chicken (an average of four servings daily) had a 21% lower risk for colorectal adenomas (growths that can be precursors of colon cancer) than those who ate the least chicken (less than one serving daily).

Theory: Chicken eaters may consume smaller amounts of processed meat, which has been found to increase colon cancer risk.

Self-defense: Substitute chicken for processed meats, such as cold cuts and hot dogs.

Douglas J. Robertson, MD, MPH, assistant professor of medicine, Dartmouth Medical School, Hanover, NH.

The Shocking Truth About Deodorants and Cancer

Philippa D. Darbre, PhD, senior lecturer on oncology, University of Reading, England.
Bert Petersen, MD, breast surgeon and director, Family Risk Program, Beth Israel Medical Center, New York City.
Cosmetic, Toiletry and Fragrance Association.
Journal of Applied Toxicology.

The most common group of chemical preservatives that are in cosmetics and deodorants has been found in human breast cancer tissue.

Although the discovery links breast tumors and this group of chemicals, called parabens, it is not clear what the relationship is and whether the use of these products might be hazardous.

The US Food and Drug Administration (FDA) has called parabens the most widely used preservatives in the United States. They are common in shampoos, foundations, facial masks, hair-grooming aids, nail creams and permanent-wave products.

Previous studies on animals and in the laboratory have shown that parabens can mimic the actions of the hormone estrogen. That has raised red flags because estrogen is known to fuel breast cancer.

The latest research takes those findings one step further.

"We have always been assured that parabens could not get into the body. This study shows that they do," says Philippa D. Darbre, lead author of the study and a cancer specialist at the University of Reading, England.

"It's one more nail in the coffin, or one more piece in the jigsaw," adds Darbre.

RESULTS CAN'T BE IGNORED

"It's preliminary, but I think that it's a little worrisome. And I think there's definitely enough data here to suggest that more work needs to be done to look at this issue," adds Dr. Bert Petersen, a breast surgeon and director of the Family Risk Program at Beth Israel Medical Center in New York City. "I don't think it can be dismissed."

THE STUDY

Darbre has been studying breast cancer for 20 years, but could not get funding for a study on parabens.

"I was told that I wouldn't find anything," Darbre recalls. So, she galvanized friends and colleagues in the medical community, who helped her gain access to analytic machinery and to breast tissue.

Eventually, Darbre was able to analyze samples of 20 human breast tumors with high-pressure liquid chromatography followed by tandem mass spectrometry.

In four of the 20 tumors, the total concentration of parabens was more than twice the average level.

The form the chemicals were found in suggests that they entered the body topically, not orally, the researchers add.

DON'T TOSS YOUR DEODORANT...YET

Of particular concern to many people are underarm products, such as deodorants and antiperspirants, which are applied topically and absorbed through the skin.

But the Cosmetic, Toiletry and Fragrance Association defends the safety of parabens.

"There is no evidence of harm from the use of deodorants or antiperspirants. Consumers should not be unnecessarily alarmed," according to the Association.

The study authors acknowledge that many issues need to be resolved before any definitive conclusions can be reached.

Researchers need to determine levels of parabens in normal breast tissue as well as in other parts of the body. Also, more samples should be examined.

"It would be interesting to see if women [who do not have breast cancer] have very low levels of parabens," Petersen says. "Then you might start to believe maybe this isn't just an association. It might be cause and effect here."

■■■■

Teflon and Cancer?

Teflon has not been found to cause cancer. *Perfluorooctanoic acid* (PFOA), a chemical used in the synthesis of Teflon, has been labeled a "likely carcinogen" by a panel advising the Environmental Protection Agency. But Teflon pans do not emit PFOA when used properly.

Teflon cookware might emit a small amount of PFOA when heated to extreme temperatures—for example, when a frying pan has been left empty on a heated burner for an extended period. Even then, it has not been established that overheated Teflon produces a dangerous amount of PFOA. Still, it wouldn't be unreasonable to dispose of a Teflon pan that has been left empty on a heated burner.

Approximately 95% of the population has some amount of PFOA in their bloodstream—but most of this PFOA likely comes from stain- and water-repelling treatments used on carpets and fabrics. Grease-resistant food packaging, such as microwave popcorn bags and cardboard fast-food boxes, also might contain small amounts of PFOA.

The fact that PFOA is in our bodies does not mean that we're all going to die from PFOA-related cancers. Individuals who have worked in factories where PFOA is produced, and perhaps some people who live in neighboring areas, seem to have the highest levels of PFOA.

Ronald Melnick, PhD, senior toxicologist with National Institute of Environmental Health Sciences, a division of the National Institutes of Health, Research Triangle Park, North Carolina.

■■■■

Supplement Lowers Colon Cancer Risk

High magnesium consumption may help prevent colorectal cancer. In a recent analysis of 61,433 women ages 40 to 75, those with the highest daily intakes of the mineral had a 40% lower risk of developing the disease than those with the lowest daily intakes.

Theory: Magnesium lowers levels of insulin (a hormone produced in the pancreas that regulates blood glucose). Elevated insulin levels are associated with colorectal cancer risk.

Self-defense: Eat food containing 300 mg to 400 mg of magnesium daily. Good sources, which contain 50 mg of magnesium per serving, include one cup of cooked or one-half cup of raw spinach...one large banana...one-half cup of cooked oatmeal...two slices of whole-grain bread...and one-half cup of beans. If you include magnesium-rich foods in your diet, there is no need to take a magnesium supplement.

Susanna C. Larsson, researcher, division of nutritional epidemiology, National Institute of Environmental Medicine, Karolinska Institute, Stockholm, Sweden. Her study was published in the *Journal of the American Medical Association*.

Massage as Effective as Drugs For Cancer?

In a three-year study of the effect of massage on more than 1,000 cancer patients—the largest study to date of massage used for cancer patients—patients rated their symptoms immediately before and after a single treatment of massage therapy.

Result: Anxiety declined by 52%...pain, 40% ...fatigue, 41%...depression, 31%...and nausea, 21%. Massage was as effective as standard drug therapy for these symptoms.

Helpful: Insurance companies are more likely to pay for massage therapy if a doctor writes a referral to a certified therapist or if treatment is part of a hospital in-patient therapy.

To locate a massage therapist in your area, contact the American Massage Therapy Association, 877-905-2700, or visit *www.amtamassage.org*.

Barrie R. Cassileth, PhD, chief, Integrative Medicine Service, Memorial Sloan-Kettering Cancer Center, New York City.

Alcohol and Colon Cancer

Some research suggests that alcohol is a factor in developing colon cancer, but the evidence has not been consistent and the mechanism of alcohol-induced colon cancer risk is not clear.

Theory: Heavy drinkers (typically more than two drinks daily) may be more susceptible to colon cancer due to a general immune deficiency and poor dietary intake of cancer-preventing foods. Also, alcohol by-products may build up to high concentrations in the colon and interfere with the absorption of cancer-preventing substances. Several dietary factors may be involved in the development of colon cancer, including diets low in fresh vegetables and fruits and high in red meat. A deficiency of the B vitamin folic acid is thought to play a role in the development of colon cancer.

Self-defense: Get 400 micrograms of folic acid daily in your diet or through the use of a supplement.

Samuel Meyers, MD, clinical professor of medicine, Mount Sinai School of Medicine, New York City.

Mushrooms for Cancer Prevention

Mushroom extracts are used by health practitioners around the world to prevent cancer and enhance immune function in people who already have cancer. Some mushroom extracts, such as Coriolus versicolor (*Trametes versicolor*) and maitake (*Grifola frondosa*), are considered cancer drugs in China and Japan, since they have been so well studied. Various mushroom extracts are used to treat and prevent different cancers. Coriolus, for instance, is used specifically as an adjunct treatment along with chemotherapy, radiation and surgery, and as a preventive for esophageal, lung, stomach and colon cancers. Many studies support its use. Maitake is used specifically to support conventional treatment of breast, prostate, liver and lung cancers. Be sure to tell your primary care doctor and your oncologist if you are taking mushroom extracts. In some cases, they may interfere with immune-suppressing drugs, such as those taken after a transplant.

Mark A. Stengler, ND, naturopathic physician in private practice, La Jolla, California...adjunct associate clinical professor at the National College of Natural Medicine, Portland, Oregon...author of many books, including *The Natural Physician's Healing Therapies* and coauthor of *Prescription for Natural Cures* (both from Bottom Line Books)...and author of the *Bottom Line/Natural Healing* newsletter.

7 Foods Proven to Fight Cancer

David Grotto, RD, LDN, a registered dietitian and former spokesperson for the American Dietetic Association. He is founder and president of Nutrition Housecall, LLC, a Chicago-area consulting firm specializing in family nutrition programs. He serves on the scientific advisory board of *Men's Health* and is author of *101 Foods That Could Save Your Life*. Bantam.

Up to one-third of all cancers could be prevented if people adopted healthier lifestyles, including eating healthier foods. *For even better odds, choose these seven specific foods that have been proven to prevent cancer...*

CABBAGE

It's high in anticarcinogenic compounds called *glucosinolates*. Raw cabbage, particularly when it is fermented as sauerkraut, also is a good source of *indole-3-carbinol* (I3C), a substance that promotes the elimination of carcinogens from the body.

The Polish Women's Health Study, which looked at hundreds of Polish women in the US, found that those who had eaten four or more servings per week of raw, lightly cooked or fermented cabbage during adolescence were 72% less likely to develop breast cancer than women who had eaten only one-and-a-half servings per week. High consumption of cabbage during adulthood also provided significant protection even if little cabbage was eaten at a young age.

Recommended: Three or more one-half-cup servings per week of cabbage, cooked or raw.

Alternatives: Any cruciferous vegetable, including brussels sprouts, cauliflower, kale and broccoli. A recent study found that men who ate at least three servings per week of broccoli or other cruciferous vegetables were 41% less likely to get prostate cancer than men who ate less than one serving per week. Kimchi, a Korean pickled dish that is similar to sauerkraut, also is a good choice.

FLAXSEEDS

Little seeds with a nutty flavor, flaxseeds contain lignans, compounds that act like a weak form of estrogen. One study found that women with high levels of *enterolactone* (linked to a high intake of lignans) had a 58% lower risk for breast cancer. Flaxseeds also contain omega-3 fatty acids, which appear to inhibit colon cancer in both men and women.

Recommended: One to two tablespoons of ground flaxseed daily. You can sprinkle it on cereal or yogurt or add it to soups or stews.

Alternatives: Two or more servings per week of cold-water fish, such as mackerel or salmon, provide cancer-fighting amounts of omega-3s.

For more lignans: Eat walnuts, and cook with canola oil.

MUSHROOMS

The common white button mushroom found in supermarkets contains anticancer compounds. Scientists who compared vegetable extracts in the lab found that an extract made from white button mushrooms was the most effective at blocking *aromatase*, an enzyme that promotes breast cancer. Button mushrooms also appear to suppress the growth of prostate cancer cells.

Recommended: One-half cup of button mushrooms, three or four times per week.

Alternatives: Porcinis or chanterelles, wild mushrooms with a nuttier taste.

OLIVES

A Spanish laboratory study found that two compounds in olives—*maslinic acid* and *oleanolic acid*—inhibit the proliferation of cancer cells and promote *apoptosis*, the death of these cells. Other studies suggest that people who eat olives as part of a classic Mediterranean diet have lower rates of a variety of cancers, including colon cancer.

Recommended: Eight olives a day, green or black.

Alternative: One to two tablespoons of extra-virgin olive oil daily. Drizzle it on salad or vegetables to enhance absorption of their healthy nutrients.

ONIONS

When researchers compared the 10 vegetables most frequently consumed in the US, onions had the third-highest level of phenolic compounds, which are thought to be among the most potent anticancer substances found in foods.

In a Finnish study, men who frequently ate onions, apples and other foods high in *quercetin* (a phenolic compound) were 60% less likely to develop lung cancer than men who ate smaller amounts. Quercetin also appears to reduce the risk for liver and colon cancers.

Recommended: One-half cup of onions, cooked or raw, three times per week. Yellow and red onions contain the most cancer-preventing substances.

Alternatives: Apples, capers and green and black tea, all of which are high in quercetin. Garlic, a botanical relative of onions, provides many of the same active ingredients.

PUMPKIN

Pumpkin, like all winter squash, is extremely high in *carotenoids*, including beta-carotene. A long-running Japanese study that looked at more than 57,000 participants found that people who ate the most pumpkin had lower rates of gastric, breast, lung and colorectal cancers. There also is some evidence that pumpkin seeds can help reduce the risk for prostate cancer.

Recommended: Three or more one-half-cup servings per week. Pumpkin can be baked like any winter squash. (To learn how to make Baby Roasted Pumpkins with Pink Potatoes, go to *www.BottomLineSecrets.com/Pumpkin*.)

Alternatives: Carrots, broccoli and all of the winter squashes, including acorn, butternut and spaghetti squash.

RASPBERRIES

All of the foods that end with "erry"—including cherry, blueberry and strawberry—contain anti-inflammatory compounds that reduce cell damage that can lead to cancer. Raspberries are higher in fiber than most berries and are an excellent source of *ellagic acid* and *selenium*, both of which protect against a variety of cancers.

Recent studies have shown that raspberries (or raspberry extract) inhibit both oral and liver cancer cells. The responses in these studies were dose-dependent—the more raspberry extract used, the greater the effect.

Recommended: One-and-a-half cups of raspberries, two or three times per week.

Alternative: Cherries (and cherry juice) contain about as much ellagic acid as raspberries. Frozen berries and cherries, which contain less water, provide a higher concentration of protective compounds than fresh ones.

The Anticancer Diet

Timothy C. Birdsall, ND, vice president of integrative medicine for Cancer Treatment Centers of America, a national network of cancer care facilities. Based in Zion, Illinois, he is the coauthor of *How to Prevent and Treat Cancer with Natural Medicine*. Riverhead. *www.cancercenter.com*.

Take healthy cells and expose them to a damaging substance—a toxic chemical, tobacco, radiation, a virus or a bacterium—and the result may be a *mutation*, a permanent change in cell DNA. Expose the cells again, and you get more mutations. Eventually, the healthy cells can turn into cancer cells.

Mutations also can be triggered by breathing, digesting, moving—in other words, living. As part of metabolism, our bodies create harmful molecules called *free radicals*, which can damage cell DNA, cause mutations and induce cancer.

First line of defense: An anticancer diet.

FREE RADICAL WEAKENERS

To combat free radicals, we need beneficial nutrients known as antioxidants. *How they work...*

A free radical is an unstable molecule that's missing an electron. To stabilize it, an antioxidant donates one of its own electrons, neutralizing the free radical. Problem solved...except now the antioxidant is missing an electron, so it becomes a free radical. This new free radical is less dangerous than the original one, but it still can damage cells. So you need another antioxidant to give up its electron—and so on. *To get enough antioxidants, eat...*

•**A rainbow of produce.** Varied colors of fruits and vegetables come from antioxidant pigments called phytochemicals. Each plant food contains hundreds of *phytochemicals* in different combinations.

Remember "Roy G. Biv": The old mnemonic for the colors of the rainbow helps you shop for variety. Go for *red* raspberries, cranberries, tomatoes...*orange* pumpkin, papayas, yams...*yellow* peppers, pineapple, corn...*green* grapes, asparagus, kale...*blue, indigo* and *violet* blueberries, plums and eggplant.

•**Green tea.** These leaves contain antioxidants called *flavonoids.* Consuming green tea daily may reduce risk for various cancers, including bladder and pancreatic cancers.

Recommended: Decaffeination removes flavonoids, so opt for regular green tea rather than decaf. Aim for at least three cups daily, or take green tea extract capsules.

ESTROGEN CONNECTION

The hormone estrogen affects many body functions, including menstruation and cognition. It also may promote some types of breast, ovarian and uterine cancers, although the exact mechanisms are not known. *Protective foods include...*

•**Cruciferous vegetables.** After being used by the body, estrogen is broken down and excreted. The breakdown produces two *metabolites*, or chemical compounds—one that promotes breast cancer and one that does not. Cruciferous vegetables contain the phytochemical *indole-3-carbinol* (I3C), which promotes formation of estrogen's harmless metabolite instead of its carcinogenic one.

I3C foods: Cabbage, broccoli, cauliflower, kale, brussels sprouts. Have four or five half-cup servings weekly.

•**Soy foods.** Soy contains *phytoestrogens* (compounds that mimic natural estrogen in the body), including isoflavones.

Paradox: Some test-tube studies indicate that concentrated phytoestrogens promote breast cancer cell growth—but in real life, soy seems to protect against breast cancer. In Japan and China, where the typical diet is rich in soy isoflavones, breast cancer incidence is about one-third of the US rate.

Theory: Lifelong intake of isoflavones may reduce levels of natural estrogen in breast tissue.

Isoflavone sources: Soy milk, tofu, miso (soybean paste), tempeh (soybean cake), edamame (green soybeans), soy nuts (roasted soybeans).

Goal: One cup of soy milk or one-half cup of another soy food daily.

Caution: Limit soy foods to three servings weekly if you have a history of breast cancer, or are pregnant or nursing. Women with thyroid problems should consult their doctors before eating soy.

•**Fiber.** Estrogen metabolites and toxins pass through the colon on their way out of the body. If they linger there, they can be reabsorbed by the body and cause damage. Fiber may bind to estrogen metabolites and toxins, so they are excreted before they can be reabsorbed.

Goal: Five or more servings per day.

Good sources: Whole-grain bread (one slice) or cereal (typically three-quarters of a cup) ...fruit (one piece or one-half cup)...vegetables and legumes (one-half cup)...nuts and seeds (one-quarter cup).

INFLAMMATION FIGHTERS

Inflammation is part of the normal healing process. However, when this mechanism does not turn itself off properly, inflammation becomes chronic.

Result: More free radicals and cell damage that can lead to cancer. *To reduce inflammation, eat...*

•**Fish.** Many fish are rich in beneficial omega-3 fatty acids. Omega-3s contain an inflammation-fighting component called *eicosapentaenoic acid* (EPA). They also create substances called *prostaglandins* that further reduce inflammation.

Best: Three four-ounce servings weekly of cold-water fatty fish, such as salmon, mackerel, herring and sardines.

Alternative: Take fish oil supplements that provide 1,500 mg daily of combined EPA and *docosahexaenoic acid* (DHA).

•**Flaxseeds.** Ground flaxseeds also provide anti-inflammatory omega-3s.

Bonus: Flaxseeds contain compounds called lignans that may kill some types of cancer cells.

Smart: Add one tablespoon of ground flaxseeds to your daily diet. Sprinkle on cereal or salad, or add to a fruit smoothie.

•**Turmeric.** This yellow spice, commonly used in curry, contains *curcumin*, a compound that neutralizes free radicals and shuts down proteins that promote an abnormal inflammatory response.

Use liberally: Sprinkle turmeric on pasta and rice...add it to fish...stir into soups and salad dressings.

■ **More from Dr. Birdsall...**

Beware the Beef...and Poultry And Pork

A diet high in meat and poultry increases cancer risk. *Here's why...*

•**Sedentary farm animals tend to have more body fat than wild or free-range animals.** High-fat meat and poultry contain more *arachidonic acid*, a fatty acid that promotes cell-damaging inflammation.

•**Cattle often are given hormones to make them bigger.** When we eat their meat, we ingest residual hormones that may stimulate cancer growth.

•**Preserved, cured and smoked meats—** such as hot dogs, ham, bacon, salami and smoked turkey—contain preservatives called *nitrites*, which the body can convert into carcinogenic nitrosamines.

•**Grilling meat or poultry allows fat to drip onto coals,** forming carcinogenic *polycyclic aromatic hydrocarbons* (PAHs)—which smoke then deposits onto the food.

To decrease your risk...

•**Choose meats and poultry labeled "free-range,"** which generally contain less fat.

•**To avoid hormones, opt for poultry or pork** (the USDA prohibits hormone use in these animals)...or buy beef labeled "hormone-free."

•**Select nitrite-free brands of deli meats, hot dogs and bacon.**

•**When grilling, stick to vegetables, which do not form PAHs.** If you do grill meat, cut off charred bits.

•**Limit serving sizes of meat and poultry to three or four ounces—**about the size of a woman's palm.

Optimal Cancer Care

Lise Alschuler, ND, president of the American Association of Naturopathic Physicians. She is a board-certified naturopathic oncologist with a private practice in Scottsdale, Arizona, and is coauthor of *Definitive Guide to Cancer: An Integrative Approach to Prevention, Treatment, and Healing.* Celestial Arts.

W hen a person is diagnosed with cancer, conventional doctors typically recommend surgery, chemotherapy and/or radiation.

Latest development: A growing body of research shows that complementary and alternative medicine (CAM) therapies benefit cancer patients in a number of ways, such as by reducing the adverse effects of conventional cancer treatments.*

AN ATTACK ON CANCER CELLS

Normal cells divide in a predictable and orderly fashion—for example, in the growth of a fetus. When the DNA within cells is damaged—due to genetic abnormalities, for example, or lifestyle factors, such as smoking or getting too much sun exposure—the cells may become cancerous.

The cornerstone of integrative cancer care is to mobilize the body's natural ability to stimulate *apoptosis*—the selective destruction of cells, including cancer cells. Most patients still require surgery, chemotherapy and/or radiation. The integrative component—including dietary changes and the use of supplements simultaneously with conventional treatments—improves the patient's odds of living a longer and healthier life by altering the body processes closely linked with cancer.

*Integrative cancer centers can be found at major US medical institutions, such as Memorial Sloan-Kettering Cancer Center and M.D. Anderson Cancer Center. To find an integrative medicine program at a National Cancer Institute (NCI)–designated cancer center, contact the NCI (800-422-6237, *www.cancer.gov/cam/health_designated_centers.html*).

IMPROVED IMMUNITY

The immune system is the first line of defense against cancer. For example, natural killer cells produce an estimated 100 biochemical poisons that attack foreign proteins, including those on the surface of cancer cells.

Key recommendations...**

•**Load up on antioxidants.** The average cell is subjected to 10,000 daily assaults from free radicals (unstable, negatively charged molecules that can harm DNA), and the resulting damage can overwhelm the ability of immune T cells (including natural killer cells) to destroy cancer cells.

Recommended: Antioxidant-rich fresh produce (at least five servings daily) and supplements, such as vitamin C (1,000 mg to 2,000 mg daily)...selenium (100 mcg to 200 mcg daily)... and zinc (30 mg to 45 mg daily).

•**Take mushroom extracts.** When scientists recently reviewed the results from several randomized clinical trials in Japan, Korea and China, they found that the use of mushroom extracts (which contain a chemical compound that stimulates the immune system to destroy tumors) significantly improved survival rates for patients with malignancies of the stomach, colon, esophagus or breast.

A commonly recommended medicinal mushroom is Coriolus versicolor (or its chemical compound, PSK).

Typical dose: 3,000 mg daily.

CONTROL HORMONES

All cells have *hormone receptors*, molecular sites where hormones attach and cause biochemical reactions. One of the primary reactions is growth, which can be dangerous if a cell is cancerous.

Hormone-dependent cancers—such as some forms of breast cancer as well as many ovarian and prostate cancers—are most likely to be stimulated by certain hormones. But other cancers, such as malignancies of the lung or pancreas, are also influenced by hormones, particularly estrogen and cortisol, that compromise immunity or directly stimulate the growth of tumor cells. *My advice...*

**Important: Consult an integrative health-care practitioner before taking any new supplements.

•**Consume phytoestrogens.** The estrogen-like compounds in plants (phytoestrogens) can reduce the potentially carcinogenic effects of estrogen in the body. Phytoestrogens occupy the estrogen receptor sites, thereby preventing the body's estrogens from binding to those sites. Foods such as soy and flaxseed are rich in phytoestrogens.

Recommended: One tablespoon daily of ground flaxseed and one to two servings weekly of soy foods.

Caution: Women with a previous or current diagnosis of breast or ovarian cancer should talk to their doctors before consuming high doses of phytoestrogens—in such cases, they may trigger the growth of estrogen-dependent cancer cells.

•**Eat leafy greens.** They promote the health of hormone-producing glands, including the thyroid, and support the liver's detoxification of hormones.

Recommended: At least one cup of dark, leafy greens, such as kale and chard, daily.

•**Eat organic.** Many of the herbicides and pesticides used in commercial produce have strong hormonal and genotoxic (DNA-damaging) effects that can increase the risk of getting or having a recurrence of cancers of the breast, kidney, lung and prostate.

•**Exercise regularly.** It regulates the body's production of insulin as well as cortisol and other stress hormones, which, if elevated for too long, can have cancer-causing effects.

Recommended: Six 30-minute sessions weekly.

REMOVE TOXINS

The body is constantly removing potentially carcinogenic toxins, such as *benzene* (commonly found in gasoline and tobacco).

One of the best herbs for detoxification is green tea. It supports the liver's elimination of toxins. Drink at least five cups of green tea daily.

■ **More from Dr. Alschuler...**

Curb Chemo Side Effects

Chemotherapy, a standard part of conventional cancer therapy, often causes side

effects that can be treated with supplements.*
For example...

•**Melatonin,** 20 mg nightly, is a hormone that has been shown in several human trials to reduce chemotherapy side effects, such as immune suppression and decreased appetite, while also improving response to those drugs.

Important: When taken as a sleep aid (a common use of melatonin), the typical dose is 1 mg to 3 mg nightly.

•**Ginger,** 500 mg (in capsules) as needed, is an herb that may help reduce chemotherapy-induced nausea. Ginger also can be consumed in tea form.

•**Glutamine,** an amino acid, 10 g to 30 g daily, can reduce numbness and tingling in the hands and feet (neuropathy) that can be caused by certain chemotherapy drugs.

■ ■ ■ ■

Antioxidants May Lower Pancreatic Cancer Risk

In an analysis of dietary data for 183,518 men and women, those who had the highest

*Consult your doctor before trying supplements.

overall intake of *flavonols* (antioxidant compounds)—found in such foods as black tea, onions and apples—had a 23% lower risk for pancreatic cancer than those who had the lowest intake.

Theory: Flavonols help eliminate unhealthy cells that may develop into pancreatic cancer.

Self-defense: Aim to eat several weekly servings of flavonol-rich foods.

Ute Nöthlings, PhD, researcher, German Institute of Human Nutrition, Potsdam-Rehbruecke, Nuthetal, Germany.

■ ■ ■ ■

C "Suffocates" Cancer

Researchers once thought that vitamin C and other antioxidants helped prevent cancer by neutralizing free radicals.

Recent finding: Vitamin C appears to block a protein that allows cancers to survive in a low-oxygen environment.

Johns Hopkins Medical Institution

15

Men's Health

The Secret to Keeping Men Healthy

Most people know that men tend to develop heart disease at a younger age than women do, but medical researchers now are uncovering other important gender-specific risks that can have a profound effect on men's health.

What you need to know...

COLORECTAL CANCER

Colorectal cancer is slightly more common in men than it is in women. Most of these malignancies begin as small masses of precancerous cells (polyps). By removing these growths before they become cancerous, doctors can prevent most colorectal malignancies.

Interesting fact: Men are most likely to develop polyps in the rectum (the last few inches of the large intestine) and the left side of the colon (the major part of the large intestine, above the rectum), while in women, polyps tend to develop in the right side of the colon.

How men can protect themselves: Starting at age 50, all men should have an annual fecal occult blood test (FOBT). This test can detect hidden blood in the stool, which may signal cancer.

Important: To ensure accurate test results, about three days prior to the FOBT, avoid certain foods, including red meat, radishes, cauliflower and cantaloupe (these foods contain a chemical that can affect test results).

The FOBT should be performed each year in addition to a colonoscopy (the "gold standard" for detecting polyps and early-stage malignancies in the large intestine) every five years. If a polyp is found, a repeat colonoscopy in three years is advisable.

Marianne J. Legato, MD, founder of the Partnership for Gender-Specific Medicine at Columbia University, professor of clinical medicine at Columbia University College of Physicians and Surgeons, both in New York City, and adjunct professor of medicine at Johns Hopkins School of Medicine in Baltimore. She is the author of *Why Men Die First: How to Lengthen Your Lifespan* (Macmillan), and a member of the *Bottom Line/Health* Board of Advisers.

DEMENTIA

Stroke prevention may be especially important for reducing dementia risk in men, according to a new study published in the *Journal of Neurology, Neurosurgery and Psychiatry.* Researchers found that a history of stroke was a major predictor of dementia in men but not in women, even though stroke rates are similar for both sexes. Researchers theorize that this disparity may be due, in part, to diet.

How men can protect themselves: Pay close attention to blood pressure. High blood pressure (hypertension) is the single most important controllable risk factor for stroke.

In my opinion, all men over age 40 should consider an ultrasound (at least every two years) of their carotid (neck) arteries, which deliver blood to the brain. Excessive fatty buildup (plaque) in these arteries may increase stroke risk. If necessary, plaque can be removed with a surgical procedure known as *endarterectomy*—a doctor makes an incision in the affected artery and uses a specially designed tool to remove plaque. In some cases, cholesterol-lowering statin drugs can reduce plaque.

DEPRESSION

Research has shown that a history of depression is an independent risk factor for heart disease in men but not in women. Another study found that men who had suffered depression in their 20s were twice as likely to develop heart disease later in life as those without a history of depression.

Why does depression have such a dramatic effect on men's health?

One theory points to the fact that depression goes undiagnosed and untreated more often in men than in women.

Important: Treatment with prescription antidepressants and/or psychotherapy probably lowers the chance of developing heart disease in people with depression, though this has not been proven in studies.

How men can protect themselves: Any man who suffers symptoms of depression should see his doctor.

Caution: Classic depression symptoms, such as expressing sadness or hopelessness to others, are more likely to occur in women than in men.

In men, depression is usually characterized by persistent irritability, increased use of alcohol, disturbed sleep patterns (insomnia or sleeping too much) and an inability to function effectively at work.

Also helpful: Any man who has ever been diagnosed with depression should have a baseline stress echocardiogram (which uses sound waves to produce images of the heart) or a stress thallium test (which involves the use of a radioactive dye to show how well blood flows to the heart).

HIGH BLOOD PRESSURE

One-third of American adults have high blood pressure. In men, the condition can be affected by such factors as...

•**Lack of treatment.** Men with high blood pressure are less likely than women to have the problem successfully treated—possibly because of an unwillingness to take medication that has been prescribed for the condition. One study found that only 19% of men with high blood pressure had the condition controlled, compared with 28% of women.

How men can protect themselves: Men over age 40 should have an annual physical that includes a blood pressure check. A reading above 130/80 mmHg may require treatment, including lifestyle measures (such as following a healthful diet, maintaining a normal weight, exercising regularly, not smoking and limiting sodium and alcohol intake) and, in many cases, medication.

Important: Men with high blood pressure should be rechecked after three months if blood pressure medication is prescribed—drug therapy often must be adjusted. Subsequent checks should occur every six months.

•**Obstructive sleep apnea.** This condition, marked by brief interruptions in breathing during sleep, can cause or aggravate high blood pressure. Sleep apnea is more common in men than in women.

How men can protect themselves: If you have symptoms of sleep apnea, such as loud snoring, gasping for air during the night and/ or excessive daytime sleepiness, see your doctor. The condition can be treated with lifestyle changes, such as losing weight, and/or the use of a face mask that delivers air pressure to help keep the sufferer's airways open during sleep.

LUNG CANCER

Smoking is the most common culprit in lung cancer, the leading cause of cancer deaths in the US.

Important study: National Cancer Institute researchers recently compared lung cancer risk in male and female smokers, taking into account not only whether people smoke, but also how much. In men and women who smoked about the same amount, men had a slightly higher risk for lung cancer. Also, male *former* smokers were more likely to develop lung cancer than female former smokers with similar smoking histories.

Interesting fact: Lung cancer usually produces symptoms at an earlier stage in men than in women—perhaps because men's cancers tend to cluster in the center of the lung, whereas women's are more often located at the periphery of the lung. A centrally located lung malignancy is more likely to cause a blood-producing cough.

How men can protect themselves: In addition to not smoking, any man who has ever smoked—no matter how long ago—should have a chest X-ray to screen for lung cancer even if he has no symptoms of the disease. He should ask to be tested for lung cancer (with a CT scan, for example) if he has symptoms of a lung malignancy, including lung infections more than once a year, hoarseness, shortness of breath, cough or chest pain.

TESTICULAR CANCER

Most people think that testicular cancer is a young man's disease, since most cases occur between ages 15 and 34, but it is also relatively common between ages 50 and 60. The risk is highest in men who have a father or brother who has had testicular cancer and in those with a history of an undescended testicle, in which one of the testes failed to move down from the abdomen into the scrotal sac after birth.

How men can protect themselves: All men should examine their testicles monthly for any hard lumps—the most common warning sign of testicular cancer. Most testicular malignancies are painless, but they may produce a dull ache

or a feeling of heaviness in the affected testicle or groin area or cause the affected testicle to enlarge. Breast tenderness or an increase in breast size also can occur with testicular cancer.

■ ■ ■ ■

Reduce Prostate Cancer Risk

In a recent finding, men who engaged in at least three hours weekly of vigorous physical activity, such as jogging, swimming or bicycling, had a nearly 70% lower risk of being diagnosed with advanced prostate cancer.

Theory: Exercise reduces levels of hormones, such as *insulin* and *leptin*, that may contribute to the development of prostate cancer.

For optimal prostate cancer prevention: Men should aim for at least three hours of vigorous exercise per week. Walking or other types of milder exercise have cardiovascular and other benefits.

Edward L. Giovannucci, MD, ScD, professor of nutrition and epidemiology, Harvard School of Public Health, Boston.

Prostate Cancer: Diagnosis and Treatment

J. Stephen Jones, MD, chairman of the Glickman Urological Institute at the Cleveland Clinic, Ohio, is the author of The Complete Prostate Book: What Every Man Needs to Know *and* Overcoming Impotence *(both from Prometheus).*

Since its introduction more than 20 years ago, the prostate-specific antigen (PSA) blood test has become a key tool in screening men for prostate cancer.

Until the PSA test, men received only a digital rectal exam (DRE), in which the doctor inserts a gloved, lubricated finger into the rectum to feel the prostate for lumps and thickenings that suggest a tumor.

The PSA test became popular because it can help detect some prostate cancers earlier than the DRE alone. An elevated level of the PSA enzyme doesn't necessarily mean that cancer is present, but it can indicate the need for a biopsy.

Yet now, after years of use, experts disagree about whether men should receive routine PSA testing. Some medical groups, such as the American Urological Society and the American Cancer Society, advocate annual screening for all men age 50 and over—and starting at age 40 or 45 for those at high risk (African-Americans and men with a family history of the disease). Other groups, including the American Medical Association, advise doctors to spell out the risks and benefits of PSA testing and let the patients decide. Unfortunately, few men have all the facts about PSA testing. *What men need to know…*

INTERPRETING TEST RESULTS

PSA is produced by the walnut-sized prostate gland. When cancer is present, the prostate secretes more PSA than usual. But cancer isn't the *only* reason for increased PSA levels. Infection or the enlargement of the prostate that accompanies aging, known as benign prostatic hyperplasia (BPH), can do the same thing. Even ejaculation within 48 hours of the test can affect PSA levels. That's why PSA levels can be difficult to interpret.

What's a "normal" PSA level? Until the last several years, it was defined as below 4.0 ng/ml, but newer data on prostate cancer have made it clear that a man's risk often rises at lower PSA levels. Many experts now say that 2.5 or below is normal for men in their 40s…up to 3.5 for those in their 50s…up to 4.5 for men in their 60s…and up to 6.5 for men 70 and older. (PSA levels naturally rise with age—even in the absence of cancer.)

Another way of looking at PSA is a matter of percentages—one-third of men with a PSA level between 2 and 4 have prostate cancer…44% when the level is 4.1 to 7…and one-half have the disease at a PSA level of 7.1 to 10. Above 10, the chance that a man has prostate cancer rises to two-thirds.

WHAT'S WRONG WITH THE PSA?

Since screening with the PSA test (followed by other tests, such as biopsy, when indicated) catches most cancers—and early detection is generally desirable—why do many experts question whether men should have the PSA test?

The answer isn't simple, because prostate cancer isn't simple. Most prostate tumors grow very slowly, if at all—and are best left alone because they are unlikely to lead to death. Other prostate cancers need aggressive treatment to keep them from spreading. In these cases, early detection can mean the difference between life and death.

How can you tell the difference? You can't with certainty. That's why a substantial number of prostate cancers—found with the help of PSA testing—will be treated even though they are not life threatening. Treatment generally means surgery to remove the prostate and/or radiation to kill the tumor. These treatments carry significant risks for impotence and urinary incontinence.

Proponents of the PSA test point out that prostate cancer deaths have declined in the years since the test has been widely used. However, PSA skeptics say that this trend could also be the result of better treatment, not just better diagnosis.

IMPROVING ACCURACY

In recent years, several variations on the PSA test have been used to improve its accuracy at indicating prostate cancer and limit the number of men who are advised to receive a biopsy.

•**Free vs. bound PSA.** Most PSA floats through the bloodstream bound to protein molecules, while a smaller portion is free. Evidence has shown that when PSA is produced by cancer, higher levels than usual are in the bound form, and a smaller proportion is free. Less free PSA (15% or below) means a greater chance that it's cancer. This test is recommended for men who have abnormal results from the standard PSA test.

•**PSA velocity.** The rate at which PSA changes over the course of three or more annual readings is a significant predictor. The PSA level shouldn't rise more than 0.75 per year, according to the National Cancer Care Network, a consortium of cancer specialists. The group recommends a biopsy if levels rise faster.

•**PSA density.** The larger a noncancerous prostate is, the more PSA it will normally produce. So density—the amount of PSA divided by the size of the gland—also may indicate whether prostate cancer is present. High density—that is, a big number in a man with a small prostate—means more risk. A range of 0.10 to 0.15 and above indicates increased risk.

Drawback: Measuring the prostate requires rectal ultrasound, an invasive procedure that involves placing a thumb-sized probe into the rectum.

WHAT TO EXPECT FROM A BIOPSY

If your PSA results are abnormal, the next step is a biopsy. Some men receive one as soon as possible, while others wait several months and repeat the PSA test. The results of a second PSA test are different enough to warrant a third PSA test in less than 20% of cases, but it is often worth waiting for this confirmation.

Important: If your doctor suspects a prostate infection (from a clinical exam and bacterial culture), he/she should prescribe a course of antibiotics before repeating the PSA test.

If a biopsy is indicated, your doctor will refer you to a surgeon, who will perform the procedure.

What the biopsy involves: While you lie on your side, the surgeon inserts an ultrasound probe through your rectum. A needle-like device is guided through a hole in the probe to take tiny tissue samples from the prostate for examination under a microscope. An estimated 40% of surgeons only take six tissue samples, which allows cancer to be missed 30% to 50% of the time. That's why it's crucial for the surgeon to take at least 12 tissue samples, which decreases the false-negative rate to less than 20%.

Important: Injecting local anesthesia into nerves at the base of the prostate makes the procedure less painful. Not all surgeons are familiar with this technique. Before the biopsy, make sure that local anesthesia is available.

Following the biopsy, there may be slight soreness in the area around the rectum for a few days.

The risk for infection from the biopsy is 1%. To minimize this risk, surgeons should give an antibiotic beforehand.

TREATMENT

Most of the 230,000 prostate cancers diagnosed in the US each year are found when the malignancy is still confined to the prostate. Choosing a treatment at this stage isn't simple.

Active treatment—surgery and/or radiation—is highly effective, but side effects, including impotence and urinary incontinence, are common.

A majority of men who undergo treatment will develop impotence either immediately or within five years. On the other hand, treatment may not even be required. While some prostate cancers are indeed dangerous and must be treated quickly and aggressively, others cause no harm. Unfortunately, it's impossible to say with certainty whether treatment—or no treatment—is more desirable.

WATCHFUL WAITING

The most misunderstood option in treating prostate cancer is "watchful waiting." Many men believe that it means "doing nothing." It does not. Watchful waiting means following the cancer very closely. It aims to minimize unnecessary treatment of tumors that cause no trouble while taking precautions to avoid giving an aggressive cancer a dangerous head start.

The most obvious candidates for watchful waiting are men whose age (typically 70 and older) and other illnesses (heart disease, for example) make it unlikely that they will live long enough to suffer ill effects from the prostate malignancy. But refinements in diagnosis have made watchful waiting a reasonable choice for some younger men as well—if it's done properly. *Here's how…*

•**Fully evaluate the tumor.** Watchful waiting should be considered only for a tumor that appears unlikely to grow quickly. The key measure is the Gleason score, which refers to the tumor "grade" (how abnormal the cells are, and how likely they are to spread). Grades are assigned to the two areas that make up the highest and second highest concentrations of cancer cells. The Gleason score (a number from 2 to 10) is expressed as the sum of the two grades (for example, 3 + 4 = 7). The lower the score, the better.

Prostate-specific antigen, the protein produced in excess by prostate tumors, also may be taken into account. When the PSA is under 10, watchful waiting may be a possibility. Past 20, few doctors would advocate it. A PSA of 10 to 20 falls in a gray zone.

•**Repeat biopsy within a year.** If the cancer has gotten worse (a PSA or Gleason score that has risen significantly) within one year of the first biopsy, it will probably continue to worsen.

How often to biopsy after that depends on age and other factors. A 55-year-old man may want to have a biopsy each year, to discover quickly if treatment is necessary. A 75-year-old with a low-grade tumor may not want a third biopsy for years. In both cases, a rectal exam and PSA testing should be done at least every year.

SURGERY AND RADIATION

The most common treatments for localized prostate cancer (surgery and radiation) are comparably effective—the cancer doesn't come back in the vast majority of cases—and they both carry similar (and substantial) risks for impotence and urinary incontinence.

•**Surgery** involves removal of the entire prostate (prostatectomy). Technical advances have improved *nerve-sparing surgery*, which aims to protect potency and reduce incontinence risk by leaving the nerve bundle next to the prostate intact. It is only possible for some tumors and not always successful in preserving function.

With *laparoscopic surgery*, the entire prostate is removed, but the operation is done through a thin tube, or laparoscope. It's less invasive than conventional surgery and involves less blood loss.

Men seem to recover quicker with laparoscopic surgery (about three weeks versus six weeks for standard prostatectomy), and some reports suggest that there's a better chance of preserving potency—but neither has been definitively shown.

Latest development: With *robotic laparoscopic surgery*, the surgeon watches the operating field on a screen and manipulates surgical instruments with precision controls. It takes years of training and experience to become truly adept at robotic laparoscopic surgery—there are few such experts nationwide. But most surgeons skilled in conventional prostatectomy can quickly master the robotic technique. It appears to be as effective as other types of surgery, but studies are ongoing.

•**Radiation therapy** includes e*xternal beam therapy* (the oldest type, which focuses intense energy on the tumor from a number of angles to destroy it while limiting exposure of normal tissues). With brachytherapy, "seeds," or tiny pellets of radioactive material, are implanted within the prostate itself to deliver radiation to the tumor.

Latest development: *Intensity-modulated radiation therapy* (IMRT) finely adjusts an external radiation beam to conform to the shape of the tumor. And seeds now can be targeted more precisely with ultrasound imaging. Side effects include irritation to the bladder or rectum.

AN IMPROVED ALTERNATIVE

•**Cryotherapy,** which involves freezing the prostate to destroy it, is an alternative to surgery that was developed decades ago. Only recently have advances made cryotherapy a reasonable option.

The tissue-freezing instrument (cryoprobe) is smaller than before (the diameter of a pencil lead rather than a pencil), and the temperature can be adjusted more precisely, which reduces damage to other tissues.

Cryotherapy is far less invasive than surgery, and recovery is much shorter—only a week or two. For five to seven years after the procedure, studies show, survival and cancer control with cryotherapy are comparable to that offered by surgery or radiation. Cryosurgery is less likely to cause lasting urinary incontinence than other procedures.

■ ■ ■ ■

Prostate Screening

In a recent study, 647 men were tested for prostate cancer. Researchers found that for those whose body mass index (BMI) was 25 or above, a lower threshold for the prostate-specific antigen (PSA) density test—a measure of PSA divided by prostate volume—was necessary to accurately predict who had cancer. Researchers don't know why BMI may be linked to prostate cancer.

If you are an overweight or obese man: Ask your doctor whether you need additional screening tests for prostate cancer.

Mark Garzotto, MD, associate professor of urology, Oregon Health & Science University Cancer Institute, Portland, and director of urologic oncology at the Portland Veterans Affairs Medical Center.

How to Beat Advanced Prostate Cancer

Celestia Higano, MD, associate professor of medicine and urology, University of Washington, Seattle.

Bruce Roth, MD, professor of medicine and urologic surgery and section chief, solid tumor oncology, Vanderbilt University, Nashville.

Multidisciplinary Prostate Cancer Symposium, Orlando, Florida.

American Society of Clinical Oncology news release.

Prostate Cancer Foundation news release.

For the first time, a vaccine therapy that harnesses the power of the body's own immune system is proving successful in the fight against metastatic prostate cancer.

Scientists say the compound, called APC8015 (Provenge), primes patients' immune systems to recognize and kill prostate cancer cells that have spread throughout the body.

THE STUDY

The Seattle study looked at 127 men who had cancer that had spread beyond the prostate and grown resistant to hormonal therapy. Eighty-two of the men received Provenge, while the remaining 45 received a placebo. The researchers tracked patient outcomes for three years.

The patients taking Provenge survived an average of 25.9 months, compared with 22 months for those not taking the vaccine, an 18% increase in survival. By the three-year mark, 34% of the men on Provenge remained alive, compared with just 11% in the placebo group.

The side effects were minimal—"some fever and shaking for a few days at the beginning of therapy, but that was transient," says study coresearcher Dr. Celestia Higano, an associate professor of medicine and urology at the University of Washington in Seattle.

THE SCIENCE OF THE VACCINE

"The vaccine is composed of a person's own immune cells that have been isolated from the blood and then sensitized to prostatic acid phosphotase, which is found on 95% of prostate cancer cells," Higano says. Once infused back into the patient, these sensitized cells prime the patient's immune system to recognize and destroy prostate cancer cells that are roaming throughout the body, she adds.

GREAT NEWS

"For those of us doing research into metastatic prostate cancer, it looks pretty great," says Higano. "We prolonged survival—that's great news. It's the first time we've seen it with a vaccine in prostate cancer," she adds.

The therapy also gives "proof of principle" to the theory that immune-based treatments can have a real impact on prostate cancer and other malignancies, experts say.

"It's the first immunological therapy to have some efficacy against metastatic prostate cancer, after years of trying," says Dr. Bruce Roth, a prostate cancer researcher at Vanderbilt University in Nashville. "There have been many failures with this kind of approach, and many have wondered if we shouldn't set the bar lower, somehow lower our expectations, and not hope for extended survival.

"But these findings are saying, 'No, looking for a survival advantage is a valid endpoint to look at for these agents,'" he says.

The US Food and Drug Administration has not approved Provenge. Additional research and clinical trials by Provenge's developer, the Seattle-based Dendreon, are under way.

PROSTATE CANCER RECURRENCE

When caught early, prostate cancer remains very curable. However, despite advances in early detection, the disease remains the second-leading cancer killer of men in the US, according to the American Cancer Society.

Several recent breakthroughs highlight the medical advances in prostate cancer treatment.

EXTENDING SURVIVAL WITH TAXOTERE

Because prostate cells depend heavily on testosterone to grow, therapies that reduce levels of circulating testosterone are often the first course of action in men who experience a recurrence.

However, prostate cancer cells gradually grow resistant to hormonal therapy, so relapse is almost inevitable. Even among men who develop the disease while it is still confined to the prostate, between 30% and 40% will experience a recurrence in years to come, experts say.

Until very recently, doctors could only offer palliative therapies once relapse occurred. However, one chemotherapy agent—*docetaxel* (Taxotere)—was found to improve survival in patients who had metastatic disease by an extra six months, on average.

STUDY 1:
VITAMIN D AND PROSTATE CANCER

A study by researchers at Brigham and Women's Hospital and the Harvard School of Public Health suggests that higher levels of vitamin D may help protect against prostate cancer.

Comparing vitamin D levels in blood samples from more than 2,400 men, the Boston team discovered that men who had high levels of two vitamin D metabolites were at a 45% lower risk of developing prostate cancer, compared with men who had lower levels of these two metabolites or those who had a high level of only one metabolite.

"Our finding suggests that vitamin D plays an important protective role against prostate cancer," says lead investigator Dr. Haojie Li. Vitamin D is best obtained through exposure to sunlight or certain foods.

STUDY 2:
OBESITY AND PROSTATE CANCER

In another study, also from Brigham and Women's Hospital, Dr. Jing Ma and colleagues report that obesity may increase risks for death from prostate cancer. They found that, even after adjusting for other risk factors, obese men who have a body mass index (BMI) of 30 or above were twice as likely to die of the disease than normal weight men.

According to the researchers, obesity also doubled the risk of being diagnosed with metastatic prostate cancer—19% among obese men compared with 8% among normal-weight men.

"There are two possible explanations for these findings," Dr. Ma says. "First, that being obese may delay the diagnosis of prostate cancer, or, second, that being overweight or obese is associated with a biologically more aggressive form of prostate cancer."

To learn more about detecting and treating prostate cancer, visit the American Cancer Society at *www.cancer.org*.

Natural Ways to Fight Prostate Enlargement

Mark A. Stengler, ND, naturopathic physician in private practice, La Jolla, California…adjunct associate clinical professor at the National College of Natural Medicine, Portland, Oregon…author of many books, including *The Natural Physician's Healing Therapies* and coauthor of *Prescription for Natural Cures* (both from Bottom Line Books)…and author of the *Bottom Line/Natural Healing* newsletter.

If you're a man approaching age 45, you have a nearly 50% chance of having an enlarged prostate. By age 70, the chances are almost nine in 10 that you'll have it. Called *benign prostatic hyperplasia* (BPH), the condition involves an enlarged prostate that compresses the urethra and partially blocks urine flow. BPH is the most common prostate problem among men. While it's not life-threatening—it is not, for example, related to the development of prostate cancer—symptoms can be troublesome. Fortunately, there are natural ways to prevent and treat it.

THE PROSTATE PRESSURE POINT

The job of the prostate is to produce fluid that nourishes and transports sperm. This walnut-sized gland weighs approximately 20 grams. Located in front of the rectum and below the bladder, the prostate surrounds the urethra, the passageway that carries urine away from the bladder and into the penis.

A swollen prostate can compress the urethra like a clamp on a garden hose, restricting urine flow. It also may press upward, irritating the outer wall of the bladder. This irritation makes the bladder wall thicker and even more easily irritated. A man with BPH might start having bladder contractions, making him feel the need to urinate frequently even when there's not much urine. Over time, the bladder may lose the ability to completely empty, increasing discomfort.

POSSIBLE CAUSES

There remains a lot to be answered when it comes to the causes of BPH. One thing researchers can agree on is that hormonal factors play the largest role.

Research has focused on the hormone *testosterone* and a related substance called *dihydrotestosterone* (DHT). Some researchers believe that testosterone, an anabolic (growth-promoting) hormone, is the main culprit. Others disagree because prostate growth tends to be a problem later in a man's life, while the amount of testosterone is at its highest when males are in their late teens or early 20s.

The conversion of testosterone to DHT increases as men get older—and DHT is very potent. It stimulates the proliferation of new prostate cells and slows the death of older ones. But if DHT is a cause, why do some men with prostate enlargement have normal DHT levels? Could another hormone be involved?

Now researchers are looking at the effect of the hormone *estrogen* (especially the kind called *estradiol*) on prostate growth. Estrogen isn't just a "female" hormone. Men have it as well, and as they age, estrogen levels increase. High estrogen-to-testosterone ratios could increase the effects of DHT on prostate cells.

LOOKING FOR TROUBLE

The most common test to diagnose BPH and other prostate-related problems is a digital rectal exam. Your physician inserts a gloved finger into the rectum and feels the part of the prostate next to the rectum for any enlargement or hardness. All men over age 40 should have this test once a year.

A variety of pharmaceuticals can help relieve BPH symptoms, but each has potential side effects. Many doctors prescribe alpha-blockers, such as *terazosin* (Hytrin) or *doxazosin* (Cardura), which relax the neck of the bladder, making urination easier—but these can cause fatigue, weakness, headaches and dizziness. Another prescription drug, *finasteride* (Proscar), relieves symptoms by shrinking the prostate gland, but it can cause impotence and reduced sexual desire.

For men who have serious BPH problems that are interfering with their lifestyle, some doctors recommend surgical procedures—but surgery can lead to impotence or incontinence.

I find that drugs and surgery usually are unnecessary. As long as a man is getting his prostate checked at least once a year and there are no signs of tumor growth or urinary blockage, BPH can be treated with natural therapies. These include improved diet and supplements. Also, 30 minutes of daily exercise has been shown to reduce BPH symptoms quite significantly.

HEALING FOODS

•**Avocados** contain *beta sitosterol*, a phytonutrient that protects against prostate enlargement by inhibiting growth factors that cause prostate swelling. Avocados also are a good source of *oleic acid*, a monounsaturated fatty acid that is thought to reduce inflammation, which can contribute to BPH. Have at least two weekly servings (one-fifth of a medium avocado per serving). If you don't like avocados, you can have three half-cup servings a week of peanuts, rice bran or wheat germ.

•**Fish** is a good source of *eicosapentaenoic acid* (EPA), a powerful omega-3 fatty acid that helps reduce swelling and inflammation. Eat at least two three-ounce servings of trout, salmon or sardines each week.

•**Ground flaxseed** has been shown to reduce estrogen levels, and it contains anti-inflammatory omega-3 fatty acids. I advise men to take one or two tablespoons daily along with 10 ounces of water (to prevent constipation). Ground flaxseed has a mild, nutty flavor and can be added to salads, cereals, yogurt, smoothies and protein shakes or just eaten plain.

•**Pumpkin seeds** are natural sources of zinc. This mineral helps keep your prostate healthy by reducing the activity of the enzyme *5-alpha-reductase*, which produces DHT. Sprinkle a tablespoon or two of pumpkin seeds—raw or roasted, with or without the hulls—on salad, yogurt, cereal, etc. four times weekly.

•**Soy** contains a number of phytoestrogens (plant chemicals that balance estrogen), including *genistein*, which can help control prostate enlargement. I prefer fermented soy foods, such as miso, tempeh and fermented soy protein powder, which provide a form of genistein that can be readily absorbed by the body. Have at least one-half cup serving daily.

•**Tomatoes** are rich in the disease-fighting antioxidants known as *carotenoids*. Preliminary scientific research has suggested that tomatoes and tomato products help prevent prostate cancer. They also may have a beneficial effect on prostate enlargement. Consume two servings of fresh tomatoes and two servings of cooked tomatoes (e.g., tomato paste/sauce) weekly (one serving equals one-half to one cup of tomatoes and/or tomato sauce). If you don't like tomatoes, eat watermelon or cantaloupe.

Foods to avoid: Men with BPH should avoid caffeinated beverages and alcohol—they irritate and inflame the prostate. Also reduce your intake of foods that contain harmful fats, such as hydrogenated or partially hydrogenated oils, that promote inflammation. Stay away from packaged foods that are high in sugar, which also can worsen inflammation.

NATURAL SUPPLEMENTS

The following supplements are listed in order of importance—start with the first and move down the list until you find what works best for you. Many formulas contain a blend of two or three of the ones listed.

•**Saw palmetto berry extract** is a mainstay in the natural treatment of BPH and alleviates most symptoms. It was first used medicinally by Native Americans for prostate and urinary tract problems. Recently, researchers have found that saw palmetto helps the prostate by reducing activity of the DHT-producing enzyme 5-alpha-reductase. A review of 18 randomized, controlled trials involving 2,939 men found saw palmetto to be as effective as the BPH drug *finasteride*.

It can take six to eight weeks before this natural prostate protector begins to fully take effect. I recommend a product that is standardized to contain 80% to 95% fatty acids (check the label) and a total daily dosage of 320 mg, which can be taken all at once. Two brands I recommend are Nature's Way Standardized Saw Palmetto Extract and Enzymatic Therapy Super Saw Palmetto, which are widely available at health-food stores. It is best to take it on an empty stomach. A small percentage of men get stomach upset from saw palmetto. If this occurs, try taking it with meals.

•**Pygeum africanum,** an extract that comes from the bark of the African plum tree, decreases the need to urinate at night and improves urine flow during the day. I prefer a formula that combines pygeum with saw palmetto, such as Ultra Saw Palmetto and Pygeum by Jarrow Formulas (800-726-0886, *www.jarrow.com*). The daily pygeum dosage is 100 mg.

•**Nettle root** can provide modest benefits. The nettle-containing product from Nutrilite, Saw Palmetto with Nettle Root, produced good

results in a UCLA study. Over six months, the 44 men in the study showed modest improvements in BPH symptoms. The Nutrilite formula includes saw palmetto, nettle root, beta-carotene, pumpkin seed oil and lemon bioflavonoid concentrate (Amway Global, 800-253-6500, *www.quixtar. com*). Take one softgel three times daily.

•**Rye grass pollen extracts** seem to relax the muscles of the urethra and improve the ability of the bladder to contract. The extract most widely tested is from Graminex (877-472-6469, *www.graminex.com*). Take three 63-mg tablets twice daily for a total of 378 mg.

•**Fish oil** can help reduce prostate swelling and inflammation. Take 3,000 mg to 5,000 mg daily in addition to two weekly servings of fish. If you prefer a vegetarian source of omega-3 fatty acids, use one to two tablespoons of flax-seed oil.

Caution: Fish oil should not be used by anyone who takes blood-thinning medications such as *warfarin* (Coumadin).

COMMON SYMPTOMS OF BPH

•**A need to urinate frequently.**

•**Urination that is hard to start or stop.**

•**Weak urination or "dribbling."**

•**Sensation of an incompletely emptied bladder.**

•**Increased need to urinate at night.**

•**Burning pain accompanying urination.**

•**Recurring bladder infections.**

■ ■ ■ ■

Enough Saw Palmetto?

Saw palmetto doesn't help enlarged prostate symptoms when taken at a typical dosage, a new study shows. It doesn't reduce the frequent urge to urinate or other enlarged prostate symptoms, such as a weak urinary stream. The typical dosage is 160 milligrams twice a day. A higher dose might alleviate mild symptoms—a new study on this is in the final planning stages.

Best: For now, don't stop taking saw palmetto if it seems to help.

Stephen W. Bent, MD, assistant professor of medicine, University of California, San Francisco.

■ ■ ■ ■

Prostate Cancer Warning

Men with low-risk prostate cancer that hasn't spread should not have hormone therapy, warns Nancy Keating, MD, MPH.

Reason: Hormone therapy lowers levels of testosterone that feed prostate cancer—but it also can quickly raise risk of heart disease and diabetes. For younger men who have been treated for tumors confined to the prostate or nearby lymph nodes and who have no signs of the disease other than a rise in *prostate-specific antigen* (PSA), hormone therapy may be riskier than monitoring the cancer. Hormone therapy remains the treatment of choice if the cancer has spread to the bone.

Nancy Keating, MD, MPH, is associate professor of health-care policy and of medicine, Harvard Medical School, Boston, and leader of a study of 73,000 prostate cancer patients, published in *Journal of Clinical Oncology*.

■ ■ ■ ■

Osteoporosis Drug Helps Prostate

Prostate cancer patients being treated with hormones may benefit from an osteoporosis drug to maintain healthy bones.

Study: More than 100 prostate cancer patients treated with androgen deprivation therapy, which lowers testosterone levels and often causes bone loss, took either the osteoporosis drug *alendronate* (Fosamax) or a placebo for one year.

Result: Bone mass in the spine increased by 3.7% in those taking alendronate compared with a decline in the placebo group.

Susan L. Greenspan, MD, director, Osteoporosis Prevention and Treatment Center, and associate program director General Clinical Research Center, University of Pittsburgh.

■ ■ ■ ■

Safe Surgery

Prostate surgery is safe for older men. Men over age 70 who have prostate cancer are less likely to undergo radical prostatectomy to remove the prostate gland.

Recent finding: Age alone does not make prostate surgery more risky.

But: Men who have heart disease or high blood pressure or who are obese are more likely to die of complications after prostate surgery. Other alternatives for early-stage prostate cancer include radiation treatment, which some studies have indicated has similar outcomes to surgery…and watchful waiting (also known as active surveillance), in which the patient is monitored for signs that the cancer is worsening before any treatment is begun.

Durado Brooks, MD, MPH, director of prostate and colorectal cancers, American Cancer Society, Atlanta.

■ ■ ■ ■

Prostate Risks

Prostate cancer survivors should watch their weight. Prostate cancer progressed more rapidly in obese patients, according to a study of prostate cancer surgery patients.

Also: The disease was more likely to recur in men who had gained an average of three and a half pounds a year, starting at age 25 (the mean age of diagnosis was 60 years).

Sara S. Strom, PhD, associate professor of epidemiology, M.D. Anderson Cancer Center, University of Texas, Houston, and leader of a study of 526 prostate cancer patients, published in *Clinical Cancer Research*.

■ ■ ■ ■

New Prostate Cancer Test 94% Accurate

The current test for prostate cancer, which measures blood levels of prostate-specific antigen (PSA), detects 85% of prostate cancer cases but gives a "false positive" (a test result that wrongly indicates the presence of disease) in 80% of cases.

Recent study: Researchers tested 330 men for elevated levels of early prostate cancer antigen-2 (EPCA-2).

Result: EPCA-2 detected 94% of prostate cancer cases with only a 3% false-positive rate. It is not yet known when the test might be available for public use.

Robert H. Getzenberg, PhD, director of urology research, Johns Hopkins University School of Medicine, Baltimore.

Prostate Cancer Research Is Saving Lives

Peter T. Scardino, MD, chairman of the department of surgery at Memorial Sloan-Kettering Cancer Center in New York City and head of the center's prostate cancer program. He is a professor in the department of urology at Weill Medical College of Cornell University and at the State University of New York Downstate Medical Center. He is coauthor of *Dr. Peter Scardino's Prostate Book: The Complete Guide to Overcoming Prostate Cancer, Prostatitis, and BPH*. Avery.

One man out of six in the US will be diagnosed with prostate cancer during his lifetime—more than 230,000 American men a year—and 30,000 men die every year from the disease. Recent scientific findings could dramatically change this situation, preventing tens of thousands of cases of prostate cancer and saving thousands of lives...

FINASTERIDE UPDATE

Finasteride (Proscar) is used to treat *benign prostatic hyperplasia* (BPH), a noncancerous form of prostate enlargement. It limits the production of an enzyme that converts testosterone to *dihydrotestosterone,* a male hormone that stimulates the growth of prostate cells. (The baldness drug Propecia is also finasteride, but it contains one-fifth the amount used to treat BPH.)

Landmark study: In 2003, an article in *The New England Journal of Medicine* announced the results of the seven-year Prostate Cancer Prevention Trial (PCPT), involving nearly 19,000 men ages 55 and older. Those taking five milligrams (mg) a day of finasteride were 25% less likely to develop prostate cancer than those taking a placebo.

However, biopsies showed that those taking finasteride who did develop prostate cancer (18% of the finasteride group) were slightly more likely to have "high-grade" cancer, an aggressive form that can spread quickly. Because of this, the medical community did not endorse the drug for cancer prevention.

Latest development: In a study published in the August 2008 issue of *Cancer Prevention Research*, scientists from the Fred Hutchinson Cancer Research Center in Seattle revisited the trial results, conducting three new and careful analyses of the data. *They found...*

•**Men taking finasteride did not have a significantly higher rate of aggressive prostate cancer.** In fact, one analysis showed that men on the drug had 27% less high-grade prostate cancer than men on the placebo.

•**The original finding that finasteride increased the risk for high-grade cancer was due to what scientists call a "sampling error."** Finasteride shrinks the size of the prostate by 20% to 30%, making it much more likely that a six-needle biopsy (the type used in the original study) will find a "nest" of high-grade cancer cells.

•**Finasteride has greater cancer-preventing power than previously estimated.** It reduces the risk for prostate cancer by 30%. In other words, it could prevent three out of every 10 cases of prostate cancer—nearly 70,000 cases a year.

Bottom line: "Men undergoing regular prostate cancer screening or who express an interest in cancer prevention should be informed of the opportunity to take finasteride for preventing prostate cancer," concluded the researchers.

That conclusion is particularly important for men with a higher-than-normal risk for the disease. These include men with a family history of prostate cancer (two or more first-degree relatives diagnosed with the disease, such as a grandfather, father or brother)...African-American men (who, compared with Caucasians, have more than twice the risk for dying from prostate cancer)...and men with a level of *prostate specific antigen* (PSA) that is 2.5 nanograms per milliliter (ng/mL) or higher. (PSA is the primary biomarker for prostate cancer.)

EARLIER PSA TESTING

In a recent major study, researchers in Sweden analyzed data from more than 21,000 men who had their PSA measured for the first time (a baseline measurement) in the 1970s and 1980s, when they were 44 to 50 years old.

Twenty-five years later, higher baseline PSA levels were the best predictor of whether or not a man would subsequently develop prostate cancer. In fact, PSA was the only accurate predictor among 90 different factors, including

467

family history and various lifestyle, biochemical and medical parameters.

Latest development: Later, the researchers showed that an early baseline PSA also is the most accurate predictor of who will develop high-grade prostate cancer.

Bottom line: Earlier PSA tests can identify men at higher risk for developing prostate cancer. Those men can have more intensive screening (such as biopsies), improving the odds of finding and treating the disease at an early stage when a cure is more likely.

Every man should have his first PSA test at the age of 40, which is typically covered by insurance. (The American Cancer Society recommends annual PSA screening starting at age 50 for most men.) Men should be tested again at the age of 45. If the result at age 45 is 0.9 or higher, have a PSA test annually.

PSA TEST AFTER 75?

Approximately half of American men 75 and older have had a PSA test in the past two years.

Latest development: In August, the government's US Preventive Services Task Force recommended that men age 75 and over should not receive routine PSA screening for prostate cancer.

Reason: Most prostate cancers found with PSA are slow-growing, taking 10 years or more to cause death—and most 75-year-old men have a life expectancy of about 10 years. That means the potential harm from treating the cancer with surgery, radiation or other types of therapy—including erectile dysfunction, incontinence and bowel difficulties—is likely to be greater than the harm from the cancer itself.

Bottom line: Routine PSA tests for men over 75 are not necessary. However, it's reasonable for your doctor to order a test if you're healthy and active, free of a life-shortening disease, such as heart failure or type 2 diabetes...and you have a concern about prostate cancer or an interest in receiving a PSA test.

COMPUTER PREDICTION

Once prostate cancer is diagnosed, treatment decisions are difficult. *That's because it's hard to determine whether the cancer is...*

• **Slow-growing and unlikely to invade areas outside the prostate,** a situation that may call for avoiding or delaying treatment or...

• **Fast-growing and potentially invasive,** a situation that may call for immediate treatment, such as surgery, radiation and/or hormonal therapy. These treatments can result in side effects that diminish the quality of life, such as erectile dysfunction, urinary incontinence and bowel difficulties.

Doctors use many factors to determine whether prostate cancer is slow- or fast-growing. These include PSA...digital rectal exam...the amount of cancer in a biopsy...the Gleason grade (the microscopic appearance, including size and shape of the cells, with high-grade cells being more aggressive)...and the size of the prostate (the larger the prostate, the less likely that cancer will spread beyond it).

Problem: Physicians tend to recommend immediate treatment based on one worrisome factor, such as high-grade cancer cells.

Solution: The nomogram—a sophisticated computer-based prostate cancer prediction tool that takes into account all the factors that determine the likely outcome of a case of prostate cancer.

Latest development: Using data from nearly 2,000 men (average age 70) diagnosed with local (confined to the prostate) cancer, researchers at the Cleveland Clinic evaluated a nomogram that predicts whether a man will survive for at least five years if he doesn't immediately receive aggressive treatment. The nomogram was determined to be 73% accurate. The findings were published in the January 2008 issue of *Cancer,* the journal of the American Cancer Society.

Bottom line: If you are diagnosed with prostate cancer, ask your doctor about a nomogram. There are prostate cancer nomograms to analyze many different scenarios, such as the likely effectiveness of using radiation after a recurrence or using hormonal therapy after surgery and radiation.

You and/or your doctor can download free prostate cancer nomograms developed by the Memorial Sloan-Kettering Cancer Center at *www.mskcc.org/mskcc/html/10088.cfm.*

THE SURGEON MATTERS

Researchers at Memorial Sloan-Kettering Cancer Center studied results from 72 surgeons at four major medical centers who performed 7,765 radical prostatectomies (removal of the prostate) over 16 years.

The patients of surgeons who had performed 10 or fewer radical prostatectomies over their professional lifetimes had a 17.9% prostate cancer recurrence rate within five years. The patients of surgeons who had performed 250 or more radical prostatectomies had a recurrence rate of 10.7%. The study appeared in the August 2007 issue of *Journal of the National Cancer Institute.*

Latest development: In a subsequent analysis of the same data, published in the September 2008 issue of *Journal of Urology,* the researchers found that patients with low-grade cancer had nearly 100% freedom from recurrence when they were operated on by the most experienced surgeons.

Bottom line: If you're having a radical prostatectomy, seek out the most experienced surgeon available.

RADIATION AFTER RECURRENCE

If you had a radical prostatectomy for prostate cancer, but your cancer returned and your PSA is rising rapidly, what should you do? To save your life, consider radiation.

Latest development: Men who got radiation therapy within two years of surgery had an 86% chance of surviving 10 years, compared with 62% among those who did not have radiation, reported researchers from The Johns Hopkins School of Medicine in the June 18, 2008, issue of *The Journal of the American Medical Association.*

Bottom line: In the past, radiation therapy was not always recommended for men with a fast-growing recurrence and a high PSA. After this study, it should be.

WARNING: NEWER ISN'T ALWAYS BETTER

Many American men with prostate cancer are traveling to Canada, Mexico and other foreign locales to receive high-intensity focused ultrasound (HIFU).

This treatment—available in other countries for the past several years but not yet approved in the US—destroys prostate cancer cells by heating them to between 176°F and 212°F via a probe inserted into the rectum.

Red flag: There is not enough clinical data to show that HIFU is an effective way to treat prostate cancer. In fact, doctors in the US are beginning to see recurrences in men treated with HIFU—men who might have been cured with standard therapy.

Bottom line: New treatments for prostate cancer may be popular, but that doesn't mean they work. Only clinical data from large and rigorous studies can provide proof of effectiveness.

■■■■

Fertility Danger

Insecticides reduce male fertility, according to new research.

Recent finding: Men with higher levels of exposure to the lawn and garden insecticide *chlorpyrifos* or its metabolite (TCPY) were found to have lower levels of testosterone, which may affect reproductive health.

Best: Limit exposure to pesticides.

John D. Meeker, PhD, assistant professor, environmental health sciences, University of Michigan, Ann Arbor, and author of a study of 336 men, published in *Epidemiology.*

Testosterone: Is Yours Too Low?

Culley C. Carson III, MD, Rhodes Distinguished Professor and chief of urology, University of North Carolina School of Medicine, Chapel Hill, is editor in chief of *Contemporary Urology.*

If you're a middle-aged or older man and feel irritable, depressed or fatigued…have trouble concentrating…if you are losing muscle mass and strength and/or putting on more body fat…losing bone density, as indicated by a bone-density test…or experiencing a decreased sex drive or difficulty achieving or maintaining an erection…you might be one of the estimated five million men in the US with abnormally low testosterone levels, or hypogonadism.

It's estimated that only one out of 20 men with low testosterone is currently being treated.

Good news: All it takes is a simple blood test to determine if you have low testosterone. If you do have low testosterone, the latest form of testosterone-replacement therapy (TRT), in which the hormone is applied to the skin as a gel, is effective and at least in the short term safe. In cases where symptoms are due to low testosterone, TRT gel can begin to reverse the above symptoms almost immediately.

WHY IS TESTOSTERONE IMPORTANT?

The most powerful of a group of male hormones known as androgens, testosterone is largely responsible for men's growth of facial and pubic hair, deepening of the voice, increased muscle and bone mass, sex drive and, to some extent, aggressiveness. Although testosterone is present in both sexes, women typically have only one-tenth the amount of testosterone that men do.

In men, a normal blood testosterone level is generally considered to be between 300 and 1,000 nanograms per deciliter (ng/dl). Testosterone levels tend to be highest in the early morning hours, then go down somewhat as the day wears on.

As men get older, however, testosterone levels gradually decline. This occurs most acutely after age 65, but the decline can also be noticeable among men in their 50s and even 40s. Testosterone levels vary greatly from patient to patient, and drops are relative to each patient's starting level—which is usually not known. There can be many causes for decreasing levels, but the most common is testicular failure—the testicles "wear out" and fail to produce enough testosterone.

Low testosterone has long been associated with decreased sex drive, but researchers are now discovering that low testosterone levels can cause numerous other negative health effects (in addition to those already mentioned), including reduced fertility, loss of body hair, reduced muscle mass and strength, problems sleeping and increased risk of depression.

In addition, men with a number of chronic conditions are also much more likely to have low testosterone levels. These conditions include type 2 diabetes, cardiovascular disease, chronic renal failure, obesity, hypertension, insulin resistance (prediabetes) and HIV/AIDS. If you have any of these conditions, it's important to get treatment for the underlying medical problem and a blood testosterone test to see if you might benefit from TRT as well.

DIAGNOSIS AND TREATMENT

You can visit your doctor specifically to get a screening testosterone level blood test, or you can request to have it done as part of your annual checkup. The accuracy of lab tests is far better than it used to be, and testing of free circulating testosterone (not the testosterone that is bound to protein in the body) is also now available. Your doctor may also do this test if your levels in the screening test indicate a problem. Among men with low testosterone, what we typically see are levels in the 150 ng/dl range—about half of what is considered the minimum normal level. These men are prime candidates for TRT to bring blood levels into the normal range (above 300 ng/dl).

In addition to ordering a blood test, your primary care doctor can also prescribe TRT treatments. If he/she is unfamiliar or uncomfortable with TRT, however, you should consider seeing a urologist or endocrinologist for treatment.

OLDER TREATMENT METHODS

One older treatment, injection therapy, requires frequent visits to the doctor for shots and produces uneven testosterone levels, which spike drastically after injection, then decline steadily afterward. Testosterone pills carry a high risk of liver damage because of the strain put on the liver as it breaks down the testosterone. And the earliest testosterone treatment, patches (introduced in the early 1990s), were safer than pills but caused skin irritation in many patients.

The latest testosterone treatment, gels (which have been on the market for about three years), have proven to be very safe and nonirritating. They are very effective at raising testosterone levels back into the normal range. Gels are more effective than patches, which are rarely used anymore, and have fewer side effects. An added benefit of these gels is that, when applied in the morning, they come close to mimicking the normal daily fluctuations in testosterone levels—high in the morning, lower at night.

There are currently two FDA-approved gels. AndroGel is scent-free but takes up to two hours to dry completely. Testim has a slightly musky scent and dries a little more quickly on the skin.

The recommended method is to apply a five-gram packet of gel (about the size of a fast-food ketchup packet) containing 50 mg of testosterone in the morning to the shoulders, upper arms and/or abdomen. After applying, wash your hands carefully, cover the treated area with clothing and avoid bathing or swimming for six hours.

After applying either type of gel, avoid skin-to-skin contact of that area with your partner or any other family members until the gel has dried completely. Otherwise, they may experience elevated testosterone levels as well. (If your female partner experiences any unusual acne or body hair growth, she should see her doctor immediately.)

What to expect: Initial benefits of TRT tend to be seen quickly, especially improvements in libido, mood and mental sharpness.

Example: One of my patients, a university professor, had been depressed and very forgetful, and was convinced that he had early Alzheimer's. After his blood test showed a testosterone level of 100 ng/dl, he was placed on TRT—and found that within a few weeks his mood and his mental abilities were fully restored.

Increases in muscle and bone mass occur more slowly and can be enhanced by strength training (for muscle and bone development), calcium/vitamin D supplements (for bone growth) and, if necessary, osteoporosis medication.

No long-term studies have been done on TRT —the longest was three years. But, in the three-year study, there was no indication of any risk or side effects.

Prostate alert: While TRT doesn't appear to increase the risk of prostate cancer or benign prostate enlargement, testosterone supplements may spur the growth of existing prostate tumors. For this reason, TRT should never be taken by anyone who has been diagnosed with prostate cancer.

Men on TRT should be given both a prostate-specific antigen (PSA) test for prostate cancer and a digital rectal exam twice a year. As testosterone levels move from low to normal, it's typical to experience a slight rise in PSA levels and a slight increase in prostate size, but these changes usually present no problem.

Low-Testosterone Men Prone to Falls

In a recent finding, older men with the lowest levels of the hormone testosterone had a 40% greater risk of falling than those with the highest levels. It is too soon to say whether testosterone replacement would help prevent falls. Testosterone declines naturally with age. Older men can lower the risk of falling by increasing leg strength and coordination and by avoiding alcohol and sedatives, which may increase the risk of falls.

Eric Orwoll, MD, is professor of medicine, associate vice president and associate dean for research, School of Medicine, Oregon Health & Science University, Portland. He is leader of a study of 2,587 men, published in *Archives of Internal Medicine.*

Alcoholism Reduces Men's Fertility

Men being treated for alcoholism as in a recent study had lower levels of testosterone and more sperm abnormalities than men who did not drink at all.

Also: 71% of alcoholics had erectile dysfunction, compared with 7% of men who abstained from alcohol.

K.R. Muthusami, PhD, senior biochemist and laboratory manager, Institute of Laboratory Medicine, Kovai Medical Center and Hospital, Coimbatore, India, and leader of a study of 96 men, published in *Fertility & Sterility.*

Incontinence Aid

Male urinary incontinence may be relieved by collagen injections. Incontinence is a frequent side effect of prostate surgery.

Recent finding: Transurethral collagen injections after prostate surgery improve short-term bladder control for six to seven months, at which time injections can be repeated. Injections are administered via the urethra, under local anesthesia. Collagen helps control urine leakage by bulking up the area around the urethra, compressing the sphincter.

O. Lenaine Westney, MD, associate professor, department of urologic surgery, University of Texas M.D. Anderson Cancer Center, Houston.

■ ■ ■ ■

Cancer Risk

Cure rates for testicular cancer are high, but the treatments may lead to an increased likelihood of tumors elsewhere in the body for at least 35 years. Most patients are diagnosed with the disease in their 20s or early 30s and treated with radiation or chemotherapy. A man diagnosed at age 35 who survives the cancer for 10 years has nearly twice the risk of the general population of developing a malignant tumor elsewhere.

Self-defense: Testicular cancer survivors should adopt a healthy lifestyle, follow screening guidelines and seek medical consultation for any changes in health status.

Lois B. Travis, MD, ScD, senior investigator, National Cancer Institute, Bethesda, Maryland, and leader of a study of 40,576 testicular cancer patients, published in *Journal of the National Cancer Institute* of the National Institutes of Health.

■ ■ ■ ■

Warning Sign

Male infertility could be a warning sign for testicular cancer.

Recent study: Men with low sperm counts were 20 times more likely to develop testicular cancer than men with normal counts.

Self-defense: Men whose sperm counts are low should schedule a semen analysis and cancer screening and do regular self-examinations. Speak to your doctor for information on performing testicle self-exams.

Marc Goldstein, MD, professor of urology and reproductive medicine, Weill Cornell Medical Center, New York City, and leader of a study of 4,000 infertile men, published in *Journal of Urology.*

■ ■ ■ ■

Cell Phones Zap Sperm

Excessive cell-phone use may affect a man's sperm production.

Recent finding: Radio waves such as those emitted by cell phones damaged sperm DNA in mice. DNA damage in sperm correlates to poor fertility and increased rates of miscarriage and childhood disease, including cancer. More study is needed to determine the effects in humans.

R. John Aitken, PhD, ScD, director, Australian Research Council Centre of Excellence in Biotechnology and Development, discipline of biological sciences, School of Life and Environmental Sciences, University of Newcastle, Callaghan, New South Wales, and leader of a study of 22 mice, published in *International Journal of Andrology.*

■ ■ ■ ■

No-Rush Hernia

Men whose hernias are not causing pain can wait to have them repaired, according to the late Olga Jonasson, MD. Their outcomes are similar to those of men who have them repaired immediately. A hernia occurs when part of the intestine bulges through a weak area of the abdomen's muscle wall.

Caution: In rare cases, when you are unable to push the hernia back and it is accompanied by cramps and vomiting, the hernia requires immediate repair.

Also: Watchful waiting is appropriate for men only. When women get hernias, the condition is more dangerous.

The late Olga Jonasson, MD, was professor, department of surgery, University of Illinois at Chicago, and coauthor of a study of 720 men with hernias, published in *The Journal of the American Medical Association.*

■ ■ ■ ■

Exercise Cuts Risk of Dying

Exercise greatly cuts a man's risk of dying from heart disease.

New finding: Men at high risk for heart disease (due to hypertension, high cholesterol and/or other risk factors) who exercised for 30 minutes four to five days per week reduced their risk of dying from a heart attack or stroke by 50%.

Self-defense: Everyone—especially those who are at risk for heart disease—should perform aerobic exercise, such as walking or swimming, for at least 30 minutes four to five days a week.

Peter T. Katzmarzyk, PhD, associate professor, School of Kinesiology and Health Studies, Queens University, Kingston, Ontario, Canada.

Viagra Curbs Urinary Problems

An enlarged prostate is common in men who also experience erectile dysfunction (ED).

Recent finding: In a study of 370 men age 45 or older, those who took the ED drug *sildenafil* (Viagra) for 12 weeks reported improvement in symptoms associated with an enlarged prostate, such as decreased urinary flow.

Theory: The enzyme that Viagra acts on in the penis also relaxes cells in the bladder and prostate that promote urinary flow and emptying of the bladder.

Kevin T. McVary, MD, professor of urology, Northwestern University Feinberg School of Medicine, Chicago.

Statins May Help Men's Bones

Statins may help prevent osteoporosis, says Richard E. Scranton, MD, MPH.

Finding: In a study of more than 91,000 men, those who took a cholesterol-lowering statin had an overall 36% lower risk for fractures.

Theory: Statins improve the function of small blood vessels, which may promote bone growth and remodeling.

If you have high cholesterol: Ask your doctor about taking a statin to lower cholesterol —and to help prevent osteoporosis.

Richard E. Scranton, MD, MPH, director of projects, Massachusetts Veterans Epidemiology Research and Information Center, Boston.

Double Trouble

Erectile dysfunction (ED) may mean heart trouble, a new study says. There is a strong association between ED and cardiovascular disease. In a clinical trial, men older than 55 who reported a new problem with ED had a 25% increased risk of suffering a cardiovascular "event," such as a heart attack, stroke or angina, than men who had no problem with ED.

Precaution: When you seek help for ED, ask your doctor to check for heart trouble.

Ian Murchie Thompson, Jr., MD, professor and chairman, department of urology, University of Texas Health Science Center, San Antonio.

The Secret of Half-Priced Viagra

Carmen Reitano, founder and president, Three Chestnuts Technologies Inc., Newburyport, Massachusetts.
Ira Sharlip, MD, president, Sexual Medicine Society of North America, and urologist, San Francisco.
US Patent and Trademark Office, Alexandria, Virginia.

Each diamond-shaped Viagra pill costs the same (almost $10) whether you get the 25-milligram (mg), 50-mg or 100-mg version. This flat-pricing strategy has led many in the older-than-50 crowd to buy the larger pill and try to break it up into smaller pieces.

The patient should take the dose the doctor recommends, says Dr. Ira Sharlip, president of the Sexual Medicine Society of North America. "But I can tell you it's common practice for physicians to recommend a dose of 50 mg and write a prescription for a 100-mg tablet." Carmen Reitano, inventor and Viagra user, was involved in a conversation about the difficulties of splitting a Viagra pill.

"It explodes," complained one man.

"You cut it with a knife and it splits apart with such fury it bounces off the wall," said another.

Reitano had never tried splitting his Viagra pills, but he decided to give it a try. He went home, took out the kitchen knife and tried to cut open one of his Viagra pills. Nothing happened. He went at it with an X-Acto® knife blade. Nothing. A hammer. Still, nothing.

"It's not flat. It's awkward to hold. There's no scoring on the covering," Reitano discovered. So, to help the many frustrated Viagra users, Reitano designed the V2 Pill Splitter, for which he was awarded a patent.

Pfizer, which manufactures Viagra, did not specifically comment, but advises against pill-splitting.

To buy Viagra pill splitters directly, visit *www.forgettingthepill.com* or *www.pillcutter.com*.

Millions of Men Have "Silent"Osteoporosis

Angela J. Shepherd, MD, associate professor in the department of family medicine at University of Texas Medical Branch, Galveston. She specializes in osteoporosis screening and prevention, and recently published in *Annals of Family Medicine* a system that physicians can use to identify men with an elevated risk for osteoporosis.

Virtually every woman knows about osteoporosis, the main cause of weakened bones and fractures as women age. Few men, however, realize that they face similar risks.

Fact: About 30% of men 50 years and older will suffer an osteoporosis-related bone fracture at some time in their lives. Yet only about 10% of men with osteoporosis ever get diagnosed.

According to the National Osteoporosis Foundation, more than two million men have osteoporosis. Nearly 12 million more have osteopenia, a precursor condition that commonly leads to full-fledged osteoporosis.

Few doctors take the time to investigate bone loss in men. They, too, tend to think of osteoporosis as a "woman's disease," even though men are twice as likely as women to die following a hip fracture or hip-replacement procedure due to osteoporosis.

WHO GETS IT?

The strength and density of bones largely depend on the amount of calcium and other minerals that are present. The body is constantly creating and breaking down bone, a process called *remodeling.* For both men and women, the formation of new bone exceeds bone breakdown until about age 35. After age 35, the reverse happens. Men and women lose more bone than they create, leading to an overall loss of bone strength.

Women experience a precipitous loss of bone mass when estrogen declines after menopause. They also have smaller bones to begin with, which means they have fewer bone reserves. It's not unusual for women in their 70s to have lost up to 50% of their total bone mass.

Men experience a similar process, but without the rapid "bone drain" caused by declining estrogen. They lose bone more slowly than women—and because they start out with more

bone mass, it takes them longer to start getting fractures. But once a man reaches his mid-70s, his risk for getting osteoporosis is about the same as a woman's.

Men with osteoporosis often are diagnosed only when they suffer a low-impact fracture. This is when even a minor impact or movement —falling down or bumping into something— causes a bone to break. Most fractures occur in the wrists or hips. Spinal fractures also are common, although they're typically asymptomatic and thus less likely to be diagnosed.

MALE RISKS

A sedentary lifestyle and nutritional deficiencies—mainly of calcium and vitamin D—are among the main causes of osteoporosis in men as well as women. Also, people who have taken oral steroids for a six-month period over their lifetime (for severe asthma, rheumatoid arthritis or some other condition) are at increased risk. *Additional risk factors for men...*

•**Low body weight.** Older men who weigh less than 154 pounds are more than 20 times more likely to get osteoporosis than heavier men— partly because they have smaller bones and possibly because men with other osteoporosis risk factors, such as smoking and heavy alcohol consumption, tend to be thinner.

•**Prostate cancer.** The disease itself doesn't increase a man's risk of osteoporosis but some of the treatments do. For example, the drug *leuprolide* (Lupron) reduces levels of androgens, male hormones that play a protective role in bone strength. Men who are given antihormone drugs for prostate cancer—or who have undergone actual castration—are now assumed to be at high risk for osteoporosis.

•**COPD.** Men with chronic obstructive pulmonary disease (COPD) often develop osteoporosis. Smoking, the main cause of COPD, weakens bones. Also, COPD is commonly treated with steroids, drugs that decrease bone strength.

DIAGNOSIS

The dual-energy X-ray absorptiometry (DEXA) test measures bone density at the hip and spine, and sometimes at the wrist. The test gives a T-score—your bone density compared with what normally is expected in a healthy young adult with peak bone mass. *Any reading with a "minus" sign indicates that bone density is lower than average...*

• **-1** indicates some bone loss.

• **-2.5** is a borderline reading that indicates a significant problem.

• **Below -2.5** is diagnosed as osteoporosis. It's not unusual for older men to have a T-score of –4, which indicates their bones are almost like paper.

Who should get tested? Men over age 60 with low weight and/or COPD should get a bone-density test—as should anyone who has taken steroids for six months.

TREATMENT AND PREVENTION

In February 2008, the National Osteoporosis Foundation issued official guidelines for treating and preventing osteoporosis in women and men age 50 and older. *These include...*

• **Get regular exercise.** It's among the best ways to increase bone mass during peak bone-building years. It also can increase bone density and strength in men who already have osteoporosis and improve overall health.

Bonus: Exercise increases balance and muscle strength—important for avoiding falls.

Any exercise is beneficial, but weight-bearing aerobic workouts, such as walking or lifting weights, may be superior to swimming or biking for stimulating bone growth.

• **Supplement with calcium and vitamin D.** Both are essential for bone strength. Dietary sources probably aren't enough. The body's ability to absorb calcium declines with age. There's also an age-related decline in vitamin D synthesis from sunshine.

Men need 1,000 milligrams (mg) to 1,200 mg of calcium daily until age 65 and 1,500 mg thereafter. After age 40, men should take 200 international units (IU) of vitamin D daily...400 IU after age 50...and 600 IU at age 71 and older.

• **Ask your doctor about bone-building drugs.** Many drugs that treat osteoporosis in women also are effective in men. These include the *bisphosphonates* (such as Fosamax and Actonel), *calcitonin* (Miacalcin) and *parathyroid hormone* (Forteo). Each of these drugs slows bone loss, and some increase the body's ability to build new bone. Your doctor can tell you if you need drugs and, if so, which one is right for you.

A T-score of –2.5 or worse may warrant drug intervention, and many doctors think a score of –2.0 is reason for a "drug discussion" with patients.

• **Don't smoke.** Nicotine is toxic to bone marrow. Also, men who smoke tend to weigh less than those who don't.

• **Limit alcohol.** Heavy alcohol use in men is one of the main risk factors for osteoporosis. Excessive alcohol inhibits the body's ability to form new bone, and men who are alcoholics often eat poorly.

• **Deal with depression.** People who are depressed tend to have lower-than-normal bone density, possibly because they exercise less and eat less.

Caution: Some research has linked SSRI antidepressants, such as Prozac, Paxil and Zoloft, with lower bone density. People should not stop taking these drugs because of concerns about osteoporosis—but they should ask their doctors if they need to be screened for osteoporosis.

■ ■ ■ ■

A High-Sugar Diet May Lower A Man's Sex Drive

Foods that are high in simple sugars, such as candy and soda pop, reduce blood levels of the protein that carries testosterone—an effect that occurs rapidly after high sugar consumption and may continue as long as the high-sugar diet does. Men whose sex drive has dropped should consider eating fewer sweets—that may be enough to increase testosterone levels and restore sex drive.

Geoffrey Hammond, PhD, scientific director, Child & Family Research Institute, and professor, department of obstetrics and gynecology, University of British Columbia, both in Vancouver, Canada, and leader of a study of the effect of a high-sugar diet on mice and human liver cells, published in *Journal of Clinical Investigation*.

■ ■ ■ ■

Coffee Reduces Risk of Gout in Men

Men who drank four to five cups of coffee a day had a 40% lower risk of gout than men who drank none. Men who drank six or more cups daily had a 59% decreased risk.

Reason: Gout—a painful inflammatory disease characterized by attacks of arthritis—is caused by excessive buildup of uric acid. Coffee tends to lower *uric acid* levels.

Hyon K. Choi, MD, associate professor, department of rheumatology, University of British Columbia, Vancouver, Canada, and Brigham and Women's Hospital, Boston, and leader of a study of 45,869 men, published in *Arthritis & Rheumatism*.

■ ■ ■ ■

Pomegranate and Prostate Cancer

Pomegranate juice may fight prostate cancer, reports Kelly Morrow, RD.

Recent study: Drinking eight ounces of pomegranate juice daily increases the doubling time of *prostate specific antigen* (PSA) by more than 300% (more research is needed to determine why). The longer the doubling time, the slower the tumor growth.

Extra benefit: Pomegranate juice may slow the progression of breast, testicular and lung cancers, as well as help reduce blood pressure and protect against heart disease.

Kelly Morrow, MS, RD, assistant professor of nutrition, Bastyr University, Kenmore, Washington.

■ ■ ■ ■

Red Meat and Prostate Cancer

There is no strong scientific evidence linking red-meat consumption to prostate cancer. Some studies have found that people who eat lots of red meat are more likely to develop prostate cancer—but these people also have other unhealthy dietary habits.

We do know that eating large quantities of red meat has other negative effects, such as increasing risk for heart disease and atherosclerosis.

Best: Follow five dietary rules if you have or had prostate cancer—maintain a low-fat diet… high in soy…high in cooked tomatoes…and containing *resveratrol*, which is found in red

wine. And take vitamin E and selenium supplements. Specifics of the best diet vary for each individual—consult your doctor.

J. Stephen Jones, MD, vice-chair, Glickman Urological and Kidney Institute, The Cleveland Clinic, Ohio.

Alternative Approaches To Prostate Cancer Care

Mark A. Stengler, ND, naturopathic physician in private practice, La Jolla, California…adjunct associate clinical professor at the National College of Natural Medicine, Portland, Oregon…author of many books, including *The Natural Physician's Healing Therapies* and coauthor of *Prescription for Natural Cures* (both from Bottom Line Books)…and author of the *Bottom Line/Natural Healing* newsletter.

Over the course of a lifetime, one man in six eventually will be diagnosed with prostate cancer…one in 35 will die from it. Despite how common the disease is, the treatment path for prostate cancer is seldom clear. Even conventional doctors who specialize in prostate cancer frequently disagree about the best course of action.

Surgery to remove the prostate gland and perhaps the nearby lymph nodes often is recommended, yet it can have onerous side effects—including incontinence that lasts for months or years and lifelong erectile dysfunction. What's more, statistics show that surgery does not necessarily increase a man's life span.

For these and other reasons, doctors sometimes recommend a "watch and wait" approach rather than surgery. Prostate cancer usually is slow-growing, and more than 70% of the men who develop it are over age 65. The older a man is, the more likely he is to die of some other condition before his prostate cancer becomes a real threat. The American Cancer Society (*www.cancer.org*) states, "At this time, watchful waiting is a reasonable option for some men with slow-growing cancers because it is not known whether active treatment, such as surgery, radiation therapy and hormone therapy, prolongs survival."

The holistic view: For prostate cancer patients age 65 and older, as well as for some younger men whose cancer does not appear to be fast-growing, I support the decision to watch and wait before pursuing aggressive conventional treatment—with one important caveat. Instead of waiting passively while doing nothing, I recommend a proactive approach using natural therapies that may slow or halt cancer growth or even cause the cancer to diminish.

My regimen includes various nutritional supplements—including two new ones being researched at major university medical centers. Several of my patients with localized prostate cancer are using these natural therapies under my care—and now, up to 12 years after diagnosis, they continue to do well.

Unless noted otherwise, all supplements described below are available at health-food stores, generally are safe to take indefinitely and cause few side effects.

Important: It is vital that men who have prostate cancer be monitored by an oncologist. Show your doctor this article, and discuss your desire to incorporate these natural therapies.

CUTTING-EDGE PROSTATE CARE

Aaron E. Katz, MD, associate professor of clinical urology and director of the Center of Holistic Urology at Columbia University Medical Center in New York City, is heading the research on two new supplements that are showing promise in the fight against prostate cancer. Studies are still in progress. *Here is what we know so far...*

•**Zyflamend.** This unique formula from New Chapter (800-543-7279, *www.newchapter. com*, about $50 for 120 capsules) combines *phytochemicals* (beneficial plant chemicals) with herbal extracts from turmeric, ginger, green tea, rosemary, *hu zhang* (Japanese knotweed), Chinese goldthread, barberry, oregano, baikal skullcap and holy basil.

Dr. Katz's laboratory study, published in 2005, found that Zyflamend reduced prostate cancer cell proliferation and may even have killed some existing prostate cancer cells.

How it works: Chronic inflammation is linked to the formation of cancerous cells...and Zyflamend inhibits activity of two enzymes (COX-1 and COX-2) that promote inflammation.

Researchers at The University of Texas MD Anderson Cancer Center published their own laboratory study showing that Zyflamend reduces activity of a family of proteins called *NF-kappa B*. When overactive, these proteins stimulate abnormal prostate cell growth.

Dr. Katz's team continues to analyze Zyflamend. Preliminary findings of a clinical trial among men at high risk for prostate cancer are encouraging. The trial included 23 men, ages 46 to 75, who were diagnosed via biopsy with a type of precancerous cell proliferation called high-grade *prostatic intraepithelial neoplasia* (PIN)—a marker suggesting an 80% chance that cancer will develop within 10 years. The men also had elevated levels of *prostate specific antigen* (PSA)—a substance produced by prostate gland cells and often elevated when cancer exists. Participants took one Zyflamend pill three times a day for 18 months. *Blood tests and biopsies then showed...*

•**The marker disappeared in 62% of patients.**

•**Half of the men had decreases in PSA levels**—some by more than 50%—indicating a return to more normal prostate cell activity.

•**For all of the nine patients who did develop cancer,** the disease was the slow-growing type and confined to a small area.

If you are at risk: Based on the evidence that Zyflamend can reverse PIN and reduce PSA, I recommend taking three Zyflamend capsules daily (with meals to avoid gastric upset), continuing indefinitely, if you have any of the following...

•**An enlarged prostate** (as detected during a doctor's exam)

•**Any abnormal prostate PIN**

•**PSA that is elevated for your age.** PSA is considered elevated if it is at or above 2.5 nanograms per milliliter (ng/ml) in your 40s...3.5 ng/ml in your 50s...4.5 ng/ml in your 60s...or 6.5 ng/ml in your 70s.

•**An ultrasound or other imaging test showing prostate lesions**

•**One or more immediate family members with a history of prostate cancer,** if you are over age 50.

If you have high-grade PIN or prostate cancer: In addition to taking Zyflamend, consider taking a second new supplement, Prostabel, described below…

•**Prostabel.** Available on-line from Natural Source International (888-308-7066, *www.natural-source.com*, $145 for 100 capsules), Prostabel combines extracts from the barks of the Amazonian *Pao pereira* tree and the sub-Saharan plant *Rauwolfia vomitoria*.

In 1980, scientists from the Pasteur Institute in France identified the cancer-fighting properties of these substances.

Dr. Katz's team at Columbia also conducts clinical trials on Prostabel. A recent study has 25 men, ages 40 to 75, with negative biopsy reports but elevated PSA levels. Participants were assigned to take from two to eight capsules of Prostabel daily for 12 months.

Findings are preliminary. Prostabel significantly lowered PSA in five of eight men who completed the 12-month course.

While four of the men have developed cancer, their cancers are small and slow-growing. Researchers are waiting to see if Prostabel suppresses cancer cell growth in the remaining 17 participants. Just one patient, who was on the highest dosage, developed liver enzyme problems as a side effect.

Surprising: Patients experienced significant improvements in urination problems common among older men, such as frequent need to urinate and slowed stream.

Recommended dosage: Three Prostabel capsules daily. Take on an empty stomach to maximize absorption.

Helpful: If it causes digestive upset, take with meals instead.

MORE CANCER FIGHTERS

In addition to taking Zyflamend and/or Prostabel, I recommend that men who have had a diagnosis of prostate cancer take all of the following, continuing indefinitely…

•**Zinc.** The prostate gland is extremely sensitive to hormones, especially estrogen. Although estrogen is primarily a female hormone, as men age and their testosterone levels decrease, an enzyme called *aromatase* converts some of the remaining testosterone to estrogen, thereby increasing risk for prostate cancer. Zinc helps to slow the activity of aromatase.

Dosage: 50 mg daily.

Caution: Check with your doctor before taking zinc if you are undergoing chemotherapy —zinc may not be compatible with some chemotherapy drugs.

•**Copper.** Long-term zinc supplementation can lead to a copper deficiency, so also take 2 mg of copper daily.

•**Selenium.** This mineral appears to protect against prostate cancer, perhaps by providing *antioxidants* (chemical compounds that protect cells from free radicals that can damage cell DNA).

Dosage: 200 micrograms (mcg) daily.

Note: Although evidence is not conclusive, selenium has been linked to increased risk for diabetes—so have your blood sugar monitored regularly.

•**Vitamin E.** This provides antioxidants that guard against cell damage.

Dosage: 200 international units (IU) daily of "mixed" vitamin E (as indicated on label).

•**Calcium limit.** Take no more than 500 mg of supplemental calcium daily. Some evidence links high doses to increased prostate cancer risk.

Men who have been diagnosed with prostate cancer and who want a more aggressive approach can add the following and continue taking them indefinitely…

•**Indole 3-carbinol.** Supplementing with this plant chemical found in cruciferous vegetables helps the liver metabolize and excrete estrogen.

Dosage: 400 mg daily.

•**Maitake mushroom extract.** This enhances immune function. Use capsules or tincture labeled "standardized MD-fraction."

Dosage: 1 mg per day for every 2.2 pounds of body weight (for instance, a 165-pound man would take 75 mg daily…a 200-pound man would take 90 mg daily).

Note: Take in two divided doses on an empty stomach.

•**Beta glucan.** Beta glucan is a complex sugar. The most beneficial form is derived from baker's yeast and sold under the brand name WPG 3-6. It boosts the immune system's effectiveness against cancer and other diseases.

Dosage: 500 mg twice daily. The brand I recommend is ImmunotiX 3-6, the potent and purified WGP 3-6 product from Xymogen (800-647-6100, *www.xymogen.com*).

CHECKLIST: WHAT TO DISCUSS WITH YOUR DOCTOR

A man diagnosed with prostate cancer faces a significant challenge in deciding what treatment regimen is most appropriate. *It is essential that he work closely with his oncologist and other health-care providers, being sure to discuss the following matters...*

•**Stage of the disease.** Is it localized (confined to the prostate gland), or has it spread?

•**Grading of the disease.** The key measure is the Gleason score (a number from 2 to 10), which refers to how abnormal the tumor cells are and how likely they are to spread. The lower the score, the better.

•**Prostate-specific antigen (PSA) velocity.** New research shows that the speed at which PSA increases—for instance, as measured three times over an 18-month period—is more significant than the initial reading.

•**Age of the patient.** The younger the patient, the more aggressive the cancer is likely to be.

•**Benefits and side effects of treatment options.**

■ ■ ■ ■

Frequent Sex Is Good For the Prostate

In one recent finding, men who ejaculated at least 21 times per month had one-third lower risk of prostate cancer than men who averaged four to seven ejaculations monthly.

Possible reason: Frequent ejaculation may remove potentially cancerous cells from the body.

It does not matter whether a man has intercourse or masturbates.

Michael Leitzmann, MD, DrPH, investigator, National Cancer Institute, Bethesda, Maryland.

16

Women's Health

Natural Ways to Ease Menopause Symptoms

For decades, women relied on hormone-replacement therapy (HRT) to relieve symptoms of menopause —hot flashes, sleep disturbance, anxiety and mood swings. But several large studies have linked long-term HRT with increased risk of breast cancer, dementia, heart attack and stroke.

Fortunately, there are safer, natural alternatives to HRT.

MORE THAN JUST ESTROGEN

People typically attribute menopausal symptoms to declining production of the female hormones *estrogen* and *progesterone*. But poor eating and lifestyle habits also play a role, by overtaxing the adrenal glands. For women who are going through menopause, the adrenal glands are nature's backup system. When the ovaries decrease their production of estrogen and progesterone, the adrenals have the ability

to produce hormones to compensate. Poor diet and lifestyle choices put stress on the adrenals, creating an imbalance in body chemistry and contributing to the uncomfortable symptoms that we associate with menopause.

If you are a woman with menopausal symptoms, adopting healthier habits can help to even out these imbalances.

If you are a man and the woman you love is going through menopause, you can help by understanding that she is experiencing a profound physiological change. Your kindness and patience can ease her transition through a time that is confusing—for her as well as for you.

Common symptoms and natural solutions…

HOT FLASHES

As many as 80% of women experience hot flashes during menopause. One theory is that the hypothalamus, which controls body temperature, is triggered in some way by hormonal fluctuations.

Ann Louise Gittleman, PhD, nutritionist based in Post Falls, ID, is author of many books, including *Hot Times: How to Eat Well, Live Healthy, and Feel Sexy During the Change*. Avery.

•**Avoid spicy foods.** Foods containing cayenne or other peppers have a thermogenic effect, meaning that they raise body temperature.

•**Cook with garlic, onion, thyme, oregano and sage.** These seasonings contain very small amounts of phyto-estrogens (plant-based estrogens such as lignans and isoflavones that occur naturally in certain foods) and can help restore hormone balance.

•**Cut down on caffeine.** Caffeine stimulates the adrenal glands, leading to a spike in blood sugar levels followed by a plunge in blood sugar to even lower levels than before. This stresses the body and aggravates menopause woes.

If you don't want to give up coffee completely, have one cup a day with food. Don't use coffee as a stimulant between meals. Instead, eat frequent small meals for energy.

Better than coffee: Green, white and black teas have less caffeine and are high in disease-fighting antioxidants. Try substituting tea for coffee. Then transition to herbal tea or hot water with lemon.

•**Add flaxseed.** Ground flaxseed contains lignans, which seem to modulate fluctuating estrogen and progesterone levels. Aim for two tablespoons a day. Ground flaxseed has a pleasant nutty flavor—sprinkle it on cereal, yogurt and salads.

Bonus: Flaxseed reduces cholesterol, helps prevent certain cancers and relieves constipation (be sure to drink plenty of water).

•**Eat soy foods in moderation.** Some countries with diets high in soy report low rates of menopausal symptoms and breast cancer. But I'm cautious about soy. Preliminary research suggests that while isoflavones in soy appear to protect against some breast cancers, they may stimulate growth of other types of breast cancer.

I'm especially concerned about isolated soy protein, which often is added to protein powder, energy bars and supplements. This puts far more soy isoflavones into the diet than other cultures typically consume—and these high amounts may not be healthful.

If you enjoy soy foods, limit your consumption to two servings a week, and eat them in their whole-food form—as tofu, tempeh, miso and edamame.

•**Be wary of herbal remedies.** I'm cautious about black cohosh, red clover and other plant remedies with estrogen-like properties. Research has not demonstrated clearly that they help, and some can have harmful side effects if not properly monitored. However, some women do report good results from these remedies. Check with your doctor first. If you don't notice a clear change in symptoms after two to three weeks of trying a new remedy, ask your doctor about trying something else.

What men can do: Buy a dual-control electric blanket so that you both will be comfortable. Make her a cup of herbal tea. Join her in eating flaxseed—it is good for your colon and prostate.

INSOMNIA

During menopause, elevated levels of the stress hormone *cortisol* make it difficult to fall asleep and can trigger intermittent awakening throughout the night. *Natural sleep aids...*

•**Wild yam cream.** This topical cream extracted from yams grown in Mexico is a source of natural progesterone. It's available at most health-food stores and some pharmacies. Applying small amounts of wild yam cream daily may help to balance cortisol levels and enhance sleep. (The cream also helps reduce anxiety and hot flashes.)

Apply one-quarter teaspoon once in the morning and once at night. Gently rub the cream into areas where you see capillaries, such as the wrist, back of the knee and neck—these are the places where skin is thinnest and the cream is easily absorbed. Rotate where you apply the cream on a daily basis.

•**Magnesium.** Levels of magnesium, a natural sleep aid, are depleted when you consume too much coffee, cola, alcohol, sugar or salt. Foods high in magnesium include halibut...whole-wheat bread...leafy green vegetables such as spinach...nuts...and dried beans (soaked and cooked). If your diet is low in magnesium, take 200 milligrams (mg) to 400 mg in supplement form at bedtime.

•**Zinc.** This mineral can help quiet an overactive mind. Foods rich in zinc include poultry, red meat and nuts, but it is hard to get enough zinc from food. Take 25 mg to 45 mg in supplement form before bed.

•**Exercise.** One study found that women over age 50 who walked, biked or did stretching exercises every morning fell asleep more easily. Try to get a half-hour of exercise most mornings. Avoid working out in the evening—you may have trouble winding down. And don't go to extremes. Overexercising (more than two hours of strenuous, nonstop activity every day) can lead to hormonal imbalance.

What men can do: Exercise with her in the morning. Make sure there is a bottle of magnesium tablets by the bedside at home and when traveling.

MOOD SWINGS

Drinking less coffee and eating frequent small meals will go a long way toward balancing your moods by reducing spikes in blood sugar and stress on adrenals. *In addition…*

•**Eat a balanced diet.** The emotional and mental stress of menopause can lead to a vicious cycle in which stress depletes important mineral stores, further taxing the adrenals.

Among the minerals depleted by stress are copper, calcium, magnesium, potassium, sodium and zinc. To restore these minerals, eat an adrenal-supportive diet rich in bright-colored fruits and vegetables, legumes, lean meats and whole grains. Avoid sugar and other refined carbohydrates.

Recommended: Sea vegetables, such as nori, arame, wakame and hijiki. These are especially high in key minerals. Health-food stores sell them in dried form. They can be crumbled into soup and over fish, salad and vegetables.

•**Get the right kind of fat.** Though you should avoid saturated fats (found in pork, beef and high-fat dairy products) and hydrogenated fats (in margarine, shortening and many packaged baked goods), certain fats are necessary for hormonal regulation and proper functioning of the nervous system. Known as *essential fatty acids* (EFAs), these healthy fats help to stabilize blood sugar.

Strive to consume two tablespoons a day of healthy oil (use it in cooking, salad dressings, etc.). Olive, sesame, almond, macadamia and flaxseed oils are especially high in EFAs. (Flaxseed oil does not cook well.)

•**Take B-complex vitamins.** B vitamins are known as the antistress vitamins because they nourish the adrenals. Good sources of B vitamins include whole grains and dried beans (soaked and cooked). Most diets are too low in these vitamins, so supplements usually are needed to make up the deficit. Take 50 mg to 100 mg of a vitamin-B complex daily.

What men can do: Make it easy for her to avoid sugar and caffeine by cutting back on them yourself—your health will benefit, too. If she seems distant or on edge, don't take it personally. Remind yourself that it is not you—it is her biochemistry that is acting up.

WEIGHT GAIN

One reason why so many women gain weight during menopause is that the ovulation process burns calories—as many as 300 per day during the first 10 days of the menstrual cycle. When ovulation stops, fewer calories are burned and metabolism slows. *Foods to counter the slowdown…*

•**Protein.** Increasing protein intake can raise the body's metabolic rate by as much as 25%. Aim for three to four ounces of lean protein from fish, poultry, beef or lamb twice a day. Eggs and beans also are good sources.

•**Healthy carbohydrates.** Whole grains, vegetables and fruits metabolize slowly and give you energy throughout the day. Try to consume daily at least two servings of fruits, three servings of vegetables and three servings of whole grains.

What men can do: Don't nag her about her weight. Support her by not buying high-calorie foods, such as potato chips and rich desserts.

At-Home, Handheld Scanner Helps Women Spot Cancer Early

Britton Chance, PhD, ScD, professor emeritus of biophysics, physical chemistry and radiologic physics, University of Pennsylvania School of Medicine, Philadelphia.

Juri Gelovani, MD, professor and chair, experimental diagnostic imaging, M.D. Anderson Cancer Center, Houston.

US Department of Defense Breast Cancer Research Program. *http://cdmrp.army.mil/bcrp/*.

A n experimental handheld imaging device designed for home use appears effective in detecting breast cancer in its early stages, according to a small study.

If future, larger studies prove successful, the device—tentatively called *iFind*—could be available commercially within a few years.

HOW IT WORKS

The size of a deck of cards, iFind uses near-infrared light to measure how much blood is flowing in different locations in the breast, says creator Britton Chance, PhD, ScD, professor emeritus of biophysics, physical chemistry and radiologic physics, University of Pennsylvania School of Medicine, Philadelphia.

Scientists believe that tumors require new blood vessels to grow, so those areas will have more blood. iFind monitors differences in blood oxygen ratios in growing cancer tissue compared with normal tissues. In this way, it detects "hypermetabolism"—the more rapid growth rate of malignant cells. When a certain threshold is passed, the device emits a light, tone or beep, indicating a woman needs to go to her doctor for further breast screening, says Chance.

THE EVIDENCE

Chance's team tested the device on 116 women over a five-year period. The device, which takes five minutes to use, was 96% accurate when someone had breast cancer. In other words, 96% of the women who actually had cancer had an abnormal reading. All had been diagnosed by standard methods.

iFind is not meant as a substitute for mammograms or biopsies, Chance says, but might supplement those detection methods.

"The [purpose] of this device is to get the women to go to the doctor if something is wrong," says Chance. "It records what it finds on a chip when she scans it across her breasts."

He estimates iFind would cost several hundred dollars and could be especially valuable for women who have a family history of cancer or those who have the breast cancer genes, BRCA1 and BRCA2.

THE REACTION

"The results of this initial study are very encouraging," says Dr. Juri Gelovani, professor and chair of the department of experimental diagnostic imaging at M.D. Anderson Cancer Center in Houston. "Yet, large population-based studies are required to reproduce the findings to validate the technology."

For more information about breast cancer, visit the American Cancer Society Web site at *www.cancer.org*.

■ ■ ■ ■

Birth Control Risk

Women who take low-dose birth control pills are twice as likely to have heart attacks or strokes as women who don't take them. Especially at risk are women who are over 35 years old...have a high risk of heart disease or diabetes...are overweight...or have polycystic ovary syndrome—a condition characterized by menstrual disturbances, reduced ovulation rates and increased testosterone levels. Researchers believe that the risk disappears after birth control pills are discontinued.

Jean-Patrice Baillargeon, MD, professor of internal medicine, department of medicine, endocrine division, University of Sherbrooke, Quebec, Canada, and lead researcher of a meta-analysis of 14 studies of women taking oral contraceptives between 1980 and 2002, published in Journal of Clinical Endocrinology & Metabolism.

■ ■ ■ ■

Pill Warning

Birth control pills can cause migraines during menstruation.

Recent study: Women taking oral contraceptives containing estrogen have a 40% greater risk of suffering migraine headaches during menstruation than women who don't take oral contraceptives.

Reason: When one is on oral contraceptives, the hormone-free week causes a steep drop in estrogen levels right before menstruation, which increases the risk of migraines.

Better for migraine sufferers: Use estrogen patches during the hormone-free week, or use the oral contraceptive Mircette, which allows for a gradual decrease in estrogen. Women who get migraines with auras should avoid hormone birth control entirely.

Karen Aegidius, MD, researcher, department of clinical neuroscience, Norwegian National Headache Center, Trondheim, and leader of a study of 13,944 premenopausal women, published in Neurology.

What Low Testosterone Means for Women

Culley C. Carson III, MD, Rhodes Distinguished Professor and chief of urology, University of North Carolina School of Medicine, Chapel Hill.

Some 30 million American women are thought to have low levels of the androgens (so-called male hormones) they need, including testosterone and DHEA.

Common causes include diminished ovarian function, estrogen supplementation (either in birth control pills or in hormone replacement therapy) and impaired adrenal function.

Symptoms include: Osteoporosis, reduced sex drive (which could be due to diminished libido or lack of interest due to pain or dryness), loss of muscle tone, low energy, lack of mental clarity and decreased enjoyment of life.

Diagnosis: To check for androgen deficiency in women, it's best to measure levels of testosterone and DHEA-sulfate (DHEA-S), another androgen. Total testosterone below 30 nanograms per deciliter and/or DHEA-S levels below 100 micrograms per deciliter may be cause to consider supplementation.

Treatment: Among women with sexual dysfunction due to low androgens, treatment with low-dose testosterone or low-dose DHEA significantly increases sex drive about 70% of the time. While the FDA has not yet approved testosterone supplements for use in women, many doctors are prescribing them anyway.

Warning: Unnecessary supplementation can lead to excessive androgen levels, resulting in heavier pubic hair growth, clitoral enlargement, acne, increased facial hair growth, lowered voice and reduced levels of HDL (good) cholesterol. Close monitoring of testosterone levels is advised.

■ ■ ■ ■

Morning-After Pill Warning

Mifeprex (*mifepristone*) can cause a rare, fatal infection in women who use it incorrectly.

More than four deaths from *sepsis*—an infection of the bloodstream—have been reported since 2000, when the so-called "abortion pill" went on the US market. These infections occurred in women who inserted the second course of two pills vaginally, as some clinics recommend, rather than swallowing them, as the instructions state. The Food and Drug Administration says that the pill is safe when used properly and it will stay on the market.

Center for Drug Evaluation and Research, US Food and Drug Administration, Washington, DC.

■ ■ ■ ■

Drugs Affect Women Differently

Women respond differently than men to certain drugs and should be aggressive in researching their medications. Women have been underrepresented in clinical drug studies, which long assumed that they respond to drugs as men do. But in fact, women suffer more adverse drug events than men do.

Steps: Understand the need for a drug. Ask a doctor or pharmacist about side effects and potential interactions with other drugs and be sure to understand correct dosage amounts and timing of doses.

Rosaly Correa-de-Araujo, MD, MSc, PhD, director, women's health and gender-based research, Agency for Healthcare Research and Quality (AHRQ), Rockville, MD, *www.ahrq.gov.*

■ ■ ■ ■

Depression and Menopause

As they approach menopause, women who have premenstrual syndrome (PMS) are more likely to suffer depression than women who don't suffer from PMS, a recent study found.

Self-defense: Seek medical treatment if you are approaching menopause and suffering from symptoms of depression.

Ellen Freeman, PhD, research professor, department of obstetrics and gynecology, University of Pennsylvania School of Medicine, Philadelphia, and leader of a study of 231 women, published in the *Archives of General Psychiatry* journal.

Finally, Good News About Menopause and Memory

Peter Meyer, PhD, assistant professor of preventive medicine and director, section of biostatistics, Rush University, Chicago.
Neurology.

When women going through the "change of life" experience a memory lapse, they often blame it on a "menopausal moment." But researchers have found that the working memory and perceptual speed of women improve with age, even during menopause.

Peter Meyer, assistant professor of preventive medicine at Rush University in Chicago, and his colleagues tested the memories of 803 women each year for six years.

The women who were included in Meyer's study were aged 42 to 52 years and were tested annually on their working memory and perceptual speed. They also answered questions about their health, menopausal status, ethnicity and education.

The subjects were in different stages of pre- and postmenopause.

Premenopause is the reproductive stage just prior to menopause. Perimenopause is the stage prior to menopause, when physical changes begin to accelerate due to declines in hormone production.

The working memory test asked the women to repeat increasingly long lists of numbers backward. In the perceptual speed test, the women were shown a series of symbols and a corresponding number. They were asked to match as many symbols with their corresponding number as they could in 90 seconds.

Meyer found that perceptual speed and working memory improved slightly over time for women in premenopause and early perimenopause.

Only for the perceptual speed tests was there a decrease in scores, and that was for postmenopausal women. Working memory scores for postmenopausal women did not change greatly over time.

Meyer says that, although the results are surprising, they do not indicate that women don't have problems with forgetfulness as they age.

WHAT CHANGE?

Women in the age group studied often say they have trouble remembering someone's name or coming up with the proper word, Meyer says. Why? "Verbal processing skills might be different, but not worse" with age, he says, somehow accounting for the forgetfulness.

Meyer also says that one explanation for the improvement on the tests might be that the women got better with practice.

■ ■ ■ ■

Hot Flash Relief

A drug used to control pain and epilepsy can sharply reduce the intensity and frequency of hot flashes in women with breast cancer, we hear from Kishan J. Pandya, MD. When breast cancer patients with chemotherapy-induced hot flashes took 900 mg daily of the anticonvulsant *gabapentin* (Neurontin), they reported a 46% reduction in the frequency and severity of hot flashes.

Self-defense: Chemotherapy patients who experience hot flashes should ask their doctors if gabapentin is right for them.

Kishan J. Pandya, MD, is professor of medicine and oncology and clinical director of hematology-oncology, James P. Wilmot Cancer Center, University of Rochester, Rochester, NY, and leader of a study of 420 women with breast cancer, published in *The Lancet.*

Fight the Weight Gain

Jana Klauer, MD, former research fellow, New York Obesity Research Center, St. Luke's-Roosevelt Hospital, New York City, and weight reduction physician in private practice.

For many women, as they get older, weight seems to go on more quickly and come off more slowly—no matter how much you exercise. Many women's once-lean bodies turn matronly as they reach menopause. The good news, though, is that several recent studies prove that weight gain at menopause is not inevitable.

RECENT STUDIES

The National Institutes of Health sponsored the Study of Women's Health Across the Nation (SWAN) in which researchers tracked 3,064 ethnically diverse women ages 42 to 52 over a three-year period. None had yet gone through menopause at the time the study began. At the end of the three years, the women had gained an average of 4.5 pounds, or 3% of their body weight, and increased waist circumference by about one inch. However—and this is what's really intriguing—whether or not the women had gone through menopause made no difference in their weight gain. Furthermore, the study found that women who were highly active or who became active during the course of the study did not gain weight. In fact, with activity, some lost both weight *and* inches from their waistlines.

In the second study, Harvard's famous ongoing Nurses' Health Study, researchers measured 116,686 young and middle-aged women several times during an eight-year period. They discovered that women who drank no more than one sugar-sweetened soft drink per week did not gain weight, but women who drank more put on weight. So, is it simply the age-old issue of "too much *in* results in too much *on*"?

A DIFFERENT PACE

Jana Klauer, MD, former research fellow at the New York Obesity Research Center at St. Luke's-Roosevelt Hospital in New York City and physician in private practice teaching weight control says that weight gain does not necessarily accompany menopause. In turn, it is crucial to avoid gaining weight at this time because postmenopausal women's cardiovascular risks go up—extra weight is an additional risk.

She acknowledges that weight can be harder to control in middle age—not because of hormones, but because metabolism slows by about 10% in these years. If unchecked, this can result in a gain of 10 or so pounds. You can indeed stop and even easily reverse that slowdown. Tests for metabolism are largely based on the body's resting rate (when the body is not in motion), she says, and the determiner of that is mostly the amount of muscle mass a person has. The more muscle you have, the higher your metabolic rate will be. The way to obtain more muscle mass is through exercise, especially strength training.

EXERCISE, A MUST

Working with weights several times a week isn't nearly enough when it comes to exercise, says Dr. Klauer. She emphasizes that exercise after age 40 is no longer an option—to stay healthy, it is a daily imperative. She recommends an hour each day of a weight-bearing exercise such as walking, jogging, dancing and the like—whatever takes you beyond the level you experience walking around your house or office. Although this may seem like a lot, if you can manage 15-minute spurts of activity throughout your day, it adds up. Be sure the activity you choose helps you build strength in your legs. Dr. Klauer points out that if the legs aren't strong, people begin to slow in their movements and balance problems set in.

SMART DIET CHOICES

After women pass age 40, their food choices also begin to play an ever-bigger role, says Dr. Klauer. Diet should be one that is heart-healthy and nutrient-rich. In fact, she points out that if you are eating all the nutrients you need, there won't be room in your diet for what she considers junk foods—processed foods, simple carbs, including high-sugar foods, and anything more than one drink of alcohol a day.

She reminds people that large quantities of fruits and vegetables are a wonderful way to keep weight under control because they are filling and provide much-needed fiber. She also advises eating about 60 g a day of high-quality protein.

Example: 3.5 ounces of fish has about 21 g of protein...a similar amount of chicken has 25 g...and a pint of milk has 19 g.

To get started on a healthy diet that will help you reduce or maintain a proper weight, Dr. Klauer says to record everything you eat until your new way of eating is firmly entrenched. She finds that most people are shocked to see how many little extras have crept into their daily diet, small splurges that add up to big numbers on the scale. Keeping a record will make you aware of what extra treats you are eating and help protect you from falling back into those bad habits.

No doubt, following the high level of exercise and healthy diet that Dr. Klauer describes is the surest way to control weight in and past middle age. It is also the best guarantee of a long and healthy life. And that's not a bad trade-off, not bad at all.

■ ■ ■ ■

Hot Flash Help

Hot flashes may be eased by acupuncture, says a new study.

Recent study: After seven weeks, post-menopausal women who had acupuncture twice a week for the first two weeks and once a week thereafter had a greater reduction in nocturnal hot flashes than women who had a treatment that felt like acupuncture but wasn't. Some women getting acupuncture had minor side effects, such as pain, redness and itching where needles were inserted.

Mary I. Huang, MS, is clinical research coordinator of a Stanford University School of Medicine study, led by Rachel Manber, PhD, of the effectiveness of acupuncture for nocturnal hot flashes, published in *Fertility and Sterility*.

Chasteberry for Women

Mark A. Stengler, ND, naturopathic physician in private practice, La Jolla, California…adjunct associate clinical professor at the National College of Natural Medicine, Portland, Oregon…author of many books, including *The Natural Physician's Healing Therapies* and coauthor of *Prescription for Natural Cures* (both from Bottom Line Books)…and author of the *Bottom Line/Natural Healing* newsletter.

If you were to examine some of the many "women's hormone-balancing" products in health-food stores and pharmacies, you would most likely see chasteberry (also known as *Vitex agnus castus*) listed as an ingredient. It has been recommended for female conditions, including hormone-related acne, fibrocystic breast syndrome, endometriosis, infertility, lactation difficulties, menopausal hot flashes, menstrual disorders, ovarian cysts and uterine fibroids. In other words, it is touted as helping almost all major female conditions.

The herb comes from the berries of the chasteberry tree, actually a shrub found in subtropical climates. The ancient Greeks used chasteberry as a symbol of chastity in young women, hence the name "chaste berry" or "chaste tree."

HOW IT WORKS

Chasteberry does not contain hormones. It acts on the pituitary gland in the brain to increase the production of *luteinizing hormone* (LH). LH stimulates the ovaries to release eggs, as occurs with ovulation. Ovulation triggers a surge in levels of the hormone *progesterone*. This release of progesterone is important in maintaining a balance with the other major female hormone, *estrogen*. Research has shown that some premenopausal women do not ovulate regularly. This sets the stage for what is known as "estrogen dominance"—too much estrogen relative to progesterone. By helping to normalize progesterone levels, chasteberry promotes hormone balance. This is why it is effective for so many female conditions, including premenstrual syndrome and fibrocystic breast disease as well as uterine fibroids in women of all ages, which are in large part caused by estrogen dominance.

Chasteberry also has been shown to lower levels of the hormone *prolactin*. When elevated, this hormone, which is secreted by the pituitary gland, is associated with premenstrual syndrome, irregular menstrual cycles and infertility.

DOSAGE

For all of these conditions, I commonly recommend 160 mg to 240 mg daily of a 0.6% *aucubin* or 0.5% *agnuside* extract (important active ingredients) in capsule form—available from Enzymatic Therapy (800-783-2286, *www.enzy.com*) and Natural Factors (sold by Vitacost, 800-381-0759, *www.vitacost.com*). Or I suggest 40 drops of the tincture in four ounces of water, taken once daily.

For best results, chasteberry should be used until the problem is alleviated and then for an additional three months. Women may notice improvements within two menstrual cycles.

Chasteberry often needs to be taken for four to six months or longer for long-standing cases of hormone imbalance that have resulted in infertility, amenorrhea (no menstrual cycles), irregular menstrual cycles or endometriosis.

Mild digestive upset, nausea, headaches and skin rash are infrequent side effects of chasteberry. Stop taking it if they occur.

Chasteberry should not be used by women taking birth control pills or injections. It also should be avoided by those taking drugs that block dopamine receptors, such as the antipsychotic medication *haloperidol* (Haldol).

As with most herbs, chasteberry should be avoided during pregnancy, although it is helpful for lactation in nursing mothers.

Lastly, some women experience an "adjustment phase" during the first few months of taking chasteberry. It is not uncommon for the menstrual cycle to shorten or lengthen, and flow can become lighter or heavier than what it was previously. This adjustment phase almost always normalizes after two to three months of use.

■■■■

Postmenopausal Incontinence

Postmenopausal women have a high prevalence of urinary incontinence.

Recent finding: 60% of postmenopausal women experience one or more episodes of incontinence in a month. Postmenopausal women with diabetes are more likely to report severe incontinence—difficulty controlling urination, inability to completely empty the bladder and discomfort during urination. Treatment options for incontinence include Kegel (pelvic floor) exercises, medication and surgery.

Sara Jackson, MD, MPH, senior fellow, VA Puget Sound Health Care Center, department of medicine, University of Washington, Seattle, and lead author of a study of 1,017 postmenopausal women, published in *Diabetes Care*.

Natural Remedies For Menopause Relief

Mark A. Stengler, ND, naturopathic physician in private practice, La Jolla, California...adjunct associate clinical professor at the National College of Natural Medicine, Portland, Oregon...author of many books, including *The Natural Physician's Healing Therapies* and coauthor of *Prescription for Natural Cures* (both from Bottom Line Books)...and author of the *Bottom Line/Natural Healing* newsletter.

Nearly 38 million American women are between the ages of 40 and 54, according to the US Census Bureau. Most are in some stage of menopause. If you're among them, you may be wondering about the best ways to deal with the symptoms. Fortunately, several natural remedies and medicines can help. They are safe and effective—and some work quickly, particularly if you have mild to moderate symptoms.

Menopause is a normal stage in a woman's life. Unless a woman has another reason such as low body weight or vigorous athletic training, if a woman hasn't had a period for 12 consecutive months, she is considered to have reached menopause. In the US, the average age is 51. During menopause, ovaries produce less of the hormones estrogen, progesterone and testosterone. Meanwhile, there's an increase in the release of two hormones produced by the pituitary gland—*follicle stimulating hormone* (FSH) and *luteinizing hormone* (LH). Doctors believe the surge of these latter two hormones trigger menopausal symptoms, including hot flashes (which affect three-quarters of American menopausal women) and vaginal dryness. You also may experience insomnia, depression and mood swings.

In the year or two before menopause, many women go through perimenopause, or premenopause, during which hot flashes and other symptoms usually begin. The menstrual cycle becomes irregular. A period of lingering symptoms after menopause is called postmenopause. The therapies I recommend are effective for women in any stage, from perimenopause to postmenopause—but not one of these therapies includes typical pharmaceuticals. *Here's why...*

THE HORMONE HERESY

Sixty years ago, doctors started giving women equine estrogen along with a synthetic form of progesterone known as progestin to control menopausal symptoms. Premarin, made from the urine of pregnant mares, has been one of the best-selling drugs in recent history—but I view it as one of the biggest scams of all time.

Premarin, and drugs like it, were said to offer many benefits, including prolonged youthfulness, a sound mind, improved libido, strong bones and a healthy heart. I never believed the hype, nor did many other holistic doctors.

The dangers of taking hormone formulas came to light a few years ago. Doctors and female patients were alarmed at the results of a study on the drug Prempro, a combination of Premarin and a synthetic progesterone called Provera. Prempro had been touted as a panacea for menopausal problems, but views changed in July 2002, when results of the Women's Health Initiative study, which included more than 16,000 women, showed unexpected dangers from the drug. Investigators found significant increases in risk of heart disease, stroke, blood clots and breast cancer among women taking Prempro.

In 2003, the Women's Health Initiative Memory Study revealed that women 65 and older who had been taking Prempro had an increased risk of dementia. Premarin has also been shown to increase gallbladder disease risk.

Additionally, the British Million Women Study found that the use of hormone-replacement therapy by women ages 50 to 64 over the past decade had resulted in an estimated 20,000 additional breast cancers and an increased incidence of fatal breast malignancies.

LOWER DOSAGE

The response of pharmaceutical giants makes my hair stand on end—they recommended lower dosages of the drugs, even though there were no studies showing that lower doses were safer. Companies also started promoting pharmaceutical antidepressants, such as *venlataxine* (Effexor), *fluoxetine* (Prozac), *paroxetine* (Paxil) and *sertraline* (Zoloft), for relief of menopausal symptoms, especially hot flashes. All these drugs have potential side effects—including fatigue, headache and weight gain.

Fortunately, many natural therapies are readily available. Natural therapy's goal is to alleviate or reduce symptoms quickly without harmful side effects. I recommend starting with nutritional supplements—including various herbal and homeopathic therapies.

MILD TO MODERATE SYMPTOMS

Women with "mild" symptoms may be annoyed by occasional hot flashes. Those in the "moderate" category have hot flashes along with other symptoms. For example, if a woman experiences three or four hot flashes a day, doesn't sleep at night and has reduced sex drive, I consider her symptoms to be moderate. You can take these remedies one at a time or use a formula that contains some or all of the ingredients.

- **Black cohosh.** This shrub was used by Native Americans for hormonal problems. At least six studies have shown that it can help relieve hot flashes, night sweats and depression. One popular brand of black cohosh is Remifemin, which is available at pharmacies and at *www.drugstore.com*. Choose an extract standardized to 2.5% *triterpene glycosides* (an ingredient that helps control luteinizing hormone). Start by taking a dose of 80 mg daily and increase to 160 mg daily if necessary. Many women notice improvement within two to four weeks. You can take black cohosh for four to six months, then stop to see if your symptoms return. If they do, resume taking it. In rare cases, black cohosh can cause digestive upset, headache and/or dizziness.

- **Vitex (chasteberry).** This hormone-regulating herb has been recommended since the days of Hippocrates. Use vitex during perimenopause to reduce heavy bleeding and hot flashes. Take 160 mg to 240 mg of a 0.6% *aucubin* standardized extract or 40 drops of the tincture daily. Vitanica (800-572-4712, *www.vitanica.com*) offers a 0.6% aucubin extract, which is available at health-food stores. You can take it for as long as you have symptoms. Vitex should not be taken with birth control pills.

HOMEOPATHIC FORMULAS

Work with a practitioner trained in homeopathy who can match your symptoms to appropriate compounds. The following remedies are available at most health-food stores. For each, start with two pellets of a 30C potency twice daily. You should notice positive results within two weeks. After symptoms improve, stop taking the remedy unless symptoms return.

- **Sepia** helps with hot flashes, night sweats and vaginal dryness. It is recommended for women who feel short-tempered, irritable, have a low libido or when symptoms include incontinence or uterine prolapse (falling or sliding of the uterus from its normal position in the pelvic cavity into the vaginal canal).

- **Lachesis** eases hot flashes, anxiety, headaches, insomnia, palpitations and irritability.

- **Pulsatilla** is for women who feel much worse in a warm room. It also is recommended if you have mood swings, weepiness or a strong craving for sweets.

•**Sulphur** relieves insomnia and helps women who are constantly overheated, sweat easily and have a strong thirst for ice-cold drinks.

MODERATE TO SEVERE SYMPTOMS

•**Natural progesterone cream** is helpful for women with stronger symptoms. I advise perimenopausal women to apply 20 mg of the cream (about one-quarter teaspoon) on the inside of their wrists and forearms or other areas of the body one to two times daily for the last two weeks of their menstrual cycles. Do not use it during your period. If you're menopausal, apply the same amount one to two times daily. Stop using it five to seven days each month unless your symptoms return during this time. Postmenopausal women should apply 10 mg (about one-eighth teaspoon) one to two times daily, and be sure to take five to seven days off each month.

■ **More from Mark A. Stengler…**

Help for Yeast Infections

Menopausal women are susceptible to yeast infections because of the changes in their hormones. The use of natural estrogen (*estriol*) inserted vaginally can help prevent such infections in some women. Increasing estrogen levels locally in the vaginal area works to favorably change the pH level, so that microbes cannot grow as easily. Estriol requires a prescription from your general doctor or gynecologist. Also, some researchers think that yeast infections may be transmitted sexually, so cleanse the genital area before intercourse and make sure your partner uses a condom. Finally, certain homeopathic remedies work very well to reduce susceptibility to yeast infections. Consult a local practitioner of homeopathy for an individualized treatment plan. For acute infections, consider using Kreosotum, a remedy derived from beechwood. It is widely available at health-food stores and on-line. At the first sign of symptoms (itching and/or creamy discharge), take two pellets of a 30C potency up to four times daily.

Less Invasive Alternatives To Hysterectomy

Esther Eisenberg, MD, MPH, professor of obstetrics and gynecology and director of reproductive endocrinology and infertility at the Vanderbilt University School of Medicine in Nashville, is coauthor of Hysterectomy: Exploring Your Options. *Johns Hopkins University Press.*

Over the past 25 years, advances in gynecologic surgery have caused a steady decline in the number of hysterectomies (removal of the entire uterus) performed in the US.

Now: A variety of new surgical techniques are giving women even more options for treating abnormal uterine bleeding and fibroid tumors.

ABNORMAL UTERINE BLEEDING

This condition typically occurs in women over age 45. It results from a high level of estrogen that is not balanced by progesterone. Ovulation does not occur, but the lining of the uterus (endometrium) thickens and is then shed incompletely and irregularly, causing bleeding.

In the past, abnormal uterine bleeding was treated with complete hysterectomy.

Alternatives to hysterectomy…

•**Endometrial ablation.** This approach, which requires no incision and is performed on an outpatient basis, stops uterine bleeding in up to 80% of women.

How it works: A hysteroscope (a thin, fiber optic tube) is introduced through the vagina and cervix into the uterus. An electric current or laser is then used to heat and destroy the endometrium. Scar tissue may develop, which is likely to impair a woman's ability to become pregnant. Other potential risks include perforation of the uterine wall and injury to adjacent structures, such as burns to the bowel.

•**Thermal balloon ablation.** This newer technique appears to be as effective as endometrial ablation, and it typically has fewer risks. However, not all hospitals have the equipment that is required to perform thermal balloon ablation.

How it works: A balloon placed in the uterus and filled with fluid is heated until it destroys the endometrium without damaging surrounding tissue.

UTERINE FIBROIDS

Up to 40% of hysterectomies are performed to remove uterine fibroids. Although the cause of these tumors is unknown, recent research has linked them to a genetic mutation. Fibroids are almost always benign and often produce no symptoms.

However, fibroids can cause extremely heavy or frequent menstrual flow (sometimes leading to anemia)…chronic pain…bloating…pressure on the bladder and other internal organs…infertility…and/or abdominal swelling. In these cases, surgery is often the best solution. *Procedures to consider…*

•**Myomectomy.** Currently the preferred treatment for women who want to keep their reproductive options open, this procedure removes fibroids but retains the woman's uterus to allow for pregnancy.

How it works: A surgeon makes an abdominal incision, cuts the fibroid out and repairs the wall of the uterus with sutures.

•**Laparoscopic myomectomy.** This procedure is less invasive than standard myomectomy, but it may not be advisable if the fibroid is too large.

How it works: A laparoscope (a thin, lighted viewing tube) and other instruments are introduced through a small (less than one inch) abdominal incision. The fibroids are cut into fragments small enough to be removed through the abdominal incision or another small incision made through the vaginal wall. Most women can sustain a pregnancy following laparoscopic myomectomy. However, there is increased risk for uterine rupture at delivery because the laparoscopic closure of the uterine muscle may not be as effective as in a standard myomectomy.

In one out of three women who receive standard or laparoscopic myomectomy, fibroid tumors eventually recur.

•**Hysteroscopy.** An even less invasive technique than laparoscopic myomectomy, hysteroscopy is now being used for some submucous fibroids, which protrude inside the uterine cavity.

(Many fibroids are embedded in the uterine muscle.)

How it works: After the cervix is dilated, a hysteroscope is passed through the cervix into the uterus, which is inflated with gas or fluid to give a better view. Because dilation is painful, local or regional anesthesia is usually administered. With hysteroscopy, fibroids are removed with an electrosurgical tool that burns the tissue so that the fibroids can be removed in pieces. The procedure, which requires no incision, is performed on an outpatient basis, and recovery occurs within two to three days.

•**High-frequency ultrasound.** This is a promising experimental procedure.

How it works: While the patient lies in a magnetic resonance imaging (MRI) scanner, a doctor uses the MRI image to aim heat-producing, high-frequency ultrasound beams at the tumor to destroy it.

The patient is awake throughout high-frequency ultrasound, and no incisions are required. Currently available at The Johns Hopkins Hospital in Baltimore, Brigham and Women's Hospital in Boston and Mayo Clinic in Rochester, Minnesota, this procedure has been found to be safe and effective in preliminary studies.

NEW HYSTERECTOMY OPTIONS

Despite the availability of newer treatments, up to 600,000 women each year still choose a hysterectomy for their gynecologic condition.

Reason: A hysterectomy provides a permanent cure for abnormal uterine bleeding and fibroid tumors and eliminates risk for uterine cancer.

Newer, less-invasive types of hysterectomy have sharply reduced hospitalization—to just two to three days for many patients—and hastened recovery to as little as a week.

•**Supracervical hysterectomy.** The uterus, but not the cervix, is removed through an abdominal incision. This surgery has fewer complications than total hysterectomy, but it still leaves a woman at risk for cervical cancer.

•**Laparoscopic hysterectomy.** The uterus is removed using a laparoscope inserted through a small abdominal incision.

•**Vaginal hysterectomy.** The uterus is removed through an incision inside the vagina.

The procedure includes removal of both the cervix and the uterus. It can only be performed on fibroids that are small enough to pass through the vagina. Vaginal hysterectomy can also be performed with laparoscopic assistance.

■ ■ ■ ■

Preventing Breast Cancer

Nearly 20,000 women in a recent study took either *tamoxifen* (Nolvadex), the only drug currently approved to reduce breast cancer incidence in high-risk women, or the osteoporosis drug *raloxifene* (Evista) daily for five years.

Result: Both drugs cut invasive breast cancer incidence by 50%. However, the raloxifene group developed 36% fewer uterine cancers and 29% fewer blood clots than the tamoxifen group.

Theory: Like tamoxifen, raloxifene helps moderate the hormone estrogen, but with fewer side effects. Raloxifene received FDA approval in September 2007 for breast cancer prevention.

Kathy S. Albain, MD, director, breast clinical research program, Cardinal Bernardin Cancer Center, Loyola University Health System, Maywood, Illinois.

■ ■ ■ ■

Breast Cancer Screening Critical for Women 70+

Breast cancer screening and treatment for older women should be the same as that for younger women, we hear from Len Lichtenfeld, MD. Breast cancer is most commonly diagnosed between the ages of 75 and 79, yet many women over age 70 fail to have regular mammograms.

Also: Some physicians discourage chemotherapy because they believe older women can't tolerate it well, but this usually is not the case.

Helpful: When discussing treatment options with your physician, ask whether he/she would recommend a different treatment if you were younger and, if so, why he is not suggesting it.

J. Leonard Lichtenfeld, MD, is deputy chief medical officer, American Cancer Society, Atlanta. Dr. Len's Cancer Blog can be viewed at *www.cancer.org/aspx/blog.*

Breakthrough— A Therapy That Beats Tamoxifen

Anthony Howell, the United Kingdom's first professor of cancer prevention, Christie Hospital, Manchester.

Otis W. Brawley, MD, professor of oncology, Emory University Winship Cancer Institute, Atlanta.

M.D. Anderson Cancer Center news release.

Loyola University, Chicago Stritch School of Medicine news release.

San Antonio Breast Cancer Symposium.

A newer drug called *anastrozole* could soon replace *tamoxifen* as the standard treatment for postmenopausal breast cancer patients whose cancer is fueled by estrogen, according to an international study.

Anastrozole (Arimidex) is one of a class of drugs called *aromatase inhibitors* and was significantly more effective than tamoxifen in a number of areas. More women taking anastrozole remained free of cancer than those taking tamoxifen. If cancer did recur, more time elapsed before the recurrence in patients taking anastrozole. In addition, anastrozole reduced the incidence of cancer spreading, particularly to the other breast.

THE STUDY

The study included nearly 10,000 postmenopausal women who had *localized* breast cancer—it had not spread to the lymph nodes or beyond—and had been treated with surgery.

The women were placed in three groups: those who took tamoxifen, those who took anastrozole, and those who took both drugs. The women were followed up for five years following their initial treatment. However, after three years, the group taking both drugs was disbanded because the treatment appeared to be not as effective.

THE RESULTS

After five years, researchers found that 10% more women taking anastrozole were disease-free compared with the women taking tamoxifen. The anastrozole group also had a 20% longer period of time until the cancer recurred and 40% fewer instances of cancer spreading to the other breast than the group taking tamoxifen. In addition, the women taking anastrozole were 14% less likely to have their cancer spread to other sites in the body.

In addition, compliance rates were higher for those women taking anastrozole compared with tamoxifen perhaps because anastrozole produced fewer side effects, although bone fractures and joint pain were more common than among women given tamoxifen, the study found.

The study did not show any significant improvement in the overall survival rates among those women who took anastrozole compared with the women who took tamoxifen. However, more time is necessary to determine if anastrozole will produce better long-term survival rates.

IMPLICATIONS

The researchers found that prescribing anastrozole immediately after surgery significantly improved results for patients, and they recommend giving anastrozole instead of tamoxifen to women for five years following their initial cancer treatment.

Currently, postmenopausal women whose breast cancer is hormone-receptor-positive—approximately 75% of all patients—take tamoxifen for five years after breast cancer surgery. The drug blunts estrogen's ability to fuel cancer growth. In contrast, anastrozole prevents estrogen from being produced. It is often prescribed for women following tamoxifen therapy.

"Results from studies suggest that it is reasonable to switch patients currently on tamoxifen to an aromatase inhibitor," say the researchers. The study was led by Anthony Howell, a professor at Christie Hospital NHS Trust, in Manchester, England.

However, some cancer experts note that aromatase inhibitors can have significant side effects, including an increased risk of osteoporosis.

Dr. Otis W. Brawley, professor of oncology at Emory University's Winship Cancer Institute in Atlanta, says, "This is the strongest of the studies I've seen so far that aromatase inhibitors are more effective than tamoxifen, and it will

sway a lot of people. But the problem is that aromatase inhibitors cause significant osteoporosis, and one worries that you might be buying a woman worse problems down the road."

Another issue, Brawley adds, is the higher cost of aromatase inhibitors compared with tamoxifen. That cost differential might lead some women to stop taking the drugs before the therapy is completed.

■ ■ ■ ■

Benign Breast Lesion Danger

Papillary lesions (benign growths in the milk-producing ducts) account for 1% to 3% of lesions sampled by core needle biopsies.

New finding: More than 20% of patients diagnosed with papillary lesions who underwent surgery or further imaging tests were found to harbor adjacent cells that increase breast cancer risk.

If you are diagnosed with a breast lesion: Ask your doctor what type it is and discuss whether removal is appropriate. If you have a papillary lesion that has not been surgically removed, monitor it closely with imaging tests.

Cecilia L. Mercado, MD, assistant professor of radiology, New York University Medical Center, New York City.

■ ■ ■ ■

Breast Asymmetry And Cancer

Researchers examined the mammograms of 252 women who later developed breast cancer and 252 women of the same age who did not develop the disease.

Result: Those who developed breast cancer had higher breast volume asymmetry (difference in volume between left and right breasts) than other women.

Theory: Estrogen, which has been linked to breast cancer, may also play a role in breast asymmetry.

Diane Scutt, PhD, director of research, School of Health Sciences, University of Liverpool, England.

Freezing Shrinks Benign Breast Tumors By 73%

Peter J. Littrup, MD, professor of radiology, urology and radiation oncology, Wayne State University, and director, image-guided therapy program, Karmanos Cancer Institute, both in Detroit.

George Hermann, MD, professor of radiology, Mount Sinai Medical Center, New York City.

Radiological Society of North America annual meeting, Chicago.

Doctors are able to sharply shrink the size of benign breast tumors by using a small probe that freezes abnormal breast cells.

The procedure, called *cryotherapy*, combines ultrasound and the probe in a type of image-guided therapy that is a painless, quick and noninvasive alternative to surgery, says Dr. Peter J. Littrup, a radiologist at Wayne State University and director of the image-guided therapy program at Karmanos Cancer Institute, both in Detroit.

"We can treat major tumors on an outpatient basis with minimum discomfort. It is a great boon for patients and patient care," says Littrup, who performed the procedure in 27 women, reducing the size of their noncancerous tumors by an average of 73%.

Benign breast lumps affect approximately 10% of women, most in their late teens and early 20s, and they are twice as common in African-American women as Caucasian women, Littrup says. Although most lumps aren't removed, approximately one million are excised annually because of their size, continued growth or for cosmetic reasons, he says.

Cryotherapy is currently used to treat cancerous tumors in the prostate, Littrup says. He is also involved in trials using the procedure to remove malignant tumors in the lung and kidney.

LETHAL ICE

To perform the procedure, doctors will first numb the area around the tumor, which is visible through ultrasound.

Next, they insert a cryoprobe—similar to a large needle—into the middle of the lesion and inject liquid nitrogen into it.

An ice ball forms at the tip of the probe and continues to grow until the ultrasound confirms the entire lump has been engulfed, killing the tissue around the tumor, Littrup says.

The benefits of the procedure, according to Littrup, are that the ice is easily visible in the ultrasound so doctors can be precise in seeing the tumor, the method is painless and it doesn't affect the collagen in the breast, so it keeps its shape. Also, there is no significant scarring.

Insurers don't automatically pay for the procedure for benign lumps. "It depends on the insurers," Littrup says. But because the patients don't have to stay overnight, the procedure is cost effective, he says.

ANOTHER VIEW

Dr. George Hermann, a radiologist at Mount Sinai Medical Center in New York City, says the procedure is interesting, but he questions its use for benign breast lumps.

He says that physicians still need to do a biopsy, and then decide whether to remove any benign lumps.

Further, he says, if cryotherapy is used to remove a cancerous tumor, it's impossible to evaluate the mass afterward because it's gone. When a lump is surgically removed, you can study it, which is important to treatment, Hermann says.

But Littrup says cryotherapy has already been shown to be effective as a way to treat cancerous tumors (such as in the prostate) without surgical intervention.

Breast Cancer Patients, Walk for Your Life!

Michelle D. Holmes, MD, DrPH, assistant professor of medicine, Harvard Medical School, and associate physician, Brigham and Women's Hospital, both in Boston.

Whoever coined the phrase "walk for life" for fundraising and awareness-raising may not have realized how meaningful his/her efforts were. Many studies have established that regular exercise reduces the risk of developing breast cancer, but a recent study suggests that women battling breast cancer who exercise regularly may significantly lower their risk of dying from the disease.

THE RESEARCH

The study, led by Michelle D. Holmes, MD, DrPH, assistant professor at Harvard Medical School, analyzed data from 2,987 women with breast cancer who took part in the long-range Nurses' Health Study. This study revealed that female breast cancer patients who walked one to three hours a week at a moderate pace were 20% less likely to die from the disease, compared with those who didn't exercise at all. Those who walked three to five hours weekly reduced their risk by 50%. Interestingly, participants who walked five to eight hours a week had a reduced risk of 44%...and more than eight hours a week had a reduced risk of 40%. Most important is that, with exercise, there was significant improvement in risk for cancer death.

The immediate question, of course, is whether the women who were healthy enough to walk were more likely to survive anyway. Dr. Holmes explained that this was clearly their concern while conducting the study. Accordingly, they also conducted an analysis based on the stage of cancer, from one to three (women with stage-four cancer, in which the disease has spread, were not included in the study).

THE THEORY

Exercise lowers hormone levels, which suppresses cancer growth recurrence.

THE FINDINGS

Surprisingly, they discovered that the group that had the maximum benefit from walking was the stage-three group—their risk was 68% lower, apparently disproving the idea that those with more advanced disease and so poorer health wouldn't do as well. However, she cautions that there were fewer women in this group (about 260 total), and further studies are important. A contributing factor might be that women diagnosed with more advanced cancer may be more motivated to adopt a healthy lifestyle generally.

OTHER SPORTS

Although the study focused on walking, the women participated in a number of equivalent aerobic activities, including bicycling, hiking, tennis, swimming and jogging, as well as aerobics classes. The study designers evaluated these in terms of activity units and translated that to the equivalent number of hours of walking.

MODERATE AMOUNT OF EXERTION

It's encouraging for women in treatment to learn that they don't need to walk a great deal to gain benefit. Remember, a mere three to five hours a week was the optimum amount of time associated with decreased risk for death. Right now, there are many theories for why walking is so beneficial for breast cancer patients. The good news is that it does seem to be beneficial.

WALK FOR A CURE

Save more lives by walking to raise money for breast cancer research. For information on upcoming events, visit the following Web sites...

- *www.The3Day.org*
- *http://makingstrides.acsevents.org*
- *www.avonwalk.org*

■ ■ ■ ■

Ginkgo and Ovarian Cancer

Taking a standard dose of ginkgo daily for at least six months decreased ovarian cancer risk by 60% or more and slowed growth of cancer cells in the lab by up to 80%. If you have a personal or family history of cancer, ask your physician about ginkgo.

Caution: Ginkgo may interact with blood thinners such as aspirin and *warfarin*.

Daniel William Cramer, MD, ScD, is professor of obstetrics, gynecology and reproductive biology, Brigham and Women's Hospital/Harvard Medical School, Boston. His study of 1,389 women was presented at the American Association for Cancer Research annual meeting.

Breast Implants Linked To Higher Suicide Rates

Veronica Cornelia Maria Koot, MD, PhD, clinician, University Medical Center, Utrecht, the Netherlands.

David L. Feldman, MD, director of plastic surgery, Maimonides Medical Center, Brooklyn, New York.

James Wells, MD, former president, American Society of Plastic Surgeons, based in Long Beach, California.

British Medical Journal.

Does having surgically enhanced breasts make women happier? Researchers found that Swedish women who had breast implants were 50% more likely to commit suicide than women without them.

The study showed that deaths of women with breast implants were higher than expected in the categories of suicide and lung cancer due to smoking. The authors suggested the extra deaths might be attributable to underlying psychiatric problems, something that plastic surgeons are generally on guard for. Dr. Veronica Koot, one of the study's authors and a clinician at the University Medical Center in Utrecht, the Netherlands, said that "very low self-esteem" might be to blame.

"This is not the first study to suggest that suicide rates might be higher [in women who have had breast enlargement surgery]," according to Dr. David L. Feldman, director of plastic surgery at Maimonides Medical Center in Brooklyn, New York. "Women are deluded into thinking that having larger breasts will change their life. It won't. It'll change their breasts."

A DIFFERENT VIEWPOINT

Not everyone agrees that the suicides can be linked to the breast implants. "That just doesn't compute with the information that we have in this country," says Dr. James Wells, former president of the American Society of Plastic Surgeons. "We don't know that we have a cause-and-effect relationship."

Part of the problem, Wells suggests, is inherent in looking at people from two different societies—in this case, the United States and Sweden.

Wells estimates that US plastic surgeons turn away clients roughly 2% to 5% of the time. "There's an evaluation process by the physicians to try to identify those patients who seem a little unstable. Their job history isn't stable, they're bouncing from relationship to relationship," he says. "We need to spend time listening to the patient. Surgeons have a responsibility to say no just as much as they have a responsibility to say yes."

EVALUATING THE PATIENTS

Koot agreed that different screening procedures could account for a difference in risk, depending on the country.

The typical woman seeking breast augmentation in the US is happily married and has several children, Wells says. "She is looking to reverse what pregnancy did in terms of her breasts and appearance," he says.

Still, identifying the "right" person can be as much art as science. "We try to avoid operating on somebody who has a propensity for suicide, but this is a tough call and some people will slip through the cracks," Feldman says. "It does point out our obligation to do a full evaluation and not just rush a person off to the operating room."

The American Society of Plastic Surgeons at *www.plasticsurgery.org* and The American Society for Aesthetic Plastic Surgery at *http://surgery.org* provide extensive overviews for women thinking about breast enlargement.

■ ■ ■ ■

Painkiller Benefit

Painkillers may reduce ovarian cancer risk. Women who regularly used nonsteroidal anti-inflammatory drugs (NSAIDs), such as aspirin, ibuprofen and naproxen, had a 28% risk reduction over a five-year period. Acetaminophen was associated with a 22% risk reduction. Not enough is known yet to recommend painkillers as a preventive. Consult your physician.

Joellen Schildkraut, PhD, is associate professor of community and family medicine, Duke University Medical Center, Durham, North Carolina, and leader of a study published in *Epidemiology.*

Nonsurgical Technique Shrinks Fibroids

Society of Interventional Radiology.

Anonsurgical treatment for uterine fibroids, known as *uterine fibroid embolization* (UFE), has a five-year success rate of 73%, according to a new study of 182 women.

UFE is an interventional radiology treatment that blocks the blood supply to fibroid tumors, causing them to shrink and die. Because it is minimally invasive, the treatment offers a faster recovery time than surgery and preserves the uterus—two factors that have made UFE increasingly popular.

THE FUTURE IS NOW?

"Some gynecologists have been waiting for long-term data before being comfortable recommending the UFE procedure, and now that we have that data, I think patients will be hearing more about UFE as a nonsurgical option," says principal investigator Dr. James B. Spies, professor of interventional radiology at Georgetown University Medical Center.

"The [study] results are comparable to *myomectomy*, a procedure in which the fibroids are surgically removed. However, UFE is less invasive, and women recover from it more quickly," Spies explains.

Myomectomy may be performed laparoscopically or through an abdominal incision.

"With any of the uterine-sparing treatments, growth of new fibroids is possible," he notes. However, the rate of recurrence after UFE is similar to that of myomectomy.

The next step is to determine which patients are best suited for each treatment, Spies says.

Uterine fibroids are common benign growths that develop in the muscular wall of the uterus. Fibroids result in approximately 200,000 hysterectomies annually.

The National Uterine Fibroids Foundation has more about uterine fibroids at *www.nuff.org*.

■ ■ ■ ■

Better Fibroid Treatment

The most common treatment for symptomatic fibroids (benign growths inside the uterus), which can result in excessive menstrual bleeding, pain and frequent urination, is hysterectomy (removal of the uterus).

Now: Magnetic resonance-guided, focused ultrasound surgery (MRgFUS) allows radiologists to precisely target fibroids without hysterectomy. The new outpatient procedure uses high-intensity ultrasound waves to heat and destroy uterine fibroid tissue. Side effects include slight cramping. The procedure is FDA-approved for premenopausal women who do not plan to become pregnant.

To locate an MRgFUS treatment center in your area, go to the Center for Uterine Fibroids Web site at *www.fibroids.net*.

Fiona M. Fennessy, MD, PhD, assistant professor of radiology, Brigham and Women's Hospital, Dana Farber Cancer Institute, Harvard Medical School, Boston.

■ ■ ■ ■

Ovarian Cancer Treatment

Researchers compared the care that gynecologic oncologists, gynecologists and general surgeons provided to 3,000 women ages 65 or older who had surgery for early-stage ovarian cancer. Patients treated by the gynecologic oncologists and gynecologists had half the mortality rate (2.1% versus 4%) of those treated by general surgeons. Women diagnosed with ovarian cancer should seek treatment by a gynecologic oncologist. To find one, contact the Society of Gynecologic Oncologists, 312-235-4060, *www.sgo.org*.

C.C. Earle, MD, associate professor of medicine, Brigham and Women's Hospital, Dana Farber Cancer Institute, Harvard Medical School, Boston.

■ ■ ■ ■

Cancer Vaccine

New cervical cancer vaccine will save many women's lives. The vaccine Gardasil protects against sexually transmitted human papilloma virus (HPV), which is responsible for 70% of cervical cancer cases. Gardasil, which is given in three doses over a six-month period, also helps prevent most types of genital warts. The vaccine is recommended for girls and young women ages nine through 26.

Important: Vaccinated individuals should still have regular Pap tests to check for cervical cell changes caused by HPV.

William Schaffner, MD, chairman of the department of preventive medicine at Vanderbilt University School of Medicine, Nashville is a fellow of the Infectious Diseases Society of America, and a liaison member of the Advisory Committee on Immunization Practices of the Centers for Disease Control and Prevention.

■ ■ ■ ■

Thinning Hair? What to Try

Most common type of hair loss among women is *androgenetic alopecia*, in which hair thins over several months in a predictable triangle pattern. It may be caused by a hormonal imbalance and can be treated with a hair transplant or topical medication, such as Rogaine. *Telogen effluvium* occurs suddenly and strikes different parts of the scalp randomly. It often occurs after women have gone on or off hormone therapy for menopause or birth control, after pregnancy or illness, during periods of stress or when certain medications, such as blood pressure medication, are started or stopped. *Traction alopecia* is caused by tight braids or ponytails that pull on the scalp.

If your hair is falling out or thinning: See a dermatologist—simple diagnostic tests should reveal the problem.

Sandra Johnson, MD, dermatologist in private practice, Dublin, Ohio.

■ ■ ■ ■

Trying to Stop Hormone Therapy?

Stopping abruptly after menopause results in more hot flashes within the first three months than stopping gradually. Gradual stopping—reducing the dose by one tablet per week per month, so hormones are stopped in six months—reduces short-term hot flashes but makes them more likely after six months.

Fast or slow stopping makes no difference after nine or 12 months.

Best: Work with your doctor to find the best approach for you.

Ronit Haimov-Kochman, MD, reproductive endocrinologist, obstetrics and gynecology department, Hadassah University Hospital, Jerusalem, and leader of a study of 91 postmenopausal women who had been on hormone therapy for more than eight years, published in *Menopause*.

■ ■ ■ ■

Post-Cancer Fertility

Breast cancer survivors may be able to preserve their ability to have children. Chemotherapy often leaves ovaries unable to produce eggs, and doctors are cautious about prescribing fertility hormones to breast cancer patients because estrogen can fuel tumor growth.

Recent study: Future pregnancies became possible when doctors prescribed two common cancer-fighting drugs that also stimulate ovulation—*tamoxifen* and *letrozole*—before chemotherapy. Harvested eggs were used to produce healthy embryos that could be frozen for future pregnancies. Cancer recurrence was not increased in women undergoing in vitro fertilization using these drugs. Experts say it may be too soon to know whether the procedure is completely safe for women with breast cancer —patients are being monitored for relapses. This procedure also can be used in women with endometrial cancer.

Best: Young women who have breast cancer and who want to be able to have children should contact a fertility specialist.

Kutluk Oktay, MD, associate professor of reproductive medicine and obstetrics and gynecology, director of Fertility Preservation Program, Weill Cornell Medical College, New York City, and leader of the study of 60 women, published in *Journal of Clinical Oncology*.

■ ■ ■ ■

Breast Cancer Disguise

Breast cancer may look like a skin irritation. This rare type of cancer is known as Paget's disease of the breast. Symptoms include a rash or flaking or a crusty area on a nipple.

Self-defense: Perform breast self-exams every month, and report to your physician any change—in the nipple or elsewhere—that persists for more than one month.

Carolyn M. Kaelin, MD, MPH, founding director of the Comprehensive Breast Health Center at Brigham and Women's Hospital, surgical oncologist at Dana Farber Cancer Institute and an assistant professor of surgery at Harvard Medical School, all in Boston. Dr. Kaelin is the author of *Living Through Breast Cancer* and coauthor of *The Breast Cancer Survivor's Fitness Plan* (both from McGraw-Hill).

■■■■

Phantom Risk

A dangerous heart disorder often does not show up on an angiogram.

New study: At least half of women with chest pain who showed no evidence of blocked arteries on an angiogram had cholesterol build-up that restricted blood flow to the heart. This disorder, *coronary microvascular syndrome*, which affects women 80% of the time, can more than triple heart attack risk.

Self-defense: If you have recurrent chest pain and an angiogram shows no blockage, ask your physician about further testing.

C. Noel Bairey Merz, MD, is director of the women's heart center, Cedars-Sinai Medical Center, Los Angeles, and coleader of a study of more than 1,000 women, published in *Journal of the American College of Cardiology*.

Mastectomy Survival Rates No Better Than Alternative Surgeries

B. Jay Brooks, Jr., MD, chief of hematology/oncology, Ochsner Clinic Foundation, Baton Rouge, Louisiana.
The New England Journal of Medicine.

According to recent research, two types of breast-conserving surgeries have the same 20-year survival rates as the radical mastectomy. As a result of these trials, authors of an Italian study believe that approximately 300,000 women worldwide who have early-stage breast cancer will undergo breast-conserving surgery each year, rather than radical mastectomy, the previous gold standard.

"Whether a woman decides to preserve her breast or not, the chances of being alive and free of cancer 20 years from now is the same," says Dr. B. Jay Brooks, Jr., chief of hematology/oncology at the Ochsner Clinic Foundation in Baton Rouge, Louisiana.

STUDIES IN ITALY AND PITTSBURGH

The first 20-year study, led by Dr. Umberto Veronesi of the European Institute of Oncology in Milan, Italy, looked at 701 women who had either received a radical mastectomy or a procedure known as a *quadrantectomy*, in which the quadrant of the breast containing the tumor is removed.

The result: There was little difference in the incidence of *metastasis*, or spread, of the cancer. As a result, the overall survival rate was virtually identical among women in the two groups.

Veronesi says the study shows that if breast cancer is diagnosed early enough, there's no need for radical surgery. "I believe that today the treatment of a woman with early breast cancer with a mastectomy must be considered unethical," he maintains.

The second study, conducted by the National Surgical Adjuvant Breast and Bowel Project in Pittsburgh, also used a 20-year follow-up. It compared a radical mastectomy with a *lumpectomy*, in which the tumor and a margin of tissue are removed.

Among 1,851 women, those receiving lumpectomy with radiation had the lowest incidence of a recurrence in the same breast.

The authors of the Pittsburgh study say it's unclear which of the two breast-conserving surgeries is better. The lumpectomy removed tumors that were no more than four centimeters in diameter, while the quadrantectomy excised tumors that were no more than two centimeters in diameter.

Brooks believes that the lumpectomy is the better of the two options because "it gives a better cosmetic result."

The Smarter Breast Cancer Drugs

Paul Goss, MD, PhD. He is professor of Medicine at Harvard Medical School and Massachusetts General Hospital, Boston, formerly at Princess Margaret Hospital, Toronto, Ontario, Canada.
The New England Journal of Medicine.

The results of a major international trial of the cancer drug *letrozole* were so promising that investigators decided to stop the trial early.

Breast cancer patients taking letrozole, one of a new class of drugs called aromatase inhibitors, had about half the rate of cancer recurrences as women taking a placebo.

"The results are absolute, confirmed and credible," says study investigator Dr. Paul Goss. "An independent monitoring committee recommended that we stop the study by preset statistical boundaries, which we exceeded by at least tenfold."

TAMOXIFEN BENEFITS AND RISKS

An older drug called *tamoxifen* has helped women who have estrogen-receptor-positive breast cancer; that is, cancer fueled by the hormone estrogen.

Tamoxifen reduces the risk of recurrence by 47% and the risk of death by 26% for five years after surgery.

Unfortunately, when tamoxifen is used for longer than five years, it may actually promote the growth of cancer cells.

Women who are more than five years past surgery represent the largest subgroup of women with breast cancer, Goss says.

"What is unrecognized is that over 50% of recurrences unfortunately occur beyond five years after diagnosis," Goss says. "Because it continues to relapse almost indefinitely, there is no limit to the disease."

Doctors have lacked any appropriate tools for the hundreds of thousands of women who enter that critical post-five-year period every year. Until now.

THE STUDY

The letrozole trial started enrolling participants in 1998 and ended up with 5,187 women in Canada, the United States and Europe who were postmenopausal, had hormone-receptor-positive tumors and had been taking tamoxifen for approximately five years. All of the women had to be within three months of stopping tamoxifen and all were disease-free when enrolled. The trial was coordinated by the National Cancer Institute of Canada.

The participants in Goss's study received either 2.5 milligrams (mg) of letrozole or a matching placebo daily for five years. Letrozole reduced the risk of recurrence by 43%.

SIDE EFFECTS

The median follow-up was only 2.4 years when the trial was stopped. There are some drawbacks to stopping a trial early, including questions about side effects and the effectiveness of the drug over time.

At the time of the study's early closure, the number of women who were experiencing side effects in the placebo and the letrozole groups was approximately the same, except in the rate of bone thinning, which was slightly higher in the letrozole group.

Tamoxifen provides protection against bone fractures, but it contributes to endometrial cancer and blood clots. Women considering letrozole therapy need to discuss with their doctor ways to mitigate the risk of osteoporosis.

Letrozole has been approved by the US Food and Drug Administration (FDA) for the treatment of some forms of breast cancer.

The American Cancer Society has more information on cancer drugs at *www.cancer.org*.

What Most Women Still Don't Know About Breast Cancer

Carolyn M. Kaelin, MD, MPH, founding director of the Comprehensive Breast Health Center at Brigham and Women's Hospital, surgical oncologist at Dana Farber Cancer Institute and an assistant professor of surgery at Harvard Medical School, all in Boston. Dr. Kaelin is the author of *Living Through Breast Cancer* and coauthor of *The Breast Cancer Survivor's Fitness Plan* (both from McGraw-Hill).

Most women know to tell their doctors about any new breast lumps. But a lump is not the only potential warning sign of breast cancer. As a breast cancer surgeon who also has survived this disease, I know many subtle signs of breast cancer that initially may go unnoticed.

In my own case, the first clue was not a lump—but rather a tiny area of retracted skin on my breast. The mammogram I received the next day appeared normal, but I knew to follow up with an ultrasound (an imaging test using high-frequency sound waves). This test revealed a tumor, which a biopsy later confirmed was malignant.

Important facts that could save your life—or that of a loved one…

•**A swollen, red, warm and/or tender breast can indicate breast cancer.** Such symptoms can mean an infection, but they also can be caused by inflammatory breast cancer, a rare condition in which cancer cells clog the lymphatic channels in the breast skin, preventing the lymph fluid from draining.

Self-defense: If you're diagnosed with a breast infection that doesn't clear within one week of antibiotic treatment, your doctor should order a mammogram and arrange for a skin biopsy to check for inflammatory breast cancer.

•**Mammograms miss about 10% to 20% of breast cancers.** Even so, studies suggest that among women who undergo annual screenings, mammograms may reduce the breast cancer death rate by as much as 65%. And the technology continues to improve. According to a study published recently in *The New England Journal of Medicine*, newer digital mammography (which provides computer-generated images that can be enlarged and/or enhanced) is up to 28% more accurate than film mammography in detecting cancers in women who are under age 50, premenopausal or who have dense breast tissue (breasts that have a much greater proportion of non-fatty tissue than fat). Digital mammography is not yet widely available in the US.

Self-defense: If you have a lump or another suspicious symptom and have already had a normal mammogram, request an ultrasound. This test can distinguish between fluid-filled and solid masses. It's a rare breast cancer that eludes both a mammogram and ultrasound.

•**Some breast cancer risk factors are not well-known.** More than 75% of breast cancers occur in women over age 50. You're at higher risk if you've been taking combination estrogen/progesterone hormone replacement therapy for at least five years…if you began menstruating before age 12 or stopped after age 55…if you've never had children or had your first child after age 30…and/or if you consume more than one to two alcoholic drinks daily. Dense breast tissue on a mammogram has recently been identified as an independent risk factor.

You also are at higher risk for breast cancer if one or more of the following is true: A first-degree relative (mother, sister or daughter) has had breast cancer…a family member was diagnosed with breast cancer when younger than age 40 or before menopause…a family member had cancer in both breasts…or you have a family history of ovarian cancer. This constellation of factors could suggest the presence of a mutated gene, such as the BRCA1 or BRCA2, which may be inherited.

STAY-WELL STRATEGIES

There's no way to predict or prevent every breast cancer, but you can lower your chances of developing or dying from the disease.

Here's how…

•**Maintain a healthy weight.** Gaining weight and being overweight raise the likelihood of developing a breast malignancy—and worsen your prognosis if you already have this type of cancer.

Reason: Body fat produces estrogen, which is one of the factors that increase breast cancer risk.

•**Stay active.** Exercise helps prevent breast cancer—probably by decreasing circulating estrogen. Newer research suggests that it also may improve long-term survival odds for those previously treated for the disease. In a recently published *Journal of the American Medical Association* study, breast cancer patients who walked or engaged in another moderate exercise three to five hours weekly were 50% less likely to have a recurrence or to die prematurely than women who exercised less than one hour weekly.

Best choice: Aerobic exercises, such as walking, jogging or cycling.

501

Weight-bearing exercises, such as walking or weight-lifting, also help to minimize bone loss—a significant advantage, since chemotherapy can lead to osteoporosis. (Chemotherapy can damage the ovaries, reducing estrogen levels and inducing early menopause in premenopausal women, which greatly accelerates bone loss.)

Self-defense: In addition to performing regular weight-bearing exercise, women with breast cancer should take a daily calcium supplement (1,000 mg for those ages 31 to 50…and 1,200 mg for those ages 51 or older) plus at least 200 international units (IU) of vitamin D. If you've had chemotherapy, experienced premature menopause or take an aromatase inhibitor (a drug used to treat postmenopausal breast cancer patients), ask your doctor what levels of calcium and vitamin D intake are right for you.

Tamoxifen (Nolvadex), the FDA-approved breast cancer preventive drug, also has been shown to conserve bone while reducing malignancies in high-risk women by as much as 50%.

Downside: Tamoxifen increases risk for blood clots, stroke and uterine cancer.

Some recent studies have shown the osteoporosis drug *raloxifene* (Evista) to be as effective as tamoxifen for preventing breast cancer and preserving bone in postmenopausal women—with lower risk for uterine cancer. Evista has been approved by the FDA as a breast cancer preventive and for preserving bone in premenopausal women.

Best: Ask your doctor if either drug may be appropriate for you.

LATEST ADVANCES

•**Aromatase inhibitors (AIs)** may offer even more powerful protection against breast cancer recurrence and death for postmenopausal women than tamoxifen. Whereas tamoxifen works by blocking estrogen from binding with cancer cells, AIs work by inhibiting estrogen production in fat tissues—our primary source of the hormone after menopause.

In a recent British study, breast cancer patients who switched from tamoxifen to an AI called *exemestane* (Aromasin) were 17% less likely to see their breast cancer spread to other organs, had a 15% lower chance of dying within about five years than women who stayed on tamoxifen, and had a 44% lower risk of developing cancer in the opposite breast. AIs do not appear to raise risk for endometrial cancer as tamoxifen does, but AIs do speed bone loss and are not effective for premenopausal women.

•**Newly developed tests** are enabling doctors to look at the genetic makeup of tumors and predict with increasing accuracy which are likely to recur or metastasize.

In the past, breast cancer patients had been routinely prescribed chemotherapy, usually following surgery, since doctors had no way of knowing which cancers would return and become fatal. New tests, which include "tumor profiling" (a more detailed analysis of the tumor than biopsy alone), take some of the guesswork out of deciding who will benefit most from chemotherapy and who is most likely to do just fine without it.

■ **More from Carolyn M. Kaelin, MD…**

Signs of Breast Cancer

A newly developed lump in the breast is the most common sign of breast cancer, but other red flags include…

•**Thickened, red skin in one breast.**

•**Any dimpling, puckering or retraction** (small depression) of breast skin.

•**Nipple scaling, flaking or ulceration.**

•**A newly inverted nipple.**

•**Spontaneous discharge from one nipple.**

•**A lump in the underarm.**

•**Persistent pain in one breast** (this usually indicates a benign cyst, but it should be assessed).

■ ■ ■ ■

Coffee and Tea Slow Cognitive Decline in Women

A recent study shows that women who drank three cups of caffeinated coffee or six cups of caffeinated tea a day had 18% less decline in memory than those who drank one cup or less of coffee or tea daily.

Theory: Caffeine may protect cognitive function.

Karen Ritchie, PhD, lead researcher, INSERM, French National Institute of Health and Medical Research, Montpellier, France, and leader of a study of 7,017 people, published in *Neurology*.

■ ■ ■ ■

Women Who Do Yoga Stand Taller

Older women walked more quickly, had better balance and gained an average of one centimeter in height after a nine-week yoga program—because they stood more upright as a result of practicing yoga. Twice a week, for 90 minutes each time, the women did a series of basic poses developed especially for older people. After nine weeks, participants used longer strides when walking and could stand for a longer time on one leg. They also felt more confident in their ability to balance while standing or walking.

Jinsup Song, DPM, PhD, director, Gait Study Center, Temple University Institute on Aging, Philadelphia, and principal investigator of a study presented at a recent meeting of the Gait and Clinical Movement Analysis Society.

How to Get Unfrazzled

Georgia Witkin, PhD, assistant clinical professor of psychiatry and director of the stress program at Mount Sinai School of Medicine in New York City. She appears on the Fox News Channel and is the author of numerous books, including *The Female Stress Syndrome Survival Guide*. Newmarket.

As women's options have increased over the past few decades, our expectations of ourselves have increased as well. We've added new roles, responsibilities and opportunities—without dropping others.

Result: Our to-do lists are longer than ever. We play catch-up late at night—doing the family's laundry, finishing work assignments, counseling our kids, paying bills for aging parents, e-mailing friends—when what we really need to do is rest.

Being on-call around the clock makes us susceptible to the emotional and the physical costs of stress—from irritability, anxiety and depression to insomnia, headaches, digestive problems and even heart disease.

To keep stress symptoms from becoming chronic, we need to take care of ourselves the same way we take care of others. Of course, when we are pressed for time, it is hard to invest additional time in ourselves. Here's how to feel less overwhelmed—in as little as five seconds.

IF YOU HAVE 5 SECONDS: BREATHE

Focusing on your breathing is the quickest way to interrupt the body's stress reaction. Increased heart rate and blood pressure—two physical stress reactions—are not under voluntary control. But by changing your breathing pattern from fast and shallow to slow and deep, you signal your body to calm down.

Practice belly breathing: Place one hand on your chest and one on your belly button. The hand on your chest should stay still—only the bottom hand should rise and fall. Breathe in…out…and pause. This sequence should take about five seconds. For greater benefit, repeat 10 times.

Option: Close your eyes and imagine your breath as a mist of your favorite color. This engages the visual part of your brain, switching attention away from the worrying words inside your head.

IF YOU HAVE 5 MINUTES: MOVE

Physical activity burns off *adrenaline* that floods your body when you're overwhelmed.

Best: Dancing, which restores a stress-relieving sense of control—you hear the rhythm of the music and know the next beat will follow a predictable pattern.

Keep a portable music player and earphones handy, and move to your favorite music for five minutes.

Important: The music should be fast—faster than the average heartbeat of 72 beats a minute. Although slow music can be calming when you're already relaxed, it's likely to frustrate you when you're frantic.

IF YOU HAVE 5 HOURS: PLAY

Regularly set aside a few hours to do whatever helps you feel renewed. Browse in a bookstore...get a massage or facial...go for a long walk in the woods...take an art class. Once a week is ideal, but even once a month helps. Don't feel guilty—these breaks promote physical and emotional health and give you more energy to tackle whatever tasks await you afterward.

Trap to avoid: Using scheduled playtime to catch up with chores, errands or correspondence. If you can't resist the temptation to work instead of play, take your break outside the house, away from reminders of all that needs to be done. You can include family as long as the activity is genuinely fun for you and easy to arrange. If you can't spare five hours, take an hour or two this week and promise yourself extra playtime next week.

IF YOU HAVE 5 DAYS: ESCAPE

Family outings and extended trips can be fun but often add to stress—because wives and mothers usually wind up planning, packing and keeping track of everyone's needs during the trip.

Solution: Take a mini-vacation with a girlfriend or by yourself. At least five days is ideal because it takes most people a few days to wind down and let go of work and home concerns. What if you can only manage a weekend or long weekend? For several days beforehand, take a few minutes each morning and evening to visualize yourself at your destination—stretched out on the beach, strolling through a museum or enjoying a fabulous meal.

IN 5 WEEKS: FORM NEW HABITS

For a long-term approach to strengthening your self-care skills, develop a new stress-reducing behavior each week.

Week 1: **Practice saying no.** Turn down all nonemergency requests for help. Don't

apologize. Say graciously but matter-of-factly, "Thanks for asking, but I'm overextended and have to say no." At the end of the week, when and if you start to say yes again, you'll be more discriminating about the responsibilities you agree to take on.

Week 2: **Prune your to-do list.** Whenever you add a task to your list, cross off another either by delegating it or letting it go. Each evening, erase one nonessential uncompleted task. When an unexpected hassle arises, such as the car breaking down, cross off two or three items—it doesn't matter if your closets stay cluttered or your dinner-party desserts aren't homemade.

Week 3: **Mother yourself.** Whatever loving care you would provide for a child, do for yourself. Feed yourself well...take a nap...enjoy some physical activity...get eight hours of sleep every night...pay yourself a compliment when you need one.

Week 4: **Act "as if."** It's not necessary to feel comfortable with a change before you can shift behavior—when you change behavior first, feelings follow. The more you treat yourself as if you're entitled to play and take breaks and say no, the more genuinely entitled you'll feel. Act as though other people are delighted to treat you the way you want to be treated. Soon you'll feel comfortable asking for what you need and will respond to others' helpfulness with appreciation rather than guilt.

Week 5: **Change your internal dialog.** Every time you catch yourself thinking *"I should..."* substitute, *"It would be nice if I could..."* or *"How terrific that my sister is able to..."* Then follow with, *"It's okay for me not to..."* With practice, you'll start to believe it—and you'll stop feeling so frazzled.

17

Healthy Relationships

Natural Ways to Much Better Sex

It's true that drugs can help with the mechanics of sex. A man with erectile dysfunction (ED) may have better erections when he takes Viagra. A woman with low libido may benefit from testosterone cream. Medications are only a temporary solution. They don't solve the underlying problems. Natural remedies often can.

CAUSES

Millions of men and women have impaired circulation, which can reduce the ability to have erections and diminish sexual sensation. Chronic stress dampens libido and sexual performance. Insomnia and low energy can make people too tired to enjoy sex.

Certain herbs and other natural products address these problems and have been used safely and successfully for hundreds of years. Natural remedies, taken alone or in combination, can improve all aspects of sexual energy and performance. They promote better blood flow, increase libido and make erections stronger.

Start with one supplement. Take it for a week or two. If you don't notice a difference, add a second or third supplement that works slightly differently.

Example: Combine ginkgo biloba (which enhances blood flow) with ginseng (which improves overall energy). Always check with your doctor before taking any supplement.

Best choices…

GINKGO BILOBA

Function: Dilates blood vessels and improves circulation to the penis or vagina and clitoris. Impaired circulation is the most common cause of ED in men. In women, reduced blood flow can result in diminished sexual sensation and responsiveness. Ginkgo biloba is a very effective vasodilator, which means it opens

Chris D. Meletis, ND, executive director, the Institute for Healthy Aging (*www.theiha.org*). He is author of several books, including *Better Sex Naturally* (HarperResource), *Complete Guide to Safe Herbs* (DK Publishing) and *Instant Guide to Drug-Herb Interactions* (DK Publishing).

(dilates) blood vessels. In one study, more than 70% of men with ED who took ginkgo improved their ability to have erections.

Anyone who is taking a selective serotonin reuptake inhibitor (SSRI) antidepressant, such as Prozac, should consider taking ginkgo. It offsets the libido-dampening side effect that often occurs in people taking these drugs.

Suggested dose: 40 mg three times daily. It usually takes one to three weeks to work.

Caution: Ginkgo reduces the ability of blood to clot. Do not use ginkgo if you are taking *coumadin* (Warfarin) or other blood-thinning drugs. Patients taking daily aspirin, which also inhibits clotting, should be sure to talk to their doctors before using ginkgo.

ARGININE

Function: Increases pelvic circulation...improves erections...boosts libido and clitoral sensation. Arginine is an amino acid that is used by the body to produce *nitric oxide*, a chemical that relaxes blood vessels and promotes better circulation.

Suggested dose: 1,000 mg to 2,000 mg twice daily. People who take arginine typically notice the effects within a few days.

Caution: Patients with heart problems who are taking *nitroglycerin* should not take arginine. The combination could result in excessive vasodilation.

Also: Don't take arginine if you get cold sores from the herpes virus or have genital herpes. Arginine promotes viral replication and can increase flare-ups.

GINSENG

Function: Supports the adrenal glands, which produce hormones that affect genital circulation and the ability to have erections... modulates emotional stress...increases overall energy and libido. Ginseng safely increases levels of testosterone, the hormone that stimulates sexual response in men and women.

Suggested dose: 10 mg twice daily. People who take ginseng usually notice an increase in energy after about one week.

Caution: Ginseng is a mild stimulant that can increase blood pressure. Don't take it if you have been diagnosed with hypertension or heart disease.

YOHIMBE

Function: Improves libido and sexual response in women...promotes firmer erections in men.

Yohimbe is the only herb approved by the Food and Drug Administration for treating low libido and sexual dysfunction in men. It stimulates the release of *norepinephrine* from the adrenal glands, improving genital circulation and the ability to have erections. Women who take yohimbe experience greater sexual arousal.

Suggested dose: Follow directions on the label. Yohimbe works more rapidly than most natural products, so take it one to two hours before sex.

Caution: Yohimbe can cause sharp rises in blood pressure in some patients. It also can cause headaches and nausea. Use yohimbe only under medical supervision.

DHEA

Function: Increases sexual arousal in women...improves erections in men.

Dehydroepiandrosterone (DHEA) is a naturally occurring hormone that is converted to testosterone in the body. Testosterone and other androgens stimulate libido and sexual performance in men and women. The body's production of DHEA declines by about 1% annually after age 30, which can result in diminished sexual desire, performance and satisfaction.

Suggested dose: 5 mg daily for no more than three days a month.

Caution: Patients should take DHEA only if blood tests show that they have lower-than-normal levels. An excessive amount increases risk of side effects, such as acne, facial hair growth in women and sometimes heart palpitations. It also increases risk of tumors in the prostate gland. Men with a history of prostate cancer should not take DHEA.

WATER

Function: Increases blood volume...improves erections in men and sexual responsiveness in women.

How can good old water be an aphrodisiac? Because millions of Americans are chronically dehydrated—they don't drink enough water or they consume excessive amounts of caffeine, a diuretic that removes water from the body.

Dehydration can result in diminished blood flow to the pelvis and genitals. Adequate hydration improves blood flow and makes it easier for men to have erections. Women who stay hydrated experience greater sexual comfort and satisfaction.

Suggested dose: Drink at least eight full glasses of water daily. Limit coffee and other caffeinated beverages to one or two servings daily.

Sex After 50— Better Than Ever

Dagmar O'Connor, PhD, a sex therapist in private practice in New York City. The first woman trained in New York City by Masters and Johnson, she has been practicing for more than 30 years and gives workshops around the world, and is the creator of a self-help sex therapy video and book packet: *How to Make Love to the Same Person for the Rest of Your Life—and Still Love It.* www.dagmaroconnor.com.

Most older Americans grew up not talking about sex. Through others' silence, they were taught to believe that sex was shameful and taboo. Any mention of sex between "old folks," in particular, made people shudder.

Sexual activity is a natural and healthy part of life. In fact, you can get better at sex and enjoy it more—at any age. I treat couples in their 80s and 90s who wouldn't dare tell their children or grandchildren that they're seeing a sex therapist. Typically, whatever the state of their sex life, therapy improves it.

With retirement's gift of time, you can learn how the aging body works differently from its younger self, what pleases you individually and how to please each other in new ways.

PRACTICAL MATTERS

Yes, bodies change with age. Many women start to feel old and asexual at menopause. Men may develop erectile problems. But most difficulties can be overcome.

Physical change: Chronic conditions, such as diabetes, thyroid disease, cancer, Parkinson's disease and depression, can affect sexual function. With heart disease, sex can cause chest pain, and with asthma, breathlessness.

Remember, intercourse is the equivalent of walking two city blocks. Check with your doctor first.

Physical change: Joint pain and stiffness from arthritis makes sex difficult.

Solution: Relax in a Jacuzzi or bath before sex…vacation together in a warm climate…find new positions that won't stress your sore spots.

Physical change: Many drugs—antidepressant, hypertension, heart disease and some cancer medications, as well as alcohol—can affect sexual function.

Solution: If your sex drive is down or you're having other sexual problems, ask your doctor whether your medications could be the cause and if switching might help.

Physical change: After menopause, vaginal tissue becomes less elastic, the vaginal opening becomes smaller and lubrication decreases.

Result: Discomfort during intercourse.

Solution: Don't avoid sex—increase it. The more tissue is exercised, the more it stretches and the more you relax your muscles. Using your finger or a dildo, gently widen the vaginal opening every day. If the problem persists for more than two months, see a gynecologist or sex therapist.

Meanwhile, smooth the way with a nonprescription water-based lubricant, such as Astroglide or K-Y Jelly.

Not as good: Oil-based lubricants or petroleum products such as Vaseline. They may linger in the vagina and irritate it.

Bonus: Applying lubricant may get you in the mood for sex. Or let your partner apply it as part of lovemaking. Good foreplay makes lubrication flow naturally.

Physical change: With age, men require more manual stimulation for erections, take longer to ejaculate and have a longer refractory period—the amount of time between an orgasm and the next erection.

Solution: Patience. These changes are an invitation to discover the slow, loving sex that many women, in particular, have always wanted but haven't received.

Erectile problems can be treated medically, too. Discuss the situation with your doctor. You may be referred to a urologist for medication or other treatment.

BEYOND INTERCOURSE

Couples in their 60s and 70s and older often ask me what to do about erectile problems and other issues that interfere with intercourse. I tell them to slow down—expand their sexual horizons, develop new sexual habits and start all over again. The goal is simply to feel more.

Our society fears low-level arousal—pleasurable excitement that doesn't lead to penetration or orgasm. But those who have always resisted "just touching" become gluttons for such physical connection once they realize how great it is.

Exercise: During the day or with a light on at night, one partner lies back and is touched by the other—but not on the breasts or genitals —for 15 minutes to an hour. The person being touched stipulates what's wanted in a nonverbal way. If you would like your partner to touch more slowly, put your hand over your partner's and slow it down. When the "touchee" is finished, switch places.

Simple interludes set a loving, sensual tone and encourage you both to overcome shyness about requesting what pleases you. Prolonged sensual touching without genital contact removes sexual anxieties…helps you become relaxed, sensitized and responsive…revives a sense of trust and well-being that you may not have experienced since you were stroked as a child.

You'll emerge from the interlude feeling wonderful about each other. Resentments and recriminations will evaporate. Making sensual, uninhibited love often follows naturally. If not, there's always next time.

LOVE YOUR BODY AS IT IS

Our society presumes that only the young and skinny are (or should be) sexually active. As a result, many older people avoid sex out of embarrassment about spotted skin, a protruding stomach, wrinkles and flab. (Do remember that while you are ashamed of your wrinkles and protruding belly, your partner's eyesight has probably also diminished!) A mastectomy or other surgery can interfere with self-esteem, too, especially with a new partner.

Your body is miraculous. Learn to love it the way it really looks. One woman attending my sexual self-esteem workshop said, "I did not learn to love my body until I lost it." But your body at any age is a gift. Value it for itself…not as it compares with anyone else's or to how you looked when younger.

Exercise: Stand together before a full-length mirror. Say what you like about your own body out loud. Do this exercise alone first, before sharing it with your partner. Then try the exercise with your partner, taking turns. Listen, but don't respond.

To learn to appreciate your body, admire it often. Come away from this event loving five things about your body.

If you look better, you'll feel better. I recommend exercise—walking, swimming, Pilates— to couples of all ages. Getting stronger makes both women and men look better and feel more powerful…more sexual.

EDUCATE YOUR PARTNER

The young body works without thought. As you grow older, you can—and may need to— benefit from learning more about your body and your lover's. The key to intimacy is to express your needs—once you have learned what they are—and to insist on knowing the needs of your partner so that you can try to fulfill them.

Special note to women: If you rarely initiated sex but would like to, take baby steps. Try asking for different ways of being touched, or take his hand and show him how you like to be touched.

Exercise: Turn up the thermostat, and hang out nude together. Sleep nude in the same bed even if you haven't done so for years.

Increasing Your Sex Drive—With Light!

Daniel Kripke, MD, professor emeritus of psychiatry, University of California, San Diego.

Ronald Swerdloff, MD, professor of medicine, and chief of the division of endocrinology, department of medicine, Harbor-UCLA Medical Center, Torrance, California.

Neuroscience Letters.

Ultra-bright lamps may boost the body's ability to produce sex hormones, particularly for men, say researchers who studied the effects of light therapy on mood.

The importance of the finding is not fully established, but it's possible that light therapy could one day be used to control ovulation in women or treat people who take antidepressants and find themselves with low sex drives, the researchers say.

"It's a very promising lead," says study coauthor Dr. Daniel Kripke, a professor emeritus of psychiatry at the University of California at San Diego.

Researchers have known for decades that exposure to light affects the way animals live. Changes in the light from the sun, for example, set off hibernation in some mammals. Seasonal changes in light also control reproduction in rats and mice; they only mate during warmer months, Kripke says.

THE HUMAN FACTOR

Researchers are still working to understand how exposure to light affects humans. Kripke and colleagues discovered two decades ago that light therapy—shining powerful lamps at people's eyes—affects mood. Light therapy has become a common treatment for seasonal affective disorder, a type of depression that strikes when days grow shorter.

In his study, Kripke enlisted 11 healthy men, aged 19 to 30 years, to test whether light affects the body levels of luteinizing hormone, which is produced by the pituitary gland and also leads to the release of other hormones, such as testosterone in men. The men woke at 5 am for five days and spent an hour in front of a light box giving off 1,000 lux, much more brightness than typical indoor lighting. Later, they spent five days in front of a light box that only gave out 10 lux.

The result: Body levels of luteinizing hormone grew by nearly 70% while the men were exposed to the higher levels of light.

The researchers didn't look at women because the rapidly cycling hormones in their bodies would make it difficult to study the effect, Kripke says. However, luteinizing hormone does affect ovulation, he adds, and "we think light is potentially a very promising treatment for women who have ovulatory problems or long and irregular menstrual cycles."

TESTOSTERONE INCREASE?

Light therapy could also boost testosterone in men, potentially increasing sexual potency and muscle mass, he says. Researchers, however, did not monitor testosterone levels in the men.

A hormone expert cautioned that research is still needed. The study was small, and it's not clear whether the changes in the level of the hormone are significant enough to actually cause changes in the body, says Dr. Ronald Swerdloff, chief of the division of endocrinology at Harbor UCLA Medical Center, part of the University of California at Los Angeles School of Medicine.

For more information, visit the Society for Light Treatment & Biological Rhythms at *www. websciences.org/sltbr.*

■ ■ ■ ■

Stress Reducer?

Nervous about stressful situations, such as public speaking? Have sexual intercourse the night before.

Recent finding: Participants who engaged in intercourse before stressful events had lower blood pressure levels and felt less stressed the next day than those who abstained from intercourse.

Stuart Brody, PhD, full professor of psychology, University of Paisley, Scotland, and leader of a study of 50 people, published in *Biological Psychology.*

■ ■ ■ ■

Sexy Nasal Spray

Sex drive may be enhanced with a nasal spray? *PT-141*, also called *bremelanotide*, is a hormone that stimulates regions of the brain responsible for arousal. PT-141 nasal spray is undergoing clinical trials and may be available in 2009.

Michael A. Perelman, PhD, codirector, human sexuality program, NewYork-Presbyterian Hospital, and clinical associate professor of psychiatry, reproductive medicine and urology, Weill-Cornell Medical College, both in New York City.

Heart Disease Patients Need Not Fear Intimacy

Holly S. Andersen, MD, department of cardiology, NewYork-Presbyterian Weill/Cornell Medical Center, New York City.

Exercise and sex are two aspects of normal living that men with heart disease often fear. However, a study from Italy shows that moderate exercise boosts sexual function in these men, including the quality of their erections...and they also reported improvements in their relationships with their partners.

The study included 59 men whose chronic heart failure had been stable for at least three months. Half of the men took part in a supervised exercise program of riding a stationary bicycle and stretching three times a week over an eight-week period...the other group did nothing. The couch potato group showed no improvement in either their heart disease or sexual functioning at the end of the two months, while the exercisers showed an increase in oxygen uptake during exercise (measured by a sophisticated test that shows how well the patient is absorbing oxygen) and the aforementioned improvement in sexual function. Researchers theorize that this might be because exercise improves blood vessel function and blood vessel lining (the endothelium).

IS THE STUDY BELIEVABLE?

Cardiologist Holly S. Andersen, MD, at the New York-Presbyterian Weill/Cornell Medical Center in New York City, spoke about the study. She points out that there is a much larger population of people who are living with coronary disease because medicine has become so good at keeping them alive...and that the quality-of-life issue has become especially important now. Dr. Andersen is enthusiastic about exercise for all of her patients, encouraging even the sickest ones to have some form of modest exercise. However, she specifies that they should do aerobic or stretch exercise only. Strength training increases pressure on the cardiovascular system and strains it—and it is definitely not recommended.

Dr. Andersen says that patients must start slowly and gradually build up their activity. Warming up and cooling down are also important. She stresses that patients plan their exercise activity with guidelines from the doctor who may well recommend supervised exercise to start. By performing aerobic activities such as walking, swimming or riding the stationary bike, she explains that patients allow their blood vessels to dilate, have better oxygen uptake and increase their heart performance.

Dr. Andersen says the rule of thumb is that when a patient can climb two flights of stairs

(à la Jack Nicholson in the movie *Something's Gotta Give*), he is ready for sex with a familiar partner. Interestingly, relations with someone new is considerably more stressful, and likely needs a doctor's okay. She adds that patients who resume physical intimacy should be sure to continue to get some regular aerobic exercise out of bed.

Good Friends May Promote Good Health

Laverne Bardy-Pollak, author of the humor column "Laverne's View" for *50 Plus Monthly*, and a columnist for the nationally syndicated Senior Wire news service.

All the way through school, we live in constant proximity to our age peers and make friends almost without effort. Later on, especially after marriage, many adults grow apart from their friends and fail to renew or replace them.

Friends can cheer us up, provide a sense of community and continuity, share memories, offer tips for living better in a thousand ways, rejoice in our triumphs and commiserate in our sorrows. Having friends can even fortify our health. *Here's how...*

HAVING FRIENDS BOOSTS YOUR HEALTH

Considering the good feelings and stress relief that friendship brings, it's not surprising that having friends can improve your health.

In a 10-year Australian study of nearly 1,500 people age 70 and older, those with the strongest networks of friends and confidants (as measured by the degree of closeness and the number of friends, even if far away) lived longest. Contact with relatives, including children, barely affected survival rates.

A Harvard School of Public Health study of more than 3,200 people (average age 62) examined health-related effects of friendship by assessing levels in the blood of a marker for inflammation that's linked to cardiovascular disease. This was part of the ongoing, more-than-50-year-old Framingham (Massachusetts) Heart Study, supported in part by the National Heart, Lung, and Blood Institute.

Results: Marker levels were lowest in the most socially active men…highest in the least socially active men. No such connection was found in women.

Another Harvard School of Public Health study, done in conjunction with the David Geffen School of Medicine, University of California, Los Angeles, found that socially active men ages 70 to 79 produced more fibrinogen, a desirable protein that aids blood clotting, than less social men (not in women).

Still, friendships may reduce heart disease in women. In a federally supported study, 503 women with risk factors for heart disease were assessed for the extent of their social relationships, tested for coronary artery disease and followed for several years to track who had died and why. Those with larger social circles had less severe disease than those with fewer friends—and were less than half as likely to die within a few years.

Conclusion: Having friends may help you to live better…and longer.

FRIENDS FOR REASONS AND SEASONS

It's unrealistic to believe that one friend can meet all our needs. Each friend meets some…or just one.

Examples: To commiserate with…see movies with…shop or dine out (or in) with…discuss troublesome issues with…and especially to laugh with.

It's fortunate that there's no limit on the number of friends we can have.

A few treasured friends—some, if we're lucky, are relatives, too—may be life-long, adding texture and richness to our lives, bolstered by decades of shared memories. Other friends enter our lives for a reason and then are gone. But even brief friendships can have purpose and value.

"DIVORCING" A FRIEND

As vital as good friends are, less-than-good friends can suffocate you and may need to be jettisoned. *How to tell the difference…*

•**Friendship should reduce your stress,** not add to it. A friendship that's hard work or feels bad is not a true friendship.

•**Real friends support you…**and help without being asked. They never judge you, belittle you or act superior to you.

•**Friends listen.** I dropped one so-called friend because her eyes always glazed over while I was talking as she waited for her next chance to speak.

•**Friends needn't agree** about politics or religion, but they must share the same values—what's important in life—or at least respect each other's.

Example: One friend that lived 20 minutes away phoned me countless times with minor problems, demanding my instant presence. I was forced to break with her. Later she insisted that she had reformed. I gave her another chance—and had to "break up" again.

Reevaluate your friendships periodically. You may have outgrown some. If any have become toxic, fix them or end them.

To fix a broken friendship: Identify what's wrong. Maybe your needs have changed. Then articulate your concerns (not easy!). If that doesn't work, give up and move on.

TRACKING DOWN LONG-LOST FRIENDS

There are no friends like old friends who knew you "when"…met your parents…matured into adulthood with you. If you miss chums from the old neighborhood, why not look them up? *Here's how…*

•**Ask mutual friends for contact information…**call their college, high school or summer camp alumni organization or visit its Web site…look on the Internet through Google or another search engine.

•**On-line phone books can help**—visit Whitepages.com…Switchboard.com…Anywho.com…Addresses.com…Reunion.com…Classmates.com…SchoolNews.com.

International: Visit Infobel.com.

•**Go to reunions.** Last year, I attended my 50th high school reunion, accompanied by my brand-new second husband. We had a blast—and I reconnected with a few old buddies. We've stayed in touch.

KEEPING FRIENDSHIPS AFTER WIDOWHOOD OR DIVORCE

When my first husband and I divorced after 23 years of marriage, I wondered which of our mutual friends would stick by me. After initial awkwardness, and to their credit, all remained loyal to both of us. To my credit, I worked at it. *Lessons I learned…*

• **Widows and divorcées pose a perceived threat** to married women friends. The suddenly single woman must put those wives at ease.

No longer appropriate: Hello and goodbye hugs and kisses with other women's husbands…playful banter…sexy clothing…double entendres. Over time, you may, selectively and judiciously, resume your playful behavior.

Common mistake: Asking girlfriends' husbands for help with home repairs or chores. Hire a handyman.

• **Relationships with couples change** when you're no longer half of a couple yourself. After divorce or widowhood, many men's social activities consist of golf or poker games. Women's get-togethers may be restricted to matinees, lunch and shopping.

Tip: If you miss your friends' spouses, invite couples for dinner occasionally.

• **When your life changes, your social circle alters, too.** In the latter decades, many people are single. Seek out unattached comrades to complement your stable of friends. You can't have too many good friends…but unless you work at it, you can easily have too few.

IDENTIFYING TRUE FRIENDSHIP

Potential friends are attracted much as lovers are—through chemistry and body language…the recognition of similar temperaments, intelligence, sense of humor, experiences, tastes and interests. The more two people have in common, the deeper their relationship promises to be. *How you'll know a true friend…*

• **Friends are people you genuinely look forward to sharing time with** and miss when you're apart for too long.

• **Friends reveal their weaknesses.** At our age, we (finally) know we're not perfect. Recognizing the same faults in ourselves strengthens the bond.

• **Friends accept each other's quirks and value their strengths.**

Example: My friends know that as a writer, I have an inordinate personal and professional craving for solitude. An old pal confided, "It's a

good thing I understand your needs. Otherwise, this relationship wouldn't have lasted so long."

• **Friends reveal truths that you may not want to hear.** In turn, you can say what's on your mind without being hurtful or insulting. A solid friendship withstands well-intended criticism.

Bonus: Those who know us best may offer better personal advice than anyone else could.

• **Friends are generous and flexible.**

Example: Two old pals and I choose activities to share on our own birthdays. They love museums, plays and visits to the big city…I prefer craft shows, antiquing and being pampered at a spa. Obliging each other is part of the fun—and opens us to new experiences.

■ ■ ■ ■

Partner Up

Living with a partner is better for your health. People ages 30 to 69 who live alone are almost twice as likely to develop angina, have a heart attack or suffer sudden cardiac death as people who live with others. The risk is even greater for women over age 60 and men over 50. Living alone itself is not the reason for the increased risk. People who live by themselves eat more fat, are more likely to smoke and are less likely to exercise.

Kirsten Melgaard Nielsen, MD, internist, Aarhus Sygehus University Hospital, Aarhus, Denmark.

"All You Need Is Love" …And Other Lies About Marriage

John W. Jacobs, MD, a psychiatrist and couples therapist in private practice in New York City, is an associate clinical professor at New York University School of Medicine and author of *All You Need Is Love, And Other Lies About Marriage*. HarperCollins.

Marriage is more fragile today than ever before. With so many marriages breaking up, it is clear that some of our basic assumptions about the modern institution are misguided—and even outright wrong. Understanding the realities of marriage today can help make your relationship more satisfying...

Myth: All you need is love.

Reality: Love is not enough to keep you together. Marital love is conditional and based on how you behave toward one another day after day.

What to do: First, be clear to your spouse about what you need from the relationship—what you can live with and what you cannot live with.

Ask your partner to think about that, too. Then share your views and negotiate how you each can fulfill each other's wishes.

Example: You may feel the need to go out with friends regularly without your partner, but your partner may feel hurt by this. You might negotiate to go out one night with friends in exchange for one night out with your partner.

Myth: Talking things out always resolves problems.

Reality: Communication has been oversold as the key to a good marriage, but many couples actually make things worse by talking things out. Brutal honesty often backfires, causing a spouse to dig in his/her heels instead of making changes in behavior.

What to do: Learn how to communicate skillfully by focusing on problems rather than fault. Use "I language," not "you language." With "I language," you take responsibility for your emotional experience rather than blaming it on your partner.

Example: "I feel anxious when we don't have things planned in advance, and it would be a big help to me if we could make dates with friends as far in advance as possible." That's better than making accusatory statements such as, "You always wait until the last minute to make plans, and then our friends are too busy to see us."

Myth: People don't change.

Reality: Change is always possible, and small changes often can produce big results. But most people go about trying to change their relationships in unproductive ways—by trying to get their spouses to change. Marital problems are rarely the fault of just one partner, and the biggest impediment to change is the belief that you aren't the one who needs to change.

What to do: Change your own behavior—this often is the best way to prompt shifts in your partner's behavior.

Example: If your spouse always seems to criticize you, try praising his actions on a regular basis. Eventually, he may reciprocate by praising you.

Myth: Our culture's shift in gender roles has made marriage easier.

Reality: The modern marital arrangement—in which both husband and wife work outside the home, and family responsibilities and decisions are handled by both partners—may be "fairer," but it has created its own problems. Confusion about roles, as well as mutual feelings of being taken for granted, can lead to resentment and conflict.

What to do: When discussing your expectations of your relationship, be on the alert for gender stereotypes, such as the idea that women cook and men take out the garbage. Apportion your duties and responsibilities fairly.

Example: You cook two days a week, and your spouse cooks two days a week. Order takeout on the other days.

Myth: Children solidify a marriage.

Reality: The stress of having children is a serious threat to a couple's harmony. Even when you feel that you are prepared for their impact on your relationship, your natural devotion to them will leave little time and energy for your marriage.

What to do: If you want to preserve your marriage, your children cannot always come first. Commit to regular alone time as a couple with weekly or biweekly date nights and occasional trips away from the kids.

Myth: The sexual revolution has made great sex easier.

Reality: Movies, television shows and advertisements have raised our expectations about sex, making it seem like everyone is having great sex on a regular basis and you're abnormal if you're not. But many married couples have sexual problems—they just don't talk openly about them.

What to do: Expect ebbs and flows in your sex life, and don't buy into the Hollywood image of what your sex life should be. Consider seeking help from a couples counselor or sex therapist if you can't resolve sexual problems on your own.

To locate a qualified practitioner, contact…

•American Association for Marriage and Family Therapy, 703-838-9808, *www.aamft.org.*

•American Association of Sexuality Educators, Counselors, and Therapists, 804-752-0026, *www.aasect.org.*

How to Deal with Defensive People

James Tamm, former judge and current adjunct law professor, Santa Clara University School of Law, is co-author of *Radical Collaboration: Five Essential Skills to Overcome Defensiveness and Build Successful Relationships.* HarperCollins.

A coworker responds with anger whenever someone disagrees with him. A husband retreats into silence whenever he gets into an argument with his wife. An employee buries her boss in piles of irrelevant information whenever she is asked a question.

These behaviors might appear different, but they're all just variations of the same problem—defensiveness. Additional forms of defensive behavior include habitually claiming, "I already knew that," when corrected…rationalizing or explaining away every misstep…or chronically making fun of others to deflect criticism from oneself.

Defensive people believe that their reactions protect them from outside attack. In fact, defensive people are unconsciously trying to shield themselves from their own doubts about their significance, competence or likeability.

We all get defensive sometimes and to some degree, but most of us learn to limit our defensive tendencies. Those who don't curb their defensiveness make life difficult for themselves and those who live and work with them. Their chronically defensive behavior promotes conflict and divisiveness…encourages rigid thinking that stifles creativity…and brings out the defensiveness in others.

Here's how to control your defensiveness—and better deal with the defensiveness of those around you…

DEALING WITH DEFENSIVE PEOPLE

The best way to blunt other people's defensiveness is to not become defensive yourself, even when provoked (more on that later). If you start to get upset, remind yourself that this person's defensiveness is rooted in his/her insecurities and has little to do with you. Arguing back will only make the person more insecure. *Instead…*

•**Be a good listener.** After the emotional moment has passed, offer the defensive person a chance to speak with you about the situation that led to the defensiveness. During the conversation, resist the urge to evaluate, criticize or suggest. Just listen intently, and take both the words and emotional content into account. Every now and then, summarize what you're hearing to make sure you understand—and to make sure the person knows that you're really listening.

Example: A coworker is upset with you because you criticized his proposal in a meeting. Rather than defend your position, listen to what your coworker has to say, then summarize —"You felt I misunderstood your recommendations" or "You were embarrassed in front of your colleagues."

By listening, you help the defensive person feel understood and accepted, easing his insecurities and making future defensive reactions less likely.

•**Change the way you argue.** Try "interest-based negotiation." With this strategy, your first goal is to state your opponent's underlying interests to his satisfaction. Your second goal is for him to do the same to you. Only then do you start proposing solutions. This creates an atmosphere of understanding that makes defensiveness less likely.

Example: I once mediated a labor strike in which the union insisted on a 7% raise, though the union leaders knew that management couldn't go past 4%. The discussions became adversarial. Through interest-based negotiation, management learned that the underlying goal of the union negotiators was not the 7% raise itself, but to make good on a promise they had made to their members to deliver a 7% raise. The parties agreed to a 7% raise for six months of the year, the equivalent of a 3.5% annual raise, which was within management's budget. Union members were happy with the 3.5% increase overall and pleased to have the negotiations resolved.

MANAGING YOUR OWN DEFENSIVENESS

The most difficult step in overcoming defensiveness in yourself is acknowledging that you are indeed defensive.

You probably consider your responses to perceived criticisms to be rational and justified when they occur. Reconsider them after the moment of confrontation has passed. Do they still seem appropriate, or were they unwarranted and unhelpful? If you're not certain, ask your spouse or a trusted friend—and try not to get defensive at the reply.

If you feel you tend to be defensive, identify the form your defensiveness takes. Are you belligerent? Uncommunicative? Overly talkative?

Other warning signs: Tightening in the gut...general sense of paranoia...adrenaline rush ...feeling that you lack allies...a sense that you have been personally rejected, though the subject under discussion is only tangentially related to you.

To cut off defensive reactions...

•**Intercept the physical symptoms of defensiveness,** such as rapid, shallow breathing and a quickened pulse. It will be easier to alter your behavior if you can alter these physical reactions. Head to the rest room and splash cool water on your face...take a short walk to calm down...or if there's no time for a break, take a few long, deep breaths.

•**Monitor your thoughts.** If your mind is telling you, "This guy is out to get me," or "She doesn't think I'm very smart," you're likely to become increasingly defensive. Respond to negative thoughts with positive self-talk.

Examples: "I know this is difficult, but I can get through it"..."They're entitled to a different opinion"..."If I listen carefully enough, maybe I can learn something."

•**Develop a reaction appropriate to your particular form of defensiveness.** If you tend to flood others with information when you feel attacked, force yourself to remain quiet for a full minute. If you tend to shut down, push yourself to say something. If you counterattack when you feel confronted, take a few deep breaths and find something that you can agree with in what's being said.

There are times when we must defend ourselves against verbal attacks, but these times are rare—and knee-jerk defensiveness isn't effective anyway. Defensive reactions make us feel temporarily better about ourselves but rarely paint us or our opinions in a favorable light. Defensiveness provides no defense—it only makes us seem less credible.

■ ■ ■ ■

To Wake Up Your Libido

Combine and drink equal parts of the tincture form of the herbs damiana and Panax ginseng to stimulate arousal and increase levels of the hormone testosterone. Works for women and men. Consult a health-care professional knowledgeable in herbal medicine to determine if the formula is right for you and what dosage you should use.

If that doesn't work: Ask your doctor to check you for a deficiency in *dehydroepiandrosterone* (DHEA). The steroid hormone is available at health-food stores and is a precursor to such hormones as *estrogen* and *androgen*. Ask your doctor if this is right for you.

Jane Guiltinan, ND, clinical professor, Bastyr Center for Natural Health, Bastyr University, Seattle.

Why Men Never Remember and Women Never Forget

Marianne Legato, MD, FACP, a physician and professor of clinical medicine at Columbia University, New York City, and founder of Columbia's Partnership for Gender-Specific Medicine, is author of several books, including Why Men Never Remember and Women Never Forget. *Rodale.*

Neither men nor women can claim that their brains are "better." While men's brains are 10% larger on average, women's brains have more elaborate connections that make them more efficient. Male and female brains unquestionably are different, in terms of both structure and chemistry, and that can cause problems when we try to communicate with one another.

Most of us speak to our spouses just as we would speak to members of our own sex—then wonder why they don't seem to understand.

Here's how to communicate more effectively with the opposite sex…

NONVERBAL CUES

The female brain is good at decoding nonverbal signals, including facial expressions and tone of voice, perhaps because mothers must understand the needs of children too young to speak. When women send nonverbal signals to men, women are often dismayed to find that these signals are ignored.

Women don't realize that the typical male brain is not skilled at interpreting nonverbal communications. Men are particularly bad at identifying signs of sadness in women—though men are pretty good at spotting signs of anger and aggression.

Women: Tell him verbally when something is bothering you. A sad expression or the silent treatment won't get you anywhere. It's not that he is ignoring your feelings—he is just unaware of them.

If a man asks you what he can do to make you feel better, tell him. If you say "nothing," he'll assume that you mean nothing and he'll do nothing. He isn't trying to hurt you—men's brains just work in a more linear, literal manner. Because men often like to be left alone when they're upset, he might conclude that he is doing you a favor by giving you some space.

Men: Search for clues beyond her words when she seems unusually quiet or terse. She might be sending signals that you're not picking up. If you can't figure out the signals and she won't tell you what she needs, remind her that you really want to help, but it's hard for you to pick up her nonverbal cues.

LISTENING

The female brain seems to be better at listening than the male brain—women have more nerve cells in the areas that process language

and put a larger percentage of their brains to work when they hear someone speak.

The more elaborate wiring of the female brain also makes women better multitaskers than men. Evolution likely made women this way so that mothers could keep an eye on the children and still get other things done. Evolution shaped the male brain to focus on one very difficult task at a time. Tiger hunts were more successful when the hunters could focus all their attention on the tiger.

Add men's inferior listening ability to their superior focus, and the result is a phenomenon most wives know well. Tell a man something important while he's watching a ball game, and he might not remember a word of it. He isn't purposely ignoring you—his brain simply isn't wired to hear what you said.

Women: Put him on alert that what you're about to say is important. If it's particularly vital information, begin with a gentle "I need you to look me in the eyes." If there are too many distractions in your present location, ask him to go with you for a walk or out to a quiet restaurant.

Men: Don't be insulted if she doesn't stop what she is doing when you want to talk. Chances are that she can pay attention to you even if she's occupied. If you want her undivided attention, ask for it.

PROBLEM SOLVING

The structure of the male brain makes men straight-ahead thinkers—when they see a problem, their instinct is to try to solve it.

Women are more likely to ruminate over decisions. They'll verbalize a problem and talk though all the implications and issues before they proceed. When women try to talk through their problems with men, they're often dismayed and insulted that the men try to tell them what to do. This confuses the men, who thought they were being asked for a solution.

Women: Tell a man the specific type of response you want before you share a problem. Are you asking the man for a solution, or do you just want to talk through the issue so it's clear in your mind? If you don't specifically tell him that it's the latter, he'll assume it's the former. If he tries to solve your problem anyway, understand that this is just how his brain responds.

As for how to respond to a man's problems, this rarely comes up. Men tend not to share their problems with anyone.

Men: Understand that women like to verbalize their thinking and don't always want you to solve their problems.

Instead, wait for a question before providing an answer. Ask what you can do to help rather than assume you know. And if your wife starts crying, holding her quietly works better than telling her she's being too emotional.

DIFFERENT INTERESTS

Women tend to expect their male partners to be interested in every subject they wish to discuss. That isn't fair. A woman wouldn't expect her female friends to chat about a subject that she knows bores them.

Women: Tailor your conversation to your partner's interests. (Men should do this, too, but because men talk less, it isn't as often an issue.) Find other conversation partners for topics that don't interest him.

Men: Encourage your partner to spend time with female friends so there's another outlet for the conversations that don't interest you. Don't get upset if she's busy with friends when you want to see her.

BETTER ARGUMENTS

During an argument, women are more likely to bring up past events. Estrogen increases the amount of cortisol, a memory-boosting hormone, released by the adrenal glands during stressful moments. Because the female brain has more estrogen, memories of old fights remain fresher in a woman's mind. The male brain finds it easier to forget emotional situations and move on. Maybe forgetting a close call on a tiger hunt made it easier for men of the past to continue to hunt.

Women: Use simple, declarative sentences, and state what you want in outline form when imparting important information to men. Leave out anecdotes and unnecessary adjectives. Take advantage of your ability to read his emotions to spot the signs of boredom. When you see them, sum up your argument with a closing statement and end the conversation. Try not to rehash old arguments.

Men: Try to keep women focused on the point under discussion. If during an argument she brings up a fight you had five years ago, tell her, "We've discussed that already and it isn't going to help to go over it again. Let's focus on the current problem."

Beat Bad Breath

Mark A. Stengler, ND, naturopathic physician in private practice, La Jolla, California...adjunct associate clinical professor at the National College of Natural Medicine, Portland, Oregon...author of many books, including *The Natural Physician's Healing Therapies* and coauthor of *Prescription for Natural Cures* (both from Bottom Line Books)...and author of the *Bottom Line/Natural Healing* newsletter.

About half of Americans have bad breath (halitosis). Fortunately, a simple natural approach often is all it takes to eradicate the problem.

Several conditions may contribute to bad breath, including gum disease, degrading silver fillings, chronic dental and/or throat infections and ulcers and other digestive problems. It is important to work with your dentist to determine the cause because bad breath may indicate a bigger problem. *If your dentist can't find a problem, try these suggestions...*

Take one teaspoon of liquid *chlorophyll* (the green pigment in plants) straight or diluted in a glass of water after meals. Chlorophyll (available at most health-food stores) freshens breath immediately and supports detoxification of the digestive tract.

Many people who have bad breath have an overgrowth of bacteria in the mouth, which is typically caused by certain foods, sugar, lack of good bacteria and/or infection. For these cases, I recommend rinsing with *xylitol*, a natural sugar alcohol found in many fruits, berries, vegetables and mushrooms. Xylitol prevents bacteria from adhering to teeth and gums. I have seen good results with a product called Spry Coolmint Oral Rinse, which should be used twice daily. A 16-ounce bottle sells for $4.79. It is available at many health-food stores and some dentists' offices.

When Adult Children Don't Get Along

Peter Goldenthal, PhD, a psychologist and family therapist in Wayne, Pennsylvania, is author of several books on family relations, including *Why Can't We Get Along? Healing Adult Sibling Relationships*. Wiley.

Many adults don't get along with their siblings—and sometimes it's not even clear where the bad blood began. Rivalries and hostilities among adult siblings can often be traced back deep into childhood, obscuring their origins. It's likely that your parents could be a significant contributing factor.

You're likely to have trouble getting along with your adult siblings if…

• **Your parents paid more attention** to one child than another.

Examples: A father shows more interest in the son who is active in sports than the one who prefers acting. A mother devotes more time to her son who has a serious health problem than to her healthy daughter.

• **Your parents implied that one sibling was better** than the other. There are few surer ways for parents to sabotage relations between children than to say things like, "Why can't you be more like your sister?" Even subtler, well-intentioned comments can drive a wedge between siblings.

Examples: "I'm proud of you. It's okay that you're not as successful as your brother." Or, "We should talk about money management," followed 20 minutes later by, "Your sister is saving a lot of money."

• **One sibling persistently bullied,** taunted or threatened the other, and your parents did nothing to stop it.

Sometimes these troublesome parental behaviors continue during the siblings' adult lives, sometimes they don't. Either way, the seeds of sibling rivalry have been planted.

Once siblings are grown, nothing their parents do is likely to cause a major rift between them—unless this animosity dates back to childhood.

Example: You might be unhappy that your parents visited your sister's home for the holidays this year instead of yours, but this probably won't create significant hostility unless you've always felt that your parents favored your sister.

WHAT PARENTS CAN DO

Most parents don't believe that they're to blame for problems between their grown children, but if one or more of the kids hold you responsible, citing perceived favoritism or some other reason, you might be able to help heal the situation with an apology. Say something like, "I know we made some mistakes, and we're sorry for them. It's too late to change the past, but understand that we do love you every bit as much as your sibling."

If the issue is favoritism, you might also point out that any unequal treatment that did exist was your fault, not the sibling's, so there's no reason why it should keep siblings from getting along.

It's worth noting that people who believe they were the victims of parental favoritism as children often see evidence of ongoing parental favoritism during their adult lives. Parents can keep the strained family relations from getting even worse by balancing their visits to their grown kids' homes…treating their grandchildren exactly the same (adults who feel they received less parental attention or praise growing up tend to believe that their children now get the short end of the stick from their grandparents)…and never telling a child who feels he doesn't measure up how well his siblings are doing.

WHAT ADULT CHILDREN CAN DO

If you or your sibling thinks, "My brother/sister needs to change before we can get along," your relationship is doomed. There's hope only if you can ask, "What do I need to do to make this relationship work?"

Call your sibling and say you would like your relationship to be closer. Suggest that the two of you get together and try to work through your problems. If you think your parents have poisoned the waters between you, share this idea with your sibling, but don't be shocked if the sibling doesn't agree. Siblings often remember childhood very differently.

Example: Your sibling might think that you were the golden child. While your parents were comparing you unfavorably with your sibling, they might have been doing the same to him/her.

Whatever your sibling has to say, listen without interrupting. Then, before responding, summarize what he said to make sure you understand. Discuss what you can do to improve the relationship before suggesting things your sibling can do.

Helpful: If your relationship with your sibling is so strained that you can't even call him to try to reconcile, start by seeing a family therapist. Let the therapist decide when and how to involve the sibling in the healing process.

If your parents continue to feed your competition, explain to them that they're preventing the family from being as close as it might be. Even if your parents don't agree that they're part of the problem, they might agree to be more careful about their behavior in the future for the good of the family.

Whether or not you're able to change your parents, be careful to treat your own kids as equitably as possible. People who feel that their parents treated one kid better than another often unintentionally repeat this behavior with their own children.

Is Your Parents' Marriage In Trouble? How to Help

Joseph Ilardo, PhD, and Carole Rothman, PhD, mental-health professionals specializing in elder care and family communication issues, Somers, New York, and coauthors of the recently expanded and reissued *Are Your Parents Driving You Crazy?* VanderWyk & Burnham.

Your parents have been arguing for decades—but now their marriage seems worse than ever. Or maybe they have always seemed happy together, but the marriage suddenly is on the rocks. A marriage can hit rough spots even late in the journey. When that happens, the couple's adult children typically wish to help their parents save the relationship, but what can they do to help?

STRATEGIES

When a marriage falters after decades, the best question to ask yourself is "What's changed?" *Cer-*

tain changes are particularly likely to create problems for older married couples, including...

•**Increased togetherness.** Your mother and father probably spent many hours apart each week for most of their married lives. Retired couples often are together 24 hours a day, which can be a difficult adjustment.

What to do: Help your parents find individual hobbies. Suggest they return to activities enjoyed long ago...join clubs on their own...or spend more time with their own same-sex friends.

•**Different plans.** Perhaps one of your parents wants to travel, but the other just wants to be near the grandkids.

What to do: Help them reach a compromise by suggesting, for example, that they travel for a few months each year but spend the rest of the time at home.

•**Depression.** If one of your parents isn't happy—perhaps because of a health problem, adjusting to retirement or a child moving away—that unhappiness can taint the whole marriage.

What to do: Help this parent see that his/her marriage isn't to blame for the unhappiness. Suggest that he seek help—a therapist or support group, perhaps.

•**Financial difficulties.** Your parents' retirement savings might not have lasted as long as they had expected. Money problems can strain even the strongest relationship.

What to do: Remind your parents that they're not unhappy with each other—they're just tense about money. Help them find ways to trim expenses...offer financial support if you're able ...and point out that living separately is even pricier than living together.

•**Medication side effects.** Has either of your parents changed medications recently? Drugs sometimes cause changes in behavior or personality, potentially resulting in marital conflicts.

What to do: Consult a doctor about possible behavioral side effects of your parent's medications and alternative drug options.

•**Chronic illness or dementia.** The onset of dementia, perhaps as yet undiagnosed, can alter a person in ways that might frustrate his spouse. Illness or dementia can alter your parents' roles in ways that strain a marriage, forcing one spouse to become the caregiver and the other the dependent.

What to do: Help your parents locate appropriate support groups. If acceptable to your parents and financially feasible, consider hiring someone to ease the caregiver's burden.

•**Loss of friends.** Parents may be dealing with friends dying or retiring to different parts of the country. This can alter their social circles and outlook on life.

What to do: Encourage your parents to continue to expand their social circle by joining clubs or other groups.

•**Declining driving ability.** The loss of the ability to drive safely is a common source of arguments in older couples.

What to do: Ask a family doctor to decide if a parent can still drive safely, or let a driver's test decide so that it isn't just one parent telling the other he's not capable. Look into senior transport programs in your area, or arrange for family, friends or volunteer drivers to provide rides on a regular basis so that your parent isn't stranded.

YOUR PROPER ROLE

If your parents don't want your help with their marital problems, don't force the issue. Some parents aren't comfortable sharing their problems with their kids. When that's the case, you'll only make things worse by interfering. If you're not confident that your input will be welcomed, ask, "Is this something you would like my help with?" If the answer is no, let your parents know that you love them both…that you're there for them if they change their minds…and that you can help them find a third party to help, such as a professional marriage counselor, if they would prefer.

You won't help your parents' marriage by taking sides in their arguments. As soon as you side with one parent, the other will feel ganged up on and become wary of your continued involvement. Even if you're certain one parent is completely to blame, remember that you might not know the whole story.

Exception: If one parent is suffering from dementia or serious depression, you may need to take a more active role in helping both parents find appropriate medical and psychological help.

If your parents burden you with their problems but won't listen to your advice, tell them

they must let you help or leave you out of it. Make it clear that you'll cut visits short if they can't be civil to each other. Keep in mind that you're not responsible for their marriage. If you have offered assistance and a sympathetic ear, you have done all you can do.

Do You Have a Short Fuse? Five Ways to Break the Anger Habit

Brenda Shoshanna, PhD, a psychologist and therapist for more than 25 years, is author of *The Anger Diet: 30 Days to Stress-Free Living* (Andrews McMeel) and *Zen Miracles: Finding Peace in an Insane World* (Wiley).

Expressing anger at your spouse, your boss or the driver in front of you may make you feel more powerful and less vulnerable—but only for a short time. It rarely resolves feelings and often intensifies them. Over time, anger can become addictive. You don't even recognize that you are angry or investigate why.

Even if you don't outwardly express your anger, it can be destructive. Repressed anger can be a root cause of anxiety, depression, overeating and other problems. *To reduce anger…*

1. GAIN CONTROL

The moment you begin to sense anger rising in you…

•**Regain your physical equilibrium.** Stop talking, break eye contact with the other person and/or breathe deeply.

•**Avoid personalizing the situation.** That cashier isn't just being rude to you—she is rude to everybody. If her parents, teachers and bosses couldn't teach her to be polite, how are a few words from you going to change anything? It's a waste of your emotional and intellectual energy to confront her.

•**Gain perspective** by placing your anger in a larger context. Imagine yourself looking back at the incident a year from now. Would it matter?

Example: I had a patient who had a wonderful new wife. She had a habit of talking to her friends on the phone late at night. He felt she was taking time away from him, and he would blow up at her. The next morning, he would apologize profusely, but she was left feeling wounded. He had tried asking his wife to spend less time on the phone, but she felt he was being unreasonable. I suggested that whenever he was in a rage, he write down five great things he got out of their relationship. This helped remind him of what was really important.

2. TURN A FOE INTO A FRIEND

Change your perceptions by thinking about what you can do to turn a perceived "enemy" into a friend.

Example: I had a patient who was furious because a particular employee of his kept showing up late for work. My patient saw this as a conscious refusal to be a team member and submit to the established channels of authority.

I suggested that instead of reprimanding the employee, my patient ask what he could do to help the employee arrive at work on time. It turned out that the employee was a single parent who was struggling with child-care issues but was too proud to admit it. My patient altered the man's working hours and earned an ally in his office.

3. STOP OBSESSING

Anger builds when you dwell on an incident, playing it over and over in your mind in an obsessive loop. Instead, direct your mental attention elsewhere.

Example: One patient was a hardworking manager at an insurance company. He was convinced that his boss didn't like him. The loop in his head kept saying, "You're going to be passed over for promotion." His resulting anger expressed itself in cold and distant behavior toward the boss. He turned down social invitations, kept conversations short and never smiled. In reality, his boss valued my patient's work but was turned off by his curt actions. When my patient realized how he was fueling this negative situation, he changed his self-talk. He told himself that he was doing a fine job and that his boss recognized it. He also became aware of the boss's needs and began to reach out to him and offer support. A promotion followed naturally.

4. TAKE THE HIGH ROAD

Avoid responding to an insult with an insult. It only escalates situations and can inflict long-term wounds. Realize that the other person is probably acting out of pain, fear or weakness. Respond with, "What do you need from me right now?" This cuts through the other person's anger.

Example: I worked with a couple whose arguments would escalate quickly and viciously. I suggested to the woman that the next time her husband insulted her, she not lash out but ask her husband what he needed. The next week, the woman agreed to meet her husband at a cocktail party after work. When she arrived, he snapped, "You're late." Instead of snapping back, she asked her husband what he needed. That stopped the argument cold. It turned out that he was angry because he had been uncomfortable waiting at the party alone. He didn't feel as capable as she did in social situations. He wanted her company and the warm, engaging manner in which she met people. Simply communicating this defused the anger between them.

5. LET GO OF A GRUDGE

We like to nurture old hurts because it legitimizes our ill thoughts or bad behavior.

Example: One patient had held a grudge against her husband for decades. At their engagement party more than 20 years earlier, her husband had commented in front of the entire family how beautiful her sister looked that night, but he hadn't commented on my patient's appearance. She felt deeply hurt and thought that forgiving her husband would mean she was weak and lacked self-esteem. I told her that dropping the grudge would be healing, giving her the freedom and clarity to improve their relationship. *How to let go of a grudge...*

•**Think about times when you might have behaved in a similar way.** My patient realized that she had hurt her husband's feelings in the past by talking negatively about him in front of his own family.

•**Figure out what you need to do to release your grudge.** My patient wanted her husband to acknowledge that she was beautiful to him.

•**Ask for what you want.** Express your needs clearly. My patient discussed her grudge with her husband. He responded, "I think you are the most beautiful woman in the world!" After hearing that, her anger disappeared.

The Sex-Starved Marriage

Michele Weiner-Davis, MSW, a social worker and relationship expert who is founder and director of The Divorce Busting Center in Boulder, Colorado. A regular guest on *Oprah*, *48 Hours* and the *Today* show, she is author of numerous books, including her most recent, *The Sex-Starved Wife: What to Do When He's Lost Desire.* Simon & Schuster. *www.divorcebusting.com.*

One out of five marriages is virtually sexless—these couples have sex 10 or fewer times a year. In about one in three marriages, one spouse has a considerably larger sexual appetite than the other. If you see yourself in these statistics, don't despair—there's a great deal that can be done to boost your marriage's libido.

WHO'S SEX-STARVED?

A sex-starved marriage occurs when one spouse is desperately longing for more physical affection. Sex-starved marriages can't be defined by the number of times per week or month that a couple has sex, because there are no daily or weekly minimum requirements to ensure a healthy sex life. What works for one couple is grounds for divorce for another.

Most people believe that it is principally women who struggle with low sexual desire. While it's true that more men than women complain about the frequency of sex, the difference between genders isn't great. In fact, low desire in men is one of America's best-kept secrets. Too many men are simply unwilling to discuss their low desire with doctors, therapists or even their wives.

In a sex-starved marriage, the less interested spouse, whether male or female, typically thinks, *Why are you making such a big deal out of this? It's just sex.* But to the spouse wanting more physical closeness, sex is extremely important because it's not just a physical act. It's about feeling wanted, attractive, appreciated and emotionally connected. When the low-desire spouse doesn't understand sex's significance and continues to reject sexual advances, intimacy on many different levels tends to fall off. The couple stops cuddling on the couch, laughing at each other's jokes, going on dates together. In short, they stop being friends. This places their marriage in jeopardy.

CATCH-22

Frequently, the lower-desire spouse needs to feel close and connected on an emotional level before he/she is interested in being sexual. This usually entails spending quality time together and talking about intimate issues.

The catch-22 is that typically the higher-desire spouse needs to feel connected physically in order to open up with conversation or feel that spending time together is a priority.

One spouse waits for time together and heart-to-heart talks before investing in the physical relationship, while the other spouse waits to be touched before initiating time together or intimate conversation.

Each waits for the other to change.

THE NOs HAVE VETO POWER

The spouse with the lower sexual drive usually controls the frequency of sex—if he doesn't want it, it generally doesn't happen. This is not due to maliciousness or a desire for power—it just seems unimaginable to be sexual if one partner is not in the mood.

Furthermore, there is an unspoken and often unconscious expectation that the higher-desire spouse must accept the no-sex verdict, not complain about it—and, of course, remain monogamous. After decades of working with couples, I can attest that this is an unfair and unworkable arrangement. This is not to say that infidelity is a solution, but as with all relationship conflicts, being willing to find middle ground is the best way to ensure love's longevity.

If you're in a sex-starved marriage, you and your spouse need to make some changes. Don't worry about who takes the lead. Relationships are such that if one person changes, the relationship changes.

ADVICE FOR HIGH-DESIRE SPOUSES

•**Tune in to your spouse's needs outside the bedroom.** High-desire people usually try to boost their spouses' desire by doing things that would turn themselves on, such as buying sexy lingerie and renting X-rated videos. However, these actions often don't work for their spouses, who are more likely to be responsive to loving behaviors outside the bedroom, such as helping more with housework and offering more compliments and fewer criticisms.

•**Talk from the heart.** Some people talk to their spouses about their sexual unhappiness, but instead of speaking from their hearts—which might prompt their spouses' empathy—harsh words are exchanged and tempers flare. Although it's understandable that unending rejection might lead to anger and resentment, these emotions are not aphrodisiacs. Instead of complaining, say, "I miss being close to you physically. We seem to get along so much better after we make love. I'm hoping that we can be more affectionate this week."

ADVICE FOR LOW-DESIRE SPOUSES

•**Don't ignore the problem.** If you and your spouse have been arguing about sex, don't stick your head in the sand. Your differences won't disappear—the only thing that will disappear is your intimate connection and friendship. There are many excellent resources to help you feel more sexual. Good books include *Hot Monogamy* by Patricia Love, MD, and Jo Robinson …*Rekindling Desire: A Step-by-Step Program to Help Low-Sex and No-Sex Marriages* by Barry and Emily McCarthy…and my book, *The Sex-Starved Marriage*. Also, licensed sex therapists can be found through the American Association of Sexuality Educators, Counselors and Therapists (*www.aasect.org*).

•**Just do it.** Perhaps you've had the experience of not being in the mood when your spouse approached you, but you gave it a try, and once you got into it, you enjoyed it. You're not alone. There are millions of people who simply don't experience out-of-the-blue sexy thoughts—unlike their more highly sexed spouses who may have lusty thoughts many times every day.

Try this: For the next two weeks, initiate sex twice each week. Also, flirt, call your spouse pet names, dress more provocatively and be more physically affectionate. Do this whether you feel like it or not. Then carefully watch your spouse for any changes in his behavior. An irritable, withdrawn, uncooperative spouse most likely will become much more fun to be around.

Is Your Marriage Making You Sick?

Theodore Robles, PhD, assistant professor of health psychology in the department of psychology at the University of California, Los Angeles. Robles' research focuses on the effects of marital conflict on endocrine and immune functioning in healthy adults.

Researchers have long known that marriage can improve one's health. But only recently has scientific evidence emerged indicating that serious health consequences can result from a chronically stressful marriage.

Important new findings…

•**Increased heart disease risk.** Negative marital interactions have been convincingly linked by studies at the University of Utah to increases in heart rate and blood pressure, coronary artery fatty deposits (plaques) and decreased elasticity in the arteries—all of which contribute to heart disease.

•**Weakened immunity.** Married couples who were more hostile or angry during a single interaction were found by an Ohio State University study to have decreased function of infection-fighting natural killer cells and, in a later study, slower rates of wound healing.

As a health risk, marital stress is on par with social isolation, high cholesterol, poor diet and lack of exercise, according to these and other findings. For unknown reasons, women seem to be particularly hard hit by marital woes—studies consistently show that wives experience stronger cardiovascular, hormonal and immunological reactions to marital stress.

Good news: While virtually all marriages endure some degree of conflict, studies suggest that it's how we *deal with* disagreements—not just whether we have them—that largely determines the effects on our health. For example, University of Utah researchers have shown that a couple's demeanor during disputes—warm, hostile, controlling, submissive—is as good an indicator of underlying heart disease as cholesterol levels.

To minimize the health impact of marital stress…

•**Break the tension.** Ohio State University researchers recently measured blood levels of the stress hormones *cortisol* and *adrenocorticotropic hormone* (ACTH) in 90 newlywed couples before, during and after a 30-minute discussion about sensitive marital issues. When both partners were consistently negative, the wives' cortisol and ACTH levels escalated.

However, when one or both partners were supportive and constructive—even during heated discussions—the wives' stress hormones declined throughout the discussion. (Men's hormone levels were unaffected by both the negative and supportive behaviors.)

What both spouses can do: Agree with your partner on some points…accept responsibility for your shortcomings…and propose compromises.

Research involving women with high blood pressure suggests that more hostile behaviors during marital discussions are associated with elevated blood pressure during the exchanges, and more supportive behaviors are associated with lower blood pressure during the discussions.

•**Watch your words.** While husbands appear less physiologically affected by their wives' hostility, they do react—with increased heart rate and blood pressure—to perceived challenges to their competency or skills.

What both spouses can do: Avoid controlling statements such as "You're never on time… why don't you wear your watch?" or "Why can't you just do what I ask?"

Replace comments such as: "You're spending us into bankruptcy!" with: "I know you love to shop for the grandkids, but we need to stick to a budget."

Helpful: Because we cannot control everything about our spouses, look for something to value even in those things you may not readily admire. For example, if you resent your spouse's messiness but value his/her easygoing nature, try viewing these qualities as flip sides of the same coin. You may find you have greater tolerance for—and less need to control—the clutter.

•**Trust your spouse.** In a University of Utah study involving 300 middle-aged and older couples, researchers found no correlation between self-reports of anger or antagonism and calcium buildup in their coronary arteries (a risk factor for cardiovascular disease). However, partners whose spouses had rated them high on scales of anger and antagonism were more likely to have significant calcium buildup.

What both spouses can do: Pay attention if your partner says you are being angry, hostile, unreasonable or cold. While you may be unaware of your negativity, your arteries could be paying the price.

•**Speak your mind.** In a University of Michigan study involving 192 older couples, those in which both spouses clammed up to avoid confrontation were much more likely to experience the death of one or both partners over a 17-year period. In fact, among 26 such "dual-suppressor" marriages, 27% suffered the loss of one spouse, and 23% experienced the death of both partners, while among the 166 more communicative couples, a significantly lower 19% experienced one death, and only 6% experienced the death of both partners.

Shocking new finding: In a recent study involving nearly 4,000 married adults from Framingham, Massachusetts, women who reported regularly stifling themselves during marital disagreements were *four times* more likely than outspoken wives to die during a 10-year period.

The culprit could be stress—when husbands respond with silence to their wives' anger, studies show that wives' cortisol levels go up and stay up for the day. Chronically elevated cortisol has been linked to impaired cognitive and immune functioning, heart disease, diabetes and other ills.

What both spouses can do: Communicate openly.

•**Relax.** Studies have shown that the higher a woman's levels of stress hormones before she and her husband engage in a discussion about their relationship, the more likely she and her husband are to be critical, defensive or hostile to one another during conflict. Unfortunately, these negative behaviors only exacerbate the wife's already elevated ACTH and cortisol levels.

What both spouses can do: Make time daily to relax, whether with exercise, meditation, hobbies or spending time with friends. By lowering stress, women, in particular, may be able to keep hostility—and their stress hormones—from escalating during marital conflict.

The Four Love Personalities

Helen Fisher, PhD, research professsor of anthropology at Rutgers University, New Brunswick, New Jersey, and chief scientific adviser to the on-line dating site Chemistry.com. She is author of several books on human sexual and social behavior, including, *Why We Love: The Nature and Chemistry of Romantic Love*. Holt. *www.helenfisher.com*

When your spouse does things that mystify you or drive you crazy, you probably wish he/she would behave more reasonably. Yet your partner may not be "programmed" to behave any other way.

My research suggests that each of us has a "love personality"—how we are naturally inclined to behave with a romantic partner—that may depend on the particular chemicals dominant in one's brain. This research comes from my analysis of existing genetic and pharmaceutical studies, as well as from my work as chief scientific adviser to the Internet dating site Chemistry.com. I devised a series of questions to establish to what degree we express specific chemicals in the brain and collected data on 28,000 men and women.

I determined that love personalities can be divided into four main types, based on which brain chemicals—*serotonin, dopamine, estrogen* and *testosterone*—are predominant. Some people show characteristics of one type...others are a combination. *The four types...*

BUILDERS

Serotonin promotes orderly, cautious behavior and respect for authority. More than the other three types, Builders enjoy planning far ahead. They are literal and predictable, fastidious about their possessions, conscientious and dutiful. They tolerate routine well.

What the Builder brings to a relationship: Builders are good at forming strong networks and run businesses and households with great efficiency. A Builder will never keep you waiting, forget to fill the gas tank or write down the wrong flight departure time.

Sources of stress: Builders are stubborn—if you helpfully suggest to a Builder a better way to mop the floor, you may find yourself in an argument. Builders can be moralistic and overly rule-bound. They are suspicious of new experiences and ideas—in fact, they will be quick to point out all the reasons why an idea might not work.

Sex and fidelity: Builders are most likely to be attracted to other Builders. They are serious when they court. Sex may become routine, but Builders like routines, and two Builders will rarely fight about their life in the bedroom. Highly loyal, Builders are unlikely even to consider divorce.

Living with a Builder: Let the Builder do things his way, even if you're convinced there is a better way. If you crave more adventure than the Builder, map out a new experience beforehand so that it doesn't look like a risk...or let the Builder plan the details.

EXPLORERS

High dopamine activity is associated with curiosity, spontaneity, risk-taking, novelty-seeking, irreverence, mental flexibility and optimism.

What the Explorer brings to a relationship: Explorers are enthusiastic and full of energy. Charming and creative, Explorers don't like to be told what to do—they chafe at rules, plans and schedules. They can be extravagant gift givers.

Sources of stress: The Explorer's impulsiveness can grate on someone who would like to know what time to be ready for dinner or who prefers to buy theater tickets in advance. An Explorer doesn't like repetitive tasks, so you shouldn't depend on an Explorer to take out the garbage every night.

Sex and fidelity: Explorers tend to be attracted to other Explorers, and they make exciting sex partners. Instead of discussing the deep meaning of a relationship, an Explorer would rather make love or go out together for a good time. Big fights may be followed by passionate lovemaking. It is important to have adventures with an Explorer, lest he decide to find someone else to share his experiences with.

Living with an Explorer: Don't try to keep an Explorer from doing what interests him. Instead of imposing rules, find parameters that the Explorer can live with.

Example: A Builder husband and Explorer wife had repeated showdowns over the Explorer's chronic lateness. They finally agreed that the Explorer would call her husband when she was running late…and that the Builder would go ahead with plans instead of waiting for his wife, who would join him later.

NEGOTIATORS

Men, as well as women, can have high estrogen activity in the brain, promoting connection-seeking.

What the Negotiator brings to a relationship: Negotiators are highly verbal, agreeable and good at reading people. They are skilled at coming up with the right thing to say to make others feel valued. Negotiators have rich imaginations and think holistically—they see creative and unusual connections between disparate pieces of information. They are flexible and willing to change their minds.

Sources of stress: The ability to see many sides of an issue can make it difficult for Negotiators to reach decisions. They are so imaginative about possibilities that they may create constant anxiety for themselves. Because Negotiators want everyone to be happy, they don't always say clearly what they need or mean, leading to confusion and misunderstanding.

Sex and fidelity: Negotiators tend to be most attracted to Directors (see right). The Negotiator needs the Director's logic, forthrightness and decisiveness to get things done.

Negotiators seek deep intimacy with their partners—they want a soul mate—so they will be patient, forgiving and compassionate. But if a Negotiator feels that he won't ever "reach" you to share an intimate life together, he may eventually turn elsewhere for the romance he craves.

Living with a Negotiator: Recognize that what sounds to you like endless processing is a way for the Negotiator to address the needs of everyone involved. Don't rush the Negotiator's decision. Trust that once he has examined all the angles, the solution will make a lot of people happy, including you.

DIRECTORS

Both women and men can have high testosterone activity in the brain, leading them to be competitive, straight-forward, logical and pragmatic.

What the Director brings to a relationship: You don't have to second-guess Directors—they say what they mean without nuance. Because of their ambition and competitiveness, they are dedicated to their work and typically well-paid. Directors like to focus very deeply on a few subjects and learn everything about them.

Sources of stress: Directors can alienate people with their bluntness, coming across as dictatorial and aloof. They get impatient when others are not as focused as they are or don't immediately grasp their ideas. They have a hard time leaving work behind—at the beach, the Director is the one checking e-mail.

Sex and fidelity: Directors are most likely to be attracted to Negotiators. The Director relies on the Negotiator's people skills. Sex is a genuine form of intimacy for them. They tend to be loyal, but if they cannot get the physical connectedness they need, they will seek it elsewhere.

Living with a Director: Don't give a Director hints or make gentle requests—the message will not get through. Instead of "Would you have time to…" say, "I need you to do this by Friday." During disagreements, appeal to logic ("This would be more efficient") rather than emotion ("This makes me frustrated").

To get Directors to relax outside work hours, encourage activities that are absorbing, challenging or competitive enough to distract them, such as joining a tennis league or a book club.

18

Your Skin and Senses

Look Younger Without Surgery

Recently, the science of reducing wrinkles has been transformed by the introduction of remarkable new devices and treatments that don't involve surgery. *Here are the latest developments that could help men and women alike look and feel better if they are concerned about wrinkles...*

•**Digital imaging machine** that provides a computerized analysis of your skin. A device called Visia, made by Canfield Clinical Systems, uses a computer-aided digital camera to analyze facial skin in minute detail.

It gives doctors an unprecedented ability to diagnose skin conditions and monitor the effectiveness of various treatments.

How it works: While the patient's head is immobilized, digital photographs are taken under different types of light to identify the precise location and depth of various skin features, including wrinkles, brown spots, enlarged pores and acne. Ultraviolet light is used to scan for latent sun damage, which will emerge as the patient gets older.

When the analysis is complete, the patient's profile is matched against a database containing thousands of profiles.

A percentile score shows how the patient's skin compares with that of people of similar age, gender and skin type. This analysis can then be used to guide doctors in prescribing and administering treatments. On subsequent visits, new digital images are taken to measure how well the skin is responding.

•**Laser treatment** that stimulates skin to renew itself. *Intense pulsed light (IPL) photorejuvenation* is becoming the treatment of choice for

Barry DiBernardo, MD, a board-certified surgeon; director, New Jersey Plastic Surgery, a private practice, Montclair; chief, aesthetic surgery program, Mountainside Hospital, Montclair; and clinical assistant professor of plastic surgery, University of Medicine and Dentistry of New Jersey, Newark. He is a spokesperson for the American Society for Aesthetic Plastic Surgery, and past president of the New Jersey Society of Plastic Surgeons.

eliminating fine wrinkles, brown spots, broken capillaries and birthmarks—all without any recovery time.

How it works: This treatment produces light pulses at a variety of wavelengths, which penetrate the skin to different depths, depending on the problem being treated (brown spots tend to lie near the surface, for example, while broken capillaries are slightly below).

This allows blemishes to be treated precisely without damaging surrounding tissue. Even better, IPL can penetrate below the top layer of skin (epidermis) to stimulate the cells that produce *collagen* and *elastin*—naturally occurring tissues that make skin more firm and elastic, and which we all tend to lose as we get older. IPL photorejuvenation reverses this aging effect, making skin tighter and plumper.

While IPL has been around for a number of years, a new machine called the Lumenis One (manufactured by Lumenis) represents a significant advance over previous IPL devices.

Among other things, its computer has an improved ability to deliver light at exactly the right location. This new device is so good at removing difficult-to-treat blemishes—and rejuvenating the skin—that even longtime patients praise its effectiveness.

This treatment is available in most states. To find a practitioner in your area, call Lumenis at 877-586-3647.

Sessions last approximately 20 minutes. Typically, patients undergo a series of IPL treatments over several weeks, followed by a maintenance treatment every six months.

With older IPL technology, treatments lasted 45 minutes, but the maintenance intervals were the same.

Cost: $200 to $500 per treatment.

•**Radio frequency devices** that use radio frequency to tighten the skin have been available for approximately two years, but a new device called Titan (manufactured by Cutera) represents a big improvement over previous machines—it is safer, more effective and less costly. It is available throughout the US and abroad. Radio frequency devices operate in the infrared range to heat the tissue under the skin surface, causing loose skin and its underlying collagen to contract and tighten. The treatment is effective even on large wrinkles.

Since it doesn't remove any layers of skin, there is no flaking or redness following the treatment, eliminating the need for recovery time.

Radio frequency treatment is currently approved by the US Food and Drug Administration (FDA) for use on the forehead, cheek, neck and around the eyes.

A series of treatments may be needed for optimal results. It is not yet known how long the results will last.

Cost: $500 to $2,500 per treatment, depending on the area covered and the amount of time involved.

•**Hyaluronic filler** that replaces collagen. Deeper lines can be temporarily eliminated by injecting a filler material into the fat layer directly beneath the depressed area.

Until recently, the only filler approved for use in the US was *bovine collagen*, which is derived from cattle.

Collagen injections last approximately three months and require allergy testing before use.

The FDA has approved Restylane, a hyaluronic acid product already available in approximately 60 countries.

Because hyaluronic acid occurs naturally in humans, it's nonallergenic, and no skin test is necessary.

In addition, Restylane injections last much longer than collagen injections—typically up to one year.

Many dermatologists and aesthetic surgeons now use Restylane exclusively, while others continue to offer both Restylane and collagen.

Cost: $500 to $1,000 per treatment.

MULTI-TREATMENT SKIN MAINTENANCE

Taking advantage of the array of new tools described above, many people are now adopting a maintenance program where they see a doctor (either a plastic surgeon, dermatologist or other medical doctor who has been trained to perform aesthetic services) every six months for IPL treatment and Botox® injections, and on every second visit—once a year—they get a Restylane touch-up. Other procedures are done as needed, including radio frequency treatment and *CO₂ laser resurfacing* (which produces more dramatic results than IPL, but also requires recovery time).

The final component of the program is a good home-care regimen—including regular use of sunblock to prevent ultraviolet (UV) damage, as well as products that speed up the turnover of the skin cells.

Bottom line: People who decide to follow this skin rejuvenation program not only have great-looking skin, but they also have a less invasive alternative to cosmetic surgery as they get older.

Caution: Botox has risks. Ask your doctor.

Cures for Adult Acne

Richard G. Fried, MD, PhD, clinical director of Yardley Dermatology Associates, a skin-enhancement and wellness center in Yardley, Pennsylvania, is author of *Healing Adult Acne.* New Harbinger Publications.

Acne used to be rare in adults. No more. It can occur in people in their 20s and 30s—and some people continue to have acne into their 40s and 50s. In a recent study, 34% of participants who experienced adult-onset acne never had it during adolescence.

Doctors don't know why adult acne is on the rise, but one factor could be that we have busier lives and experience more stress than in the past. Stress triggers the release of hormones, such as testosterone (in women and men), and chemicals, such as neuropeptides, that increase skin oils and impair facial circulation. Contrary to popular belief, food has little effect on acne.

Adult acne tends to affect deeper skin layers than adolescent acne. There's more inflammation and a greater risk of scarring.

THE ROOT OF ACNE

Acne occurs when hair follicles become plugged with oil and abnormally thick, sticky dead skin cells. Follicles are bulblike structures that encase hair roots and are attached to oil-producing glands. The oil travels up the hair shaft to the skin surface. Adults who produce excessive oil—due to high levels of testosterone, for example—may experience blockages in the follicles. The trapped oil (sebum) provides a haven for bacteria, which can cause inflammation and infection, resulting in acne.

About 54% of adults with acne are women, probably because their skin is more sensitive to testosterone's effects.

BEST TREATMENTS

To treat acne, start with step one, then move on to subsequent steps if there isn't substantial clearing in two to four weeks…

•**Step 1.** Benzoyl peroxide is the main ingredient in dozens of acne lotions, many of which are available over-the-counter. It has antibacterial/anti-inflammatory effects that usually work for mild acne. Use a 2.5% formula (such as PanOxyl AQ 2.5% Gel) for dry or sensitive skin…a 7% to 10% formula (such as Clearasil Maximum Strength medicated cream) for oily skin. Apply to affected areas once daily.

Helpful: Also apply a salicylic acid product (such as Salacid), which reduces swelling and inflammation. Use benzoyl peroxide and salicylic acid at different times of day, perhaps benzoyl peroxide at night and salicylic acid in the morning. The combination gives better results.

•**Step 2.** Retinoids, prescription topical products, such as Retin-A, Renova and Avita, help unblock hair follicles. These products may cause irritation. Apply twice weekly initially, then increase to once daily as skin adjusts.

Important: Benzoyl peroxide reduces the effects of retinoids. You can use them both, but not at the same time.

•**Step 3.** Combination ointment. Prescription products, such as Duac, contain both benzoyl peroxide and an antibiotic. Patients with mild-to-moderate acne who don't respond to other products usually do well with these.

•**Step 4.** Periostat. Available by prescription, this oral drug contains a low dose of the antibiotic *doxycycline.* It doesn't have antibiotic properties at this dose but does act as an anti-inflammatory. When used in combination with acne ointments, such as benzoyl peroxide or topical retinoids, it is very effective in most patients (though it may need to be taken for months).

•**Step 5.** *Isotretinoin* is a prescription vitamin-A derivative, taken in pill form, that can eliminate acne in most patients. It helps normalize hair follicles, so cells don't thicken and clog the pores, and can prevent acne from coming back.

Women who are pregnant or planning to become pregnant cannot take isotretinoin (Accutane, Claravis) because it increases the risk of birth defects.

•**Step 6.** Smoothbeam laser. About 40% of adults with severe acne experience substantial improvements with laser therapy. The 1,450-nanometer laser wavelength targets the sebaceous glands and can eliminate excess oil.

The procedure takes 15 to 20 minutes and is relatively painless—although there may be some irritation/redness for several days. Most patients require four to six treatments, usually given one month apart.

Cost: About $150–$500/treatment depending on the size of the area treated, not covered by insurance.

■ ■ ■ ■

Green Tea for Acne?

Green tea provides better acne control than traditional medication.

Recent finding: Patients with moderate to severe acne showed significant improvement after applying a specially formulated 3% green tea solution to their skin twice daily for 12 weeks. The solution cleared skin as effectively as the conventional acne medication benzoyl peroxide but with less itching, peeling and other side effects. Green tea cream is available at health-food stores.

Jennifer Gan-Wong, MD, dermatologist, Memorial Medical Center, Manila, the Philippines.

■ ■ ■ ■

Antibiotics Risk for Acne Sufferers

Acne sufferers who use antibiotics are more likely to get upper-respiratory tract infections than those who don't use antibiotics.

Recent finding: Patients who use oral or topical antibiotics, such as any of the tetracyclines, for more than six weeks at a time to treat acne have about twice the risk of developing an upper-respiratory tract infection, compared with those who don't take antibiotics.

David J. Margolis, MD, PhD, associate professor of dermatology and epidemiology, Center for Education and Research in Therapeutics and director, cutaneous ulcer program, University of Pennsylvania, Philadelphia.

Two New Psoriasis Treatments May Hold Key to Real Relief

University of Michigan.
M.D. Anderson Cancer Center.

Two separate approaches to treating psoriasis, a painful condition that attacks the skin, have shown promise in the lab and may be ready for human testing.

SUPPRESSING CELL GROWTH

The first treatment is an experimental drug called *benzodiazepine-423* (Bz-423)—a chemical cousin of the well-known anti-anxiety drugs Valium and Xanax.

In human skin cultures designed to model psoriasis, University of Michigan researchers found the drug suppressed the unchecked cell growth that characterizes psoriasis.

"Currently, the best treatments for skin lesions that are associated with psoriasis are topical steroids, but they affect normal cells as well," says Gary Glick, a professor of biological chemistry at the University of Michigan. "And repeated use over time can lead to tissue destruction.

"What makes our compound particularly exciting is that it has the potential to be applied topically," and it can distinguish between disease-causing cells and normal cells, adds Glick.

"So we believe the problems associated with repeated topical steroid use could possibly be alleviated with compounds like this," he says.

Glick and his colleagues hope to begin human clinical trials with Bz-423 in the near future.

EASING THE ITCH

The second treatment under study addresses the cause of psoriasis itself.

At the University of Texas' M.D. Anderson Cancer Center in Houston, scientists say they have identified a protein called STAT3 that leads to psoriasis when the body's immune system is activated to fight off a wound, burn or some other type of invasion.

That discovery led to developing a skin cream that cured the itching, redness and scaling of psoriasis—at least in study mice.

The ointment may also be able to prevent recurrence.

"We may have found an entirely new treatment option for psoriasis," says John DiGiovanni, the lead investigator of the study, who is also the director of the M.D. Anderson department of carcinogenesis.

The American Academy of Dermatology has information specifically for people who have psoriasis at *www.skincarephysicians.com.*

What Your Scent Says About Your Health

Jamison Starbuck, ND, a naturopathic physician in family practice in Missoula, Montana. She is past president of the American Association of Naturopathic Physicians.

As a physician, I pay attention to many details about my patients, including body odor. If I detect anything other than a mild, almost neutral scent, my medical curiosity is piqued. Body odor tells me about a patient's health status, dietary habits and hygiene. People with liver disease may have a musty odor...infections anywhere on the body usually emit a foul smell...uncontrolled diabetes often creates a smell best labeled as sweet fermentation. People who are on high-protein diets or who eat a lot of fatty and/or fried foods, onions, garlic or curry, or drink coffee or alcohol excessively, also have particular body odors. Poor hygiene leads to its own recognizable scent.

If you're worried about your body odor, ask a trusted friend or family member to do a sniff test.

What to do: Ask the person to stand within one inch of you and inhale. If the body odor is new, quite strong or confined to a specific part of your body—for example, your mouth, ears or genitals—see your doctor for an exam and evaluation. *If body odor is a familiar, long-standing problem that's not related to an illness, try the following suggestions for 10 days (if they help, continue as needed)...*

•**Eat right.** Fresh, whole foods give your body a fresh, wholesome scent. Eat a salad daily made with dark, leafy lettuce, sprouts, raw veggies and two tablespoons of olive oil. Avoid mayonnaise and cheese-based dressings, which contain odor-producing fat. Choose brown rice or a baked potato instead of fried potatoes. Reduce protein putrification in the digestive tract by eliminating meat—or consuming no more than three ounces of red meat or poultry per day. Drink one-half ounce of water for every pound of your body weight daily.

•**Take three saunas.** Saunas make you perspire, which has a detoxifying effect that reduces body odor.

What to do: Brush your dry skin with a loofah or other skin brush. Enter the sauna and stay there until you perspire all over your body, then leave the sauna and rinse with cold water for 30 seconds. Brush your skin again and return to the sauna. End with a brisk 30-second skin brush, then wrap up in soft, warm clothing. Repeat this process two more times over the next several days.

Caution: People with high blood pressure or heart disease should avoid saunas.

•**Use chlorophyll.** This chemical compound, which is responsible for the green pigment in plants, has astringent properties and can help control the type of body odor that comes from the fermentation of food in the digestive tract. Add one tablespoon of chlorophyll (available at health-food stores) to four ounces of water and drink it at the end of each meal. If you prefer, you can eat one-eighth cup of fresh parsley daily as a substitute for liquid chlorophyll.

•**Eliminate oral bacteria.** In addition to brushing your teeth at least twice daily and flossing at least once a day, gargle each morning with a cup of warm chamomile tea mixed with one teaspoon of hydrogen peroxide. This mixture will kill bacteria living in the throat and

without sunscreen while the sun is high in the sky, such as before or after lunch, to get enough sunlight to meet your body's vitamin-D needs.

Ralph W. Moss, PhD, cancer researcher based in Lemont, PA, and author of *Cancer Therapy*. Equinox. His Moss Reports service offers alternative cancer treatment information to clients, *www.cancerdecisions.com.*

Amazing Remedy Eases Pain, Swelling And Bruising

Mark A. Stengler, ND, naturopathic physician in private practice, La Jolla, California...adjunct associate clinical professor at the National College of Natural Medicine, Portland, Oregon...author of many books, including *The Natural Physician's Healing Therapies* and coauthor of *Prescription for Natural Cures* (both from Bottom Line Books)...and author of the *Bottom Line/Natural Healing* newsletter.

The homeopathic remedy *arnica montana* significantly reduces bruising. In a recent double-blind clinical trial involving 29 women who were undergoing face-lifts, participants were randomly assigned to receive homeopathic arnica (12C potency) or a placebo beginning the morning of surgery. The treatment was repeated every eight hours for four days. Facial bruising and swelling were evaluated by doctors and nurses, as well as through a computerized digital-image analysis of photographs taken before and after surgery. Subjective symptoms—those observed by the patients and professional staff—and the degree of discoloration were not significantly improved by the arnica. However, the area of bruising was significantly smaller for the group of subjects who took arnica. Although the study was on women, I would expect the same results for men and for other types of bruising.

Arnica montana, also known as leopard's bane, is a widely used homeopathic remedy for injury to soft tissues. Arnica preparations have been used in homeopathic medicine for two centuries. Sesquiterpene lactones, major active compounds in arnica, are known to reduce inflammation, decrease pain and improve circulation.

I can attest to hundreds of cases in which arnica has reduced pain and swelling. I also have seen this benefit with infants and animals—where a placebo effect is unlikely. You can use arnica for any soft-tissue injury, such as bruising after a fall or a sprained ankle. The most common dose is two pellets of 30C strength taken two to four times daily for two days. Or apply homeopathic arnica cream two to three times daily until healed. Arnica is sold at most health-food stores and some pharmacies.

Caution: Do not use topical arnica on broken skin or open wounds.

■ **More from Mark A. Stengler ND...**

Breakthrough Treatments for Hair Loss

Why do some men go bald in their 30s while others have a full head of hair until their final days? Why do some women have ever-thinning hair, while others never seem to lose a single strand?

Blame your genes, first of all. If your mom, dad or a grandparent had hair loss, chances are greater that you will, too. Even so, there are ways to slow hair loss and stimulate growth.

THE HORMONE FACTOR

You grow and shed hair all the time. Of the 100,000-plus strands of hair on your head, it is perfectly normal to lose 50 to 100 every day. Once a hair is shed, a new hair grows from the same follicle. Hair grows at a rate of nearly one-half inch per month (faster in warm weather, slower when frost is on the vine). Baldness results when the rate of shedding exceeds the rate of regrowth.

Hair loss usually accelerates when you're over age 50. One hormone, *dihydrotestosterone* (DHT), seems to be the chief culprit. DHT is a derivative of *testosterone* (the sex-determining hormone that is more abundant in men than women). In both men and women, DHT increases in the presence of the enzyme *5-alpha reductase*, which is produced in the prostate, adrenal glands and the scalp. 5-alpha reductase is more likely to proliferate after age 50. When DHT is overproduced, hair follicles are damaged. Some follicles die, but most shrink and produce thinner, weaker hairs—and the weak hairs are the ones that fall out.

533

An oily skin substance called *sebum*—produced by the sebaceous glands—makes matters worse. Excess sebum clogs follicles and contributes to high 5-alpha reductase activity, which stimulates production of DHT.

STRESS

Among my own patients, stress is a factor for both men and women. I have found that highly stressed women, in particular, have higher-than-normal levels of *cortisol*, a stress hormone that can contribute to hair loss.

A study published in the *Journal of Clinical Biochemistry* confirms that cortisol is indeed elevated in some women who suffer hair loss—and that when they learn to cope better with stress, hair growth improves.

For stress relief, I recommend daily exercise, such as brisk walking, as well as relaxation techniques, including deep breathing and meditation. B vitamins and ashwagandha (a stress-reducing herb from India) also can help counteract the effects of cortisol.

A regular daily dose of 100 mg of a B-vitamin complex and 250 mg to 500 mg of ashwagandha can help control cortisol levels. Look for Sensoril Ashwagandha, a patented extract formula by Jarrow Formulas, available at many health-food stores or by calling 800-726-0886 or at *www.jarrow.com*.

A PROMISING FORMULA

Taking a daily multivitamin and mineral supplement as well as the herbal remedy saw palmetto also can help slow hair loss. A daily scalp massage with essential oils is beneficial, too.

•**Saw palmetto** helps block the effects of DHT on hair follicles, strengthening hair. In a study in the *Journal of Alternative and Complementary Medicine*, researchers used a product containing saw palmetto and a plant compound called *beta-sitosterol* that is found in saw palmetto and other plants. The study included 19 men between ages 23 and 64 who had mild-to-moderate hair loss. Men in one group were given a placebo daily… and men in the other group received the saw palmetto/beta-sitosterol combination (none of the participants knew which group they were in). After five months, researchers found that 60% of the men who received the saw palmetto/beta-sitosterol combination showed improvement,

while only 11% of the men receiving a placebo had more hair growth.

In my clinical experience, saw palmetto is helpful for both men and women. I recommend 320 mg to 400 mg daily of an 85% liposterolic extract. It is safe to use long term but should not be taken if you are pregnant or nursing.

For a more aggressive approach, you should also take beta-sitosterol. Source Naturals (800-815-2333, *www.sourcenaturals.com*) offers a 113-mg tablet that can be taken daily. It is available at health-food stores and at *www.iherb.com*.

•**The essential oils of rosemary and lavender** have been shown to improve hair growth when applied to the scalp. My own belief is that they improve blood flow to the scalp, ensuring that nutrients get to the sites where they're needed.

You can purchase these essential oils in separate containers. Pour some of your regular shampoo into the lid of the shampoo bottle, then add five to 10 drops of each essential oil. Massage into the scalp and leave on three to five minutes before rinsing thoroughly.

OTHER SUPPLEMENTS

If you have tried these approaches for two to three months and still aren't satisfied with the growth of your locks, here are some other supplements that can help both men and women…

•**Biotin,** a nutrient that is required for hair growth, is particularly good for brittle hair. Food sources of biotin include brewer's yeast, soybeans, eggs, mushrooms and whole wheat. For supplementation, take 3,000 micrograms daily for at least two months or use a biotin-enriched shampoo daily.

•**MSM (methylsulfonylmethane)** is a great source of sulfur, an integral component of the amino acids that are the building blocks of hair protein. MSM improves the strength, sheen and health of hair. In one study, 21 adults (16 men and five women) who were assessed by a certified cosmetologist under the direction of a medical doctor were given MSM or a placebo and then were reassessed at the end of six weeks. The participants did not know who was given MSM and who was given a placebo.

Those given MSM showed significant improvement in hair health, while those taking a placebo showed few or no changes. I recommend a

3,000-mg daily dose of MSM. Look for Opti-MSM or Lignisul MSM, available from many manufacturers and at health-food stores.

Essential fatty acids keep hair from becoming dry and lifeless by decreasing inflammation. Inflammation worsens the quality of hair follicles, and essential fatty acids are needed for the proper development of hair. Food sources include walnuts, eggs, fish, olive oil, flaxseed and hempseed and flax oils. Or you can take a formula like Udo's Choice Oil Blend, produced by Flora (800-446-2110, *www.florahealth.com*). Follow directions on the label. The formula contains both omega-3 fatty acids (from flax oil or fish oil) and omega-6 fatty acids from evening primrose oil or borage oil. Don't expect immediate results, however. It can take four to six weeks to see improvement.

Not Just Wrinkles: Secrets to Younger-Looking Skin

Neal B. Schultz, MD, dermatologist in private practice, assistant clinical professor at Mount Sinai School of Medicine and assistant adjunct physician at Lenox Hill Hospital. Dr. Schultz is coauthor, with Laura Morton, of *It's Not Just About Wrinkles*. Stewart, Tabori & Chang.

When people complain about looking older, they usually talk about lines and wrinkles. However, most people who are dissatisfied with their appearance have color or texture problems as well that make them look older than they should.

Well-known treatments, such as Botox and collagen, are very effective for lines and wrinkles, but they don't affect color and texture issues. About three-quarters of patients will notice a dramatic improvement when they treat these two important factors, too.

COLOR

Color problems are among the easiest skin defects to correct. They basically fall into two categories—browns (such as age spots and freckles) and reds (usually due to engorged or broken capillaries).

•**Browns.** Brown spots go by many different names—sunspots, liver spots, age spots, etc. They're almost always caused by sun exposure, which triggers excessive activity in some of the skin's pigment-producing cells. Most brown spots appear on exposed areas of the skin, such as the face, arms and back of the hands.

On the other hand, blotchy brown areas that don't have a clear border are usually caused by an imbalance of female hormones, such as during pregnancy or in women taking birth control pills.

Virtually all brown defects can be removed with laser treatments, which cost $400 to $1,200 per treatment. A less expensive but more time-consuming approach is to lighten the brown areas with exfoliation.

Best home treatment: A product with 8% *glycolic acid* used daily. Glycolic acid is one of the alpha hydroxy acids (AHAs). It dissolves *keratin*, the uppermost layer of dead skin. Over-the-counter products, such as Aqua Glycolic Face Cream, Glytone Day Cream for Dry Skin and Kinerase Cream, lighten brown spots and stop the formation of new pigment cells.

Glycolic acid begins to work within two weeks —and will significantly reduce brownness in four to six weeks.

Important: Continue to apply a sunscreen whenever you are going outdoors. Repeated sun exposure will cause the brownness to return.

Also helpful: Twice-daily applications of over-the-counter topical vitamin C, such as Stallex C Complex Rescue Serum or SkinMedica Vitamin C Complex. Topical vitamin C lightens brown spots and blocks cell-damaging free radicals. It can be used in addition to glycolic acid.

Skin cancer warning: If there is a change in a brown spot's or a mole's size, shape or color (other than lightening from treatment) or if it bleeds, itches or becomes painful, contact your dermatologist immediately.

•**Reds.** Most people have one or more red spots or lines on their faces. They're often present on the cheeks or alongside the nose and usually are due to dilated or broken capillaries.

Common types: Telangiectasias, which appear as tiny straight or curved red lines…*spider hemangiomas*, which are raised red bumps with red lines emanating from the center…*or cherry hemangiomas*, flat or dome-shaped spots. Another type of redness is caused by *rosacea*—an acne-like condition that's characterized by red blotches (telangiectasias) that appear intermittently on the cheeks and nose.

Best home treatment: An over-the-counter topical sulfur preparation—such as Rezamid Acne Treatment Lotion or Sulforcin Acne Treatment Lotion. Sulfur shrinks blood vessels and helps reduce redness. This can work for rosacea, too, but test an area the size of a dime first to see how your skin reacts.

Because it's difficult to eliminate skin redness entirely, I usually advise patients to conceal it by using color-correcting makeup—a green-tinted foundation works best. Neutrogena makes a good one.

Diet: Certain foods have dilating effects on blood vessels, causing them to temporarily increase in diameter. The most common perpetrators are alcohol and spicy foods. Also, certain medications and vitamins (the most common of which is any form of *niacin*, one of the B vitamins) are known to cause dilation of facial blood vessels and thus to increase their conspicuousness.

TEXTURE

Young skin is smooth, with a noticeable "slip factor" when you run a finger across the face. Older "dull" skin feels rough, or there are "bumps" when the finger passes over enlarged pores.

Both of the main texture problems—enlarged pores and dull, flaky skin—are caused by the retention of dead skin cells. Skin cells shed every 28 days—but not all cells do this. This results in an uneven accumulation of dead cells.

Best home treatment: Exfoliation with glycolic acid. People should start with a product that has 8% glycolic acid. The concentration can be increased to 10% or 15% if needed.

Bonus: Exfoliating can remove early precancerous cells along with the dead skin cells.

In-office exfoliation treatments: There are two types of in-office exfoliation—chemical, with a prescription glycolic acid treatment…and mechanical with microdermabrasion. The latter involves the use of a machine by a properly trained doctor, nurse or esthetician that bombards the skin with sterilized aluminum-oxide crystals. It immediately strips away dead cells and leaves the skin looking uniform and fresh.

In-office treatments cost $100 to $200 per treatment. You will need six to 10 treatments done at one- to two-week intervals.

CONTOUR

After about age 40, just about everyone notices an increase in lines, wrinkles and sagging skin. These and other contour problems usually are treated with products such as Botox* and/or "filler" materials, such as collagen.

Botox can cost $400 to $1,600 per treatment, depending on the area done, and lasts about three months. Fillers are $600 to $2,000 per treatment and last three to nine months, depending on the area done and the filler used.

The main problems and best treatments…

• **Frown lines** (the vertical lines between the eyes) and forehead lines (horizontal lines across the forehead) are known as dynamic lines because they're most visible when the underlying muscles move. Injections of Botox often can eliminate these types of lines, but when the injections wear off in about three months, they have to be repeated.

• **Marionette lines** run from the nose down to the corner of the mouth. They're caused mainly by the age-related loss of fat and skin elasticity. Botox can't be used for these lines because it can paralyze the entire cheek muscle and prevent smiling. A better approach is to inject collagen or another filler, such as Restylane. These products add volume to the skin and fill out the hollow contours.

• **Crow's feet,** the lines that radiate from the corners of the eyes, often can be improved or eliminated with Botox. In about 20% of cases, patients require a combination of Botox plus collagen.

• **Smoker's lines** on the lips (also called "lipstick lines" because lipstick can "bleed" into the tiny crevices) will disappear when injected with a very fine form of collagen. Most patients also are given injections of Botox to reduce muscle contractions that cause the lines.

*Botox has risks. Consult your doctor.

FOUR STEPS TO BEAUTIFUL SKIN

Getting enough sleep, eating a healthy diet and finding time to relax all contribute to younger-looking skin.

In addition, everyone can have smoother, more lustrous skin with this simple, twice-a-day program, done in the morning and evening. The first three steps are the same for both times of day…the fourth is different in the morning and evening.

Step 1: Cleanse the skin to remove oils and debris. Doing this also allows the active ingredients in other products to penetrate the skin. Never scrub with a washcloth. Use your fingertips to massage a small amount of cleanser onto the face for 10 to 15 seconds, then rinse with warm water.

Step 2: Apply a toner to a soft, thin cotton makeup pad, and gently wipe. Toner removes leftover debris, along with any cleanser that wasn't removed by rinsing.

Step 3: Use the right active ingredient for your skin-care issues—glycolic acid for brown spots, sulfur for reds, etc.

Step 4 (morning): Apply sunscreen after completing the first three steps but before applying makeup. A sunscreen with an SPF of about 30 is right for most people.

Step 4 (evening): Apply a moisturizer that is right for your skin. An oil-based moisturizer is good for extremely dry skin…a water-and-oil moisturizer is good for "normal" skin…and an oil-free, water-based moisturizer is best for oily skin.

■ ■ ■ ■

Telltale Link?

Psoriasis is linked to heart attack risk. In a study of patients ages 20 to 90, a patient who is 30 years old with severe psoriasis has more than three times the risk of heart attack as a person the same age without psoriasis. Risk also is elevated—but not as much—in older patients and people with mild psoriasis.

Likely link: Both psoriasis and heart disease are associated with high levels of inflammation. If you have psoriasis, ask your doctor to evaluate your risk factors.

Joel M. Gelfand, MD, is medical director of the clinical studies unit and assistant professor of dermatology, University of Pennsylvania School of Medicine, Philadelphia. His study of 130,976 people was published in *The Journal of the American Medical Association.*

■ ■ ■ ■

Psoriasis Relief

Natural remedy for psoriasis, *Reliéva,* a homeopathic product containing Oregon grape extract, reduces skin redness and scaly patches associated with mild-to-moderate psoriasis, reports Mark A. Stengler, ND. Because it has no side effects, Reliéva is worth trying even for severe psoriasis before moving on to stronger treatments. Oregon grapes contain an alkaloid chemical that fights cell proliferation, which is what occurs in psoriasis. Reliéva now is being studied for eczema, too.

Mark A. Stengler, ND, naturopathic physician in private practice, La Jolla, California…adjunct associate clinical professor at the National College of Natural Medicine, Portland, Oregon…author of many books, including *The Natural Physician's Healing Therapies* and coauthor of *Prescription for Natural Cures* (both from Bottom Line Books)…and author of the *Bottom Line/Natural Healing* newsletter.

■ ■ ■ ■

Better Block

New sunscreen protects against UVA rays longer than traditional sunscreens, says Nelson Lee Novick, MD. Anthelios SX, made by L'Oréal, is also effective against UVB rays.

Downside: It costs more than other sunscreens and washes off in water.

However: Sweat doesn't interfere with its effectiveness. It is available at *www.anthelios.com.*

Nelson Lee Novick, MD, is clinical professor of dermatology, Mount Sinai Medical Center, New York City, and author of *Super Skin.* iUniverse.

■ ■ ■ ■

Acne Aid

Over-the-counter acne creams are just as effective for mild to moderate acne as prescription oral antibiotics.

Bonus: Use of topical creams—such as Clearasil and Oxyderm—does not lead to antibiotic resistance.

Hywel C. Williams, PhD, professor of dermatology, University of Nottingham, England, and leader of a study comparing commonly used acne treatments, published in *The Lancet.*

■ ■ ■ ■

Hair Restoration?

Fight hair loss by getting more iron. You normally shed about 100 hairs a day, but if hair comes out in clumps, get screened for iron deficiency. Getting more iron (through diet or supplements) may limit shedding and promote regrowth.

Caution: Do not take supplements without consulting a physician—too much iron can lead to heart disease, liver disease and diabetes.

Leonid Trost, MD, is resident physician in dermatology at Cleveland Clinic, OH, and coauthor of a research review published in *Journal of the American Academy of Dermatology.*

How I Won the War on Toenail Fungus

Dwight Thomas, PhD, a medical writer and former toenail fungus sufferer in Savannah, is author of *The War Against Toenail Fungus,* a book about his battle to cure his own toenail problems. Monterey Square Press.

I contracted toenail fungus and spent nearly four years and several thousand dollars searching for a cure. Eventually, I found a treatment that worked, and my toenails now have been healthy for more than three years.

Millions of Americans suffer from toenail fungus. It's caused by *Trichophyton rubrum* (T. rubrum), the fungus responsible for athlete's foot. Affected toenails thicken and become discolored and crumbly. The nail bed can become so scarred after a few years of infection that the nail won't grow at all. People with diabetes who suffer from toenail fungus face increased risk of ulcerations on the toes and even gangrene.

Older people are more likely to get toenail fungus. Young people's toenails tend to be strong enough to prevent the fungus from getting into the nail bed below. But as we age, our toenails and the surrounding skin are increasingly likely to develop cracks or cuts that offer a point of entry—and the heat and moisture in our shoes allow the fungus to thrive.

Also, some people seem genetically predisposed to the fungus—if you have had athlete's foot, you also may be susceptible to toenail fungus. I had athlete's foot many times before I got toenail fungus.

THE CURE

I tried several different medications. The two most effective are Lamisil tablets and a topical nail lacquer called Penlac. Both are prescription drugs, and they are expensive for those like me who don't have health insurance—a full regimen of either can cost well into the hundreds of dollars.

I tried both medications individually, but my toenail fungus wasn't cured until I used Lamisil and Penlac at the same time for a full year. Studies in Europe have reported success rates as high as 88% for people who combine a systemic treatment (that is, a pill) with a topical treatment.

The good news is that you don't have to use both of these expensive medications each day for the full course of treatment.

Penlac is effective when applied three times a week for the first month, twice a week for the second month and once a week thereafter. Lamisil is effective when taken once each day for the first month, followed by daily doses one week in four thereafter, with three weeks off between. Neither medication has significant side effects for most people, though Lamisil can be dangerous for those suffering from severe liver problems.

If you don't have health insurance and/or aren't willing to spend hundreds of dollars on expensive medications, consider asking your podiatrist to grind the damaged nails down to a normal thickness, a process known as "debridement." I did this. It won't cure the infection, but it can make the nails more presentable and allow shoes to fit more comfortably.

PREVENTION

Take these steps to prevent the fungus, especially if you have had toenail fungus before or you have had athlete's foot and you're past age 40...

•**Apply antifungal powder to your feet each day before you put on your shoes.** Zeasorb Powder (available over-the-counter) is particularly effective, I have found.

•**Choose loose, breathable shoes** such as canvas sneakers or sandals. Avoid tight, pointed shoes as well as leather shoes, such as boots and dress shoes.

Shingles Prevention: New Strategies

Albert Lefkovits, MD, associate clinical professor of dermatology and codirector of the cosmetic dermatological surgery training program at Mount Sinai School of Medicine in New York City, lectures widely at national and international medical conferences.

Few people realize that a severe case of shingles—a viral infection characterized by a rash, blisters and sometimes excruciating pain—can lead to serious complications, such as blindness or hearing impairment.

That's why physicians are doggedly pursuing new ways to prevent shingles, and stressing the importance of early treatment to lessen its severity and duration.

Latest development: This past May, the FDA approved a new vaccine, called Zostavax, that promises to reduce the risk of developing shingles in adults age 60 or older. However, the vaccine may not be appropriate for everyone who is at risk for the condition.

Here's what you need to know...

SIGNS AND SYMPTOMS

Shingles is caused by the varicella-zoster virus, the same virus that causes chicken pox. After an attack of chicken pox (usually in childhood), the virus remains dormant in nerve tissue until it is reactivated by the onset of a serious illness, such as leukemia or lymphoma...weakened immunity, even from a bad cold...or normal aging.

Each year, approximately 1 million Americans develop shingles. The virus primarily attacks people over age 60, but it also can occur in children and teenagers. Half of all people age 80 or older can expect to develop shingles.

The first signs of shingles are easy to miss because they can mimic flu symptoms—chills, fever, nausea, headache, even difficulty urinating. Within a week, the virus spreads to the skin, causing the emergence of fluid-filled blisters in a band on one side of the body. The location of the blisters and pain correlates with the area of skin served by the infected nerve. While the rash and blisters usually appear on the trunk, they can appear on the face, near an eye, in the genital area or anywhere else on the body. The blisters usually dry and begin to scab about five days later. But the pain can continue for weeks, months or even years.

Shingles itself is not contagious. However, anyone who has never had chicken pox can develop chicken pox if he/she is exposed to the live virus in the skin of a shingles patient. The virus primarily is transmitted via direct contact with blisters that haven't completely dried. Airborne transmission, while rare, may occur.

Although the reason is unclear, doctors tend to see multiple patients with shingles at the same time—coinciding with a seasonal outbreak of chicken pox in grade-school children, typically in the fall or spring.

IF SHINGLES IS SUSPECTED

If you suspect that you may have shingles (based on the signs and symptoms already described), you should seek prompt medical attention (within 72 hours) either from your family doctor, a dermatologist or a neurologist.

Antiviral medication, which is generally taken for seven to 10 days, can be an extremely effective treatment for shingles. The antiviral agent *acyclovir* (Zovirax) is now available in a generic form, so it is the least expensive antiviral available. However, some people find acyclovir inconvenient to use because it must be taken five times a day. Both *famciclovir* (Famvir) and *valacyclovir* (Valtrex) can be taken three times a day. They are not available in generic forms and cost about $250 for a seven-day supply. If you start the medication right away, you'll decrease the odds of needing a painkiller later on. Side effects of antivirals may include nausea, headache and diarrhea.

When shingles pain does occur, sufferers describe it as itching, burning or cutting. At its extreme, the pain can be so severe that people contemplate suicide or are willing to undergo radical surgery (which entails cutting the infected nerve's roots) to relieve it. The standard painkillers used for shingles include topical and systemic steroids, the antidepressant *amitriptyline* (Elavil) and the antiseizure drug *gabapentin* (Neurontin).

A NEW VACCINE

As people grow older, their immunity tends to decrease. The new shingles vaccine contains a small dose of a live but weakened varicella-zoster virus. With exposure to the varicella-zoster virus, the recipient's immune system is stimulated to create antibodies against it. This helps protect people who receive the vaccine from developing shingles. The vaccine costs about $150 per dose, not including your physician's fee for the office visit.

Recent finding: In a study of almost 40,000 people age 60 or older, half of whom received a placebo, the vaccine reduced the occurrence of the virus by about 50%. The vaccine reduced postherpetic neuralgia (PHN), extreme nerve pain that can last for months or years after the rash is healed, by 66%. About 20% of shingles patients develop PHN, according to the Varicella-Zoster Virus (VZV) Research Foundation. However, in my experience, the incidence rate and the severity of PHN symptoms have decreased since the introduction of antiviral drugs to treat them.

Who should get the vaccine? That still hasn't been clearly established. The chance for a recurrence is low (about 5%), so people who have already had shingles do not need the shingles vaccine.

Because shingles responds well to treatment when it is initiated within the first 72 hours, I recommend using the new vaccine for adults over age 80 who are generally in good health but very frail. They are most likely to contract shingles and develop PHN.

The studies conducted thus far suggest that the vaccine has only mild side effects, such as redness, pain and tenderness, swelling at the site of the injection, itching and headache. However, many doctors—myself included—are prescribing cautiously because, like other live-virus vaccines used for other conditions, the live varicella-zoster virus can infect others.

Those who are at greatest risk of becoming infected after exposure to a person who has received the varicella-zoster virus vaccine include people with weakened immune systems due to cancer or AIDS and pregnant women, whose fetus could be harmed by a chicken pox infection. Anyone who gets the shingles vaccine should avoid the people mentioned above for about three months following vaccination.

Although doctors are optimistic about the potential of Zostavax, many of us are waiting to see whether widespread use results in yet-unreported adverse side effects.

BEST PAIN RELIEF

Shingles often causes severe pain. In a new survey conducted by the American Pain Foundation, 35% of 401 shingles sufferers reported "severe" pain...11% said it was "very severe"...and 6% called the pain "intolerable" during the first few weeks of the illness.

Dr. Lefkovits recommends...

•**Take an over-the-counter (OTC) painkiller.** Some doctors recommend a nonsteroidal anti-inflammatory drug (NSAID), such as aspirin or *ibuprofen* (Advil), to help curb skin and nerve cell inflammation as well as pain. Because these medications are known to cause stomach problems, I tell most of my shingles patients to try *acetaminophen* (Tylenol). It has little effect on inflammation but is a very effective pain reliever.

To avoid possible liver damage: Do not exceed the maximum daily dose of 4 g (eight extra-strength tablets)—or 2 g daily if you're age 70 or older.

•**Use topical steroids.** Skin inflammation as well as burning and itching can be relieved with OTC creams and lotions that contain hydrocortisone (1%). These treatments can be used up to three times daily and do not cause side effects, such as weight gain, that are generally associated with oral steroids. If you must take oral steroids for an extended period, you should be closely supervised by your doctor.

•**Take warm baths.** Do this several times daily, if necessary. Warm baths are soothing and help relieve pain.

•**Go to a pain clinic.** People who cannot get adequate pain relief on their own should consider going to a pain clinic, where anesthesiologists, neurologists and other specialists will recommend different pain relief methods. Acupuncture also may be helpful.

For more information, contact the Varicella-Zoster Virus (VZV) Research Foundation, 212-222-3390, *www.vzvfoundation.org*.

Surprising Causes of Fungal Infections

John R. Perfect, MD is an infectious disease specialist and professor of medicine at Duke University School of Medicine in Durham, North Carolina. Dr. Perfect is director of Duke's mycology research unit and leads the antibiotic trials unit. He has authored over 250 publications in the field of medical mycology.

Most people blame viruses or bacteria when they get an infection. Fungi is another—often-overlooked—possibility. Fungal infection is more common than most people realize.

Example: *Candida*, a fungus that causes yeast infections, is the fourth most common microorganism found in the blood of hospitalized patients. Candida can infect the mouth, causing white, painful patches on the tongue and inside the cheeks (thrush). In the hospital or during serious illnesses, these mild fungal infections can develop into potentially fatal ones, which can affect the heart or brain.

Fungi are normally present on the skin and in the intestinal tract. Local fungal infections, such as athlete's foot, are common and relatively easy to treat. Mild infections also can occur in the other places that fungi normally inhabit, such as the vagina, mouth, groin area or in fingernails or toenails.

It's rare for someone who's healthy to get a serious fungal infection. Those at greatest risk include people with compromised immune systems, such as hospitalized patients and individuals with diabetes, lung disease, kidney failure, cancer, human immunodeficiency virus (HIV) or some other chronic illness…as well as anyone who has undergone an organ or bone-marrow transplant.

•**How difficult is it to diagnose a fungal infection?** Infections of the skin usually can be diagnosed just by looking at them. *Dermatophytosis* (ringworm), for example, usually appears as scaly, red ring-shaped patches. Systemic infections (that have spread into several organs) usually require taking a sample of body fluid, such as sputum from the lungs or blood, and culturing it in a laboratory and/or examining specimens under a microscope for fungal forms.

Caution: Fungal infection in the lungs can be mistaken for cancer on an X-ray. The only way to distinguish the two is by taking a biopsy.

•**Are fungal infections contagious?** Some fungal infections of the skin, such as ringworm, can be passed from one person to another by sharing towels or clothing or having direct contact with a rash. Most other fungal infections occur when microscopic spores in the air come in contact with the skin or are inhaled. Many fungi reproduce and spread through these microscopic spores.

•**Is there any way to protect yourself from developing a fungal infection?** We live in a virtual "sea of fungi," so it is impossible to avoid them. The vast majority cannot cause disease. The best prevention is for your doctor to be aware of these infections and for you to get treatment early if one develops.

•**Does a skin/nail infection indicate that there's a more serious underlying problem?** Usually not. It's possible that someone with a serious, underlying illness will get a nail or skin fungal infection—but it's unlikely that the infection would be the first sign. The most dangerous fungal infections, such as *aspergillosis* and *cryptococcosis*, tend to occur in patients who are already sick and perhaps undergoing extensive medical treatments. Both of these infections primarily affect the lungs but occasionally spread to other areas of the body.

Someone with cancer or diabetes might be more likely to develop a severe Candida infection because he/she may be in a hospital receiving intravenous antibiotics or chemotherapy, which may allow fungi to proliferate in the body. Although Candida most often causes yeast infections, in more serious cases, it can invade the bloodstream or certain organs.

Some fungal infections may be important warning signs. Therefore, anyone who's getting fungal infections more than twice a year or has an infection that doesn't respond to treatments needs to consider the possibility that his/her immune system isn't working well—and see his doctor right away.

•**Aren't fungal infections difficult to treat?** Fungi are very hard to kill. Like humans, fungi are eukaryotes (single-celled or multicellular organisms whose cells contain a distinct membrane-bound nucleus). This means that we share the same kinds of "cellular machinery." It's difficult to develop drugs that will kill a fungus without killing human cells at the same time. Fungi grow slowly and protect themselves inside host cells. Despite this, there has been great improvement in the drugs we have for invasive fungal infections. However, some antifungal medications can be costly—about $300 for a month's treatment.

Latest development: The newest class of antifungal drugs, known as candins, include *caspofungin* (Cancidas), *micafungin* (Mycamine) and *anidulafungin* (Eraxis), which are used to treat aspergillosis and serious Candida infections. These medications inhibit a component that fungi require to create cell walls. Since human cells don't have that component, they aren't affected by these drugs. Because of this, the candins are less likely to cause toxicity and/or side effects than older antifungal agents, such as polyene drugs, including *amphotericin B* (Fungizone).

Topical antifungal drugs are effective, but they don't necessarily work quickly. It's common for patients with athlete's foot to apply the creams for weeks or months. Treating a nail fungus may require oral antifungal drugs.

•**What happens if a fungal infection goes untreated?** That depends on the severity of the infection. Mild skin fungal infections sometimes clear up on their own—and even if they don't, they may require minimal treatment. A patient with a nail fungus, for example, might choose to ignore it, since the only symptom—usually yellow, green or brown nail discoloration—is cosmetic.

Athlete's foot, jock itch and vaginal yeast infections, on the other hand, can be itchy and uncomfortable. They respond well to over-the-counter topical agents, such as *clotrimazole* (Gyne-Lotrimin or Mycelex) or *miconazole* (Monistat).

An invasive fungal infection, which usually begins in the lungs or bloodstream, can spread rapidly to other parts of the body and always requires treatment. The drugs may be given orally or intravenously. In the highest-risk patients, such as those getting chemotherapy, an antifungal drug can be given prophylactically—that is, to prevent an infection from occurring.

■ ■ ■ ■

Cellulite Creams Don't Work

Clinical experiments have found that anticellulite formulations are no more successful than placebos at reducing cellulite, the fatty dimples that make skin on the hips and thighs appear lumpy. The only treatment proven to temporarily reduce cellulite is *endermologie*—a somewhat painful process in which a suction device squeezes and kneads the affected skin between two rollers. A course of 15 to 20 treatments over several months produces a temporary visible reduction in cellulite. Monthly sessions are required to maintain results. Each treatment can cost up to $125. Some physicians are testing a new procedure called *thermage*, which attempts to eliminate cellulite by the application of heat.

Barney J. Kenet, MD, dermatologic surgeon, NewYork-Presbyterian Hospital/Weill Cornell Medical Center, New York City. Dr. Kenet is the president and founder of the American Melanoma Foundation and coauthored (with his wife, Patricia Lawler) *Saving Your Skin*. Four Walls Eight Windows.

Natural Ways to Protect Your Vision

Mark A. Stengler, ND, naturopathic physician in private practice, La Jolla, California…adjunct associate clinical professor at the National College of Natural Medicine, Portland, Oregon…author of many books, including *The Natural Physician's Healing Therapies* and coauthor of *Prescription for Natural Cures* (both from Bottom Line Books)…and author of the *Bottom Line/Natural Healing* newsletter.

Millions of Americans have lost some or all of their sight to cataracts, glaucoma, macular degeneration and other eye diseases. Medications and surgical procedures can help, but the results are rarely optimal.

Fact: Up to 80% of all diseases can be prevented with natural approaches—and there is evidence that nutritional treatments can halt or even reverse underlying vision problems.

Sun exposure is one of the main causes of vision loss. Everyone should wear sunglasses that block the sun's damaging ultraviolet (UV) rays.

Other measures to combat vision loss include eating certain foods and taking supplements. The antioxidants described below (*lutein, zeaxanthin* and the recommended vitamin supplements) help prevent and treat most eye conditions. The other remedies described can help specific problems. You can take all the supplements listed here (available at health-food stores), but it is always wise to consult with your physician before taking any supplement.

LUTEIN

Spinach, kale and other leafy greens contain an antioxidant called lutein, which reduces damage caused by unstable molecules known as free radicals. Smoking and exposure to UV light are two common sources of free radicals. Decreasing damage from free radicals can reduce the risk of cataracts and macular degeneration.

Recommended: One to two servings of leafy greens daily, or supplement with 15 mg of lutein daily. I usually have my patients take a daily supplement that combines lutein (15 mg) with zeaxanthin (3 mg), another antioxidant. A study of 876 older adults found that those with the highest levels of these antioxidants were less likely to develop age-related macular degeneration.

VITAMINS C & E

Individually, these vitamins are among the most potent antioxidants. Taken together, they're very effective at preventing vision loss. Vitamin E blocks free radicals in the fatty parts of cells, such as in the macula of the eye, while vitamin C fortifies the watery portions in the cornea and retina.

For optimal protection, I recommend to my patients supplements of vitamins C and E, along with zinc and beta-carotene. Patients who take this combination daily can reduce their risk of vision loss. In patients who have age-related macular degeneration, these supplements can slow the disease's progression.

Recommended: Daily supplements with 400 IU of mixed natural vitamin E (a mixture of tocopherols and tocotrienols), 500 mg of vitamin C, 80 mg of zinc and 15 mg of beta-carotene.

GINKGO BILOBA

The herb ginkgo biloba blocks free radicals and dilates blood vessels, increasing circulation to the optic nerve. There is some evidence that it can improve peripheral vision in patients with glaucoma.

Recommended: 120 mg of ginkgo daily. Choose an extract that is standardized to 24% flavone glycosides.

Caution: Do not take a supplement with ginkgo if you are taking a prescription blood-thinning medication, such as *warfarin* (Coumadin).

N-ACETYL CARNOSINE

This naturally occurring molecule is composed of two amino acids.

A recent study found that N-acetyl carnosine (NAC) eyedrops improved visual acuity and glare sensitivity in patients with cataracts. During the two-year study, 90% of the eyes treated with NAC had significant improvements in vision.

Recommended: Patients with cataracts should ask their doctors about using topical NAC drops.

FISH OIL

About half of the retina consists of *docosahexaenoic acid* (DHA), a component in fish oil that provides the main structural support in cell membranes. DHA causes a significant drop in intraocular pressure—important for patients with glaucoma. Another component in fish oil, *eicosapentaenoic acid* (EPA), has anti-inflammatory effects and is thought to play an important role in maintaining visual acuity.

Recommended: Eat fish twice a week. Avoid fish high in mercury, including shark, swordfish, tilefish, king mackerel and large tuna, such as albacore, yellowfin, bigeye and bluefin. Or take a fish-oil formula daily that includes 600 mg of EPA and 400 mg of DHA. Check with your doctor if you are on a blood thinner, such as *warfarin*.

MAGNESIUM AND CHROMIUM

Each of these minerals dilates blood vessels in the eye and reduces pressure from glaucoma. Chromium is particularly important for patients with diabetes, a common cause of vision loss. Chromium supplements help maintain an optimal blood-sugar balance and reduce the risk of glaucoma.

Recommended: Take 250 mg of magnesium (citrate or chelate) and 200 mcg of chromium (polynicotinate or picolinate) twice daily.

DIGESTIVE ENZYMES

Cells in the retina have an extremely high rate of metabolism. They require high levels of nutrients (along with blood and oxygen) for optimal function and to repair normal damage. Older adults often get insufficient nutrients, in part because levels of stomach acid decline with age and impair normal digestion.

Supplements that contain *betaine hydrochloride* mimic the hydrochloric acid normally produced by the stomach and can improve the digestion/absorption of eye-protecting nutrients, which are particularly helpful in the prevention and treatment of macular degeneration.

Recommended: One or two capsules of betaine hydrochloride with each meal.

Also helpful: One or two capsules of a full-spectrum plant-based enzyme (such as Longevity Science Total Gest) during or at the end of meals.

Caution: Patients who have active ulcers should not take digestive enzymes.

Devices Improve Eyesight

Eleanor E. Faye, MD, an ophthalmologist in private practice and ophthalmic surgeon emeritus at the Manhattan Eye, Ear and Throat Hospital in New York City, is the author of Clinical Low Vision. *Little, Brown & Company. Dr. Faye is medical director of Lighthouse International, has two Merit Awards from the American Academy of Ophthalmology, and the Distinguished Service Award from the American Optometric Association.*

Low vision, a permanent vision impairment that cannot be improved by standard eyeglasses, surgery or medical treatment, affects approximately 14 million Americans. Ninety percent of the eye diseases that lead to low vision —macular degeneration, diabetic retinopathy, glaucoma and cataracts accompanied by additional eye problems—occur in people over age 50.

Now: Vision aids—devices that provide magnification, light and/or contrast—can help people with low vision perform tasks that otherwise would be difficult or even impossible. Few doctors prescribe these aids for their patients—so only about 20% to 25% of people with low vision are using them.

GET A PROPER EVALUATION

If you have vision loss due to macular degeneration, diabetic retinopathy, glaucoma or cataracts, it is a good idea to consult an ophthalmologist (a medical doctor who diagnoses and treats eye diseases) or optometrist (a doctor who treats eye conditions not needing surgery) who specializes in low vision.

To find a low-vision specialist in your area, consult the free referral service sponsored by the American Academy of Ophthalmology, the American Optometric Association and Lighthouse International, a not-for-profit organization that provides education, research, advocacy and rehabilitation services, 800-829-0500, *www.lighthouse.org* (click on "Vision Services," then "Find Help Near You").

The doctor will perform a detailed evaluation of your visual function, including your contrast sensitivity and visual field. Based on his/her findings—and your lifestyle needs—the doctor will prescribe vision aids that best suit you. The products most widely used for low vision—including aids that do not require a prescription— are available at Maxi-Aids, 800-522-6294, *www.maxiaids.com*…and Independent Living Aids, 800-537-2118, *www.independentliving.com*.

Best vision aids for the following eye conditions…

MACULAR DEGENERATION

The most common cause of low vision, macular degeneration occurs when the macula (the central part of the retina, which is responsible for sharpness, color and daylight vision) is damaged by gradual degeneration of retinal cells or hemorrhaging of underlying blood cells into the retina.

Best vision aids: Macular degeneration destroys central vision, so magnification is necessary for most people who have this disease. Magnifiers can be handheld ($10 to $150)… placed on a stand ($20 to $150)…or even attached to your television or computer screen ($50 to $200). Tiny telescopes ($50 to $300) that magnify objects ranging from reading distance to far away can be held up to the eye or mounted on eyeglasses (by prescription only) to help you see better at the movies or the opera or while watching television.

Computer screen magnification is available with software such as Zoomware ($150), which enlarges on-screen text up to two times its original size. The software can be purchased at Enable Mart, 888-640-1999, *www.enablemart.com.*

DIABETIC RETINOPATHY

A complication of advanced or long-term diabetes, diabetic retinopathy results in peripheral and central vision loss. It is caused by leaking blood vessels that damage the entire retina, including the macula.

Best vision aids: Diabetic retinopathy affects each individual differently, but most require a variety of aids, such as magnifiers and large-print books and periodicals.

Vision aids that help patients administer insulin are good for those with moderate vision loss from diabetic retinopathy. The Count-a-Dose syringe-filling device ($55) makes a clicking sound that can be heard for each dosage increment. The Magni-Guide Magnifier and Needle Guide ($7.95) magnifies syringe markings and helps guide the syringe needle into an insulin vial.

GLAUCOMA

Increased eye pressure, resulting from a buildup of fluid in the eyes that damages the optic nerves, often leads to the progressive eye disease known as glaucoma. In late-stage glaucoma, the optic nerve damage can cause an irreversible loss of peripheral vision.

Although glaucoma patients typically retain their central vision, it is impaired because their ability to see contrast is significantly reduced. This makes it difficult to distinguish edges, such as those on a curb or steps.

Best vision aids: Good lighting and contrast enhancement are crucial for people with glaucoma. They usually need double or triple the amount of light that a person with normal vision would use. For reading, good options are lighting that simulates the full spectrum of daylight, increasing clarity and reducing glare.

Warning: Regardless of whether you have low vision, never use halogen light for reading. Halogen is fine as an incidental light, but it is too intense as a direct reading light and can potentially damage the retina.

CATARACTS

Although cataracts can be surgically removed, some people must delay or even forgo surgery because of other health problems, such as stroke or a broken hip. For these cataract patients, low-vision aids can be helpful until surgery can be performed.

Best vision aids: Magnification makes reading easier, and polarized sunglasses ($12 to $35) eliminate glare and are helpful for people who have had cataract surgery.

Also helpful: To increase contrast on steps, sinks and bathtubs, mark the edges with brightly colored tape. Reduce glare by installing adjustable blinds on windows and covering shiny surfaces with dark tablecloths or towels.

Protect Your Vision

Melvin Schrier, OD, an optometrist who practiced in New York City for 40 years. A past president of the New York Academy of Optometry, he is now a vision consultant based in Rancho Palos Verdes, California.

Every person over age 45 should have an annual eye exam—even if you don't have any apparent eye problems. Cataracts, macular degeneration and glaucoma often cause no symptoms in the early stages but can be detected with an exam. Our eyes also can indicate hypertension, diabetes and some types of tumors. Even dizziness or clumsiness can be related to an eye disorder.

Schedule a checkup with an optometrist (a doctor of optometry, or OD, who examines, diagnoses, treats and manages eye disorders) or ophthalmologist (a medical doctor, or MD, who specializes in eye diseases and surgery).

GETTING STARTED

Many people experience episodic eye problems that they forget to mention during an exam.

What you can do: Make a list. Is your vision occasionally blurry? You may have cataracts. Do you sometimes feel dizzy? You may have *hyperphoria*, a condition in which one eye sees higher than the other.

Also, don't allow your doctor to depend solely on an intake form that you fill out in the waiting room.

What you can do: Even if your doctor doesn't ask, tell him/her how you use your eyes. Do you golf? Drive? Use a computer? Read a lot?

EYE EXAM

Your doctor should carefully assess the health of your eyes using various instruments, including an ophthalmoscope (an instrument for examining the interior of the eye). The cornea (the front of the eye), the lens (the central part of the eye) and the retina (which consists of nerve tissue and blood vessels at the back of the eye) are evaluated. A cloudy lens may indicate cataracts, and abnormal nerve tissue could suggest diabetes, macular degeneration or, in rare cases, a tumor.

What you can do: If your doctor says that the blood vessels in your eyes are unhealthy, you may have problems in the vessels throughout your body. This could indicate high blood pressure, which could lead to a heart attack or a stroke. See your primary care doctor.

You also should be tested for glaucoma (loss of vision due to abnormally high pressure in the eye). The test measures the pressure in your eyes. Eye pressure of 10 to 18 millimeters of mercury (mm/Hg) is considered normal…25 and higher can indicate glaucoma.

What you can do: If you have a borderline reading of 19 to 24, get your eye pressure rechecked approximately every three months if your doctor doesn't prescribe follow-up care (usually eye drops).

Eye-muscle tests (there are six muscles that move each eye) determine if your eyes are working in tandem. If they are not, you may have eye discomfort or a headache.

What you can do: If your doctor does not perform eye-muscle tests during your exam, ask for them.

VISION EXAM

Your eyes should be tested for near visual acuity (for activities such as reading, sewing and looking at a map)…and distance visual acuity (for driving, watching movies and playing golf). People in their 50s may begin to have trouble with their middle-distance vision (for using a computer, shopping and seeing the dashboard on their cars).

What you can do: Before going to your appointment, measure the distance from your eye to the object you view most frequently from an intermediate distance. Is it 20, 25 or 30 inches away? You may want a pair of glasses for intermediate distance alone. Or you may prefer trifocals (lenses with three vision zones—the top for distance, middle for intermediate distances and the bottom for reading).

Important: If you are not seeing clearly and comfortably within a week of receiving any new vision prescription, insist on a recheck from your doctor.

To locate an optometrist in your area, contact the American Academy of Optometry, *www. aaopt.org.* To find a local ophthalmologist, contact the American Academy of Ophthalmology, *www.aao.org.*

New Treatments to Save Your Sight

Lylas G. Mogk, MD, founding director of the Visual Rehabilitation and Research Center of the Henry Ford Health System in Detroit, and chair of the American Academy of Ophthalmology's Vision Rehabilitation Committee, is coauthor of *Macular Degeneration—The Complete Guide to Saving and Maximizing Your Sight.* Ballantine Books.

The leading cause of vision impairment in adults is age-related macular degeneration (AMD). It's terrifying to think about, much less have.

Good news: In its very early stages, damage from wet AMD can be minimized and new treatments are now available.

AMD is a gradual, progressive eye disease. It affects the macula, which sits at the center of the retina and is responsible for central vision. AMD affects the sight of more adults than glaucoma, cataracts and diabetes combined. One out of 25 Americans over 65—nearly 1.75 million people—already have significant vision loss from AMD, and another 200,000 Americans' vision is significantly affected each year.

HOW IT WORKS

Doctors don't know for sure what causes AMD. But contributing factors include exposure to (nonultraviolet) blue light, which passes through the lens into the retina, where it creates free radicals—destructive, electrically charged particles. (People with blue or light-colored eyes are at greater risk of AMD.) Other stresses that cause free radical formation in the retina include air pollution, pesticides and, particularly, cigarette smoke. Studies have shown that smoking doubles the risk of developing AMD—and living with a smoker increases the risk, even if you don't smoke.

AMD occurs when the layers of tissue beneath the retina—the retinal pigment epithelium (RPE), Bruch's membrane and the third layer, called the choroid—stop functioning properly. The macula's cells then become deprived of oxygen and clogged with waste particles, causing them to die.

Result: Central vision gradually diminishes, making it difficult to read, make out faces or read signs.

Most cases of AMD are the so-called "dry" version, characterized by deposits of small, fatty particles, called drusen, in the macula. Over time, these deposits can enlarge and coalesce, forming a scar in the center of the retina. Ten percent to 15% of people with dry AMD go on to develop "wet" AMD, in which abnormal blood vessels form in the underlying layers and leak fluid into the retina. This fluid reduces vision in and of itself, and also contributes further to cell damage in the macula. Late-stage wet AMD can also cause retinal scarring.

MONITORING AMD

If you get examined every two years after age 40 by an ophthalmologist—as recommended by medical experts—he/she should spot telltale signs of drusen in the macula (indicating early-stage AMD) before any vision loss. The first symptom is often difficulty reading, recognizing faces and seeing in low light or low contrast conditions, such as reading ATM screens or a car dashboard.

If you have AMD, the best tool for checking subtle changes in your central vision is an Amsler grid (right, with instructions).

SELF-CHECK FOR MACULAR DEGENERATION

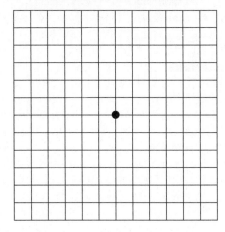

1. Put on your regular reading glasses, and use adequate lighting each time.

2. Cover your right eye, and look only at the dot in the center of the grid.

3. If any lines around the dot appear wavy, choppy or distorted, tell your ophthalmologist immediately.

4. Cover your left eye and repeat the same steps.

Important: See an ophthalmologist every two years.

TREATING WET AMD

The primary treatment for wet AMD used to be photodynamic therapy (PDT), in which a laser is used to cauterize the blood vessels leaking fluid into the retina. This method has been in use for about eight years, and was a big improvement on the older "hot laser" treatment.

How it works: A photosensitive dye is injected into the patient's arm and gravitates to the newly formed blood vessels beneath the retina. A cool laser is then focused on one blood vessel at a time, and the light of the laser activates the dye, causing it to destroy the vessel without damaging the retina—unlike with a hot laser.

While PDT can eliminate existing blood vessels, it can't stop more from forming. So, patients may need to come back for repeated treatments, ranging from every year to as often as every six weeks, depending on frequency of new blood vessel formation.

Your doctor may want a fluorescein angiogram or indocyanine green angiogram (ICG)

547

before laser treatment. These both involve injecting dyes that make the offending blood vessels show up clearly in photographs, allowing the doctor to "map" the blood vessels before treating them.

Good news: Two newly approved drugs can help prevent new blood vessels from forming beneath the retina—Macugen (*pegaptanib sodium*), in use for slightly over a year, and Lucentis (*ranibizumab*), approved by the FDA just a few months ago. Both drugs block the effects of endothelial growth factor, a naturally occurring chemical that triggers the growth of new blood vessels. In the studies, Lucentis did restore some newly lost vision as long as the cells in the macula had not already died. Macugen could stop new vessels from forming but couldn't restore vision.

Avastin (*bevacizumab*), a much cheaper drug currently approved for colorectal cancer, is being used and may work just as well as Lucentis, even though it has not been studied for macular degeneration specifically.

The medication is injected through the white of the eye, with supplemental injections every six to 12 weeks. This is not painful.

Downside: Macugen and Lucentis cost around $2,000 per dose. Although Medicare typically covers 80%, this still leaves the patient with a sizable monthly expense. Avastin, on the other hand, is about $60 per dose.

Latest: Research on gene interference for macular degeneration is currently in clinical trials.

TREATING DRY AMD

For the 85% of patients with dry AMD, the progression of the disease is slower, but vision loss can eventually become significant. About 20% of people with dry AMD develop a blind spot in the shape of a ring or donut at the center of their vision. While dry AMD can't be reversed, trials are under way to see if its progress can be slowed by using low-intensity lasers to destroy the drusen particles in the retina. One preliminary study found that when 64 patients had their drusen lasered, progression of dry AMD was halted for at least two years.

THE RIGHT NUTRITION

Evidence also suggests that nutritional supplements can help. A large National Institutes of Health study found that loss of visual acuity was slowed in 30% of people who had either wet or dry AMD who took the following combination of over-the-counter nutrients each day—25,000 international units (IU) beta carotene (only recommended for non-smokers), 500 milligrams (mg) vitamin C, 400 IU vitamin E, 80 mg zinc and 2 mg copper. This full combination is sold in pill form. Ask your doctor.

Other studies suggest that progression of wet and dry AMD may be slowed by taking six grams to 20 grams per day of lutein—a nutrient, found mainly in kale, that's active in the retina—and 1,000 mg daily of the omega-3 fatty acids DHA and EPA (contained in fish oil and flaxseed oil). I recommend taking daily capsules of both lutein and either fish oil or flaxseed oil, since it's difficult to eat enough kale or oily fish each day to get the needed amounts.

Also promising are dried wolfberries, available in some health food stores and on-line. I recommend sprinkling a handful each day into dry cereal or oatmeal. These berries, taken for centuries by the Chinese for eye health, contain high amounts of zeaxanthin, a nutrient similar to lutein that's particularly active in the macula.

PROTECTING YOUR RETINA

Finally, in addition to the precautions listed earlier, you should wear sunglasses that screen out ultraviolet (UV) rays to protect against cataracts. For protection against AMD, use amber, orange or yellow tints to screen out blue light, which contributes to damage to the retina. Those tints also provide high contrast.

KEEP LIVING FULLY!

It's important to keep up your normal activities. Vision rehabilitation—training and counseling to maximize existing sight—can help.

For services in your area, visit Lighthouse International (800-829-0500, *www.lighthouse.org*).

■ ■ ■ ■

Beware of Glare

Open wide—squinting causes itchy, tired, dry eyes.

Reason: It reduces blinking, which allows eyes to rewet themselves with tears and reduces eyestrain. Even slight squinting can cut blinking rates by half. Many computer users squint while looking at the screen.

To reduce squinting: Reduce glare by positioning monitors so windows are to the side, not behind…use lower-wattage bulbs in lamps.

James E. Sheedy, OD, PhD, dean of Pacific University's College of Optometry, Forest Grove, Oregon, and leader of a study of computer users, published in *Optometry and Vision*.

The Whys of Dry Eyes— And How to Get Relief

J. Daniel Nelson, MD, professor of ophthalmology at the University of Minnesota in Minneapolis.

A healthy adult produces tears every minute during waking hours. Tears protect and lubricate the surfaces of the eyes (corneas), remove dust and other particles, and flush out inflammatory chemicals that accumulate when the eyes are irritated.

But about 15% of Americans over age 65 suffer from dry eyes. The problem occurs most often after age 50, as our tear production declines with age. Symptoms of dry eyes include stinging or burning sensations…eye fatigue when reading…mucus in or around the eyes…or the sensation that there's sand or gravel in the eyes.

What most people don't know: Tears help people see. By spreading across the eye surface to create a "tear film," tears work in tandem with the cornea to provide the major optical surface. That's why long-distance vision may be impaired in people who have chronic dry eyes.

If you think you have dry eyes, see an ophthalmologist (a medical doctor who specializes in eye diseases and surgery). He/she usually can diagnose dry eyes after taking a medical history and noting your symptoms. There may not be a cure for dry eyes, but treatment can minimize discomfort and help protect your vision.

CAUSES OF DRY EYES

Tears are composed of 90% water and small amounts of salts or electrolytes and proteins that are secreted by the lacrimal glands located at the top outer edge of each eye. Tears also contain mucus and blood fats (lipids) produced by the *meibomian glands* located on the edge of the eyelids.

Main causes of dry eyes…

•**Blepharitis.** This inflammation of the eyelids is often caused by a blockage of the lipid-producing meibomian glands or by the secretion of oils that are unusually thick and don't flow properly.

•**Medications.** Many prescription and over-the-counter (OTC) drugs cause dry eyes.

Main offenders: Antihistamines, decongestants, diuretics and some antidepressants, such as *amitriptyline* (Elavil). If you experience dry eyes after starting a new medication, talk to your doctor about alternatives.

•**Inflammation.** When allergies or exposure to environmental irritants, such as dust or wind, or chemicals found in household cleaning products irritate the eyes, cells release inflammatory chemicals called cytokines. In normal eyes, the flow of tears dilutes the concentration of inflammatory cytokines and may counteract their effect, thereby reducing irritation. But in allergy sufferers and other people with chronic inflammation, there aren't enough tears to dilute the cytokines. Treating allergies or other sources of eye irritation may eliminate dry eyes—but not always.

•**Sjögren's syndrome.** This autoimmune disease occurs when a person's antibodies damage the lacrimal glands, which reduces tear production. Drug treatments for Sjögren's help relieve dry eyes, but do not cure them.

DIAGNOSIS AND TREATMENTS

If you've been diagnosed with dry eyes, here are the best ways to treat the condition…

•**Lubricate the eyes.** Patients who experience only mild dryness of the eyes usually can get relief by using "artificial tears" one to four times daily. These OTC products are available in liquid and gel forms. Both are equally effective.

Caution: The preservatives, such as benzalkonium chloride, added to many products can damage eye cells if used more than four times daily.

For more frequent use, choose a preservative-free product, such as Refresh Liquigel, Systane or Tears Naturale Free, or one with a "vanishing preservative," such as GenTeal. The preservative disappears as soon as the drops come into contact with the tear film.

•**Reduce inflammation.** People with inflammatory conditions, including Sjögren's syndrome, may require anti-inflammatory medications to diminish dryness. Steroid or immunosuppressant eye drops, such as *cyclosporine* (Restasis), control the inflammation response and significantly reduce dry eye symptoms in many patients. These drugs are typically used for a few months to several years.

Caution: Because topical steroids can cause an increase in eye pressure and cataracts, patients must have their eye pressure measured monthly while using these drops.

•**Wear "moisture chamber" eyeglasses.** They are designed to create a high-humidity environment by fitting snugly to prevent moisture in the eyes from evaporating. They also minimize exposure to wind or dust. Some patients can get by with tight-fitting, wrap-around sunglasses. If these don't help, an eye-care professional can make special moisture-chamber glasses.

Cost: As high as $250 in addition to the cost of the lenses and frames. Many insurance policies pay for them.

Also helpful: Put a humidifier or vaporizer beside your bed, desk or any area where you spend a lot of time.

•**Practice blinking.** Four times a day, blink 20 times. Many people with dry eyes experience subconscious discomfort when they blink—as a result, they get in the habit of not blinking completely. Blinking is essential because it causes the eyes to secrete protective oils...wipes away dead skin cells...and increases tear production.

•**Take an omega-3 supplement.** The omega-3 fatty acids found in cold-water fish and flaxseed have anti-inflammatory effects and often reduce eye dryness. Because it can be difficult to get adequate amounts of these essential fatty acids in your diet, I recommend taking TheraTears Nutrition or ProOmega capsules, formulas that contain a good mix of fatty acids for eye health. Such products are usually found in the eye-care section of pharmacies. Take two capsules twice daily.

If your dry eyes don't improve enough with these therapies, you may be advised to undergo *punctal occlusion*, a simple outpatient procedure in which the tear drainage ducts are either sealed with silicone plugs or permanently closed. This causes tears to remain in the eyes longer and can reduce dry eye symptoms by up to 50%. Possible side effects include watery eyes and increased inflammation.

Caution: This procedure should only be done if your doctor determines there is no eye inflammation. Otherwise, inflammatory chemicals stay in contact with the eyes longer and *increase* irritation.

■ ■ ■ ■

Cataract Breakthrough

New lens implants allow people with cataracts to see near, far and in between, we hear from Gina Gladstein, MD. Previous lenses corrected for either distance or reading. Multifocal intraocular implants could cost from $2,000 to $3,000 more per eye than traditional ones. Health insurers pay only up to the cost of traditional implants.

Gina Gladstein, MD, is section head of ophthalmology, Greenwich Hospital, Greenwich, Connecticut.

■ ■ ■ ■

Children's Vision

Distance glasses can worsen nearsightedness in children. They are prescribed routinely by some doctors when children start to become nearsighted. Some children can become nearsighted because they spend excessive time on computers or playing video games. That can cause eyestrain and focusing problems. Most nearsightedness (myopia), however, is genetic in nature. Doctors often prescribe distance lenses to clear the blur, but the lenses may aggravate the problem by bringing everything closer, forcing the child's vision to refocus and strain. This may lead to a need for stronger lenses every year or two. If other visual tests show that the eyes are under stress, children should be given nearpoint, or "plus," lenses for reading, using the computer and playing video games. Reading

550

lenses tend to push things farther away, allowing the focusing muscles to relax.

Also: Don't be afraid of bifocals for children if your optometrist recommends them—they can play a big part in limiting myopic changes.

Melvin Schrier, OD, an optometrist who practiced in New York City for 40 years. A past president of the New York Academy of Optometry, he is now a vision consultant based in Rancho Palos Verdes, California.

■ ■ ■ ■

Contact Lens Risk

Contact lenses can increase the risk of eye infections.

Recent finding: One of every 2,500 contact lens wearers will develop an infection.

Especially risky: Wearing contacts while sleeping—they impede the flow of oxygen to corneas.

If you don't often remove your lenses before bed: Switch to the new silicone hydrogel lenses, which allow more oxygen to reach the eyes and reduce risk of infection fivefold over traditional lenses.

Thomas Steinemann, MD, associate professor of ophthalmology, Case Western Reserve University, and cornea and external eye disease specialist, MetroHealth Medical Center, both in Cleveland.

■ ■ ■ ■

Carbs Can Cause Cataracts!

Carbohydrates can increase the chances of developing cataracts.

Recent study: People who consumed 200 grams or more per day of any kind of carbohydrate for more than 14 years had more than twice the risk of developing cataracts as those who consumed the USDA-recommended 130 grams per day. Carbohydrates are found in such foods as bread, cookies, white potatoes and rice.

Theory: The excess glucose liberated within the body from the digestion of dietary carbohydrates may damage proteins in the lens of the eye and lead to cataracts.

Allen Taylor, PhD, professor of nutrition, biochemistry and ophthalmology, USDA Human Nutrition Research Center on Aging, Tufts University, Boston, and leader of a study of 417 women, published in *The American Journal of Clinical Nutrition*.

■ ■ ■ ■

Glaucoma Link

High blood pressure and glaucoma may be related.

Recent study: Among people with glaucoma, 29% also had high blood pressure—a significantly higher percentage than in the population as a whole. If you have hypertension, watch your weight, eat healthful foods, exercise regularly and ask your doctor about medication.

Michael J. S. Langman, MD, professor of medicine, University of Birmingham, Queen Elizabeth Hospital, Birmingham, England.

■ ■ ■ ■

Eye Strain

New animated 3-D films can cause eye pain, headaches and visual discomfort in children and adults. Watching a 3-D movie can be stressful to the eyes if a person's prescription is significantly different in one eye than the other. Images do not fuse easily or at all, causing the brain to use extra effort to focus.

Melvin Schrier, OD, an optometrist who practiced in New York City for 40 years. A past president of the New York Academy of Optometry, he is now a vision consultant based in Rancho Palos Verdes, California.

Natural Cures for Nasal Congestion

Jamison Starbuck, ND, a naturopathic physician in family practice in Missoula, Montana. She is past president of the American Association of Naturopathic Physicians.

When cold weather arrives, decongestants and boxes of tissue are familiar standbys for people with stuffy, runny noses. The common cold is often the culprit. With a cold, the nose can become congested as the body tries to eliminate the virus that is causing the illness. But there are other irritants that also cause nasal congestion. *Fortunately, you can get at the root cause of your nasal congestion and avoid taking decongestants, which only temporarily mask symptoms, by following these steps...*

•**Identify respiratory irritants.** One of my patients recently complained of congestion when she vacuumed her house. Although she has a cat, she claimed to not be allergic since she does not sneeze or get congested when she spends time with her pet. As an experiment, I asked her to visit a friend who doesn't have pets and spend a little time vacuuming. When she did not become congested, my patient agreed that the cat dander released in the air from the vacuum could be the problem. A simple dust mask worn while vacuuming prevented any other bouts of congestion. Dust masks made of paper (less than $1 each) work nicely for reducing sneezing and/or runny noses triggered by dust, pollen, pet dander, smoke, grass, hay or fallen leaves. If potentially harmful vapors, such as fumes from paint, varnish or cleaning compounds, bother your nose, use a carbon-filtration mask, available in paint stores from $40–$42. They trap vapors, removing them from the air breathed.

•**Test for food allergies.** If you're chronically congested, or regularly get a stuffy nose after eating, ask your doctor for a food allergy blood test to check for IgG-mediated—or delayed sensitivity—food allergens. These allergies cause generalized inflammation, leading to congestion.

Most common food allergens: Dairy, wheat, peanuts and soy.

•**Eat the right foods.** To soothe and strengthen the mucous membranes of your nose and upper-respiratory tract, eat lots of *proanthocyanidins*, a type of plant pigment with anti-inflammatory, antiviral and antiallergenic properties. Blueberries, blackberries, Marion berries or raspberries (fresh or frozen) are great sources of proanthocyanidins. If you suffer from chronic nasal congestion, eat one-half cup daily.

•**Drink hot tea.** For a gentle decongestant, try a tea made from equal parts dried linden, elder and chamomile flowers. Combine the herbs and use three teaspoons of the mix per 10 ounces of boiling water. Steep, covered, for 10 minutes. Strain and flavor the tea with honey and lemon, if desired. Drink one cup twice daily until congestion is eliminated.

•**Use a neti pot.** In Ayurvedic (Indian) medicine, neti pots, which cost less than $20 and resemble small watering cans, are used to pour a saline solution through each nostril, to reduce congestion. You can buy saline solution at drugstores or make your own (follow the instructions that accompany the pot). Use once or twice daily —upon waking and/or at bedtime, when congested or exposed to allergens.

■ ■ ■ ■

Hearing Loss

Hearing loss may be caused by the brain, not the ears. In some older people, when sound reaches the brain, it is not processed correctly due to various factors, including aging itself. Specialized hearing tests can determine where the problem occurs.

Robert D. Frisina, PhD, associate chair for research and professor, otolaryngology department, University of Rochester Medical Center, Rochester, New York.

Sudden Hearing Loss: The Symptom You Should Never Ignore

Gordon B. Hughes, MD, professor and head of the otology and neurotology section of the Head and Neck Institute at Cleveland Clinic. Dr. Hughes is coeditor of a landmark book, *Clinical Otology*. Thieme Medical Publishers.

Don't confuse a temporary, normal loss of hearing—the kind you get from a head cold or an airplane's descent—with sudden hearing loss (SHL), in which your hearing gets worse over a few hours or days without an obvious cause. SHL is an emergency that can result in permanent ear damage. SHL usually affects just one ear. Approximately half of patients with SHL also experience dizziness, light-headedness, a sensation of spinning and/or ringing in the ear (tinnitus).

•**See a doctor immediately.** The optimal window for treatment is within two weeks. About one-third of SHL patients experience significant improvement if they are treated within this period. Even with rapid treatment, however, less than 20% of patients return completely to normal.

It's estimated that more than 80 conditions can cause SHL. *Main causes…*

VIRAL INFECTIONS

Viruses, particularly the herpes viruses, can cause SHL. Mumps, measles and chicken pox/shingles viruses have been linked to SHL. A viral infection affecting the inner ear can cause inflammation that damages the *organ of Corti*, the structure that generates hearing impulses and sends them to the brain.

Red flag: SHL accompanied by a cold sore may be due to the *herpes simplex* virus. SHL patients who also have herpes symptoms may be treated with antiviral drugs, such as *acyclovir* (Zovirax), *valacyclovir* (Valtrex) or *famciclovir* (Famvir)—but it's not known for sure if antivirals affect the outcome of SHL.

Primary treatment: Oral *prednisone* for 10 to 14 days. About one-third of patients given this powerful anti-inflammatory steroid experience significant improvement, even if the underlying causes are not known. It's a first-line treatment for most cases of SHL. Side effects can include excitability, increased appetite, increased urination and facial flushing.

New treatment: A national study is under way to determine whether inner-ear injections of *methylprednisolone*, a prednisone-like drug, work as well as, or better than, oral treatments for SHL.

CIRCULATORY PROBLEMS

The cochlea, a snail-shaped structure in the inner ear that translates sound vibrations into signals to the brain, requires a steady flow of blood. Reductions in blood flow can disrupt cochlear function in as little as one hour.

Treatment: People who have circulatory disorders may be given drugs to improve circulation—as well as prednisone.

ACOUSTIC NEUROMA

About 3% of SHL cases are caused by a slow-growing, noncancerous tumor (neuroma) that puts pressure on the acoustic nerve. It is not known why hearing loss is sudden when the tumor is slow-growing.

SHL accompanied by dizziness, tinnitus and/or unsteadiness may be due to a neuroma. An MRI of the brain stem and hearing nerve will show if an acoustic neuroma is present. Hearing loss caused by a neuroma usually can't be reversed. Treatment is recommended if the tumor continues to grow…hearing loss gets progressively worse…or other symptoms are present. Otherwise, your doctor may recommend watchful waiting—having an MRI once or twice a year to check the neuroma's progress.

Treatment: Surgery or radiation therapy.

EXCESSIVE FLUID

Fluid buildup in the inner ear is usually due to Meniere's disease, in which excessive fluid causes fluctuating SHL along with vertigo and balance difficulties. Meniere's disease can be diagnosed from a health history (two or more episodes of vertigo lasting at least 20 minutes…ringing in the ears…and hearing loss), along with a hearing test and electronystagmography (ENG), a diagnostic test that evaluates balance by detecting abnormal eye movements.

Treatment: Most patients are put on a low-salt diet and given diuretics for 10 to 14 days. Those with Meniere's disease continue treatments indefinitely.

EARWAX

Some SHL cases are caused by compacted wax in the ear canal.

Common cause: Cleaning inside the canal with a cotton swab. Wax naturally migrates from the inner to the outer canal. Cleaning inside the canal pushes wax downward and compresses it into a plug that prevents sound waves from reaching the eardrum.

Treatment: Over-the-counter solutions containing *hydrogen peroxide* or *carbamyl peroxide* soften wax and make it easier to flush out with a bulb irrigator. If home treatments don't help, the wax has to be removed by a doctor with a curette (a small metal loop at the end of a metal handle) or a suction device.

MEDICATION SIDE EFFECTS

Approximately 200 drugs can cause SHL, including aspirin, quinine and the aminoglycoside antibiotics *gentamicin* and *neomycin* (usually prescribed for serious infections and given intravenously). SHL caused by these "ototoxic" drugs can range from mild to severe—and may be permanent in some cases.

Red flag: Hearing loss that occurs in both ears simultaneously following the use of these or other medications.

Hearing can improve when patients discontinue or take lower doses of certain drugs. The risk of permanent hearing loss is higher with aminoglycoside antibiotics.

■ ■ ■ ■

Ear Infections

Kids with recurrent ear infections may benefit from seeing an osteopathic physician (DO) trained to perform osteopathic manipulation to relieve pressure in the eustachian tube. Osteopaths are licensed to practice medicine just as MDs are.

Recent study: Children who received osteopathic manipulations in addition to routine care—antibiotics, ibuprofen, ear tubes, etc.—had fewer ear infections and were less likely to need antibiotics or surgery than ones given routine pediatric care only.

Miriam V. Mills, MD, pediatrician in private practice in Tulsa, Oklahoma.

■ ■ ■ ■

Hearing Aid News

Invisible hearing aids are here, says Paul Pessis, AuD. *Completely in the Canal* models fit deeply into the ear. The microphone picks up less wind noise than other hearing aids do. Controls can be hard to adjust, but some models come with remote controls. Open ear fit models are placed behind the ear and are barely noticeable. In *Behind the Ear* (BTE) models, the casing is concealed by hair. Sound ID (866-768-6343, *www.soundid.com*) makes a unit that doubles as a wireless cell-phone headset.

Paul Pessis, AuD, is past president of the American Academy of Audiology, Reston, Virginia, and founder of North Shore Audio-Vestibular Lab, Highland Park, Illinois.

■ ■ ■ ■

Easier Dentistry

Afraid of the dentist? Some dentists with special training now use sedation pills, such as *triazolam*, to treat patients who are afraid of having dental work done. The pills lead to conscious sedation—relaxation so deep that even patients with strong fear of the dentist can relax while work is being done. Such sedation does not reduce pain, so there is still a need for a local anesthetic, such as novocaine.

For information, contact Dental Organization for Conscious Sedation, 877-325-3627, *www.sedationdocs.com*.

Matt Smith, DDS, The Center for Esthetic Dentistry, Commack, New York.

■ ■ ■ ■

Quick Fixes for Tooth Trouble

Consider these temporary fixes for dental problems.

If a tooth is sensitive to cold or sweets: Rinse with warm water.

If you have swelling from an injury: Apply ice—a half-hour on, a half-hour off.

If swelling is from infection: Apply a heating pad or hot washcloth, or hold hot salty water in your mouth—the heat stimulates blood flow to the area, which helps remove toxins.

If you lose a filling: Rinse your mouth with warm water and place cotton dipped in oil of cloves in the cavity—the clove oil eases pain.

If a crown pops off: Use denture adhesive or tooth cement—available at most drugstores—to reattach it temporarily. See a dentist as soon as possible for any of these problems.

Irwin Smigel, DDS, president and founder, American Society for Dental Aesthetics, and a dentist in private practice, New York City.

■ ■ ■ ■

Filling Alert

Mercury fillings are not safe, despite recent reports that they are, warns naturopathic physician Mark A. Stengler, ND. Studies at the University of Calgary have found that mercury vapor from fillings enters the body and may cause brain-cell degeneration and immune suppression, among other problems.

Self-defense: Have your dentist use mercury-free white composite fillings, and try to have existing amalgam ones replaced over time by a "biological dentist."

Mark A. Stengler, ND, naturopathic physician in private practice, La Jolla, California…adjunct associate clinical professor at the National College of Natural Medicine, Portland, Oregon…author of many books, including *The Natural Physician's Healing Therapies* and coauthor of *Prescription for Natural Cures* (both from Bottom Line Books)…and author of the *Bottom Line/Natural Healing* newsletter.

Natural Ways to Care for Your Gums

Jamison Starbuck, ND, a naturopathic physician in family practice in Missoula, Montana. She is past president of the American Association of Naturopathic Physicians.

For years, I've observed that far too many otherwise health-conscious people neglect their oral health. That's a mistake. Gum (periodontal) disease occurs in 50% of people over age 55. Even though we all know the importance of regular brushing and flossing, it often takes more than conventional tooth and gum care to keep our mouth tissues healthy. The mildest form of periodontal disease is gingivitis. This inflammatory condition, which is primarily caused by poor oral hygiene, typically leads to red, swollen gum tissue that often bleeds.

If you have these symptoms, see your dentist for a checkup. If you've got periodontal disease, and it is left untreated, surgery may be needed. The first step I recommend is to reduce your sugar intake. Sugar increases plaque formation and feeds the harmful bacteria that dwell in your gums.

Taking the right nutritional supplements also can help reverse gingivitis, often within three months. This could eliminate the need for costly periodontal surgery. *My favorite supplements for gum health…*

•**Vitamin C.** It strengthens gum tissue and enhances your white blood cells' ability to fight inflammation-promoting microorganisms in your mouth. To restore gum health, take 3,000 mg daily in divided doses for three months. If this amount of vitamin C causes diarrhea, cut back on the dose. If you have high iron levels, do not take a vitamin C supplement—it increases iron absorption. For healthy gum maintenance, take 1,500 mg of vitamin C daily.

•**Zinc.** Like vitamin C, zinc improves gum health by enhancing white blood cell activity. This mineral also inhibits plaque buildup (which increases inflammation) and speeds the healing of bleeding gums. To treat gingivitis, take 40 mg of zinc daily for three months. For healthy gum maintenance, take a daily dose of 20 mg of zinc.

•**Folate.** A deficiency of this B vitamin is common and increases risk for gingivitis. To treat gingivitis, add a daily dose of 1 mg of folic acid along with 500 micrograms (mcg) of vitamin B-12 to your supplement regimen for three months. Taking folic acid alone can mask a possible B-12 deficiency. Bleeding gums also improve with a 0.1% solution of liquid folic acid, which is available at health-food stores. Brush your teeth, then swish one-half ounce of the solution in your mouth twice daily for 60 seconds and then spit it out. For optimal gum absorption, do not eat or drink anything for at least 15 minutes after swishing. To maintain gum health, take 800 mcg of folic acid along with 400 mcg of vitamin B-12 daily.

•**Coenzyme Q10.** This powerful antioxidant helps our cells function efficiently. Studies show that CoQ10 not only protects the heart and brain, but also the gums. For periodontal disease, take 100 mg of CoQ10 daily for three months. Take 60 mg for gum maintenance. It is available wherever vitamins are sold.

Good Oral Health Lowers Risk for Heart Disease, Arthritis, Cancer and More

Robert J. Genco, DDS, PhD, distinguished professor in the department of oral biology, School of Dental Medicine, and in the department of microbiology, School of Medicine and Biomedical Sciences at the State University of New York at Buffalo. He is also a professor in the department of immunology at the Roswell Park Cancer Institute and a recipient of the American Dental Association's Gold Medal for Excellence in Research.

Until recently, most people who took good care of their teeth and gums did so to ensure appealing smiles and to perhaps avoid dentures. Now, a significant body of research shows that oral health may play a key role in preventing a wide range of serious health conditions, including heart disease, diabetes, some types of cancer and perhaps even dementia.

Healthy teeth and gums also may improve longevity. Swedish scientists recently tracked 3,273 adults for 16 years and found that those with chronic gum infections were significantly more likely to die before age 50, on average, than were people without gum disease.

What's the connection? Periodontal disease (called *gingivitis* in mild stages…and *periodontitis* when it becomes more severe) is caused mainly by bacteria that accumulate on the teeth and gums. As the body attempts to battle the bacteria, inflammatory molecules are released (as demonstrated by redness and swelling of the gums). Over time, this complex biological response affects the entire body, causing systemic inflammation that promotes the development of many serious diseases. *Scientific evidence links poor oral health to…*

•**Heart disease.** At least 20 scientific studies have shown links between chronic periodontal disease and an increased risk for heart disease.

Most recently, Boston University researchers found that periodontal disease in men younger than age 60 was associated with a twofold increase in angina (chest pain), or nonfatal or fatal heart attack, when compared with men whose teeth and gums are healthy.

•**Diabetes.** State University of New York at Buffalo studies and other research show that people with diabetes have an associated risk for periodontitis that is two to three times greater than that of people without diabetes. Conversely, diabetics with periodontal disease generally have poorer control of their blood sugar than diabetics without periodontal disease—a factor that contributes to their having twice the risk of dying of a heart attack and three times the risk of dying of kidney failure.

•**Cancer.** Chronic gum disease may raise your risk for tongue cancer. State University of New York at Buffalo researchers recently compared men with and without tongue cancer and found that those with cancer had a 65% greater loss of alveolar bone (which supports the teeth)—a common measure of periodontitis. Meanwhile, a Harvard School of Public Health study shows that periodontal disease is associated with a 63% higher risk for pancreatic cancer.

•**Rheumatoid arthritis.** In people with rheumatoid arthritis, the condition is linked to an 82% increased risk for periodontal disease, compared with people who do not have rheumatoid arthritis.

Good news: Treating the periodontitis appears to ease rheumatoid arthritis symptoms. In a recent study, nearly 59% of patients with rheumatoid arthritis and chronic periodontal disease who had their gums treated experienced less severe arthritis symptoms—possibly because eliminating the periodontitis reduced their systemic inflammation.

•**Dementia.** When Swedish researchers recently reviewed dental and cognitive records for 638 women, they found that tooth loss (a sign of severe gum disease) was linked to a 30% to 40% increased risk for dementia over a 32-year period, with the highest dementia rates suffered by women who had the fewest teeth at middle age. More research is needed to confirm and explain this link.

DO YOU HAVE GUM DISEASE?

At least half of adults over age 55 have gum (periodontal) disease, inflammation of the soft tissues (gums) surrounding the teeth. It results primarily from the accumulation of plaque (a sticky substance comprised mainly of bacteria) around the teeth and along the gum line.

What to watch for…

•**Red, swollen gums that bleed easily during brushing or flossing.**

•**A change in the appearance of your teeth.**

•**Chronic bad breath.**

•**Gum recession (loss of gum tissue at the base of a tooth).**

Important: With advanced gum disease, gums seldom bleed because they become firmer due to the disease.

STEPS TO IMPROVE YOUR ORAL HEALTH

Even though the rate of gum disease significantly increases with age, it's not inevitable. To promote oral health, brush (twice daily with a soft-bristled brush, using gentle, short strokes starting at a 45-degree angle to the gums) and floss (once daily, using gentle rubbing motions —do not snap against the gums). *In addition…*

•**See your dentist at least twice yearly.** Ask at every exam, "Do I have gum disease?" This will serve as a gentle reminder to dentists that you want to be carefully screened for the condition. Most mild-to-moderate infections can be treated with a nonsurgical procedure that removes plaque and tartar from tooth pockets and smooths the root surfaces. For more severe periodontal disease, your dentist may refer you to a periodontist (a dentist who specializes in the treatment of gum disease).

Note: Patients with gum disease often need to see a dentist three to four times a year to prevent recurrence of gum disease after the initial treatment.

Good news: Modern techniques to regenerate bone and soft tissue can reverse much of the damage and halt progression of periodontitis, particularly in patients who have lost no more than 30% of the bone to which the teeth are attached.

•**Boost your calcium intake.** Research conducted at the State University of New York at Buffalo has shown that postmenopausal women with osteoporosis typically have more alveolar bone loss and weaker attachments between their teeth and bone, putting them at substantially higher risk for periodontal disease. Other studies have linked low dietary calcium with heightened periodontal risk in both men and women.

Self-defense: Postmenopausal women, and men over age 65, should consume 1,000 mg to 1,200 mg of calcium daily to preserve teeth and bones. Aim for two to three daily servings of dairy products (providing a total of 600 mg of calcium), plus a 600-mg calcium supplement with added vitamin D for maximum absorption.

Helpful: Yogurt may offer an edge over other calcium sources. In a recent Japanese study involving 942 adults, ages 40 to 79, those who ate at least 55 grams (about two ounces) of yogurt daily were 40% less likely to suffer from severe periodontal disease—perhaps because the "friendly" bacteria and calcium in yogurt make a powerful combination against the infection-causing bacteria of dental disease.

•**Control your weight.** Obesity is also associated with periodontitis, probably because fat cells release chemicals that may contribute to inflammatory conditions anywhere in the body, including the gums.

•**Don't ignore dry mouth.** Aging and many medications, including some antidepressants, antihistamines, high blood pressure drugs and steroids, can decrease saliva flow, allowing plaque to build up on teeth and gums. If you're taking a drug that leaves your mouth dry, talk to your doctor about possible alternatives. Prescription artificial saliva products—for example, Caphosol or Numoisyn—also can provide some temporary moistening, as can chewing sugarless gum.

•**Relax.** Recent studies reveal a strong link between periodontal disease and stress, depression, anxiety and loneliness. Researchers are focusing on the stress hormone *cortisol* as a possible culprit—high levels of cortisol may exacerbate the gum and jawbone destruction caused by oral infections.

•**Sleep.** Japanese researchers recently studied 219 factory workers for four years and found that those who slept seven to eight hours nightly suffered significantly less periodontal disease progression than those who slept six hours or less. The scientists speculated that lack of sleep lowers the body's ability to fend off infections. However, more research is needed to confirm the results of this small study.

■ **More from Robert J. Genco, DDS...**

If You Dread Going To the Dentist

Studies show that up to 20% of Americans suffer "dental anxiety"—many to the point of avoidance.

To overcome this problem, find a dentist who makes you feel comfortable. *Then...*

•**Don't delay seeing your dentist** for tooth or gum problems. Generally, earlier diagnosis means less troublesome and more successful treatment.

•**Schedule appointments** for times when you won't be harried or rushed.

•**Admit that you're anxious.** In a study conducted by researchers at the University of Liverpool School of Dentistry, highly anxious patients who told their dentists about their fears at the beginning of the appointment experienced significantly less anxiety during treatment than patients who kept mum.

•**If you have sensitive teeth,** request a topical numbing agent, such as Oraqix, before cleanings or other procedures.

•**Ask about using a throat-numbing spray** if a strong gag reflex makes getting dental impressions or X-rays difficult.

•**Agree on a hand signal** that you can use to alert the dentist when you need to take a break.

•**Consider conscious sedation.** If you're extremely anxious or need extensive work, consult a dentist who specializes in "relaxation" dentistry. He/she may prescribe a tranquilizer, such as *diazepam* (Valium), and/or sedative, such as *triazolam* (Halcion), to be taken prior to (and/or during) your visit.

Important: Many states require dentists to meet certain requirements, including at least 18 hours of training, before using conscious sedation in their practices.

■ ■ ■ ■

Raisins Good for Your Teeth

Oleanolic acid, a plant chemical found in raisins, was shown to inhibit the growth of two species of oral bacteria, Streptococcus mutans, which causes cavities, and Porphyromonas gingivalis, which is associated with gum disease. This finding refutes the long-standing belief that raisins promote tooth decay.

Christine D. Wu, PhD, professor and associate dean for research, periodontics department, University of Illinois at Chicago College of Dentistry.

■ ■ ■ ■

Best for Your Teeth

Avoid all-natural toothbrushes, made with boars' hairs. The hairs are hollow and retain bacteria. Beyond that, it doesn't matter if you use a manual or electric nylon, rounded-bristle brush.

Also: Any toothpaste will clean teeth and remove bacteria—just be sure it has fluoride to help prevent decay—but some have minor enhancements.

Examples: Tartar-control toothpaste may be slightly better at preventing the formation of tartar...sensitivity toothpastes contain ingredients that may be helpful if your teeth are extremely sensitive to heat and cold...whitening toothpastes may make teeth slightly whiter if used according to the manufacturers' directions.

Sheldon Nadler, DMD, dentist in private practice in New York City.

■ ■ ■ ■

Hiccup Cures That Work

Stick a finger into each ear—this stimulates the vagus nerve, which runs from the brain to the abdomen and controls hiccups. Use a cotton swab to draw a line gently down the roof of your mouth—the tickling stops the throat spasm that causes hiccups. Breathe into a paper bag to produce carbon dioxide, which helps calm the diaphragm—but do this only if someone is with you, in case you get light-headed. Get distracted—have someone ask you a nonsensical question or try to make you hiccup at an exact moment.

Health, 2100 Lake Shore Drive, Birmingham, Alabama 35209.

■ ■ ■ ■

Wait for Nasal Surgery

Cosmetic nasal surgery for teenagers should be done only after the nose is structurally stable and the teenager is psychologically mature. For most girls, this means at least age 15… for boys, who tend to develop later than girls, at least age 17. Be sure the teen is comfortable altering his/her appearance and is not being pushed into surgery by peers or family members.

Robert Kotler, MD, FACS, clinical instructor, University of California, Los Angeles, and author of *Secrets of a Beverly Hills Cosmetic Surgeon*. Ernest Mitchell.

■ ■ ■ ■

Dry Eye Self-Test

To determine if your eyes have adequate lubrication, buy a vision test card (available online for $10 to $20) and a small bottle of artificial tears, such as Refresh Tears or HypoTears. Then…

•**Stand the test card on a table or shelf.*** Next, step backward until the top line of letters is just blurry enough that you can't read it.

•**Put two drops of artificial tears in each eye.**

•**Look again at the blurry line of letters.** If you can see the letters clearly—even if only for a split second—you're probably suffering from dry eye.

If this test indicates that you may have dry eye, see an ophthalmologist for further evaluation.

Robert Latkany, MD, an ophthalmologist and founder and director of the Dry Eye Clinic at the New York Eye and Ear Infirmary and the Dry Eye Center of New York, both in New York City. He is actively involved in dry eye research and is the author of *The Dry Eye Remedy*. Hatherleigh. *www.dryeyedoctor.com*.

*If you prefer, use this publication.

Easy Ways to Protect Your Eyes

Jamison Starbuck, ND, a naturopathic physician in family practice in Missoula, Montana. She is past president of the American Association of Naturopathic Physicians.

Researchers have identified a wide range of foods that help protect the eyes—leafy greens, such as spinach, chard and kale, have received the most attention, but there are plenty of other choices if you don't like those foods. *To optimize your eye health…**

•**Eat *enough* of the right foods.** The carotenoids *lutein* and *zeaxanthin,* found in leafy greens (as well as in green peas, corn, zucchini and eggs), have been rightly touted for their ability to act as disease-preventing antioxidants in the retina of the eye. For example, research has found that women ages 50 to 79 whose diets were rich in lutein and zeaxanthin were 32% less likely to develop cataracts (clouding of the eyes' lenses, resulting in blurred vision) than those whose diets contained less. Other studies have shown that these nutrients may reduce the incidence of macular degeneration (an eye disorder that gradually destroys central vision). To get these benefits, be sure to eat enough of these foods—aim for at least two servings daily. One serving equals one ear of corn, one egg or one-half cup of leafy greens, peas or zucchini.

•**Take coenzyme Q10 (CoQ10).** This nutrient, widely recognized for its heart-protective properties, also helps prevent and treat cataracts and macular degeneration. If you have either of these eye conditions—or a family history (parent or sibling) of them—take 100 mg of CoQ10 daily.

•**Get your berries, too.** The botanical medicine bilberry has long been used to treat retinal diseases. For my patients with cataracts or macular degeneration, I recommend that they take a daily 400-mg bilberry supplement—and eat one-half cup of blueberries or blackberries. These berries contain antioxidants that help

*If you have a serious eye condition, such as macular degeneration, see an ophthalmologist. I also recommend annual eye examinations.

protect the eyes. To help prevent eye disease, eat one-half cup of dark berries (fresh or frozen) daily.

Caution: If you take diabetes medication, do not use bilberry.

• **Use fish oil.** Fish oil, which contains *docosahexaenoic acid* (DHA) and *eicosapentaenoic acid* (EPA), is known to improve heart and immune health. These fatty acids also reduce dry eye symptoms and the risk for macular degeneration. For dry eye, cataracts or macular degeneration, ask your doctor about taking a total of 1,750 mg of EPA and DHA daily.

• **Make an herbal eye compress.** The herb eyebright has been widely used to treat eye ailments, particularly the itchy, watery, red eyes that accompany allergies, colds and sinusitis. For relief from these symptoms, make a cold compress (to be used externally on your eyes) with eyebright tea. Use two teaspoons of dried eyebright leaf (available at health-food stores) per eight ounces of boiling water. Steep covered for five minutes, strain and refrigerate in a closed jar. When cool, pour the tea over a clean cotton cloth and place it over your closed eyes for 10 minutes. For additional relief from symptoms, drink a mixture of 60 drops of eyebright tincture in one ounce of water, three times a day.

Warning: Do not put eyebright tea or extract directly into your eyes.

■■■■

Do You Need a Hearing Test?

The American Speech, Language and Hearing Association recommends a hearing test every 10 years for adults up to age 50 and every three years thereafter. A hearing test may be recommended sooner if you or your family are worried about your hearing loss…you have a family history of hearing loss…you have a loud hobby, such as woodworking or recreational shooting…and/or you work in an environment with loud music or noise. Hearing tests can be performed by an audiologist (specialist in hearing disorders) or an ear, nose and throat (ENT)

doctor.* Some insurance plans cover hearing tests. Check with your provider.

Important: Tinnitus—random ringing or chirping in the ears when there is no actual sound—is often a sign of impending hearing loss, so people who experience this condition should consider getting their hearing tested.

John M. Burkey, CCC/A, FAAA, a certified audiologist and director of audiology at the Lippy Group for Ear, Nose & Throat in Warren, Ohio. A fellow of the American Academy of Audiology, he is the author of *Baby Boomers and Hearing Loss* and *Overcoming Hearing Aid Fears* (both published by Rutgers University).

*To find an audiologist near you, go to the Web site of the American Academy of Audiology (*www.audiology. org*). For an ENT, consult the American Academy of Otolaryngology (*www.entnet.org*).

Younger Look with No Face-Lift

David Colbert, MD, FAAD, founder of New York Dermatology Group, a private dermatological practice and research facility in New York City, is on the teaching staffs of several New York hospitals. His patients include many people in the film and television industry.

Not long ago, men and women who wanted a more youthful appearance assumed that they would have to have a face-lift. A face-lift smooths sagging skin by pulling it up and tightening it, but the surgery doesn't give the skin itself a younger look.

Cosmetic dermatologists, on the other hand, have a number of options to create younger-looking skin by getting rid of many lines and age spots. Some of these techniques make it possible to "plump" the face to reverse the sunken look that age can cause. These techniques are all nonsurgical and safe.

FILLERS

Fillers are materials that create volume to make up for the tablespoons of facial fat people lose as they age. The filler is injected directly into deep wrinkles to plump them. The materials are effective for many people over age 60, assuming that their skin is reasonably taut. Fillers can decrease facial lines and wrinkles, treat frown lines between the eyes and also plump hollow cheeks and thinning lips.

Although there are a number of fillers, Restylane is one of the most popular along with Perlane (a thicker form of Restylane), which is used for deeper wrinkles. Procedures take about an hour. The results are immediate and last for three to six months, after which the body absorbs the material. The procedure can be a bit uncomfortable, but the only side effects are a few hours of slight puffiness in the area and sometimes small, barely visible lumps that will disappear within a few days to a few weeks. Restylane is an FDA-approved, bioengineered, non-animal, stabilized hyaluronic acid, a substance almost identical to one naturally found in the body, making it safe to have repeat procedures.

I like to combine Restylane treatments with Botox. Although many people associate Botox skin injections with the "frozen" look sometimes seen on the faces of film stars, I prefer to use it more judiciously to relax muscles and give the face a de-stressed look.

Note: I don't advocate silicone injections to smooth the skin. Unlike other fillers, silicone is permanent. You are stuck with the result and your face may not age well around it. Botox also has risks as the material may spread from the injection site.

Cost: Restylane and Perlane costs range from $350 to $800 per syringe with some discount for additional syringes used during the same treatment.* Most people need more than one syringe. The cost of Botox may range from $125 to $400 per treatment area.

A patient's own fat is a good filler, as well, because it gives the face an especially soft, natural look. For such fat transfer, the person's own fat is taken from another area of the body, usually the thighs or buttocks. Because this requires a micro liposuction procedure, exceptionally thin people are not candidates. Once the fat is harvested, it is frozen and remains usable for the next three years.

Fat transfer requires several treatments over a few months. Although this procedure hasn't been in use long enough for us to give a definitive time frame for the results, we are finding it

*All costs are approximate and are not covered by insurance.

to be semipermanent. And unlike synthetic fillers, natural fat tends to build up and stay—eventually eliminating the need for more injections. You may experience some bruising and swelling for a week or so after the procedure. There is a slight risk of infection. While this is a more expensive treatment (total cost is around $5,000), it is cost-effective because it is so long lasting.

PEELS

Peels are available in gentle, medium and strong intensities. All peels chemically remove skin on the face and/or hands, which exposes the under layer—new skin that has been sheltered from the sun and other elements and so looks better. The difference among peels is how deeply they penetrate.

•**Gentle peels** affect only the top layer and diminish fine lines and fade age spots. Ideally, you would have gentle peels about once a month. Many spas offer these, but technicians there may not have adequate training and use weaker chemicals than dermatologists do. You can resume normal activities immediately after gentle peels.

•**Medium peels** go deeper and more effectively remove age spots and fine lines and improve skin color and texture. They require two or three sessions over three to five weeks. You can resume normal activities immediately afterward. Results last about a year.

•**Deep (or strong) peels.** The strongest peel—either a phenol or a TCA (*trichloroacetic acid*) peel—penetrates deep into the skin. It dramatically rids the face of moderately deep lines and age spots in just one treatment. Often, just specific wrinkled or discolored areas of the face are deep-peeled.

This peel is relatively painful because it destroys the upper layer of skin and results in temporary blisters and scabbing. There is some risk of infection, so meticulous post-procedure care is necessary. People with darker skin are not candidates because these peels lighten the skin and would create too much contrast with the neck. Also, anyone who has taken the drug Accutane in the last year is not a candidate because the skin would be too sensitive for a deep peel. The recovery process takes at least three weeks.

Cost: Gentle peels run from $200 to $400 each...medium peels, from $1,200 to $2,000, depending on how much of the face is peeled...phenol or TCA peels up to $4,000, also depending on the amount of skin treated.

LASER AND PHOTO REJUVENATION

Laser treatment tones skin and improves texture.

Photo rejuvenation uses pulsed light to rid the face and body of age spots and undesirable pigmentation.

Laser therapy also stimulates production of collagen, the natural substance in the skin that helps keep it plump and unlined. This stimulation continues several months after the treatment, giving ever-improving results. These treatments are painless and it takes from one to three treatments to achieve desirable results.

For skin that appears leathery and discolored by sun exposure, a topical photosensitizing solution called Levulan is applied an hour before the light-based therapy session begins. Levulan allows the light to go deeper into the skin, thereby enhancing the effect of the treatment. We have not found any risks or side effects for laser or photo rejuvenation treatments.

Cost: Laser and photo rejuvenation treatments run from $200 to $1,200 depending on how much skin is treated. Adding Levulan brings the cost to $500 to $1,500.

INTENSE REJUVENATION

The most intense form of skin rejuvenation comes from an infrared light machine called the Titan.

Skin rests on support collagen that keeps it firm, but this collagen collapses and loses elasticity with age. The heat from the Titan's infrared light contracts and tightens collagen deep in the dermis (the second of the three major layers of the skin) and at the same time stimulates collagen production. The result is an overall tightening of the skin on the face, jawline, arms and/or legs with an effect that lasts from one to three years.

One to three treatments are needed, depending on the patient's age, previous sun exposure and general skin condition. I prefer to combine mild photo rejuvenation for the outer layers of skin with the Titan to tighten up the underlayer of skin.

Cost: $1,500 to $2,500 per treatment. There are no currently known risks or side effects for Titan treatments.

Look Years Younger... Lunchtime "Face-Lifts" For Men & Women

Nelson Lee Novick, MD, clinical professor of dermatology, Mount Sinai Medical Center, New York City. He is author of *Super Skin: A Leading Dermatologist's Guide to the Latest Breakthroughs in Skin Care.* iUniverse.com.

A decade ago, aggressive cosmetic surgery was the main treatment for wrinkles, sagging jowls and other signs of aging. Patients experienced significant bruising and swelling, and the full effects of the procedures weren't visible for at least six months.

Today, cosmetic surgeons perform three times as many noninvasive cosmetic procedures as aggressive surgeries. More than half of the procedures are done in doctors' offices instead of hospitals—and some can be completed during a lunch break. In many cases, patients see the final results immediately.

Botox has gotten most of the headlines, but there are a number of other "instant" cosmetic procedures. All of the following procedures are safe for most people and cause no scarring.

VOLUME FILLING FOR WRINKLES AND LINES

Synthetic collagen-like substances are injected into the skin to plump up depressed areas, including wrinkles and worry and smile lines. Collagen itself, one of the first filling agents, rarely lasted more than three to six months and sometimes caused allergic reactions. The new synthetic fillers last longer and are hypoallergenic.

The patient is given a local anesthetic, then fillers are injected into the problem spots. One syringe usually can treat the entire face. It only takes a few minutes, and changes in appearance are immediately apparent.

Different fillers...

•**Restylane** is chemically similar to the gelatinous material that supports skin collagen and elastic fibers. It retains water and plumps skin. It is especially good for smile lines, lips that have gotten thinner with age and "smoker's lines" on the upper lip. One treatment usually lasts eight to 18 months.

Approximate cost: $350 to $800 per syringe.

•**Perlane** is similar to Restylane. It's used for deeper depressions and/or furrows and costs about the same as Restylane. It lasts about six months.

•**Radiesse** (formerly Radiance) is the newest filler. It's made of *calcium hydroxylapatite,* the same material that makes up teeth and bone. It is ideal for deeper smile lines and sunken cheeks. One treatment may last two to five years. It is slightly more likely than other fillers to cause temporary bruising.

Approximate cost: $650 to $800 per syringe.

DERMASPACING FOR ACNE SCARS AND FURROWS

This new technique uses the body's natural healing mechanisms to add volume to depressed areas such as acne scars and furrows. It also is effective for cellulite on other parts of the body.

The patient is given a local anesthetic. A needle-like cutting instrument is used to break up fibrous bands and create a hollow area beneath the skin. The area fills with body fluids, and within a few weeks, natural collagen is created that fills the pocket and plumps and smoothes the skin surface.

Dermaspacing, also called subcision, may be enough by itself to restore younger-looking skin, or it can be used in combination with fillers.

Approximate cost: $400 per treatment.

Dermaspacing causes minor bruising that can last several weeks. Also, some patients need more than one treatment. It takes about a month to gauge how effectively the body will repair the area. For acne and other scars, the results may be permanent. For furrows, the results may last several months.

CHEMICAL PEEL FOR LEATHERY SKIN

Skin loses luster and gets leathery with age, especially in people who spend a lot of time in the sun. Resurfacing uses concentrated acids to restore youthful luster and texture to skin. *Main approaches...*

•**Alpha hydroxy acids,** also called *fruit washes*, are applied to the skin. Dermatologists use products with a 70% concentration—home-use chemical peels usually don't exceed 15%. These acids diminish mottling as well as fine wrinkles, in part by stimulating the production of gelatinous tissue under the skin. Most patients require six to 12 treatments (two to four weeks apart), with occasional touch-ups.

Approximate cost: $150 per 10-minute treatment.

•**Beta hydroxy acids** are used in the same way, but they are somewhat more effective. Most patients require two to four treatments.

Approximate cost: $500 per treatment.

THREAD LIFT FOR SAGGING JAW, BROW, CHEEKS

Also called a "feather lift" or "loop lift," this technique can diminish sagging—in the jaw, brows and cheeks—without the extensive surgery used in traditional face-lifts. The patient is given a local anesthetic. A needle is used to insert a fine thread under the skin. The thread loops under the loose tissue and then is pulled taut and anchored to fibrous tissue under the skin or within the hairline. Depending on the area, a single thread or multiple threads are used.

The results can last anywhere from three to 10 years—about the same as a traditional face-lift. Adjustments may be made later by tightening the thread or adding additional threads. If the patient doesn't like the results, the thread can be removed and the face will return to its previous appearance.

When treating multiple areas, the procedure takes about 60 minutes. When doing one area, such as the brow, it takes about 30 minutes.

Approximate cost: $2,500 for the brow or lower face.

RADIOSURGERY FOR VISIBLE BLOOD VESSELS

A small wand directs high-energy radio waves through the skin to eliminate the tiny networks of blood vessels that appear on the cheeks or around the nose, mostly in people who have rosacea or those exposed to too much sun.

The patient is given a topical anesthetic, then radio waves penetrate deeply into the skin without damaging the surface or adjoining tissues. The treatment takes about five minutes.

Approximate cost: $300 to treat the face.

SCALPEL SCULPTING FOR REMOVING MOLES

In the past, moles were excised from the skin and the resulting wound was sutured. The wound could take weeks to heal, and many patients were left with small scars from the stitches.

Scalpel sculpting doesn't require stitches. A drop of local anesthetic is placed on the mole. The mole is then "sculpted"—cut flush with the face. Normal skin grows to cover the area, usually with no scarring. In 90% of cases, the mole never comes back.

Approximate cost: $300.

There may be a darkening (repigmenting) of the area. Radio waves can often eliminate this.

SANDING FOR SCARS AND FINE WRINKLES

A sterilized sanding material is used to buff away scars—from acne, injuries, etc.—as well as fine wrinkles. Normal skin covers the area once the scar tissue is removed.

Approximate cost: $400.

Scar abrasion can be combined with dermaspacing or filling. One patient had a deep scar between his eyes after being hit by a crate. I did dermaspacing to fill the area, then buffed the surface. Now he has no visible mark.

Important: Scar abrasion is most effective when performed within eight to 12 weeks after an injury/surgery to prevent long-term scarring.

■ More from Nelson Lee Novick, MD...

No-Surgery Nose Job— In Minutes

Using new, safe and practically painless nonsurgical techniques, a dermatologist now can reshape a nose in less than 10 minutes, giving immediate results that last about a year or longer.

Average cost: $750 to $1,500. *Options...*

•**Smooth a bump or straighten a bend.** Radiesse, a synthetic gel of tiny bone-like calcium-based spheres, is injected beneath the skin where desired—for instance, above or below a bump on the bridge or along the side of the nose. Then it is quickly molded like clay to the desired shape and fully retains its shape within about a day. For more precise shaping, the doctor also may inject Juvéderm or Restylane, fillers made of synthetic *hyaluronic acid.* (In the body, one function of natural hyaluronic acid is to provide volume to the skin.)

•**Lift a long, drooping tip.** Botox (a purified form of a protein produced by the *Clostridium botulinum* bacterium) is injected into the crevices on each side and at the base of the nose, weakening the muscles that pull the nose tip downward and permitting muscles higher up on the nose to draw the tip upward. Next, Radiesse is injected at the base of the nose to buttress the tip, providing longer-lasting effects than from Botox alone.

With either procedure: Prior to treatment, the area is injected with a local anesthetic plus *epinephrine* (a blood vessel constrictor).

Recovery: There are no restrictions on activities. You may have minor swelling and bruising for a few days. Risk for infection is very slight. Generally, results last 12 to 18 months with Radiesse...eight to 12 months with Juvéderm and Restylane...and three to six months with Botox. After that, touch-ups may be desirable.

Botox can spread from the injection site. Consult your doctor.

■ ■ ■ ■

Quick Fix

Nonsurgical nose jobs are quick, relatively inexpensive and effective for small bumps, dents and irregularities. A doctor injects an FDA-approved cosmetic filler called *Radiesse* into the nose to contour it and hide bumps. The procedure takes about 15 minutes. The patient remains awake during the procedure so he/she can guide the doctor while looking in a mirror.

Cost: $750 to $1,500, compared with $15,000 for a surgical nose job. The effects last about a year.

Cameron K. Rokhsar, MD, assistant clinical professor of dermatology, Albert Einstein College of Medicine of Yeshiva University, New York City. *www.cosmeticlaserskin surgery.com*

How to Prevent or Minimize Scars

James Spencer, MD, clinical professor of medicine in the department of dermatology at Mount Sinai School of Medicine, New York City. He is a spokesperson for the American Academy of Dermatology and director of Spencer Dermatology Mohs Skin Surgery Center in St. Petersburg, Florida. *www.spencerdermatology.com*

If you have a shallow wound—a skinned knee, a paper cut, a minor burn—new skin grows back, filling the injured area with fresh tissue that is virtually identical to the original.

If a wound has a depth of one-half inch or more—piercing the skin's outermost layer (the *epidermis*) and penetrating the dermis beneath it—the repair won't be perfect. To heal a deeper wound, your body relies on *collagen,* an elongated protein that provides structural support, like girders in a building—which often results in a scar.

Here's how to prevent scars and minimize the ones you have…

TYPES OF SCARS

Scars are categorized by shape…

• **Indented**—typically caused by acne or chicken pox.

• **Hypertrophic.** These red, thick scars stay within the boundary of the wound but rise above the skin's surface.

• **Keloid.** The scar tissue is raised but also pours out beyond the outline of the wound, over the surrounding skin.

Many factors can affect how a scar develops, including…

• **Age**—younger skin tends to heal more vigorously, producing larger scars.

• **Skin color**—keloids are more common among dark-skinned people.

• **Location**—tighter skin, such as that along the jawbone, makes a scar more visible.

• **Size of wound**—larger wounds typically produce larger scars.

PREVENTING SCARS

Proper self-care after sustaining a wound is crucial in either preventing a scar or achieving the smallest, least noticeable scar possible.

Important: Many people believe that a dry, uncovered wound heals best, but scientific studies show that keeping a wound moist is ideal for minimizing scars as wounds heal. *What to do…*

• **Apply an over-the-counter antibiotic ointment.** Use enough to moisten the wound. This also helps prevent infection, which may create a deeper wound that is more likely to scar.

• **Cover the wound.** Use a bandage of some kind. Hundreds of products are available. Choose one that you find comfortable and easy to use.

• **Keep the wound covered until it's healed.** Change the ointment and covering every day or two. When showering, remove the bandage and replace with a clean one after the shower.

• **Don't pick at the wound.** Don't squeeze acne bumps, scratch mosquito bites or dig at scabs—you may increase the chances of a scar.

• **Try massage.** Just after healing is complete, if there is a scar, cover it with petroleum jelly and massage it gently but firmly with the tips of your fingers for 10 minutes or so every day for one to two months. This will soften the scar and help minimize its appearance.

• **Ask your doctor about silicone sheeting and gels.** Although scientists don't know why it works, applying a bandagelike sheet of silicone gel can help stop a new scar from becoming hypertrophic or keloidal, or it can help reduce an old scar. For new scars, the sheeting should be applied about one week after the injury or removal of sutures.

MINIMIZING EXISTING SCARS

Many medical treatments may minimize an old scar—but none can completely remove it. A dermatologist and/or a plastic surgeon can recommend the best treatment(s) for the scar you have. *Here, the most effective ways...*

•Keloid and hypertrophic scars.

•Pulsed dye laser. Although many types of laser treatments are available (and widely advertised) for scar reduction, the pulsed dye laser (PDL)—which focuses ultrashort pulses of high-energy yellow light on the scar—is the gold standard. It can remove redness, flatten the scar and relieve itching (which often accompanies a scar). Two or three treatments are typical, once every one to two months.

•Cortisone injections. Injecting *cortisone*—a synthetic version of a hormone produced by the adrenal gland—can shrink and flatten a scar. (How it works is unknown.) Typically, three or four injections are needed, every two to four weeks.

•Interferon. The immune system produces this protein when battling viruses, bacteria and other infectious agents. When injected, it can flatten a scar and reduce redness. The number and timing of injections are the same as for cortisone.

•Aldara. A keloid scar can be surgically removed, but it's a risky procedure—chances are 50-50 it will grow back, perhaps even larger. Aldara cream is an immune response modulator that stimulates the production of interferon. Applied after surgery, it may help keep a keloid from returning. It is best for surgically removed keloids.

•Indented scars.

•Laser resurfacing. This intense treatment employs the high-energy light of a carbon dioxide laser, which literally burns off the layers of damaged skin, creating an even, smooth surface. The procedure often requires local anesthesia and takes about a week to heal. The skin may remain red for months.

•Fillers. Made from a material such as collagen, a filler is injected with a fine needle two to three times over three months into one or more indented scar areas, temporarily lifting the area. It typically takes more than one treatment to see results, which last six to eight months. Popular fillers include Dermalogen, Restylane, Juvederm, Hylaform, Cosmoderm, Cymetra and Artecoll.

•Other scars.

•Surgical scar revision. The body has skin tension lines—creases where wrinkles form, such as where the nose meets the cheek. Scars falling along a tension line are less prominent than scars at an angle to a line. In this technique, the doctor surgically repositions the scar to within a tension line.

Best for: Wide or long scars, scars in prominent places (such as the forehead) and scars with irregular, rather than straight, patterns.

•Botox. The muscle-paralyzing toxin, used cosmetically to relax wrinkles, also can minimize scars from forehead wounds.

Recent study: Injections of Botox around a forehead wound from injury or surgery improved the appearance of the wound six months later by 20%, compared with noninjected wounds.

Best for: Scars on the forehead.

Caution: Botox has risks. Ask your doctor.

WHAT DOESN'T WORK

•**Mederma.** This over-the-counter topical gel, made from onion extract, often is recommended to minimize scars.

Recent study: Dermatological surgeons at Harvard Medical School studied 24 surgical patients, treating half of their scars with onion extract and the other half with petroleum-based gel. There was no difference between the two areas in appearance, redness or size of scar.

•**Vitamin E.** In a study conducted at the University of Miami reported in *Dermatological Surgery,* dermatologists found no difference in scarring of wounds treated with or without topical vitamin E.

Skin Care from the Inside Out

Joy Bauer, MS, RD, CDN, a nutritionist/dietitian in private practice in New York City. She is the nutrition expert for the *Today* show and nutritionist for the New York City Ballet, the American Ballet Theatre and several Olympic athletes. She is author of several books, including the best seller *Joy Bauer's Food Cures: Treat Common Health Concerns, Look Younger & Live Longer.* Rodale. *www.joybauernutrition.com.*

To take care of their skin, most people reach for sunscreen, lotions and creams to protect, smooth and moisturize. These products can help, but beautiful, healthy skin starts with what goes into your body, not what you rub on it. Research shows that good nutrition may reduce the effects of sun damage… minimize redness and wrinkling…and even protect against some skin cancers.

FIRST STEP: HYDRATE

The single most important nutritional factor for keeping skin healthy is water. Staying hydrated keeps cells plump, making skin look firmer and clearer. When cells are dehydrated, they shrivel and can make your skin look wrinkled. Think of it this way—when you dehydrate a juicy grape, you get a raisin. In addition, water transports nutrients into skin cells and helps flush toxins out of the body.

To stay hydrated, drink whenever you feel thirsty.

Helpful sign: If your urine is pale yellow, you are adequately hydrated—but if it is bright or dark yellow, you may need to boost your fluid intake.

Good news: Drinking unsweetened tea helps keep you hydrated, plus you get the benefit of antioxidant nutrients called *polyphenols,* which may help prevent sun-related skin cancers. Green, white, black and oolong teas provide more polyphenols than herbal teas. It is your choice whether to drink caffeinated or decaffeinated tea. Although caffeine is a mild diuretic (increasing the amount of urine that is passed from the body), the relatively small amount in tea doesn't affect its ability to keep skin hydrated and healthy.

Avoid: Teas sweetened with a lot of sugar—excess sugar can make skin dull and wrinkled.

For extra hydration: Eat "juicy foods" that are at least 75% water by weight—fruits such as apples, berries, cherries, grapes, grapefruit, mangoes, melons, oranges, peaches, plums… and vegetables such as asparagus, beets, carrots, celery, cucumbers and tomatoes.

SKIN-HEALTHY FOODS

Everything we eat is reflected in the health of our skin—for better or for worse. *Among the best nutrients for the skin…*

•**Beta-carotene,** a powerful antioxidant which, once ingested, is converted to vitamin A, a nutrient necessary for skin tissue growth and repair.

Skin-smart: Have at least one serving per day of beta-carotene–rich foods—for instance, orange carrots, sweet potatoes and tomatoes… green arugula, asparagus and spinach…and fruits such as cherries, grapefruit, mangoes and watermelon.

•**Omega-3 fatty acids,** healthful fats that are important building blocks of the membranes that make up cell walls, allowing water and nutrients to enter and keeping out waste and toxins.

Skin-smart: Eat at least three servings of omega-3–rich foods each week—such as wild salmon (farm-raised salmon may have higher levels of potentially dangerous contaminants)… mackerel (not king mackerel, which has too much mercury)…anchovies, herring and sardines. Good fats also are found in smaller amounts in flaxseed, soybeans and walnuts. If you don't eat enough of these omega-3 foods, consider taking daily supplements of fish oil providing 1,000 mg of combined *eicosapentaenoic acid* (EPA) and *docosahexaenoic acid* (DHA), the most biologically active and beneficial components. Look for brands that have been tested for purity, such as VitalOils 1000 (877-342-3721, *www.myvitalremedymd. com*) and Ultimate Omega by Nordic Naturals (800-662-2544, *www.nordicnaturals.com*).

•**Selenium,** a mineral with antioxidant activity thought to help skin elasticity (which means you'll look younger longer) and prevent sun-related skin damage and cancers.

Skin-smart: Eat at least one serving a day of a selenium-rich food—canned light tuna (which has less mercury than canned albacore or white tuna), crab, tilapia…whole-wheat breads and pasta…lean beef…chicken and turkey (breast meat is lowest in fat).

Caution: Taking selenium in supplement form may increase the risk for squamous cell skin cancer in people with a personal or family history of the disease. Selenium in food is safe and healthful.

•**Vitamin C,** an antioxidant that helps build collagen and elastin (proteins that comprise the skin's underlying structure)…and also protects against free radicals (molecules in the body that damage cells) when the skin is exposed to sunlight.

Skin-smart: *Eat at least one serving a day of any of these vitamin C-rich foods*—cantaloupe, citrus fruits, kiwifruit, papaya, pineapple, strawberries, watermelon...and bell peppers, broccoli, brussels sprouts, cabbage, cauliflower, kale and kidney beans.

•**Zinc,** a mineral that helps maintain collagen. People with zinc deficiencies often develop skin redness and lesions.

Skin-smart: *Eat at least one serving of a zinc-rich food daily*—chicken or turkey breast, crab, lean beef, pork tenderloin (lower in fat than other cuts)...peanuts and peanut butter...fat-free dairy products (cheese, milk and yogurt).

Wise for everyone: A daily multivitamin that contains 100% of the daily value for vitamins A, C, E and zinc and no more than 70 mcg of selenium.

WHAT TO AVOID

•**Sugar.** Research suggests that sugary foods (such as soda and cookies) may contribute to skin blemishes. These "bad carbs" may promote harmful inflammation throughout the body, which can trigger breakouts. Limit your indulgence in sweet treats to no more than one small serving per day.

•**White flour.** Minimize white-flour foods (such as white bread and pasta) in your diet by choosing whole-grain breads and rolls, cereals, crackers and pasta.

•**Dairy foods.** Milk may contain hormones (especially if cows are pregnant) and iodine from iodine-fortified feed. Although uncommon, both of these components can cause pimples. If you are prone to acne, try going off dairy for a while to see if your skin improves.

•**Cigarette smoke, including second-hand smoke.** It fills your body with toxins, inflammation-causing irritants and free radicals that damage every cell they touch...and also limits blood flow, so skin cells don't receive the oxygen and nutrients they need.

■ **More from Joy Bauer, MS, RD, CDN...**

Hair Care from the Inside Out

Foods that are healthy for skin also are healthy for hair. *In addition, hair requires...*

•**Iron-rich protein.** Hair is made primarily of protein. Without enough of it, hair can weaken, grow more slowly or fall out. Iron helps red blood cells carry oxygen throughout the body, including to hair-growth cells. Eat at least one serving per day of protein foods high in iron, such as clams, oysters, shrimp...duck, lamb, lean beef, pork, turkey...eggs...fortified whole-grain breads and cereals...tofu and legumes (beans, peas, etc.).

•**B vitamins.** Folate, biotin, vitamin B-6 and vitamin B-12 are needed to make red blood cells. Without enough of these vitamins, hair follicles can become starved for nutrients and oxygen, and your hair can fall out. Eat two servings a day of foods that contain one or more of these nutrients.

Good choices: Fortified whole-grain breads and cereals...broccoli, leafy dark green vegetables and legumes...eggs and fat-free dairy products...peanut butter...and salmon.

My Secrets to Better Foot Care

Jamison Starbuck, ND, a naturopathic physician in family practice in Missoula, Montana. She is past president of the American Association of Naturopathic Physicians.

"Honestly, I don't pay much attention to them, doctor." That's how Bill, a 70-year-old man I once treated, summed up the condition of his feet. Upon close inspection of Bill's feet, however, I found several clues to his overall health. I always include a foot exam during the routine physicals I perform, and I encourage my patients to examine their own feet.

To take care of your feet, spend at least 15 minutes on foot care once a week.

What to do: Palpate (feel with your hands and fingertips) the soles of your feet, the skin and tissue surrounding your ankles, and each toe, feeling for tender areas or other changes… note the color of your feet (for example, blue or purple may mean bruising or circulatory problems)…clean between each toe…and trim your toe nails.

See your primary care doctor or a podiatrist if any of these problems persists for more than two weeks…

•**Discolored nails** may be due to a fungus, poor-fitting shoes or a circulatory disorder.

•**Persistently cold feet** can indicate circulatory problems.

•**Chronic foot pain or immobility** can be due to arthritis or a bone spur (a sharp protrusion of bone).

See your primary care doctor immediately if you experience significant pain or changes as well as…

•**"Hot spots"** (areas of warm tissue), which may be a sign of an injury or inflammation related to gout (a condition marked by painful joints).

•**Swelling or numbness,** which can be a sign of problems with an organ, such as the kidneys or heart, or the nervous system or spine.

Smart idea: If you're not flexible enough to comfortably examine and care for your own feet, ask your spouse or a family member to help. As an alternative, most podiatrists offer medical pedicures (for about $50). Check with your health insurer to see whether the cost is covered.

If your feet or ankles hurt or they are swollen (due to arthritis or overuse), you may want to soak them in hot and cold water alternately, which promotes circulation.

What to do: Put one cup of Epsom salts in a dishpan, and fill it with hot tap water. Fill a second pan with cold tap water. Place your feet in the hot water, making sure the water covers the ankles. Soak for two minutes. Then put both feet in the cold-water pan for 30 seconds. Switch back and forth—from hot to cold, two minutes to 30 seconds, respectively—three times. Be sure to end the process with cold water, which closes the pores and reduces swelling. Dry your feet thoroughly, and then massage each foot with massage oil (containing wintergreen or peppermint oil to promote circulation) for five minutes.

Caution: Do not do the alternating hot/cold foot bath if you have diabetes or lack of sensation in your feet—you may scald or chill your feet.

Also helpful for foot pain: Orthotics are custom-made shoe inserts that firmly support the foot, reducing discomfort. See a podiatrist to be fitted for orthotics (about $100 to more than $200 each).

19

Surprising Food Cures

The Healing Power Of Spices

Traditional medicine has recognized the medicinal benefits of spices for thousands of years.

Now: A growing body of scientific evidence supports the use of spices to prevent—and even help treat—various diseases, such as arthritis, diabetes, cancer and Alzheimer's.* *New findings…*

CAYENNE PEPPER

What it does: Lowers cholesterol…helps prevent atherosclerosis…and reduces allergic responses. An extract from the pepper, called capsaicin, can be used in a topical cream to treat pain from arthritis, shingles, bursitis, low-back ache and neuropathy (nerve pain). Cayenne's benefits can be attributed to the antioxidants, flavonoids and carotenoids it contains, all of which have anti-inflammatory effects and enhance circulation. Capsaicin depletes nerve endings of *substance P*, a neurotransmitter that facilitates nerve transmission of pain.

Scientific evidence: A four-week study published in the *Journal of Rheumatology* found that patients with osteoarthritis of the hands who applied capsaicin cream four times a day experienced reduced pain and tenderness.

Typical dose: Cayenne is available as a supplement in capsules and tincture. Take one capsule of cayenne pepper up to three times a day…or add three to eight drops of cayenne tincture to four ounces of water and drink two to four times a day. Apply topical cream containing capsaicin to painful areas, as directed on the label. You also can season your food with powdered cayenne pepper or hot sauce.

Possible side effects: Cayenne pepper can cause gastric upset. To avoid pain and burning,

---

*Check with your doctor before using spices for medicinal purposes. They can interact with prescription medication.

David Winston, a Washington, New Jersey–based registered herbalist (RH) and professional member of the American Herbalist Guild, is coauthor of *Herbal Therapy and Supplements: A Scientific and Traditional Approach*. Lippincott.

do not let topical capsaicin come in contact with your eyes or other mucous membranes. If you take *warfarin* (Coumadin), do not use cayenne pepper supplements.

CINNAMON

What it does: Helps prevent heart disease and type 2 diabetes.

Due to its antioxidant properties, cinnamon helps people with metabolic syndrome (a cluster of factors, including excessive abdominal fat, high blood sugar and elevated blood pressure, which increase the risk for cardiovascular disease and type 2 diabetes) use the hormone insulin in their bodies more efficiently.

Scientific evidence: A US Department of Agriculture clinical study found that consuming capsules containing 1 g, 3 g or 6 g of cinnamon daily (about ¼ teaspoon, ¾ teaspoon or 1¼ teaspoons, respectively) for 40 days lowered blood levels of glucose and triglycerides (fats in the blood) by about 25% in adults with type 2 diabetes. It also reduced LDL "bad" cholesterol by up to 27%.

Typical dose: Use one-half to one teaspoon of powdered cinnamon daily on cereal or toast or mix into yogurt…take one capsule twice a day…or add 20 to 40 drops of tincture to one ounce of water and drink three times daily.

For tea, mix one-fourth to one-half teaspoon of powdered cinnamon with eight ounces of boiling water. Steep for 10 to 15 minutes, covered. Drink a four-ounce cup up to three times a day.

Possible side effects: Because cinnamon can affect blood glucose levels, people with diabetes should carefully monitor their blood sugar and ask their doctors if their medication needs to be adjusted.

GINGER

What it does: Reduces the pain and swelling caused by rheumatoid arthritis and osteoarthritis…helps prevent the nausea and vomiting associated with motion sickness or pregnancy…enhances digestion and circulation…and eases intestinal gas.

Scientific evidence: Two clinical studies found that ginger relieved pain and/or swelling in 75% of arthritis patients.

Typical dose: Take one to two capsules with meals two to three times daily…or add 10 to 30 drops of the tincture to one ounce of water and drink three to four times daily.

For tea, mix one-fourth to one-half teaspoon of powdered ginger (or use a ginger tea bag) with eight ounces of boiling water. Steep for 10 to 15 minutes, covered. Drink four ounces up to three times daily.

Possible side effects: Ginger can have a blood-thinning effect, so check with your doctor before using it if you take an anticoagulant, such as *warfarin* (Coumadin). Ginger may cause an upset stomach in people who take larger doses than those described above.

TURMERIC

What it does: Helps prevent atherosclerosis, some types of cancer and Alzheimer's disease…reduces the pain and stiffness of rheumatoid arthritis and osteoarthritis…eliminates indigestion…and eases the symptoms of inflammatory bowel disease and irritable bowel syndrome. The beneficial effects of turmeric (also found in curry) are due to its anti-inflammatory compounds known as *curcuminoids*, as well as the essential oils and carotenoids it contains.

Scientific evidence: In a double-blind, placebo-controlled study, 116 people with indigestion took either a 500-mg capsule of curcumin (the substance that gives turmeric its yellow color) or a placebo four times a day. Nearly 90% of those taking curcumin experienced full or partial relief after seven days.

Typical dose: Take 250 mg to 500 mg of curcumin (standardized to 80% to 90% curcumin) three times daily…or add 40 to 60 drops of the tincture to one ounce of water and drink three to four times daily.

For tea, mix one-half teaspoon of powdered turmeric with eight ounces of boiling water. Steep for 10 to 15 minutes, covered. Drink four ounces up to four times a day.

Possible side effects: Turmeric stimulates liver function, so it should be avoided by anyone with gallstones or any other bile-duct obstruction. Preliminary studies show that curcumin may lessen the effectiveness of chemotherapy drugs, such as *doxorubicin* (Rubex) and *cyclophosphamide* (Cytoxan). If you are undergoing chemotherapy, talk to your doctor before taking curcumin.

■ ■ ■ ■

Spices Fight Cancer

Adding fresh rosemary leaves to ground beef has been found to lower production of cancer-causing compounds during cooking by up to 60%.

Theory: Antioxidants in rosemary reduce levels of heterocyclic amines, known carcinogens found in protein-rich meat that has been grilled, broiled or fried. Basil, oregano and thyme also are believed to confer this benefit.

J. Scott Smith, PhD, professor, Animal Sciences & Industry, Food Science Institute, Kansas State University, Manhattan, KS.

Best Ways to Get the Nutrients You Need

C. Leigh Broadhurst, PhD, research scientist at the University of Maryland in College Park, and a research geochemist at the US Department of Agriculture, has published scientific research on diabetes, polyunsaturated fats and medicinal plants.

With all the processed food now consumed in the US, getting the necessary nutrients from our diet has become increasingly difficult. Of course, we can turn to nutritional supplements, but research has consistently shown that fresh food—with an abundance of healthful compounds that are believed to work synergistically—is usually our best source of valuable nutrients.

What most people don't realize: Choosing the right foods and food combinations allows you to consume these vital nutrients in a form that is most bioavailable, meaning the food components are efficiently digested, absorbed and assimilated.

What you must know to maximize the bioavailability of nutrients in your food…

•**Iron.** This mineral is critical for brain function and helps your immune system function normally by increasing your resistance to stress and disease. Iron can help you avoid symptoms of fatigue, weakness and irritability.

Plant foods are rarely a good source of iron. For example, the iron from spinach is a net loss. Even though spinach is a good source of magnesium, bone-building vitamin K and other important nutrients, the fiber and plant chemicals in the spinach leaf bind to iron, inhibiting the mineral's bioavailability.

Helpful: When shopping for meat, look for dark meat products, such as liver, beef or dark meat turkey. They are the best sources of iron. Tofu and seafood (especially clams and shrimp) also are rich in iron.

•**Zinc.** This mineral is essential for a healthy immune system. It is highly bioavailable in red meat, though some zinc also is found in nuts (almonds and walnuts). Poultry is another good source of zinc.

Helpful: Consider adding oysters to your diet. They are one of the richest sources of zinc.

Caution: Raw oysters are often contaminated with bacteria.

•**Magnesium.** Up to 75% of Americans are deficient in this vital mineral, which is needed for heart health, strong bones and blood sugar control.

Helpful: Vegetables are among the richest sources of magnesium. Eat raw or lightly steamed vegetables—highly processed or overcooked veggies lose their magnesium content. Whole grains are also much richer sources of magnesium than refined grains.

•**Calcium.** Many people advocate green, leafy vegetables for calcium, but these foods do not provide ample amounts of the mineral in a bioavailable form.

Sardines are an often-overlooked source of calcium, but they are not standard fare for many Americans.

Dairy foods remain the best regular source of calcium. Milk with 1% or 2% fat is a good choice. Skim milk is not recommended. That's because the bioavailability of fat-soluble vitamins, such as vitamin D, is diminished when you remove all the fat from milk.

Helpful: Avoid "fat-free half and half." This product provides no nutritional value—it is usually filled with corn syrup and other sugars to give it the creamy feel of real half and half.

•**Selenium.** The number-one source of this cancer-fighting mineral is the soil in which plants are grown. Soil in the Great Plains states contains adequate levels of selenium, so products made from whole-grain wheat, which is typically harvested in this area, are generally good sources of selenium.

Helpful: If you are at increased risk for cancer (due to family history, exposure to second-hand smoke or other carcinogens), consider taking a 50-microgram (mcg) to 200-mcg selenium supplement.

Important: If you are currently undergoing treatment for cancer, talk to your doctor before taking selenium.

•**Chromium.** This mineral, shown in dozens of studies to help control blood sugar levels, is poorly absorbed. Unless you eat organ meats, such as liver, it's best consumed in a supplement.

Helpful: Everyone should consider taking a 200-mcg chromium supplement daily for general health. If you have diabetes, ask your doctor about taking 1,000 mcg of chromium daily.

•**Carotenoids.** More than 600 nutritious plant compounds known as carotenoids can be found in vegetables and fruits.

Examples: Lycopene, found in tomatoes, watermelon and pink grapefruit, may help prevent prostate cancer...and lutein and zeaxanthin, found in dark green, leafy vegetables and corn, may help prevent and treat macular degeneration. This disease is the leading cause of vision loss in people over age 65.

Helpful: Because carotenoids are fat-soluble nutrients (that is, they require some amount of dietary fat for optimal absorption), consume carotenoid-rich foods with olive oil or other healthful fat sources. Low-fat salad dressings can be used, but try to stay away from no-fat versions.

Also helpful: Steam or lightly simmer vegetables. Raw fruits and vegetables contain valuable enzymes, but cooking breaks the cell walls, increasing the bioavailability of many valuable nutrients.

Examples: To maximize the amount of cancer-fighting lycopene from tomatoes, cook them in a sauce.

•**Protein.** On the bioavailability scale, meat, poultry, fish and eggs are among the best sources of protein. Although the protein found in lunch meats, such as ham and bologna, is bioavailable, these foods typically contain high levels of sodium and harmful fillers and preservatives known as nitrates.

Aim for 50 g to 120 g of protein daily (one-half of a salmon fillet contains 42 g...one-half of a chicken breast contains 27 g...three ounces of top sirloin contains 25 g).

Helpful: To maximize the bioavailability of nutrients found in beef, prepare it medium rare.

For a convenient protein source that lasts for several days, roast a turkey breast or chicken in an oven cooking bag, slice it up and use it during the week.

As an alternative to meat, consider using whey protein powder—an excellent source of protein derived from milk. Look for "cold filtered" and "ion exchanged" on the label, which indicates that the processing has removed lactose (milk sugar) and casein (a highly allergenic protein found in milk). This breaks down the whey, making it more absorbable. Next Nutrition as well as Jarrow each make excellent whey products. Only 2% of people with dairy allergies are allergic to whey protein.

Whey protein powder can be easily added to a smoothie.

What to do: Mix one scoop of protein powder (typically 20 g of protein) with eight ounces of water, milk or juice and ice in a blender. Add frozen blueberries or other fruit, if desired.

If you are allergic to whey protein, consider soy powder—the protein in soy powder is more easily utilized than that in other soy foods. Soy powder also can be used in smoothies.

Important: If you eat a vegan diet (no animal products of any kind), take a multivitamin as nutritional insurance. Plant-based diets do not contain adequate amounts of all nutrients.

Maca—The Super Food

Mark A. Stengler, ND, naturopathic physician in private practice, La Jolla, California…adjunct associate clinical professor at the National College of Natural Medicine, Portland, Oregon…author of many books, including The Natural Physician's Healing Therapies and coauthor of Prescription for Natural Cures (both from Bottom Line Books)…and author of the Bottom Line/Natural Healing newsletter.

Super foods are foods and herbs considered to be especially healthful due to their hefty nutritional content. The list includes familiar favorites, such as blueberries, broccoli and beans. Now a more exotic super food you may never have heard of is generating excitement in the world of natural health—a Peruvian root vegetable called maca (*Lepidium meyenii* or *peruvianum*), pronounced MACK-ah.

The root of the maca is shaped like a large radish. It is a cousin to other cruciferous plants, such as cauliflower and brussels sprouts. Peruvians traditionally boil or roast the maca root or grind it into flour for baking. However, despite maca's popular description as a "super food," you won't see it in food form in this country. Instead, the root is dried and ground into a fine powder. It then is distributed primarily in capsules, although you also can buy the powder to blend into beverages or sprinkle on foods.

I began looking into maca for my patients about seven years ago. In addition to its healthful fiber, complex carbohydrates and protein, maca provides numerous minerals, including calcium, magnesium, phosphorous, potassium, sulfur, iron, zinc, iodine and copper…vitamins B-1, B-2, C and E…nearly 20 amino acids, including *linoleic acid, palmitic acid* and *oleic acid*…as well as various plant sterols, which are natural cholesterol-lowering agents. All of these nutrients have been shown to promote health in a multitude of ways.

Here is what this super food can do to help you…

BOOST SEX DRIVE

Legend holds that in the era of the Inca empire, battle leaders provided maca to warriors to enhance their strength—then cut off the supply after the fighting ended to protect women from the warriors' maca-heightened libidos.

Modern research has suggested that maca does indeed increase sex drive in men. One double-blind, randomized study published in the journal *Andrologia* examined the effect of maca on sexual desire in 57 men, ages 21 to 56. Participants took either placebos or 1,500 mg or 3,000 mg of maca daily. After four, eight and 12 weeks, they reported on their sex drive levels. Placebo users experienced no change in libido, while the men taking either quantity of maca reported heightened sexual desire starting at eight weeks and continuing throughout the study.

How it works: Maca's libido-enhancing powers are attributed primarily to its amino acids and sterols. Blood tests indicated that maca did not affect the men's levels of the hormones testosterone or estradiol (a form of estrogen present in women and men). This is just one of maca's virtues—it does not change hormone regulation in men.

A small study published in the *Asian Journal of Andrology* yielded some interesting results, indicating that maca also improves male fertility. Nine men, ages 24 to 44, received either 1,500 mg or 3,000 mg of maca per day. Compared with tests done at the outset of the study, semen analysis performed at the end of the four-month research period demonstrated that maca increased semen volume, sperm count and sperm motility at both dosage levels. Again, maca achieved these results by unknown mechanisms that were not related to increases in testosterone or other hormones.

SOOTHE MENOPAUSAL SYMPTOMS

For women, maca has a long-standing reputation for soothing menopausal symptoms. A recent study in the *International Journal of Biomedical Science* details research at five sites in Poland, focusing on 124 women, ages 49 to 58, in the early stages of menopause.

During the study, the women took varied combinations of either a placebo or 2,000 mg of maca every day.

Results: Compared with placebo users, those taking maca experienced significant reductions—84%, on average—in the frequency and severity of menopausal symptoms, particularly hot flashes and night sweats. The participants also reported that maca reduced nervousness, mood swings, fatigue, stress, headaches and depression, as well as improved sleep patterns and libido.

Bonus: In a substudy of the trial, researchers found that the women taking maca had a notable increase in bone density.

How it works: Blood tests showed that maca reduced *follicle-stimulating hormone*, which normally increases during menopause and is thought to be one cause of troublesome symptoms, such as hot flashes and night sweats. Study authors speculate that maca stimulates the regulatory mechanism responsible for optimizing ovarian function and estrogen secretion, significantly increasing the level of estradiol in a woman's body.

It appears, then, that maca offers a safe and effective way to reduce menopausal symptoms —and it is unlikely to increase a woman's risk for breast cancer, heart disease and stroke, as can non-bioidentical hormone replacement therapy.

We don't know this for certain, but the fact that breast cancer is not among the leading causes of death in Peruvian women, despite a diet rich in maca, supports the assumption. In addition, increases in estradiol as a result of taking maca supplements may be safer than adding a hormone to a woman's system because maca appears to stimulate the body's natural estrogen production.

Historically, maca also has been used to improve libido in women. We don't have conclusive data on this, but the National Institutes of Health (NIH) is conducting a study to determine if maca can effectively address female sexual dysfunction caused by antidepressant drugs. The study is expected to be completed in November of 2009.

FIGHT STRESS AND DISEASE

Any kind of stress—from work, personal problems, illness, injury, toxins, hormonal imbalances or any other source—can negatively affect how our bodies function. Maca is what holistic doctors call an *adaptogen*, a plant or herb that boosts the body's ability to resist, deal with and recover from emotional and physical stress.

Practitioners of traditional medicine from China and India have known about and made use of adaptogens for centuries, though the term itself was not coined until the middle of the 20th century. Well-known adaptogens include the herbs ashwagandha, ginseng, rhodiola and licorice root, all of which I have prescribed to my patients with much success over the years.

How it works: To be classified as an adaptogen, a natural substance must meet specific criteria. It must be nontoxic…normalize levels of chemicals raised during periods of stress… and produce physical, chemical and/or biological responses that increase the body's resistance to stress.

Although all adaptogenic plants contain antioxidants, researchers do not believe that antioxidants alone account for adaptogens' normalizing powers. Rather, it is thought that a variety of phytochemicals helps balance the dozens of endocrine, digestive and neural hormones that operate throughout the body—including *insulin* (which regulates blood sugar levels) and *dopamine* (which enhances and stabilizes mood). Many adaptogens also stimulate immune system components, leading to better immune function.

MORE OF MACA'S SUPER POWERS

In addition to its documented beneficial effects on the human reproductive system, laboratory tests and animal studies suggest that maca may reduce the risk for…

• **Arthritis**—by promoting cartilage growth.

• **Blood contamination**—by improving liver function.

• **Diabetes**—by allowing for better control over blood sugar levels and body weight.

• **Digestive health**—by combating ulcers.

• **Fatigue**—by increasing overall energy and endurance.

• **Heart disease**—by lowering levels of LDL "bad" cholesterol and triglycerides (a type of blood fat).

• **Infertility**—by stimulating production of estrogen and other hormones in women and boosting sperm count in men.

• **Memory and mood**—by enhancing certain brain chemicals.

• **Osteoporosis**—by increasing bone density.

• **Premenstrual syndrome (PMS)**—by regulating hormone levels.

• **Prostate problems**—by reducing prostate enlargement.

THE SAFEST WAY TO START

Maca generally appears to be safe, given its long history of use by Peruvians…but there are a few guidelines to bear in mind. Women who take estrogen to ease menopausal symptoms should talk to their doctors about using maca. They may be able to wean off hormone therapy or at least lower the estrogen dosage under a doctor's supervision.

Breast cancer patients taking *tamoxifen* or other estrogen blockers and women who have had breast cancer must not use maca, because it raises estrogen levels. Women in a family with a strong history of breast cancer should discuss maca use with their doctors first. People who take thyroid medication should be monitored by their doctors because maca may increase thyroid activity. Women who are pregnant or breast-feeding should not take maca, as a general precaution.

Since its long-term effects have not been scientifically studied, I recommend taking a break from maca now and then in order to give the body's cell receptors a break from any hormone stimulation. People who want to try maca to see if it is a "super food" for them should take supplements for three months (six months for women with severe menopausal symptoms), then stop using maca for one or two weeks. They may then continue this regimen as needed for symptom relief.

HOW MUCH TO TAKE

Maca is available in supplement and powder form.

The average dose of maca supplements is 1,000 mg to 2,000 mg daily—which you can take with or without food at any time of day.

Or you can get your maca by adding powder to your favorite foods and drinks. It has a slightly nutty flavor, so you may enjoy mixing it with almond milk. *Other ways to incoporate maca into your diet…*

• **Sprinkle on cereal (hot or cold).**

• **Mix into your favorite smoothie or protein shake.**

• **Add to yogurt or applesauce,** perhaps with a little cinnamon.

• **Stir into tea**—especially chai blends, as the flavors complement each other.

• **Use in baking**—substitute maca powder for one-quarter of the flour in any recipe (no more, or it might affect texture or consistency).

Be aware: Maca powder has a high fiber content and may initially cause gassiness. I suggest beginning with one teaspoon a day, then gradually increasing your intake by one teaspoon every five days until you find your comfort zone. The optimum dosage is three to six teaspoons daily.

WHERE TO GET MACA

Maca capsules and powder are widely available at many supplement and health-food stores…

Maca powder typically costs about $17 per pound. Reliable on-line sources include *www.iherb.com*, which sells a brand called Maca Power. You also can buy Maca Power from its manufacturer, Navitas Naturals (888-645-4282, *www.navitasnaturals.com*).

There is a maca capsule made for post-menopausal women that is similar to the formulation used in the Polish study of menopausal women. It is called Femmenessence MacaPause and is made by Natural Health International (888-668-3661, *www.naturalhi.com*).

Cost: $35 for 120 capsules of 500 mg each.

SuperFoods That Prevent Heart Disease, Cancer, Diabetes, More

Steven G. Pratt, MD, senior staff ophthalmologist at Scripps Memorial Hospital in La Jolla, California, is coauthor of the best-selling book, *Bottom Line's SuperFoods Rx.* Bottom Line Books.

You know that spinach and broccoli are good for you. But did you know that dark chocolate can lower blood pressure? Or that avocados can prevent migraine headaches?

Steven G. Pratt, MD, has added dark chocolate, avocados and seven other foods to the original list of 14 that he presented in his best-selling *Bottom Line's SuperFoods Rx*.

Together with exercise, weight control, healthy sleep habits and stress reduction, these foods can help you live a long and healthy life…

APPLES

Apples can reduce your risk of heart disease, certain cancers, high blood pressure and type 2 diabetes. They are particularly good for the respiratory system, helping to prevent lung cancer and asthma.

Why are apples so beneficial? They are a great source of fiber, potassium and disease-fighting antioxidants, such as vitamin C and polyphenols. But evidence suggests that it is the complex synergistic interactions among these various elements that make the fruit so healthful.

Eat as wide a variety of apples as possible—and don't remove the peels. A study in *Journal of Agricultural and Food Chemistry* confirmed that the concentration of antioxidants in an apple's skin is several times greater than in its flesh.

Best: An apple a day, just as the saying goes.

AVOCADOS

Avocados have a remarkable ability to help the body absorb nutrients from food. You'll get substantially more health benefits from the carrots and tomatoes in your salad if you toss in half an avocado as well. This is probably because the monounsaturated fat of the avocado increases the body's absorption of fat-soluble carotenoid phytonutrients, such as beta-carotene.

Avocados also contain lots of magnesium, which helps prevent type 2 diabetes and migraine headaches, as well as plenty of potassium, which promotes low blood pressure and good circulation.

Though relatively high in calories (48 calories per ounce), avocados help fight obesity because they boost satiety—the feeling of fullness that signals us to stop eating and thus helps control calorie intake.

Best: One-third to one-half an avocado two to three times a week.

DARK CHOCOLATE

Dark chocolate contains plenty of polyphenols, such as flavonols, which lower blood pressure. (Milk chocolate does not appear to lower blood pressure.) Chocolate also is a natural anti-inflammatory.

A study published in *American Journal of Clinical Nutrition* showed that the effects on blood flow from drinking one cup of cocoa rich in flavonol were comparable to those from taking a low-dose aspirin (though the benefits didn't last quite as long). This suggests that a bar of dark chocolate can be used to treat a mild headache or other minor pains.

Newman's Own Sweet Dark Chocolate has significantly more polyphenols than many other dark chocolates. Next on the list are Dove Silky Dark Chocolate…Endangered Species Chocolate Company Wolf Bar…Cadbury Royal Dark Indulgent Dark Chocolate…and Hershey's Special Dark Mildly Sweet Chocolate. The higher the percentage of cocoa solids in your dark chocolate, the more polyphenols it contains.

Despite its high fat content, dark chocolate does not seem to increase blood cholesterol levels.

Best: Chocolate is a high-calorie food, so consume no more than 100 calories of chocolate per day—that's about half of a 2.8-ounce Newman's Own Sweet Dark Chocolate bar.

OLIVE OIL

The single most healthful change people can make to their cooking habits is to use extra-virgin olive oil in place of other oils and fats. While most fats and oils are bad for us, olive oil has been shown to reduce the risk of breast and colon cancer, lower blood pressure and improve cardiovascular health. Select an extra-virgin olive oil that is cold pressed and greenish in color—this suggests that it has a high level of polyphenols.

Best: One tablespoon most days.

GARLIC

Eating garlic on a regular basis helps reduce blood pressure, triglyceride levels and your LDL (bad) cholesterol—and it may increase HDL (good) cholesterol. Garlic is an anti-inflammatory that can help control arthritis. It has been shown to have significant antibiotic properties, decreasing the incidence and severity of bacterial infections.

There's even some evidence that garlic consumption might reduce the risk of certain cancers, including colorectal, gastric and prostate cancer, though more research is needed on this subject.

Best: About one clove of garlic several times a week. Fresh garlic is better than dried garlic or garlic supplements. Raw garlic offers the most health benefits, but cooked is fine, too.

HONEY

Daily honey consumption increases the amount of antioxidants in the blood, which appears to reduce the risk of heart disease and cancer. It also helps prevent constipation and reduces cholesterol and blood pressure.

Honey even does a better job of maintaining energy levels than other sweeteners. While consuming sugar typically provides only a very brief spike in blood sugar, a study found that athletes given honey after a workout maintained optimal blood sugar levels for a full two hours—and their muscles recovered faster from the workout than those who consumed other sweeteners.

Darker honeys tend to have more antioxidants—and more flavor.

Best: One to two teaspoons, taken several times a week.

KIWIS

Kiwis contain massive amounts of vitamins C and E. Vitamin C can reduce our risk of asthma, osteoarthritis and colon cancer. It also can boost our immune systems. Dietary vitamin E appears to lower the risk of Alzheimer's disease—and unlike most vitamin E–rich foods (nuts, oils), kiwis aren't high in fat or calories.

Kiwis are an excellent source of the antioxidant *lutein*, which is associated with lower risk of cataracts and macular degeneration. And they have been shown to reduce the risk of blood clots.

Best: One kiwi two to three times a week.

ONIONS

Onions deliver many of the same benefits as garlic. They can help reduce blood pressure, cholesterol levels and the risk of heart disease. They're useful as anti-inflammatories and have antibiotic properties. There's some research to suggest that onions might reduce the risk of colon cancer.

After you cut open an onion, let it sit for five to 10 minutes before cooking. Applying heat sooner will deactivate the *thiopropanal sulfoxide* in the onion. That's the compound that contributes to the onion's ability to help our hearts, among other health benefits. In general, you will get the greatest benefits by eating the most pungent onions.

Best: Dishes containing onions at least three times a week.

POMEGRANATES

Pomegranates are phytochemical powerhouses, and they are packed with potassium, which can help lower your blood pressure. Studies even suggest that pomegranates can slow the progression of prostate cancer and reduce the risk of atherosclerosis, the narrowing and hardening of the arteries.

Best: Four to eight ounces of 100% pomegranate juice several times each week. Avoid brands that contain added sugar.

■ ■ ■ ■

Dr. Pratt's SuperFoods

Here are 14 tasty superfoods that can keep us healthy...

Beans	Soy
Blueberries	Spinach
Broccoli	Tea
Oats	Tomatoes
Oranges	Turkey
Pumpkin	Walnuts
Wild salmon	Yogurt

Six Incredible Cancer-Fighting Foods

Karen Collins, RD, a registered dietitian and nutrition adviser to the American Institute for Cancer Research (AICR) in Washington, DC, is the author of *Planning Meals That Lower Cancer Risk*. AICR.

Only about 10% of all cancers are due to genetics. The remaining 90% of malignancies are related to diet, weight and exercise...smoking...and/or environmental factors.

Even though most people realize that diet can affect cancer risk, few regularly consume a variety of the foods that contain large amounts of *phytochemicals*, substances that actually can inhibit the cellular damage that leads to cancer.

Eating a combination of cancer-fighting foods is the best approach because no single food supplies all the available protective substances—vitamins, minerals, phytochemicals and fiber.

BLACK BEANS

Beans (legumes) have high levels of the cancer-fighting compound phytic acid. They're also rich in fiber and saponins, chemical compounds that reduce the ability of cancer cells to proliferate.

The landmark Nurses' Health study found that women who ate four or more servings of legumes weekly were 33% less likely to develop colon polyps than those who consumed one or fewer weekly servings. In people already diagnosed with colon polyps, those who ate more beans reduced their risk for a recurrence by 45%, compared with those who ate fewer beans.

Bonus: Beans are very high in protein. They're a good substitute for people who want to reduce their consumption of red meat—a major source of saturated fat, which can increase cancer risk.

Other cancer-fighting legumes: Small red beans, red kidney beans, pinto beans and garbanzo beans.

Helpful: If you don't want to spend time cooking dried beans, you can get many of the same benefits by eating canned. To reduce the sodium in canned beans, empty them into a colander and rinse thoroughly with cold water.

Recommended: Eat one-half cup of beans at least four times weekly.

BLUEBERRIES

Berries are rich sources of vitamin C and other antioxidants. People who regularly eat berries have a lower risk for malignancies of the colon, bladder, esophagus and prostate. Berries also may lower the risk for lymphoma and premenopausal breast cancer.

Blueberries are an ideal choice for cancer prevention because they are among the richest sources of antioxidants, chemical compounds that protect cells from free radicals that can damage DNA—the first step in cancer development.

Much of this nutritional power comes from their high levels of *anthocyanidins*, a type of antioxidant that reduces the ability of carcinogens to damage DNA.

Bonus: Because berries are both filling and low in calories, they can be substituted for other sweet snacks to promote weight loss—which further reduces the risk for many cancers.

Other cancer-fighting berries: Blackberries, strawberries, raspberries and cranberries.

Helpful: Keep frozen berries in the freezer. They can be kept almost indefinitely without spoiling and provide virtually the same nutritional benefits as fresh berries.

Recommended: Aim for at least one half-cup serving of berries per week.

BROCCOLI

Broccoli is a cruciferous vegetable that is rich in *isothiocyanates*, a family of phytochemicals linked to a reduced risk for colon, prostate, lung and premenopausal breast cancer. One of these phytochemicals, *sulforaphane*, reduces the ability of carcinogens to cause cell damage—and may increase the tendency of cancer cells to self-destruct, a process called apoptosis.

A study published in the *Journal of the National Cancer Institute* reports that men who consumed three or more weekly servings of broccoli (raw or cooked) were 41% less likely to get prostate cancer than those who consumed less than one weekly serving.

Other cancer-fighting cruciferous vegetables: Cauliflower, brussels sprouts, cabbage and kale.

Helpful: If you don't like the strong taste (and smell) of cooked broccoli and other cruciferous vegetables, eat them raw or lightly sautéed in olive or canola oil for three to four minutes.

You also can microwave or steam them. (Long cooking, such as boiling for 15 minutes or more, causes the release of strong-smelling/tasting sulfur compounds.)

Recommended: Aim for three to five half-cup servings per week of cruciferous vegetables.

GARLIC

Garlic is an allium, which is a family of plants that contain *allyl sulfides*, phytochemicals not found in any other foods.

The Iowa Women's Health Study found that people with the highest intake of garlic (at least one serving weekly) had a 32% lower risk of developing colon cancer than those who never ate garlic. Garlic has also been linked to a lower risk for prostate, lung, breast and skin cancers.

Bonus: Garlic can be used as a flavor enhancer to make healthful foods—vegetables, beans, whole grains, etc.—more enjoyable… and it reduces the need for unhealthful flavorings, such as salt and butter.

Other cancer-fighting alliums: Onions (all types), leeks and chives.

Helpful: To reduce the strong taste, use cooked garlic (by sautéing or roasting it, for example) rather than raw. The flavors mellow with long cooking. Wait 10 to 15 minutes after chopping garlic before cooking, to allow the active form of the protective phytochemicals to form. The cancer-fighting properties of jarred garlic are unknown.

Recommended: Aim to eat one to three cloves of garlic per week.

WALNUTS

Walnuts provide fiber and are rich in omega-3 fatty acids, the same healthful, anti-inflammatory fats that are found in fish. Reducing inflammation in the body helps prevent cell damage that can lead to cancer.

Other cancer-fighters: Almonds and hazelnuts.

Helpful: Buy packaged or bulk shelled, unsalted nuts (raw or roasted). Substituting nuts for other snacks improves the body's ratio of omega-3 to omega-6 fatty acids—important for lowering inflammation and cancer risk.

Recommended: Eat three to five one-third-cup servings weekly.

WHOLE-GRAIN BREAD

Whole-grain bread is high in fiber. As fiber and certain starches resistant to digestion are fermented in the colon, substances are produced that block the cancer-promoting effects of bile acids. In addition, whole grains are higher in antioxidant vitamins (including vitamin E) and phytochemicals called *phenols* than are refined grains.

When scientists analyzed and combined the results from 40 different studies, they found that people who ate the most whole-grain bread and/or other whole grains had a 34% lower risk for cancer overall than those who consumed less.

Other cancer-fighting whole grains: Whole-wheat pasta, whole-grain breakfast cereal, brown rice, bulgur, kasha and quinoa.

Helpful: When shopping for whole-grain bread or cereal, don't be misled by terms like multigrain, which merely means that more than one type of grain is included…and don't judge by brown color, which can result from added caramel coloring. Check the ingredients list to make sure a whole grain is listed first, such as whole wheat or whole rye. "Flour" or "wheat flour" means that the product contains refined flour made from wheat—not whole-grain flour.

Recommended: Aim for three daily servings —one-half cup of whole grains or a slice of whole-grain bread counts as one serving.

■ ■ ■ ■

The Truth About "Healthier" Snacks

Food companies are marketing candies and snacks that they say are better for your health, but only a few are truly worthwhile…

Best: Snacks that have less salt, trans fats and high-fructose corn syrup. *Examples…*

•**LesserEvil popcorn snacks,** 99 cents for a 1.75-ounce single-serving pouch and $3.49 for a 3.65-ounce carton.

•**Bearitos Tortilla Chips,** $3.50 for a 16-ounce bag.

•**Barbara's Bakery Fig Bars,** $3.50 for a 12-ounce package.

Worst: Fortified candies, including jellybeans, that have vitamins C and E and electrolytes. Electrolyte-replacement products, including sports drinks, are of little use to all but elite athletes. Added C and E are of questionable value for anyone who eats well or takes a multivitamin/mineral supplement.

Suzanne Havala Hobbs, DrPH, RD, clinical assistant professor, School of Public Health, University of North Carolina at Chapel Hill. She is the author of *Get the Trans Fat Out: 601 Simple Ways to Cut the Trans Fat Out of Any Diet*. Three Rivers.

Best Breads for Your Health

Evelyn Tribole, RD, a nutritionist in private practice in Irvine, California, is the author of *Stealth Health* (Penguin) and coauthor of *Intuitive Eating: A Revolutionary Program That Works* (St. Martin's).

The new USDA dietary guidelines recommend that most Americans get six ounces of grains daily, and that half of that—at least three one-ounce servings (one slice of bread equals about one ounce)—should be from whole-grain sources. Of course, eating only whole grains to meet the quota is even better.

Breads can be a source of whole grains, but knowing which ones are most healthful is difficult.

WHOLE VERSUS REFINED

Grain products, including pasta, oatmeal, hot and cold breakfast cereals and bread, are divided into two subgroups—whole and refined. Whole grains, by definition, contain the entire grain—the bran (outer coating), germ (seed embryo) and endosperm (also called the kernel, it makes up most of the seed). Examples include whole-wheat flour, cracked wheat (bulgur) and brown rice.

Whole grains are rich in fiber, which has been shown to reduce risk for heart disease, diabetes and some cancers. They provide large amounts of vitamins and minerals that are sometimes lacking in our diet, including magnesium, selenium, potassium, zinc, vitamin E and chromium.

Refined grains are milled to remove the bran and germ, which gives them a finer texture and lengthens their shelf life. This process is also nutritionally devastating—it removes the healthful fiber, iron and many B vitamins and other vitamins and minerals found in whole grains.

Since refined grains are digested more quickly than whole grains, they can cause spikes in blood sugar and insulin secretion, which can increase hunger—and diabetes risk. Refined grains include white flour, white rice and white bread.

IS IT WHOLE GRAIN?

When buying any type of bread, look for whole-grain flours in the list of ingredients.

These include bulgur, whole wheat, whole rye, whole oats, barley, brown rice and buckwheat. Less common whole grains include amaranth, millet, quinoa, sorghum and triticale (a hybrid of wheat and rye). One of these flours should appear first in the list of ingredients—this means it is the primary ingredient by weight.

Caution: Just because a bread package says "multigrain," "stone-ground," "100% wheat," "seven-grain" or "bran," it does not mean it is made from whole grains.

Important: Serving sizes can be deceiving. Some breads list one serving as one slice, others as two slices.

White bread, which is made from refined grains, will list enriched wheat flour as the first ingredient.

Typical nutritional data per slice: 66 calories, 0.6 g fat, 0.6 g fiber, 170 mg sodium.

Important: Sourdough bread does not cause the spikes in blood sugar that result from eating other refined breads. That's because it has a lower glycemic index, an indicator of how quickly carbohydrates are digested.

The following breads can be among the most healthful available. Just check the ingredients to ensure that they're made from whole grain.

Nutrient-dense breads...

WHOLE WHEAT

What to look for: Whole wheat is typically the first ingredient, but it could be whole oats, whole rye or millet.

Typical nutritional data per slice: 90 calories, 1 g fat, 3 g fiber, 180 mg sodium.

Good brands: Arnold Natural 100% Whole Wheat...Oroweat 100% Whole Wheat...Stroehmann Dutch Country 100% Whole Wheat.

Important: Some "wheat" breads are made with enriched wheat flour. Enriched means that after the grain was refined, only five nutrients that were removed in the refining process were added back in—thiamin, riboflavin, niacin, iron and folic acid. However, fiber, magnesium and other vitamins and minerals are not restored to the flour.

RYE

What to look for: Whole rye should be the first ingredient.

Typical nutritional data per slice: 100 calories, 0.5 g fat, 3 g fiber, 200 mg sodium.

Good brands: Rubschlager 100% Rye, Rye-Ola Black Rye...Genuine Bavarian Organic Whole Rye.

PUMPERNICKEL

What to look for: Whole rye should be the first ingredient. Long, slow cooking causes the natural sugar in rye flour to darken and sweeten the bread.

Typical nutritional data per slice: 100 calories, 0.5 g fat, 3 g fiber, 200 mg sodium.

Good brands: Mestemacher Genuine West-phalian Pumpernickel...Rubschlager 100% Rye, Rye-Ola Pumpernickel.

■ ■ ■ ■

What "Whole Grain" Really Means on Food Labels

Don't be misled by labels on cereals, bread and other foods made from grain...

• **"Made with whole grain"** means that the food contains some whole grain, either a little or a lot.

• **"Good source of whole grain"** on a cereal box means as little as eight grams of whole grain per serving, and "excellent source" means as little as 16 grams. Since the typical cereal serving is as large as 55 grams, a "good source" may be as little as 15% whole grain, and an "excellent source" as little as 30%.

• **"Whole grain"** means that at least 51% of the flour is whole grain—up to 49% may not be.

• **"100% whole grain"** means that no refined flour is used.

Note: These terms are being used this way voluntarily by cereal makers until the government makes an official rule.

Michael F. Jacobson, PhD, executive director, Center for Science in the Public Interest, and executive editor, *Nutrition Action Healthletter*, 1875 Connecticut Ave. NW, Washington, DC 20009.

■ ■ ■ ■

Get More from Food

Ounce for ounce, the drying process used for fruit nearly doubles the antioxidant content and increases levels of fiber.

Smart idea: Mix chopped prunes into your morning oatmeal...sprinkle dried cranberries into salads. Important: Dried fruit contains twice the calories of regular fruit.

Caution: Dried fruit may contain sulfites, preservatives that may trigger allergic reactions, especially in asthmatics.

Joe A. Vinson, PhD, professor of chemistry, University of Scranton, Pennsylvania, and leader of a study of 100 different foods, presented at the 230th national meeting of the American Chemical Society.

Don't Be Fooled by Food Labels

Suzanne Havala Hobbs, DrPH, RD, clinical assistant professor, School of Public Health, University of North Carolina at Chapel Hill. She is the author of *Get the Trans Fat Out: 601 Simple Ways to Cut the Trans Fat Out of Any Diet*. Three Rivers.

If you are confused about the claims that manufacturers are now making on food labels, you are not alone.

"ORGANIC"

The term organic is hotly debated. The US Department of Agriculture's (USDA) current definition states that organic foods are those plants produced without the use of pesticides, sewage sludge (for fertilization) or synthetic fertilizer...or those animals raised without hormones or antibiotics.

To read the complete definition, go to the USDA's Web site at *www.ams.usda.gov/nop/NOP/standards.html*.

Organic foods, including produce, meat, milk and other dairy products, typically cost more than nonorganic varieties.

The FDA has linked pesticides to some types of cancer, and numerous other studies have linked them to Parkinson's disease. There's also strong evidence from the American Medical Association that bacteria are becoming resistant to some antibiotics because they are used in meat production.

What you may not know: In October 2005, the Agricultural Appropriations Conference Committee voted to allow synthetic ingredients into foods labeled "organic." Therefore, yogurt, pudding and other items may be considered organic even if they contain synthetic additives.

What you can do: Whenever possible, buy organic meats and dairy products.

For produce, choose organic varieties if you're buying one of the items found by the Environmental Working Group (a nonprofit group of researchers who investigate environmental health threats) to be among the most contaminated.

If you must buy nonorganic, choose produce that is least likely to be contaminated. Wash the nonorganic produce vigorously under running water to remove as much potentially harmful residue as possible. (Organic produce also should be washed.)

If you must buy nonorganic meat, choose the leanest cuts available and, whenever possible, remove the skin from poultry (toxins from hormones and antibiotics tend to accumulate in fatty tissue).

"NATURAL"

"Natural" is a word used for marketing purposes—it is not a term that is defined by the government.

What you may not know: Natural does not mean that a food product is necessarily "healthful."

Example: Breyers labels its ice cream "all natural," but it is high in fat and saturated fat.

What you can do: Read food labels carefully to determine the levels of fat and saturated fat as well as other ingredients in products that are labeled natural.

"LOW"

Many dairy products and some processed foods, such as soup, frozen entrees and snacks, use the term "low" or some variation thereof. *What these terms mean…*

Low fat: 3 grams (g) or less of total fat per serving.

Low saturated fat: 1 g or less of saturated fat per serving.

Low calorie: 40 calories or less per serving.

Low cholesterol: 20 milligrams (mg) or less of cholesterol and 2 g or less of saturated fat per serving.

Low sodium: 140 mg or less of sodium per serving.

Very low sodium: 35 mg or less of sodium per serving.

Nonfat: Less than 0.5 g of fat per serving.

"LEAN" AND "EXTRA-LEAN"

"Lean" and "extra-lean" refer to the fat content of meat, poultry and seafood. *What these two terms mean…*

Lean: Less than 10 g of fat, including no more than 4 g of saturated fat and less than 95 mg of cholesterol per 3.5-ounce serving.

Extra-lean: Less than 5 g of fat, including no more than 2 g of saturated fat and less than 95 mg of cholesterol per 3.5-ounce serving.

OTHER TERMS

Reduced: The food contains at least 25% less of an ingredient (such as fat, cholesterol, sodium or added sugar) or calories than the regular product.

Example: Reduced Fat Fig Newtons have at least 25% less fat than the original recipe.

High: The food contains at least 20% of the Daily Value (recommended daily intake) for a particular nutrient.

Example: The Daily Value for fiber is 25 g. If a food product contains 5 g of fiber per serving, it might say "high fiber" on its label.

■ ■ ■ ■

When to Buy Organic

When does it make sense to spend the extra money for organic produce? Take a look at the lists of the most—and least—contaminated fruits and vegetables, and spend your money wisely.

MOST CONTAMINATED PRODUCE

Apples	Peaches
Bell peppers	Pears
Celery	Potatoes
Cherries	Red raspberries
Imported grapes	Spinach
Nectarines	Strawberries

583

LEAST CONTAMINATED PRODUCE

Asparagus	Kiwi
Avocados	Mangoes
Bananas	Onions
Broccoli	Papaya
Cauliflower	Peas (sweet)
Corn (sweet)	Pineapples

Environmental Working Group. *www.ewg.org.*

How to Save Money on Organic Food

Ronnie Cummins, national director of the Organic Consumers Association, a nonprofit organization that promotes food safety, children's health and environmental sustainability, Finland, MN, is the author of *Genetically Engineered Food: A Self-Defense Guide for Consumers.* Marlowe & Company.

Many people who would like to eat organic fruits, vegetables, dairy, meat and poultry are put off by the high prices. Organic foods can cost 25% to 100% more than regular foods—but if you're willing to do a bit of sleuthing and look beyond traditional grocery stores, you can find organic products for much less.

My organization's interactive Web site, *www. organicconsumers.org*, has links to most of the resources suggested below...

•**Compare prices of conventional and organic foods** when shopping at regular grocery stores. Occasionally, the price gap narrows dramatically, or organic foods may even be cheaper.

•**Shop at a farmers' market.** You can find bargains if you prowl around the stalls of your local farmers' market. You'll save even more if you haggle. Farmers may be especially willing to negotiate prices if produce is misshapen or closing time is approaching.

Sample savings: Organic apples at a farmers' market often are 25% to 50% cheaper than organic apples at grocery or natural-food stores.

•**Consider purchasing a share in a community-supported agriculture program (CSA).** There are more than 1,000 of these programs around the US. Through a CSA, you purchase produce from an organic farmer in a region near you. You'll receive a weekly basket that contains produce, flowers and perhaps even eggs and milk. A share in a CSA typically costs several hundred dollars for one growing season, which could last half a year (prices vary dramatically depending on location). In mild regions, such as California, you can receive just-picked produce year-round. Each week, it's fun to discover what goodies are in the basket.

Sample savings: In rural Minnesota, where I live, I pay $450 for the season and split my weekly harvest with another family. This is at least 50% cheaper than store prices.

Helpful: Most CSAs deliver produce orders to a central location. You may be able to reduce the price of your weekly delivery if you allow your front porch to serve as a delivery spot for your neighborhood.

CSAs can be found at the Web site of Local Harvest (*www.localharvest.org*), as well as on my Web site.

•**Join a food co-op.** Co-ops typically offer high-quality organic food and produce at a discount for members. You may be required to volunteer your time for a certain number of hours each month. For a list of co-ops, see my group's Web site.

•**Buy in bulk.** This is a great way to save money on long-lasting and nonperishable organic food, such as dried beans, lentils, pasta, rice, cereals, trail mix, nuts and even peanut butter. Health-food stores, Whole Foods, and even some supermarkets sell bulk items.

Cheaper still: Join a wholesale buying club (regular yearly membership fee is between $35 and $50). The minimum order for the club I belong to is $1,000 every three months, so I share a membership with several families in my area.

Typical savings: 30% to 50% off retail.

There is no national directory of buying clubs. Ask your local natural-food store for the names of its organic-food suppliers and contact them.

•**Eat seasonally.** You're sure to overpay if you buy organic fruits and vegetables off-season. That's when you want to buy frozen or canned. When produce is bountiful and cheap, you may want to can, freeze or dry it for the coming months.

Those Amazing Bananas

Ara DerMarderosian, PhD, professor of pharmacognosy (the study of natural products used in medicine) and Roth chair of natural products at the University of the Sciences in Philadelphia. He also is the scientific director of the university's Complementary and Alternative Medicines Institute. Dr. DerMarderosian has published more than 100 scientific papers and chapters in books as well as two books.

Most people know that bananas are an excellent source of potassium (one ripe banana supplies more than 10% of an adult's daily requirement of the mineral). That's important because people with a low dietary intake of potassium are 28% more likely to suffer a stroke than those who consume higher levels, according to a study conducted at Tulane University.

Lesser-known medicinal uses of bananas…

•**Depression.** Bananas are a good source of tryptophan (a precursor to serotonin, a brain chemical that helps regulate mood).

•**Diarrhea.** Unripe bananas and plantains (high-starch, green bananas that are typically cooked) are a rich source of tannins, astringent plant compounds that help stop water accumulation in the intestines, thus diminishing diarrhea.

•**Heartburn and ulcers.** Bananas neutralize acidity and soothe and coat esophageal tissue with pectin (a substance used as a thickener and stabilizer in jellies).

Important: In rare cases, bananas may cause an allergic reaction. Bananas with blackened skin can increase blood sugar levels. Because bananas have high levels of potassium, people with kidney problems should check with their doctors before eating this fruit.

■ ■ ■ ■

Berry Good

Blueberries protect the heart. Of all fruits, blueberries have the highest level of antioxidants. Antioxidants relax blood vessels, improving blood flow and keeping blood pressure

down. Eat between one-half and one cup every day for maximum benefit.

Dorothy Klimis-Zacas, PhD, professor of clinical nutrition, University of Maine, Orono, reported in *The Federation of American Societies for Experimental Biology Journal.*

■ ■ ■ ■

Broccoli May Prevent Blindness

Sulforaphane, the naturally occurring antioxidant in broccoli and its sprouts, protects the eye from injury caused by the sun's UV rays. This damage is believed to be a primary cause of age-related macular degeneration.

Paul Talalay, MD, professor of pharmacology and molecular sciences at Johns Hopkins University School of Medicine, Baltimore, and coauthor of a study of antioxidant protection in cells, published in *Proceedings of the National Academy of Sciences of the USA.*

■ ■ ■ ■

A "Latte" Antioxidants!

Coffee has more antioxidants than any other food or beverage in the American diet. The average adult receives more than four times the amount of antioxidants from coffee—regular or decaf—daily than from black tea (the second-most consumed source) followed by chocolate, bananas, beans and corn.

Joe A. Vinson, PhD, professor of chemistry, University of Scranton, Pennsylvania, and leader of a study of 100 different foods, presented at the 230th national meeting of the American Chemical Society.

■ ■ ■ ■

A Cup or Two

Coffee may help prevent cirrhosis. Common in heavy drinkers, cirrhosis is the irreversible scarring that prevents the liver from filtering toxins properly. On average, coffee reduces the risk of cirrhosis by 20% for people who drink one cup per day…and reduces risk by 80% for those who have four cups daily. Coffee drinkers —whether or not they drink alcohol—also score better on liver function tests.

Reason: Unknown.

Arthur Klatsky, MD, adjunct investigator, Kaiser Permanente Division of Research, Oakland, California, and leader of a study of more than 125,000 people, published in *Archives of Internal Medicine.*

■ ■ ■ ■

Figs Protect Your Heart

Dried figs safeguard your heart, says J.A. Vinson, PhD. They can help you meet daily fruit and fiber recommendations and, like all dried fruits, provide a big dose of polyphenols, potent antioxidants that help prevent the formation of artery-clogging plaque.

Best: Eat five or six dried figs a day. Add them to sweet potato and squash dishes, oatmeal and salad, or enjoy them just as they are.

Joe A. Vinson, PhD, professor of chemistry, University of Scranton, Pennsylvania, and leader of a study of 100 different foods, presented at the 230th national meeting of the American Chemical Society.

■ ■ ■ ■

Ginger Helps Arthritis Pain

Ginger relieves arthritis pain, we hear from Sung Woo Kim, PhD. Ginger supplements soothe osteoarthritic joints by inhibiting production of pain-causing prostaglandins.

Best: Take a 100-mg supplement, such as Gingerforce, one to three times a day.

Sung Woo Kim, PhD, is associate professor of animal nutrition and digestive physiology, department of animal science, North Carolina State University, Raleigh, and leader of a study published in *Journal of Medicinal Food.*

■ ■ ■ ■

Ginger Eases Nausea

In a review of studies involving a total of 363 people, those who were given at least 1 g of powdered gingerroot capsules one hour prior to surgery were one-third less likely to suffer nausea and vomiting during the first 24 hours after the operation than those who got a placebo capsule.

Theory: Ginger may suppress the neurotransmitter serotonin, which plays a role in triggering nausea and vomiting.

Nathorn Chaiyakunapruk, PhD, assistant professor, department of pharmacy practice, Naresuan University, Phitsanulok, Thailand.

■ ■ ■ ■

Grapefruit Lowers Cholesterol

Heart disease patients who were nonresponsive to cholesterol-lowering drugs ate balanced meals that included one grapefruit daily. Those who ate red grapefruit lowered their total cholesterol by 15.5%, and white-grapefruit eaters reduced cholesterol by 7.6%. Those not eating grapefruit showed no cholesterol decrease.

Caution: Grapefruit can adversely interact with certain medications. See your doctor.

Shela Gorinstein, PhD, chief scientist, The Hebrew University of Jerusalem.

■ ■ ■ ■

Put the Squeeze on Alzheimer's

Juice may ward off Alzheimer's, according to Qi Dai, MD, PhD.

Recent finding: People who drank three or more servings a week of fruit and/or vegetable juice had 76% lower risk than those who drank less (the risk reduction was greatest in people with a family history of Alzheimer's).

Likely reason: Polyphenols—antioxidants that protect brain tissue—are in fruits and vegetables. Apples, grapes and oranges have high concentrations.

Qi Dai, MD, PhD, is assistant professor of medicine, Vanderbilt University Medical Center, Nashville, and leader of a study of 1,836 people, published in *The American Journal of Medicine.*

Is It Time to Become A Vegetarian?

Neal D. Barnard, MD, president and founder of the Physicians Committee for Responsible Medicine, Washington, DC.

The average American consumes 220 pounds of meat each year, but the recent mad cow disease scare has made many people think twice about this practice.

Even before the latest questions were raised regarding the safety of the US meat supply, 10 million Americans identified themselves as vegetarians.

Here are answers to some commonly asked questions about vegetarianism from Dr. Neal D. Barnard, president and founder of the Physicians Committee for Responsible Medicine, an independent, nonprofit health research and advocacy group...

•**Why do you favor a meat-free diet?** It's been scientifically proven—in epidemiological studies of people who selected their own diets, and in clinical trials where people were assigned vegetarian diets—that a vegetarian regimen is the most healthful diet.

Studies of Seventh-day Adventists—people who don't smoke, use alcohol or eat meat and who exercise regularly—have shown that a vegetarian diet (excluding their other healthful lifestyle practices) allows them to live about 10 years longer than nonvegetarians.

Other studies show that vegetarians have a lower incidence of cardiovascular disease, diabetes and hypertension. Vegetarians also are 40% less likely to develop cancer, especially of the colon and prostate.

•**In your opinion, what are the greatest health risks associated with eating meat?** Many factors should discourage you from eating meat. Cooking meat at higher temperatures, such as those used during grilling or broiling, generates *heterocyclic amines*, carcinogens that can be formed when animal tissue is heated. Because of these carcinogens as well as the harmful effects of fat and cholesterol, a meateater has three times the risk for colon cancer as a person who rarely eats meat.

Meat also is devoid of key nutrients, like fiber and vitamin C. Because it consists of little more than fat and protein, meat is one of the most calorie-dense foods. Fat contains nine calories per gram of weight, whereas protein, such as beans, and carbohydrates, such as breads and pasta, have only four calories per gram.

•**What do you consider to be the most healthful type of vegetarian diet?** A vegan diet—one that includes no animal or dairy products whatsoever—is the most healthful.

From a health standpoint, there is no reason to add these foods to your diet. They typically are high in cholesterol and fat, and can be easily replaced with healthier alternatives, such as soy products or rice milk.

There's plenty of protein in most types of beans...and grains, such as rice and oats. If your concern is calcium, green vegetables and beans are a better source than milk because they also provide antioxidants and fiber.

As for meat being "low-fat," that's simply not true. The leanest beef is 28% fat. The leanest chicken—breast, with the skin removed—is 23% fat. The fat content of fish varies widely, from 10% to more than 50%. Compare that with beans, at 4%.

In a study of 59 people who ate either a vegan diet or less than six ounces of meat per day, the vegans got more iron from eating green vegetables and beans.

•**What foods are allowed on a vegan diet?** If you adopt this form of vegetarianism, you'll be eating from four food groups—whole grains, vegetables, fruits and legumes, such as beans and peas. Eat these in whatever proportions you like, and you'll lose weight as well.

Eat spaghetti marinara, bean burritos, vegetarian chili, many kinds of Asian dishes—the list of possibilities is almost endless. If you're time-pressured, have a Veggie Delite (on Italian bread) at Subway or a veggie burger (without mayonnaise) at Burger King.

To ensure that you're consuming all your essential nutrients, take a multivitamin specifically formulated for vegetarians (marked on the label). Also take a vitamin B-12 supplement (six micrograms daily) or eat B-12–fortified foods, including some cereals and some meat substitutes.

•**What's the best way to start a vegetarian diet?** First, speak to your doctor. If you get his/her OK, then jump in all at once, rather than simply cutting back on meat. This is safe to do, but be aware that you may experience intestinal gas if you eat a lot of beans.

Within three weeks, your taste buds will have adjusted, you'll have lost a few pounds and you'll be glad you made the change.

•**What basic food items should be included in a vegetarian's pantry?** Pasta, rice and couscous are good staples to have on hand. For legumes, I recommend dried lentils, split peas and pinto beans, as well as canned chick peas and black beans.

My favorite produce items include potatoes, carrots, celery, yellow onions and raisins.

Baked tofu, vegetarian hot dogs and veggie burgers are delicious meat substitutes. Tortillas and pita bread also are convenient. If you want snack foods, try rice cakes, popcorn or pretzels.

■ ■ ■ ■

Diet Lowers Alzheimer's Risk

The Mediterranean diet reduces Alzheimer's risk, we hear from Nikolaos Scarmeas, MD. Elderly patients who strictly followed the diet were 40% less likely to develop the disease than similar patients who did not.

Theory: The diet—which is high in mono-unsaturated fats (such as olive oil), produce, fish and legumes and low in meat and dairy—is associated with lower rates of cardiovascular disease and inflammation, both of which increase risk of Alzheimer's.

Nikolaos Scarmeas, MD, is assistant professor of neurology, Columbia University Medical Center, New York City, and lead author of a study of 2,258 elderly patients.

■ ■ ■ ■

Eating Oranges Reduces Disease Risk

A review of the literature finds that eating citrus fruits can reduce risk of mouth, larynx and stomach cancers by up to 50%. Moreover, one extra serving of citrus fruit a day (on top of the recommended minimum five daily servings of fruits and vegetables) can reduce risk of stroke by almost 20% while reducing risk of cardiovascular disease and diabetes.

Key: Citrus fruits are high in antioxidants, which strengthen the immune system and inhibit tumor growth.

Best: Oranges have the most antioxidants.

Katrine Baghurst, PhD, Commonwealth Scientific and Industrial Research Organization, Adelaide, Australia.

■ ■ ■ ■

Why OJ Is Best!

Frozen orange juice has about 25% more vitamin C than ready-to-drink juice.

Reason: At refrigerator temperatures, oxygen slowly destroys vitamin C in ready-to-drink juice. This reaction is prevented by the colder temperatures needed to store frozen juice. Once a container of any type of citrus juice is opened and exposed to air, it may lose all of the vitamin C within a month.

Carol Johnston, PhD, RD, professor of nutrition, Arizona State University, Mesa.

■ ■ ■ ■

Light Ruins Olive Oil

After 12 months under supermarket lighting, levels of tocopherols and carotenoids, two disease-fighting antioxidants found in extra-virgin olive oil, were found to be reduced by 30%.

Reason: Exposure to light allows oxygen molecules to attack nutritive properties.

Self-defense: Buy olive oil sold in tinted glass or in metal containers…and store in a cool, dark place. Do not use past the expiration date on the label.

Francesco Caponio, associate professor of food technology, University of Bari, Italy.

■ ■ ■ ■

Hot Cancer Fighter!

Red chili pepper fights cancer. It contains *capsaicin*, an anti-inflammatory that is effective against cancer cells. In tests, capsaicin caused cancer cells to die without damaging normal ones. Though clinical trials are needed before a recommendation to eat chili pepper can be made, it can be enjoyed as part of your regular diet.

Sanjay K. Srivastava, PhD, is assistant professor of pharmacology, University of Pittsburgh School of Medicine, and leader of a study of capsaicin and pancreatic cancer cells.

Tomato Extract
Lowers Blood Pressure

In a study of 54 adults with moderately high blood pressure (above 135 mmHg/80 mmHg), a dietary supplement derived from tomatoes reduced average systolic (top number) readings by 12 mmHg and diastolic (bottom number) readings by 6 mmHg after two to four weeks. The 250-mg capsule given daily was equivalent to eating four medium tomatoes.

Theory: High levels of lycopene and vitamins C and E improve function of the arterial wall, which can lower blood pressure.

Esther Paran, MD, head, hypertension unit, Soroka University Hospital, Ben-Gurion University of the Negev, Israel.

Whole Truth About Coffee, Eggs, Sweeteners ...And More

Marion Nestle, PhD, MPH, professor of nutrition, food studies and public health at New York University, New York City, is author of *What to Eat*. North Point.

We're bombarded with conflicting information about foods and health. The result is confusion. Is milk good for our bones or bad for our hearts? Is fish a source of healthful fats or dangerous toxins? Are artificial sweeteners smart low-calorie alternatives to sugar or dangerous chemicals?

Here, a closer look at the controversies about common foods...

FISH

Fish is a wonderful source of protein, vitamins, minerals and omega-3 fatty acids, but the nutritional benefits of omega-3 fatty acids fall short of their hype. Some scientists claim that they are great for the heart as well as for children's ability to learn, but all we can say for sure is that omega-3s may be beneficial.

Also, because of water pollution and some fish-farming techniques, fish can contain *methylmercury* and PCBs. High amounts of these chemicals can cause children to have muscle weakness, fatigue, headaches and severe developmental problems.

Bottom line: Eat fish if you enjoy it, with certain caveats...

•**Limit consumption of large predatory fish** likely to contain the most methylmercury (shark, swordfish, king mackerel, albacore tuna and tilefish) to no more than twice a week. Do not eat the fish at all if you are or might become pregnant—and don't feed these fish to children.

•**Select wild fish over farm-raised.** Farm-raised fish, salmon in particular, can have higher concentrations of PCBs than the same fish raised in the wild.

•**Don't regularly eat fish caught in freshwater** without checking first with state health or wildlife officials. Unless you know that the water the fish came from is safe, assume it's not. Consuming a few fish a year from a local lake or stream should be fine, but the health risks climb the more you eat.

COFFEE

It's full of caffeine, a mild "upper," and millions of people down it by the quart every day—surely coffee must be bad for us. In fact, there's little evidence that there's anything in coffee that's harmful to our health, and it may even be good for us. Coffee contains antioxidants believed to promote good health.

Bottom line: You can enjoy coffee without guilt, but don't load it with sugar, milk or cream. A 12-ounce caffe latte breve at Starbucks has 420 calories and 23 grams of saturated fat—more fat than you should consume in a day. If you become nervous or shaky when you drink coffee, you may be sensitive to caffeine. Reduce your intake or switch to decaf.

EGGS

Eggs are widely considered unhealthy because they're high in cholesterol—higher than any other food. But when eaten in limited quantities, eggs are good for you. They're relatively low in calories and are a good source of protein.

Some producers feed the hens flaxseed and fish oil to boost the eggs' omega-3 content—but these "omega-3 eggs" cost more, and it's not clear that they actually are any better for you. *Note:* There's no difference between a brown egg and a white egg aside from the color of the shell.

589

Bottom line: The American Heart Association recommends no more than one egg per day from all sources. If your doctor has warned you to watch your cholesterol, cut down on eggs or eat egg whites, which have no cholesterol.

MARGARINE

Margarines do have significantly less saturated fat and cholesterol than butter, so a nonhydrogenated (no trans fats) margarine is a healthy alternative. It certainly is cheaper than butter. But if you are not eating much of either, this decision isn't going to have a major effect on your health. Personally, I prefer butter. I just don't eat much of it. If you like margarine, you can choose from vegan or organic margarines, omega-3 margarines and "light" low-calorie/low-fat margarines—but these cost significantly more than standard margarines, and the difference they make to your health will be small, at best.

Bottom line: If you like margarine, choose one with no trans fats.

ARTIFICIAL SWEETENERS

The FDA has approved artificial sweeteners because there is no compelling evidence that they cause harm at current levels of intake. But I am not a fan of them. I can't believe any food with that kind of chemical taste can be good for you. Their single virtue is the absence of calories, but there is not much evidence that their use has helped people lose weight. Perhaps people who use them compensate by eating more calories from other sources, or artificial sweeteners reinforce our preference for sweets. Personally, I prefer sugar—just not much of it.

Bottom line: If you are trying to lose weight, it is best to eat less, move around more and avoid junk foods.

MILK

For decades, dairy trade associations and lobbying groups have told Americans that drinking milk strengthens bones. Now they claim that dairy helps us lose weight. As with many aspects of nutrition, the evidence linking dairy foods to health conditions is complicated and contradictory. Dairy foods may have lots of calcium and other nutrients, but they are high in saturated fat (the bad kind) and calories.

Bottom line: If you want to avoid the fat and saturated fat, choose nonfat options. If you don't like or can't tolerate milk, you can get the nutrients it contains from other foods. Consuming dairy foods is not the key to bone health. The best advice for bone health—and for just about any other health condition—is to eat a diet with plenty of fruits, vegetables and whole grains, don't smoke cigarettes, be active and don't drink alcohol to excess.

These good habits mean more to your health than the effects of any one food that you might choose.

■ ■ ■ ■

Free Food Facts!

Check what's in your food using software from the US Department of Agriculture's free database at *www.ars.usda.gov/ba/bhnrc/ndl* (click on "Download Software"). The information, which can be kept on a PC or handheld device, provides a detailed listing of nutrients—such as calories, protein, fat, carbs, sugars, vitamins and minerals—in almost 7,000 foods, including processed and fast foods.

Examples: Oscar Mayer fat-free hot dogs (per serving of one hot dog), 36 calories, 6.3 g protein, 0.3 g fat, 2.15 g carbs...General Mills Cheerios cereal (per cup), 111 calories, 3.6 g protein, 1.8 g fat, 22.2 g carbs.

Sneaky Places Sodium Hides

Mark Houston, MD, clinical professor of medicine at Vanderbilt University Medical School and medical director at the Hypertension and Vascular Biology Institute and the Life Extension Institute at Saint Thomas Hospital and Medical Center, all in Nashville, Tennessee, is the author of *What Your Doctor May Not Tell You About Hypertension: The Revolutionary Nutrition and Lifestyle Program to Help Fight High Blood Pressure*. Warner.

For years, Americans have been warned that excessive use of salt (sodium chloride) can elevate blood pressure in some otherwise healthy people.

Now: Doctors are becoming increasingly concerned about the amount of salt consumed by Americans and fear that it is contributing to even more health problems than previously believed.

Latest development: The American Medical Association has recommended that the FDA require food manufacturers to place warning labels on high-sodium foods.

SOURCES OF SODIUM

Sodium is a mineral that is found naturally in most foods. Everyone is aware of high-sodium foods, such as soy sauce, pickles, potato chips, most canned foods, frozen dinners and lunch meats.

However, few people realize that sodium is found in most carbonated drinks, including many diet sodas. Many brands of tomato juice contain significant amounts of sodium.

Example: Campbell's V8 contains 590 mg of sodium (more than one-quarter of the recommended daily total) per eight-ounce serving. Small amounts of sodium are even found in the tap water of many US municipalities.

Healthful foods, including poultry, dairy products and vegetables, also contain sodium.

Caution: Sodium is found in many over-the-counter medications.

Examples: Alka Seltzer (567 mg per tablet) …and Bromo Seltzer (959 mg per packet).

Our bodies require sodium to help regulate fluid balance. The mineral also is essential for nerve and muscle function. Sodium works with the mineral potassium, which counters the adverse effects of sodium, to keep the proper amount of liquid and electrolytes (minerals needed for proper functioning of the body) inside the body's cells. These minerals are excreted via sweat and urine. Imbalances can occur when too much sodium remains in the body in relation to potassium.

DANGERS OF TOO MUCH SODIUM

Even though high blood pressure (hypertension) is the most commonly recognized health risk associated with excessive sodium intake, there are other potentially serious conditions that can result.

Even in someone who does not have hypertension, excessive sodium intake increases risk for congestive heart failure (inadequate pumping action of the heart)…kidney disease…hardening of the arteries (arteriosclerosis)…swelling of the lower legs, ankles and feet (edema)…and ischemic stroke (impaired blood flow to the brain) as well as hemorrhagic stroke (bleeding into or around the brain).

Consuming too much sodium also may increase your risk for osteoporosis. That's because sodium and bone-strengthening calcium metabolism are linked. High sodium intake may increase the excretion of calcium, which is removed from the body—along with excess sodium—via urine. Over time, calcium stores in the bones will be reduced. This can lead to a calcium deficiency that often results in osteoporosis.

SAFE SODIUM LEVELS

The average American consumes at least 4,000 mg of sodium daily, but research shows that this is far too much. Our bodies require only about 500 mg of sodium daily to maintain normal functioning.

To avoid potential dangers, healthy adults should limit their sodium intake to 2,300 mg (approximately one teaspoon) daily, according to the American Heart Association (AHA).

In my opinion, everyone should limit sodium intake to 1,500 mg daily—especially older adults (age 65 or older), people with hypertension (blood pressure of 140/90 or above) or prehypertension (blood pressure of 120/80 to 139/89), diabetics, obese patients and people with kidney disease or a history of heart failure.

SALT SENSITIVITY

Salt sensitivity is a measure of how blood pressure responds to changes in salt intake. An estimated 60% of Americans with high blood pressure—and 25% of Americans with normal blood pressure—are salt sensitive.

In a recent study, salt sensitivity was found to increase a person's risk for death as much as high blood pressure, regardless of whether blood pressure actually was elevated.

In the study, salt sensitivity was measured by giving study participants a saline solution followed by a diuretic (a water- and salt-excreting drug) and testing blood pressure volume (the fluid content within blood vessels) over a two-day period as salt in the body was increased and then decreased. Unfortunately, there is no test available to the public for salt sensitivity.

Simply putting away the salt shaker is not the full solution. Salt added to food by the eaters themselves accounts for only about 15% of the average American's total daily sodium intake. About 75% comes from sodium in processed and restaurant food, while the remaining 10% of a person's total sodium intake comes from the natural sodium content of food.

Cutting back on canned and processed foods, including fast food, while increasing your intake of fresh fruits and vegetables can substantially lower your sodium intake—most produce contains small amounts of sodium and increases levels of sodium-balancing potassium. To reduce sodium intake when dining in a restaurant, ask that no salt be added to your food.

SALT SUBSTITUTES

Our bodies function most efficiently when we maintain a five-to-one ratio of potassium to sodium. In addition to fruits and vegetables, most unprocessed natural foods, including whole grains and legumes, contain more potassium than sodium. Maintaining this dietary ratio promotes healthy blood pressure.

Some salt substitutes, such as Nu-Salt and NoSalt, contain potassium chloride rather than sodium chloride. These substitutes, available at most grocery stores, taste much like table salt and can be used without potential health risks by most people.

Caution: Potassium chloride-based salt substitutes can be harmful to people who have kidney disease, which can inhibit the proper excretion of potassium and lead to heart and nerve problems. In addition, if you're taking drugs that cause potassium retention, including those for high blood pressure or congestive heart failure, consult your doctor before using a salt substitute. Good alternative: A seasoning blend such as Mrs. Dash, which does not contain potassium chloride.

Herbs and spices also add flavor to food. Instead of mimicking the taste of sodium with salt substitutes, try using garlic, lemon juice, flavored vinegar, cumin, pepper, tarragon and/or oregano in food. After a few weeks of reducing salt intake, most people no longer miss it.

■ ■ ■ ■

Honeycomb Helper

Honeycomb prevents hay fever, we hear from Joan Wilen and Lydia Wilen, experts on folk medicine. Honeycomb works as a desensitizer and antiallergen. About two months before hay fever season begins for you—and that depends on which plants you are allergic to—chew a one-inch square of local honeycomb for 10 to 15 minutes (then discard) twice a day. Purchase honeycomb from a local beekeeper or at your neighborhood health-food store.

Caution: People who are allergic to bee stings or honey should consult a physician first.

Joan Wilen and Lydia Wilen, authorities on folk remedies, New York City, and authors of *Bottom Line's Healing Remedies.* Bottom Line Books.

■ ■ ■ ■

Best Yogurt

To find yogurts that have live active cultures, look for the *Live & Active Cultures* (LAC) seal from the National Yogurt Association. The seal is an easy way for consumers to identify yogurts that have significant levels of live and active cultures, which can help to boost the immune system.

Note: Some yogurt products may have live cultures but don't display the seal, so always check labels. Look for the words *contains active yogurt cultures* or *living yogurt cultures.* Among brands with live cultures are Stonyfield Farm, Yoplait, Dannon and Nancy's.

Visit the National Yogurt Association's Web site, *www.aboutyogurt.com* for more information.

■ ■ ■ ■

Healthy Wine Trend

Natural wines—made with as little technological intervention as possible—are becoming popular. Grapes for these wines are generally —but not always—organically grown without chemical pesticides and herbicides and usually are picked by hand. Enzymes usually are not added, although some sulfites may be included late in the process as a preservative. If properly stored— at cool temperatures, like any other wine—they will last as long. Many natural wines are available nationally. Two of the better ones: Pierre Breton Bourgueil (red) and Huet Vouvray (white).

David Lille, owner, Chambers Street Wines, New York City. *www.chambersstwines.com.*

■■■■

Beer Builds Better Bones!

Dietary silicon, found in whole grains and their products (such as beer), reduces bone loss and promotes bone formation. Beer is an especially good source because it is readily absorbed. Other sources of silicon include oat bran, barley and rice.

Warning: More than two drinks per day for men or one for women is considered harmful.

Ravin Jugdaohsingh, PhD, senior research fellow, gastrointestinal laboratory, Rayne Institute, St. Thomas's Hospital, London.

The Healing Power Of Herbal Teas

Brigitte Mars, an adjunct professor of herbal medicine at Naropa University in Boulder, Colorado, is the author of numerous books, including *Healing Herbal Teas* (Basic Health) and a professional member of the American Herbalist Guild (AHG).

Herbal teas, which are generally rich in vitamins, minerals and other healthful compounds, have been used as healing agents for thousands of years.

However, because of the prevalence of over-the-counter and prescription medications, most Americans don't think of drinking tea to treat common ailments. That's a mistake.

Dozens of scientific studies have supported the use of herbals for a wide variety of health problems.* Herbal teas have the same active ingredients as herbs sold in capsules, powders and extracts. Herbal teas also have fewer side effects than medication and can be much less expensive.

Loose tea herbs, which are available at health-food stores, tend to be more potent than tea

*Check with your health-care practitioner before drinking herbal tea, especially if you are a pregnant woman, nursing mother or have a chronic medical condition. Some herbal teas should not be combined with certain drugs.

bags. To prepare tea with loose herbs, use one heaping tablespoon of dried herb or three tablespoons of fresh herb in eight ounces of boiling water. Steep for 10 minutes.

For best results, drink four eight-ounce cups of herbal tea per day until the problem subsides. If you are age 65 or older, do not exceed three cups daily...or two cups daily if you are age 70 or older.

Best teas for treating common health conditions...

COLDS AND FLU

Echinacea, which has an aromatic, earthy flavor, promotes white blood cell production... acts as an anti-infection agent...and stimulates the immune system.

How to use: Echinacea should be used for no more than 10 consecutive days, because it loses its effectiveness when taken continually. Drink echinacea tea at the onset of cold or flu symptoms, such as sore throat, sneezing and/or nasal congestion.

Caution: Echinacea stimulates the immune system, so people with autoimmune diseases, such as lupus, should consult a doctor before using this herb. People who are allergic to plants in the daisy family, such as ragweed, are more likely to have an allergic reaction to echinacea.

Other teas that fight colds and flu: Elderflower and elderberry.

DIGESTIVE DISORDERS

Peppermint, which has a zesty, fresh taste, calms muscle spasms...eases intestinal cramping ...contains antibacterial compounds...soothes ulcers...and freshens breath after a meal.

Caution: Do not drink peppermint tea if you are suffering from an acute episode of a digestive disorder, such as a gallstone attack. Seek immediate medical attention.

Other teas that fight digestive disorders: Cardamom, ginger and cinnamon.

HEADACHE

Lemon balm, which has a gentle lemon flavor and aroma, acts as an anti-inflammatory and antispasmodic...and contains magnesium, which acts as a muscle relaxant.

Caution: This herb may inhibit thyroid function. If you have low thyroid function (hypothyroidism), avoid lemon balm tea.

Other teas that fight headache: Feverfew and rosemary.

INSOMNIA

Linden flower, which has a sweet flavor and jasminelike aroma, is rich in vitamin C...calms nerves...and promotes rest. In Europe, linden flower tea often is given to patients before surgery to help them relax.

Other teas that fight insomnia: Chamomile and passionflower.

LOW LIBIDO

Oat seed, which has a slightly sweet, milky flavor, relaxes the nerves...and is often used as an aphrodisiac.

Caution: Oat seed contains gluten, so this herb should be avoided by people with gluten intolerance.

Other teas that fight low libido: Cinnamon and raspberry leaf.

■ ■ ■ ■

More Than Milk

Drinking milk isn't enough to build strong and healthy bones.

Recent finding: Women who drank one or more glasses of milk per day were just as likely to fracture a hip or wrist as those who drank less than one glass of milk per week.

Reason: Most women don't get enough vitamin D, which is necessary for calcium absorption.

Best way to get adequate vitamin D: Sit in the sun for 15 minutes a day, without sunscreen—sunlight is necessary for the skin to manufacture the body's own supply of vitamin D. Vitamin D also can be found in fortified orange juice, certain fortified cereals and fatty fish, such as salmon and sardines. The recommended daily intake for vitamin D is 400 international units (IU), but many researchers now believe that much higher daily intakes are necessary.

Diane Feskanich, ScD, assistant professor, Channing Laboratory, department of medicine, Brigham and Women's Hospital and Harvard Medical School, both in Boston, and leader of an 18-year study of 72,000 women, published in *The American Journal of Clinical Nutrition*.

Sweetener Alert

Rebecca Shannonhouse, editor of the *Bottom Line/Health* newsletter, Boardroom Inc., 281 Tresser Blvd., Stamford, Connecticut 06901.

Splenda, which has been in use in the US for nearly 10 years, is the nation's best-selling artificial sweetener—and one of the most controversial.

Some consumer groups argue that Splenda was given FDA approval without adequate toxicity studies and that it may increase the risk for cancer.

Sucralose (the main ingredient in Splenda) is an amalgam of sugar molecules spliced together with chlorine—and chlorine can potentially damage cellular DNA. Yet there's no evidence—either from case reports or scientific studies—that sucralose poses any real increased risk for cancer.

"When you consider the number of people who consume Splenda, the fact that cancer hasn't appeared suggests that the risk, if any, would likely be very modest," explains David L. Katz, MD, founder of the Yale Prevention Research Center in New Haven, Connecticut.

But there are other reasons to be concerned about—and to avoid—any artificial sweetener, Dr. Katz says. For example, some studies indicate that people who use artificial sweeteners (or products that contain them) consume more—rather than fewer—calories.

Possible reason: Artificial sweeteners are 300 to 600 times sweeter than sugar. People who consume them can develop a higher "threshold for satisfaction"—and wind up consuming excess amounts of regular sugar-rich foods.

Splenda and other artificial sweeteners don't appear to pose significant health risks—but they don't ensure calorie control either.

Best: If you're trying to lose weight, avoid artificial sweeteners and curtail your intake of regular sugar.

Best Wines for Your Health

Roger Corder, PhD, professor of experimental therapeutics at the William Harvey Research Institute, Queen Mary's School of Medicine and Dentistry in London. The author or coauthor of more than 100 scientific studies, his primary research interests are the relationship between diabetes and heart disease, and the health benefits of wine.

For years, scientists theorized that the "French Paradox"—the phenomenon of relatively low rates of heart disease among the French, who are known for their rich, fatty foods—may be due, in part, to the daily consumption of red wine.

Now: The cumulative body of scientific evidence shows that moderate consumption of red wine not only reduces the risk for heart disease, but also for stroke and metabolic syndrome (a constellation of health problems that can lead to heart disease and diabetes). Wine also helps people live longer and avoid dementia. Only recently, however, have scientists begun to identify the specific compounds in red wine that confer health benefits.

Trap: Mass-produced, sweet red wines with high alcohol content (above 14%) do *not* offer high levels of health-promoting chemicals.

What you must know to choose the most healthful wines—and the best options for non-drinkers…

WINE'S PROTECTIVE EFFECTS

Recent research shows that white wine may offer some of the same health benefits of red wine, such as protection from heart disease, but the bulk of scientific evidence focuses on red wine.

Latest developments: Animal experiments show that *polyphenols*—chemicals found abundantly in dark and/or colorful foods, such as red and purple grapes, cocoa and pomegranates—can stop atherosclerosis (fatty buildup in the arteries). That's because polyphenols affect the *endothelium* (cells lining the arteries), causing blood vessels to widen (vasodilate), increasing blood flow.

Breakthrough: English scientists published a paper in *Nature*—a renowned scientific journal—showing that…

•**The most potent polyphenols in red wines** are *procyanidins*, healthful plant substances that over time become condensed *tannins*, compounds that give an astringent taste to wine. The more procyanidins consumed, the greater degree of vasodilation that occurs.

•**Regions in Europe with the highest rates of proven longevity** produce wines with two to four times more procyanidins than do other regions.

Examples: Many varieties of Bordeaux wines from France and Chianti wines from Italy.

What you may not know: *Resveratrol* is often mentioned as the key heart-protecting component of red wine. But to get enough resveratrol to benefit the heart, you would need to drink 1,000 quarts of wine a day. Resveratrol supplements haven't been proven safe or effective.

HEART-FRIENDLY WINES

Many factors influence the level of procyanidins in red wine.

Certain varieties of grapes, including cabernet sauvignon and malbec, are higher in procyanidins than other red and white grapes. Other positive factors include the altitude of the vineyard (the higher, the better)…a slower ripening process…a lower yield (the amount of grapes produced per vine)…and older vines.

Useful: Wines described as having "firm" tannins are more likely to have high levels of procyanidins than wines with "soft" or "ripe" tannins. Look for this description in wine reviews and at the Web sites of wine retailers, such as K&L Wine Merchants (*www.klwines.com*) and Wine.com, Inc. (*www.wine.com*).

DRINK WITH MEALS

The most healthful way to drink red wine is in the classic French style—one or two small glasses at lunch and/or with dinner, as food slows alcohol absorption. Most research shows that women should not exceed five ounces of wine per day, and men should limit their daily consumption to 10 ounces.

When red wine is consumed in excess, its health benefits are outweighed by the risks associated with alcohol abuse, including increased risks for many types of cancer, as well as heart disease, obesity and diabetes.

Caution: Drinking wine quickly or on an empty stomach speeds alcohol absorption, increasing the risk for high blood pressure.

NONALCOHOLIC PROCYANIDINS

If you prefer not to drink red wine, consider these procyanidin-rich foods...

•**Dark chocolate.** Look for a bittersweet or extra-dark chocolate, with 70% to 85% cacao. One ounce of dark chocolate delivers the amount of procyanidins in four ounces of red wine.

Caution: To limit calories, don't eat more than one ounce to one-and-a-half ounces of dark chocolate daily.

•**Apples.** Red Delicious and Granny Smith have high levels of procyanidins. One medium-sized apple is equivalent to four ounces of red wine.

•**Cranberry juice.** An eight-ounce serving of juice containing 25% cranberry is roughly equivalent to a four-ounce glass of red wine. Choose low-sugar versions with at least 25% cranberry content.

Other sources of heart-healthy procyanidins: Raspberries, blackberries and strawberries, Concord grape juice, pomegranates, walnuts, pinto beans and cinnamon.

HEALTHFUL WINES

Laboratory analyses of more than 400 red wines at William Harvey Research Institute show that the following have high levels of healthful procyanidins...

•**Argentina.** Cabernet sauvignon, from Bodegas Catena Zapata.

•**Australia.** Cabernet sauvignon, from Wynns.

•**California.** Cabernet sauvignon, from Robert Mondavi Napa Valley Reserve...and many other Napa Valley cabernets.

•**Chile.** Cabernet sauvignons from Veramonte.

•**France.** Large numbers of Bordeaux wines —both at the top end of the market and modestly priced—have high or better-than-average procyanidin levels.

•**Italy.** In Tuscany, wines made from the Sangiovese grape that tested well include II Colombaio di Cencio's Chianti Classico Riserva.

In Sardinia, where wine drinkers are particularly long-lived, a good choice is Rosso Superiore del Mandrolisai.

■■■■

New Power Food!

Orange tomatoes pack an antioxidant punch, according to Steven J. Schwartz, PhD.

New finding: When 12 people ate spaghetti with sauce made from red tomatoes on one day and from orange tomatoes on another day, blood tests showed that participants absorbed two-and-a-half times more *lycopene* (a disease-fighting antioxidant) from the orange tomato sauce than from the red sauce.

Theory: Orange tomatoes contain a form of *lycopene* that is more readily absorbed than that in red varieties.

Self-defense: Try adding orange tomatoes to your diet.

Steven J. Schwartz, PhD, professor of food science, Ohio State University, Columbus.

Healthful Juices

Lisa R. Young, PhD, RD, is a nutritionist in private practice and an adjunct professor of nutrition at New York University, both in New York City. She is the author of *The Portion Teller Plan*. Morgan Road.

If you can't get enough whole fruits and vegetables in your daily diet, drinking juice may be the next best thing. And you don't have to squeeze your own if you shop wisely. *What to look for...*

•**Choose pure juice.** Avoid "juices" with added sweeteners, such as sugar and high fructose corn syrup. Blends of different juices are okay, but be aware that many naturally tart juices, such as pomegranate, are often diluted with sweeter, less nutritious juices, such as apple juice. Read the ingredient labels—ingredients appear in descending order by their amounts.

•**Limit calories.** All juices tend to be high in calories, so look for products with no more than 110 calories per eight-ounce serving and limit yourself to one serving a day—this equals two servings of fruits or vegetables. *My top picks...*

V8
- **Low-sodium Vegetable Juice.**

Per eight-ounce serving: 50 calories. The sodium content of the low-sodium variety is 140 mg versus 590 mg for the regular V8. This 100% vegetable juice blend is rich in lycopene, vitamin C and potassium.

TROPICANA
- **100% pure orange juice with calcium and vitamin D.**

Per eight-ounce serving: 110 calories. This OJ is rich in vitamin C, potassium, folate and bone-building calcium and vitamin D.

TRADER JOE'S
- **Triple berry juice.**

Per eight-ounce serving: 110 calories. This 100% juice blend is an antioxidant-rich mix of pomegranate, blueberry and cranberry juice.

■ ■ ■ ■

Sardines May Be the Healthiest Seafood

They are nearly the richest in heart-healthy omega-3 fat—richer than tuna and many fish-oil supplements. They contain fewer contaminants than tuna, swordfish, farmed salmon and most other fatty fish. They are a good source of calcium if you eat the bones.

Caution: Canned sardines may be high in salt, so if you are on a sodium-restricted diet, check the can label.

UC Berkeley Wellness Letter, 6 Trowbridge Dr., Bethel, Connecticut 06801.

Iron Out Anemia

Helen Rasmussen, PhD, RD, LDN, senior research dietician, Jean Mayer Human Nutrition Research Center for Aging, Tufts University, Boston.

If you have been diagnosed with iron-deficiency anemia, you want to get as much iron as possible from food. *Some suggestions...*

If you haven't done so already, talk to your doctor about taking a daily iron supplement, the standard treatment for this condition. In addition, when deciding which foods to eat, there are two types of foods that contain iron. *Heme* foods come from animal sources (such as red meat and poultry), and *non-heme* foods are plant-based iron-containing foods (such as grains, beans and certain vegetables, including Swiss chard and spinach). Some non-heme foods contain compounds that interfere with iron absorption. Non-heme foods have enhanced absorption if you add vitamin C (ideally from food sources, including citrus fruits and/or vegetables, such as broccoli) to your meal.

Because teas and coffee contain *tannins,* components that also block iron uptake, these beverages should be drunk between meals to maximize iron absorption. If you take iron supplements, be sure to take no more than the recommended amount (45 mg per day is the tolerable upper level), as it can cause an upset stomach.

Sneak More Nutrition Into Every Meal

Missy Chase Lapine, who is on the Culinary Arts faculty at The New School in New York City. She is author of the forthcoming book *The Sneaky Chef: How to Cheat on Your Man (in the Kitchen).* Running Press. Her Web site is *www.thesneakychef.com.*

Children aren't the only picky eaters. About 90% of adults don't eat the recommended five daily servings of fruits and vegetables.

The solution: "Sneaky" cooking. You can sneak produce and other healthy ingredients into foods that everyone enjoys. One great way to do this is with purées—cooked or raw vegetables, fruits and beans that are mixed with a little water and processed in a blender or a food processor.

GARLIC MASHED POTATOES

You don't need butter and milk for great mashed potatoes.

Healthier: Assuming that you're using about two pounds of potatoes, replace the butter with two tablespoons of olive oil, and add about one cup of puréed cauliflower and zucchini. Steam the cauliflower until very tender (about 10 to 12 minutes) before puréeing. The zucchini is peeled and puréed raw, then blended with the cauliflower purée. Instead of milk, add one-half cup of plain, low-fat yogurt. Then add three heads of roasted garlic. Most people like garlic —and it provides a "decoy" flavor that masks the taste of the vegetables.

TUNA SWAP

Sardines are rich in omega-3 fatty acids, important for cardiovascular and neurological health. Many people prefer the milder taste of tuna, which is high in omega-3s but also may have toxic mercury. Sardines are smaller than tuna and are less likely to accumulate mercury.

Healthier: Make a traditional tuna salad, but replace some of the tuna with mashed skinless, boneless sardines. My husband can't stand sardines, but he likes my tuna salad. At first, I replaced just a little bit of the tuna with sardines. Now I'm at a 50-50 ratio.

MEGA-MARINARA SAUCE

A tomato-based red sauce—for meat loaf, pasta, etc.—is the ideal hiding place for sneaky additions. Vegetable purées reduce the natural acidity of tomatoes, helping to prevent heartburn, and the strong flavor of the sauce makes the vegetable flavors disappear.

Healthier: Replace about one-third of your sauce with either a carrot–sweet potato purée (cook the vegetables until soft before puréeing) or the purée made with cauliflower and zucchini.

BEANS 'N' MUFFINS

Traditional muffins are high in fat. You can make a leaner version with a white bean purée. Beans are an excellent source of protein, and they also are high in fiber and antioxidants.

Healthier: Add one-half cup of white bean purée in place of about half the fat. A 15-ounce can of white beans, rinsed, makes about one cup of purée. Store the rest in the refrigerator for up to three days, or freeze.

BETTER BROWNIES

Traditional brownie recipes contain a lot of butter and sugar.

Healthier: Substitute one-half cup of "purple purée," made with wild, frozen blueberries, organic raw baby spinach and lemon juice, for up to half the butter or oil and half the sugar. Baby spinach has a milder flavor than the mature leaves.

CHILIS AND SOUPS

Chilis and soups are among the best foods for substitutions because you can add healthy ingredients without significantly changing the flavor.

Healthier: Add two tablespoons of oat bran or wheat germ. You also can add purées, such as white bean or "green purée" made with raw baby spinach and steamed broccoli and peas.

Delicious Ways to Get More Fruits, Vegetables

Marjorie Fitch-Hilgenberg, PhD, RD, LD, an associate professor and director of the dietetics program at the University of Arkansas, Fayetteville.

Sauces, marinades and sandwich spreads (commonly known as condiments) have long been relegated to the "bad-for-you" category of foods. But it doesn't have to be that way. Condiments actually can be good for you—if you choose the right ones. When made from fruits and vegetables, condiments can provide essential vitamins, minerals and other antioxidants that help protect the body from chronic diseases, such as arthritis, heart disease and cancer. Combined with a well-balanced diet, healthful condiments can shore up one's total daily intake of fruits and vegetables.

My favorite condiments (made from ingredients available at most grocery stores)…

• **Cranberry relish.** Cranberries are packed with vitamin C and the flavonoids *anthocyanins* and *proanthocyanidins*—a disease-fighting combination that lowers LDL "bad" cholesterol, helps prevent blood clots that cause heart attacks and stroke, and may fight certain cancers, such as oral and esophageal cancers.

Best uses: Makes a delicious spread for turkey, chicken or pork tenderloin sandwiches, or it can be mixed into sauces and marinades (such as barbecue sauce or a spicy citrus marinade) as a tart counterpart to meat, fish or poultry dishes. Mix cranberry relish with orange juice (enough to create a syruplike consistency) for a delicious glaze on chicken, turkey or pork.

CRANBERRY RELISH

2 pounds fresh cranberries
1 cup sugar or Splenda (a sugar
   substitute)
3 tablespoons Grand Marnier liqueur
   or orange juice
1 orange, zested and juiced

Place all the ingredients in the bowl of a food processor, pulse several times to chop cranberries (until chunky) and mix ingredients. Let relish stand at room temperature for 30 minutes to allow flavor to develop. Relish can be made the day before and stored in the refrigerator until served.

• **Curry.** Long used in south Asian cooking, curry (available in powder form or as a sauce) is a mixture of several pungent spices, including turmeric, a perennial herb that has been found to lower blood levels of LDL cholesterol and raise levels of HDL "good" cholesterol. Turmeric contains *curcumin*, a substance that may slow the progression of Alzheimer's disease.

Best uses: For a spicy kick, sprinkle curry powder on egg salad or on top of baked chicken. Use curry sauce on beef, pork, chicken, fish or shrimp dishes, or to add "zip" to rice or vegetables.

• **Guacamole.** This Mexican dip combines mashed avocados with tomatoes, onions, spices, lime juice and heart-healthy garlic. Avocados contain nearly 20 vitamins (such as folate and vitamins C and E), minerals (iron and potassium) as well as fiber. Avocados are rich in cholesterol-lowering monounsaturated fat. Avocados also contain phytonutrients, such as the antioxidant *lutein*, which may promote eye health.

Best uses: On sandwiches (such as turkey or chicken breast), try guacamole as a low-cholesterol alternative to mayonnaise.

GUACAMOLE

3 avocados
2 tablespoons fresh lime juice
   (juice from one lime)
½ teaspoon salt
½ cup diced onion
2 tablespoons chopped fresh cilantro
2 plum tomatoes, diced
1 clove garlic, minced (about
   1 teaspoon)
Ground cayenne pepper, to taste

Cut avocados in half, remove pit. Scoop avocado into a medium bowl. Add lime juice and salt. Mix while mashing avocados. Add onion, cilantro, tomatoes and garlic. Mix. Season with cayenne pepper. Refrigerate for one hour for best flavor, or serve immediately.

• **Mustard.** An excellent source of iron, calcium, zinc, magnesium and niacin, mustard is an incredibly versatile, low-calorie condiment. Mustard also contains protective phytochemicals called *glucosinolates* that research suggests may help fight prostate, esophageal, gastrointestinal and colorectal cancers.

Best uses: Prepared mustards, such as store-bought yellow mustard—and especially coarse-ground, spicy, brown Dijon—are delicious when used on meat sandwiches, as a base for salad dressing or in marinades and sauces for beef or fish, such as salmon or swordfish. Add honey to mustard to create a sweet-and-sour marinade for pork or chicken or a dipping sauce for finger foods. (Start with two tablespoons of honey to one-half cup of mustard, then add more honey to taste.) For an extra kick, add some horseradish to mustard. Wasabi mustard, a hot mustard available at gourmet food shops, is great on beef or on tuna or salmon fillets. (A little goes a long way.)

Caution: People with high blood pressure should limit their consumption of mustard, which generally is high in sodium (about 50 mg to 120 mg per teaspoon).

WASABI MUSTARD SAUCE

¼ cup rice wine vinegar
3 tablespoons canola oil
2 teaspoons Dijon mustard
1 teaspoon wasabi paste

Mix all ingredients. Try it on flank steak.

• **Yogurt.** Yogurt contains probiotics, the live, beneficial bacteria that occur naturally in the digestive tract. The most common probiotics in yogurt are *Lactobacillus bulgaricus* and *Streptococcus thermophilus*, which studies show improve intestinal function, fight infection, reduce risk for colon cancer, ease symptoms of irritable bowel syndrome and decrease inflammation associated with arthritis.

Best uses: A healthful, low-fat alternative to mayonnaise or sour cream, plain low-fat yogurt also can be used as a tangy sandwich spread if you add just a little mustard. Yogurt can be used in place of heavy cream to thicken a variety of sauces and stews.

TANGY YOGURT MUSTARD DILL SAUCE

1 cup plain low-fat yogurt

3 tablespoons fresh minced parsley

2 tablespoons Dijon mustard

2 tablespoons fresh dill weed

2 to 3 teaspoons fresh lemon juice

⅛ teaspoon ground pepper, preferably white pepper

Salt to taste

Mix all ingredients. Refrigerate 30 minutes or longer before using. Try it on salmon.

Seven Seemingly Healthy Foods—That Aren't

David Grotto, RD, president and founder of Nutrition Housecall, LLC, a consulting firm specializing in family nutrition programs, Chicago. He serves on the scientific advisory board of *Men's Health* magazine and is author of *101 Foods That Could Save Your Life*. Bantam. He is past spokesman for the American Dietetic Association.

Nearly everyone wants to eat healthier. The food industry, which keeps a close eye on America's changing tastes, has introduced thousands of foods that purport to be healthy—but are they really?

Too many people assume that anything that comes from a health-food store is good for you or that quantities don't matter when you're eating a "good" food.

Personal story: One of my first clients was a strict vegetarian, but this woman was 5'2" and weighed 250 pounds. Something was clearly amiss. She told me that she used nearly a pint of olive oil in recipes because it's a "healthy" fat.

Some foods, such as vegetables, whole grains, legumes, etc., are almost always good for you. But many of the foods that are promoted with healthy-sounding terms, such as "natural" or "vitamin-packed," actually are loaded with sugar and/or fat and are unacceptably high in calories.

Common offenders—and healthier alternatives...

SMOOTHIES

Some smoothies can have more calories than sodas, making them an unhealthy choice to have regularly. My daughter once bought a peanut butter smoothie. I did the calculations and found that it had about 1,000 calories.

Healthier: Make your own smoothie using just fresh fruit and adding skim milk if you want. Or mix four ounces of fruit juice with four ounces of sparkling water. It tastes delicious, is relatively low in calories and has the same nutrients as a serving of whole fruit (though less fiber).

PROTEIN BARS

Millions of Americans replace one or more meals daily with bars—granola bars, high-protein bars, meal-replacement bars, etc. Many of these are high in sugar and/or fat and deliver 300 calories or more. It's fine to occasionally use one of these bars as a meal replacement, but they're too high in calories to have in addition to meals.

Healthier: Make up your own healthy snacks, using a mixture of nuts, seeds and dried fruit. One-half ounce of almonds (about 12) and one tablespoon of dried fruit totals about 140 calories. When you do crave a bar, have one that has at least three grams of fiber, with no more than 150 calories. Try Luna small-size organic bars.

FROZEN YOGURT

Healthier than ice cream? Not necessarily. Yogurt is one of the healthiest foods you can eat, but most frozen brands have more in common with desserts than with health foods.

Check the label: Some frozen yogurts have the same number of calories as ice cream. They may even have similar amounts of sugar and fat. Also, it's rare to find live and active cultures—

600

the probiotic organisms that make natural yogurt so healthy—in frozen products.

Healthier: One of the newer versions of frozen yogurt. For example, Berry Chill, a yogurt chain based in Chicago, is producing products that are relatively low in fat and sugar and contain live and active cultures. Other manufacturers are following suit, such as New England–based Brigham's with its premium frozen yogurt, élan. Look for the LAC seal on frozen yogurt containers—it means that the product has at least 10 million live and active cultures.

PRETZELS

They're often touted as a healthier alternative to potato chips because they have less fat. A one-ounce pretzel serving usually has about one gram of fat, compared to up to 10 grams in a one-ounce serving of some potato chips. However, most pretzels are high in salt. They also have a high glycemic index because they consist mostly of refined wheat flour and cornstarch—they're quickly transformed to sugar during digestion, which can increase blood glucose levels and lead to weight gain.

Be wary of pretzels with added wheat or oat bran—these often are just "window dressing" and not a significant source of whole grains.

Healthier: Satisfy your "crunch craving" with a mix of nuts, seeds and dried fruit (see Protein Bars, on previous page).

FAKE WHOLE-WHEAT BREAD

Real whole-wheat bread is among the healthiest foods you can eat. Some brands, however, only look like whole wheat—manufacturers often add a brown color to make them look more wholesome.

Another trick: Manufacturers super-size the slices so that they can make higher fiber claims on the label.

Healthier: A bread with normal-size slices that contains at least three grams of fiber per serving. Read the ingredient label. The word "whole"—whole wheat, whole grain, etc.—should be first in the list.

MUFFINS

Today's big muffins often seem like they're loaded with nutritious ingredients, such as fruit or bran, but many muffins that are sold in supermarkets or coffee shops, such as Starbucks, are loaded with fat and sugar and range from 400 to 500 calories each.

Healthier: A small one-and-a-half ounce muffin that's made with bran or a whole grain. A muffin this size that's not loaded with sugar and/or fat usually contains about 100 calories.

RICE MIXES

Brown rice has more fiber and disease-fighting phytochemicals than white rice, but people don't always want to take the time to cook brown rice. Instead, they buy a packaged rice pilaf, both for convenience and extra flavor. Most of these products are very high in sodium, as well as fat.

Healthier: Uncle Ben's microwavable brown rice. It's ready in just a few minutes, and you can season it to your own taste—without adding salt or oil.

Alcohol Helps Your Heart

Charles Bamforth, PhD, chair of the department of food science & technology and Anheuser-Busch Endowed Professor of Malting & Brewing Sciences at University of California, Davis, and special professor in the school of biosciences at University of Nottingham, England. He is editor in chief of *Journal of the American Society of Brewing Chemists*, and author of *Grape versus Grain* (Cambridge University), a comparison of wine and beer.

Maybe you drink a glass or two of red wine every day because you've heard about its high levels of heart-protecting antioxidants such as resveratrol.

What you may not know: The main heart-helping ingredient in alcoholic drinks is ethanol—alcohol itself.

Landmark study: An international team of scientists led by researchers in the department of nutrition at Harvard School of Public Health analyzed 10 studies that linked moderate intake of alcohol with a lower risk of heart disease.

Four studies showed that wine lowered risk, four showed beer lowered risk, and four showed spirits lowered risk. All alcoholic drinks are linked with lower risk of heart disease, concluded the authors, in *British Medical Journal*.

That study and others led the American Heart Association to declare, "There is no clear evidence that wine is more beneficial than other forms of alcohol."

Why it works: Scientists don't yet know the exact mechanism by which ethanol helps the heart, but it's probably by boosting "good" HDL cholesterol...decreasing levels of the clotting protein *fibrinogen*, thereby reducing the risk of artery-clogging blood clots...and normalizing blood sugar levels (diabetes is a risk factor for heart disease).

LIFESTYLE FACTORS

But, you might ask, isn't it true that many studies have found that wine drinkers are healthier than beer drinkers? *Yes, but it might not be the wine...*

Recent finding: Researchers in Denmark analyzed more than 3.5 million checkout receipts from 98 outlets of two large supermarket chains. They found that wine buyers bought more fruits, vegetables, olives, poultry, milk and low-fat cheese than beer buyers. On the other hand, beer buyers bought more chips, soft drinks, cold cuts, sausages and sugar. Other studies show that, compared with beer drinkers, wine drinkers consume less saturated fat, exercise more and smoke less.

New thinking: It might not be wine but the overall lifestyle of wine drinkers that accounts for their better health.

There is no reason why you can't drink moderate amounts of beer and/or spirits as part of a healthy lifestyle.

BENEFITS OF BEER

In fact, beer may be a healthier choice than wine because beer has...

●**B vitamins, particularly folate,** which may help protect against heart disease, stroke, Alzheimer's and various cancers.

●**Silicon.** Beer is one of the richest dietary sources of silicon, a mineral that helps counter the bone-eroding disease of osteoporosis.

●**Effective antioxidants.** Red wine has more antioxidants than beer—in the test tube— but studies show that antioxidants in beer may be more effective in raising blood levels of antioxidants. In fact, beer is better than a tomato at

raising blood levels of *ferulic acid,* a potent antioxidant that scientists say may help fight heart disease, diabetes, cancer and Alzheimer's.

●**Fiber.** Beer contains healthful levels of soluble fiber.

Studies also show that moderate drinking does not contribute to a "beer belly"—it is the calories in alcohol that are fattening, not in any particular component of beer, such as the carbohydrate maltose. In fact, many wines contain more carbohydrates and more calories than beer.

MODERATION IS KEY

The health benefits from drinking alcoholic beverages depend on moderation—on average, no more than one drink a day for women and two drinks a day for men.

Example: A drink is five ounces of wine, 12 ounces of beer, or 1½ ounces of distilled spirits or liquor, such as vodka or whiskey.

The benefits also depend on frequency. Studies show that it is healthier to have one or two daily drinks than one or two on just a couple of days a week. Binge drinking, of course, is not healthful—and alcoholics and those with a family history of alcoholism should avoid alcohol.

Also, alcohol and many medications, including sedatives, don't mix. If you're taking a medication, ask your doctor if moderate drinking is okay.

Red flag: There are fewer large-scale studies on the health benefits of spirits, because in nations where spirits are the drink of choice (such as Russia), people tend to drink heavily. Heavy drinking is associated with a range of health problems from cirrhosis to cancer.

DRINK TO YOUR HEALTH

Preventing heart disease may be the primary benefit of moderate alcohol intake, but studies show alcohol can benefit health in many other ways...

●**Aging and longevity.** Italian researchers analyzed data from 34 scientific investigations into alcohol and health conducted in the US, Europe, Australia, Japan and China, and involving more than one million people. They found that moderate drinking of any kind—wine, beer or spirits—lowered the risk of death by 18% in women and 17% in men. However, death rates were higher among men drinking more than four drinks a day and women drinking more than two.

●**Dementia.** Scientists who study memory loss and dementia divide the process into three stages of advancing severity—age-related memory loss, mild cognitive impairment and, finally, dementia.

Recent studies: Italian researchers studied 121 people ages 65 to 84 with mild cognitive impairment. Those who had at least one drink of alcohol a day developed dementia at an 85% slower rate than those who didn't drink. And Harvard researchers, in a study published in *The Journal of the American Medical Association*, found that moderate drinking decreased the risk of developing Alzheimer's by 54% compared with not drinking.

●**Diabetes.** Researchers at the Albert Einstein College of Medicine in New York City analyzed 32 studies on alcohol intake and diabetes and found that moderate consumption of alcohol (one to three drinks a day) lowered the risk of developing diabetes by 33% to 56% and the risk of developing diabetes-related heart disease by 34% to 55%.

●**Kidney stones.** Finnish researchers found that drinking a bottle of beer a day reduced the risk of developing kidney stones by 40%.

●**Gallstone disease.** Harvard researchers found that both wine and beer reduced the risk of gallstone disease (by speeding up the emptying the gallbladder after a meal).

●**Osteoporosis.** Researchers at California Pacific Medical Center San Francisco found that social drinking in older men was associated with higher bone mineral density.

●**Prostate cancer.** Men ages 40 to 64 who drank four or more glasses red wine a week halved their risk prostate cancer, say scientists from Fred Hutchinson Cancer Research Center in Seattle. And researchers in Australia and New Zealand found that beer intake decreases prostate specific antigen (PSA), a biomarker for prostate cancer.

Caution: The National Cancer Institute says that immoderate drinking cause cancer of the mouth, esophagus, pharynx or larynx, and the National Institute on Alcohol Abuse and Alco-

holism says that chronic alcohol intake may increase the risk of breast cancer by about 10%.

●**Rheumatoid arthritis.** People who drink alcohol regularly are 50% less likely to develop rheumatoid arthritis than nondrinkers say Scandinavian researchers in the June 5, 2008, issue *British Medical Journal.*

Possible reason: Alcohol reduces inflammation.

●**Stress.** A clinical psychologist at University of Pennsylvania reviewed the scientific literature on the psychological benefits of moderate drinking and found that it increased happiness, euphoria, conviviality and pleasant carefree feelings, and decreased tension, depression and self-consciousness. Heavy drinkers, however, had higher rates of clinical depression.

How to Eat Fruits and Vegetables Safely

Marion Nestle, PhD, the Paulette Goddard professor of nutrition, food studies and public health at New York University in New York City. She is the author or editor of several books, including *What to Eat.* North Point.

In the wake of the recent *Escherichia coli* (E. coli) outbreak from contaminated spinach, many Americans stopped eating spinach or became more rigorous in washing it. However, there are probably few people who adopted long-term strategies to protect themselves against dangerous contaminants that could be found in any fruits or vegetables.

WHY OUR FOOD IS AT RISK

Concern about safety should not prevent you from eating fruits and vegetables—the health benefits of produce far outweigh the risks. Nevertheless, health officials estimate that each year, foodborne bacteria, parasites and viruses sicken 76 million Americans, resulting in 325,000 hospitalizations and 5,000 deaths.

Contaminated fresh produce is the number-one cause of individual cases of foodborne illnesses, according to the Washington, DC–based consumer-advocacy group Center for Science in the Public Interest.

In the US, the safety of fruits and vegetables falls under the jurisdiction of the Food and Drug Administration (FDA). However, typically less than 2% of imported food products is inspected by the FDA, and domestic produce is rarely inspected at all.

FDA and US Department of Agriculture (USDA) guidelines for the safe handling of produce—known as "Good Agricultural Practices"—suggest methods to help prevent contamination with dangerous microorganisms from water, soil, manure or unhygienic food handlers.

However, these guidelines are voluntary—fruit and vegetable companies do not have to follow them. What's more, the reality is that the FDA does not have the financial resources or personnel to effectively monitor industry practices or the safety of the 741 pounds of produce that are consumed, on average, by every person in the US each year.

Fruits and vegetables are grown in what the FDA typically calls "nonsterile environments"—that is, they grow in dirt. If they come in contact with feces of grazing cattle, wild animals or birds, farm workers or any other source, they can become contaminated with potentially harmful microorganisms. This is clearly unappetizing, and fecal contamination causes health problems if the microorganisms are dangerous types.

BEST SELF-DEFENSE STRATEGIES

Most produce is safe to eat, but regardless of where you shop, there's no way to be 100% certain that the fruits and vegetables you're buying are free of contamination from dangerous microbes.

To do the best you can to protect yourself and your family from unsafe produce, follow these simple steps…

•**Be sure to remove the outer leaves of leafy greens.** That's the area that is most likely to come in contact with manure or other sources of dangerous contamination while leafy vegetables are growing in soil or processed after harvesting.

Caution: The FDA does not require food safety procedures to be followed for most produce, and this includes leafy greens, such as

spinach and lettuce, as well as tomatoes and carrots.

Sprouts are an exception. They must be grown under strict safety rules, and problems with them have declined since those precautions went into effect.

•**Store produce in the refrigerator, and wash it before eating.** Harmful microorganisms can multiply on fresh fruits and vegetables, especially when they are transported great distances, sit in supermarket produce bins for extended periods and are not kept cold enough.

Best way to wash produce: Thoroughly rinse produce under running cool tap water. In addition, carefully scrub firm-skinned fruits and vegetables, such as apples and cucumbers, with a clean vegetable brush.

Be sure to clean the vegetable brush, utensils and other kitchen tools in hot water (or the dishwasher) after each use.

Caution: It is a good idea to wash bagged lettuce, spinach and other vegetables—even if the bag says the contents have been "triple washed." If the bags were not kept cold, bacteria could have multiplied inside the package.

To be extra safe, rinse off the inedible rinds of fruits, such as cantaloupe and avocados. If microbes are on the rind, the fruit inside can become contaminated when the rind is pierced by a knife.

Helpful: Don't splurge on expensive fruit and vegetable washes sold in supermarket produce departments. There is no evidence that these special washes are more effective than chlorinated tap water.

Important: Although washing helps protect against foodborne illness from produce, the only way to *guarantee* that fruits and vegetables do not contain harmful microbes is to cook them in boiling water.

•**Buy certified organic.** Studies show that certified organic produce, which is grown in composted manure instead of chemical fertilizers, is no more likely to be contaminated with microbes than conventionally grown produce. That's because, to obtain organic certification, farmers must follow strict rules to ensure that harmful microbes in manure are destroyed (typically through a high-heat decontamination process). Growers of conventional produce are not required to follow such rules.

Organic produce also is a good option if you want to avoid synthetic pesticides and other chemicals that are typically used to kill insects in conventionally grown crops. These chemicals do not reduce your risk for contamination with bacteria and other microbes.

In addition, some research shows that organic produce may be superior to conventionally grown produce in its nutritional value.

Important: When buying organic produce, be sure that it is labeled with a "USDA organic" seal. This means that the producers follow organic growing rules established by the USDA Organic Standards Board and have been inspected by agencies licensed by the USDA to make sure the rules are followed.

Because organic produce is usually more expensive than nonorganic varieties, most people don't buy organic all the time. The Environmental Working Group (EWG), a Washington, DC–based, nonprofit environmental research organization, recommends buying organic varieties of produce whose nonorganic counterparts are typically highest in pesticides.

These include peaches, apples, sweet bell peppers, celery, nectarines, strawberries, cherries, pears, imported grapes, spinach, lettuce and potatoes. For a list of other fruits and vegetables evaluated by the EWG, go to the group's Web site, *ewg.org.*

•**Buy from local farmers.** When food is shipped from far away and/or stays in the supermarket for long periods before being sold and eaten, there is more time for microbes to multiply.

Example: If you live on the East Coast, some of the produce in your supermarket sits on a truck for 10 days to two weeks after being harvested in California.

Locally grown foods are fresher and taste better, but there are no guarantees that they are safe. Like any produce, they can come in contact with harmful microbes in the field or during handling, so washing is still essential. And as always, the only way to ensure perfect safety is to cook the foods before eating them.

Important: If you grow your own produce, use a fence to prevent pets and wild animals from defecating in your garden, and be sure to wash everything that you've grown.

If you visit pick-your-own farms for apples, berries, pumpkins or other seasonal produce, be sure to wash these foods, too.

■ ■ ■ ■

Make Your Own Bacteria-Busting Veggie Wash

Washing fruits and vegetables with water doesn't completely clean away bacteria, such as *E. coli* and *Listeria,* which can cause food poisoning.

Better: Fill one spray bottle with white or apple cider vinegar, another with 3% hydrogen peroxide, the same strength commonly available in drugstores. Spray produce with the vinegar first. Its acidity kills the majority of organisms. Then spray with peroxide, which is a strong oxidizer that helps eliminate Listeria. Rinse well with water. These precautions are recommended for all produce, including organic products.

Susan Sumner, PhD, professor and head, department of food science and technology, Virginia Polytechnic Institute and State University, Blacksburg, VA.

Best and Worst Cooking Oils

Mark Hyman, MD, board-certified family medicine physician, Lenox, Massachusetts, author of *Ultrametabolism* (Scribner), and editor in chief of *Alternative Therapies in Health and Medicine*, a peer-reviewed journal in alternative medicine.

For most health-conscious Americans, olive oil has become a dietary staple. It is a central feature of the Mediterranean diet (an eating plan that emphasizes fruits, vegetables, legumes, nuts, whole grains and fish) and has been shown in numerous studies to help guard against heart disease when used as a substitute for butter, margarine or oils that are higher in saturated fat.

The most healthful variety of olive oil is extra virgin olive oil, which is extracted from olives without the use of chemicals. It is the least processed and contains the highest levels of disease-fighting antioxidants. But olive oil is not the only oil that is good for you.

ALTERNATIVES TO OLIVE OIL

Among the oils that provide health benefits similar to those of olive oil are almond, flaxseed, walnut and macadamia nut oils. These oils are available at health-food stores (and even at many supermarkets) and can be used in cooking and/or baking as well as on salads.

Although these nut- and seed-derived oils usually are more expensive than vegetable oils —a 16-ounce bottle of flaxseed oil costs about $15 versus about $5 for the same size bottle of refined soy oil—a little goes a long way, and their distinctive flavors will add variety to your cooking.*

SOURCES OF DIETARY FAT

To function properly, our bodies require dietary fat. It serves not only as an energy source, but also helps our bodies absorb fat-soluble vitamins, including vitamins A, D, E and K, from the food we eat. When used properly, cooking oils can be an excellent source of healthful dietary fat.

Most of the fats in your diet should be monounsaturated and omega-3 fats. For the greatest health benefit, a combination of the fats described below should be consumed, since each provides a different nutritional component.

Best sources of dietary fat...

• **Omega-3 fatty acids** are found in fatty, cold-water fish (salmon, herring, sardines and anchovies)...walnuts...some seeds (pumpkin seeds, hempseeds and flaxseeds)...and flaxseed oil.

According to some studies, as many as 70% of Americans are deficient in these essential fats. Omega-3s have been shown to reduce the risk for heart attack, depression and stroke, and perhaps help protect against prostate and breast malignancies as well as some types of dementia.

• **Monounsaturated fat** is found in avocados, some nut oils and olive oil. This fat boosts immunity and helps lower blood pressure, blood sugar and cholesterol levels. Monounsaturated fat, in the form of olive oil, is the primary source of fat in the Mediterranean diet.

*Prices may vary.

• **Unrefined polyunsaturated fat** is found in walnut oil and natural vegetable oils that have not been chemically processed. This fat is a source of omega-6 fatty acids, which can be harmful when consumed in the high amounts that are typical in the American diet. However, small doses (no more than one tablespoon daily) of unrefined polyunsaturated fat provide a healthful ratio of omega-6 to omega-3.

Important: When selecting an unrefined vegetable oil, be sure that it is "expeller-pressed" or "cold-pressed"—this means that the oil has been processed without chemicals, using pressure rather than heat.

Caution: Commercially available, refined "vegetable oils," including corn and soy oils, are commonly used in restaurant food and still can be found in the kitchen cabinets of many Americans. However, these oils are best avoided, due to the harmful compounds that are produced in the process of refining.

Food products that typically should be avoided include those that contain saturated fat, which is found in beef, pork, lamb, chicken and dairy products—as well as all foods with trans fat, partially hydrogenated oil that is widely found in cookies, crackers and other processed foods.

WHAT ABOUT CANOLA OIL?

Although many Americans use canola oil, I do not recommend it at this time. There have been no long-term medical studies of canola oil, a relatively new food made from a plant similar to the rapeseed plant, which is part of the mustard family. Moreover, animal studies have linked canola oil with reduced platelet count, shorter lifespan and increased need for vitamin E. In contrast, olive and nut oils have been used for centuries...and have proven health benefits.

HOW MUCH IS ENOUGH?

Even though cooking oils can be a healthful addition to your diet, they are pure fat. All oils contain about 14 g of fat or 126 calories per tablespoon. This should be factored into your total daily intake of fat.

Helpful: Cooking oils have different smoke points—the temperature at which heated fat begins to break down, releasing smoke and giving a burned taste to food. Oils that have smoke points of about 350°F or higher, and therefore are good for sautéing and stir-frying (cooking quickly over high heat while stirring continuously) include almond oil, macadamia nut oil and sesame oil. Oils with low smoke points—about 225°F—include flaxseed oil and unrefined sunflower oil. They are best used raw and/or in baking.

The Latest Facts on Fiber

Len Marquart, PhD, RD, assistant professor, department of food science and nutrition, University of Minnesota, St. Paul and coeditor of *Whole Grains and Health*. Blackwell.

The health benefits of dietary fiber have been so highly touted that few people know where the scientific evidence ends and the hype begins.

What you may not know: Scientists who have studied the link between fiber (in both foods and supplements) and health have sometimes found only modest benefits—or none at all.

Reason: To get the optimal benefits of fiber, it must be combined with other healthful substances, such as the antioxidants, vitamins and minerals found in fiber-rich plant foods, including fruits, vegetables and whole grains.

That's why fiber supplements, in the form of powders, tablets and capsules, provide little overall health benefits, other than promoting bowel regularity.

Other important facts…

TYPES OF FIBER

Dietary fiber has long been divided into two main categories…

•**Soluble fiber,** which dissolves in liquid, is found in such foods as oats, beans, psyllium (a plant-derived product) and citrus fruits.

•**Insoluble fiber,** which does not dissolve in liquid, is mainly found in grain products, such as whole wheat…most nuts…and vegetables, such as beets, brussels sprouts and cauliflower.

Now: The National Academy of Sciences discourages the use of the terms "soluble" and "insoluble"—partly because distinctions between the two types of fiber and their physiological effects

aren't as clear-cut as scientists once thought. What's more, researchers have discovered subtypes of fiber, including *beta glucan* and *arabinoxylan*, both of which show promise for lowering both total and LDL "bad" cholesterol and reducing the risk for coronary artery disease.

DISEASE PREVENTION

Even though soluble fiber and insoluble fiber have different chemical properties and effects in the body, they both provide similar health benefits, such as reducing the risk for heart disease.

The latest research shows that everyone should get a mix of different fibers daily. Unfortunately, the average American's total daily fiber consumption is only about 15 grams (the equivalent of one medium apple and one cup each of raspberries and cooked oatmeal). The recommended daily amount is 38 g for men up to age 50…and 30 g at age 51 or older. For women, it's 25 g up to age 50…and 21 g at age 51 and older.

Because the optimal mix of the different fibers has not been determined, all adults should eat a wide variety of foods that contain both soluble and insoluble fibers, such as grains, fruits and vegetables, including beans. *Latest research on fiber's health effects…*

•**Colon cancer.** In theory, fiber *should* prevent colon cancer by speeding the elimination of stools. The faster that stools—and the bile acids and other potential carcinogens that are present in stools—exit the intestines, the less risk there is of cell damage that can lead to cancer.

Scientific evidence: The research on the effects of dietary fiber on colon cancer and polyps (growths that often turn into cancer) is mixed. Some studies have shown no benefit—although it's possible that the levels of fiber in these studies, and the length of time the studies were conducted, may have been insufficient.

New theory: As fiber is broken down by bacteria in the colon, it creates substances called *butyrates*—short-chain fatty acids that "bathe" cells in the colon and are thought to reduce the risk of cancer.

Helpful: Eat at least five servings daily of fruits and vegetables, including several servings of legumes, such as pinto beans.

• **Constipation and other digestive problems.** Fiber not only decreases the time it takes for stools to exit the body (transit time), it also absorbs water in the colon, which increases the weight and size of stools, making them softer and easier to eliminate.

Scientific evidence: Researchers agree that people who consume the recommended daily amount of fiber are far less likely to suffer from constipation than those who eat less. Fiber also reduces the constipation and diarrhea that can accompany irritable bowel syndrome.

Helpful: Eat three to six servings daily of high-fiber foods, such as bran cereals, whole-grain breads, brown rice, barley and whole-wheat pasta.

• **Diabetes.** There's very strong evidence that a high-fiber diet—particularly the fiber in whole grains—both reduces the risk of developing diabetes and improves insulin control in those who already have diabetes.

Scientific evidence: Research shows that people who eat the most whole grains (three servings daily) can reduce their risk of developing diabetes by about 26%, compared with those who eat the least (less than one serving daily).

Helpful: Eat three to four servings daily of whole grains, such as brown rice, whole-grain crackers or bread. Grains that have been processed, such as those used in white rice and white bread, don't have the same benefits.

• **Heart disease.** Whole grains may promote blood vessel health and are rich in antioxidants, which may inhibit cellular damage. Whole oats and barley are rich in soluble fiber, including beta glucans that help control levels of LDL cholesterol. The fiber binds to bile acids and pulls cholesterol out of the intestines and bloodstream. It's also thought to lower blood sugar and improve insulin sensitivity (the body's response to insulin)—both of which reduce the risk for heart disease.

Scientific evidence: People who eat whole grains and whole-grain breakfast cereals can reduce their risk for heart disease by roughly 35% or more. Other studies have shown that the fiber in oat cereals can lower blood cholesterol by around 5%, which results in about a 10% reduction in heart disease risk.

Helpful: Eat three servings daily of whole grains, such as oats and/or barley.

• **Obesity.** Fiber not only absorbs water in the stomach but also promotes a feeling of fullness (satiety)—causing people to consume fewer calories overall. High-fiber foods also appear to increase the body's production of *cholecystokinin* (CCK), a hormone involved in appetite control.

Scientific evidence: Studies at Harvard have shown that people who consume the most fiber are less likely to gain weight than those who get lower amounts. In one study, women with the greatest increase in fiber intake over 12 years had a 49% lower risk for major weight gain than did women with the lowest increase. An eight-year study of men found that for every 40 g per day of whole-grain and cereal fiber consumed, weight gain dropped by about one pound.

Helpful: Eat at least five servings daily of vegetables (including beans)...three servings of whole grains (including cereals, bread and brown rice)...and about four servings of fruits.

The Food That Lowers Cholesterol 24%...in Just Five Weeks

Andrea Chernus, RD, is a registered dietitian, certified diabetes educator and exercise physiologist who maintains a private practice in New York City. She counsels patients on high cholesterol, diabetes, weight management and sports nutrition. She was formerly the clinical nutritionist for Columbia University, New York City. *www.nutrition handouts.com*

If you're one of the millions of Americans with high cholesterol, chances are your doctor has told you what not to eat—high-fat meats and dairy, for example. But certain foods actually can lower your cholesterol and, in some cases, eliminate the need for cholesterol-lowering drugs. Regularly including these foods can have a particularly powerful effect on reducing LDL—the "bad" cholesterol that damages arteries and other blood vessels. High LDL levels are associated with an increased risk for heart attack and stroke.

OAT BRAN, BARLEY AND MORE

Soluble fiber is present in plant-based foods in the form of gums and pectins. The National Cholesterol Education Program Adult Treatment Panel states that five to 10 grams (g) of soluble fiber daily can help to lower LDL by 5%.

A specific type of soluble fiber—*beta-glucan* (found in oat bran and barley)—has an even more potent cholesterol-lowering effect…

•**In a 2004 study,** men eating 6g of soluble fiber from barley per day lowered their LDL cholesterol by an average of 24% in five weeks.

•**In a study published earlier this year,** men given 6g of beta-glucan in a fortified bread —who also were following a low-fat diet and walking 60 minutes per day—experienced an average reduction in LDL cholesterol of 28%.

How it works: In the intestines, soluble fiber attaches itself to cholesterol and bile acids. Bile acids help with fat digestion. They are made from cholesterol, so when the body needs to make more bile acids, it pulls cholesterol from the bloodstream. The process of binding soluble fiber to bile acids forces the body to make more bile and use up cholesterol from the body's supply. Because fiber is not digested, it carries the cholesterol and bile acids out of the body, lowering the body's cholesterol.

Best sources of soluble fiber: Oat bran, oatmeal, barley, apples, citrus fruits, pears, kidney and lima beans, carrots, broccoli and brussels sprouts. Psyllium seed husks also are a good source and are found in some cereals, such as Kellogg's All-Bran Buds cereal.

Hot cereal made of 100% oat bran has about 3g of soluble fiber per serving…plain oatmeal has about 2g. Most cold oat-based cereals have one gram. Fruits and vegetables have 0.5g to 1g of soluble fiber per serving.

Beware: Commercially prepared muffins, pretzels and breads made with oat bran may not contain much soluble fiber. Also, some may be high in saturated or trans fats, sugars and sodium. As a rough guide, check the label to make sure oat bran is one of the first ingredients listed on the food label. (Soluble fiber does not have to be listed separately from total fiber.)

PLANT STEROLS AND STANOLS

Plant sterols (*phytosterols*) and plant stanols (*phytostanols*) are substances that block absorption of cholesterol. They are particularly high in vegetable oils and, to a lesser degree, in fruits, vegetables, nuts and seeds. More than 25 studies have proved their effectiveness in cholesterol reduction. *Examples…*

•**In a 2001 study,** 155 adults with high cholesterol took in 1.5g per day of plant sterols from margarine. After six months, they had an average reduction in LDL cholesterol of 11% (and 9% reduction in total cholesterol).

•**In another study,** 72 adults with high cholesterol took in 2g per day of plant sterols from phytosterol-fortified orange juice. After eight weeks, their average reduction in LDL cholesterol was 12% (7% reduction in total cholesterol).

How they work: Plant sterols and stanols help block the absorption of dietary cholesterol and the reabsorption of cholesterol back into our intestinal tract. They compete with cholesterol for incorporation into mixed *micelles,* which are composite molecules that contain both water- and fat-soluble substances. In the body, micelles are used to carry fats through the bloodstream. When cholesterol is blocked from being absorbed and incorporated into these molecules, it is excreted from the body.

Best sources: To get a cholesterol-lowering dose from ordinary food, you would have to eat hundreds of calories worth of oils per day or bushels of fruits and vegetables. But researchers have isolated plant sterols and stanols, and food companies have incorporated them into "functional foods."

Until recently, only certain margarines contained these cholesterol-lowering ingredients, but food companies now have put them into lower-fat foods, such as yogurts, juices, breads and more. A dose of 2g to 3g of plant sterols and stanols per day has the greatest impact on lowering LDL cholesterol, reducing it by 6% to 15%. Higher doses of sterols and stanols are not more effective.

Foods containing effective amounts of plant sterols and stanols include Promise, Benecol and Take Control margarines…Minute Maid Heartwise Orange Juice…Nature Valley Healthy

Heart Granola Bars…Hain Celestial Rice Dream beverage…Lifetime low-fat cheese…Orowheat whole-grain bread…and VitaMuffins.

The FDA now allows foods containing sterols and stanols that meet certain criteria to put a health claim on the label that they can help reduce the risk of coronary heart disease.

Beware: Margarines and juices are dense in calories. Check food labels to see how much you need to eat to obtain 2g to 3g of sterols and stanols.

If you're worried about calories, you can take sterol/stanol supplements. Generally, they are called beta-sitosterol or sitostanol. It is safe to use these supplements along with statin drugs for an additional cholesterol-lowering effect.

NUTS

People who are trying to lower cholesterol levels often eliminate nuts from their diets because nuts are high in fat and calories. But nuts contain mostly monounsaturated fats, which, when substituted for the saturated fats found in high-fat meats and dairy, not only can lower LDL levels but also boost HDL "good" cholesterol levels.

Studies have shown the greatest effect when nuts comprise 20% of one's total calories, which typically amounts to 1.5 to 3.5 ounces of nuts daily (about one-quarter to one-half cup).

On average, LDL cholesterol levels fall 8% to 12% when walnuts or almonds are substituted for saturated fats. HDL levels may increase by 9% to 20%. Other nuts, such as peanuts (technically a legume), pistachios and pecans, have been shown to lower cholesterol, but fewer studies are available on these varieties.

How they work: The exact mechanism of nuts' healthful effects hasn't been discovered yet, but nuts contain a combination of plant sterols, fiber and healthy fats.

Beware: Because nuts are high in calories, the trick is to substitute nuts for less healthful, high-fat foods, including cheese and meat.

Feed a Cold, Starve a Fever and Other Nutrition Myths

Edward Saltzman, MD, chief of the division of clinical nutrition and medical director of the Obesity Consultation Center at Tufts–New England Medical Center, and a scientist at the Jean Mayer USDA Human Nutrition Research Center on Aging at Tufts University, both in Boston.

Many commonly held beliefs about the health impact of certain foods are based on hearsay, not on scientific research. *Here are the realities behind some often-cited nutrition myths…*

Myth: Feed a cold, starve a fever.

Reality: Both a cold and a fever—and you can have both at once—are associated with inflammation, which increases metabolic rate, allowing you to burn calories at rest more quickly. However, eating more or less will have no real effect on how long you remain sick. There is no evidence that food shortens a cold's duration or reduces symptoms.

It's often believed that vitamin C can help a cold, but there's no firm evidence to back that claim. Last year, researchers reviewed 55 previous studies. Most showed that taking vitamin C did not prevent colds—a few showed that colds were slightly shorter with vitamin supplementation, but usually by only one day or so.

Zinc may reduce a cold's duration, but it must be taken early on—before full-blown symptoms strike. The benefit comes from zinc gluconate lozenges (see the label for the correct dosage). Zinc acetate lozenges or zinc-rich foods, such as oysters and beef, have no impact on a cold's severity or duration.

Bottom line: The real goal is to stay hydrated and loosen mucus by increasing your intake of liquids, such as water, clear soups and tea.

Myth: Fiber prevents colon cancer.

Reality: A high-fiber diet keeps your bowel movements regular and can lower cholesterol and reduce risk of insulin resistance, a precursor to diabetes. But there is no consistent evidence that fiber protects against colon cancer.

A recent study in *The Journal of the American Medical Association* reviewed data on 726,000 people over 20 years and found that high-fiber diets did not reduce the risk of colon cancer. Another study determined that people eating 33 grams of fiber per day—roughly 6.5 servings of fruits and vegetables—had no fewer polyps (benign growths in the colon that may become cancerous) than those eating roughly half as much fiber. Even high-fiber cereals seem to strike out when it comes to protecting against colon cancer, although they may have benefits for cardiovascular health and prevent constipation.

Bottom line: Continue to eat fiber-rich foods, such as fruits, vegetables and whole grains, for their proven health benefits, including cardiovascular health and weight control. Also, while fiber-rich foods do not protect against colon cancer, they do protect against other types of cancer—including those of the breast, mouth, throat and esophagus—probably because of their phytochemicals, protective compounds found in some foods.

Myth: Soy relieves hot flashes.

Reality: Most scientific studies have not found that soy-rich foods or supplements offer relief from hot flashes. While soy is a good source of phytoestrogens (chemicals occurring naturally in plants that act like the hormone *estrogen*), it provides an extremely weak estrogenic effect. Some menopausal women may benefit from a soy-rich diet, but most do not—at least not on a consistent basis.

Bottom line: Soy-rich foods are nutritious, low in fat and may help lower cholesterol and improve prostate health (so far, studies have produced mixed results). And a recent analysis of 18 previous studies found that soy may slightly lower the risk of breast cancer. To control hot flashes, however, you're better off adjusting room temperature...wearing "breathable" fabrics, such as cotton...and drinking cool beverages when a flash starts. At this time, there are no dietary supplements known to be both safe and effective for hot flashes.

Myth: Olive oil is the healthiest oil.

Reality: This foundation of the Mediterranean diet is among the healthiest cooking oils—and certainly gets the best publicity—but other oils may be just as good. For example, just a few months ago, the FDA decreed that canola oil, like olive oil, can carry a health claim for its ability to reduce the risk of coronary heart disease due to its unsaturated fat content. The important thing is to limit saturated fats, which are most often found in animal products, such as red meat, poultry, butter and whole milk.

Bottom line: Choose oils high in mono- or polyunsaturated fat, such as olive, canola, safflower, flaxseed and walnut oils. If you choose olive oil, select extra-virgin. Extra-virgin olive oil comes from the first pressing of olives, so it's less processed and contains higher levels of antioxidants, substances that slow down the natural process that leads to cell and tissue damage.

Myth: Honey is more healthful than sugar.

Reality: Honey contains more fructose than sugar—and fructose is becoming public enemy number one among some cardiologists. Some studies suggest that high-fructose diets are linked to weight gain and metabolic syndrome, a group of health problems that includes excess abdominal fat, high blood pressure, high triglycerides (a type of fat in the blood), low "good" cholesterol and high blood sugar.

Bottom line: Go easy on sugar and honey. Both offer "empty calories"—a tablespoon of honey has 64 calories and a tablespoon of sugar has about 45 calories. Neither is a good source of any nutrient. You would need to overeat honey to an unhealthy level in order to benefit from its micronutrients or other purported health benefits.

20

Fitness Savvy

The Fat-Resistance Diet

Weight loss isn't only —or even mainly— about calories. Surprisingly, we gain weight when natural weight-control mechanisms are disrupted by inflammation, a low-grade inflammatory response caused by poor diet and environmental toxins.

When people gain weight, the extra fatty tissue produces *leptin*, a hormone that suppresses appetite and speeds metabolism. In theory, this should cause people to lose the extra weight.

Instead, inflammation in fat tissue and blood vessels stimulates the production of anti-inflammatory chemicals. These chemicals disable leptin's ability to suppress appetite and speed metabolism. This is called *leptin resistance*.

To combat leptin resistance, I have developed a fat-resistance diet based on cutting-edge research at premier institutions such as Harvard, Johns Hopkins and Rockefeller universities. Eating the proper foods can eliminate chronic

inflammation and reprogram the body's weight-loss mechanisms.

ANTI-INFLAMMATORY FOODS

The focus of the diet isn't calorie control. The idea is to eat foods that supply anti-inflammatory nutrients. A major problem with most weight-loss diets is the use of artificial sweeteners and fat substitutes to reduce calories. Substituting these products for real foods deprives your body of key anti-inflammatory nutrients. *Main principles...*

• **Eat fish at least three times weekly.** The omega-3 fatty acids in fish have powerful anti-inflammatory properties. Fish that are rich in omega-3s and relatively low in mercury include anchovies, conch, herring (fresh or pickled, not creamed), mackerel (Atlantic only), sablefish, salmon (fresh, canned or smoked, wild or farmed), sardines (Atlantic), sturgeon and tuna (fresh or canned bluefin—not albacore).

Leo Galland, MD, director, Foundation for Integrated Medicine, which promotes a comprehensive approach to health care, New York City. His latest book is *The Fat Resistance Diet*. Broadway. *www.fatresistancediet.com*. Dr. Galland is a recipient of the Linus Pauling Award.

•**Balance essential fatty acids.** The optimal ratio of omega-6 fatty acids to omega-3s is about 4:1. The ratio in the average American diet is closer to 20:1. A relative excess of omega-6 fats in tissues leads cells to produce excessive levels of pro-inflammatory chemicals called *prostanoids*. The best approach is to decrease intake of omega-6s and increase intake of omega-3s.

Foods high in omega-3s: Fish, flaxseed, walnuts and beans—navy, kidney and soybeans.

Foods high in omega-6s: Red meat, chicken, milk, eggs and most vegetable oils, including corn, sunflower and safflower.

•**Cut back on unhealthy fats.** Saturated fat—primarily found in beef, pork, lamb, dairy products and poultry skin—should be limited to no more than 10% of total calories. Don't eat any trans fat—this means avoiding any foods made with hydrogenated or partially hydrogenated vegetable oil. These include most commercial baked goods and some fast foods. Both saturated fat and trans fat greatly increase levels of inflammatory chemicals.

•**Get 25 grams of fiber daily.** A high-fiber diet helps control appetite and reduce inflammation. A study by the Centers for Disease Control and Prevention found that people who consume the most fiber have lower levels of *C-reactive protein* (CRP), which indicates the presence of inflammatory chemicals in the body. All plant foods contain some fiber. Among the best sources are beans, whole grains and vegetables.

•**Eat colorful fruits and vegetables.** Get at least nine servings daily. Produce with deep colors and intense flavors is high in flavonoids and carotenoids, chemical compounds that have anti-inflammatory effects.

Important: Have at least one serving of blueberries, cherries or pomegranates a day. These contain *anthocyanins*, which are among the most potent anti-inflammatory agents.

•**Choose alliums and crucifers.** Crucifers are strong-flavored vegetables, including broccoli, cauliflower, cabbage and kale. Alliums include onions and garlic. Both classes of vegetables reduce chronic inflammation and lower the risk of cancer, particularly breast cancer. Eat at least one serving of each daily.

•**Use only egg whites or unbroken egg yolks.** The cholesterol in yolks has relatively little effect on cholesterol in the blood—but if the yolk is broken, the cholesterol is oxidized and produces inflammatory by-products. Poached or boiled whole eggs are fine. Avoid scrambled eggs and whole-egg omelettes.

•**Favor herbs and spices that are potent anti-inflammatories.** These include basil, cardamom, cilantro, cinnamon, clove, ginger, parsley and turmeric. Use them every day. Avoid chiles, cayenne pepper and jalapeños, which can trigger inflammation.

THREE STAGES

The diet progresses in phases...

•**Stage 1.** Eat as much as you want of such foods as arugula, bell peppers, broccoli, cabbage, carrots, leeks, onions, romaine lettuce, scallions, shiitake mushrooms, spinach and tomatoes—as well as blueberries, cherries, grapefruit and pomegranates.

Eating three four-ounce servings of high-protein foods each day helps suppress appetite and maintain muscle mass. Choose fish, egg whites, poultry and plain, fat-free yogurt. Meat lovers can eat red meat twice a week but should marinate beef with cherry or pomegranate concentrate (this reduces inflammatory chemical compounds produced during cooking). You can have a tablespoon or two each day of nuts or seeds (especially flaxseed, walnuts and almonds). During this stage, get 25 grams of fiber, primarily from vegetables.

Avoid grains, even whole grains, because they tend to raise insulin levels, increasing leptin resistance. Most people stay in this stage for two weeks and lose six to 10 pounds.

•**Stage 2.** The long-term weight-loss part of the diet. Stay on this until you reach your goal weight. Expect to lose one to two pounds per week.

In addition to the Stage 1 foods, add some whole grains, such as oats and brown rice, and beans, lentils and other legumes (about two to three cups a week of each).

•**Stage 3.** The lifelong maintenance phase. Increase variety by adding potatoes, pasta and whole-grain breads.

How to Break the Weight-Gain Cycle

Ray D. Strand, MD, author of *Healthy for Life* (Real Life) and *What Your Doctor Doesn't Know About Nutritional Medicine May Be Killing You* (Thomas Nelson). Dr. Strand has devised a 15-month wellness program that is available on-line at *www.healthyandleanforlife.com.* More about his work at *www.raystrand.com.*

In a country obsessed with dieting and weight loss, we have a disproportionately large number of overweight people. In fact, two-thirds of American adults and nearly one-third of children are overweight or obese, putting them at increased risk for an array of health risks.

Ironically, according to Ray D. Strand, MD, we continue to ignore the root cause of obesity—insulin resistance and the inability to properly process glucose and fat stores. He believes that if people were able to tame insulin resistance, they would lose weight and at the same time prevent obesity-related health problems.

The earlier you get on top of insulin resistance, the greater the chance you have of reversing it and avoiding diabetes or high blood pressure. How to go about this?

It's simple: Develop a healthy lifestyle.

INSULIN RESISTANCE— A PRIMER

In order to get to the bottom of insulin resistance, let's first take a closer look at insulin's proper role in the body. Insulin is normally released into the bloodstream in response to elevated glucose (blood sugar) levels after you eat. Its role is to push glucose out of the bloodstream and into the cells of the body, where it is converted into energy. When you develop insulin resistance, however, this system goes awry and the body no longer can make efficient use of insulin. The result is uncontrollable food cravings, increased emotional eating and an inability to lose weight no matter how hard you try.

When you suffer from insulin resistance, it is as if your body holds on to fat like a sponge holds on to water, says Dr. Strand. He adds that insulin resistance and its devastating consequences are no sudden, random occurrence.

They sneak up over the course of many years, gradually eroding your health. Their roots lie in the way most Americans eat.

A VICIOUS CYCLE—CARBOHYDRATE ADDICTION AND INSULIN ABUSE

The typical American diet includes far too many fast foods, chips, cookies, doughnuts, bread and soft drinks. Atkins high-protein craze aside, we've become carbohydrate addicts in this country, warns Dr. Strand. Simple sugars quickly flood the bloodstream, and in response, the body furiously pumps out insulin. This, in turn, leads to an abrupt crash in blood sugar and a drop in energy that leaves you craving more carbs, and the vicious cycle continues—more carbs, more blood sugar, more insulin, etc.

As time goes on and insulin converts excess glucose into fat, you put on weight, which makes the body's cells more resistant to insulin. The pancreas responds by pumping out still more insulin in an increasingly vain attempt to try to force glucose into cells. The bloodstream is left awash in excess glucose.

In people with insulin resistance, blood sugar is not high enough (yet) to constitute diabetes, but it is higher than normal. If you do nothing to change your ways and break the cycle, eventually you will tip over into the abnormal metabolic state known as metabolic syndrome (also called Syndrome X). Characteristics of this devastating syndrome—shared by 25% of the adult population of the US—include obesity, diabetes, high blood pressure, abnormal cholesterol, elevated triglycerides, cardiovascular disease and, in women, polycystic ovarian syndrome (PCOS).

HOW TO TAME INSULIN RESISTANCE

Full-blown metabolic syndrome doesn't develop overnight, emphasizes Dr. Strand. It is a result of years and years of poor daily food and activity choices. The good news is that you can break the vicious cycle of carbohydrate addiction and insulin abuse, slowing down and even reversing the development of obesity and type 2 diabetes. However, there's no quick fix, no easy pill to pop—the only way you can overcome these obstacles is by developing and following a healthy lifestyle.

WATCH THE WARNING SIGNS

According to Dr. Strand, there are a number of measurable warning signs for insulin resistance, in which case you need to take action. *Warning signs of insulin resistance are...*

•**Expanding waist size.** Beware of a waist circumference of 29 or more inches in women and 34 or more inches in men.

•**Any slight elevation in blood pressure.** Even a measurement of 130/85 can be an early sign of insulin resistance.

•**Elevated blood sugar.** Ask your doctor to give you a fasting blood sugar test. A result above 100 (or even approaching 100) is a red flag.

•**A decrease in HDL or good cholesterol** (below 50 for women, or below 40 for men), which is often accompanied by increasing triglyceride levels. Dr. Strand calculates a simple ratio by dividing a person's triglyceride level by his/her HDL level. If the resulting triglyceride/HDL ratio is greater than two, this is another warning sign.

**THREE STEPS TO REVERSING
INSULIN SENSITIVITY**

Once you and your physician have identified the problem, the answer is to promote a healthy lifestyle that enhances insulin sensitivity and works to reverse the problem and reduce long-term health risks. *Dr. Strand advises...*

1. Follow a healthy diet that does not spike blood sugar. Generally, 40% to 50% of calories should come from low-glycemic carbohydrates ...30% from fat...and 20% to 30% from protein.

While you don't need to weigh your food or starve yourself, you do need to make healthy food choices. *This means...*

•Eat good complex carbs such as antioxidant-rich fruits, veggies and whole grains, and avoid high-glycemic carbs that send your blood sugar soaring, including white bread, white rice, highly processed cereal and white potatoes.

•Replace the bad saturated and trans-fats in hamburgers and french fries with good alternatives such as monounsaturated fats (for example, olive oil, avocado and macadamia nuts) and essential fatty acids (EFAs), including cold-water fish (salmon, sardines, etc.), flaxseed oil and walnuts.

•Choose good sources of protein such as nuts, hard-boiled eggs, avocados, beans, soy, legumes, fowl with the skin removed and cold-water fish. Dr. Strand notes that the poorest sources of protein are red meats and dairy products.

•Drink eight to 10 glasses of purified water every day.

•Never go hungry. Small, frequent meals will help control spikes in blood sugar. As you feel better, you should decrease meal frequency and increase content. If you're still hungry between meals, snack on an apple, a hard-boiled egg or a handful of raw almonds.

2. Develop a moderate, consistent exercise program. Physical activity is the second step to insulin sensitivity. It doesn't matter what you choose to do, says Dr. Strand. At first, consistency is the most important thing.

Your ultimate goal: Gradually work your way up to 30 to 40 minutes of aerobic exercise such as brisk walking five days a week. Every step you take will bring you one step closer to improved insulin sensitivity. To be on the safe side, Dr. Strand recommends consulting your physician before beginning an exercise program.

3. Take high-quality nutritional supplements. To boost cellular nutrition, Dr. Strand recommends taking a high-quality antioxidant with each meal. He explains that we require antioxidants to protect our bodies from oxidative stress and free radical cell damage that lie at the bottom of chronic degenerative diseases such as diabetes and cardiovascular disease. Dr. Strand in particular recommends vitamins C and E to ward off oxidative stress created by elevated levels of insulin and glucose following a rich meal high in bad fats and carbs (for example, steak and mashed potatoes). Other beneficial supplements are chromium, magnesium and selenium. Consult your physician about exact dosages.

**MORE EFFECTIVE THAN A PILL—
A HEALTHIER LIFESTYLE**

As Dr. Strand sees it, modern medicine relies too much on drugs to control the consequences of elevated insulin levels without addressing the underlying problem—insulin resistance. He speculates that this may be because there is no FDA-approved pill to cure insulin resistance. In the parlance of conventional medicine, where there's no pill, there's no disease.

However, if you follow these three simple steps to a healthier lifestyle, says Dr. Strand, your body will gradually begin to release fat, and you will see triglyceride and blood pressure numbers start to drop. It won't happen overnight, any more than insulin resistance develops overnight...but over the months, you'll find that you feel better overall and have more energy. Without a pill, without drugs or their side effects, you will have taken charge of your health and brought your body back into balance.

Shocking Reasons People Overeat

Brian Wansink, PhD, director of the Food and Brand Lab at Cornell University, Ithaca, New York, is author of *Mindless Eating: Why We Eat More Than We Think.* Bantam. *www.mindlesseating.org.*

Our minds, not our stomachs, control our eating habits—but our minds don't always do a good job of making food decisions. Most people put on weight because their minds don't accurately keep track of how much they have eaten, not because they lack the willpower to put down their forks.

Surprisingly, when our minds tell us which foods we enjoy, it's often for reasons that have little to do with how they taste.

Example: Approximately one-third of World War II veterans who served in the South Pacific love Chinese food 50 years later. A similar percentage hate it. It turns out that almost all the veterans who love Chinese food did not experience frequent heavy combat when in Asia, but those who hate it did.

Brian Wansink, PhD, a noted food psychologist, has done extensive research on how our minds trick us into unhealthy eating habits. *Here are some of the ways...*

•**If it looks like a small meal, it feels like a small meal.** Our eyes, not our stomachs, tell us when we're full. In a study conducted by our research team, when we replaced eight-inch dinner plates with 12-inch plates, diners consumed 20% to 35% more because their portions looked smaller on the larger plates. After the

meal, they were certain that they hadn't eaten any more than usual.

What to do: Use smaller plates, bowls and spoons if you want to eat less. Drink from tall, thin glasses—not short, fat ones—so you will think you are drinking more. When possible, serve food over a bed of lettuce so that the plate looks full.

•**We feel full when there's visual evidence that we have had a lot to eat.** In one study, we gave chicken wings to graduate students while they watched the Super Bowl. When we left the bones in front of the students, they ate an average of four wings apiece. When we cleared the bones away frequently—removing the visual evidence of earlier consumption—each student ate an average of six wings. After the game, students in both groups estimated that they had only four wings each.

What to do: When you're eating—particularly when you're snacking—leave out candy wrappers, peanut shells and other evidence of snacking so that your eyes can warn you about how much you have eaten.

•**When there's no distance to the food, there's no thinking before eating.** Office workers consumed an average of nine Hershey's Kisses per day when we put bowls of the chocolate candies on their desks. Their consumption dropped by more than 50% when these bowls were positioned just six feet away. Six feet is only two steps, but even a short distance forces us to think twice before we eat.

What to do: At home, fill individual plates at the stove, and leave the leftovers on the stove or a sideboard. The more hassle it is to eat, the less we eat. You will have fewer additional helpings if you must stand up to get them. A bowl of salad or vegetables can be brought to the dinner table because second helpings of these foods won't add many calories.

With snack foods, pour a serving into a bowl rather than eating straight from the bag. Then if you want more, you have to go to the kitchen to get it.

•**"Comfort foods" cause overconsumption.** Comfort foods improve our moods. These foods pick us up when we're feeling stressed or unhappy and serve as rewards when we're feeling good.

Women's comfort foods tend to be unhealthy dessert or snack items, while men's comfort foods are more likely to be hot meals. Why the difference? Men tend to associate home-cooked meals with someone taking care of them, because men's meals often are prepared by their wives. Women associate home-cooked meals with the chore of cooking, so they prefer prepared snack foods and desserts.

What to do: We get nearly as much emotional benefit from a small serving of a comfort food as from a large one—for example, a single scoop of ice cream instead of a pint.

Also, we get nearly as much emotional benefit from our second- or third-favorite comfort food as from our absolute favorite. If your top comfort food is chocolate ice cream but tomato soup is a close second, keep plenty of microwavable tomato soup in the house so that low-calorie comfort is just seconds away.

•**We underestimate beverage calories.** When people are asked to gauge the calories in a drink, they typically undershoot by 30% or more. Beverages don't seem to be filling, so we don't assume that they have as many calories as they actually do.

What to do: As a rule of thumb, estimate that you're consuming 10 calories per ounce for "thin" beverages, such as juice, soda and milk…and 20 calories per ounce for "thick" beverages, such as smoothies and meal-replacement shakes. That adds up quickly when you're drinking a 32-ounce soda—to an estimated 320 calories.

Interestingly, if you load that drink with ice, you'll actually burn off a few of those calories. Since your body has to use energy to heat up an iced beverage, you actually burn about one calorie for every ice-cold ounce you drink. If you drink the recommended eight eight-ounce glasses of water a day and if you fill those 64 ounces with ice, you'll burn about 70 extra calories a day, the equivalent of about seven pounds a year.

•**Exercise might make you fatter.** You have forced yourself to jog three miles every day for months—yet you weigh just as much as when you started. What are you doing wrong?

Most exercisers overestimate the calories their exercise burns and reward themselves with high-calorie foods after their workouts because they think they've earned it. They don't realize that the six Oreo cookies they treat themselves to as a reward have more calories (around 320) than the number of calories they burned while running three miles (around 300).

What to do: If you need a reward, opt for nonfood treats, perhaps a half-hour doing something you enjoy, such as reading a good book or watching a favorite TV show.

•**Birth order might affect your eating habits.** Oldest children and only children tend to save their favorite foods for last. Give them a chocolate chip cookie, and it might become a special treat for after dinner.

Youngest children and middle children of large families are more likely to polish off favorite foods as soon as they receive them—probably to ensure that older siblings won't snatch the food away. These birth-order eating patterns tend to continue into adulthood.

For adults who are the youngest or middle children, the result can be unnecessary pounds. Favorite foods tend to be unhealthy foods, and people who eat unhealthy foods as soon as they get them may be inclined to eat larger quantities in the long run.

What to do: Don't bring favorite snacks into the house in large quantities, especially if you are a youngest or middle child. You might polish off a box in a single sitting.

The Skinny on Thin People

Stephen Gullo, PhD, health psychologist and president of the Center for Healthful Living at the Institute for Health and Weight Sciences, New York City, is former chairman of the National Obesity and Weight Control Education Program of the American Institute for Life-Threatening Illness at Columbia-Presbyterian Medical Center and author of *The Thin Commandments Diet*. Rodale.

Do you know people who never gain an ounce and yet don't seem to have to watch what they eat? Good genes play a role—if your parents were thin, more than likely you will be, too. But in helping thousands of patients slim down, Stephen Gullo, PhD, author of *The Thin Commandments Diet*, has found that though most of us assume thin people never give their weight a second thought, they actually rely on a number of strategies to keep the pounds from accumulating. *Here, the secrets of thin people, which can help anyone who is trying to lose weight or maintain a healthy weight…*

•**Thin people don't skip meals.** They don't allow themselves to get so hungry that they become compulsive eaters rather than selective eaters. Thin people have structured eating habits. They eat three meals and one to two healthful snacks a day to keep blood sugar stable and prevent the body from secreting large amounts of *insulin*, the hunger hormone. Stable blood sugar levels also help the body metabolize calories efficiently and prevent cravings for sweets.

•**Thin people eat the right breakfast.** The National Weight Control Registry, which monitors people who have lost weight and successfully kept it off, found that 78% of those who have maintained their weight loss eat breakfast every day. But the wrong breakfast isn't helpful. A breakfast high in simple carbohydrates, such as a sugary cereal, stimulates appetite. That's because blood sugar is low in the morning. If you eat a sugary breakfast, blood sugar levels rise and then crash rapidly, making you hungry. A breakfast that contains protein and fiber—such as oatmeal and skim milk or low-fat yogurt with fresh fruit—is better. It satisfies your appetite, keeps blood sugar levels on an even keel and helps you feel full longer.

•**Thin people act quickly.** If they gain a few pounds, they immediately cut back on portion sizes and exercise more. I tell my patients that a mark of a winner at weight control is to own only one size of clothing. When thin people think their clothing is getting too tight, they don't buy larger clothes. They change the habits that are creating the problem. It's far easier to lose three or four pounds than it is to lose 20.

•**Thin people weigh themselves regularly.** Most people who have lost weight and kept it off weigh themselves at least once a week. A gain of even two to three pounds motivates them to shift into a more restricted eating plan for a few days. I weigh myself on Monday, right after the weekend, when my eating habits tend to be more liberal, and again on Friday. If I don't

like what I see on Monday, I make changes in my diet. I eat lighter meals, such as broiled fish and chicken, egg white omelets and steamed vegetables without oil or butter, and I don't eat sweets. I weigh myself again on Wednesday to see if my weight is coming down.

•**Thin people don't deprive themselves.** They devise creative strategies to limit consumption of high-calorie foods. They don't stock the house with them. When they do buy them, they select individual portions or serve them only when they have company or on weekends. A patient of mine only buys her children cookies containing peanuts because she doesn't like peanuts. Other people eat desserts only in restaurants.

•**Thin people get enough sleep.** Being sleep-deprived stimulates the appetite, especially carbohydrate cravings. Researchers at the University of Chicago studied young men who got only four hours of sleep per night for two nights. The researchers measured levels of the hormone *leptin*. An increase in leptin signals the brain that no more food is needed…a decrease triggers hunger. The sleep-deprived men had an 18% *decrease* in leptin. The researchers also found that levels of *ghrelin*, a hormone that causes hunger, increased by 28%.

The sleep-deprived men were not only hungrier, they also craved carbohydrates, such as sweets, and salty foods, such as chips. They may have wanted sweets because of lower blood sugar levels. The salt cravings may have been because sleep-deprivation lowers blood pressure. Salty foods raise blood pressure and may have temporarily made the young men feel more energetic.

•**Thin people move a lot.** Studies show that people who lose weight and keep it off exercise regularly. They may not work out in a gym or have a structured program, but they walk a lot, garden or take the stairs instead of the elevator. The National Weight Control Registry found that people who keep off weight burn about 11,830 calories per week through physical activity—the equivalent of walking more than 20 miles.

Researchers at the Mayo Clinic have reported that lean people expend about 350 more calories per day, on average, than sedentary obese people—and not just through exercise, such as walking. They fidget, tap their toes and so on.

•**Thin people exercise portion control.** They know which foods they can eat in generous amounts, such as lean protein, fruits and vegetables. If they overeat, they do it at a special restaurant or on a holiday. There's nothing wrong with overeating on Thanksgiving, but there is something destructive about consuming a pint of ice cream every night. Thin people also consider how food is prepared. They know that a healthy, low-calorie filet of sole, for example, is neither healthy nor low-calorie if it's fried in oil or sautéed in butter.

•**Thin people don't use food to deal with emotion.** Many of my patients don't really enjoy the foods that are making them heavy. They use food to cope with anger, depression and stress. People who stay trim over a lifetime don't use food as therapy. They also don't eat because of boredom or out of habit, such as when they go to the movies or they're watching TV.

Instead, they have other ways to deal with their emotions. They may go for a walk, take a bath, play a computer game or browse in a store. Mental diversion turns off the food switch. If they associate watching television with food, they chew on a stick of gum or eat cut-up vegetables. Or they allow themselves a sensible portion of a low-cal snack, such as a small bag of low-fat popcorn.

■ ■ ■ ■

Diet Myth

The commonly held belief that eating after 8 pm causes weight gain is a misconception.

Reality: It's not *when* you eat that causes weight gain—it's how much. There is no evidence that calorie "burn" is slower at night. Weight gain results from overeating and lack of activity, whether that occurs in the morning, afternoon or night.

This myth likely stems from the fact that many people eat little during the day but then overeat at night, when they're relaxing at home—but these people won't gain any more weight than those who overeat earlier in the day. Some research has suggested that people who eat breakfast are less likely to gain weight

or become obese—though the reason for this is unclear.

Bottom line: Watch portion sizes more than the clock. Don't go for long periods without eating, because you are more likely to overeat when you are ravenously hungry.

Edward Saltzman, MD, chief of the division of clinical nutrition and medical director of the Obesity Consultation Center, Tufts–New England Medical Center, and scientist at the Jean Mayer USDA Human Nutrition Research Center on Aging at Tufts University, Boston.

■ ■ ■ ■

Diet Soda Backfire?

Diet soda drinkers in a long-term study were more likely to become overweight than people who drank full-calorie beverages.

Recent finding: 57% of normal-weight people who drank two or more cans of diet soda a day became overweight after eight years, versus 47% of those who drank regular soda.

Possible reasons: Diet soda drinkers may feel that they're saving enough calories, so they can splurge elsewhere in their diet...or diet sodas may—in some as yet undetermined way—increase hunger in some people.

Sharon Parten Fowler, MPH, faculty associate, clinical epidemiology, University of Texas Health Science Center, San Antonio, and coauthor of the review of data from the San Antonio Heart Study of 1,177 people, presented at a recent meeting of the American Diabetes Association.

Is There a 'Magic Bullet' For Weight Loss?

Sandra Woodruff, RD, author of *Secrets of Fat-Free Cooking, The Good Carb Cookbook* and *Secrets of Good-Carb/Low-Carb Living.* Avery.

Some dieters put their hopes in pills that promise to "burn," "block," "flush" or otherwise eliminate fat from the system.

But science has yet to come up with a low-risk "magic bullet" for weight loss. Some pills may help control the appetite, but they can have serious side effects. Amphetamines, for example, are highly addictive and can have an adverse impact on the heart and central nervous system. Other pills are utterly worthless.

The Federal Trade Commission (FTC) and a number of state attorneys general have successfully brought cases against marketers of pills claiming to absorb or burn fat.

The US Food and Drug Administration (FDA) has banned 111 ingredients once found in over-the-counter diet products. None of these substances, which include alcohol, caffeine, dextrose and guar gum, have proved effective in weight-loss or appetite suppression.

Beware of the following products that are touted as weight-loss wonders...

• **Diet patches.** Worn on the skin, these have not been proven safe or effective. The FDA has seized millions of these products from manufacturers and promoters.

• **"Fat blockers"** purport to absorb the fat and mechanically interfere with the fat that a person might eat.

• **"Starch blockers"** promise to block or impede starch digestion. Not only is the claim unproven, but users have complained of nausea, vomiting, diarrhea and stomach pains.

• **"Magnet" diet pills** allegedly "flush fat out of the body." The FTC has brought legal action against several marketers of these pills.

• **Glucomannan** is advertised as the "weight loss secret that's been in the Orient for more than 500 years." There is little evidence supporting the effectiveness of this plant root in helping people lose weight.

• **Some bulk producers or fillers,** such as fiber-based products, may absorb liquid and swell in the stomach, thereby reducing hunger. But some fillers, such as guar gum, can prove harmful, causing obstructions in the intestines, stomach or esophagus.

• **Spirulina,** a species of blue-green algae, has not been proven effective for losing weight.

PHONY DEVICES AND GADGETS

Phony weight-loss devices range from those that are simply ineffective to those that are truly dangerous to your health.

Some of the fraudulent gadgets that have been marketed to hopeful dieters over the years include...

• **Electrical muscle stimulators,** which have a legitimate use in physical therapy treatment, do not help weight loss or body toning. In fact, when used incorrectly, they can cause electrical shocks and burns. The FDA has even taken a number of them off the market.

• **Appetite-suppressing eyeglasses** are common eyeglasses that have colored lenses that claim to project an image to the retina that decreases the desire to eat. There is no evidence that these work.

• **Magic weight-loss earrings** and devices that are custom-fitted to the purchaser's ear purport to stimulate acupuncture points that control hunger. These claims, of course, have never been proven.

---

10 Surprising Ways to Stay Healthy and Control Your Weight

Mehmet C. Oz, MD, medical director of the Integrated Medical Center and director of the Cardiovascular Institute at NewYork–Presbyterian Medical Center and professor and vice chairman of surgery at Columbia University, both in New York City, is coauthor, with Michael F. Roizen, MD, of *You on a Diet: The Owner's Manual for Waist Management*. Free Press.

Whether you're trying to lose weight or simply find a healthful eating plan you can stick with, you're bound to fail if you try to stay on a diet. Invariably, people on diets end up depriving themselves of certain foods and/or scrupulously counting calories.

Problem: Virtually no one can maintain long-term deprivation because our bodies are programmed to avoid this type of ongoing discomfort. And calorie restriction causes your metabolism to slow down in order to preserve energy, often resulting in more stored fat.

The secret is to work with your body's chemistry rather than against it, so healthful eating becomes automatic, not forced.

Recent development: Body weight used to be considered one of the best indicators of overall health.

Now: Research has shown that your waist measurement (at or just below your navel) may be more reliable. That's because abdominal fat is especially harmful due to its proximity to your vital organs, where it can lead to harmful increases in cholesterol and triglyceride levels. Fat in this area has been linked to heart disease, cancer and diabetes. Studies have found that men should strive for a waist measurement of 35 inches or less, while women should aim for 32½ inches or less. When these measurements are exceeded, health risks increase. For example, risk for metabolic syndrome (a group of conditions, including hypertension and abdominal obesity, that raises diabetes and cardiovascular disease risk) increases by 40% at 40 inches for men and 37 inches for women.

Important: Even if your weight is ideal, you can benefit from the strategies described below because they promote healthy cholesterol and blood pressure levels. *My recommendations…*

1. Spice up your morning eggs. Cayenne and other forms of red pepper contain capsaicin, a substance that suppresses appetite signals, increases metabolism and decreases the desire for food later in the day. In addition, eggs are high in protein, which tends to induce feelings of fullness.

2. Consume fiber early in the day. Fiber increases levels of appetite-suppressing signals in the small intestine. Eating fiber early in the day makes people less hungry in the afternoon—the time when most of us tend to eat snacks and other calorie-dense foods. Consume about 30 g of fiber daily in the form of high-fiber cereals, fruits and vegetables, and 100% whole grains.

3. Eat nuts. The monounsaturated fat in nuts stimulates the production of cholecystokinin (CCK), a chemical messenger that slows the rate at which the stomach empties and reduces appetite without putting your body into starvation mode—that is, the point at which it starts conserving calories, rather than burning them. Before lunch and/or dinner, have about six walnuts, 12 almonds or 12 hazelnuts.

4. Drink coffee instead of soft drinks. Coffee (caffeinated and decaffeinated) is a rich source of antioxidants, and Americans consume more of it than any other antioxidant-rich food. Coffee is much lower in calories (if you don't add a lot of sugar and/or creamer) than sugary soft drinks.

Bonus: Caffeine stimulates the release of norepinephrine, a hormone that suppresses appetite and promotes calorie burning by increasing heart rate and metabolism. Green tea also is a rich source of antioxidants and caffeine.

5. Supplement with 5-hydroxytryptophan (5-HTP). Related to the amino acid tryptophan and sold as a weight-loss supplement, 5-HTP increases brain levels of serotonin, a neurotransmitter that controls appetite. In one study, people taking 5-HTP for six weeks lost an average of 12 pounds, compared with only four pounds in a control group.

Recommended dose: 300 mg daily.

Bonus: 5-HTP has mood-enhancing benefits.

6. Turn up the thermostat. One reason that people tend to eat more during the cold months is that cold temperatures stimulate appetite. Also, people with naturally low body temperatures tend to have a slower metabolism and are more prone to weight gain. Staying warm may be a natural form of appetite control, particularly if you increase body temperature with exercise. Every one degree increase in body temperature increases metabolism by 14%.

7. Ask your doctor about Tagamet. The active ingredient (cimetidine) in this heartburn drug is thought to activate appetite-suppressing CCK. One 12-week study found that people taking a prescription form of Tagamet (400 mg, three times daily) had about a 5% decrease in waist size.

Important: Tagamet is unlikely to cause significant side effects, but should be taken to aid weight loss only if you have heartburn symptoms.

8. Consider using nicotine. It's common for people who quit smoking to gain weight, probably because the nicotine in tobacco suppresses appetite, increases metabolism and damages taste buds, which makes food less appealing. Studies have shown that nicotine—in the form of patches and gum, not from cigarettes—when combined with small amounts of caffeine, can help some people lose weight.

If you've hit a weight plateau: Talk to your doctor about combining a nicotine patch with two cups of coffee daily. Even for non-smokers, this approach can be used temporarily (to avoid possible addiction risk) to jump-start weight-loss efforts.

9. Smell grapefruit. Grapefruit oil, available from aromatherapy shops, emits an aroma that is thought to affect liver enzymes and help promote weight loss. In preliminary research, animals exposed to grapefruit scent for 15 minutes, three times weekly, had a reduction in appetite and body weight.

10. Control emotional stress. People who live with chronic stress (due to family pressures, a fast-paced job, etc.) produce high levels of cortisol, a stress hormone that increases the propensity for the *omentum*—a structure located near the stomach—to store fat. Excessive fat in the omentum can significantly increase waist size.

Important: Exercise is among the best ways to lower stress—and curb accumulations of omentum fat.

Recommended: A 30-minute walk and five minutes' worth of stretching daily...and three weekly sessions that include basic exercises, such as push-ups, shoulder shrugs, abdominal crunches, etc.

■■■■

Vitamin that Burns Fat

Vitamin C can help you burn more fat when you exercise.

Recent study: People who took 500 milligrams (mg) of vitamin C daily burned 39% more fat while exercising than people who took less. Since it is difficult to get enough vitamin C just from fruits and vegetables, take a vitamin C supplement to be sure you get at least 500 mg per day.

Carol Johnston, PhD, professor and chair, department of nutrition, Arizona State University, Mesa, and leader of a study published in *Journal of the American College of Nutrition.*

■■■■

Yoga May Slow Midlife Weight Gain

People in their 50s who regularly practiced yoga lost about five pounds over 10 years, while those who did not practice yoga gained about 13 pounds. Most yoga exercises do not burn enough calories to account for the weight loss, but some practitioners believe that yoga keeps people aware of their bodies and eating habits.

Alan Kristal, DrPH, researcher, Fred Hutchinson Cancer Research Center, Seattle, and leader of a study of 15,550 people, published in *Alternative Therapies in Health and Medicine.*

■■■■

Smart Snacks

One hard-boiled egg with half a slice of toasted wheat bread—total 109 calories... one-half cup of ice milk or sherbet—100 calories...a large rectangular graham cracker with one-and-a-half teaspoons of peanut butter— 105 calories...one-ounce slice of angel-food cake with half a cup of fresh strawberries—95 calories...one cup of chicken noodle soup with two saltine crackers—100 calories...these are all healthier than 100-calorie packaged snacks.

Woman's Day, 1633 Broadway, New York City 10019.

■■■■

The Fresh Fruit Advantage

Canned and dried fruit have twice as many calories from sugar as their fresh counterparts.

Best: Eat fresh fruit or canned fruit that is packed in its own juice or extra-light syrup to limit added sugars. Eat at least one-and-a-half to two cups of fruit each day.

Environmental Nutrition, 52 Riverside Dr., New York City 10024.

The 5 Most Common Exercise Mistakes— How to Avoid Injury

Wayne Westcott, PhD, fitness research director at South Shore YMCA and adjunct instructor of exercise science at Quincy College, both in Quincy, Massachusetts. He is the author or coauthor of more than 20 books, including *No More Cellulite* (Perigee) and *Get Stronger, Feel Younger* (Rodale).

More people start an exercise program in January than at any other time of the year. Within weeks or months, most of them have called it quits—often because of injury. Unfortunately, many people exercise in such a way that almost guarantees injuries or even chronic pain. But this common problem can be avoided.

How much exercise do you need? Opinions differ, but the American College of Sports Medicine recommends 20 minutes of aerobic exercise three days a week…and two 20-minute weight-lifting sessions a week. This level of exercise—along with ordinary activities such as going for occasional walks and working in the yard—is sufficient for fitness as well as disease prevention.

Avoid these exercise mistakes…

Mistake 1: **Stretching before workouts.** At one time, trainers advised everyone to stretch before exercise. It doesn't help—and actually increases the risk for injury.

Tendons have a limited blood supply. It takes them longer to warm up than muscles. Performing stretches before a workout—when tendons are cold—increases the risk for microtears in the connective tissue in or around the tendon. These tears are painful and slow to heal.

Recommended: Stretch after—not before—vigorous activities. Warm up by performing the exercise at a slower pace and reduced resistance for three to six minutes. For example, if you plan to bike for 35 minutes, begin by riding at a slow, comfortable pace for three to six minutes.

Mistake 2: **Using a barbell** (a bar with an adjustable weighted disk attached to each end and held with two hands). Experienced weight lifters can safely use barbells, but a dumbbell (a short bar with weight at each end and held in each hand) is better for injury prevention. That's because the wrists are less likely to move into a fully supinated (palms facing up) or pronated (palms facing down) position, which may strain your elbows. Just about every exercise that you perform with a barbell can be done with dumbbells.

Recommended: If you're using a barbell, keep your hands in your peripheral vision. If they're so far apart that you can't see them, the wrist will be cocked at an angle and more vulnerable to strain.

Mistake 3: **Performing repetitions too quickly.** People who use weight machines or lift free weights tend to go too fast—either to minimize time spent in the gym, or because accelerating the pace generates momentum and makes it easier to lift heavy loads. Fast lifting greatly increases stress on the joints, especially when people neglect proper form.

Recommended: A six-second repetition speed. When lifting weights, take about two seconds to raise the weight, then lower it to a count of four. This pace is slow enough to maintain good form throughout the movement, and fast enough to complete about 10 repetitions in one minute—the recommended number of repetitions for most workouts.

Mistake 4: **Lifting too much weight.** This is among the most common causes of joint, muscle and tendon injuries.

Recommended: Warm up by lifting lighter-than-usual weights. For example, if you are going to do curls with 15-pound dumbbells, begin with eight to 12 repetitions with five-pound dumbbells. After warming up, lift no more than 70% to 80% of your *one-repetition maximum*. That's the heaviest weight you can lift one time.

Example: If the most you can lift one time with dumbbell bench presses is 20 pounds in each hand, use 75% of that—about 15-pound weights. You'll know you're in the right range if you can complete eight to 12 repetitions. If you can't complete eight repetitions, the weight is too heavy…if you can easily complete 12 or more, the weight is too light.

Mistake 5: **Neglecting to cool down.** The cool-down period is even more important than the warmup period—not just for injury prevention, but also to protect the heart.

The elevation in heart rate that occurs during exercise continues for several minutes after you stop.

A larger-than-usual volume of blood is being pumped from the heart throughout the body. Without continued muscle activity to help pump it back into circulation, the blood tends to pool in the legs and feet. The heart has to work harder to restore normal circulation, which can trigger high blood pressure.

Recommended: After finishing any exercise or vigorous activity, keep moving for a few minutes at a slower rate—by walking in place or biking at a reduced resistance or slower pace, for example.

Bonus: Activity during cool-down helps flush lactic acid from the muscles. This metabolic byproduct increases during exercise and can result in muscle discomfort.

Since muscles and tendons have the best blood flow and elasticity during cool-down, it is a good time to stretch. A basic gentle stretch that targets many of the body's muscles is the "Figure 4." It stretches the muscles of the calves, hamstrings, hips, lower back, upper back and shoulders.

What to do: Sit on the floor with your legs extended. Bend your right knee and place your right foot just below your left knee. Bending at the waist, reach forward with your arms as far as you comfortably can toward your left ankle or foot. Hold for 20 seconds. Repeat with the opposite leg. The full cool-down should last about four to eight minutes.

■ ■ ■ ■

More Reason to Exercise

Exercise controls triglyceride levels. Eating high-fat foods, such as whipped cream and chocolate, causes triglyceride levels to spike, increasing heart disease risk.

Recent study: Triglyceride levels of all participants who ate high-fat foods rose, but the levels of those who exercised for 90 minutes before eating were 25% lower than the levels of non-exercisers.

Jason M.R. Gill, PhD, researcher, department of vascular biochemistry, University of Glasgow, Glasgow Royal Infirmary, Scotland, and leader of a study of triglycerides, published in *Journal of the American College of Cardiology.*

Proven Depression Buster—Regular Exercise

Madhukar Trivedi, MD, director, UT Southwestern Medical Center mood disorders research program, professor of psychiatry, Dallas.

For many people, exercise is a surefire way to get energized and even beat vague feelings of depression. Given that fact, the question for some researchers has been, "How far can exercise go in improving symptoms of depression for those who have been diagnosed as clinically depressed and who are undergoing treatment with either a form of psychotherapy, medication or both?"

The answer: Quite far.

RECENT STUDY RESULTS

Psychiatrist Madhukar Trivedi, MD, director of UT Southwestern Medical Center's mood disorders research program, conducted the study with 80 people, all of whom had been diagnosed as clinically depressed with mild to moderate levels of the disorder and were not physically active. The researchers separated the participants into five groups: Two groups did moderately intense aerobics on the treadmill or stationary bicycle for either three or five days a week…two groups did lower-intensity aerobics, either three or five days a week…and the last group did 15 to 20 minutes of stretching and flexibility exercises three days per week.

After 12 weeks, the group doing the higher intensity level of aerobics, whether three or five days a week, had an average 47% decline in depressive symptoms. The low-intensity aerobics group had a 30% reduction in depressive symptoms…and the stretching/flexibility group had a 29% reduction.

INSIDE THE RESULTS

Dr. Trivedi explained that public health guidelines were used to determine the intensity for the higher level aerobics group. These guidelines recommend 30 minutes a day three times a week…but this is based on the amount of physical activity needed to burn an additional 1,200 calories a week if you weigh about 155 pounds. Because the formula is derived from a calorie-to-weight ratio, heavier people must burn more calories per week. Dr. Trivedi clarified that only members in the group who worked at this higher level experienced more meaningful relief of depression. Furthermore, whether they accomplished that in three days or five depended on how intensely they worked out at each session.

This is very encouraging news for those suffering from depression. However, Dr. Trivedi is emphatic about the need for depressed people to work with a health-care professional on building exercise into their treatment regimen. In particular, those taking prescription medications to assist their depression should have their medication and performance monitored closely when starting an exercise program. Exercise—yes. But do it with guidance.

Healthy-Back Exercise

Karl Knopf, PhD, executive director, Fitness Educators of Older Adults Association, and author of five books. His latest is *Weights for 50 Plus: Building Strength, Staying Healthy and Enjoying an Active Lifestyle.* Ulysses.

Eighty percent of Americans have some form of a back problem—leading to $24 billion spent in medical costs each year directly related to low-back pain. Karl Knopf, PhD, a leading authority on exercise for baby boomers and author of *Weights for 50 Plus: Building Strength, Staying Healthy and Enjoying an Active Lifestyle* (Ulysses), explains exercises that are easy on the back.

POSTURE FIRST

Poor posture is a major contributor to back pain. Dr. Knopf believes that the first order of business for strengthening and rehabilitating the back are posture exercises, which can be practiced absolutely anywhere. "Stand upright with your weight evenly distributed over the balls of your feet and heels, with legs slightly bent. Then tilt your pelvis slightly forward so your tailbone is slightly tucked under your hips. Make the distance from your belly button to your sternum as far as possible by letting the chest rise and open, countering the "hunched over" effect. Your chin, sternum and belly button should be lined up from the front. From the side it should look like your earlobes are over your shoulders, which are over your hips." Practice that alignment whenever you are standing. When you sit, the alignment should be the same. Make sure you sit on the "sit bones" of the buttocks, not on the tailbone.

GUIDE WIRES FOR YOUR BACK

The back alone can't hold your body upright. "Think of standing a pencil upright on your desk balanced on the eraser," Dr. Knopf instructs. "You could make it stand—but it would take a lot of work and balance. How much more efficient to have guide wires? Well, the guide wires are the muscles that help keep the back aligned. These need strengthening to build a strong support system for the back."

The three basic "guide wire" muscle groups for the back are the abdominals, the gluteals (buttocks) and the perispinals (the muscles that run up and down the spine). "While many baby boomers are aware of the importance of training their abs, they often neglect the buttocks muscles, which are the other side of the guide wires." *To strengthen the abs, back and glutes, Dr. Knopf recommends the following exercises…*

Buttocks strengthener: Lie on your back with knees bent and feet flat on the floor. Tighten butt muscles and lift the butt off the floor slowly. Hold for a few seconds, return. Do 10 repetitions.

Hamstring stretch: Lie on your back, feet straight out. Pull your right knee into the chest and hold it there for a few seconds. Then gently extend the leg toward the ceiling until you feel a stretch in the hamstrings. Hold, return to start and repeat with the other leg.

This stretches the hamstrings.

Mad cat: Get on your hands and knees. Arch your back like a cat. Keep your neck in a relaxed neutral position. Hold for 10 seconds, then release.

Note: Don't do this if you have a ruptured disc.

OTHER GENTLE EXERCISES

When choosing other exercises that are gentle on the back, Dr. Knopf recommends exercises that are done with the back supported and no "load" (or weight) on the spine.

Dr. Knopf has high praise for two specific forms of exercise. "The recumbent bike is my all-time favorite," he maintains. The recumbent bike, found in almost all gyms, is a bicycle (in either stationary or outdoor road versions) that allows you to sit on the bicycle as you would in a chair with your back supported, instead of upright or hunched over the way traditional bicycles do. Dr. Knopf also loves water exercise. "Vertical water exercise allows you to work all muscle groups without putting any stress or strain on the back whatsoever," he stresses.

As for strength-training exercises, again, Dr. Knopf recommends those in which the back is supported and that avoid putting any "load" on it. *His favorites...*

1. Seated chest press.

2. Lat pulldowns to the front.

3. Sit-to-stands.

Avoid: Military or shoulder press...squats.

CAUTIONS

"You have to be careful with leg exercises," Dr. Knopf insists. "If there's injury or pain, I'd prefer you do *sit-to-stands.*" In this exercise, you sit on the edge of a chair, then stand up and sit down again. It's a "no load" version of the squat that works the front of the legs without putting any strain on the spine. You could work up to holding dumbbells in your hands to increase the resistance and build more strength.

For anyone with chronic back pain who wants to exercise and eliminate pain, Dr. Knopf strongly suggests finding a physiatrist. "They are the most underused medical specialty I know of," he says. A physiatrist is a medical doctor who treats chronic pain and chronic conditions using a nonsurgical approach that often includes exercise. "They have no vested interest in doing surgery, and are usually very open minded to medical interventions such as chiropractic and acupuncture," says Dr. Knopf. "I've had back pain for years, and I always make the physiatrist the captain of my ship when it comes to back-pain treatment."

Exercise Secrets from Jack LaLanne

Jack LaLanne, author of *Revitalize Your Life: Improve Your Health, Your Sex Life & Your Looks After Fifty* (Hastings House) and creator of exercise videos and DVDs. His recent book of healthy recipes is *Cooking with Jack—Eat Right and You Can't Go Wrong.* His Web site is *www.jacklalanne.com.*

When Jack LaLanne began his fitness career more than 70 years ago, most Americans were not even aware of the health benefits of exercise. LaLanne, now a legend in the fitness world, opened the first modern health club in 1936, invented many of the kinds of equipment used in gyms today, such as the first leg extension machine and pulley machine using cables, starred in his own fitness show on television for 34 years and became known as the "Godfather of Fitness." Today, his goal remains the same as it always was—to help people stay fit and healthy.

Jack LaLanne's latest secrets to staying fit...

YOU DON'T HAVE TO GO TO THE GYM

It's great to belong to a gym and have a personal trainer, but many people don't have the time or money for this. Fortunately, there are many activities you can do at home that take only minutes to complete.*

What you can do: Walk up and down the stairs until your muscles tire. This is one of my favorite exercises. It works your leg muscles and

*Check with your doctor before starting this—or any—exercise program.

your heart and lungs. If you feel unsteady, use a handrail.

•**Standing around?** Run or walk in place by bringing your knees as high as you can toward your chest. This gets your heart beating and targets your abdominal muscles.

•**Do you sit in a chair behind a desk?** Stand up and sit back down 10 times quickly. Now, slow it down and do it five more times.

Also: Stand up with your feet shoulder-width apart. Make a fist with your fingers and raise your fists to shoulder height. Punch your arms toward the ceiling, bring your fists back to your shoulders and repeat. Start with 10 repetitions and work up gradually until you can do three sets of 10.

•**Watching television?** Scoot down in your chair and hold on to the sides. Bring one knee to your chest, then the other, alternating and pumping like you're riding a bicycle. This works your abs, back, thighs, heart and lungs. Remember to start slowly and rest when your muscles tire.

Also: Do sit-ups. Lie on the floor or your bed so that your back is flat. Bend your knees, keeping your heels as close to your buttocks as possible. With your hands either behind your head or across your chest, try to sit up. Exhale as you raise up. Inhale as you lie down. Start slowly with five repetitions and work up to 10.

Important: Increase your workout intensity gradually.

MIX UP YOUR WORKOUTS

Sticking to the same old routine can become boring, making it harder to stick to regular exercise. Also, by doing the same routine your muscles eventually stop getting stronger.

What you can do: Change your workouts every three to four weeks, so that you are challenging your muscles to work harder. Without resistance, your muscles become complacent.

Example: If you walk regularly, walk up hills after you become used to walking on a level surface.

Also helpful: Try walking a short distance with your feet turned inward. Then repeat with your feet turned outward. All of these strategies provide resistance, which strengthens your muscles.

ADOPT HEALTHFUL EATING HABITS

You are never too old to learn to eat more nutritiously. You must replace bad habits with good ones.

What you can do: Avoid foods with added sugar and salt.

Also: Instead of cooking with oil, sauté in chicken or vegetable broth to cut calories. If you use oils, canola, olive and peanut oils are the best—they have low cholesterol. Eat plenty of whole grains, fresh fruits and raw vegetables. If raw vegetables are difficult for you to digest, lightly steam them.

How I do it: My wife, Lala, and I eat out regularly. For lunch, I usually have four hard-boiled eggs and eat only the egg whites. I also have soup with no cream and four pieces of fresh fruit. For dinner, a usual meal consists of a salad with eight to 10 raw vegetables, fresh fish and brown rice. Whenever I can, I bring my own salad dressing—a mixture of vinegar, canola oil, honey, soy sauce and a little sesame oil. On the road, we stick to oil and vinegar.

SET NEW GOALS

Keep challenging yourself by making gradual increases in your fitness routine. For example, if you don't get much exercise, aim to walk a block the first day, a block and a half or two the second day, etc. Each day, walk a little farther, and before you know it, you'll be walking a mile. If you miss a day, reset your goals.

Exercising for 20 to 30 minutes three to four days a week is adequate to keep most people healthy and fit. Remember, our body is the only machine where the more you work it, the stronger it gets.

How I do it: My personal workout consists of one hour of weight lifting in my gym and one-half hour of exercises and/or lap swimming in the pool each day. I do not expect everyone to follow my regimen—but I have been doing this for more than 70 years, so I want to see how long I can continue.

JACK'S CARROT AND GINGER SOUP

I love soup and have it at least once a day, sometimes twice. My mother made delicious soup, and her specialty was carrot soup. *Her recipe, which follows, is my favorite...*

1 medium onion, diced

4 garlic cloves, minced

2 Tbsp. olive oil

2 lbs. carrots, cut into 1-inch chunks

2 Tbsp. gingerroot, peeled and chopped

1 quart chicken stock, defatted

Plain yogurt and sesame seeds for garnish

Sauté the onion and garlic in oil for five minutes. Add carrots, cover and cook for 15 minutes. Add half of the ginger and all of the stock. Simmer 15 minutes. Add the rest of the ginger. Purée soup in a food processor or blender. Pour into bowls and garnish with yogurt and sesame seeds. Serves six.

■ ■ ■ ■

Coffee and Your Workout

Drinking coffee before exercise may be dangerous, finds Philipp Kaufmann, MD.

New finding: The equivalent of two cups of coffee 50 minutes before exercise reduces by 22% the body's ability to boost blood flow to heart muscles.

Theory: Caffeine blocks the release of adenosine, a compound produced during exercise that opens the arteries. This finding is especially important if you have coronary artery disease or other conditions that reduce blood flow to the heart.

Philipp Kaufmann, MD, professor of nuclear medicine and cardiology, University Hospital, Zurich, Switzerland.

■ ■ ■ ■

10,000 Steps the Easy Way

By walking 10,000 steps or more each day, you'll be able to build and maintain fitness. *Here's how...*

•**Measure** how much you walk everywhere with a pedometer.

Cost: $15 to $30. Less expensive ones are often not accurate, and more costly ones are unnecessary.

•**Take a walk** at lunchtime every day.

•**Park** in an inconvenient spot.

•**Get together** with friends to walk, not to drink coffee.

•**Use stairs** instead of an escalator or elevator.

•**If you bike, row or swim,** count every 10 minutes of exercise as 1,000 steps.

Katrien De Cocker, staff academic assistant, department of movement and sports sciences, Ghent University, Belgium.

Home Exercise Equipment Basics

Colin Milner, health and fitness expert for more than 23 years, and chief executive officer of the International Council on Active Aging, in Vancouver, British Columbia, which promotes healthier lifestyles for adults. www.icaa.cc.

Not long ago, home-exercise equipment was for young guys preparing for a summer at the beach. Today, men and women of every age are benefiting from treadmills, dumbbells and other home-exercise equipment.

Bulging biceps are no longer the main objective, though building up arm strength can indeed be helpful to people over age 50. Exercise equipment can also help improve your cardiovascular system, strengthen respiratory functions and help you lose weight.

Exercising on home equipment can have big advantages for people who don't enjoy the atmosphere of health clubs or for those without a club nearby. It's also a plus for people who live in areas with cold winters, where outdoor sports—or even walking—are difficult.

Even if you're a member of a health club and live in a warm climate, home equipment has the benefit of convenience. It allows you to exercise in the middle of the night, before breakfast or any other time you want.

Important: Be sure to consult your physician before you start an exercise program.

BUILDING A HOME GYM

Don't make the mistake of buying lots of equipment right away. Start with basic devices to gain strength, and then—if you still enjoy exercising at home—work up to more demanding and sophisticated equipment. *Road map...*

•**Step 1.** If you haven't exercised regularly in a few years, start again by increasing your strength. That type of exercise is relatively easy, the equipment is inexpensive and building strength will give you the ability to go to the next step—cardiovascular exercise.

•Resistance bands are the simplest type of upper-body equipment. These are bands of expandable materials with hand clasps at both ends. Stretching the band builds up strength in your arms and upper body.

•Dumbbells are also effective in building up muscles in this area, and they're usually preferable to barbells.

Reason: Dumbbells are weights lifted individually by each arm. Since you're probably stronger in one arm than the other, a dumbbell lets you concentrate on the weaker arm.

That's nearly impossible with a barbell, which is one long bar with weights at each end. Moreover, if you lose control of a barbell, it could fall on your chest and even roll back on your throat. If you have problems lifting a dumbbell, you can simply drop it on the floor.

Weight-lifting guideline: Start with about 70% of the greatest amount of weight you can lift. Then increase the amount slowly—one pound a week, for example.

As you improve your fitness, also consider a "multigym," a device with one or two weight stacks, plus attachments that let you exercise arms as well as legs in many different ways.

•**Step 2.** Once you've increased your upper-body strength, work also on improving your cardiovascular system.

•Pedometers aren't usually thought of as a piece of gym equipment, but they can serve in that role by encouraging you to take more steps, even around the house.

Some pedometers, including Digi-Walker, record the number of steps you take and estimate how many calories you burn. Most people over 50 take about 2,000 to 4,000 steps a day, and only 1,000 steps more are known to improve heart and lung functions.

•Treadmills can be an even better way to burn calories and improve the cardiovascular system. You can adjust a treadmill to move at varying speeds, so you can start at, say, one mile per hour (mph) and slowly increase the pace and/or the length of your exercise.

•Stationary bicycles and recumbent steppers (which exercise your muscular and cardiovascular systems from a sitting position) also help improve the cardiovascular system. They are safer than treadmills, which entail the risk—however slight—of falling.

General rule: If you have a problem with balance or if you haven't exercised in several years, opt for a stationary bike or recumbent stepper.

•Elliptical machines (motion is similar to a bike but you pedal while in a standing position) are a good addition to your home gym once you've worked out for several months—or if you're already physically fit. By requiring you to move in elliptical patterns, this relatively new device gives you the opportunity to improve your cardiovascular system while also getting a particularly safe workout as you stand.

If you doubt that you're exercising at the right level, use the "talk test." If you can't talk comfortably while exercising, you're probably pushing yourself too hard.

TEST, THEN BUY

With so many different types of exercise equipment on the market, it's easy to spend big bucks for a device that winds up as a coatrack. The solution is to visit retailers that sell exercise apparatus, and try out different types of equipment.

Major retailers are usually listed in the Yellow Pages under "Exercise Equipment" and include Gym Source and OMNI Fitness Equipment, Inc. Exercise devices are also sold by Sports Authority and other large sporting-goods outlets, as well as by Sears and Walmart.

Most stores have several types of exercise equipment set up on the floor and allow customers to try them out there.

Look for equipment that challenges you but doesn't cause pain or require exertion that you can't perform. Be cautious of machines with expensive gadgets that you're unlikely to use, such as a treadmill device that tells you "how far you've gone," just as though you were on a track. All you really need is a timer and speed indicator so that you can pace yourself at, say, four mph for 20 minutes.

But, if you enjoy using gadgets, they could be valuable motivators that inspire you to work out.

Don't fall into the trap of buying equipment that's difficult to use on the theory that you won't benefit much without a major challenge.

In fact, equipment that's overly demanding often falls into disuse.

Instead, consider devices that let you start with easy exercises and then work up incrementally to more demanding ones.

Example: A weight-training machine that starts at 10 or 15 pounds and allows you to work up in five-pound increments.

What about exercise equipment advertised on TV? The problem is that you can't test it like you can at a store where you can compare three or four types of equipment.

My advice: Never buy anything advertised on TV unless you have the right to return it and get a complete refund, including shipping charges.

Regardless of where you shop, the cheapest equipment will rarely be as long-lasting as more expensive models, but the most costly devices will probably have unneeded bells and whistles. Even though you don't need to buy the most expensive equipment you can find, it's still worth investing in good quality. So expect to pay up to $2,000 or $3,000 to get something durable that has what you need.

Be sure that you have room for the equipment in your home. It's easy to underestimate the space you'll need, especially when you try out equipment on a large showroom floor. For a treadmill, make sure that you have at least five feet between the device and the wall behind it. That will prevent the treadmill from pinning you against the wall in case you should fall down on it.

Tai Chi—In a Chair!

Cynthia Quarta is a tai chi instructor based in Montana, and the author of *Tai Chi in a Chair*. Fair Winds Press.

Western doctors have long dismissed the ancient Chinese concept of chi (life energy) as mere superstition.

But a growing body of scientific evidence supports the salutary effects of Eastern healing techniques—especially the traditional exercise known as tai chi. By stimulating the body's nervous system, tai chi triggers a biochemical cascade of beneficial endorphins.

Tai chi combines slow, rhythmic movements with deep breathing and visualization techniques to enhance the flow of chi. Disruption of chi flow is thought to be the source of illness and pain.

People often think of tai chi as a group activity that is best performed in a park. In reality, you can practice it anywhere, anytime. Here is a 15-minute tai chi program that can be performed while seated.

The exercises can be done on their own or as a warm-up or cool-down to your normal exercise routine.

Tai chi in a chair will tone and stretch your muscles without putting stress on your knees, feet, hips or back. The movements are less complex and easier to maintain than traditional tai chi postures. That's why it's a good form of exercise for everyone, regardless of age or fitness level.

Like traditional tai chi, the chair exercises often produce surprising gains in muscular tone, endurance and coordination.

In fact, a recent University of Connecticut study showed that older adults who practiced tai chi had greater balance and strength gains than a similar group who performed strength training.

Begin each movement sitting in a chair. Press your back against the back of the chair and place your feet flat on the floor, shoulder-width apart. Perform each movement slowly and smoothly while breathing in through your nose and out through your mouth.

You can do the exercises in the morning while you wait for coffee to brew, at your desk during the day or while watching TV at night.

BALLOON BREATHING

This exercise strengthens the diaphragm.

Close your eyes, and place both palms on your lower abdomen. Feel your diaphragm expand and contract as you breathe.

As you inhale deeply, visualize a disk in your lower abdomen (just below your belly button) spinning faster and faster as it releases energy into your body. Mentally guide these sparks of energy up into your chest. Picture them circling around your lungs. While exhaling, envision the toxins that have collected in your lungs exiting through your mouth. Repeat nine times.

BRUSHING TREE TRUNK

This pose stretches your neck muscles.

Extend your arms and reach for the ceiling as you breathe in deeply. Swing your right arm down and across your chest to your left side while turning your head in the opposite direction, looking as far toward the ceiling as you can.

As you twist, visualize your internal organs being squeezed and massaged. Exhale as you bend forward and tighten your abdomen. Return to the starting position. Repeat nine times on each side.

CENTERING CHI

This movement focuses energy.

As you do this exercise, imagine that you're collecting bits of energy from all over your body and returning them to your lower abdomen.

Hold your hands above your lap, palms upward. Breathe in deeply as you pull your abdomen inward, contracting your diaphragm. (This is the only exercise in which your diaphragm is not expanding as you inhale.) As you tighten your abdomen, raise your arms out to the side, and then extend them up over the center of your head so that your palms are facing the ceiling.

Allow your arms to drop gently to the side in an arc. As they drop downward, exhale until there is no breath left in your lungs and relax your abdomen.

Return to the starting position. Repeat three times.

FLOWER BUD OPENS

This is a great way to achieve deeper inhalation.

Hold your hands in front of your chest with palms facing each other. Raise your arms upward, inhaling deeply and visualizing energy circulating through your shoulders, arms, neck and head. As you lift your arms above your head, arch your back away from the chair and extend your arms outward. Then press your arms down to the side, palms facing the floor. Finish the inhalation by relaxing your arms and pulling them behind you.

Exhale and return to the starting position. Repeat nine times.

GREEN DRAGON

This exercise strengthens the shoulders and arms. It is especially good for firming up the backs of your upper arms.

Bring both arms over your left shoulder so that your right palm is almost touching your left shoulder, and your left hand is next to your left ear.

Move your right hand across your chest and down, until it rests just outside your right thigh, palm facing down. At the same time, move your left hand in front of your upper chest so that it is perpendicular to the floor, with the palm facing to the right. By the time your left hand reaches this position, the muscles in your left arm should be taut.

Repeat on the opposite side. Move your arms so that your left palm almost touches your right shoulder and your right hand is next to your right ear. Sweep your left arm downward so that it is alongside your left thigh, and position your right hand in front of your chest.

Repeat nine times on each side.

NEEDLE AT THE BOTTOM OF THE SEA

This movement stretches back muscles and helps tone your legs. During this exercise, visualize energy circulating from the top of your head to the bottoms of your feet.

Inhale deeply while extending your left leg so that your knee is straight. Keeping your leg straight, relax and exhale, bending forward from your hips while extending your right hand between your legs and reaching for the floor. Allow your left arm to hang totally relaxed. Repeat nine times on each side.

■ ■ ■ ■

Muscle Up

Muscles don't turn to fat when you stop working out. When people stop exercising, their muscles begin to shrink. This makes some people believe that muscle turns to fat. In reality, the ratio of fat to muscle simply changes.

Gerard P. Varlotta, DO, clinical associate professor, department of rehabilitation medicine, New York University Medical Center, New York City.

Oprah's Trainer Tells How Very Busy People Can Find Time to Exercise

Bob Greene is an exercise physiologist and personal trainer. He is the author of *Bob Greene's Total Body Makeover*. Simon & Schuster.

Over the past two decades, I have worked with many incredibly busy people to help them lose weight and get in shape.

All of them have overcome their weight and fitness "demons." They became aware of what they truly wanted—and what they were willing to do to achieve it.

No single fitness plan works for everybody, but there are steps all busy people can take to begin an exercise program and stick with it.

DESIGNING YOUR FITNESS PLAN

If your goal is to lose weight and keep it off, you don't have to give up everything else in your life to reach your fitness goals. The key to getting into better shape is to regularly challenge the body to improve strength.

You simply need to engage in a physical activity that exercises the heart muscles for 15 to 20 minutes, five times a week. In fact, many of my clients get in better shape when they cut their workout time in half because they exercise at a much higher intensity.

Any time you start or modify an exercise program, consult your doctor to be sure that program is safe for you.

Next, select a "primary" aerobic exercise that is relatively convenient and enjoyable to perform. The most effective ones are those in which you support most of your own weight.

Best: Power walking, jogging, aerobic dance and stair-stepping.

Also choose one or two alternative exercises that can help tone different muscles and prevent boredom on intermittent days. If power walking is your primary exercise on three days, do stair-stepping on the other two.

Good alternatives: Outdoor or stationary cycling, rowing, cross-country skiing or swimming—although they are a bit less intensive aerobically.

To lower risk of injury, warm up for three to five minutes…followed by about five minutes of stretching. Do each stretch twice, and hold it for four seconds. Have a two-second interval in between. After your workout, it is important to stretch for another five to 10 minutes.

Hamstrings: Lie on your back with one leg bent and the corresponding foot on the floor. Raise the other leg until you feel a gentle tension. Repeat with the other side.

Buttocks and lower back: While on your back, grab the backs of both legs just above the knee and pull them toward your chest. Hold and repeat.

Shoulders and chest: Stand with your head, shoulders and hips aligned, hands clasped behind you and knees slightly bent. Bring your hands up toward the ceiling until you feel a gentle tension.

OTHER CONSIDERATIONS

•**Exercise in the morning.** Your place of exercise should be within a few minutes of your home or work. This eliminates excuses not to exercise that inevitably arise during a busy schedule.

•**Do some physical activity on your days off.** Consistency is an important key to maintaining interest in exercise. Although the body needs a rest from vigorous training, I ask my clients to add an enjoyable activity, such as a stroll or bike ride, on their days off.

•**Work toward your results zone.** To lose weight and strengthen your body, perform aerobic exercise at a level of intensity that pushes your physical limits without causing injury. This level is what I call the results zone.

Strategy: Picture a scale from 0 to 10, with 0 equal to the feeling you have at rest and 10 equal to the feeling of all-out exercise—fatigue, labored breathing, etc.

Aim for a 7—a feeling of fatigue, deep breathing with the ability to carry on a conversation, although you don't necessarily want to. If you are physically able, you can shoot for an 8—exercising very vigorously with very deep breathing.

•**Weight training can be added in two or three months.** The greatest benefit of resistance training is to combat the effects of aging. It prevents muscle and bone loss, strengthens the body and helps control excess weight.

Surprisingly, lifting weights can significantly increase your appetite, while aerobic exercise suppresses appetite. Add weights only after your eating is under control and aerobic exercise is fully incorporated into your schedule.

STICKING WITH IT

Busy people often find it difficult to stick with an exercise program. The secret to maintaining a high motivational level is to become more self-aware.

•**Take responsibility.** All my busy clients who have changed their lives have stopped blaming external causes, such as demanding careers, their kids, etc. Instead, they have taken responsibility for their actions and made time for exercise. Positive change is possible only through conscious decisions.

To change your mind-set: Think about the three best decisions you've ever made. For each decision, write down if it was difficult, if you considered other options and why you valued your decision.

Think about how the decision affected your life and how your life would be different if you hadn't made it. Do the same for the three worst decisions you've made.

•**Anticipate setbacks.** As you embark on a new fitness program, expect the following to occur...

•Aches and pains are part of training and demonstrate that you are working hard. If they are extreme, back off a bit and do a similar activity at a lighter level.

Example: Walking can help alleviate sore muscles that come from stair-stepping.

•Physical fatigue can occur from time to time and usually indicates your body needs rest. After a rest day, you can come back stronger and resume your training.

•Mental fatigue is often a sign of stress or boredom. Varying your fitness routine, refocusing your goals or taking a day off can help eliminate it.

•**Remember why exercise is important.** This will help you define your level of commitment and keep you motivated to strive continuously for positive change.

To prioritize your life, draw a large circle and divide it into eight equal sections.

Within each section, write the eight most important areas of your life. These will likely include family, health, fitness, community, etc.

Next to each section, write down three things you can do daily to improve that area. Even if you are able to do only one of these daily steps, you will significantly improve your life.

Gentle Exercises That Ease Arthritis

Ian Fraser is a Victoria, Australia–based writer and coauthor of *Exercise Beats Arthritis.* Bell Publishing Company.

If you have arthritis—discomfort and stiffness may make you want to sit down and stop moving. But that only leads to disability.

Better idea: Do gentle exercises designed specifically for people with arthritis.

When I developed osteoarthritis years ago, one of the most helpful things I did was to follow a program of simple exercises done at home or in a pool. They worked so well that I wanted to spread the word.

My coauthor—skilled physical therapist Valerie Sayce—and I wrote a book describing and depicting exercises that have helped many people with arthritis.

These exercises are also useful as light exercise for anyone who wants to remain supple, active and mobile in later years.

The exercises shown here were developed for long-term mild-to-moderate arthritic problems. They may not be suitable for people with severe joint deformities or for those whose arthritis greatly hinders normal daily activities. To adapt these exercises for more severe arthritis, consult your doctor or a physical therapist.

GROUND RULES

•**Exercise for an uninterrupted 15 to 30 minutes a day.**

•**Choose a time when you're feeling near your best,** not tired or in pain.

•**Wear comfortable clothes that allow full movement.**

•**Don't exercise right after you have eaten.**

•**If you take pain medication,** exercise half an hour after a regular dose, when the medication is working best.

•**If you feel pain, stop.** Consult your doctor or a physical therapist. Don't take extra medication to mask pain during exercise. If your exercise-induced pain lasts for more than two hours, do fewer repetitions next time.

•**Clear a wide space.**

•**Begin with two to four repetitions of each exercise,** gradually adding one repetition a week until you reach five or six—as long as your joint doesn't become too tender.

•**For floor exercises, use a mat.** For exercise involving a chair or stool, use one whose seat is at the right height to support your thighs with your feet flat on the floor.

LEAP OVER THESE ROADBLOCKS

Occasional discouragement is normal, but don't stop just because you…

•**Lose enthusiasm.** Progress may be slow, but it will be sure. Keep plugging away.

•**Fear physical effort.** Deep down, you may believe that exertion is harmful. If you feel pain when exercising, stop. See your health professional or call the local chapter of the Arthritis Foundation.

•**Get bored.** Try exercising to medium-speed music that you like. Tired of exercising by yourself? Join a water exercise class or similar group.

MOVE IT OR LOSE IT

Once you start to exercise, keep going. You are making a lifestyle commitment—and a commitment to improving your own life. What better incentive could you have?

HANDS

1. Tuck in your elbows. Place your palms facing each other. *Then…*

•Bend your wrists forward, bringing the fingers of one hand toward the matching fingers of the other hand.

•Bend your wrists back so that your palms face front.

2. Place your hands in front of you. Look at your palms. *Then, one hand at a time…*

•Stretch your thumb across your palm. Gently close your fingers over it.

•Stretch open your fingers and thumb.

•Gently fold your fingers into your palm and close your thumb over them. Do not make a tight fist.

•Stretch open your fingers and thumb again.

3. Do each hand individually.

Touch the tip of your thumb to the tip of each other finger in turn. Make the circle as round as you can. Straighten your fingers after touching each finger.

HIPS

1. Stand, holding onto the back of a chair with both hands. Keep your body upright as you lift one leg out to the side, with your foot flexed and toes pointing out. Lower slowly and repeat with the other leg.

2. Stand, holding onto the back of a chair with one hand.

Caution: If you have had a hip replacement, do not lift your leg above hip level.

Keep your back straight and lift your outside knee.

Straighten your knee as you stretch your leg behind you, with your toes just off the floor. Turn around to work the other leg.

3. Lie on your back with your knees bent and your feet and knees comfortably apart. Push through your feet and slowly lift your buttocks off the floor. Lower slowly, rolling your spine onto the floor from the top down.

KNEES

1. Sit up straight on a chair with your thighs fully supported.

Flex your foot back and straighten your knee. Keep your back straight and your thigh on the chair. Hold for three to five seconds, then lower slowly.

2. Lie on your back with one leg bent. Flex back the other foot and tighten your knee. Lift your straight leg about two feet off the floor. Lower it slowly, touching the floor with your calf first.

Contact the Arthritis Foundation, 1330 W. Peachtree St., Atlanta 30309, 800-283-7800. To find an Arthritis Foundation chapter by zip code, visit *www.arthritis.org.* Click on "Questions & Answers" for additional information and materials.

■ ■ ■ ■

Eggs for Weight Loss

In a recent study, overweight women ages 24 to 60 ate either eggs or a bagel-based breakfast of equal calories followed by a lunch of pasta with marinara sauce and sliced apples.

Result: The women who ate eggs at breakfast reported feeling more satisfied and consumed an average of 420 fewer calories than the bagel group over the next 28 hours.

Theory: High-protein foods, such as eggs, tend to induce feelings of fullness better than foods rich in simple sugars, carbohydrates and fats.

Caution: Eggs should be thoroughly cooked.

Jillon S. Vander Wal, PhD, assistant professor, department of psychology, St. Louis University, St. Louis, Missouri.

Low-Calorie Ways To Satisfy a Sweet Tooth...Naturally

Mark A. Stengler, ND, naturopathic physician in private practice, La Jolla, California...adjunct associate clinical professor at the National College of Natural Medicine, Portland, Oregon...author of many books, including *The Natural Physician's Healing Therapies* and coauthor of *Prescription for Natural Cures* (both from Bottom Line Books)...and author of the *Bottom Line/Natural Healing* newsletter.

Consumers have deluded themselves by pretending there's no risk in using artificial sweeteners to cut calories without sacrificing sweetness. From soft drinks to salad dressings, cakes to cough drops—all manner of foods contain artificial sweeteners these days. But it's time to stop believing the fairy tale.

The facts: In some people, artificial sweeteners may be associated with a variety of health problems, from headaches to mood changes to cancer. Why take risks? All-natural alternatives can satisfy the sweetest tooth, without adding unwanted calories.

FAKE SWEETS, REAL CONCERNS

Three artificial sweeteners dominate the market today.

•**Sucralose (Splenda)** is currently the top-selling artificial sweetener in the US. In addition to its little yellow packets, it is found in more than 4,500 products, including fruit juices, protein bars, baked goods and even some so-called "natural" foods and supplements. It is 600 times sweeter than sugar (as rated by taste-testers) but has no calories. Because the body doesn't recognize sucralose as a carbohydrate, very little is absorbed during digestion. Marketers trumpet Splenda as "the only sugar substitute made from real sugar." This is done by substituting three chlorine atoms for three hydrogen-oxygen groups in sugar molecules.

Given its ubiquity, you would expect many studies to support Splenda's safety—but no long-term human studies have been done. Studies on animals show effects that include reduced growth rate...liver and brain enlargement...decreased red blood cell count...and increased risk of cataracts. (Admittedly, the quantities of sucralose fed to the study animals were very high.)

Responding to public complaints of side effects—including headaches, skin rashes, bloating, diarrhea, wheezing, cough, heart palpitations, dizziness and mood swings—some retailers have banned sucralose products. (For more information, see the Whole Foods Market Web site at *www.wholefoods.com/wholebody/ingredients/sucralose.html.)*

•**Aspartame (Equal, NutraSweet)** is sold worldwide. It comes in blue packets and is used in diet soda, instant tea, sugarless candy and gum, as well as over-the-counter cough syrups and liquid pain relievers. It loses its sweetness when heated, so it isn't used in baked goods.

Aspartame is made of the amino acids *aspartic acid* and *phenylalanine,* combined in a chemical sequence not found in natural foods. Critics say it acts as an *excitotoxin*—a substance that damages nerve cells by stimulating excess activity.

During digestion, aspartame breaks down into *methanol* (an alcohol) and then into the chemical compound *formaldehyde.* Unlike other foods that contain methanol, such as natural fruit juices—in which the methanol is bound to *pectin* (a fiber) and excreted out of the body—the methanol from aspartame is not bound, so it does not get excreted before it breaks down into formaldehyde. As reported in the journal *Toxicology* in 2005, formaldehyde can be toxic to the nervous system…can cause cell death…and is potentially carcinogenic. By 1995, the Food and Drug Administration (FDA) had received more than 10,000 complaints about adverse effects from aspartame—including headaches, concentration problems and seizures. (That year, the agency stopped tallying such reports.)

•**Saccharin (Sweet'N Low, Necta Sweet)** was banned in the US in 1912 due to safety concerns, then reinstated during World War I, when demand for sugar substitutes increased. Some users report itching, hives, headaches, nausea and diarrhea. After studies in the late 1970s showed that high doses could cause bladder cancer in rats, saccharin was banned in Canada—but it is still sold in the US (in pink packets and in tablets). It is also used to sweeten oral medications. The amount of saccharin in a child's dose of chewable aspirin or *acetaminophen* (Tylenol) equals that in a can of diet soda—though the American Medical Association recommends that children avoid saccharin.

Many people ignore the health concerns about artificial sweeteners, convinced that these products help to prevent weight gain—but in fact, they may *promote* weight gain. Researchers at the University of Texas Health Science Center followed 622 adults of normal weight for more than eight years. Participants who drank one to two cans of regular soda daily had a 33% chance of becoming overweight—but 55% of those who drank an equal amount of diet soda became overweight.

NATURE'S LOW-CALORIE OPTIONS

Natural products provide low-cal sweetness.

•**Stevia rebaudiana (stevia)** has gained popularity recently in the US. This plant grows in South America and Asia. Paraguayans have used stevia for centuries to sweeten teas and medicinal potions. In the 1970s, stevia became popular in Japan. I find it strange that, while no side effects have ever been reported, the FDA banned the use of stevia as a food additive in 1987, claiming insufficient evidence of its safety. It wasn't until December 2008 that the FDA approved its use as a general sweetener and food additive. Stevia has been available as a dietary supplement in natural food stores.

Stevia may reduce blood sugar levels in people with type-2 diabetes…lower blood pressure in people with hypertension…and prevent cavities by reducing plaque on teeth. Although stevia has almost no calories, it is 300 times sweeter than sugar—so a little goes a long way. Some people detect a licorice-type of aftertaste. A brand I enjoy is from NOW Foods (888-669-3663, *www.nowfoods com*), available at health-food stores.

•**Xylitol** is a white crystalline substance that looks and tastes like sugar. It is found naturally in fruits, vegetables and some tree bark. Birch trees and corncobs are commercial sources. The human body also produces xylitol naturally. Used in foods since the 1960s, it is approved as a food additive by the World Health Organization and the FDA. Xylitol has half the calories of sugar and is safe for people with diabetes. It works well in beverages and for baking (but not for yeast breads). Xylitol comes in powder form. One manufacturer is Xlear, which makes the Xylosweet brand (877-599-5327, *www.xlear.com*). In some people, xylitol can trigger diarrhea. To avoid this, start with a small amount and let your digestive tract adjust gradually.

Important: Unlike sugar, which is bad for teeth, xylitol reduces cavity-causing plaque…prevents bacteria buildup in the mouth…and strengthens tooth enamel. Because Xylitol reduces tooth decay by up to 80%, it has the support of six national dental associations. Xylitol is used in sugar-free chewing gums, mouthwashes and toothpastes. I like Spry Dental products (877-599-5327, *www.sprydental.com*), available at health-food stores.

•**Lo han kuo** (or luo han guo) is the fruit of the *Momordica grosvenori* plant, a member of the cucumber family. It has been used for centuries in Chinese medicine to treat coughs, sore throats, skin conditions, digestive problems and anxiety. From the dried fruits, the Chinese make juice, soup, candy and cake.

Lo han kuo is 300 times sweeter than sugar. It contains no calories and is safe for people with diabetes or low blood sugar. There is no known toxicity with this fruit extract. The lo han kuo products I have used taste like maple syrup. A liquid extract product I like is Lo Han Supreme (800-753-4372, *www.nunaturals.com*). Jarrow makes a powdered product called Lo Han Sweet, available at health-food stores, that combines lo han kuo and xylitol.

The Cellulite Solution

Wayne Westcott, PhD, fitness research director at South Shore YMCA and adjunct instructor of exercise science at Quincy College, both in Quincy, Massachusetts. He is the author or coauthor of more than 20 books, including *No More Cellulite* (Perigee) and *Get Stronger, Feel Younger* (Rodale).

When scientists say there's "no such thing" as cellulite, they mean that cellulite is not a distinct type of body tissue, but it is ordinary fat. Yet for nearly nine out of 10 women, that unwanted dimpling on the hips and thighs is undeniably real.

How it got there: Fibrous cords connect the skin to the underlying muscle. When the fat layer that lies between the skin and the muscle is too thick, the cords are pulled tight and fat cells bulge out between them, causing that "cottage cheese" look. *And cellulite gets worse with age...*

•**The typical woman loses muscle mass** at an average rate of about five pounds per decade from ages 20 to 50...and perhaps more rapidly after menopause.

•**As muscle mass decreases, metabolism slows,** the body burns fewer calories and the ratio of fat to muscle rises.

•**Supporting connective tissues** (such as collagen) break down and lose elasticity, making cellulite more pronounced.

What doesn't help: A swarm of creams, wraps, massage techniques and mechanical devices purport to eliminate cellulite, typically by "melting away fat." None addresses the underlying physiological causes. Even dieting can backfire

if you overdo it, because your body may break down muscle as well as fat to get the energy that it needs, raising your fat-to-muscle ratio.

What does help: Strength training, which rebuilds muscle, burns calories and boosts metabolism. Best: Three times a week, do the following exercises. The routine takes about 20 minutes.*

You need only three simple kinds of equipment. Go to a gym or buy your own equipment at a sporting-goods store or on-line (try *www.spriproducts.com*). Within four to six weeks, you should see a noticeable reduction in cellulite.

MEDICINE BALL

A medicine ball is a weighted ball about six to eight inches in diameter. Holding one while doing the following two moves adds extra weight that makes your lower body work harder—and as a bonus, tones the upper body, too. To start, choose a ball with which you can do eight to 12 repetitions per side. Once you work your way up to 15 reps, switch to a ball about one to two pounds heavier. Typically, a woman starts with a two- to four-pound ball and works up to six, eight or 10 pounds.

Cost: About $20 to $40 per ball.

Target zones: Front and back of thighs... buttocks.

•**Lunge.** Stand with feet shoulder-width apart, holding ball between hands at waist level, about six to eight inches in front of you. Bend elbows to bring ball up to chest level...at the same time, with right foot, lunge forward about two to three feet, bending right knee to a 90-degree angle so that it is directly above foot. Step out far enough so that your knee does not move past your ankle (left leg will be slightly bent, heel up). Hold lunge position for three seconds, keeping back straight...then push off with right foot and return to standing, bringing ball back down. Do 10 to 15 reps, then repeat on left. (Avoid lunges if you have knee problems.)

*Check with your doctor before beginning any exercise program.

•**Knee lift.** Stand with feet shoulder-width apart, holding ball between hands at waist level.

Step right foot back about two to two-and-a-half feet, keeping right leg straight and bending left knee slightly. Elbows straight, raise ball in front of you to head height.

Bring right knee forward and up as high as you can…bend elbows and bring ball down to touch knee…then step back again with right foot as you straighten arms and raise ball to head height. Do 10 to 15 reps, then repeat on left.

RESISTANCE TUBES

Resistance tubes are elastic tubes about four feet long with handles on each end. They vary in thickness—start with a tube with which you can do eight to 12 reps per side. When you can do 15 reps, switch to a thicker tube.

Cost: About $5 to $15 per tube.

Target zones: Inner and outer thighs.

•**Hip adduction.** Attach one handle to a secure anchor (such as around a bed leg). Loop other handle securely around your right foot (push past toes as far as possible so it doesn't fly off).

Sit on floor, with knees straight and legs spread, so tube is straight out to the right of your right foot. With hands on floor behind you, use inner thigh muscles to slide right leg in to meet left leg. Hold three seconds, then slowly slide right leg back out to spread-leg position. Do 10 to 15 reps, then repeat with left leg.

•**Hip abduction.** Attach one handle to a secure anchor, and loop other handle around right foot (as in the previous exercise).

Sit on floor, with knees straight and legs together, so tube is straight out to the left of your right foot, crossing over left ankle. With your hands on the floor behind you, use outer thigh muscles to slide right leg out to the right until legs are spread as much as possible. Hold three seconds, then slowly slide right leg back to meet left leg. Do 10 to 15 reps, then repeat with left leg.

DUMBBELLS

To start, use a pair of dumbbells (hand weights) with which you can do eight to 12 reps. When you are able to do 15 reps, switch to weights two to three pounds heavier. Typically a woman starts with five-pound weights, increasing to eight, then 10, then 12, then 15 pounds.

Cost: About $10 to $30 per pair.

Target zones: Front and back of thighs… buttocks.

•**Squat.** Stand with feet shoulder-width apart, one weight in each hand, arms down at sides. Keeping torso erect and head in line with spine, bend knees (as if sitting on a chair) until thighs are nearly parallel to floor. Do not allow knees to move forward past toes. Hold for three seconds, then return to standing. Do 10 to 15 reps.

•**Step-Up.** Stand at bottom of a stairway, facing steps, one weight in each hand, arms down at sides. (If you have balance problems, hold a weight in one hand and hold onto banister with the other hand.)

Place entire left foot flat on first step, then rise until you are standing on the stair. Step back down, again moving left foot first. Do 10 to 15 reps, then repeat on the right side.

Illustrations by Shawn Banner.

Subject Index

and drug interaction, 289
and exercise, 628
health benefits of, 41, 319, 394–397, 475–476, 481, 589, 621
and memory, 502–503
Cognitive ability, 311–312
Cognitive problems, from medicines, 259–260
Cognitive therapy (CT), 126–127, 336, 339
Cold sores, 44, 506, 553
Colds, 112–114
  acupressure for, 97
  and beta glucan, 120, 121
  and exercise, 114–115
  feeding (starving a fever), 610
  folk remedies for, 108–109, 130, 136, 593
  nasal congestion, 551–552
  prevention of, 99–101, 106, 120
  zinc for, 244
Colitis, 46
Collagen, 528, 535, 536, 562, 563, 565
Colon cancer, 246, 436, 447, 448–449, 607, 610–611
Colorectal cancer, 17, 456
Comfort foods, 616–617
Community health centers, 13, 18, 20
Computed tomographic angiography (CTA), 350
Computer games, 312–314
Computers, and eyestrain, 151–152, 214, 549
Condiments, 598
Constipation, 261, 414, 423–424, 608
Contact lenses, 303, 551
Cooking oils, 605–607
Copper, 235, 304, 478
Corn, 585
Corn oil, 606
Cornea, 549
Coronary angiography, 350
Coronary artery disease, 146, 351
Coronary microvascular syndrome, 499
Cortisol, 85, 93, 208, 424, 425, 534, 557
Cosmetic surgery, 26
Cosmetics, toxins in, 156–157
Coughing, 106, 113, 116, 185, 409
  allergy medicines for, 243–244
  breakthrough drugs for, 261
  folk remedies for, 109–110, 125–126
Counterirritants, 206
Cramps, 134, 228
Cranberry juice, 289, 428, 596, 597
Cranberry relish, recipe, 598–599
Crisis hotlines, 23
Critical limb ischemia (CLI), 384
Crohn's disease, 243, 445
Crossword puzzles, 308, 309, 324
Crow's feet, 536
Cryotherapy, 461, 494
CT scans, 48–49
Cucumbers, 44

Curcumin, 157, 446, 453, 571, 599
Curry, 157, 446, 453, 599
Cycling, 83–84, 155, 211, 293

D

Dairy products, 86, 96, 424, 568, 590
Dancing, 70, 503
Dark therapy, 336
Debridement, 538
Deep vein thrombosis (DVT), 50, 218, 360–362
Defibrillators, 354
Dehydration, 65, 205, 422, 506–507
Dehydroepiandrosterone (DHEA), 506, 515
Dementia, 315, 318, 457, 519–520, 556, 603
Dengue fever, 73
Dental care, 554–558
  and bad breath, 531–532
  costs of, 21–23
  exams, 150–151, 446, 557
  fears associated with, 558
  fillings and crowns, 554–555
  fluoride, 558
  for gums, 555–556
  insurance for, 21–22, 26
  and oral cancer, 446
  periodontal disease, 139, 150, 555, 556–557
  and pneumonia, 123
  and probiotics, 131
  sedation pills for, 554
  wisdom tooth extraction, 48
Deodorants, 447–448
Depression
  in bipolar disorder, 335–336
  and bone density, 475
  and Botox, 329
  and cardiovascular disease, 316
  and cognitive function, 316
  crisis hotline, 23
  and exercise, 335, 624–625
  and heart attack, 357
  and immune response, 116
  and lifestyle, 335
  in men, 457
  and menopause, 484
  misunderstandings about, 333–334
  natural remedies for, 254, 585
  and periodontal disease, 557
  treatment of, 328–329, 334, 335
Dermaspacing, 563, 564
Devil's claw, 203–204
Diabetes, 386–399
  and alpha-lipoic acid, 397–398
  and antidepressants, 388
  breakthrough drugs for, 261–262
  and cancer, 392
  clinical trials, 394
  and CoQ10, 276
  costs of, 393–394
  crisis hotline, 23
  and dental care, 150–151, 556

epidemic, 386
and exercise, 388, 390
and the eyes, 304
food and drink affecting, 240, 241, 242, 394–395, 397, 575, 603
and foot care, 383
and gastric bypass surgery, 390–391
and glucose monitoring, 392–393
and heart disease, 352, 387
pain of, 390
and pancreas transplants, 391–392
and peripheral neuropathy, 211
prediabetes, 389–390
prevention, 389–390
risk factors, 387, 389
and stroke, 381
symptoms of, 388
tests, 386–387, 388, 389, 399
treatment plan, 387, 390
and vitamins, 248
Diabetic retinopathy, 544, 545
Diarrhea, 421-422
  strategies for relief, 130, 136, 138, 414, 422, 585
Diet. See Food; Weight control
Diet patches and pills, 620
Digestive enzymes, 413, 427, 544
Digestive health
  heartburn, 405–411
  strategies for relief, 129, 131, 135, 136, 575, 593, 608, 610–611
Digital imaging machines, 527
Diphtheria shots, 115, 171
Disinfectant gels, 174, 175, 177, 179
Diuretics, 112, 256, 262–263
Doctors, 51-52, 58, 71-72
  alternative medicine, 62–63
  checkups by, 71
  costs of, 12–14, 18
  and drug companies, 256
  intensivists and hospitalists, 56
  minor surgery by, 47–48
  misdiagnoses from, 45–47
  office visits, 42
  ophthalmologists, 303–304
  overmedicating, 255–256
  primary care physicians, 15, 71
  and prostate cancer diagnosis, 479
  quality of care from, 39–40
  second opinions of, 15, 39–40
  stethoscopes of, 57
  surgeons, 53, 57
  unethical practices of, 35–36
Dog bites, and insurance, 33–34
Domestic violence, crisis hotline, 23
Dopamine, 70, 525, 575
Dreams, 279, 341–342
Drugs. See Medications
Dry eyes, 303, 549–550, 559
Dry mouth, 557
Dual-energy X-ray absorptiometry (DEXA), 399–400, 474–475

E

E. coli, 166, 178, 422, 603, 605
Ears, 119, 170, 239, 552–554, 560
Eating disorders, 336
EBCT (full-body) scans, 49
Echinacea, 238–239, 593
Eczema, 179, 219
Eggs, 166, 573, 589–590, 613, 621, 635
Elderberry/flower, 128, 552, 593
Electric shocks, 372
Endermologie, 542
Endometrial ablation, 490
Endorphins, 70, 85, 195
Endoscopy, 441
Endothelial cells, 368, 595
Energy boosters, 299–300
Epidemiology, 314
Epsom salts, 569
Epstein-Barr virus (EBV), 443
Equal, 636
Erectile dysfunction (ED), 367, 473, 505
Esophageal cancer, 407, 408, 441–442
Essential fatty acids (EFAs), 141, 535, 613
Essential oils, 228–229
Estrogen, 452, 464, 483, 487, 493, 500, 576
Evening primrose oil, 252, 535
Exercise. *See also* Exercise therapy
    adrenaline burned via, 503
    aerobic, 139, 140, 211, 311, 501
    anti-aging, 300–302
    for arthritis, 194–195, 209–210, 633–635
    and boredom, 634
    for the brain, 309–310, 315–316, 318
    and breast cancer, 494–495, 501–502
    burning calories via, 375, 617
    and cancer, 434, 458, 501–502
    and coffee, 628
    consistency in, 632
    for constipation, 424
    and depression, 335, 624–625
    and diabetes, 388, 390
    duration of, 332, 633
    equipment, 301, 623, 628–630, 640
    for gas, 412
    goals for, 627, 632–633
    and healing, 220–221
    and heart attack, 318, 348, 356–357, 362, 472
    and heartburn, 406
    and immune system, 100, 114–115, 116
    injury prevention in, 153–154
    and insulin resistance, 434, 615
    intermittent, 153
    Kegels, 418, 420, 488
    for leg pain, 383
    for men, 472
    mistakes, 623–624
    and multiple sclerosis, 402

    and nitric oxide, 368
    and osteoporosis, 475
    overtraining, 154
    and pain, 154, 188, 194, 196, 197–198, 209–211, 634
    for posture, 298–299
    progression of, 202
    and prostate cancer, 458
    resistance training, 210–211, 639
    responsibility for, 633
    for sciatica, 213, 215
    setbacks in, 633
    strength training, 300, 400, 626, 639
    for stress, 85, 331–332
    for stroke risk, 315–316, 376
    and thyroid, 182
    time for, 632–633
    warmups for, 202
    for women, 481–482, 486
Exercise therapy, 80–82, 301–302
    for abdominals, 202
    for the back, 203, 294, 625–626
    for buttocks, 294, 625, 632
    for calfs, 213, 294
    for chest muscles, 202–203, 632
    cycling, 83–84, 629
    for foot and ankle, 211, 362
    for hands, 210, 634
    for hips, 81, 210, 294, 634, 639
    for knees, 211, 634–635, 639
    for lower back, 203, 294
    for midback, 203
    for neck, 199–200, 213
    run or walk in place, 627
    for sciatica pain, 213
    for sex, 508
    for stability, 203
    on stairs, 626–627, 632, 640
    stretching, 80–82, 153, 199, 210, 294, 298–299, 623, 632
    for tennis elbow, 214
    weight lifting, 153, 629, 633
Exfoliation, 536
Exhaustion, 137
Eyeglasses, 303, 550
Eyes
    aging, 302–304
    blinking, 548–549, 550
    broccoli for, 585
    cataracts, 48, 542, 544, 545, 548, 550, 551
    contact lenses, 303, 551
    dry, 303, 549–550, 559
    exams, 303, 545, 546
    glare, 545, 548–549
    glaucoma, 303, 542, 544, 545, 546, 551
    lubrication of, 303, 549
    nutrition for, 304, 548
    protecting, 559–560
    soothing, 44, 303, 560
    sties, 130
    straining, 151–152, 548–549, 551
    tears in, 549–550
Eyesight. *See* Vision

F

Face-lift, 560–564
Falls, preventing, 64–65
Family medical history, 43, 195
Farmers' markets, 584, 605
Fat-resistance diet, 612–613
Fatigue, 137, 147, 326, 424–426, 575
Fats, dietary
    cooking oils, 605–607
    daily intake of, 426
    for immune system, 99–100
    and irritable bowel syndrome, 412
    limiting, 376, 427
    for mood swings, 482
    saturated, 368, 433, 606, 613, 615
    sources of, 583, 606, 610
Fecal occult blood test (FOBT), 436, 456
Feet, care of, 129, 146, 159, 177, 383, 568–569
Fennel seeds, 412, 426
Fermented food, probiotics in, 424
Fertility, 469, 471, 472, 498, 575
Fever, 437, 610
Feverfew tea, 594
Fiber
    for appetite control, 293, 613, 621
    bulk producer, 620
    health benefits of, 368, 374, 408, 410, 423, 452, 580, 602–609, 610–611, 621
Fibroids, 491, 497
Fibromyalgia, 197–198
Figs, 586
Fingernails, 118, 135, 532
Fish, 207, 589
    anti-inflammatory properties of, 254, 452, 464, 550, 612
    protein in, 573
    vitamin D in, 248
Fish oil, 141–143. *See also* Omega-3 fatty acids
    and blood thinners, 143, 194, 283, 335, 370, 465, 543
    for the eyes, 304, 543, 560
    for immune health, 133, 560
    supplements, 262, 283, 285, 452
Fitness, 612–640
    benefits of, 77–78, 638
    and eating habits, 612–613, 627–628, 635–637
    and exercise, *see* Exercise; Exercise therapy
    and weight, 612–622
Fitness clubs, 26
Flatulence, 411–412
Flavonoids, 70, 117, 128, 348
Flavonols, 455, 577
Flaxseed oil, 243, 304, 535, 606, 607
Flaxseeds, 142, 322, 370, 423, 450, 453, 464, 481, 550
Flu
    bird, 107
    and exercise, 115

and headaches, 189
nutrients in, 140, 369, 588, 597, 610
in smoothies, 600

K

Kale, 452, 579
Kefir, 96, 132
Kegel exercises, 418, 420, 488
Keloid scars, 565, 566
Kidney disease, 17, 404–406
Kidney stones, 402–404, 603
Kitchen, germs in, 178, 180
Kiwi fruit, 578
Knees, 197, 204, 634–635, 639
Knuckles, cracking, 44

L

L-arginine, 284, 368
L-carnitine, 139, 298, 398
L-citrulline, 368
L-glutamine, 428
Labels, reading, 169–170
Lachesis, 489
Lactobacilli, 95, 107, 131, 132, 135,
    274, 416, 422, 424, 600
Lactose intolerance, 421
Laparoscopic surgery, 461, 491
Laser therapy, for skin, 527–528, 529,
    530, 566
Latex gloves, 175
Laughter, 70, 82, 431
Laundry, germs in, 178, 179–180
Lawn mowers, 154–155
Leeks, 580
Legionnaires' disease, 107
Legs
    exercises for, 81, 302, 319, 383
    and stroke, 382–384
    uneven lengths, 218
    varicose veins, 318–319
Legumes, 579
Lemon, 109, 125, 129, 320
Lemon balm, 593
Lemonade, 403
Lentils, 189
Leopard's bane, 533
Leptin, 85, 612
Libido, 484, 515, 574, 594
Libraries, dust in, 163
Licorice, 238, 284, 407, 416–417, 427
Licorice root, 110, 425, 575
Lifestyle coach, 330
Light therapy, 336, 508–509
Lightning, airplane struck by, 165
Linden tea, 552, 594
Liquids, drinking, 119, 120, 170–171
Listening, 511, 514, 516
Liver, 397, 398, 414–416
Liver cancer, 245, 436–437
Lo han kuo (luo han guo), 637
Lockjaw, 171
Loneliness, 67–68, 557

Long-term care, 65–67, 305
Longevity. *See also* Seniors
    and alcohol, 602–603
    aspirin for, 250–251
    and oral health, 556
    RealAge concept, 291
Lumpectomy, 499
Lung cancer
    and blood clots, 361
    in men, 458
    radiofrequency ablation for, 436
    and smoking, 344, 348, 458, 474
    and vitamin A, 445–446
Lung capacity, 93, 316
Lung disease, 72
Lupus, 593
Lutein, 304, 543, 559, 573, 578
Lycopene, 292, 573, 589, 596
Lycopodium, 424
Lyme disease, 47, 155

M

Maca, 574–576
Macadamia nut oil, 606, 607
Macular degeneration, 114, 542,
    544–545, 546–548, 559, 573
Mad cow disease, 586
Magnesium, 87–88, 104, 407, 481
    and calcium, 134, 140, 298, 331
    and colon cancer, 448–449
    for constipation, 414, 423–424
    and headaches, 205
    sources of, 205, 322, 331, 423, 572
    for vision, 543
Magnet therapy, 186
Magnetic resonance imaging (MRI),
    350, 376
Malaria, 73
Malnutrition, 65
Malpractice insurance, 34
Mammograms, 501
Manicures, 532
Margarine, 590, 609, 610
Marriage
    health problems from, 523–524
    myths about, 512–514
    of parents, 519–520
    sexless, 522–523
Marriage counselor, 333
Marshmallow root, 137
Massage, 78–80, 328
    of abdomen, 412
    acupressure, 96–98, 120, 130, 344
    and cancer, 449
    qigong, 83
    reflexology, 129
    for scars, 565
Mastectomy, 499
Meadowsweet, 138
Meals. *See* Food
Measles, 115, 553
Meat
    and body odor, 531
    and cancer, 453, 572

health risks in, 167, 189, 366, 587
lean, 583
protein in, 573
raw, handling, 177
vegetarians vs., 586–587
zinc in, 572
Medicaid, 20, 22, 52, 66
Medical care. *See* Health care
Medical history, 162
Medical records, copy of, 38
Medicare, 7, 28–30, 52
Medications. *See also* Medications
    Index
    active ingredients in, 223
    advertised, 4
    age-related side effects, 40
    allergies to, 53
    bulk purchase of, 6, 14–15, 287
    caffeine in, 41
    from Canada, 9, 10–11
    clinical trials, 15, 394, 440
    cost of, 1–7, 9–10, 12–13, 14–15,
        19, 264, 286–288, 393–394
    counterfeit, 263–264
    direct sales to consumers, 4
    disposal of, 290
    dosage calculated for, 279
    drug interactions, 40, 226,
        237–238, 251–252, 272
    errors in, 64, 269–270, 273
    expiration dates for, 279
    forms, formularies, 223–224, 287
    free samples, 3, 6–7, 15, 288
    gender factor in, 270–271, 484
    generic equivalents, 4, 6, 257,
        281–283, 287
    healing powers of, 283–285
    hidden ingredients in, 170, 223
    hospital errors in, 64
    indications of use, 223
    insurance for, 5, 26
    and juices, 288–290
    labels for, 222–224
    lists of, 52
    mail-order, 280–281, 287
    management of, 40, 307
    mass-market retailers, 3, 5, 12
    measurement of, 41
    metabolism of, 289–290
    nondrug alternatives to, 287
    nutrients drained by, 274–276
    off-label use, 28
    on-line purchase, 5, 10, 11, 12
    over-the-counter, 222–254
    overmedication, 255–257
    overseas manufacturing of, 282
    overseas purchase of, 10–11
    patient advocacy groups, 3
    patient-assistance programs, 2, 4
    safety of, 10–11, 274
    side effects of, 40, 131, 170, 211,
        259–260, 519
    and snoring, 340
    split tablets, 4, 6, 8, 274, 393, 473
    storage of, 41, 288

646

and joint pain, 146–147
and osteoporosis, 474
recurrence of, 462
research, 467–469
survival of, 462–463, 466
and testosterone, 471
tests for, 16, 45, 458–460, 461, 466–468
treatment of, 460–461, 469
vaccine against, 462
and vitamins, 246, 463
Prostate-specific antigen (PSA)
density of, 459
free vs. bound, 459
and phytochemicals, 477
and prostate cancer, 239–240, 458–460, 461, 467
screening, 45, 240, 466, 467–468
velocity of, 459, 476, 479
Protein, 100, 426
and insulin resistance, 613, 615
sources, 300, 482, 573, 579
Proton-beam therapy, 435–436
Prunes, 582
Psoriasis, 118, 446, 530–531, 537
Psychotherapy, 332–333, 336
Psyllium, 423, 609
Pulmonary disease, COPD, 474
Pulmonary embolisms, 46–47, 50, 361
Pulsatilla, 489
Pumpkin, 451, 464
Punctal occlusion, 550

Q

Qigong, 82–83
Quack physicians, 35–36
Quadrantectomy, 499
Quality of care, 39–40, 55, 59
Quercetin, 112, 128, 284, 451

R

Radiation therapy, 434–435, 446–447, 461
Ragweed, 110, 111, 238–239
Raisins, 558
Rape, crisis hotline, 23
Rash, diagnoses of, 47
Raspberry leaf tea, 594
RealAge, 291–293
Recumbent bike, 626
Red spots, 535–536
Red yeast rice, 253, 370
Reflex tests, 211
Reflux, 119, 266–267, 276, 406, 407, 408, 409
Relationships, 42–43, 221, 308, 310, 332, 343, 505–526
in families, 518–520
friendship, 510–512
marriage, 512–514, 522–524
and memory, 515–517
sex, 505–510

Relaxation techniques, 129, 524
Renal disease, 405
Restaurants, 170, 180
Resveratrol, 207, 369, 476, 595
Retirement, 67, 302, 519
Reye's syndrome, 186
Rheumatoid arthritis, 190–193, 206–208, 286, 603
medication dangers, 279–280
natural remedies for, 253–254
and periodontal disease, 556
Rhinovirus, 113
Rhodiola, 134, 575
Rhus toxicodendron, 136, 219
Rice, 422, 601
Ringworm, 541
Robotic surgery, 354–355
Rocky Mountain spotted fever, 108, 155
Rosehips, 197
Rosemary, 157, 534, 572, 594
Rotation diet, 413
Rotavirus, 179
Rubella vaccination, 115
Ruta graveolens, 136
Rye grass pollen extract, 465

S

S-adenosylmethionine (SAMe), 187, 198, 208
Saccharin, 636
Sage, 109
Saliva, artificial, 557
Saliva hormone testing, 425
Salmonella, 166, 179, 422
Salt, 590–592
Sanding, 564
Sardines, 572, 597, 598
Sauerkraut, 109, 132, 189
Saunas, 100–101, 126, 531
Saw palmetto, 234–235, 239–240, 465, 534
Scams, 35–36
Scars, 564, 565–566
Sciatica, 200, 213, 214–216
Scurvy, 296
Seafood, 161–162, 197, 583
Sebum, 529, 534
Second opinions, 15, 39–40
Selenium, 104, 182, 451, 478, 573
Senior care
crisis hotline, 23, 27
drug side effects, 40, 271–274
facilities for, 63–67
herbal medicine for, 137–139
side effects from drugs, 260
Seniors
age-related macular degeneration (AMD), 546–548
and alcohol, 602–603
and Alzheimer's disease, 314–318
and arthritis, 195, 262
bones of, 262–263
brain function in, 307–310

and cardiovascular disease, 351
driving safety, 158–160, 520
dry mouth, 557
eye treatments for, 302–304
falling, 64–65
gray hair of, 44
home monitoring, 306–307
loss of friendships, 520
medication management for, 307
and memory, 310–311
metabolism in, 486
multivitamins for, 233
retirement, 67, 302, 519
scars, 565
sex for, 507–508
and sleep, 144
social networks for, 307, 310
and stroke, 382
women, 481–482
wrinkles, 562
Serotonin, 71, 130, 134, 221, 336, 525, 586, 621
Sex, 70, 357, 479, 505–510
Sex drive, 484, 515, 574, 594
Sexless marriage, 522–523
Sexual assault, crisis hotline, 23
Sexual revolution, 513–514
Sexually transmitted diseases (STDs), 17, 172
Shaped beam surgery, 435
Shaving, 174
Shiatsu, 78
Shingles, 47, 135, 136, 171–172, 219, 266, 539–540, 553
Shingles vaccine, 280
Shoulders, 146, 152–154, 210, 632
Siblings, 518–519
Sigmoidoscopies, 447
Silicon, 593, 602
Singing, 70, 89
Sinuses, 46, 85–87, 115
Sjögren's syndrome, 549, 550
Skin, 527–542
acne, 446, 529–530, 537, 563, 565
body odor, 531–532
bruising, 533
cellulite, 542, 638–640
cleansing, 537
color, 535–536
contour, 536
dryness, 139
face-lift, 560–564
fillers, 560–561, 562–563, 564, 566
fine lines removed from, 532
fungal infections, 541–542
laser treatment, 562, 566
maintenance, 528–529, 537
peels, 561–562, 563
photo rejuvenation, 562
poison ivy/oak/sumac, 155
psoriasis, 446, 530–531, 537
scars, 564, 565–566
shingles, 539–540
soaps and moisturizers, 179
texture, 536

Medications Index

Axid (*nizatidine*), 260, 426
Azithromycin, 274
Azulfidine (*sulfasalazine*), 191, 193

B

Baclofen, 120
Bactrim (*trimethoprim-sulfamethoxazole*), 117
Beclomethasone, 103, 266
Bellatal (*phenobarbital*), 259
Benadryl (*diphenhydramine*), 110, 223, 266
Benazepril, 276
Bentyl (*dicyclomine*), 259
Benzodiazepine, 267, 530
Benzoyl peroxide, 529, 530
Beta-blockers, 4, 133, 189, 261, 275–276, 356, 360, 372
Betapace (*sotalol*), 271, 372
Betaseron (*interferon beta-1b*), 402
Betaxolol, 261, 275
Betopic S (*betaxolol*), 275
Bevacizumab, 548
Bextra (*valdecoxib*), 219, 220
Bismuth subsalicylate, 223, 422
Bisoprolol, 261
Botox, 329, 528, 536, 561, 562, 564, 566
Bremelanotide, 509
Bromo Seltzer, 591
Brompheniramine, 243, 272
Bronchodilators, 289, 397
Bupropion, 260, 262, 279, 335, 345
Butorphanol tartrate, 270
Byetta (*exenatide*), 387, 398
Bystolic (*nebivolol*), 367–368
Bz-423 (*benzodiazepine-423*), 530

C

Calan (*verapamil*), 288
Calcitonin, 400, 475
Calcium channel blockers, 189, 264, 285, 372
Cancidas (*caspofungin*), 542
Candesartan, 276, 405
Candins, 542
Capoten (*captopril*), 272, 321, 405
Capsaicin
  benefits of, 570
  and cancer, 588
  for coughs, 109
  dangers with, 135, 570–571
  drug interactions with, 237
  for heart disease, 140
  for pain, 134–135, 184, 198, 206, 570
Captopril, 272, 321, 405
Carbamazepine, 282
Carbidopa, 251
Cardizem (*diltiazem*), 285, 372
Cardura (*doxazosin*), 8, 254, 370, 464
Carisoprodol, 259

Carteolol, 275
Cartrol (*carteolol*), 275
Caspofungin, 542
Catapres (*clonidine*), 260, 272
Cefdinir, 115
Cefpodoxime, 115
Celebrex. *See Celecoxib*
Celecoxib
  for arthritis, 5, 196
  and grapefruit, 371
  for pain relief, 187
  side effects of, 184, 185, 196, 206, 226, 227, 275
Celexa (*citalopram*), 8, 254, 262
Cephalosporins, 115–116
Cetirizine, 110
Chlorothiazide, 238
Chlorpheniramine, 243, 266
Chlorpropamide, 260
Chlor-Trimeton (*chlorpheniramine*), 266
Chlorzoxazone, 259
Cilostazol, 383
Cimetidine, 260, 267, 407, 409, 411, 416
Cipro (*ciprofloxacin*), 259, 272, 274, 288, 289
Ciprofloxacin, 259, 272, 274, 288, 289
Cisplatin, 442
Citalopram, 8, 254
Claravis (*isotretinoin*), 530
Clarinex (*desloratadine*), 110, 266
Claritin (*loratadine*), 86, 110, 266
Clearasil, 529, 537
Cleocin (*clindamycin*), 117
Clindamycin, 117
Clonazepam, 8, 252
Clonidine, 260, 272
Clopidogrel, 143, 266, 356, 376
Clotrimazole, 542
Codeine, 153, 184
Colace (*docusate*), 423
Copaxone (*glatiramer*), 401
Cordarone (*amiodarone*), 251, 288, 372
Corticosteroids, 110, 133, 196, 201, 209, 251, 265, 566
Cosamine DS, 194
Coumadin. *See Warfarin*
Covera-HS (*verapamil*), 285
COX-1 and COX-2 inhibitors, 5–6, 196, 226, 249
Cozaar, 387
Crestor (*rosuvastatin*), 249, 387
Cromolyn sodium, 110
Culturelle, 95
Cyclophosphamide, 571
Cyclosporine, 303, 550
Cymbalta (*duloxetine*), 184, 189, 212, 262
Cytoxan (*cyclophosphamide*), 571

D

Dalmane (*flurazepam*), 267
Deltasone (*prednisone*), 399
Depade (*naltrexone*), 336
Depakote (*valproic acid*), 189, 243, 272, 335
Desipramine, 252
Desloratadine, 110, 266
Detrol (*tolterodine*), 418
Dexedrine (*dextroamphetamine*), 330
Dextroamphetamine, 330
DiaBeta (*glyburide*), 260
Diabinese (*chlorpropamide*), 260
Diamox (*acetazolamide*), 342
Diarylquinolones, 258
Diazepam, 120, 240, 260, 288
Diclofenac, 196, 205, 417
Dicyclomine, 259
Digitek (*digoxin*), 273
Digoxin, 41, 252, 259, 273, 372
Dilantin (*phenytoin*), 41, 238, 282
Diltiazem, 285, 372
Diovan, 387
Diphenhydramine, 110, 223, 243, 266
Dipyridamole, 376
Disopyramide, 288
Ditropan (*oxybutynin*), 418
Diuril (*chlorothiazide*), 238
Divalproex, 243
DMARDs (disease-modifying anti-rheumatic drugs), 190–191
Docetaxel, 463
Docusate, 423
Donepezil, 317, 402
Dopamine, 336
Dopamine agonists, 265
Doxazosin, 8, 254, 370, 464
Doxorubicin, 571
Doxycycline, 529
Doxylamine, 272
Duloxetine, 184, 189, 212
Duragesic (*fentanyl*), 184
Dutasteride, 260
Dymelor (*acetohexamide*), 276

E

Effexor (*venlafaxine*), 184, 189, 279, 335, 489
Elavil (*amitriptyline*), 119, 271, 539
Eldepryl (*selegiline*), 289
Elixophyllin (*theophylline*), 251, 289
E-Mycin (*erythromycin*), 259
Enalapril, 276, 383
Enbrel (*etanercept*), 133, 191, 193
EpiPen, 169
Epoetin, 10, 263
Eraxis (*anidulafungin*), 542
Eryc (*erythromycin*), 274
Erythromycin, 259, 274
Escitalopram, 254, 260
Esomeprazole
  and heartburn, 266–267, 276, 407, 411, 416, 426

Methylprednisolone, 553
Metoprolol, 360, 372
Metronidazole, 211, 421
Mevacor (lovastatin), 275, 288, 356, 371, 374
Mexiletine, 397
Mexitil (mexiletine), 397
Miacalcin (calcitonin), 400, 475
Micafungin, 542
Miconazole, 542
Microzide (hydrochlorothiazide), 252
Midodrine, 369
Miglitol, 387
Misoprostol, 417
Mometasone, 111
Monistat (miconazole), 542
Monopril (fosinopril), 321
Montelukast, 284
Morphine, 184
Motrin (ibuprofen), 184, 192, 208, 223, 228, 272, 275, 427
Mycamine (micafungin), 542
Mycelex (clotrimazole), 542

N

Nabumetone, 275
Nadolol (Corgard), 261
Naltrexone, 150, 336
Namenda (memantine), 317
Naprosyn (naproxen), 184
Naproxen
    for arthritis, 190, 196, 208, 222
    and cancer, 496
    for coughs, 244
    drinking water with, 274
    gender differences in use of, 270
    for inflammation, 190, 196, 208, 215
    long-term use of, 196, 222
    for pain relief, 153, 184, 187, 199, 201, 205, 208, 275
    risks and side effects of, 185, 196, 222, 225, 228, 274, 275, 289, 416, 427
Nardil (phenelzine), 237, 239, 289
Nasacort (triamcinolone), 111
Nasalcrom (cromolyn sodium), 110
Nasalide (flunisolide), 266
Nasonex (mometasone), 111
Natalizumab, 401
Nebivolol, 367–368
Nefazodone, 8
Neomycin, 554
NeoSynephrine (phenylephrine), 110
Neurodex (dextromethorphan), 212
Neurontin (gabapentin), 184, 212, 485, 539
Nexium. See Esomeprazole
Nifedipine, 120, 288
Nimodipine, 378
Nimotop (nimodipine), 378
Nitrofurantoin, 211
Nitroglycerin, 360
Nizatidine, 260
Nolvadex (tamoxifen), 361, 492, 502

Normodyne (labetalol), 275
Norpace (disopyramide), 288
Norpramin (desipramine), 252
Nortriptyline, 271
Norvasc (amlodipine), 256
Novocaine, 554
NSAIDs
    for arthritis, 133, 190, 192, 193, 196, 206, 286
    and asthma, 101
    and blood tests, 436
    and cancer, 496
    drug and herb interactions with, 226, 237, 272, 289
    for inflammation, 540
    for pain relief, 184, 187, 205, 208–209, 417, 540
    and probiotics, 131
    reactions to, 170
    risks and side effects with, 185, 224–226, 274, 275, 416, 417, 421, 427, 540
    for women, 270
Nyquil, 230, 272

O

Ofloxacin, 274
Olanzapine, 8, 260, 335
Omacor. See Lovaza
Omalizumab, 169
Omeprazole
    and cancer, 441
    and diarrhea, 421
    for heartburn, 119, 267, 276, 277, 407, 409, 411, 426
    for hiatal hernia, 409, 411
    and hiccups, 119
    and sexual dysfunction, 260
    side effects of, 276, 277, 320, 407
Omnipen (ampicillin), 274
131 I-tositumomab, 434–435
Opioids, 184, 212
Oraqix, 558
Orencia (abatacept), 191
Orudis (ketoprofen), 286
Oseltamivir, 106
Ototoxic drugs, 554
Oxazepam, 240, 267
Oxybutynin, 418
Oxycodone, 184, 212
OxyContin (oxycodone), 184, 212
Oxyderm, 537

P

Pamelor (nortriptyline), 271
PanOxyl AQ, 529
Paraflex (chlorzoxazone), 259
Parathyroid hormone, 475
Paroxetine, 8, 238, 254, 260, 271, 328, 489
Paxil (paroxetine), 8, 238, 254, 260, 262, 271, 328, 475, 489
Pegaptanib sodium, 548

PEG-Intron (interferon), 444
Penicillin, 92, 115, 117, 263
Pentoxifylline, 383
Pepcid (famotidine), 260, 272, 407, 409, 411, 426, 441
Pepto-Bismol (bismuth subsalicylate), 422
Percocet (oxycodone and acetaminophen), 184, 230
Pergolide, 265
Periostat, 529
Perlane, 563
Phenelzine, 237, 239, 289
Phenergan (promethazine hydrochloride), 252
Phenobarbital, 259
Phenylephrine, 110, 252
Phenytoin, 41, 238, 282
Phillips Milk of Magnesia, 224
Pioglitazone, 387
Plaquenil (hydroxychloroquine), 191, 193, 253
Plavix (clopidogrel), 143, 266, 356, 376
Plendil (felodipine), 288
Pletal (cilostazol), 383
Pramipexole, 265
Pravachol (pravastatin), 8, 272, 275
Pravastatin, 8, 272, 275
Precose (acarbose), 387
Prednisone, 133, 190, 270, 399, 553
Pregabalin, 212
Premarin, 488–489
Prempro, 489
Prevacid (lansoprazole), 226, 276, 277, 320, 407, 409, 416, 421, 426
Prilosec. See Omeprazole
ProAmatine (midodrine), 369
Pro-Banthine (propantheline), 259
Procardia (nifedipine), 120, 288
Procrit (epoetin), 10, 263
Promethazine hydrochloride, 252
Propantheline, 259
Propranolol, 261, 272, 275, 285, 356, 360, 372
Proscar (finasteride), 239, 254, 260, 464, 467
Prostabel, 478
Protonix, 426
Proton pump inhibitors (PPIs)
    for heartburn, 266–267, 276, 407, 411, 416, 426, 441
    for hiatal hernias, 411
    side effects of, 189, 277
    and vitamins, 276
Provenge (APC8015), 462
Proventil (albuterol), 252, 273
Provera, 489
Prozac (fluoxetine), 4, 260, 262, 271, 279, 283, 335, 475, 489
Pseudoephedrine, 110, 222, 223, 237, 372
PT-141, 509
Pyridostigmine, 369